Toxicological Evaluation of Electronic Nicotine Delivery Products

Toxicological Evaluation of Electronic Nicotine Delivery Products

Edited by

MANUEL C. PEITSCH
PMI R&D
Philip Morris Products S.A.
Neuchâtel, Switzerland

JULIA HOENG
PMI R&D
Philip Morris Products S.A.
Neuchâtel, Switzerland

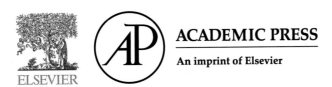

ACADEMIC PRESS
An imprint of Elsevier

ELSEVIER

Academic Press is an imprint of Elsevier
125 London Wall, London EC2Y 5AS, United Kingdom
525 B Street, Suite 1650, San Diego, CA 92101, United States
50 Hampshire Street, 5th Floor, Cambridge, MA 02139, United States
The Boulevard, Langford Lane, Kidlington, Oxford OX5 1GB, United Kingdom

Notices

Knowledge and best practice in this field are constantly changing. As new research and experience broaden our
understanding, changes in research methods, professional practices, or medical treatment may become
necessary.

Practitioners and researchers must always rely on their own experience and knowledge in evaluating and using
any information, methods, compounds, or experiments described herein. In using such information or methods
they should be mindful of their own safety and the safety of others, including parties for whom they have a
professional responsibility.

To the fullest extent of the law, neither the Publisher nor the authors, contributors, or editors, assume any
liability for any injury and/or damage to persons or property as a matter of products liability, negligence or
otherwise, or from any use or operation of any methods, products, instructions, or ideas contained in the
material herein.

Library of Congress Cataloging-in-Publication Data
A catalog record for this book is available from the Library of Congress

British Library Cataloguing-in-Publication Data
A catalogue record for this book is available from the British Library

ISBN: 978-0-12-820490-0

For information on all Academic Press publications visit our website at
https://www.elsevier.com/books-and-journals

Publisher: Andre Gerhard Wolff
Acquisitions Editor: Kattie Washington
Editorial Project Manager: Tracy I. Tufaga
Production Project Manager: Sreejith Viswanathan
Cover Designer: Alan Studholme

Typeset by TNQ Technologies

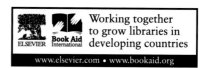

List of Contributors

Mark Bentley
PMI R&D
Philip Morris Products S.A
Neuchâtel, Switzerland

Stéphanie Boué
PMI R&D
Philip Morris Products S.A.
Neuchâtel, Switzerland

David Bovard
Philip Morris Products S.A.
Neuchâtel, Switzerland

Amin Choukrallah
PMI R&D
Philip Morris Products S.A.
Neuchâtel, Switzerland

Marc S. Firestone
Philip Morris Products S.A.
Lausanne, Switzerland

Stefan Frentzel
PMI R&D
Philip Morris Products S.A.
Neuchâtel, Switzerland

Catherine Goujon-Ginglinger
PMI R&D
Philip Morris Products S.A.
Neuchâtel, Switzerland

Christelle Haziza
PMI R&D
Philip Morris Products S.A.
Neuchâtel, Switzerland

Julia Hoeng
PMI R&D
Philip Morris Products S.A.
Neuchâtel, Switzerland

Anita R. Iskandar
PMI R&D
Philip Morris Products S.A.
Neuchâtel, Switzerland

Nikolai V. Ivanov
PMI R&D
Philip Morris Products S.A.
Neuchâtel, Switzerland

Ulrike Kogel
PMI R&D
Philip Morris Products S.A.
Neuchâtel, Switzerland

Aditya Reddy Kolli
PMI R&D
Philip Morris Products S.A.
Neuchâtel, Switzerland

Arkadiusz K. Kuczaj
PMI R&D
Philip Morris Products S.A.
Neuchâtel, Switzerland
Department of Applied Mathematics
University of Twente
Enschede, The Netherlands

Francesco Lucci
PMI R&D
Philip Morris Products S.A.
Neuchâtel, Switzerland

Karsta Luettich
PMI R&D
Philip Morris Products S.A.
Neuchâtel, Switzerland

Serge Maeder
PMI R&D
Philip Morris Products S.A.
Neuchâtel, Switzerland

Diego Marescotti
PMI R&D
Philip Morris Products S.A.
Neuchâtel, Switzerland

Florian Martin
PMI R&D
Philip Morris Products S.A.
Neuchâtel, Switzerland

Carole Mathis
PMI R&D
Philip Morris Products S.A.
Neuchâtel, Switzerland

Anne May
Consultants in Science
Epalinges, Switzerland

PMI R&D
Neuchâtel, Switzerland

Damian McHugh
PMI R&D
Philip Morris Products S.A.
Neuchâtel, Switzerland

Maya I. Mitova
PMI R&D
Philip Morris Products S.A.
Neuchâtel, Switzerland

Michael J. Peck
Scientific Consulting
Neuchâtel, Switzerland

Manuel C. Peitsch
PMI R&D
Philip Morris Products S.A.
Neuchâtel, Switzerland

Blaine W. Phillips
PMI R&D
Philip Morris International
Research Laboratories Pte Ltd
Singapore

Patrick Picavet
PMI R&D
Philip Morris Products S.A.
Neuchâtel, Switzerland

Sandrine Pouly
PMI R&D
Philip Morris Products S.A.
Neuchâtel, Switzerland

Carine Poussin
PMI R&D
Philip Morris Products S.A.
Neuchâtel, Switzerland

Pascal Pratte
PMI R&D
Philip Morris Products S.A.
Neuchâtel, Switzerland

Rebecca Savioz
Consultants in Science
Epalinges, Switzerland

Jean-Pierre Schaller
PMI R&D
Philip Morris Products S.A.
Neuchâtel, Switzerland

Walter K. Schlage
Biology Consultant
Bergisch Gladbach, Germany

Davide Sciuscio
PMI R&D
Neuchâtel, Switzerland

Daniel J. Smart
PMI R&D
Philip Morris Products S.A.
Neuchâtel, Switzerland

Maurice Smith
PMI R&D
Philip Morris Products S.A.
Neuchâtel, Switzerland

Justyna Szostak
PMI R&D
Philip Morris Products S.A.
Neuchâtel, Switzerland

Marja Talikka
PMI R&D
Philip Morris Products S.A.
Neuchâtel, Switzerland

Bjoern Titz
PMI R&D
Philip Morris Products S.A.
Neuchâtel, Switzerland

Marco van der Toorn
PMI R&D
Philip Morris Products S.A.
Neuchâtel, Switzerland

Patrick Vanscheeuwijck
PMI R&D
Philip Morris Products S.A.
Neuchâtel, Switzerland

Ee Tsin Wong
PMI R&D
Philip Morris International Research
Laboratories Pte Ltd
Singapore

Wenhao Xia
Philip Morris Products S.A.
Neuchâtel, Switzerland

Filippo Zanetti
PMI R&D
Philip Morris Products S.A.
Neuchâtel, Switzerland

Acknowledgments

This book is the result of a team effort, not only during its writing but throughout a decade of scientific assessment of innovative smoke-free nicotine delivery products that have the potential to present less risk of harm to smokers who switch to these products instead of continuing to smoke. We, the authors, would like to acknowledge those people who have been instrumental during that journey.

First we offer our sincere gratitude to the teams of scientists who conducted and published the studies referenced in this book, and to those who enabled them with their support, in particular Y Abdul Salim, I AbuTalib, S Acali, I Afandi, S Afiq, E Afolalu, V Aiyar Ganesan, A Ajithkumar, J Albino, EN Aldilla, N Ali, O Alijevic, J Almodovar, M Almstetter, M Alriquet, J Ancerewicz, S Ansari, SM Ansari, D Arndt, B Asgharian, L Astrologo, M Auberson, M Azagra Revuelta, F Azwan, M Bachmann, G Baker, M Barathiraja, M Barkhuizen, N Barozzi, J Battey, A Beguin, M Belka, M Belushkin, S Benaouag, M Benzimra, A Bergounioux, J-T Bertrand, K Bessard, P Betsch, N Bielik, J Binder, K Binte Kamsin, N Blanc, I Blaszkiewicz, P Boiteux, F Bonjour, B Bonvin, D Bornand, M Bosilkovska Weisskopf, H Bossaert, C Buchholz, J-F Bulber, T Burghart, C Burton, A Büttner, R Cabrera, L Cailleau, E Calabro, N Camille, L Cammack, PB Campelos, S Cano, S Carty Vogel, A Castellon, M Cattoni, V Chameroy, JL Chan, C Chia, C Chrea, CS Chua, J Chua, Y Chua, D Chye, C Cluse, M Colella, S Constant, CL Cooney, M Corciulo, S Corciulo, D Correia, A Cosandier, A D'Agostino, E Dargaud, M David, D de Graaf, G de La Bourdonnaye, S de la Rosa Sole, A Debrick, LR Demenescu, G Den Hartog, H Deng, I D'Errico, N Devindran, A di Fabio, M Di Franco, M Diacon, S Dijon, F Dole, A Dornier, D DosSantos, E Dossin, L Dotte, F Ducarouge, R Dulize, Q Dutertre, T Dutronc, Y Eb-Levadoux, N Edge, A Elamin, J Elcner, T Epars, M Esposito, D Etter, M Fatarova, C Favre, L Felber Medlin, J Ferrari, S Ferreira, SH Foo, D Forte, S Frederic, E Frederix, S Fredersdorf, E Garcia, S Garcia Moreno, C Gauge, L Gautier, B Geurts, D Ghosh, M Gilchrist, A Giovannini, A Giralt, A Glabasnia, S Godinho, D Goedertier, P Goh, M Gomez Lueso, L Graber, M Gremaud, F Grosjean, C Gubelmann, S Gubian, E Guedj, A Guenin, AS Gunawan, I Gunduz, A Gutleb, PA Guy, A Haiduc, M Hankins, J Havlica, P Hayden, AW Hayes, W Hays, F Helbling, A Heremans, M Hernandez, J Hirter, J Ho, I Hofer, M Hofmann-Apitius, A Huber, P Hunkeler, H Isa, S Iyer, K Jablczynska, G Jaccard, D Jacot, R Jaeger, S Jaiswal, G Janeke, V Jaquet, A Jaquier, F Jeanneret, A Jeanneret, C Jeannet, J Jedelsky, M Jicha, S Johne, M Jungo, K Kabalan, K Kaminski, D Kamperis, SWD Kang, J Kang, I Kapel-Peric, R Kaur, R Kenney, L Khachatryan, D Khalid, J Kim, A Kirchhofer, CR Kirman, S Kleinhans, A Knorr, D Koh, E Komen, A Kondylis, A Korneliou, K Koshibu, P Kozarewicz, K Kozikis, S Krishnan, K Kwok, L Lachat, A Lahrache, S Lam, ZY Lam, C Lamboley, N Lantz, C Laszlo, L Latino, P Lau, A Laurent, O Lavrynenko, M Lazzerini, S Le Bouhellec, S Lebrun, M Lee, R Lee, T Lee, R Legname, E Lemos, JY Leong, P Leroy, R Li, J Lim, J Lim, H Lin, Y-W Lin, F Lizal, G Loh, T Low, F Luedicke, SK Lwin, P Magnani, C Maier, S Majeed, JX Mak, S Malcolm, N Mamat, S Manalastras, F Maranzano, A Marchese, E Martin, C Martins Zwicky, R Matera, M Mattarella, A Mazurov, T McGrath, K Md Yusop, C Medan, S Mendes, F Mendes Castanheira, C Merg, S Merlet, D Messinis, A Mischler Profico, O Moennikes, F Moine, A Monge, C Montandon, G Mordacq, L Morris, N Mottier, R Munoz, N Murugasan, L Neau, S Neo, R Ng, WT Ng, C Nolan, M Nordlund, C Nury, M Odziomek, M Oldham, AF Omar, L Ortega Torres, S Ouadi, M Ousset, A Oviedo, C Pak, M Parel, J Park, S Pastorelli, C Pater, B Pellegrini, JM Pereira, D Peric, T Petit, R Piault, E Pierri, M Pietro, L Pigozzi, J Pijnenburg, L Pinard, D Piquard, C Pitton, G Plebani, L Poget, J Polier-Calame, M Porchet, P Pospisil, V Poux, R Punde, A Purwanti, S Quek, T Quinn, F Radtke, O Raffi, M Rahman, S Ramaiah, SK Raman, A Ramazzotti, P Reason, R Reis Pires, K Renggli, C Reyren, M Rhouma, M Rizza, M Robert-Tissot, G Rodrigo, D Rota, EGR Rouget, S Roulet, PA Ruiz Castro, M Russell, R Rytsar, NA Saini, E Salazar, A Sandoz, Y Sauser, A Saxena, E Scazzi, M Schaller, M Scherer, G Scherer, S Scheuner, B Schneider, S Schorderet Weber, M Schorpp, J Schroeter, L Schwab, K Schwach-Abdellaoui, H Sean, C

Sequeira, F Sergio, A Sester, A Sewer, M Sgandurra, A Siccama, N Sierro, SY Siew, J Simicevic, J Simko, T Sinnakalandi, V Sivalingam, J Solioz, N Soonan, T Sosnowski, A Soulan, RD Stabbert, A Stan, S Steiner, A Susz, C Taddei, D Tafin Djoko, E Tan, G Tan, S Tan, WT Tan, BV Taranu, J Tay, A Teichert, E Tekeste, C Teng, A Teo, HW Teo, S Tercier, C Tham, E Tharin, GA Thompson, T Thomson, K Tobias, WW Toh, CT Tran, T Travnickova, AR Tricker, K Trivedi, M Tsen, CK Tung, S User, F Valdez, J Valette, J-F Vallelian, E Veljkovic, M Verardo, A Voirol, F Vonmoos, C Wachsmuth, H Wahab, P Walker, J Walker, K Weber, AO Wijoyo, T Wittwer, SKC Wong, CQ Woon, K Woon, M Wronowska, J Wu, Y Xiang, R Yanuar, D Yeo, YS Yeo, J Yeo, H Yepiskoposyan, M Yerly, MK Yonchuan, D Zarro, V Zaugg, V Zdimal, C Zhang, Y Zhang, M Zielinski, and T Zivkovic-Semren, as well as to all those who no longer work with us.

We also want to acknowledge those who have supported the writing of this book, in particular S Boué for managing all aspects of the project, and I Blaszkiewicz, V Brooks, C Burton, M Chamberlain, D Ghosh, SB Gopala Reddy, N Karoglou, R Lutz, C Martins Zwicky, L Menezes, C Nolan, JB Simko, A Utan, T Wittwer, and A Zaman for their valuable comments and input.

Finally, we thank Philip Morris International's leadership for driving the development of smoke-free nicotine delivery products, and for putting science at the center of this endeavor.

Preamble

Dear Reader,

The debate around modern tobacco harm reduction has been raging for 30 years, in the face of the harms caused by cigarette smoking, even though these three statements

1. If you don't smoke, don't start
2. If you smoke, quit
3. If you don't quit, change

are supported by robust science underpinned by the natural law of toxicology.

We all know the value of this law to human health and the environment, and we all know of the net population benefits that come from reducing the use of heavy metals, endocrine disruptors, combustible fuels, pesticides, herbicides, and many other toxic substances. This knowledge comes from science, which assesses the products and corresponding opportunities, and it is policies that can, and should, maximize the net population benefits of such opportunities.

Hence our question: Are there circumstances, ever, that would justify foreclosing what the natural law of toxicology shows to be an opportunity?

The natural law of toxicology doesn't care about our needs or wants, doesn't care about our opinions and ideologies, our policies and governments, our funding sources and conflicts of interest. While, clearly, societal debates are necessary to develop sound policies that maximize the net population benefits of new opportunities, they do not override or obscure the results of the dispositive inquiry that flow from the natural law of toxicology.

Switching smokers who would otherwise not quit to noncombustible alternatives (NCAs) to cigarettes, such as electronic nicotine delivery products (ENDPs),[1] that emit significantly lower levels of toxicants than cigarettes is such an opportunity. Indeed, the natural law of toxicology fully applies to ENDPs. The science and the logic are clear, as this book summarizes: *ENDPs emit reduced levels of toxicants, which lead to reduced toxicant exposure, which, in turn, leads to reduced toxicity, and consequently reduced adverse health effects.*

If this is so clear, then why a book on the toxicological assessment of ENDPs?

First and foremost, in the search for truth it is crucial to answer scientific questions in a dispassionate manner. Modern interdisciplinary science offers, like never before in history, advanced methodologies enabling the accurate quantification of toxicant emissions and exposure, and of the biological effects of these substances at the molecular, cellular, and physiological level. Modern science also allows to control the parameters of an experiment and to verify its results. This is particularly important when testing ENDPs in the context of realistic human use. Omission of this important aspect of ENDP assessment may lead to fundamentally flawed studies and data interpretation.

Second, the concept of tobacco harm reduction is not new. Indeed, the first attempt to develop and market an NCA with reduced toxicant emissions is over 30 years old.[2] However, as reported in *The Lancet* of 1991, several medical associations combined forces to speak against this promising avenue to harm reduction, resulting in the company abandoning the project, while remaining free to promote and sell cigarettes.[1] Flawed official statements by medical associations and other interest groups result in fear and confusion; they undermine the ability of consumers to distinguish fact from fiction. Such statements incur a debt to the truth, a debt that is paid in morbidity and mortality among the large number of existing smokers who continue smoking. The editorial concludes that *"There are no good reasons why switching from tobacco products to less harmful nicotine delivery systems should not be encouraged."*[1] Imagine what could have happened over the last 30 years had this initial attempt been supported by the public health stakeholders.

---

1. As defined in Chapter 2, ENDPs include both e-vapor products, such as e-cigarettes, and electrically heated tobacco products.

2. Editorial. Nicotine use after the year 2000. Lancet. 1991 May 18;337(8751):1191−2. PMID: 1673741.

A measure of skepticism is necessary in both science and tobacco control, because it filters out ideas *not* to pursue. But skepticism should not turn into cynicism, which precludes progress.

It is disconcerting that 30 years later, the value of less harmful nicotine delivery systems is still a matter of controversy because of confusion, lack of knowledge, flawed science, and ideology. As a result, a number of countries have banned NCAs—with encouragement by a global organization—irrespective of their merit. There's no question that there need to be rigorous science-based standards to ensure that marketed products do in fact satisfy the natural law of toxicology. But preemptive bans, ones that foreclose products despite even the most compelling scientific evidence to say that, in essence, *nothing* is worthwhile, go beyond cynicism to verge on nihilism. This allows us to ask: Who ultimately bears the consequences of misinformation (or misguided policies) in tobacco harm reduction? The simple answer is the tens of millions of people who would otherwise have switched to less harmful alternatives and instead will continue smoking.

Third, history is full of cases where leaders and organizations have not listened to scientists and therefore resulted in catastrophic failures. Similarly, current guidelines and conventions that prevent the needed transparent dialog between the key stakeholders of tobacco harm reduction are preventing the development of concerted strategies and action plans to end the cigarette era. Hiding behind such guidelines and conventions is equivalent to hiding from the truth, wherever it comes from. As long as this situation prevails, progress will be limited to those who drive a genuine transformation as well as small-scale and often individual crusades. The impact of these limited endeavors is increasingly hampered by a growing ideological opposition, which will further delay the end of the cigarettes era. Therefore, we are now asking: Is it not time for all tobacco harm reduction stakeholders to join forces with the aim to end cigarettes as soon as possible? Is it not time to give NCAs (and ENDPs) a real chance to play out their harm reduction potential? Should we not focus on sound science to develop policies and measures that enable adult smoker access to these products while, at the same time, firmly restricting youth access?

Therefore, the objective of this book is to summarize the sound scientific facts that underpin the harm reduction potential of ENDPs. This clarification is clearly needed to address the confusion caused by those who are against modern tobacco harm reduction and/or ENDPs.

This book is not a literature review, but rather focuses on the evidence that links switching from cigarette smoking to ENDP use with reduced exposure and toxicity, and hence less harm than continued smoking. We describe the findings in the context of the known epidemiology of smoking and cessation as well as along the causal chain of events linking smoking to disease (CELSD). We also show that the reduction in biological impact across the CELSD is coherent with the reduction in toxicant exposure and consistent across many studies conducted by different groups.

We hope that this book will provide a useful summary of the science underpinning tobacco harm reduction, and will drive to a more open dialog among stakeholders to develop sound policies and regulation for the improvement of public health.

Manuel C. Peitsch
Julia Hoeng
Marc S. Firestone

Contents

CHAPTER 1

Tobacco Harm Reduction Concepts and Policy Approaches

MARC S. FIRESTONE • MANUEL C. PEITSCH

1.1 INTRODUCTION

Almost 30 years ago, *The Lancet* published an editorial under the title "Nicotine use after the year 2000" (The Lancet editorial, 1991). The editorial posited a strategy "*to sanction and encourage the use of purified nicotine products as substitutes for smoking, and at the same time impose stringent regulations on permissible constituents of cigarette smoke and progressively lower limits for deliveries of harmful components.*" The editorial concluded: "*There is no good reason why a switch from tobacco products to less harmful nicotine delivery systems should not be encouraged. Smoking-related deaths after the year 2000 would fall steadily and substantially if this can be achieved.*" That encouraging outcome did not, however, come to pass.

In 2007, *The Lancet* again editorialized on innovation to reduce the health burden of cigarette smoking, stating that "*efforts should be channeled into developing low-risk products capable of delivering nicotine as efficiently as cigarettes, while subjecting smoked tobacco products to increasing restrictions*" (The Lancet editorial, 2007). In its conclusion, the 2007 editorial stated: "*Given the known hazards of smoked tobacco, and the numbers of people who smoke, innovative thinking is needed. We support tobacco harm reduction alongside rigorously applied tobacco control policies*" (The Lancet editorial, 2007).

The Lancet pieces from 1991 to 2007 show that the concept of "tobacco harm reduction" is not new. For decades, there has been interest in reducing tobacco-related morbidity and mortality through measures that deter initiation, encourage cessation, and enable harm reduction.

In the past, however, the concept of tobacco harm reduction was ahead of the necessary product technology, scientific investigation, and consumer research. As such, the individual and population-wide benefits of harm reduction were more conceptual than concrete. For example, the World Health Organization (WHO) Scientific Advisory Committee on Tobacco (SACTob)

stated in 2003: "*it is possible that offering harm reduction products might induce some smokers who would not otherwise have quit to use the product and then begin a path that leads to successful long-term abstinence from tobacco. These products may also play a role in enhancing the cessation success of those who are having difficulty achieving abstinence. The potential benefits described here are theoretical, as no tobacco product has currently demonstrated such benefits.*" (WHO Scientific Advisory Committee on Tobacco Product Regulation and WHO Tobacco Free Initiative, 2003).

Further, there have been (and are) concerns that new tobacco- and nicotine-containing products—even if less harmful than conventional tobacco products at the individual level—might undermine rather than complement antismoking (or antitobacco) efforts at the population level (Institute of Medicine, 2001).

To be sure, there are complexities and controversial aspects to tobacco harm reduction, but there is also a straightforward premise: Adults who are already smoking and would otherwise keep smoking—with a corresponding increase in the risk of major diseases—should have access to and information about alternatives that would present less risk of harm (Hatsukami and Carroll, 2020). The last 10 years have seen major advances in both product technology and in the scientific means for assessing the potential health benefits of new products. There has also been an ever-larger body of expert literature with regard to the types of policies, regulatory frameworks, and decision-making methodologies that can maximize individual and population-wide opportunities while minimizing undesirable scenarios.

In short, as of 2020, the conceptual and practical aspects of harm reduction are converging. This chapter briefly introduces policy aspects of harm reduction as a prelude to the subsequent chapters, which cover the technologies and toxicological assessment of electronic nicotine delivery products (ENDPs).

Toxicological Evaluation of Electronic Nicotine Delivery Products. https://doi.org/10.1016/B978-0-12-820490-0.00001-8

1.2 A CONTINUUM OF HARM

A substantial body of epidemiology has demonstrated that the risks of serious disease, such as lung cancer, heart disease, and COPD, are substantially higher among cigarette smokers than among nonsmokers (Abrams et al., 2018a). However, products that do not combust tobacco are likely to have relative risks for major disease that are lower than those for cigarette smoking. For example, epidemiological data show that Swedish *snus*, a noncombustible product with relatively low levels of tobacco-specific nitrosamines (TSNAs) (Rutqvist et al., 2011), presents significantly less risk of harm than cigarettes (Ramström and Wikmans, 2014).

Nicotine-containing products therefore fall on a continuum of harm, with cigarettes at the highest end of the continuum. According to leading authorities in tobacco control: "[t]here is a very pronounced continuum of risk depending upon how toxicants and nicotine, the major addictive substance in tobacco, are delivered. Cigarette smoking is undoubtedly a more hazardous nicotine delivery system than various forms of non-combustible tobacco products for those who continue to use tobacco, which in turn are more hazardous than pharmaceutical nicotine products." (Zeller et al., 2009).

Of all tobacco products, cigarettes carry the greatest risk of disease and are consumed by the greatest number of people— nearly one billion. In turn, cigarette smoking is the greatest contributor of all tobacco-related morbidity and mortality. It follows that tobacco control measures should have a "laser-like focus" on cigarette smoking (Abrams et al., 2018a).

A range of products are potentially less harmful alternatives to continued cigarette smoking. Certain products, such as Swedish *snus*, are noninhalable, while others such as those that create an aerosol by heating a nicotine-containing liquid or by heating tobacco are for inhalation. The common element among the alternatives that offer the most promise for public health is the absence of combustion. This chapter therefore uses the term "noncombustible alternative" (NCA) to refer broadly to products that are (significantly) lower on the continuum of harm than cigarettes and that can, therefore, be part of a harm reduction policy. Importantly, and based on today's knowledge, NCAs will never be risk free and hence will carry a residual risk compared to cessation and total abstinence from tobacco and nicotine products. The rest of this book will be focused on the toxicological assessment of ENDPs, as defined in Chapter 2, which is aimed at comparing the effects of ENDP use with those of cigarette smoking and cessation (Chapter 3).

1.3 THE ROLE OF HARM REDUCTION

In 1997, the United Nations' (UN) Focal Point on Tobacco and Health convened a 2-day roundtable among eminent authorities, many of whom remain active in tobacco policy today, to discuss the potential role of alternative nicotine delivery systems in addressing the health consequences of smoking (UN Focal Point on Tobacco or Health et al., 1998). In his written summary of the experts' views, the rapporteur noted that: "[t]o attain a substantial reduction in tobacco-caused death and disease in existing smokers and in future generations it is important to adopt a triadic approach of coordinated (i) tobacco-use prevention; (ii) smoking cessation; and (iii) reduction of exposure to tobacco toxins in people who are unable or unwilling to completely abstain from tobacco" (UN Focal Point on Tobacco or Health et al., 1998). Further, the experts' recommendations stated: "[w]hereas total cessation remains the ultimate goal of tobacco control policy, reduction of exposure to tobacco toxins should be added to the existing treatment approaches" (UN Focal Point on Tobacco or Health et al., 1998).

A similar view is evident in the WHO Framework Convention on Tobacco Control, which was signed in 2003 and entered into force in 2005. The Convention defines tobacco control as "a range of supply, demand and harm reduction strategies that aim to improve the health of a population by eliminating or reducing the consumption of tobacco products and exposure to tobacco smoke" (World Health Organization, 2005).

Since then, concepts of tobacco harm reduction have continued to evolve. As a precautionary measure, regulators have set ceilings on "tar" (European Union, 2014), and policymakers have suggested maximum levels for selected smoke constituents (Burns et al., 2008; WHO Study Group et al., 2008). But there is great skepticism—including in light of the history of low "tar" and "light" cigarettes—that a less hazardous combustible cigarette will ever be part of tobacco control. Instead, the focus has been increasingly on NCAs that *replace* cigarettes for those who would otherwise continue to smoke and contribute to lower smoking prevalence in a way that is additive to baseline quitting rates.

A harm reduction or harm minimization policy aims to complement other measures for reducing smoking prevalence, especially those that deter initiation and encourage cessation. Doing so accommodates—*subject to various empirical conditions*—noncombustible tobacco- and nicotine-containing products as part of tobacco control. Thus, instead of a moral judgment or morality-based impulse to preclude a behavior, the policy is a pragmatic way to reduce the harm that will otherwise accompany the behavior. Abrams summarizes the key elements in this way: *"a harm minimization framework recognizes that demanding the unrealistic and unrealized utopian dream (i.e., elimination of any and all consumer nicotine or tobacco products regardless of their relative harms and the related destruction of the entire tobacco and nicotine consumer product industry) actually undercuts the realistic benefits of pragmatism. When a harmful behavior cannot be eliminated, it is necessary to reduce its adverse health consequences to the greatest extent possible among any users of nicotine or tobacco containing consumer products."* (Abrams et al., 2018b).

Moreover, a contemporary harm reduction policy recognizes the interests and, indeed, the rights of adult smokers who would otherwise keep smoking in having access to, and information about, less harmful alternatives.

1.4 BENEFIT TO THE POPULATION AS A WHOLE

Scientific evidence that a particular noncombustible product presents less risk than continued smoking demonstrates benefit to the individual and leads to a second line of inquiry: What is the expected population-wide outcome? In particular, is it reasonable to foresee a net population benefit? In that regard, the WHO's "Statement of Principles Guiding the Evaluation of New or Modified Tobacco Products," which its SACTob released in 2003, remains instructive: *"The harm to the population is the net effect of the changes in harm to the individual users and the changes in number of users who are exposed .... Population harm, therefore, is the net of the combined effects that harm reduction products and their marketing have on the use of tobacco products and resultant population exposure to toxicants"* (WHO Scientific Advisory Committee on Tobacco Product Regulation and WHO Tobacco Free Initiative, 2003).

Especially when considering new and emerging products, assessment of net population harm involves forecasts of human behavior. Under United States (US) law, therefore, when assessing premarket applications for new tobacco products, the US Food & Drug Administration (FDA) looks at risks and benefits to both users and nonusers, taking into account

a. the increased or decreased likelihood that existing users of tobacco products will stop using such products; and

b. the increased or decreased likelihood that those who do not use tobacco products will start using such products (United States Code, 2006).

There are now several sophisticated models for depicting flows toward or away from different consumer behaviors in the context of NCAs (Abrams et al., 2018a; Lee et al., 2017; Vugrin et al., 2015; Weitkunat et al., 2015). For example, Abrams and colleagues depict a Markov state transition model of cigarette and e-vapor product (EVP, a.k.a e-cigarettes) use (Abrams et al., 2018a), while Vugrin and coworkers show nine transition states in a two-product model (Vugrin et al., 2015), and Weitkunat and colleagues use 12 smoking transition probabilities to model the population health impact of introducing an NCA into the US market (Lee et al., 2017; Weitkunat et al., 2015).

For the sake of illustration, Fig. 1.1 is a simple model that focuses specifically on cigarette smoking and four states: (1) people who have never smoked or used nicotine, (2) current smokers, (3) former smokers, and (4) people who are current [exclusive] users of NCAs.

There are five pathways between the states:

a. Initiation of regular cigarette smoking by a never user

b. Cessation of cigarette smoking

c. Switching from cigarette smoking to an NCA

d. Cessation of NCA use

e. Initiation of regular NCA by a never user

By definition, pathways *a* and *e* are unidirectional because current users of cigarettes or NCAs cannot become never users. The other three are bidirectional. For example, there is a subset of former smokers who relapse (*b*).

Long-standing measures for reducing smoking prevalence focus on minimizing initiation (*a*) by never users while maximizing cessation among current smokers (*b*). A harm reduction policy adds focus on the possibility that the large subset of current adult smokers who will otherwise continue to smoke would benefit by switching completely to less harmful alternatives (*c*).

On average, in countries for which reliable data are available, approximately 5% of existing smokers will quit successfully in a given year (Substance Abuse and Mental Health Services Administration (US) and Office of the Surgeon General (US), 2020). As such, each year, approximately 19 out of 20 men and women who are already smoking will continue to smoke. This is a slice-in-time inference from annual cessation (or quit) rates, but it serves to illustrate that the intended consumer base for NCAs does not include never (1) or former users (3).

At the individual level, the policy objective is to maximize switching along pathway *c* among existing smokers who will otherwise continue to smoke. The population-level objective is to enable switching while,

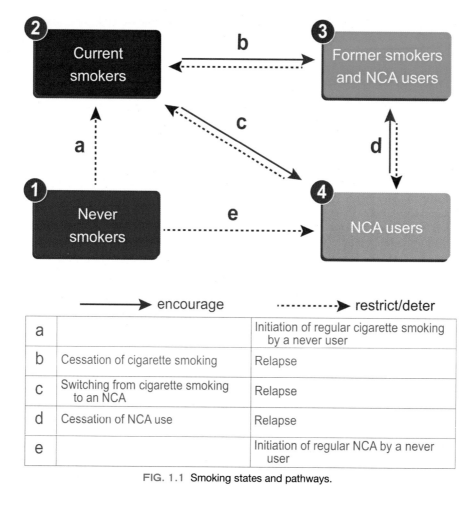

	encourage	restrict/deter
a		Initiation of regular cigarette smoking by a never user
b	Cessation of cigarette smoking	Relapse
c	Switching from cigarette smoking to an NCA	Relapse
d	Cessation of NCA use	Relapse
e		Initiation of regular NCA by a never user

FIG. 1.1 Smoking states and pathways.

at a minimum, holding baseline rates of initiation and cessation constant. Moreover, it is possible that some people might go from cigarettes to NCAs (*c*) and later give up NCAs (*d*). Finally, NCA users should be deterred from going back to smoking cigarettes (*c*).

In brief, the net population benefit increases as (**A**) smoking initiation goes down, cessation goes up, and remaining smokers switch to NCAs while (**B**) NCA initiation and relapse to smoking are held to a minimum.

As a corollary, the net contribution of NCAs to population harm reduction depends primarily on the availability of significantly less harmful NCAs that a significant number of cigarette smokers are willing to accept and switch to without there being a countervailing increase in initiation or decrease in cessation. This net contribution can be illustrated by a simple *tobacco harm reduction equation* (Fig. 1.2) (Smith et al., 2016). This equation is formulated as a "*multiplication function*" to illustrate that

the achieved population benefit is a function of how much harm can be reduced by an NCA "*multiplied*" by its acceptance by smokers and its usage among the population. This means that a significant contribution to population harm reduction would be achieved by products with very low harm (compared with cigarettes) that

i. are widely accepted by smokers—maximizes pathway *c*,
ii. do not attract persons who do not currently smoke (both never and former smokers)—minimizes pathways *d* and *e*, and
iii. do not negatively influence smokers who intend to quit—neutral to pathway *b*.

The net contribution to population harm reduction depends on the magnitude of the product harm reduction (i.e., significantly less harmful than cigarettes to the individual) and its acceptance by smokers and effect on usage among the population.

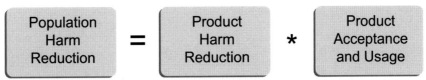

FIG. 1.2 The tobacco harm reduction equation. The net contribution to population harm reduction depends on the magnitude of the product harm reduction (i.e., significantly less harmful than cigarettes to the individual) and its acceptance by smokers and effect on usage among the population.

Conversely, low product acceptance would offset even the strongest reduced harm product profile, negating any significant population benefit. Similarly, a product with a marginal harm reduction profile but wide consumer acceptance would also not result in significant population benefit.

1.5 PARAMETERS INFLUENCING HARM REDUCTION POLICIES

There are several parameters that are crucial to the implementation of a successful harm reduction policy. Among them, one can identify product innovation, awareness, access, and price, each playing a key role in driving the reduction in smoking prevalence above and beyond the effects of policies aimed at minimizing initiation and maximizing cessation.

1.5.1 Product Harm Reduction

As expressed by the harm reduction equation, population harm reduction critically depends on the availability of significantly less harmful alternatives to cigarettes. This means that product innovation, which is key to tobacco harm reduction, is aimed at developing NCAs that are less and less harmful. Given that the harm caused by cigarette smoking is overwhelmingly due to the toxicants generated during tobacco combustion, companies leverage novel technologies to avoid combustion and, thereby, minimize the emission of toxicants.

1.5.2 Product Acceptance and Usage

1.5.2.1 Product acceptance

As NCAs are still competing with cigarettes in the marketplace, NCAs must, by definition, be acceptable to smokers and provide at least some of the ritual as well as the sensory and nicotine-based rewards associated with cigarettes. Indeed, for an NCA to be a net contributor to population harm reduction, it must be not only significantly less harmful than cigarettes but also acceptable to at least a fraction of current smokers. Product innovation is, therefore, faced with a multiobjective optimization challenge. The challenge is to

(i) minimize product harm while, at the same time, (ii) maximizing product acceptance by smokers (pathway *c* in Fig. 1.1). Moreover, the product should be minimally attractive to former (pathway *d* in Fig. 1.1) and never-smokers (pathway *e* in Fig. 1.1), especially youth. Consequently, developing a product with zero risk that is acceptable to all smokers is a *utopia*.

Over the last decade, it has become apparent that a single product category is not sufficient to address the diversity of consumer demands. Hence, different products have reached the market—ranging from oral NCAs such as Swedish *snus* and nicotine pouches to inhalable NCAs such as ENDPs (Chapter 2)—and are being further developed.

1.5.2.2 Awareness

It goes without saying that smokers, especially those who do not quit and are searching for less harmful alternatives, should be aware of the existence and availability of products that are less harmful than cigarettes. As the goal of harm reduction is to switch completely these smokers from cigarettes to NCAs, it is crucial that they are accurately informed about the harm reduction potential of NCAs. It is equally important to inform them that NCAs are not risk free, and, therefore, quitting tobacco or nicotine altogether remains the best option for reducing the risk of smoking-related disease. Moreover, and for the same reason, it is crucial to inform nonsmokers that NCAs are not for them and that they should not initiate, or reinitiate, nicotine consumption with NCAs (see red (*dashed*) *arrows* for pathways *e* and *d* in Fig. 1.1).

For consumers to receive such information, there should be a coherent sharing of information that is accurate and nonmisleading. The content of such information should be agreed upon by regulators and public health officials and based on sound scientific risk assessments (see Section 6 below). There are, however, several barriers to this:

1. There is widespread confusion among the general population and healthcare professionals about the harm of nicotine versus that of cigarette smoke. Recent studies have shown that 49%−80% (Villanti

et al., 2019) of the population believes that nicotine—rather than the hundreds of toxicants generated during tobacco combustion—is responsible for most of the cancer and health risks caused by smoking.

2. Strong antitobacco sentiment held by tobacco control advocates, medical associations, and nongovernmental organizations that overshadows the scientific underpinnings of harm reduction. These organizations generally oppose tobacco harm reduction on the basis of nonscientific and dogmatic arguments and often invoke flawed science while disregarding the large body of evidence in favor of harm reduction and NCAs because of its origin. The 1991 editorial in *The Lancet* had already reported that several medical associations combined forces to speak against this promising avenue, resulting in a company abandoning the development of an NCA, while remaining free to promote and sell cigarettes (The Lancet editorial, 1991). This has not changed (at least not dramatically) over the past 30 years and continues to be a major barrier to harm reduction, especially in a world where the press and social media are prompt to amplify sensationalist news based on flawed science aimed at equating the harms of NCAs with those of cigarettes.

1.5.2.3 Access
To enable smokers who do not quit to access NCAs, these products must be broadly and readily available to smokers in the marketplace—while reinforcing that NCAs are not for never- and former smokers. There should be appropriate sales practices, restrictions, controls, and oversight, with particularly high barriers against youth access, including effective youth access prevention measures that can be implemented through technology and regulations.

In contrast, banning NCAs, as is the case in a number of countries, effectively deprives smokers of opportunities to switch to less harmful alternatives, while not improving the rate of smoking cessation. The net result is a stagnation or slower decline in smoking prevalence and the loss of the net population benefit NCAs can bring. These bans might target a specific NCA, such as Swedish *snus* in the European Union (despite its known contribution to harm reduction) (Clarke et al., 2019; Fisher et al., 2019; Lee, 2013), certain flavors that enable smokers to switch, or all NCAs without distinction. Bans block access to existing products while also discouraging further research and development that might otherwise lead to useful innovations.

1.5.2.4 Price
Increasing the purchase price of tobacco products is a key measure used to minimize smoking initiation and maximize smoking cessation. Similarly, a positive price differential between cigarettes and NCAs is likely to encourage smokers to switch from cigarettes to NCAs. It is, therefore, important that governments, through the lever of taxation, ensure that a significant price differential is maintained between cigarettes and NCAs. There is sound argumentation in favor of excise tax policies that distinguish cigarettes and other combusted tobacco products from NCAs on the basis of relative risk (Chaloupka et al., 2015).

1.5.2.5 Sales practices
Sound sales practices are a valid means for maximizing the net population benefit of NCAs. Such practices can be implemented, both voluntarily and through regulation, to minimize NCA access to unintended audiences, while ensuring that current smokers, the intended audience, are made broadly aware of the existence of NCAs and receive transparent information about their benefits and limitations. Such sales practices should be based on principles aimed at encouraging consumers on a path of harm reduction. These principles need to address pathways *b*, *c*, *d*, and *e* in Fig. 1.1.

The first principle is that NCAs are for adult smokers who want to continue enjoying tobacco or nicotine products and would otherwise continue to smoke. Therefore, smokers must be clearly informed that NCAs are not an alternative to quitting and that the best choice is undoubtedly to quit tobacco or nicotine altogether. Furthermore, consumer messages must clearly state that NCAs are not risk-free or a safe alternative to cigarettes, but are a better choice than smoking. Consumers must also be informed that NCAs contain nicotine, which is addictive.

The second principle is that NCAs are not for people who have never smoked or who have quit smoking, which means that information about the existence and availability of NCAs is principally for existing current adult smokers. Marketing activities might, for example, use cigarette packs as a vehicle for information about NCAs or use consumer databases for appropriately targeted digital messaging.

Finally, to experience the benefit of NCAs, smokers should switch completely to them and abandon cigarettes permanently. Indeed, the harm reduction potential of an NCA is, at least in part, negated by concurrent cigarette smoking (so-called "dual use"). As it takes time for a current smoker to switch completely to an NCA, the consumer should be provided various support measures, both in person and digitally, until complete switching is achieved.

1.6 BALANCING RISK AND BENEFITS UNDER UNCERTAIN CONDITIONS

Tobacco harm reduction requires that many actors make decisions under conditions of uncertainty. As a corollary, unintended outcomes and undesirable scenarios can arise despite thoughtful, empirical decisions. An added element in making the soundest possible decisions is, therefore, to tease out—and estimate the likelihood and consequences of—specific types of erroneous decisions. To be clear, however, to characterize a decision as erroneous is neither a value judgment nor a critique of the decision-making process. Instead, the aim is to elicit a context-specific error preference as part of sound decision-making.

1.6.1 Error Types in Hypothesis Testing

In particular, the concept of type I and type II errors, which originally comes from statistics (Neyman and Pearson, 1933, 1928), is useful, even if by analogy, in many contexts. The basic terminology is that there is a type I error in *erroneously rejecting* a (true) hypothesis and a type II error in erroneously *accepting* a (false) hypothesis, which can also be described as failing to reject a false hypothesis (U.S. Department of Health and Human Services Food and Drug Administration et al., 1998). Thus, if the null hypothesis (H_0) is that substance A has *no* effect, there is a type I error in *rejecting* H_0 when there *is no* effect and a type II error in *accepting* (or, failing to reject) H_0 when there *is* an effect. In shorthand, to reject the true is a type I error and to accept the false is a type II error.

As a simple example, consider a situation in which an art appraiser must decide whether a newly discovered artwork is real or fake. Fig. 1.3 depicts four possible decisions in light of whether the painting is in reality—which is unknown to the appraiser *ex ante*—real or fake.

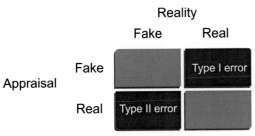

FIG. 1.3 Error types when appraising art

The appraiser might *correctly* conclude that the painting is real or *correctly* conclude that it is a fake. The two erroneous decisions are that a real painting is appraised as fake, or that a fake is appraised as real. If an auction house acts on the basis of an erroneous appraisal, it would either sell a fake painting or refrain from selling a real one, with each scenario presenting consequences. It is the difference in the *nature* of the consequences that informs a decision-maker's error preference.

1.6.2 Error Preference

Presumption of innocence is an example of an explicit preference for one type of error versus another, namely a strong preference for avoiding type I errors, in a criminal trial. The presumption corresponds to a null hypothesis (H_0) that the defendant is not guilty. In *rejecting* H_0 when the defendant is *not* guilty, there is a type I error, while the type II error lies in accepting H_0 when the defendant *is* guilty. In other words, the type I error is convicting the innocent, and the type II error is acquitting the guilty. The burden on the prosecution to prove guilt beyond reasonable doubt is analogous to setting a low α (e.g., 0.05 or 0.01) in hypothesis testing. Put differently, society has long held the view that the negative consequences of convicting the innocent are far greater than those of acquitting the guilty.

Whether or not it does so explicitly, regulatory policy also incorporates aspects of, and attitudes toward, type I and type II errors. In the context of drug and device regulation, for example, *"there is a relationship between risk tolerance and risk aversion by regulators … and the expected outcomes in terms of either avoidance of drug-induced patient harm or net public-health gains."* (Eichler et al., 2013).

Moreover, regulatory frameworks and decisions tend to focus less on the consequences of erroneously keeping useful innovation off the market (type II error) than erroneously allowing innovations with adverse effects (type I error). As the US Supreme Court Justice Stephen Breyer has noted, *"hearings are far more likely to mean criticism for leniency than for strictness."* (Breyer, 1993). Similarly, Henningfield and coauthors have described the possible role of omission bias in the context of tobacco harm reduction: *"In public health policy, medical practice, and other areas of policy, practice, and services, there has been increasing focus on errors and harms resulting from what is referred to as an 'omission bias' in human decision-making—a bias towards avoidance of commission errors and insensitivity to or an undervaluing of omission errors."* (Henningfield et al., 2018). But, type II errors (or errors of "omission") can, in fact, be significant, including in the context of measures for reducing tobacco-related morbidity and mortality. According to Eichler and coauthors, when decision-makers move *"too far … beyond a 'sweet spot' of maximum efficiency, increased risk aversion or requests for more data are anticipated to result in diminishing net health gains from drug research and development."* (Eichler et al., 2013). Their conclusion is that *"risk aversion comes with its own risks. Stakeholders, including those who are critical of regulatory standards, should be aware that a drive towards an excessive focus on avoiding risks and uncertainties will mean that patients pay a price: delay in accessing therapeutics and lost therapeutic options. Good drug regulation is more than just minimizing risks; it is about maximizing gains in public health."* (Eichler et al., 2013).

Similarly, but writing in the specific context of tobacco control, Abrams and coauthors have stated: *"During the early stages of responding to disruption, hypothetical fears about unknown consequences abound, coupled with an instinctive resistance to changing course."* (Abrams et al., 2018b). In their view, *"the opportunity lost by not changing course must also be considered. In light of the dramatic changes in the product landscape, by not taking some risks to speed the demise of deadly smoked tobacco, then worldwide over the next century the lives of a billion smokers are ultimately at stake."* (Abrams et al., 2018b).

To be sure, harm reduction policy requires great care to limit the possibility of type I errors. Given the known risks of continued smoking, however, decision-makers must also be alert to the possibility and consequences of type II errors.

1.6.3 Reducing (and Accepting) Uncertainty

As in fields ranging from space exploration to medical devices, when creating regulatory frameworks and then acting within them with respect to tobacco harm reduction, policymakers, regulators, and the private sector must make the best choices possible without perfect knowledge (*epistemic* uncertainty) and an element of chance or randomness (*aleatory* uncertainty). To quote a prominent authority on the history of science and probability: *"All-or- nothing outcomes—either everything under control or everything left to chance—are nonstarters. The debate must assay possibilities, probabilities, and desirabilities with a jeweler's balance."* (Daston, 2008).

What are the long-term health consequences of EVP use? What will be the effect of new products on youth uptake of traditional, combustible products? How will battery life over time affect aerosolization of a nicotine-containing liquid? What is the role of flavors in enabling switching? These are only a few examples of the epistemic and aleatory uncertainties that arise in the context of NCAs. When epistemic and aleatory uncertainties persist,

as they often will, decision-makers must act on the basis of the best available evidence (Warner, 2019). For example, manufacturers should follow rigorous standards of scientific investigation and empiricism to confirm product performance and reliability, and regulators must make sound inferences from available evidence in light of policy objectives.

Knowledge tends to increase as information accumulates over time—although not always in a predictable relationship. Vast quantities of additional information (data and facts) might be necessary to have a small increase in knowledge that will reduce epistemic uncertainty … or perhaps not. To illustrate, Fig. 1.4 plots knowledge on the y-axis against time and information on the x-axis. The shape of the blue curve is purely hypothetical. There is no a priori formula for the relationship between the values on the two axes.

Purely for the sake of illustration, the three zones in Fig. 1.4 show different stages of knowledge accumulation. Zone A is a phase during which knowledge is increasing but is not yet sufficient to make an informed "go/no-go" decision. Type I errors are latent in Zone A when there is a decision to proceed (i.e., a "go" decision).

Zone B depicts the range of knowledge that adequately informs a timely decision (whether "go" or "no go").

In Zone C, there is already a substantial body of knowledge, and the rate of increase is slowing: More time and more information are, at the margin, producing less knowledge. When a decision-maker in Zone C decides not to proceed ("no go")—or to await more data, which has the same implications as "no go" pending a "go"—there is a likely type II error. There is a missed opportunity to proceed under conditions of (and notwithstanding) a level of uncertainty. Additional knowledge might reduce uncertainty, but perhaps not materially or perhaps only after a long delay that carries its own risks.

The red (*straight*) *line* in Fig. 1.4 represents knowledge about the base case in the context of NCAs—that is, continued cigarette smoking. The line is illustrative only but provides a reference point for assessing uncertainty. Scientific investigation of smoking continues; but, there is already an enormous amount of knowledge, especially with respect to the correlation between increasing pack-years of smoking (i.e., the combination of amount smoked and duration of smoking) and increased risk of serious disease. Accordingly, the amount of knowledge that is appropriate to a particular decision regarding NCAs has to take account of the near certainties regarding the effects of continued cigarette smoking.

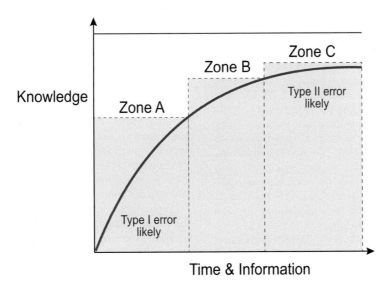

FIG. 1.4 Relationship between knowledge and time.

A measure of pragmatism in addressing the epistemic challenges does not dilute the rigorous standards of scientific investigation. Taking account of both the ideal amount of knowledge and the amount that is practicable, a policy framework can encourage a step-by-step approach. For example, in its 2003 "Statement of Principles Guiding the Evaluation of New or Modified Tobacco Products," the WHO's Scientific Advisory Committee suggested an approach that builds over time: *"More timely examination of new products is important for both regulatory oversight and for providing accurate public health advice to consumers. The data upon which this evaluation is made will, of necessity, be more limited than that which would be available from epidemiological and other observations made over a long duration of the use of the new product. Limitations of the data likely to be available make it useful to conceptualize the evaluation as a set of questions that can be answered in series and which allow a progressively more complete understanding of the actual benefits likely to be experienced by those who switch to a new product."* (WHO Scientific Advisory Committee on Tobacco Product Regulation and WHO Tobacco Free Initiative, 2003).

By contrast, some might insist on an evidentiary standard of "zero harm" or "100% less than cigarettes" for NCAs (Hall et al., 2019). To proceed without due care would lead to avoidable negative outcomes; but, an imperative to eliminate uncertainty would preclude opportunity. The task is, therefore, to find the appropriate balance. In an oft-cited paper on what they

designate as vaporized nicotine products, Levy and co-authors state: *"until clearer data are available, our ability to understand the impact of use will need to be based on careful and prudent extrapolations of their probable benefits and harms from shorter-term evidence."* (Levy et al., 2017a).

In short, policy devolves to paradox when it insists that new products have a history of long-term use before consumers can choose them instead of continued smoking, the risks of which decades of epidemiology vividly demonstrate. As Fairchild and coauthors have written: *"Harm reduction recognizes that the proposed alternatives carry uncertainties. It involves making a strategic determination when the risks are considerable—as they surely are with cigarette smoking—moving forward in the face of uncertainty is unavoidable."* (Fairchild et al., 2018).

1.7 EXAMPLES OF REGULATORY FRAMEWORKS

Policies and regulatory frameworks for tobacco products tend to date back roughly 20 years and, in any event, vary around the world. Few countries have laws and regulations that are contemporary with the substantial and growing consumer interest in less-harmful alternatives to cigarettes or with the technological and scientific developments that have enabled NCAs. Nonetheless, as experience with new products, including combustion-free alternatives, increases over time, there is likely to be a degree of convergence with respect to the core elements of regulatory frameworks.

1.7.1 Regulatory Objectives

A regulation on NCAs should be clear in stating its objectives, means, and rationale. Although that seems obvious, as Bullen has observed with regard to EVPs: *"In most jurisdictions the goal of proposed e-cigarette regulation has not been clearly articulated."* (Bullen, 2016). There is, however, a good deal of support for the proposition that regulation should aim to reduce tobacco-related morbidity and mortality, as distinct from bans or restrictions that might reflect an ideological or moralistic perspective. Thus, according to the WHO's Advisory Committee's 2003 statement, *"The major acceptable public health rationale for development of new or modified tobacco products is the potential for a reduction in the harm caused by existing tobacco products."*

With the objective of reducing tobacco-related harm, regulation would aim to encourage (and, at a minimum, enable) current smokers who would otherwise continue smoking to switch to less harmful alternatives—while maintaining measures that deter initiation and encourage cessation. More specifically, the regulatory framework would aim to

a. *Maximize* the opportunity to reduce the prevalence of cigarette smoking through exclusive switching by those who would otherwise continue smoking; *and*
b. *Minimize* potentially negative outcomes, such as (i) reduced rates of cessation and (ii) youth initiation of smoking.

Regulatory mechanisms and tools can target the factors (and their interplay) that determine the likelihood and magnitude of the desired and undesired scenarios. As Abrams and coauthors have written: *"The key challenge is to implement policies that maximize the net flow away from smoking and toward the use of safer products or to no use. A balance can and must be found to protect youth without discouraging cleaner nicotine use by smokers unable or not wishing to stop their nicotine use. Delays in harm minimization may impede the end of smoking rather than encourage smokers to switch to safer nicotine delivery products."* (Abrams et al., 2018a).

A policy that seeks the right balance—or the "sweet spot" as some authorities state (Abrams et al., 2018b; Eichler et al., 2013)—must, of course, include measures to guard against various concerns, from consumer deception to youth uptake. Preemptive bans on product categories might seem to preclude negative outcomes; but, they carry their own consequences, a point that Levy has crystalized: *"Countries whose policies discourage [vaporized nicotine products] use run the risk of neutralizing a potentially useful addition to methods of reducing tobacco use."* (Levy et al., 2017a).

Governments have a suite of tools for optimizing the overall benefit of less harmful alternatives to cigarettes. Targeted interventions can address specific concerns. For example, sales and marketing restrictions, warning notices on packaging, educational campaigns, and minimum age requirements can specifically target unintended scenarios while propelling switching by adult smokers. Moreover, postmarket surveillance that monitors actual consumer behavior and use patterns—especially with respect to the ratio between switching by existing adult smokers and youth initiation—provides valuable insights into continued oversight, and enables appropriate corrective action if necessary.

In short, the right mix of policy measures can maximize the opportunities that innovation offers. The following sections outline basic considerations in regulating NCAs.

1.7.2 Ex Ante and Ex Post Regulation

As a general matter, government oversight varies with respect to the timing of regulatory intervention relative to market (private sector) action (Kolstad et al., 1990; Stern, 2017). Broadly stated, the timing might be ex ante or it might be ex post. An ex ante mechanism requires a regulatory body's prior approval to take a certain action. Regulation of large mergers, utility rates, and new drugs is often ex ante in that the regulator's approval or authorization is necessary before a proposed action can proceed. The regulator is essentially acting as a gatekeeper to the market, with authority to make "go/no-go" decisions in advance with respect to commercial activities.

In the US, the FDA has largely ex ante oversight of novel tobacco products. A 2009 law vests the FDA with jurisdiction over tobacco products, including EVPs that contain nicotine derived from tobacco (Food and Drug Administration (FDA), 2009). "Modified risk" products and, subject to certain exceptions, "new" products require premarket authorization (Food and Drug Administration (FDA), 2009).

An ex post framework uses market surveillance and strict enforcement. For example, regulation of common carrier rates, distribution agreements, and certain medical devices is usually ex post. *Ex post* does not mean unregulated or *laissez-faire*. There are enforceable standards and corresponding government oversight. The distinction is that a regulation is not a gating mechanism for market access.

By virtue of a 2014 Directive, the European Union has an intricate set of rules that address nine categories of tobacco products (cigarettes, roll-your-own tobacco, pipe tobacco, water pipe tobacco, cigars, cigarillos, chewing tobacco, nasal tobacco, and tobacco for oral use); distinguish between products for smoking and smokeless products; and create a notification regimen, with an authorization option, for "novel" products (i.e., products that do not fall into the preceding categories and were placed on the market after May 19, 2014) (European Union, 2014). The notification regime operates at the Member State level, with largely ex post oversight of novel products and, in some jurisdictions, ex ante oversight of consumer communication.

Neither ex ante nor ex post regulation is a priori right or wrong, better or worse. The question is which timing is more likely to yield the best outcome in a specific context. Useful innovation is certainly possible within an ex ante framework, but it can easily become a highly capillary system, with a limited flow of products—somewhat analogous to a line of airliners waiting to take off at a busy airport.

The choice between ex ante and ex post oversight also bears on the institutional capabilities that a regulator requires. A regulator's ability to decide on "go/no-go" questions in a largely ex ante regime—and to do so efficiently—depends on its expertise, objectivity, funding, staffing, and infrastructure. Without those attributes, the requirement for ex ante intervention becomes counterproductive. A largely ex post regime depends on timely, vigorous enforcement of regulatory standards and penalties that are effective deterrents. Otherwise, ex post regulation can devolve into a lack of necessary and consistent regulatory oversight.

1.7.3 Product Bans

Some policymakers (and jurisdictions) endorse highly restrictive rules against NCAs, including category-wide bans that foreclose the possibility of specific products within the category irrespective of the supporting data. For example, in Australia, the Therapeutic Goods Administration (TGA) classifies nicotine as a "Schedule 7 Dangerous Poison" under the Standard for the Uniform Scheduling of Medicines and Poisons ("Poisons Standard") (Australian State, 2017). Nicotine-containing products are, therefore, unlawful unless they fall within an exemption to the classification.

One exemption covers nicotine replacement therapies, which require TGA premarket approval as prescription drugs. The other exemption is for "tobacco which is prepared and packed for smoking." (Australian State, 2017). As a result, products that are not for smoking, including EVPs (Hall et al., 2019), are not permissible as consumer products (as opposed to products for therapeutic use). Further, a 1991 statute precludes Swedish

snus despite epidemiological evidence that it presents significantly less risk than cigarette smoking (Gartner and Hall, 2008).

The TGA has the authority to expand the exemptions, and the Parliament could amend the TGA's enabling legislation (Australian Government, 1989) to exempt certain products from Schedule 7. To date, however, Australian authorities have taken the position that, inter alia, there is insufficient evidence to merit an expanded set of exemptions and that allowing EVPs risks undermining the country's tobacco control measures (Hall et al., 2019). Moreover, according to the TGA's final decision that denied a proposed exemption for EVPs, "Current government policy supports the cessation of smoking rather than harm reduction." (Australian Government, Department of Health, 2017).

Several respected tobacco control experts have questioned the rationale for Australia's ban on ENDPs. Notably, Hall and coauthors published a "critical analysis" of the ban in a 2018 article, and they describe the ban as "poorly justified," "weakly based in evidence," and "paternalistic" (Hall et al., 2019). The article recognizes "legitimate public health concerns"—including those with respect to youth initiation—while emphasizing that a "A sales ban is an incoherent form of risk management that prevents the sale of a less harmful nicotine product while allowing the sale of cigarettes, the most harmful nicotine product. A sales ban is poorly justified as a policy to prevent Australian youth from initiating smoking when there are other less restrictive policies that could achieve the same goal." (Hall et al., 2019).

In another paper, Gartner notes that a "policy that bans vaporized nicotine products in order to reduce adolescent smoking uptake may be much less effective (and possibly counterproductive) than reducing youth (and adult) access to smoked tobacco products." (Gartner, 2018). She adds that the "most important policy question often ignored in the debate about youth vaping is: what should we be doing to reduce youth access to cigarettes?" (Gartner, 2018).

1.7.4 Product Standards

Regulation can also set clear standards for critical aspects of product performance. For example, in the case of ENDPs, electrical product safety standards should be set to ensure that only high-quality products that can be operated safely reach the market. This is particularly important when considering the safety of battery operation. ENDP product standards could also be extended to ensure youth access prevention and child safety (i.e., childproofing). In the case of inhaled products, there can be standards that describe methodologies for measuring the compounds in aerosol emissions and set maximum levels for certain compounds, such as carbon monoxide, TSNAs, carbonyls, polycyclic aromatic hydrocarbons, and heavy metals. The standards can also be extended to include methodologies for comparing the toxicity of an inhaled product aerosol with that of cigarette smoke and set the minimal levels of reduction in toxicity.

1.7.5 Consumer Access to Information

Assuming a product meets relevant standards as outlined in the previous section, and is scientifically substantiated as having the potential to reduce harm compared with cigarette smoking, the next inquiry concerns consumer access to—and corresponding information about—the products. According to the UN and national policies around the world, consumers deserve access *"to adequate information to enable them to make informed choices according to individual wishes and needs."* (United Nations Conference on Trade and Development, 2016a). As a corollary, *"[b]usiness should assist consumers to develop knowledge and skills necessary to understand risks ... to take informed decisions."* (United Nations Conference on Trade and Development, 2016b). The preceding principles are critical in many areas, including the effort to reduce smoking prevalence. The EU has stated, for example, that the *"greatest possible transparency of product information should be ensured for the general public."* (European Union, 2014). Access to information is also recognized as a critical component for achieving the right to health, allowing individuals to participate in health-related decision-making (Office of the High Commissioner for Human Rights, 2000).

Manufacturers must provide truthful, nonmisleading information to consumers. Regulation, whether ex ante or ex post, should include strict rules for scientific substantiation and vigorous enforcement of consumer protection laws. At the same time, policymakers should also aim to provide the public with accurate information, including information with respect to the continuum of harm and the potential of new products. Surveys have indicated that smokers do not necessarily understand the differences between the risks of smoking versus switching to a scientifically validated NCA (McNeil et al., 2015). A regulatory framework should aim to provide accurate information as part of a harm reduction policy. As Kiviniemi and Kozlowski have written, *"[g]iven the scientific consensus that cigarettes are the most deadly form of tobacco use, the public has a right to a clear understanding of this fact and efforts should be made to impart an understanding of the differential health risks for various tobacco/nicotine products."* (Kiviniemi and Kozlowski, 2015)

Just as manufacturers should inform consumers, *"Information provided by governments and health authorities could also clearly indicate the relative harms of each product, rather than misleadingly suggesting that all tobacco products are equally hazardous."* (Gartner et al., 2010).

Regulations should take account of the latest scientific and technical developments and should have specific measures for reducing the likelihood of unintended scenarios. And, there is no question that there needs to be strict regulatory oversight by a body with the appropriate mandate, expertise, and resources. High standards and strict oversight, however, should not foreclose the benefits of innovation, especially when it is entirely possible to find a regulatory equilibrium that promotes a net population benefit. As Abrams and coauthors have written, *"if, out of an abundance of caution, tobacco control strategies fail to fully embrace movement to less harmful products (or actively discourage such movement), the result could be detrimental for smokers who are unable to quit or who do not wish to quit nicotine use completely."* (Abrams et al., 2018a). Similarly, in an article on EVPs, Fairchild and Bayer note: *"what such a strong position does not acknowledge is that this perspective also entails a cost: It only recognizes the potential benefits of erecting barriers to e-cigarettes without considering the potential toll measured by lives lost to combustible products. In a world of multiple risks ... 'precaution against one risk may induce other countervailing risks' and associated burdens."* (Fairchild and Bayer, 2015). In essence, regulations should be issued within a contemporaneous policy framework that clearly sets the objectives, means, rationale, and that is flexible enough to adapt to the specific dynamics of the market, including how the products perform in regards to their net contribution to population harm reduction. The purpose of the regulator's precaution should be *"to avoid irreversible decisions"* (Renn, 2007). If the negative outcomes or their probabilities turn out to be higher than expected, *"it is prudent to proceed in a way in which the decision can be reversed quickly"* (Renn, 2007). A contemporaneous and evidence-based framework contains the risk, sets boundaries, maximizes the opportunities, and minimizes the risks in a balanced manner by promoting evidence gathering and its assessment in a manner that continuously supports the required equilibrium.

1.8 THE ROLE OF TOBACCO COMPANIES

A final consideration in crafting policy concerns the role of tobacco companies in commercializing NCAs. From one perspective, which tends toward absolutism, there is "an irreconcilable conflict" between the interests of public health and the interests of tobacco companies (WHO FCTC, 2008). Advocates of this position call for a "war" to eliminate "Big Tobacco" (Ghebreyesus and Vázquez, 2018) and assert that *"the tobacco industry and tobacco companies cannot be seen as socially responsible corporations and should be viewed, ultimately, in the same way we view the arms industry, biochemical waste and nuclear weapons."* (da Costa e Silva, 2018).

By contrast, there is a perspective that tends toward pragmatism and does not foreclose the idea that the tobacco sector might be the source of useful innovation. For example, the 2007 *Lancet* editorial (*"Adding harm reduction to tobacco control"*) addressed the topic skeptically but with an open mind: *"Allowing tobacco companies to get yet another wedge in the tobacco market is a serious concern. But so long as there are progressively increased restrictions on smoked tobacco, effective and familiar branding of harm-reduction products may help smokers to switch."* (The Lancet editorial, 2007).

More recently, Fairchild and Bayer have written: *"Rejecting e-cigarettes because the tobacco industry will profit from them has the virtue of being uncompromising. But it also means rejecting the evidence and accepting the predictable, deadly toll of cigarette smoking. That's a virtue, we argue, the world can no longer afford."* (Fairchild and Bayer, 2017).

1.9 CONCLUSION

The word "tobacco" can so polarize a discussion of health policy that foundational questions and essential distinctions often escape proper consideration. Is there one form of tobacco product that most accounts for tobacco-related morbidity and mortality? Do risk profiles differ between combustible and noncombustible products? Should policy differentiate among products to reduce consumption of the most harmful forms? What is best for the millions of men and women who will otherwise keep smoking? These and many other questions deserve empirical, in-depth, and nuanced attention (Warner, 2019). Put differently, *"To facilitate individual and population-level behavior change, we need policies based on science, not those based on speculation, fear and bias."* (Levy et al., 2017b).

The rest of this book presents science that can indeed inform policies to reduce tobacco-related morbidity and mortality by switching the present generation of cigarette smokers to less harmful alternatives.

REFERENCES

Abrams, D.B., Glasser, A.M., Pearson, J.L., Villanti, A.C., Collins, L.K., Niaura, R.S., 2018a. Harm minimization and tobacco control: reframing societal views of nicotine use to rapidly save lives. Annu. Rev. Publ. Health 39, 193–213. https://doi.org/10.1146/annurev-publhealth-040617-013849.

Abrams, D.B., Glasser, A.M., Villanti, A.C., Pearson, J.L., Rose, S., Niaura, R.S., 2018b. Managing nicotine without smoke to save lives now: evidence for harm minimization. Prev. Med. 117, 88–97. https://doi.org/10.1016/j.ypmed.2018.06.010.

Australian Government, 1989. Federal Register of Legislation. Therapeutic Goods Act of 1989: Act No 21 of 1990 as amended.

Australian Government, Department of Health, 2017. Therapeutic goods administration. In: Final Decisions and Reasons for Decisions by Delegates of the Secretary to the Department of Health, p. 91.

Australian State, 2017. Australian State & Territory Regulatory Controls on Schedule 7 Poisons. Scheduling medicines & poisons.

Breyer, S., 1993. Breaking the Vicious Circle - toward Effective Risk Regulation.

Bullen, C., 2016. Regulatory policy and practical issues arising from a disruptive innovation a public health perspective on E-cigarettes. Am. J. Publ. Health 11.

Burns, D.M., Dybing, E., Gray, N., Hecht, S., Anderson, C., Sanner, T., O'Connor, R., Djordjevic, M., Dresler, C., Hainaut, P., Jarvis, M., Opperhuizen, A., Straif, K., 2008. Mandated lowering of toxicants in cigarette smoke: a description of the World Health Organization TobReg proposal. Tobac. Contr. 17, 132–141. https://doi.org/10.1136/tc.2007.024158.

Chaloupka, F.J., Sweanor, D., Warner, K.E., 2015. Differential taxes for differential risks–toward reduced harm from nicotine-yielding products. N. Engl. J. Med. 373, 594–597. https://doi.org/10.1056/NEJMp1505710.

Clarke, E., Thompson, K., Weaver, S., Thompson, J., O'Connell, G., 2019. Snus: a compelling harm reduction alternative to cigarettes. Harm Reduct. J. 16, 62. https://doi.org/10.1186/s12954-019-0335-1.

da Costa e Silva, V.L., 2018. Implementing the UN tobacco control treaty in the SDG's era. In: 17th World Conference on Tobacco or Health.

Daston, L., 2008. Life, chance & life chances. Daedalus 137, 5–14.

Eichler, H.-G., Bloechl-Daum, B., Brasseur, D., Breckenridge, A., Leufkens, H., Raine, J., Salmonson, T., Schneider, C.K., Rasi, G., 2013. The risks of risk aversion in drug regulation. Nat. Rev. Drug Discov. 12, 907–916. https://doi.org/10.1038/nrd4129.

European Union, 2014. Directive 2014/40/EU of the European Parliament and of the Council of 3 April 2014 on the Approximation of the Laws, Regulations and Administrative Provisions of the Member States Concerning the Manufacture, Presentation and Sale of Tobacco and Related Products and Repealing Directive 2001/37/EC Text with EEA Relevance.

Fairchild, A.L., Bayer, R., 2017. The Shadow of Big Tobacco Looms over E-Cigarettes and Harm Reduction.

Fairchild, A.L., Bayer, R., 2015. Public Health. Smoke and fire over e-cigarettes. Science 347, 375–376. https://doi.org/10.1126/science.1260761.

Fairchild, A.L., Lee, J.S., Bayer, R., Curran, J., 2018. E-cigarettes and the harm-reduction continuum. N. Engl. J. Med. 378, 216–219. https://doi.org/10.1056/NEJMp1711991.

Fisher, M.T., Tan-Torres, S.M., Gaworski, C.L., Black, R.A., Sarkar, M.A., 2019. Smokeless tobacco mortality risks: an analysis of two contemporary nationally representative longitudinal mortality studies. Harm Reduct. J. 16, 27. https://doi.org/10.1186/s12954-019-0294-6.

Food and Drug Administration (FDA), 2009. Family Smoking Prevention and Tobacco Control Act. Public Law 111-31 Section 911(b)(1), 21 U.S.C 387 k.

Gartner, C., 2018. How can we protect youth from putative vaping gateway effects without denying smokers a less harmful option? Addiction 113, 1784–1785. https://doi.org/10.1111/add.14126.

Gartner, C., Hall, W., McNeill, A., 2010. Harm reduction policies for tobacco. In: EMCDDA Monograph No. 10, Harm Reduction: Evidence, Impacts and Challenges, pp. 255–273.

Gartner, C.E., Hall, W.D., 2008. Should Australia lift its ban on low nitrosamine smokeless tobacco products? Med. J. Aust. 188, 44–46.

Ghebreyesus, T.A., Vázquez, T.R., 2018. Seeing through Big Tobacco's Smokescreen.

Hall, W., Morphett, K., Gartner, C., 2019. A Critical Analysis of Australia's Ban on the Sale of Electronic Nicotine Delivery Systems. SpringerLink, Neuroethics.

Hatsukami, D.K., Carroll, D.M., 2020. Tobacco harm reduction: past history, current controversies and a proposed approach for the future. Prev. Med. 106099. https://doi.org/10.1016/j.ypmed.2020.106099.

Henningfield, J.E., Higgins, S.T., Villanti, A.C., 2018. Are we guilty of errors of omission on the potential role of electronic nicotine delivery systems as less harmful substitutes for combusted tobacco use? Prev. Med. 117, 83–87. https://doi.org/10.1016/j.ypmed.2018.09.011.

Institute of Medicine, 2001. Clearing the Smoke: Assessing the Science Base for Tobacco Harm Reduction. The National Academies Press, Washington, DC.

Kiviniemi, M.T., Kozlowski, L.T., 2015. Deficiencies in public understanding about tobacco harm reduction: results from a United States National Survey. Harm Reduct. J. 12, 21. https://doi.org/10.1186/s12954-015-0055-0.

Kolstad, C., Ulen, T., Johnson, G., 1990. Ex post liability for harm vs. Ex ante safety regulation: substitutes or complements? Am. Econ. Rev. 80, 888–901.

Lee, P.N., 2013. The effect on health of switching from cigarettes to snus - a review. Regul. Toxicol. Pharmacol. 66, 1–5. https://doi.org/10.1016/j.yrtph.2013.02.010.

Lee, P.N., Fry, J.S., Hamling, J.F., Sponsiello-Wang, Z., Baker, G., Weitkunat, R., 2017. Estimating the effect of differing assumptions on the population health impact of introducing a Reduced Risk Tobacco Product in the USA. Regul. Toxicol. Pharmacol. 88, 192–213. https://doi.org/10.1016/j.yrtph.2017.06.009.

Levy, D.T., Cummings, K.M., Villanti, A.C., Niaura, R., Abrams, D.B., Fong, G.T., Borland, R., 2017a. A framework for evaluating the public health impact of e-cigarettes and other vaporized nicotine products. Addiction 112, 8–17. https://doi.org/10.1111/add.13394.

Levy, D.T., Fong, G.T., Cummings, K.M., Borland, R., Abrams, D.B., Villanti, A.C., Niaura, R., 2017b. The need for a comprehensive framework. Addiction 112, 22–24. https://doi.org/10.1111/add.13600.

McNeil, A., Brose, L.S., Calder, R., Hitchman, S.C., Hajek, P., McRobbie, H., 2015. E-Cigarettes: An Evidence Update A Report Commissioned by Public Health England. Public Health England, London. https://www.nicopure.com/wp-content/uploads/2016/01/Ecigarettes_an_evidence_update_A_report_commissioned_by_Public_Health_England_FINAL.pdf.

Neyman, J., Pearson, E.S., 1933. On the problem of the most efficient tests of statistical hypotheses. Philos. Trans. R. Soc. Lond. Ser. A Contain. Pap. Math. Phys. Character 231, 289–337.

Neyman, J., Pearson, E.S., 1928. On the use and interpretation of certain test criteria for purposes of statistical inference: part I. Biometrika 20A, 175–240. https://doi.org/10.2307/2331945.

Office of the High Commissioner for Human Rights, 2000. Committee on Economic Social and Cultural Rights General Comment No. 14: The Right to the Highest Attainable Standard of Health (Art. 12).

Ramström, L., Wikmans, T., 2014. Mortality attributable to tobacco among men in Sweden and other European countries: an analysis of data in a WHO report. Tob. Induc. Dis. 12, 14. https://doi.org/10.1186/1617-9625-12-14.

Renn, O., 2007. Precaution and analysis: two sides of the same coin? Introduction to talking point on the precautionary principle. EMBO Rep. 8, 303–304. https://doi.org/10.1038/sj.embor.7400950.

Rutqvist, L.E., Curvall, M., Hassler, T., Ringberger, T., Wahlberg, I., 2011. Swedish snus and the GothiaTek® standard. Harm Reduct. J. 8, 11. https://doi.org/10.1186/1477-7517-8-11.

Smith, M.R., Clark, B., Lüdicke, F., Schaller, J.-P., Vanscheeuwijck, P., Hoeng, J., Peitsch, M.C., 2016. Evaluation of the tobacco heating system 2.2. Part 1: description of the system and the scientific assessment program. Regul. Toxicol. Pharmacol. 81 (Suppl. 2), S17–S26. https://doi.org/10.1016/j.yrtph.2016.07.006.

Stern, A.D., 2017. Innovation under regulatory uncertainty: evidence from medical technology. J. Publ. Econ. 145, 181–200. https://doi.org/10.1016/j.jpubeco.2016.11.010.

Substance Abuse and Mental Health Services Administration (US), Office of the Surgeon General (US), 2020. Smoking Cessation: A Report of the Surgeon General, Publications and Reports of the Surgeon General. US Department of Health and Human Services, Washington (DC).

The Lancet editorial, 2007. Adding harm reduction to tobacco control. Lancet 370, 1189. https://doi.org/10.1016/S0140-6736(07)61519-0

The Lancet editorial, 1991. Nicotine use after the year 2000. Lancet 337, 1191–1192.

UN Focal Point on Tobacco or Health, International Council on Alcohol and Addictions, European Medical Association Smoking or Health, 1998. Social and Economic Aspects of Reduction of Tobacco Smoking by use of Alternative Nicotine Delivery Systems (ANDS): Summary Report of a Roundtable. Adis International.

United Nations Conference on Trade and Development, 2016a. United Nations Guidelines for Consumer Protection, Section 5 (e).

United Nations Conference on Trade and Development, 2016b. United Nations Guidelines for Consumer Protection, Section 11 (D).

United States Code, 2006. Edition, Supplement 5, Title 21, Chapter 9, Subchapter IX, Sec. 387j - Application for Review of Certain Tobacco Products - Paragraph (C)(4), pp 425.

U.S. Department of Health and Human Services Food and Drug Administration, Center for Drug Evaluation and Research (CDER), Center for Biologics Evaluation and Research (CBER), 1998. Guidance for Industry E9 Statistical Principles for Clinical Trials.

Villanti, A.C., Byron, M.J., Mercincavage, M., Pacek, L.R., 2019. Misperceptions of nicotine and nicotine reduction: the importance of public education to maximize the benefits of a nicotine reduction standard. Nicotine Tob. Res. 21, S88–S90. https://doi.org/10.1093/ntr/ntz103.

Vugrin, E.D., Rostron, B.L., Verzi, S.J., Brodsky, N.S., Brown, T.J., Choiniere, C.J., Coleman, B.N., Paredes, A., Apelberg, B.J., 2015. Modeling the potential effects of new tobacco products and policies: a dynamic population model for multiple product use and harm. PLoS One 10, e0121008. https://doi.org/10.1371/journal.pone.0121008.

Warner, K.E., 2019. How to think-not feel-about tobacco harm reduction. Nicotine Tob. Res. 21, 1299–1309. https://doi.org/10.1093/ntr/nty084.

Weitkunat, R., Lee, P.N., Baker, G., Sponsiello-Wang, Z., González-Zuloeta Ladd, A.M., Lüdicke, F., 2015. A novel approach to assess the population health impact of introducing a Modified Risk Tobacco Product. Regul. Toxicol. Pharmacol. 72, 87–93. https://doi.org/10.1016/j.yrtph.2015.03.011.

WHO FCTC, 2008. Guidelines for Implementation of Article 5.3 of the WHO Framework Convention on Tobacco Control on the Protection of Public Health Policies with Respect to Tobacco Control from Commercial and Other Vested Interests of the Tobacco Industry.

WHO Scientific Advisory Committee on Tobacco Product Regulation, WHO Tobacco Free Initiative, 2003. SACTob Statement of Principles Guiding the Evaluation of New or Modified Tobacco Products.

WHO Study Group, Ashley, D.L., Burns, D., Djordjevic, M., Dybing, E., Gray, N., Hammond, S.K., Henningfield, J., Jarvis, M., Reddy, K.S., Robertson, C., Zaatari, G., 2008. The Scientific Basis of Tobacco Product Regulation: Second Report of a WHO Study Group. World Health Organization Technical Report Series, pp. 1–277, 1 P Following 277.

World Health Organization, 2005. WHO Framework Convention on Tobacco Control (FCTC). World Health Organization, Geneva.

Zeller, M., Hatsukami, D., Strategic Dialogue on Tobacco Harm Reduction Group, 2009. The strategic dialogue on tobacco harm reduction: a vision and blueprint for action in the US. Tobac. Contr. 18, 324–332. https://doi.org/10.1136/tc.2008.027318.

CHAPTER 2

Electronic Nicotine Delivery Products

MAURICE SMITH • MANUEL C. PEITSCH • SERGE MAEDER

2.1 INTRODUCTION

This chapter will provide brief historical details on the development of the two main technologies that deliver nicotine to the lungs in an aerosol that is not smoke. As outlined in Chapter 1 on tobacco harm reduction, for these products to be successful as cigarette replacements for adult smokers who would otherwise continue smoking, they should provide an acceptable and pleasurable alternative to cigarettes. The additional essential requirement is that such products are scientifically assessed to substantiate their potential to reduce harm at both individual and population levels. This latter aspect is covered in great detail in the remaining chapters of this book.

2.2 CONSUMER PRODUCTS THAT DELIVER NICOTINE

Consumer products that deliver nicotine can be broadly classified into two categories. The first broad category, which includes cigarettes, cigars, and pipes, relies on tobacco combustion to generate the heat necessary for nicotine evaporation, aerosolization, and inhalation (Fig. 2.1). The products in the second broad category do not burn tobacco and are designed for either inhalation or oral/nasal use. These products can contain either tobacco or purified nicotine formulated as a liquid (products for inhalation) or as a solid matrix (products for oral use) (Fig. 2.1). Nicotine delivery products for inhalation that employ electronics to control an electrical system that heats either tobacco or a nicotine-containing liquid will hereafter be referred to as electronic nicotine delivery products (ENDPs). The product design principles of various commercially available ENDP types are provided in Fig. 2.2, and their operating principles are discussed in the text.

2.3 THE RATIONALE FOR ENDP DEVELOPMENT

A burning cigarette is a typical example of a self-sustaining smoldering (flameless) combustion process,

where the temperatures of the tobacco in the burning tip of the cigarette can exceed 850°C when air is drawn through the lit tip. The smoke aerosol produced from a lit cigarette is generated by complex combustion, pyrolysis, and pyrosynthesis processes that overlap with lower-temperature distillation and sublimation processes. The composition of the smoke aerosol formed is a complex and dynamic mixture of gases, liquid droplets, and solid particles suspended in air (Baker, 2006).

The self-sustaining smoldering combustion of the tobacco results in a region inside and behind the burning tip of the cigarette that is depleted in oxygen, where the temperatures remain high enough (300−600°C) to promote the thermal decomposition (pyrolysis) of unburned tobacco components. Directly behind the high-temperature pyrolysis and smoldering combustion regions of a burning cigarette, there is a much lower-temperature region (<300°C) where volatile constituents native to tobacco evaporate because of the heat of the encroaching burning zone.

Of the more than 6000 chemical compounds that have been identified in cigarette smoke (Rodgman and Perfetti, 2013), public health authorities and others have proposed some 100 harmful and potentially harmful constituents (HPHCs) that are causally linked to smoking-related diseases (Health Canada, 2000; US Food and Drug Administration (FDA), 2012; World Health Organisation, 2008). The formation of HPHCs in a burning cigarette has been extensively studied and is influenced by a number of factors, including the tobacco variety and high temperatures induced by the self-sustaining smoldering combustion process (US Food and Drug Administration (FDA), 2012). Different tobacco leaf constituents, such as carbohydrates, biopolymers, waxes, and proteins, that decompose at different temperatures release chemical compounds that form part of the cigarette smoke aerosol.

A number of published studies contain information on the temperature of formation of selected HPHCs from different tobacco varieties, tobacco extracts, and selected model tobacco plant components

Toxicological Evaluation of Electronic Nicotine Delivery Products. https://doi.org/10.1016/B978-0-12-820490-0.00016-X

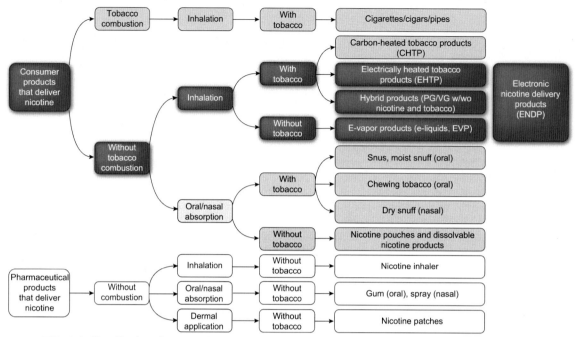

FIG. 2.1 Classification of commercially available nicotine delivery products. Products that use an electronic device are highlighted in gray and collectively termed ENDP. *ENDP*, electronic nicotine delivery product; *PG*, propylene glycol; *VG*, vegetable glycerin.

(Baker, 1987; McGrath et al., 2001, 2003, 2007; Piadé et al., 2013; Rodgman, 2001; Schlotzhauer and Chortyk, 1981; Senneca et al., 2007a,b; Torikai et al., 2004; Torikaiu et al., 2005; Yi et al., 2005). Most HPHCs result from the thermal decomposition of tobacco plant components at temperatures up to 850°C (Baker, 2006; Piadé et al., 2013; Torikaiu et al., 2005).

Nicotine is naturally present in tobacco leaves and can be evaporated from tobacco at temperatures below 300°C (Barontini et al., 2013; Forster et al., 2015). By heating rather than burning tobacco, it is possible to generate a nicotine-containing aerosol with a significant reduction in the levels of emitted HPHCs. This was the main driver for the development of heated tobacco products (HTPs) also referred to as *heat-not-burn* (HNB) tobacco products (Fig. 2.2). HTPs use blended and processed tobacco substrates that contain an added aerosol former (e.g., glycerin) and operate by heating the tobacco substrate to temperatures sufficient to release the aerosol former, nicotine, and other volatile compounds naturally present in the tobacco leaf (including naturally present flavors), but not to temperatures high enough to initiate high-temperature pyrolysis processes and the self-sustaining smoldering combustion of tobacco that would form smoke.

Electronic cigarettes (e-cigarettes) or e-vapor products deliver nicotine when the e-liquid (typically composed of a mixture of propylene glycol, vegetable glycerin, and nicotine) is heated to form an aerosol (also called "vapor"), which is then inhaled. E-cigarettes do not contain tobacco, and, therefore, no tobacco combustion product forms a part of the aerosol (Fig. 2.2). There is an emergence of hybrid products in which an e-vapor without nicotine is drawn though a tobacco plug to elute nicotine and flavors at low temperatures (Fig. 2.2).

Therefore, nicotine can be delivered to a smoker in the form of a respirable aerosol in amounts and at a rate that they are used to obtaining from their cigarettes, without the need to combust tobacco. There is an associated elimination/reduction of the HPHCs, and such products have the potential to reduce the harm associated with cigarette smoking.

2.4 BRIEF HISTORY OF PRODUCT DEVELOPMENT

2.4.1 Electronic Cigarettes

The early history of e-cigarettes has been reviewed (Knowledge-Action-Change, 2018) previously. The

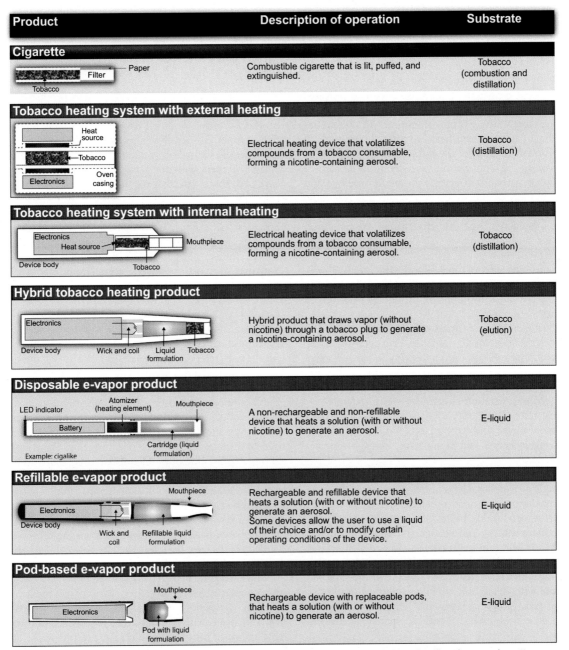

Product	Description of operation	Substrate
Cigarette		
Paper / Filter / Tobacco	Combustible cigarette that is lit, puffed, and extinguished.	Tobacco (combustion and distillation)
Tobacco heating system with external heating		
Heat source / Tobacco / Oven casing / Electronics	Electrical heating device that volatilizes compounds from a tobacco consumable, forming a nicotine-containing aerosol.	Tobacco (distillation)
Tobacco heating system with internal heating		
Electronics / Heat source / Mouthpiece / Device body / Tobacco	Electrical heating device that volatilizes compounds from a tobacco consumable, forming a nicotine-containing aerosol.	Tobacco (distillation)
Hybrid tobacco heating product		
Electronics / Device body / Wick and coil / Liquid formulation / Tobacco	Hybrid product that draws vapor (without nicotine) through a tobacco plug to generate a nicotine-containing aerosol.	Tobacco (elution)
Disposable e-vapor product		
LED indicator / Atomizer (heating element) / Mouthpiece / Battery / Cartridge (liquid formulation) / Example: cigalike	A non-rechargeable and non-refillable device that heats a solution (with or without nicotine) to generate an aerosol.	E-liquid
Refillable e-vapor product		
Mouthpiece / Electronics / Device body / Wick and coil / Refillable liquid formulation	Rechargeable and refillable device that heats a solution (with or without nicotine) to generate an aerosol. Some devices allow the user to use a liquid of their choice and/or to modify certain operating conditions of the device.	E-liquid
Pod-based e-vapor product		
Mouthpiece / Electronics / Pod with liquid formulation	Rechargeable device with replaceable pods, that heats a solution (with or without nicotine) to generate an aerosol.	E-liquid

FIG. 2.2 Schema of electronic nicotine delivery products in comparison with the scientific reference cigarette 3R4F. (Adapted from Breheny, D., Adamson, J., Azzopardi, D., Baxter, A., Bishop, E., Carr, T., Crooks, I., Hewitt, K., Jaunky, T., Larard, S., Lowe, F., Oke, O., Taylor, M., Santopietro, S., Thorne, D., Zainuddin, B., Gaça, M., Liu, C., Murphy, J., Proctor, C., 2017. A novel hybrid tobacco product that delivers a tobacco flavour note with vapour aerosol (part 2): in vitro biological assessment and comparison with different tobacco-heating products. Food Chem. Toxicol. 106, 533–546. https://doi.org/10.1016/j.fct.2017.05.023.)

person attributed with the invention of the modern e-cigarette is Hon Lik who, in 2003, came up with the idea of using a high frequency, piezoelectric, ultrasound-emitting element to vaporize a pressurized jet of liquid containing nicotine and filed the first patent in 2003. The first e-cigarette went on sale in China in 2004. Most e-cigarettes today use a battery-powered heating element rather than the earlier ultrasonic technology design. The typical components of e-cigarettes include a battery, which heats up a coil or atomizer, a wick system to transfer the e-liquid from the tank or reservoir to the atomizer and, thereby, form an aerosol through a mechanism of evaporation followed by rapid condensation of the vapor into small and respirable droplets. E-liquids are composed typically of four main ingredients: vegetable glycerin, propylene glycol, nicotine, and flavoring.

There are now many types of e-cigarettes, ranging from disposable types to user-modifiable, refillable devices. These different types have been historically broadly classified into different product generations as follows:

(a) First-generation e-cigarettes called "cigalikes," designed to closely resemble a cigarette in shape, comprise a battery and a disposable (or refillable) cartridge of e-liquid that contains a heating element or atomizer (called a cartomizer).

(b) Second-generation e-cigarettes—tank system e-cigarettes. Some offer adjustable airflow; some hold more liquid and have a larger battery capacity for longer charge; and some have adjustable power features.

(c) Third-generation e-cigarettes—mechanical mod-style e-cigarettes. Users in this group typically want maximum control over their devices, to maybe mix their own liquids, build coils, and experiment with battery wattage and voltage and tank size to optimize their vaping experience (Knowledge-Action-Change, 2018).

E-cigarettes have developed along two lines: closed systems with disposable prefilled (with e-liquid) cartridges (pods) and open systems, which allow the user to fill an e-liquid, which is sold separately or custom-made.

Such e-cigarettes are typically "wick and coil" systems, where there is a possibility—when the e-liquid reservoir is low—of "dry wicking" (where the coil is also dry and not covered with e-liquid), which leads to elevated emission of carbonyls. There are newer products on the market that do not use the "wick and coil" system, which has been replaced by a fabric-free stainless steel mesh distiller plate technology, which

heats and aerosolizes the e-liquid in a single process. Both "wick and coil" and steel mesh products have the possibility to include a mechanism that shuts off the power if the reservoir level of e-liquid is low, to prevent the heating system from operating when dry.

E-cigarettes constitute a diverse range of devices and a large range of e-liquids. Closed system products are sold ready-to-use and made from components that cannot be easily modified and are filled with liquids that cannot be easily accessed. Open system e-cigarettes allow the user to modify various components and/or fill them with any liquid, thereby, giving rise to concerns about effective regulation of such products (Eissenberg et al., 2020). However, all e-cigarettes have the same operating principle, where a liquid is heated to generate a vapor that rapidly condenses to form a respirable aerosol. The aerosol composition will be influenced by the e-liquid formulation and the design characteristics and operating conditions of the device.

2.4.2 HTPs

HTPs are also known as tobacco heating systems or HNB products. For cigarettes, tobacco is blended and cut for use (referred to as cut filler). For HTPs, the tobacco is prepared differently: For example, the tobacco is ground to a powder and mixed with glycerin, guar gum, cellulose, and other minor ingredients. The tobacco production process is designed to result in greater uniformity than that in cut filler and facilitate heat transfer through the tobacco upon heating. There are a number of methods in which tobacco is heated in an HTP. These include direct internal heating by using a ceramic heating blade inserted into the tobacco; external heating of the tobacco by electric heating; heating the air, which, in turn, heats the tobacco through a carbon-based heat source separated from the tobacco.

Early HTPs have been reviewed by Baker (2006) and Schorp et al. (2012).

Reynolds launched an early version of an HTP called the Premier cigarette in 1988, which was made of aluminum capsules containing tobacco pellets. The pellets were heated (instead of burned) by using a burning charcoal tip as the energy source. The product was withdrawn from the market a year later owing to poor uptake by smokers. Reynolds brought a second HTP to the market in 1996, called Eclipse. This product contained a tobacco mixture that was heated via a charcoal tip to distill nicotine, glycerol, and flavors from the tobacco without burning it. This product also was not commercially successful, with poor consumer acceptance, and raised health concerns because air was drawn through the heated carbon tip, resulting in relatively high levels of carbon monoxide in the inhaled aerosol. It was finally withdrawn from the market in 2008 and rebranded as Revo in 2015, which has since been withdrawn.

Philip Morris US launched Accord in 1998, which was updated and finally withdrawn in 2006. Philip Morris International (PMI) launched Heatbar (a version of Accord) in 2007, which was withdrawn in 2008 following poor consumer acceptance. PMI launched the first of the current generation of HTPs in 2014 as "IQOS." British American Tobacco (BAT) launched "glo" in 2016, and Korean Tobacco and Ginseng (KT&G) entered the HTP market with the launch of "lil" in 2017. Japan Tobacco (JT) launched the HTP "ploom" in 2016.

The latest generation of HTPs has been launched in over 40 markets around the world, and there is evidence from Japan that their presence is reducing cigarette sales (Stoklosa et al., 2020).

2.4.3 Hybrid E-cigarette Products

There is a further category of products that contain tobacco where, similar to that in an e-cigarette, heat is applied to a liquid to generate a vapor which, in turn, passes through the tobacco to pick up nicotine and flavors before the aerosol is inhaled. This product is described as a hybrid product (between an e-cigarette and HTP). For an example, see (Breheny et al., 2017; Poynton et al., 2017).

2.5 CONCLUSIONS

There are a range of products that are able to deliver nicotine in an aerosol that is not smoke. These include e-cigarettes, HTPs, and hybrid products. Together, they offer adult smokers who would otherwise continue to smoke alternative products with the potential to reduce the risk of harm associated with smoking. Such products are available in many markets around the world but face regulatory challenges in some markets, which underlines the need to share and understand the science that substantiates their potential to reduce risk at both individual and population levels.

REFERENCES

Baker, R.R., 2006. Smoke generation inside a burning cigarette: modifying combustion to develop cigarettes that may be less hazardous to health. Prog. Energy Combust. Sci. 32, 373–385. https://doi.org/10.1016/j.pecs.2006.01.001.

Baker, R.R., 1987. A review of pyrolysis studies to unravel reaction steps in burning tobacco. J. Anal. Appl. Pyrol. 11, 555–573. https://doi.org/10.1016/0165-2370(87)85054-4.

Barontini, F., Tugnoli, A., Cozzani, V., Tetteh, J., Jarriault, M., Zinovik, I., 2013. Volatile products formed in the thermal decomposition of a tobacco substrate. Ind. Eng. Chem. Res. 52, 14984–14997. https://doi.org/10.1021/ie401826u.

Breheny, D., Adamson, J., Azzopardi, D., Baxter, A., Bishop, E., Carr, T., Crooks, I., Hewitt, K., Jaunky, T., Larard, S., Lowe, F., Oke, O., Taylor, M., Santopietro, S., Thorne, D., Zainuddin, B., Gaça, M., Liu, C., Murphy, J., Proctor, C., 2017. A novel hybrid tobacco product that delivers a tobacco flavour note with vapour aerosol (part 2): in vitro biological assessment and comparison with different tobacco-heating products. Food Chem. Toxicol. 106, 533–546. https://doi.org/10.1016/j.fct.2017.05.023.

Eissenberg, T., Soule, E., Shihadeh, A., 2020. 'Open-System' electronic cigarettes cannot be regulated effectively. Tobac. Contr. 1–2. https://doi.org/10.1136/tobaccocontrol-2019-055499. In press.

Forster, M., Liu, C., Duke, M.G., McAdam, K.G., Proctor, C.J., 2015. An experimental method to study emissions from heated tobacco between 100–200°C. Chem. Cent. J. 9 https://doi.org/10.1186/s13065-015-0096-1.

Health Canada, 2000. Health Canada - Tobacco Products Information Regulations SOR/2000-273, Schedule 2. http://laws-lois.justice.gc.ca/PDF/SOR-2000-273.pdf.

Knowledge-Action-Change, 2018. No Fire, No Smoke: The Global State of Tobacco Harm Reduction. https://gsthr.org/report/full-report (Accessed 20 April 20).

McGrath, T., Sharma, R., Hajaligol, M., 2001. An experimental investigation into the formation of polycyclic-aromatic hydrocarbons (PAH) from pyrolysis of biomass materials. Fuel 80, 1787–1797. https://doi.org/10.1016/S0016-2361(01)00062-X.

McGrath, T.E., Chan, W.G., Hajaligol, M.R., 2003. Low temperature mechanism for the formation of polycyclic aromatic hydrocarbons from the pyrolysis of cellulose. J. Anal. Appl. Pyrol. 66, 51–70. https://doi.org/10.1016/S0165-2370(02)00105-5.

McGrath, T.E., Wooten, J.B., Geoffrey Chan, W., Hajaligol, M.R., 2007. Formation of polycyclic aromatic hydrocarbons from tobacco: the link between low temperature residual solid (char) and PAH formation. Food Chem. Toxicol. 45, 1039–1050. https://doi.org/10.1016/j.fct.2006.12.010.

Piadé, J.-J., Wajrock, S., Jaccard, G., Janeke, G., 2013. Formation of mainstream cigarette smoke constituents prioritized by the World Health Organization–yield patterns observed in market surveys, clustering and inverse correlations. Food Chem. Toxicol. 55, 329–347. https://doi.org/10.1016/j.fct.2013.01.016.

Poynton, S., Sutton, J., Goodall, S., Margham, J., Forster, M., Scott, K., Liu, C., McAdam, K., Murphy, J., Proctor, C., 2017. A novel hybrid tobacco product that delivers a tobacco flavour note with vapour aerosol (part 1): product operation and preliminary aerosol chemistry assessment. Food Chem. Toxicol. 106, 522–532. https://doi.org/10.1016/j.fct.2017.05.022.

Rodgman, A., 2001. Studies of polycyclic aromatic hydrocarbons in cigarette mainstream smoke: identification, tobacco precursors, control of levels: a review. Beiträge zur Tabakforschung Internat. Contrib. Tob. Res. 19, 361–379. https://doi.org/10.2478/cttr-2013-0724.

Rodgman, A., Perfetti, T.A., 2013. The Chemical Components of Tobacco and Tobacco Smoke, second ed. CRC Press, Taylor & Francis Inc (United States), Boca Raton, FL, USA.

Schlotzhauer, W.S., Chortyk, O.T., 1981. Pyrolytic studies on the origin of phenolic compounds in tobacco smoke. Tob. Sci. 25, 6–10.

Schorp, M.K., Tricker, A.R., Dempsey, R., 2012. Reduced exposure evaluation of an electrically heated cigarette smoking system. Part 1: non-clinical and clinical insights. Regul. Toxicol. Pharmacol. 64, S1–S10. https://doi.org/10.1016/j.yrtph.2012.08.008.

Senneca, O., Chirone, R., Salatino, P., Nappi, L., 2007a. Patterns and kinetics of pyrolysis of tobacco under inert and oxidative conditions. J. Anal. Appl. Pyrol. 79, 227–233. https://doi.org/10.1016/j.jaap.2006.12.011. PYROLYSIS 2006: Papers presented at the 17th International Symposium on Analytical and Applied Pyrolysis, Budapest, Hungary, 22-26 May 2006.

Senneca, O., Ciaravolo, S., Nunziata, A., 2007b. Composition of the gaseous products of pyrolysis of tobacco under inert and oxidative conditions. J. Anal. Appl. Pyrol. 79, 234–243. https://doi.org/10.1016/j.jaap.2006.09.011.

Stoklosa, M., Cahn, Z., Liber, A., Nargis, N., Drope, J., 2020. Effect of IQOS introduction on cigarette sales: evidence of decline and replacement. Tobac. Contr. 29 (4), 381–387. https://doi.org/10.1136/tobaccocontrol-2019-054998.

Torikai, K., Yoshida, S., Takahashi, H., 2004. Effects of temperature, atmosphere and pH on the generation of smoke compounds during tobacco pyrolysis. Food Chem. Toxicol. 42, 1409–1417. https://doi.org/10.1016/j.fct.2004.04.002.

Torikaiu, K., Uwano, Y., Nakamori, T., Tarora, W., Takahashi, H., 2005. Study on tobacco components involved in the pyrolytic generation of selected smoke constituents. Food Chem. Toxicol. 43, 559–568. https://doi.org/10.1016/j.fct.2004.12.011.

US Food and Drug Administration (FDA), 2012. Harmful and potentially harmful constituents in tobacco products and tobacco smoke; established list. Fed. Regist. 77, 20034–20037.

World Health Organisation, 2008. The Scientific Basis of Tobacco Product Regulation. Report of a WHO Study Group (TobReg), Geneva. WHO Technical Report Series 945.

Yi, S.-C., Hajaligol, M.R., Jeong, S.H., 2005. The prediction of the effects of tobacco type on smoke composition from the pyrolysis modeling of tobacco shreds. Pyrolysis 2004 J. Anal. & Appl. Pyrolysis 74, 181–192. https://doi.org/10.1016/j.jaap.2005.01.007.

CHAPTER 3

Scientific Basis for Assessment of Electronic Nicotine Delivery Products

JULIA HOENG • STÉPHANIE BOUÉ • MANUEL C. PEITSCH

3.1 INTRODUCTION

As outlined in Chapter 1, the potential public health benefit of electronic nicotine delivery products (ENDP) depends on their potential to reduce smoking-related disease risk and their acceptability as alternatives to cigarettes by adult smokers. Furthermore, ENDPs should not attract unintended audiences such as former smokers, never-smokers, and youth. Therefore, the assessment of new-generation tobacco products needs to take into account the following considerations:

- The focus of tobacco harm reduction (THR) is to develop products that are less harmful, and acceptable, alternatives to cigarettes. THR is not a risk-free approach, and the use of ENDPs is not risk-free. Therefore, ENDPs are only intended for current adult smokers who would otherwise continue to smoke cigarettes. The goal is to provide these smokers with less harmful alternatives.
- For this reason, ENDPs should be "less harmful" than cigarettes. Toxicological evaluation of ENDPs should, therefore, be conducted within an assessment framework defined by the principles of epidemiology and toxicology outlined below.
- Current adult smokers must have access to accurate and nonmisleading information about the relative toxicity and risk of ENDPs versus cigarettes. This is crucial for encouraging smokers to switch completely from cigarette smoking to using ENDPs if they would otherwise continue to smoke.
- It is also important that former smokers and never-smokers, including youth, are not attracted to ENDPs.

As outlined in Chapter 1, the potential for reduction of harm and smoking-related disease risk (compared with continued smoking) is a prerequisite for ENDPs to achieve their objective of reducing the burden of disease caused by cigarette smoking at the population level (see harm reduction equation in Chapter 1). The objective of this book is to describe the scientific assessment of ENDPs from a toxicological standpoint, and the focus will, therefore, be on the chemical and biological aspects of this assessment. While it is well understood that the population-level impact of any ENDP results from the combination of its toxicological profile and its use pattern by the general population (Chapter 1), we will not discuss the latter aspect in this book.

3.2 ENDP ASSESSMENT FRAMEWORK

The assessment of ENDPs is guided by two fundamental principles derived from epidemiology and toxicology.

3.2.1 First Principle: Epidemiology

The harms of cigarette smoking are well known and documented. Smoking-related harm and disease are directly caused by long-term exposure to the toxicants in cigarette smoke (Office of the Surgeon General U. S., 2010). Smokers are far more likely than nonsmokers to develop cardiovascular diseases (CVD), lung cancer, chronic obstructive pulmonary disease (COPD), and other conditions (Carter et al., 2015). The best way to avoid the harm from smoking is to never start. For current smokers, smoking cessation has been demonstrated to lead to reduced harm and risk of tobacco-related diseases (Carter et al., 2015; Jha et al., 2013). Consequently, quitting tobacco and nicotine altogether is the most effective way to reduce the risk of harm and smoking-related disease. Smoking cessation is, therefore, the "gold standard" for the scientific assessment of ENDPs (Institute of Medicine, 2012).

Fig. 3.1 presents the level of disease risk resulting from continued smoking and the changes in disease risk that occur following cessation (Smith et al., 2016). The risk of tobacco-related diseases increases with the duration and extent of exposure to cigarette

Toxicological Evaluation of Electronic Nicotine Delivery Products. https://doi.org/10.1016/B978-0-12-820490-0.00003-1

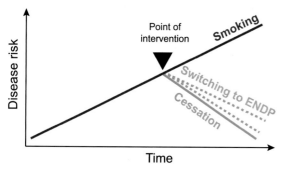

FIG. 3.1 **Epidemiological risk framework for assessment of electronic nicotine delivery products (ENDPs).** The straight lines used in this figure are for illustration purposes only as the accumulation of disease risk and the reduction upon cessation and switching to an ENDP follow different trajectories for specific diseases. These lines represent the two boundaries for assessment of ENDPs: comparing switching to an ENDP with continued smoking and benchmarking switching against smoking cessation (gold standard). Note that the straight lines used in this figure are for illustration purposes only, as the accumulation of disease risk and the reduction following cessation or switching to an ENDP follow different trajectories for specific diseases. (Adapted from Figure 4 of Smith, M.R., Clark, B., Ludicke, F., Schaller, J.P., Vanscheeuwijck, P., Hoeng, J., Peitsch, M.C., 2016. Evaluation of the tobacco heating system 2.2. Part 1: description of the system and the scientific assessment program. Regul. Toxicol. Pharmacol. 81 (Suppl. 2), S17–S26. https://doi.org/10.1016/j.yrtph.2016.07.006.)

smoke, while smoking cessation results in a gradual reduction in smoking-related disease risk over time, which, for many smokers, can fall to levels approaching those of a never-smoker if given sufficient time. The reason for this risk reduction is the elimination of exposure to the toxicants in cigarette smoke, which corresponds to elimination of the first event in the causal chain of events linking smoking to disease (CELSD). It is, therefore, critical to emphasize that

- It is the elimination of exposure to the toxicants in cigarette smoke that leads to reduced harm and risk of smoking-related disease. Smoking cessation is, therefore, the maximum achievable risk reduction modality for a smoker and, hence, represents the gold standard for ENDP assessment.
- A reduction in disease risk approaching that of cessation should be achieved by ENDPs that significantly

reduce or eliminate exposure to the high number and levels of toxicants found in cigarette smoke.

3.2.1.1 Effects of smoking cessation on disease risk

Epidemiological studies have shown that the accrued risk of smoking-related disease is reversible over time (Carter et al., 2015; Inoue-Choi et al., 2019). Smoking history, age at quitting, and type of disease must be considered in this context, as the decline in relative risk differs for each disease (Fig. 3.2). The risk of ischemic heart disease (Lee et al., 2012) and stroke (Lee et al., 2014b) declines more rapidly than that of lung cancer (Fry et al., 2013) and COPD (Lee et al., 2014a).

3.2.2 Second Principle: Toxicology

The fundamental principle of toxicology is that the degree of exposure to toxicants determines the nature and extent of adverse health effects. In addition, for toxicant exposure to occur, toxicants must be present and, hence, emitted by a product and/or process. This principle also applies to smoking (Carter et al., 2015; Jha et al., 2013), which exposes the body to the toxicants emitted by the combustion of cigarettes (Fig. 3.3, top). This exposure then leads to changes in the abundance (and sometimes composition) of a large number of the body's molecules (including mRNA, proteins, lipids, and metabolites). These molecular changes then perturb multiple healthy biological mechanisms, leading to changes at the cellular and tissue levels. Accumulation of such changes over time results in the development of smoking-related diseases and, by extension, population harm. For most smokers, the effects of smoke exposure on adverse molecular, cellular, tissue, and physiological responses are progressive with continued smoking, and, hence, the risk of smoking-related disease increases with time and dose (Inoue-Choi et al., 2019).

Smoking cessation is the elimination of the first step in this chain of events. Smoking cessation, therefore, leads to a reduction in the effects of smoking in all subsequent events of the CELSD (Fig. 3.3, middle). The principle and mechanisms of toxicology, therefore, explain the epidemiology of smoking and smoking cessation shown in Fig. 3.1 (Carter et al., 2015; Inoue-Choi et al., 2019; Jha et al., 2013). By extension, using a product with significantly reduced toxic emissions (relative to cigarettes) will result in reduced exposure

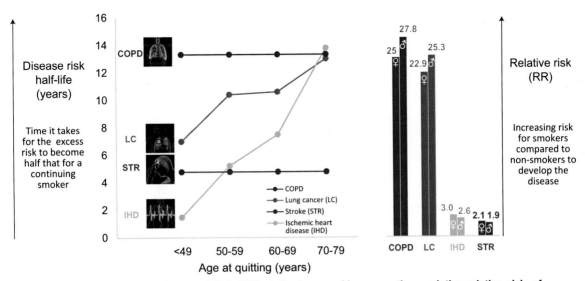

FIG. 3.2 **Half-life of disease risk half-life following smoking cessation and the relative risk of disease.** Left panel: Half-life of disease risk following smoking cessation by age at quitting. Right panel: Relative risk of disease among smokers and nonsmokers. *COPD*, chronic obstructive pulmonary disease; *IHD*, ischemic heart disease; *LC*, lung cancer; *RR*, relative risk; *STR*, stroke. (Adapted from Carter, B.D., Abnet, C.C., Feskanich, D., Freedman, N.D., Hartge, P., Lewis, C.E., Ockene, J.K., Prentice, R.L., Speizer, F.E., Thun, M.J., Jacobs, E.J., 2015. Smoking and mortality—beyond established causes. N. Engl. J. Med. 372, 631–640. https://doi.org/10.1056/NEJMsa1407211; Fry, J.S., Lee, P.N., Forey, B.A., Coombs, K.J., 2013. How rapidly does the excess risk of lung cancer decline following quitting smoking? A quantitative review using the negative exponential model. Regul. Toxicol. Pharmacol. 67, 13–26. https://doi.org/10.1016/j.yrtph.2013.06. 001; Lee, P.N., Fry, J.S., Forey, B.A., 2014a. Estimating the decline in excess risk of chronic obstructive pulmonary disease following quitting smoking – a systematic review based on the negative exponential model. Regul. Toxicol. Pharmacol. 68, 231–239. https://doi.org/10.1016/j.yrtph.2013.12.006; Lee, P.N., Fry, J.S., Thornton, A.J., 2014b. Estimating the decline in excess risk of cerebrovascular disease following quitting smoking–a systematic review based on the negative exponential model. Regul. Toxicol. Pharmacol. 68, 85–95. https://doi.org/10.1016/j.yrtph.2013.11.013, Lee, P.N., Fry, J.S., Hamling, J.S., 2012. Using the negative exponential distribution to quantitatively review the evidence on how rapidly the excess risk of ischaemic heart disease declines following quitting smoking. Regul. Toxicol. Pharmacol. 64, 51–67. https://doi.org/10.1016/j. yrtph.2012.06.009).)

to toxicants, which, in turn, would lead to a reduction in adverse health effects (Fig. 3.3, bottom).

3.3 KEY SCIENTIFIC CHALLENGES IN ASSESSMENT OF ENDPS

Several scientific challenges must be overcome in assessing the disease risk-reduction potential of ENDPs before or soon after these products are introduced into the market. The first key challenge is that the most prevalent smoking-related diseases (CVD, COPD, and lung cancer)[1] generally occur after decades of smoking and that the reduction in excess risk following smoking cessation

and, a fortiori, following switching to ENDPs is slow (Fig. 3.2). This means that clinical health outcome studies based on such definitive endpoints that aim to assess the reduction in disease risk associated with switching from cigarette smoking to the use of ENDPs are difficult to execute in a premarket setting (Chang et al., 2019; Hoeng et al., 2019). Importantly, the diseases with the shortest disease risk reduction half-life following smoking cessation (ischemic heart disease and stroke; Fig. 3.2) are also those with the lowest relative risk and are associated with important confounding factors that include diet and lifestyle. Ischemic heart disease (relative risk of 3.0 in women and 2.6 in men)[2] and stroke (relative risk of 2.1 in women and 1.9 in men)

---

[1]CVD, COPD, and lung cancer account for approximately 60% of all smoking-related mortality (Carter et al., 2015).

[2]In the US population (Carter et al., 2015).

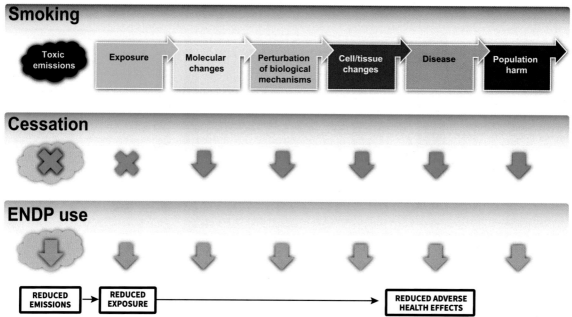

FIG. 3.3 **The principle of toxicology applied to assessment of ENDPs.** Top row, Smoking: CELSD. Smoking leads to inhalation of toxicants, which leads to exposure of the body to toxicants, which, in turn, causes molecular changes in the body that perturb biological mechanisms. These perturbations cause cell and tissue changes that lead to disease and, by extension, population harm. Middle row, Cessation: Smoking cessation is effectively the elimination of the first step in the CELSD and the gold standard in THR. Therefore, cessation causes a decrease in all subsequent events in the CELSD (arrows). Bottom row, ENDP: Switching to ENDPs with significantly reduced toxic emissions (relative to cigarettes) will also lead to a reduction in toxicant exposure. Consequently, all subsequent events in the CELSD, including adverse health effects and population harm, will be reduced (*arrows*). *CELSD*, causal chain of events linking smoking to disease; *ENDP*, electronic nicotine delivery products; *THR*, tobacco harm reduction. (Adapted from figure 5 of Smith, M.R., Clark, B., Ludicke, F., Schaller, J.P., Vanscheeuwijck, P., Hoeng, J., Peitsch, M.C., 2016. Evaluation of the tobacco heating system 2.2. Part 1: description of the system and the scientific assessment program. Regul. Toxicol. Pharmacol. 81 (Suppl. 2), S17–S26. https://doi.org/10.1016/j.yrtph.2016.07.006.)

have a much shorter disease risk half-life than COPD (relative risk of 25 in women and 27.8 in men) and lung cancer (relative risk of 22.9 in women and 25.3 in men). This presents additional challenges in conducting clinical health outcome studies, as assessing the effectiveness of both cessation and switching to ENDPs will be hampered by either a low dynamic range in relative risk and confounding factors or by very long (over a decade) risk reduction half-lives.

The second key challenge is that smoking affects several organ systems (Carter et al., 2015) and multiple biological mechanisms, so that no single endpoint can inform, on its own, about the relative risk of ENDPs in comparison with that of cigarettes. Therefore, a number of biomarkers that address the multifaceted biological impact of cigarette smoke should be considered in combination. However, there is a dearth of clinically validated biomarkers (often termed biomarkers of

potential harm; BOPHs) that can be used to assess the effects of smoking cessation and, therefore, switching to ENDPs in healthy smokers. Because the aim of ENDPs is to reduce the risk of smoking-related disease in smokers who switch instead of continue smoking, clinical studies designed to assess the biological effects of switching to ENDPs must be conducted in current adult smokers who either continue to smoke, abstain from smoking at least for the duration of the study, or switch to ENDPs. The selection of such BOPHs is driven by three main criteria:

- They must be associated with a smoking-related disease through epidemiological evidence.
- They must be affected by smoking.
- Their levels must revert upon smoking cessation, within the timeframe of the study (6–12 months).

There are, however, very few biomarkers that have been well-studied in the context of smoking and cessation that fit these criteria, and most of these are related to CVD and COPD. These biomarkers are discussed in Chapter 17.

It is, therefore, clear that only long-term epidemiological studies will eventually enable researchers to quantify the overall disease risk reduction associated with switching from cigarette smoking to ENDP use and to evaluate the excess disease risk associated with ENDP use. However, conducting epidemiological studies requires long-term market availability of ENDPs and that ENDPs are used exclusively by a large proportion of smokers who have fully switched to these products for at least a decade. This renders such studies impracticable in a premarket setting or in the early phase of market introduction.

As outlined in Chapter 1, there is an urgent need to reduce the disease burden caused by cigarette smoking, the most dangerous form of nicotine delivery, and, therefore, implement coherent THR policies to complement established tobacco control measures aimed at preventing initiation and encouraging cessation. This requires that ENDPs be assessed for their disease risk reduction potential more rapidly and that current smokers be provided with accurate and nonmisleading information about the relative risk of switching to ENDP use in comparison with that of continued cigarette smoking.

In this context, a new and more predictive scientific approach is needed to evaluate the disease risk reduction potential of ENDPs within a practicable time frame. This approach is based on the understanding of the CELSD (Fig. 3.3). This mechanism-based approach permits comparative and holistic evaluation of the effects of ENDPs on each event in the CELSD in comparison with those of cigarettes and represents a solid scientific basis for showing that switching to ENDPs is likely to significantly reduce the risk of smoking-related disease (Hoeng et al., 2019; Smith et al., 2016). This mechanism-based approach leverages the principles of systems toxicology (Hoeng et al., 2012; Sturla et al., 2014) across in vitro, in vivo, and clinical studies.

3.4 SYSTEMS TOXICOLOGY–BASED ASSESSMENT OF ENDPS

As outlined above, the pathway from smoke exposure to disease manifestation can be depicted as a causal chain of biological events (Fig. 3.3). The impact of cigarette smoke on the CELSD can be quantified by using analytical chemistry methods, advanced omics technologies (e.g., transcriptomics, proteomics, and metabolomics), cytological and histopathological analyses, physiological measurements, and, eventually, epidemiological studies.

The data generated by these measurements can then be analyzed by using statistical methods and advanced computational biology approaches. Advances in these methodologies have enabled the development and application of systems toxicology (Sturla et al., 2014), a new approach to toxicology derived from the fundamental principles of systems biology (Ideker et al., 2001).

Systems toxicology is the integration of safety and regulatory toxicology approaches with the quantitative analysis of large sets of molecular and functional measures of changes occurring across multiple levels of biological organization and along the CELSD (Hoeng et al., 2014, 2012; Sturla et al., 2014) (Chapter 9). Systems toxicology–based research enables identification of the biological mechanisms and molecular pathways that are affected by exposure to cigarette smoke and hence provides a more comprehensive understanding of the causal link between exposure-induced molecular changes and the ensuing toxicity endpoints and adverse outcomes. This knowledge can then be used to assess the biological effects of ENDPs.

Systems toxicology, like systems biology (Peitsch and de Graaf, 2014), seeks to describe and represent the knowledge of biological mechanisms as diagrams of nodes (entities such as genes or proteins) and edges (relationships such as increase or decrease), known as biological networks models (Hoeng et al., 2012; Sturla et al., 2014). These models are a core component of the systems toxicology approach, as they enable mechanism-driven analyses of large-scale molecular measurements. Therefore, the first necessary step is to conduct systems toxicology research and construct computable biological network models of the mechanisms affected by cigarette smoke. This is achieved by using experimental data and the available literature evidence (De Leon et al., 2014; Gebel et al., 2013; Park et al., 2013; Schlage et al., 2011; Westra et al., 2013, 2011). These biological network models can then be applied to a detailed, mechanism-by-mechanism assessment of the biological effects of ENDP aerosol in comparison with those of cigarette smoke. With this approach, one can also evaluate whether a reduction in toxicant exposure, caused by switching from cigarette smoking to the use of an ENDP, translates into a concomitant reduction in the perturbation of the biological mechanisms affected by cigarette smoke exposure. Importantly, the same approach can be used to compare the effects of switching with those of cessation. The mechanisms perturbed by cigarette smoke include inflammation, cell stress, cell proliferation, tissue repair and angiogenesis, and cell fate (Boue et al., 2015). These mechanisms are causally linked to downstream cigarette smoke toxicity—related events in the CELSD and have been causally linked to smoking-related diseases such as CVD, COPD, and lung cancer. Sophisticated computational biology approaches enable quantification of the perturbation of each biological mechanism as network perturbation amplitudes (Martin et al., 2014, 2012) and aggregation of these perturbations into an overall relative biological impact factor (Thomson et al., 2013). These computational approaches enable objective, data-driven, and quantitative mechanism-by-mechanism comparison of the effects of ENDP aerosols with those of cigarette smoke. If exposure to an ENDP leads to (i) a substantial reduction in the overall perturbation of all relevant biological mechanisms affected by cigarettes and (ii) an overall reduction in perturbation that is coherent with the degree of reduction in toxicant exposure, then the ENDP is associated with a lower risk of smoking-related disease than cigarettes (Chapter 9).

Importantly, in the context of ENDP assessment, this approach can be applied to large-scale molecular measurement data collected in vitro (Iskandar et al., 2013), in vivo (Hoeng et al., 2014), and in clinical samples (Iskandar et al., 2013; Talikka et al., 2017) by using the same set of biological mechanisms that have been fine-tuned to account for species differences (Boue et al., 2015) (Chapter 9). This enables coherent assessment that is based on the totality of the evidence generated by a rigorous study program of in vitro, in vivo, and clinical investigations.

3.4.1 Predictive Power of Systems Toxicology

The predictive power of systems toxicology, as applied to assessment of the effects of cigarette smoke and ENDP aerosol exposure, is probably best exemplified by an integrative analysis of two rat inhalation studies designed to evaluate the toxicity of formaldehyde (Hoeng et al., 2014; Martin et al., 2020). Formaldehyde is a known carcinogen found in cigarette smoke and to a much lesser extent in many ENDPs (Stephens, 2017) (Chapter 4). The first was a 24-month carcinogenicity study (Monticello et al., 1996) and the second was a 13-week study designed to measure gene expression changes in respiratory nasal epithelium (Andersen et al., 2010).

Although formaldehyde naturally occurs in the body, prolonged (24 months) and sustained exposure to relatively high concentrations of formaldehyde caused the development of squamous cell carcinomas in the respiratory nasal epithelium of rats (Monticello et al., 1996). An overt threshold effect was observed, as exposure for 24 months to low doses of formaldehyde did not trigger tumorigenesis (Fig. 3.4). A computational analysis of respiratory nasal epithelium gene expression data from the 13-week inhalation study (Andersen et al., 2010) by using biological network models (Boue et al., 2015) found that the relative biological impact factor values at 13 weeks were well correlated with the tumor loads at 24 months across a wide range of formaldehyde concentrations (Fig. 3.4). These results show that the relative biological impact factor values derived from integrating biological network perturbation amplitudes after 13 weeks of exposure can be predictive of a disease outcome after 24 months of sustained exposure to formaldehyde.

Deeper analysis of the biological network perturbations revealed that, although similar network models were impacted by the various exposure doses, the directionality of the mechanistic effects was, in some cases, opposite when comparing the lower and higher doses. For instance, NF-κB was inferred to be upregulated in response to the higher doses and downregulated in response to the lower doses in the context of the epithelial innate immune activation network model (Martin et al., 2020). This confirms that NF-κB, which is involved in many aspects of inflammation and cancer biology, could be the defining mechanistic switch for tumorigenesis at a later time point (Karin, 2009). The immune regulation of the tissue repair network model replicated the indication that high doses of formaldehyde induced an inflammatory response in the rat respiratory nasal epithelium after 13 weeks of exposure, whereas the two lower doses triggered an apparent downregulation of these pathways.

This example of systems toxicology—based data analysis shows that the mechanistic understanding derived from data collected at early time points can be predictive of later outcomes, as long as the exposure is sustained. This approach is, therefore, applicable to assessment of ENDPs in evaluating whether a substantial reduction in toxicant exposure leads to a substantial reduction in the biological network perturbations caused by cigarette smoke. Furthermore, the approach also allows one to estimate how these reductions in perturbation compare with those caused by the gold standard of smoking cessation. Therefore, systems toxicology (presented in more detail in Chapter 9) bridges short-term effects and long-term outcomes.

The following section describes how these principles can be implemented in a coherent ENDP assessment program that enables comparison of ENDPs with cigarettes across the CELSD.

3.5 A COMPREHENSIVE ASSESSMENT PROGRAM FOR ENDPS

To assess the risk reduction potential of ENDPs by using the framework described above, one needs to

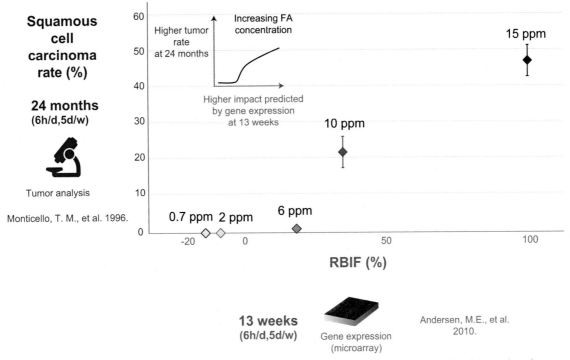

FIG. 3.4 Rat inhalation studies with FA. Nasal squamous cell carcinoma rates after 24 months of exposure to FA as a function of the RBIFs in respiratory nasal epithelium after 13 weeks of exposure. FA concentrations are expressed in parts per million. *FA*, formaldehyde; *RBIF*, relative biological impact factor. (Adapted from Martin, F., Talikka, M., Hoeng, J., Peitsch, M.C., 2020. Systems toxicology approach to unravel early indicators of squamous cell carcinoma rate in rat nasal epithelium induced by formaldehyde exposure. In: Rocha, M., Mohamad, M.S., Zaki, N., Castellanos-Garzón, J.A. (Eds.), Practical Applications of Computational Biology and Bioinformatics, 13th International Conference. Springer International Publishing, pp. 16–24.)

implement a comprehensive assessment program that addresses each event in the CELSD. For practical reasons, the assessment program (Murphy et al., 2017; Smith et al., 2016) is articulated around relevant scientific disciplines and their technical expertise: from aerosol chemistry and physics through nonclinical to clinical studies (and ultimately perception and behavior studies that are not discussed in this book). However, most studies conducted within each discipline will collect data relevant to more than one step in the CELSD (Fig. 3.5). Before describing the key steps of the assessment program, the fundamental principles of the program should be considered in the context of THR:

1. Given that the aim of ENDPs is to replace cigarettes, studies should always compare the effects of an ENDP with those of cigarettes.

2. As the effects of smoking cessation are the "gold standard" for assessing those of an ENDP, the effects of switching from cigarette smoke to ENDP aerosol exposure should be compared to those of smoking cessation, whenever possible. If this is not feasible or relevant, the effects of ENDP aerosols should be compared to those of cigarette smoke and fresh air. By combining the first and second principle, one can generally calculate (i) the dose at which an ENDP aerosol has the same effect as cigarette smoke, (ii) the effects of an ENDP aerosol relative to those of cigarette smoke as a percentage, (iii) the residual effect of switching to an ENDP aerosol over cessation, and (iv) the residual effects of ENDP aerosols over fresh air. Importantly, these results can be put into the context of realistic human exposure levels.

3. An adequate comparator product should be selected and used as systematically as possible across studies.

4. Nonclinical studies should (i) be conducted by using the most relevant and/or accepted test systems and, (ii) whenever possible, cover a dose range that includes a realistic human exposure dose. Achieving the latter objective can be challenging, and great care

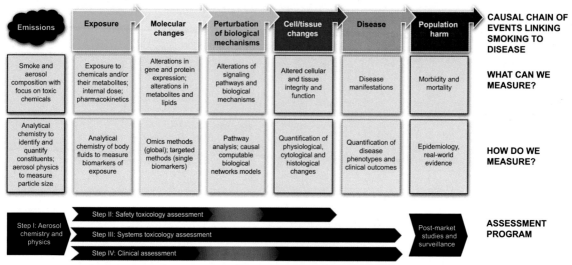

FIG. 3.5 **Causal chain of events linking smoking to disease and the assessment program.** Links between the events linking smoking to disease, what can be measured in practice, and the toxicological assessment steps described in this chapter. (Adapted from Figure 2 of Sturla, S.J., Boobis, A.R., FitzGerald, R.E., Hoeng, J., Kavlock, R.J., Schirmer, K., Whelan, M., Wilks, M.F., Peitsch, M.C., 2014. Systems toxicology: from basic research to risk assessment. Chem. Res. Toxicol. 27, 314–329. https://doi.org/10.1021/tx400410s under ACS Author Choice license. Any permission for reuse should be directed to the ACS.)

must be given when selecting exposure dose ranges, which should be based on human exposure data (Benowitz et al., 2009; Marchand et al., 2017).

5. Biomarkers linked to biological mechanisms should be selected such that they (i) are affected by smoking or smoke exposure, (ii) show positive changes (revert) upon smoking cessation, and (iii) are linked to smoking-related diseases, either through mechanistic understanding or epidemiological data.

3.5.1 Toxicological Assessment Steps
3.5.1.1 Step I
The first step of the toxicological assessment of ENDPs focuses on the first event of the CELSD—*toxic emissions*—and is, therefore, based on analysis of the chemical composition of the aerosol generated by ENDPs. The aim is to quantify the reduction in the level of toxicants, or harmful and potentially harmful constituents (HPHCs) (Center for Tobacco Products, 2019), emitted by an ENDP in comparison with those emitted by a reference cigarette (Chapter 4). This first step also evaluates whether ENDPs emit new or elevated levels of some toxicants by using advanced analytical chemistry approaches supported by computational chemistry methods (Chapter 6). Furthermore, beyond analysis of classical HPHCs, the comparative aerosol chemistry assessment should ideally be extended to solid carbon-based nanoparticles that are generated

during combustion (Lighty et al., 2000) and to free radicals (Pryor et al., 1990), as these substances are related to the toxicity of cigarette smoke (Chapter 7).

In addition, this step should also assess the influence of puffing regimens on aerosol composition to ensure that the ENDP performs in a way that results in an actual reduction in HPHCs levels across a range of realistic human puffing topographies.

Aerosol droplets are also analyzed during this step to verify that the ENDP aerosol particle size distribution is as similar as possible to that of cigarette smoke, ensuring similar delivery of nicotine by the aerosol (Chapter 5).

Finally, this step should also assess the effects of ENDPs use on indoor air chemistry, to evaluate the impact of ENDP use on air quality in comparison with that of cigarette smoking and benchmark against national and international standards for exposure to environmental toxicants (e.g., European Commission, 2006). These environmental studies can be conducted under well-controlled and realistic conditions based on accepted building standards (European Committee for Standardization. CEN European Standard EN 15251, 2006) or in real settings such as an apartment, shop, or restaurant (Chapter 8). Importantly, in all cases, such studies should be based on realistic product use to ensure their validity in the real world (Chapter 20).

Taken together, the results of this assessment step provide evidence for the first event in the CELSD and a quantification of the degree of reduction in the level of toxicants emitted by ENDPs relative to those generated by cigarettes.

3.5.1.2 Step II

The second step of the toxicological assessment—based on classical approaches that follow the widely accepted toxicity testing guidelines of the Organization for Economic Co-operation and Development (OECD) ("OECD Guidelines for the Testing of Chemicals, Section 4")—is used to determine whether the measured reductions in HPHC emissions lead to reduced toxicity in laboratory models. This step also contributes to evaluation of any new hazards. This second level of evidence, *reduced toxicity in laboratory models*, is based on in vitro and in vivo toxicology studies designed to compare the effects of ENDP aerosols with those of cigarette smoke and fresh air. First, a battery of in vitro assays designed to assess the cytotoxicity and genotoxicity of ENDP aerosols in comparison with those of cigarette smoke should be conducted (Chapter 13). Second, the systemic and respiratory organ toxicity of ENDP aerosols should be evaluated in well-designed animal inhalation studies conducted in accordance with established OECD guidelines (Chapter 14). These studies should rigorously monitor the composition of the test atmosphere and measure biomarkers of exposure (BoExps) in the urine and blood of the exposed animals. These measurements ensure that the exposure levels are verified and enable assessment of the degree of exposure reduction in laboratory models, providing an indication of what can be achieved independent of human behavior and use patterns.

This second step of the toxicological assessment provides evidence for several events along the CELSD, ranging from exposure to molecular, cellular, and tissue changes. Importantly, the level of reduction in biological effects induced by exposure to ENDP aerosols should be coherent with the degree of reduction in toxicant emissions by ENDPs within each of the events in the CELSD. Furthermore, the results of the assessment should be consistent across studies and test systems for all events.

3.5.1.3 Step III

The third step of the toxicological assessment focuses on evaluating whether the reduced emission of HPHCs by ENDPs, which results in reduced exposure to these chemicals and reduced toxicity in laboratory models, leads to a third level of evidence—*reduced risk in laboratory models*. This evidence is based on systems toxicology studies conducted both in vitro and in vivo.

In vitro systems toxicology studies compare the effects of ENDPs with those of cigarettes (and fresh air) on key

mechanisms involved in smoking-related diseases (Chapter 13). Toward this end, we have proposed a three-layer in vitro assessment framework for ENDPs (Iskandar et al., 2016) that employs both primary human cells, as they are more relevant than immortalized cell lines, and organotypic tissue cultures that mimic the structure of the human epithelial tissues exposed to ENDP aerosol/cigarette smoke. The first two layers of this assessment framework are used to compare the effects of both e-liquids and heated tobacco product aerosol fractions with the effects of cigarette smoke fractions on primary normal human airway epithelial cells and endothelial cells by high-content screening and a detailed mechanistic analysis of the changes at the transcriptome level (Iskandar et al., 2016). This type of study provides an initial assessment of an ENDP's impact on key pathways of toxicity along the CELSD. The third layer of this assessment compares the effects of the whole ENDP aerosols generated by actual products with those of whole cigarette smoke on organotypic respiratory epithelium tissue cultures (Iskandar et al., 2016); this step provides a more refined assessment of ENDP aerosols and enables evaluation of the impact of aerosol generation on both toxicity and mechanistic endpoints in vitro.

In vivo systems toxicology studies represent the most sophisticated and comprehensive nonclinical studies that can be conducted to assess the comparative toxicity of ENDPs. In their most advanced form, such studies compare the effects of ENDP aerosols with those of cigarette smoke at every step of the CELSD, from exposure to disease endpoints (Fig. 3.5) in animal models of human disease, and can be designed to include both "smoking cessation" and "ENDP switching" arms to replicate the epidemiological risk framework depicted in Fig. 3.1 (Chapter 15). However, there is also value in complementing studies conducted under the OECD guidelines for inhalation studies with systems toxicology approaches to gain a more detailed quantitative and mechanistic understanding of the differential effects of ENDPs and cigarettes on toxicity endpoints along the CELSD (Kogel et al., 2014) (Chapter 14).

3.5.1.4 Step IV

The fourth step of the assessment is based on human clinical studies and assesses three critical aspects of ENDP use (Chapter 17).

First, pharmacokinetics/pharmacodynamics studies should be conducted to evaluate whether an ENDP delivers nicotine in a way that is acceptable to smokers but does not expose the user to significantly higher levels of nicotine than cigarettes and, therefore, does not present a higher abuse liability than cigarettes (Hatsukami et al., 2009).

Second, the effect of switching to ENDP use from cigarette smoking should reflect a reduction in exposure to HPHCs (Hatsukami et al., 2009). Clinical reduced—exposure studies should assess both the maximum achievable effect of switching, which can be done in a confinement setting, and the sustained effect of switching in a more realistic ambulatory setting. Such studies should include a smoking abstinence arm to enable fair comparison between the potential of ENDPs to reduce exposure and the maximum achievable effect of cessation.

The third aspect involves assessment of the harm reduction potential of ENDPs by measuring changes in clinical markers associated with smoking-related diseases. Ideally, such studies would measure the effect of switching to ENDPs versus ongoing smoking on smoking-related disease incidence. However, smoking-related diseases may take decades to develop, and measuring health outcomes in randomized clinical trials is not practicable in a premarket setting. Therefore, these studies should measure the effect of switching from cigarette smoking to ENDP use on biomarkers of effect and potential harm (Chang et al., 2019). Importantly, no single biomarker can, in itself, address all biological mechanisms affected by smoking. Therefore, a collection of biomarkers should be selected in a way that addresses the key mechanisms of smoking-related diseases (Chang et al., 2019). The selection of these biomarkers should be based on key principles aligned with the CELSD:

a. The biomarker must be affected by smoking or smoke exposure.
b. The biomarker must revert (show a positive change), at least in part, following smoking cessation. Importantly, the dynamics of the biomarker's reversal should be aligned with the duration of the study.
c. The biomarker should be linked to smoking-related diseases, either through mechanistic understanding (CELSD) or epidemiological data.

Furthermore, the selected biomarkers should be stable, robust, and measurable with validated methods (Chang et al., 2019).

These studies should compare the effect of switching with that of continued smoking and cessation.

Once ENDPs are on the market, more long-term studies could be conducted (i) to confirm that the harm and risk reduction potential determined by the assessment program described above translates into both individual and population-level benefits and (ii) to quantify both the residual risk of ENDPs and their population-level benefits. At the time of writing this book, no such long-term studies have yet been reported. It will take many years until long-term randomized

clinical studies and real-world epidemiological evidence can be reported.

3.6 QUALITY CONSIDERATIONS

The toxicological evaluation of any product must be scientifically sound and repeatable. To ensure scientific excellence and quality in experimental execution, studies should be designed on the basis of the best available prior knowledge. Therefore, nonclinical studies should be, as much as possible, executed under a quality management system such as OECD Good Laboratory Practice.[3] Moreover, when conducting research in humans, both ethical and quality aspects of the study must be considered to ensure scientific excellence and appropriateness of the study outcomes. Therefore, clinical studies should be conducted in accordance with the Declaration of Helsinki and the principles of Good Clinical Practice.

For toxicological assessment of ENDPs, the following key aspects must be considered.

3.6.1 Comparative Studies
As the aim of ENDPs is to reduce the risk of harm and smoking-related disease relative to cigarettes, toxicology studies should always be conducted in a comparative manner to enable sound assessment of both the risk reduction potential and residual risk within the ENDP assessment framework described in this chapter.

3.6.2 Exposure and its Verification
To ensure that ENDP toxicological studies can be properly interpreted, exposure of experimental test systems must be adequately controlled and verified. This is particularly important in the context of THR. Several aspects must be taken into account.

3.6.2.1 Adequate exposure
Both in vitro and in vivo test systems must be exposed to ENDP aerosols or cigarette smoke concentrations that are well-controlled and understood in the context of realistic human exposure. This is crucial to proper interpretation of the data in the context of human toxicity (Chapters 10–12).

First, the generation, delivery, and collection of ENDP aerosols and cigarette smoke should be performed in accordance with sound methodologies to ensure that the test systems are exposed to well-understood aerosols (Chapter 12). Without proper

---

[3]https://www.oecd.org/chemicalsafety/testing/good-laboratory-practiceglp.htm.

validation of the exposure system, it is impossible to draw appropriate conclusions from the study results.

Second, in vitro and in vivo test systems must be exposed to comparable ENDP aerosols and cigarette smoke concentrations. This can be achieved by exposing the test system to an equivalent concentration of nicotine in the test atmosphere (in vivo studies), an equivalent number of puffs of known nicotine concentration (in vitro studies), or an equivalent concentration of total particulate matter of known nicotine content (in vitro studies). The method used depends on the particular study system, aim, and design, but should always enable sound comparison of the measured biological endpoints between groups exposed to equivalent nicotine concentrations or doses (Chapter 11).

Third, experimental test systems should be exposed to ENDP aerosol and cigarette smoke doses that represent realistic human exposure, or are aimed at determining the highest exposure level at which no or only very low adverse effects are observed. Such exposure doses can be derived from human pharmacokinetics studies (Benowitz et al., 2009; Marchand et al., 2017) by applying widely agreed conversion factors for in vivo studies (Alexander et al., 2008; Bide et al., 2000; Reagan-Shaw et al., 2008) and simple concentration calculations for in vitro studies.

3.6.2.2 *Exposure verification in nonclinical studies*

It is not sufficient to just control and verify exposure parameters during the studies, as other factors can influence cigarette smoke and ENDP aerosol uptake in both in vitro and in vivo experiments. These include parameters such as respiratory frequency and volume in vivo and aerosol deposition in vitro. To ensure that nonclinical studies can be properly interpreted, it is necessary to measure the system's actual exposure to aerosol and smoke constituents. These obviously include nicotine and nicotine metabolites, but they also include BoExps to HPHCs contained in cigarette smoke and, in relevant cases, BoExps to typical e-vapor constituents such as flavor ingredients, vegetable glycerol, and propylene glycol.

3.6.2.3 *Exposure verification in clinical studies*

Self-reporting of cigarette consumption and ENDP use by study participants in ambulatory clinical studies is not always reliable (Lüdicke et al., 2019) because of the frequent underreporting of cigarette use on top of

the investigated ENDPs. This can affect the interpretation of clinical study results, especially when comparing the biological effects of switching to an ENDP with continued smoking and/or cessation. It is, therefore, important to verify the study participants' actual exposure to cigarette smoke and ENDP aerosols by using biochemical measurements. Exposure verification can be made by measuring BoExps to HPHCs specifically found in cigarette smoke but (nearly) absent in ENDP aerosols. For instance, measuring a combination of the urinary levels of nicotine metabolites, 2-cyanoethylmercapturic acid (CEMA, a biomarker of exposure to acrylonitrile), and total 4-(methylnitrosamino)-1-(3-pyridyl)-1-butanol (tNNAL, a biomarker of exposure to NNK) would help verify adherence to a particular exposure regimen or self-reported product use pattern, as there is a linear relationship between the levels of these BoExps and number of cigarettes smoked. Urine from cigarette smokers will contain high levels of all three BoExps, while that of ENDP users will contain low levels of CEMA or tNNAL, as reported in a recent comparative analysis of urine from over 5000 participants in the Population Assessment of Tobacco and Health study (Goniewicz et al., 2018). This study also found that dual users had intermediate levels of these BoExps.

3.6.3 Independent Peer Review

It is critical that the evidence supporting the exposure or risk reduction potential of an ENDP is reviewed by independent experts. Regulatory agencies, for instance, rely on peer review to ensure that the quality and scientific integrity of products' risk assessments and decisions are maintained (EPA (United States Environmental Protection Agency), 2015; The National Academies, 2003; U.S. Food and Drug Administration, 2012). Many companies and agencies perform peer reviews as part of product risk assessment. For example, risk-ranking methods are available for prioritizing food safety risks (van Asselt et al., 2012). The methods that are generally used may be qualitative, semiquantitative, or quantitative, but are typically based on the concept of risk being a function of the presence of a hazard and the severity of its impact on human health (National Research Council - Division on Earth and Life Studies - Board on Environmental Studies and Toxicology - Committee on Improving Risk Analysis Approaches Used by the U.S. EPA, 2009).

Inconsistencies in peer review models and expectations across organizations (Fig. 3.6) mean that the level

A   Peer-review process

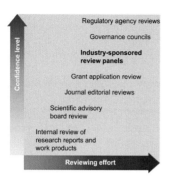

B   Tiered review of scientific research

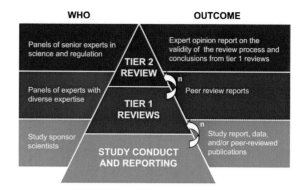

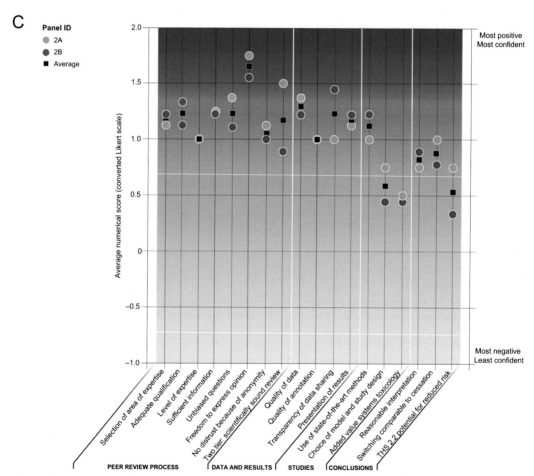

FIG. 3.6 **Two-tier review process for assessment of an ENDP.** (A). Comparison of models of peer review. (B). Tiered review of scientific research. (C). Results obtained in such a tiered review—conducted by two independent panels for tier 2 and by five panels for tier 1—of studies that have assessed the Tobacco Heating System 2.2, an electrically heated tobacco product. Responses from the two independent tier 2 panels

of expertise, depth of assessment, and consistency of recommendations vary, and the risk of bias and conflict of interest are not always adequately controlled (Manchikanti et al., 2015). Manufacturers of ENDPs may sponsor a review of their own assessment results to support risk assessment, understand which additional experiments might be needed prior to regulatory submission, provide insights into scientific plausibility to the external community, and increase confidence in the results. For example, the nonprofit organization Toxicology Excellence for Risk Assessment (https://www.tera.org) provides peer consultation and peer review services and convenes groups of experts to evaluate the scientific basis of the work products and its conclusions in accordance with United States Environmental Protection Agency peer review procedures.

Philip Morris International (PMI) commissioned a two-tiered scientific peer review of the methods, data, and results from studies that have assessed the Tobacco Heating System 2.2 (THS), an electrically heated tobacco product (Boue et al., 2019). Tier 1 panels addressed the study models and conduct, transparency of documentation, quality of data, and interpretation of results using online questionnaires with yes/no, multiple-choice, and open-ended responses. Some experts also participated in a debate (Delphi) process. In tier 2, two panels participated in three independent but concurrent rounds of review. Round 1 reviewed the data package and tier 1 responses to the online question set. Round 2 was a Delphi process with access to the summary statistics for round 1. Round 3 provided an opportunity to revise inputs. Apart from commenting on the data package, the peer reviewers were also asked to assess the reproducibility of the tier 1 panel results, assess potential bias, and provide recommendations for improving the peer review process.

Sixty-five peer reviewers with expertise levels comparable to those of reviewers on United States Food and Drug Administration advisory committees contributed to the process for THS. All positive reviews of study models and designs in tier 1 were upheld by tier 2 reviews. The peer reviewers were confident to very confident that state-of-the-art methods had been used. Overall, in tiers 1 and 2, 65% of reviewers found the data that switching to THS is likely to reduce the risk of smoking-related diseases relative to continued cigarette smoking to be convincing or very convincing. Critical findings from omics platforms were upheld. The interpretation and presentation of data were largely supported by both tier 1 and tier 2 reviews. Some questions pertaining to the use of longer study duration, multiple exposure doses and modes, and additional mouse strains and cell lines arose because the THS dataset was substantial but not complete at the time of review. Nonetheless, having access to in-depth reviews prior to submission was beneficial for the sponsor (Boue et al., 2019).

3.7 TRANSPARENT SHARING OF SCIENTIFIC DATA ON ENDP ASSESSMENT

Technology is increasingly enabling collection of "big data" (Dinov, 2016; Kahn, 2011), and this is also the case in evaluation of ENDPs. However, several challenges must be overcome to fully harness the power of big data. For example, appropriate analytical tools and statistical methods must be used to extract sound information from large datasets (Harford, 2014). Furthermore, new and better data sharing and interoperability practices must be promoted and embraced by all stakeholders to realize the potential of big data (Dinov, 2016; Rocca-Serra et al., 2010; Sansone et al., 2012). Regardless of the type or size of the data generated, adopting the best practices in data sharing is of central importance, particularly in light of the fact that some research studies cannot be reproduced (Begley and Ellis, 2012). Factors contributing to the irreproducibility of biomedical findings include inadequate attention to experimental design (such as flaws in statistical analysis or low statistical power), lack of sharing of material and methods, publication bias (Begley and Ioannidis, 2015; Button et al., 2013), and, in only a minority of cases, research misconduct (Collins and Tabak, 2014).

The reproducibility crisis is often associated with a lack of transparency, which can be defined as a "process with openness and communication, so that it is easy for others to understand and see what has been done as well as what was intended" (Skoog et al., 2015). The concept of transparency assumes an even narrower meaning when applied to scientific research, as

were converted to a Likert scale and displayed on the y-axis. *ENDP*, electronic nicotine delivery product. (Adapted from Boue, S., Schlage, W.K., Page, D., Hoeng, J., Peitsch, C.M., 2019. Toxicological assessment of tobacco heating system 2.2: findings from an independent peer review. Regul. Toxicol. Pharmacol. Revised version submitted (minor revision requested).)

scientists and physicians are ethically mandated to embrace a transparent and open culture by sharing all the findings, data, and methods associated with a study or clinical trial, thus allowing the scientific community to verify and build upon their work for valid, evidence-based decision-making (Altman and Moher, 2013; Nicholls et al., 2016).

In recent years, researchers have started sharing patient-level data in the reporting of clinical studies (Drazen, 2015; Kirillova, 2012). The status quo in clinical research still differs from that in preclinical research, and the quality of reporting is still lagging. Several reporting guidelines have been developed to assist in implementing measures for addressing reproducibility concerns, including the Transparency and Openness Promotion guidelines (Nosek and Lakens, 2014), Standard Protocol Items: Recommendations for Interventional Trials statement for preparation of clinical trial protocols (Chan et al., 2013), and Animals in Research: Reporting In Vivo Experiments guidelines for animal research (Smith et al., 2017). An overview of such guidelines is maintained by the EQUATOR network (Simera et al., 2008).

Data sharing among scientists is not yet practiced in a systematic manner that allows reanalysis and reuse, despite its benefit to the scientific community and society in general, especially when data sharing relates to the scientific assessment of consumer products, including ENDPs. Moreover, transparency in sharing findings becomes even more critical when the quality of the science is questioned because of the affiliation of the scientists, funding source, or research topic (e.g., THR).

INTERVALS (https://www.intervals.science/) is an online platform developed by PMI to demonstrate the scientific rigor, thoroughness, and precision required to assess ENDPs, by sharing datasets and testing strategies and encouraging external verification (Boue et al., 2017). To address reproducibility concerns, INTERVALS was constructed by using the latest standards in data sharing and reproducible research, including FAIR (findable, accessible, interoperable, and reusable) principles (Wilkinson et al., 2016), to gather detailed information on the design and conduct of studies. This platform enables easy review of methods and results as well as reuse of data and generation of new hypotheses. INTERVALS can serve as a hub for a community of scientists from the industry, academia, nonprofit organizations, foundations, regulatory bodies, and publishers with a common interest in harm reduction.

It should be possible to improve the reproducibility of research findings In topics as important to society as THR by adopting validated reagents and ensuring rigorous study design and analysis, adherence to standard operating procedures, verification of methods, and transparency in sharing data and methods. This can be accomplished through the cooperation and adoption of best practices by all stakeholders to enable evidence-based decision-making.

REFERENCES

Alexander, D.J., Collins, C.J., Coombs, D.W., Gilkison, I.S., Hardy, C.J., Healey, G., Karantabias, G., Johnson, N., Karlsson, A., Kilgour, J.D., McDonald, P., 2008. Association of Inhalation Toxicologists (AIT) working party recommendation for standard delivered dose calculation and expression in non-clinical aerosol inhalation toxicology studies with pharmaceuticals. Inhal. Toxicol. 20, 1179–1189. https://doi.org/10.1080/08958370802207318.

Altman, D.G., Moher, D., 2013. Declaration of transparency for each research article. Br. Med. J. 347 https://doi.org/10.1136/bmj.f4796.

Andersen, M.E., Clewell 3rd, H.J., Bermudez, E., Dodd, D.E., Willson, G.A., Campbell, J.L., Thomas, R.S., 2010. Formaldehyde: integrating dosimetry, cytotoxicity, and genomics to understand dose-dependent transitions for an endogenous compound. Toxicol. Sci. 118, 716–731. https://doi.org/10.1093/toxsci/kfq303.

Begley, C.G., Ellis, L.M., 2012. Drug development: raise standards for preclinical cancer research. Nature 483, 531–533. https://doi.org/10.1038/483531a.

Begley, C.G., Ioannidis, J.P.A., 2015. Reproducibility in science. Improv. Stand. Basic Preclin. Res. 116, 116–126. https://doi.org/10.1161/circresaha.114.303819.

Benowitz, N.L., Hukkanen, J., Jacob, P., 2009. Nicotine chemistry, metabolism, kinetics and biomarkers. Handb. Exp. Pharmacol. 29–60. https://doi.org/10.1007/978-3-540-69248-5_2.

Bide, R.W., Armour, S.J., Yee, E., 2000. Allometric respiration/body mass data for animals to be used for estimates of inhalation toxicity to young adult humans. J. Appl. Toxicol. 20, 273–290. https://doi.org/10.1002/1099-1263(200007/08)20:4<273::aid-jat657>3.0.co;2-x.

Boue, S., Exner, T., Ghosh, S., Belcastro, V., Dokler, J., Page, D., Boda, A., Bonjour, F., Hardy, B., Vanscheeuwijck, P., Hoeng, J., Peitsch, M., 2017. Supporting evidence-based analysis for modified risk tobacco products through a toxicology data-sharing infrastructure. F1000Research 6, 12. https://doi.org/10.12688/f1000research.10493.2.

Boue, S., Schlage, W.K., Page, D., Hoeng, J., Peitsch, C.M., 2019. Toxicological assessment of tobacco heating system 2.2: findings from an independent peer review. Regul. Toxicol. Pharmacol. Revised version submitted (minor revision requested).

Boue, S., Talikka, M., Westra, J.W., Hayes, W., Di Fabio, A., Park, J., Schlage, W.K., Sewer, A., Fields, B., Ansari, S., Martin, F., Veljkovic, E., Kenney, R., Peitsch, M.C.,

Hoeng, J., 2015. Causal biological network database: a comprehensive platform of causal biological network models focused on the pulmonary and vascular systems. Database Oxf. 2015, bav030. https://doi.org/10.1093/database/bav030.

Button, K.S., Ioannidis, J.P.A., Mokrysz, C., Nosek, B.A., Flint, J., Robinson, E.S.J., Munafo, M.R., 2013. Power failure: why small sample size undermines the reliability of neuroscience. Nat. Rev. Neurosci. 14, 365–376. https://doi.org/10.1038/nrn3475.

Carter, B.D., Abnet, C.C., Feskanich, D., Freedman, N.D., Hartge, P., Lewis, C.E., Ockene, J.K., Prentice, R.L., Speizer, F.E., Thun, M.J., Jacobs, E.J., 2015. Smoking and mortality—beyond established causes. N. Engl. J. Med. 372, 631–640. https://doi.org/10.1056/NEJMsa1407211.

Center for Tobacco Products, 2019. Harmful and Potentially Harmful Constituents in Tobacco Products and Tobacco Smoke: Established List [WWW Document]. FDA. URL http://www.fda.gov/tobacco-products/rules-regulations-and-guidance/harmful-and-potentially-harmful-constituents-tobacco-products-and-tobacco-smoke-established-list. (Accessed 14 2 20).

Chan, A., Tetzlaff, J.M., Altman, D.G., et al., 2013. Spirit 2013 statement: defining standard protocol items for clinical trials. Ann. Intern. Med. 158, 200–207. https://doi.org/10.7326/0003-4819-158-3-201302050-00583.

Chang, C.M., Cheng, Y.-C., Cho, T.M., Mishina, E.V., Del Valle-Pinero, A.Y., van Bemmel, D.M., Hatsukami, D.K., 2019. Biomarkers of potential harm: summary of an FDA-sponsored public workshop. Nicotine Tob. Res. 21, 3–13. https://doi.org/10.1093/ntr/ntx273.

Collins, F.S., Tabak, L.A., 2014. NIH plans to enhance reproducibility. Nature 505, 612–613.

De Leon, H., Boue, S., Schlage, W.K., Boukharov, N., Westra, J.W., Gebel, S., VanHooser, A., Talikka, M., Fields, R.B., Veljkovic, E., Peck, M.J., Mathis, C., Hoang, V., Poussin, C., Deehan, R., Stolle, K., Hoeng, J., Peitsch, M.C., 2014. A vascular biology network model focused on inflammatory processes to investigate atherogenesis and plaque instability. J. Transl. Med. 12, 185. https://doi.org/10.1186/1479-5876-12-185.

Dinov, I.D., 2016. Methodological challenges and analytic opportunities for modeling and interpreting Big Healthcare Data. GigaScience 5. https://doi.org/10.1186/s13742-016-0117-6.

Drazen, J.M., 2015. Sharing individual patient data from clinical trials. N. Engl. J. Med. 372, 201–202. https://doi.org/10.1056/NEJMp1415160.

EPA (United States Environmental Protection Agency), 2015. Peer Review Handbook, fourth ed.

European Commission, 2006. Commission Directive 2006/15/EC of 7 February 2006 Establishing a Second List of Indicative Occupational Exposure Limit Values in Implementation of Council Directive 98/24/EC and Amending Directives 91/322/EEC and 2000/39/EC (Text with EEA Relevance).

European Committee for Standardization. CEN European Standard EN 15251, 2006. Indoor Environmental Input Parameters for Design and Assessment of Energy Performance of Buildings Addressing Indoor Air Quality, Thermal Environment, Lighting, and Accoustics. Eur. Comm. Stand. Bruss.

Fry, J.S., Lee, P.N., Forey, B.A., Coombs, K.J., 2013. How rapidly does the excess risk of lung cancer decline following quitting smoking? A quantitative review using the negative exponential model. Regul. Toxicol. Pharmacol. 67, 13–26. https://doi.org/10.1016/j.yrtph.2013.06.001.

Gebel, S., Lichtner, R.B., Frushour, B., Schlage, W.K., Hoang, V., Talikka, M., Hengstermann, A., Mathis, C., Veljkovic, E., Peck, M., Peitsch, M.C., Deehan, R., Hoeng, J., Westra, J.W., 2013. Construction of a computable network model for DNA damage, autophagy, cell death, and senescence. Bioinf. Biol. Insights 7, 97–117. https://doi.org/10.4137/BBI.S11154.

Goniewicz, M.L., Smith, D.M., Edwards, K.C., Blount, B.C., Caldwell, K.L., Feng, J., Wang, L., Christensen, C., Ambrose, B., Borek, N., van Bemmel, D., Konkel, K., Erives, G., Stanton, C.A., Lambert, E., Kimmel, H.L., Hatsukami, D., Hecht, S.S., Niaura, R.S., Travers, M., Lawrence, C., Hyland, A.J., 2018. Comparison of nicotine and toxicant exposure in users of electronic cigarettes and combustible cigarettes. JAMA Netw. Open 1, e185937. https://doi.org/10.1001/jamanetworkopen.2018.5937.

Harford, T., 2014. Big data: a big mistake? Significance 11, 14–19. https://doi.org/10.1111/j.1740-9713.2014.00778.x.

Hatsukami, D.K., Hanson, K., Briggs, A., Parascandola, M., Genkinger, J.M., O'Connor, R., Shields, P.G., 2009. Clinical trials methods for evaluation of potential reduced exposure products. Cancer Epidemiol. Biomark. Prev. 18, 3143–3195. https://doi.org/10.1158/1055-9965.EPI-09-0654.

Hoeng, J., Deehan, R., Pratt, D., Martin, F., Sewer, A., Thomson, T.M., Drubin, D.A., Waters, C.A., de Graaf, D., Peitsch, M.C., 2012. A network-based approach to quantifying the impact of biologically active substances. Drug Discov. Today 17, 413–418. https://doi.org/10.1016/j.drudis.2011.11.008.

Hoeng, J., Maeder, S., Vanscheeuwijck, P., Peitsch, M.C., 2019. Assessing the lung cancer risk reduction potential of candidate modified risk tobacco products. Intern. Emerg. Med. 14, 821–834. https://doi.org/10.1007/s11739-019-02045-z.

Hoeng, J., Talikka, M., Martin, F., Sewer, A., Yang, X., Iskandar, A., Schlage, W.K., Peitsch, M.C., 2014. Case study: the role of mechanistic network models in systems toxicology. Drug Discov. Today 19, 183–192. https://doi.org/10.1016/j.drudis.2013.07.023.

Ideker, T., Galitski, T., Hood, L., 2001. A new approach to decoding life: systems biology. Annu. Rev. Genom. Hum. Genet. 2, 343–372.

Inoue-Choi, M., Hartge, P., Park, Y., Abnet, C.C., Freedman, N.D., 2019. Association between reductions of number of cigarettes smoked per day and mortality among older adults in the United States. Am. J. Epidemiol. 188, 363–371. https://doi.org/10.1093/aje/kwy227.

Institute of Medicine, 2012. Committee on Scientific Standards for Studies on Modified Risk Tobacco Products. National Academies Press.

Iskandar, A.R., Gonzalez-Suarez, I., Majeed, S., Marescotti, D., Sewer, A., Xiang, Y., Leroy, P., Guedj, E., Mathis, C., Schaller, J.-P., Vanscheeuwijck, P., Frentzel, S., Martin, F., Ivanov, N.V., Peitsch, M.C., Hoeng, J., 2016. A framework for in vitro systems toxicology assessment of e-liquids. Toxicol. Mech. Methods 26, 389−413. https://doi.org/10.3109/15376516.2016.1170251.

Iskandar, A.R., Martin, F., Talikka, M., Schlage, W.K., Kostadinova, R., Mathis, C., Hoeng, J., Peitsch, M.C., 2013. Systems approaches evaluating the perturbation of xenobiotic metabolism in response to cigarette smoke exposure in nasal and bronchial tissues. BioMed Res. Int. 512086. https://doi.org/10.1155/2013/512086.

Jha, P., Ramasundarahettige, C., Landsman, V., Rostron, B., Thun, M., Anderson, R.N., McAfee, T., Peto, R., 2013. 21st-century hazards of smoking and benefits of cessation in the United States. N. Engl. J. Med. 368, 341−350. https://doi.org/10.1056/NEJMsa1211128.

Kahn, S.D., 2011. On the future of genomic data. Science 331, 728−729. https://doi.org/10.1126/science.1197891.

Karin, M., 2009. NF-kappaB as a critical link between inflammation and cancer. Cold Spring Harb. Perspect. Biol. 1, a000141. https://doi.org/10.1101/cshperspect.a000141.

Kirillova, O., 2012. Results and outcome reporting in ClinicalTrials.gov, what makes it happen? PLoS One 7, e37847. https://doi.org/10.1371/journal.pone.0037847.

Kogel, U., Schlage, W.K., Martin, F., Xiang, Y., Ansari, S., Leroy, P., Vanscheeuwijck, P., Gebel, S., Buettner, A., Wyss, C., Esposito, M., Hoeng, J., Peitsch, M.C., 2014. A 28-day rat inhalation study with an integrated molecular toxicology endpoint demonstrates reduced exposure effects for a prototypic modified risk tobacco product compared with conventional cigarettes. Food Chem. Toxicol. 68, 204−217. https://doi.org/10.1016/j.fct.2014.02.034.

Lee, P.N., Fry, J.S., Forey, B.A., 2014a. Estimating the decline in excess risk of chronic obstructive pulmonary disease following quitting smoking − a systematic review based on the negative exponential model. Regul. Toxicol. Pharmacol. 68, 231−239. https://doi.org/10.1016/j.yrtph.2013.12.006.

Lee, P.N., Fry, J.S., Hamling, J.S., 2012. Using the negative exponential distribution to quantitatively review the evidence on how rapidly the excess risk of ischaemic heart disease declines following quitting smoking. Regul. Toxicol. Pharmacol. 64, 51−67. https://doi.org/10.1016/j.yrtph.2012.06.009.

Lee, P.N., Fry, J.S., Thornton, A.J., 2014b. Estimating the decline in excess risk of cerebrovascular disease following quitting smoking−a systematic review based on the negative exponential model. Regul. Toxicol. Pharmacol. 68, 85−95. https://doi.org/10.1016/j.yrtph.2013.11.013.

Lighty, J.S., Veranth, J.M., Sarofim, A.F., 2000. Combustion aerosols: factors governing their size and composition and implications to human health. J. Air Waste Manag. Assoc. 1995 50, 1565−1618. https://doi.org/10.1080/10473289.2000.10464197 discussion 1619-1622.

Lüdicke, F., Ansari, S.M., Lama, N., Blanc, N., Bosilkovska, M., Donelli, A., Picavet, P., Baker, G., Haziza, C., Peitsch, M., Weitkunat, R., 2019. Effects of switching to a heat-not-burn tobacco product on biologically relevant biomarkers to assess a candidate modified risk tobacco product: a randomized trial. Cancer Epidemiol. Biomark. Prev. 28, 1934−1943. https://doi.org/10.1158/1055-9965.EPI-18-0915.

Manchikanti, L., Kaye, A.D., Boswell, M.V., Hirsch, J.A., 2015. Medical journal peer review: process and bias. Pain Physician 18, E1−E14.

Marchand, M., Brossard, P., Merdjan, H., Lama, N., Weitkunat, R., Lüdicke, F., 2017. Nicotine population pharmacokinetics in healthy adult smokers: a retrospective analysis. Eur. J. Drug Metab. Pharmacokinet. 42, 943−954. https://doi.org/10.1007/s13318-017-0405-2.

Martin, F., Sewer, A., Talikka, M., Xiang, Y., Hoeng, J., Peitsch, M.C., 2014. Quantification of biological network perturbations for mechanistic insight and diagnostics using two-layer causal models. BMC Bioinf. 15, 238. https://doi.org/10.1186/1471-2105-15-238.

Martin, F., Talikka, M., Hoeng, J., Peitsch, M.C., 2020. Systems toxicology approach to unravel early indicators of squamous cell carcinoma rate in rat nasal epithelium induced by formaldehyde exposure. In: Rocha, M., Mohamad, M.S., Zaki, N., Castellanos-Garzón, J.A. (Eds.), Practical Applications of Computational Biology and Bioinformatics, 13th International Conference. Springer International Publishing, pp. 16−24.

Martin, F., Thomson, T.M., Sewer, A., Drubin, D.A., Mathis, C., Weisensee, D., Pratt, D., Hoeng, J., Peitsch, M.C., 2012. Assessment of network perturbation amplitudes by applying high-throughput data to causal biological networks. BMC Syst. Biol. 6, 54. https://doi.org/10.1186/1752-0509-6-54.

Monticello, T.M., Swenberg, J.A., Gross, E.A., Leininger, J.R., Kimbell, J.S., Seilkop, S., Starr, T.B., Gibson, J.E., Morgan, K.T., 1996. Correlation of regional and nonlinear formaldehyde-induced nasal cancer with proliferating populations of cells. Cancer Res. 56, 1012−1022.

Murphy, J., Gaca, M., Lowe, F., Minet, E., Breheny, D., Prasad, K., Camacho, O., Fearon, I.M., Liu, C., Wright, C., McAdam, K., Proctor, C., 2017. Assessing modified risk tobacco and nicotine products: description of the scientific framework and assessment of a closed modular electronic cigarette. Regul. Toxicol. Pharmacol. 90, 342−357. https://doi.org/10.1016/j.yrtph.2017.09.008.

National Research Council - Division on Earth and Life Studies - Board on Environmental Studies and Toxicology - Committee on Improving Risk Analysis Approaches Used by the U.S. EPA, 2009. Science and Decisions − Advancing Risk Assessment. The National Academies Press, Washington, DC. https://doi.org/10.17226/12209.

Nicholls, S.G., Langan, S.M., Benchimol, E.I., Moher, D., 2016. Reporting transparency: making the ethical mandate explicit. BMC Med. 14, 44. https://doi.org/10.1186/s12916-016-0587-5.

Nosek, B.A., Lakens, D., 2014. Registered reports: a method to increase the credibility of published results. Soc. Psychol. 45, 137−141. https://doi.org/10.1027/1864-9335/a000192.

OECD Guidelines for the Testing of Chemicals, Section 4: Health Effects [WWW Document], n.d. URL https://www.oecd-

ilibrary.org/environment/oecd-guidelines-for-the-testing-of-c
hemicals-section-4-health-effects_20745788 (accessed 14 2
20).

Office of the Surgeon General U. S, 2010. How Tobacco Smoke
Causes Disease: The Biology and Behavioral Basis for
Smoking-Attributable Disease : a Report of the Surgeon
General ; Executive Summary. U.S. Dept. of Health and Hu-
man Services, Public Health Service, Office of the Surgeon
General, Rockville, MD.

Park, J.S., Schlage, W.K., Frushour, B.P., Talikka, M.,
Toedter, G., Gebel, S., Deehan, R., Veljkovic, E.,
Westra, J.W., Peck, M., Boue, S., Kogel, U., Gonzalez-
Suarez, I., Hengstermann, A., Peitsch, M.C., Hoeng, J.,
2013. Construction of a computable network model of tissue repair and angiogenesis in the lung. Clin. Toxicol. S12
https://doi.org/10.4172/2161-0495.S12-002.

Peitsch, M.C., de Graaf, D., 2014. A decade of systems biology:
where are we and where are we going to? Drug Discov.
Today 19, 105–107. https://doi.org/10.1016/
j.drudis.2013.06.002.

Pryor, W.A., Church, D.F., Evans, M.D., Rice, W.Y., Hayes, J.R.,
1990. A comparison of the free radical chemistry of
tobacco-burning cigarettes and cigarettes that only heat
tobacco. Free Radic. Biol. Med. 8, 275–279. https://
doi.org/10.1016/0891-5849(90)90075-t.

Reagan-Shaw, S., Nihal, M., Ahmad, N., 2008. Dose translation
from animal to human studies revisited. FASEB J. 22,
659–661. https://doi.org/10.1096/fj.07-9574LSF.

Rocca-Serra, P., Brandizi, M., Maguire, E., Sklyar, N., Taylor, C.,
Begley, K., Field, D., Harris, S., Hide, W., Hofmann, O.,
2010. ISA software suite: supporting standards-compliant
experimental annotation and enabling curation at the community level. Bioinformatics 26, 2354–2356.

Sansone, S.A., Rocca-Serra, P., Field, D., Maguire, E., Taylor, C.,
Hofmann, O., Fang, H., Neumann, S., Tong, W., Amaral-
Zettler, L., Begley, K., Booth, T., Bougueleret, L., Burns, G.,
Chapman, B., Clark, T., Coleman, L.A., Copeland, J.,
Das, S., de Daruvar, A., de Matos, P., Dix, I., Edmunds, S.,
Evelo, C.T., Forster, M.J., Gaudet, P., Gilbert, J., Goble, C.,
Griffin, J.L., Jacob, D., Kleinjans, J., Harland, L., Haug, K.,
Hermjakob, H., Ho Sui, S.J., Laederach, A., Liang, S.,
Marshall, S., McGrath, A., Merrill, E., Reilly, D., Roux, M.,
Shamu, C.E., Shang, C.A., Steinbeck, C., Trefethen, A.,
Williams-Jones, B., Wolstencroft, K., Xenarios, I.,
Hide, W., 2012. Toward interoperable bioscience data.
Nat. Genet. 44, 121–126. https://doi.org/10.1038/
ng.1054.

Schlage, W.K., Westra, J.W., Gebel, S., Catlett, N.L., Mathis, C.,
Frushour, B.P., Hengstermann, A., Van Hooser, A.,
Poussin, C., Wong, B., Lietz, M., Park, J., Drubin, D.,
Veljkovic, E., Peitsch, M.C., Hoeng, J., Deehan, R., 2011.
A computable cellular stress network model for non-
diseased pulmonary and cardiovascular tissue. BMC Syst.
Biol. 5, 168. https://doi.org/10.1186/1752-0509-5-168.

Simera, I., Altman, D.G., Moher, D., Schulz, K.F., Hoey, J.,
2008. Guidelines for reporting health research: the EQUA-
TOR network's survey of guideline authors. PLoS Med. 5,
e139. https://doi.org/10.1371/journal.pmed.0050139.

Skoog, M., Saarimäki, J.M., Gluud, C., Scheinin, M.,
Erlendsson, K., Aamdal, S., 2015. Transparency and Regis-
tration in Clinical Research in the Nordic Countries
(Report). Nordic Trial Alliance.

Smith, A.J., Clutton, R.E., Lilley, E., Hansen, K.E.A., Brattelid, T.,
2017. PREPARE: guidelines for planning animal research
and testing. Lab. Anim. https://doi.org/10.1177/
0023677217724823.

Smith, M.R., Clark, B., Ludicke, F., Schaller, J.P.,
Vanscheeuwijck, P., Hoeng, J., Peitsch, M.C., 2016. Evaluation of the tobacco heating system 2.2. Part 1: description
of the system and the scientific assessment program. Regul.
Toxicol. Pharmacol. 81 (Suppl. 2), S17–S26. https://
doi.org/10.1016/j.yrtph.2016.07.006.

Stephens, W.E., 2017. Comparing the cancer potencies of emissions from vapourised nicotine products including e-
cigarettes with those of tobacco smoke. Tobac. Contr.
https://doi.org/10.1136/tobaccocontrol-2017-053808.

Sturla, S.J., Boobis, A.R., FitzGerald, R.E., Hoeng, J.,
Kavlock, R.J., Schirmer, K., Whelan, M., Wilks, M.F.,
Peitsch, M.C., 2014. Systems toxicology: from basic
research to risk assessment. Chem. Res. Toxicol. 27,
314–329. https://doi.org/10.1021/tx400410s.

Talikka, M., Martin, F., Sewer, A., Vuillaume, G., Leroy, P.,
Luettich, K., Chaudhary, N., Peck, M.J., Peitsch, M.C.,
Hoeng, J., 2017. Mechanistic evaluation of the impact of
smoking and chronic obstructive pulmonary disease on
the nasal epithelium. Clin. Med. Insights Circulatory,
Respir. Pulm. Med. 11 https://doi.org/10.1177/
1179548417710928.

The National Academies, 2003. Policy on Committee Composition and Balance and Conflicts of Interest for Committees
Used in the Development of Reports. Natl. Acad. Press.

Thomson, T.M., Sewer, A., Martin, F., Belcastro, V.,
Frushour, B.P., Gebel, S., Park, J., Schlage, W.K.,
Talikka, M., Vasilyev, D.M., Westra, J.W., Hoeng, J.,
Peitsch, M.C., 2013. Quantitative assessment of biological
impact using transcriptomic data and mechanistic network
models. Toxicol. Appl. Pharmacol. 272, 863–878. https://
doi.org/10.1016/j.taap.2013.07.007.

U.S. Food & Drug Administration, 2012. Agency Program Directives, Volume IV – Agency Program Directives General
or Multidiscipline Scientific Integrity Scientific Integrity at
FDA.

van Asselt, E.D., Sterrenburg, P., Noordam, M.Y., van der Fels-
Klerx, H.J., 2012. Overview of available methods for risk based
control within the European Union. Trends Food Sci. Technol.
23, 51–58. https://doi.org/10.1016/j.tifs.2011.08.009.

Westra, J.W., Schlage, W.K., Frushour, B.P., Gebel, S.,
Catlett, N.L., Han, W., Eddy, S.F., Hengstermann, A.,
Matthews, A.L., Mathis, C., Lichtner, R.B., Poussin, C.,
Talikka, M., Veljkovic, E., Van Hooser, A.A., Wong, B.,
Maria, M.J., Peitsch, M.C., Deehan, R., Hoeng, J., 2011.
Construction of a computable cell proliferation network
focused on non-diseased lung cells. BMC Syst. Biol. 5,
105. https://doi.org/10.1186/1752-0509-5-105.

Westra, J.W., Schlage, W.K., Hengstermann, A., Gebel, S.,
Mathis, C., Thomson, T., Wong, B., Hoang, V.,

Veljkovic, E., Peck, M., Lichtner, R.B., Weisensee, D., Talikka, M., Deehan, R., Hoeng, J., Peitsch, M.C., 2013. A modular cell-type focused inflammatory process network model for non-diseased pulmonary tissue. Bioinf. Biol. Insights 7, 167–192. https://doi.org/10.4137/BBI.S11509.

Wilkinson, M.D., Dumontier, M., Aalbersberg, I.J., Appleton, G., Axton, M., Baak, A., Blomberg, N., Boiten, J.W., da Silva Santos, L.B., Bourne, P.E., Bouwman, J., Brookes, A.J., Clark, T., Crosas, M., Dillo, I., Dumon, O., Edmunds, S., Evelo, C.T., Finkers, R., Gonzalez-Beltran, A., Gray, A.J., Groth, P., Goble, C., Grethe, J.S., Heringa, J., t Hoen, P.A., Hooft, R., Kuhn, T., Kok, R., Kok, J., Lusher, S.J., Martone, M.E., Mons, A., Packer, A.L., Persson, B., Rocca-Serra, P., Roos, M., van Schaik, R., Sansone, S.A., Schultes, E., Sengstag, T., Slater, T., Strawn, G., Swertz, M.A., Thompson, M., van der Lei, J., van Mulligen, E., Velterop, J., Waagmeester, A., Wittenburg, P., Wolstencroft, K., Zhao, J., Mons, B., 2016. The FAIR guiding principles for scientific data management and stewardship. Sci. Data 3, 160018. https://doi.org/10.1038/sdata.2016.18.

CHAPTER 4

Quantification of HPHCs in ENDP Aerosols

MARK BENTLEY • SERGE MAEDER

4.1 HPHCS IN TOBACCO PRODUCTS

Cigarette smoke, formed during the process of burning tobacco, is a complex mixture known to contain more than 6000 constituents, which are representative of nearly all known organic chemical classes (Rodgman and Perfetti, 2013) and include approximately 150 established toxicants (Fowles and Dybing, 2003). Within this complex mixture, a number of harmful and potentially harmful constituents (HPHCs) have been associated with disease causation in smokers, including aromatic amines (Bartsch et al., 1993; Vineis and Pirastu, 1997), gas-phase constituents (Costa et al., 1986; Penn and Snyder, 1996; Witschi et al., 1997), oxygen-centered free radicals (Pryor, 1997; Valavanidis et al., 2009), polycyclic aromatic hydrocarbons (Penn et al., 1981; Smith and Hansch, 2000), and tobacco-specific nitrosamines (TSNAs) (Hecht, 1999, 1998). However, a causal link between a specific smoke constituent and disease has yet to be conclusively established.

In 1998, a list of compounds present in tobacco smoke that were known to have biological effects was published by Hoffmann and Hoffmann (Hoffmann and Hoffmann, 1998). Commonly referred to as the "Hoffmann analytes," they were based on work performed between 1970 and 1990. This list represented the first benchmark for toxicants that should be monitored in tobacco and tobacco smoke. Various scientific bodies have since acknowledged the presence of more than 100 HPHCs in tobacco and cigarette smoke, and several priority lists of smoke toxicants in mainstream cigarette smoke have been proposed for the evaluation of commercial market cigarettes, based mainly on risk assessments (Cunningham et al., 2011; Fowles and Dybing, 2003; Haussmann, 2012; Hecht, 2006; Hoffmann et al., 1997; Pankow et al., 2007; Rodgman and Green, 2003; Smith and Hansch, 2000; Talhout et al., 2011; Vorhees and Dodson, 1999; Xie et al., 2012).

4.2 SMOKE CONSTITUENT REPORTING

Different regulatory authorities require smoke-constituent reporting and brand-by-brand disclosure, either on an annual basis (Health Canada, British Columbia, Brazil, and Taiwan) or as a one-off disclosure (Massachusetts Department of Health, UK, and Australia) (Wright, 2015). The lists of smoke constituents required to be reported by different regulatory authorities show a great deal of similarity. However, with the exception of Health Canada (Health Canada, 2000), specific test methods have not been defined or validated. In the absence of specific provisions for heated tobacco products (HTPs), it seems logical to be guided in the assessment of HTPs by the reporting requirements applicable to cigarettes.

4.3 WHO STUDY GROUP ON TOBACCO PRODUCT REGULATION

The World Health Organization (WHO) Study Group on Tobacco Product Regulation (TobReg), composed of leading public health experts and scientists, proposed a scientific basis for tobacco product regulation in 2007 (WHO, 2007). As part of their recommendation, this group concluded that chemical measurement of smoke constituents generated by a smoking machine is probably the most effective approach currently available for scientifically assessing the differences among products for regulatory assessment of product toxicity (Burns et al., 2008). It was concluded that the Health Canada Intense (HCI) machine-smoking protocol (55-mL puff volume, 30-s puff interval, 2-s puff duration, 100% vent blocking, and 23-mm butt length for nonfilter cigarettes or the length of filter overwrap plus 3 mm for filter brands) (Health Canada, 1999) offered significant advantages over both the International Organization for Standardization (ISO)/Federal Trade Commission standard machine-smoking regimen

Toxicological Evaluation of Electronic Nicotine Delivery Products. https://doi.org/10.1016/B978-0-12-820490-0.00004-3

(35-mL puff volume, 60-s puff interval, 2-s puff duration, and no vent blocking) (FTC, 1967; ISO, 2012) and the Massachusetts Department of Public Health machine-smoking regimen (45-mL puff volume, 30-s puff interval, 2-s puff duration, 50% vent blocking, and 23-mm butt length for nonfilter cigarettes or the length of filter overwrap plus 3 mm for filter brands). Cigarettes should be collected and sampled in accordance with ISO 8243 (ISO, 2013a) and conditioned prior to machine smoking for at least 48 h at $22 \pm 1°C$ and a relative humidity of $60 \pm 3\%$, in accordance with ISO 3402 (ISO, 1999). TobReg recommended that manufacturers of tobacco products use the HCI machine-smoking protocol to report to the Member States of the WHO Framework Convention on Tobacco Control (FCTC) the yields of a priority list of 25 smoke constituents in mainstream smoke, expressed on a per-milligram nicotine-free dry particulate matter (NFDPM) basis. Furthermore, it was proposed to regulate the presence of two TSNAs, namely N-nitrosonornicotine (NNN) and 4-(methylnitrosamino)-1-(3-pyridyl)-1-butanone (NNK), on the basis of ceilings of 114 and 72 ng normalized per-mg nicotine in smoke, respectively. Normalizing the levels of NNK and NNN per-mg nicotine was considered as a strategy for addressing compensatory smoking and, presumably, for making cigarette emissions more relevant to human behavior rather than expressing these emissions on a per-cigarette basis (Hammond et al., 2007).

In 2008, TobReg (WHO, 2008) reduced the previous priority list from 25 to 18 toxicants in mainstream smoke and proposed that nine priority toxicants (1,3-butadiene, acetaldehyde, acrolein, benzene, benzo[a]pyrene, carbon monoxide (CO), formaldehyde, NNK, and NNN) should be mandated for lowering and regulation. The most important criterion for the selection of priority compounds for regulation was evidence of toxicity (Fowles and Dybing, 2003). It was proposed that cigarette samples should be obtained as part of a series of at least five sub-periods from manufacturers/importers or retail locations in accordance with the ISO standard method 8243 for sampling of cigarettes (ISO, 2013a). The ISO standard method 3402 for conditioning of cigarettes prior to smoking (ISO, 1999) and the HCI machine-smoking regimen (Health Canada, 1999) were proposed. It was also proposed that nicotine and CO yields should be determined by ISO standard methods 10315 and 8454, respectively (ISO, 2013b, 2007), while other toxicants should be determined by official methods recommended by Health Canada (2000) and expressed on a per-mg nicotine basis.

In 2015, TobReg identified 39 priority toxicants in mainstream cigarette smoke (WHO, 2015). The list of 39 priority toxicants was based primarily on lists of toxicants previously identified by Health Canada (2000), the National Institute for Public Health and the Environment in the Netherlands (Talhout et al., 2011), and the United States (US) Food and Drug Administration (FDA, 2012a). Previous recommendations for standard cigarettes were extended to cover other smoked tobacco products, such as non-standard cigarettes (e.g., "slims"), cigars, water pipes, and roll-your-own and low-ignition-propensity cigarettes. However, specific recommendations on machine-smoking regimens for these products were not detailed, although it was recommended that standardized testing methods validated by the WHO Tobacco Laboratory Network (TobLabNet), a global network of government, academic, and independent laboratories, should be used. At present, TobLabNet has validated methods for determining B[a]P, CO, humectants, nicotine, tar, and TSNAs (NNK and NNN) in mainstream smoke, while validation of methods for determining ammonia, volatile organic compounds, and aldehydes is in progress. TobReg also concluded that the same principles used to set the upper limits of emissions for toxicants in foods and other consumer products should be applied to tobacco products and that tar need not be quantified, as it is not a sound basis for regulation.

In 2019, TobReg (WHO, 2019a) reported a literature review performed for HTPs, which covered all available literature up to the end of October 2017. A recommendation was made that product contents and emissions for the 39 priority toxicants and/or the FDA HPHC list (FDA, 2012a) reported by the tobacco industry should be verified. In addition, potential novel toxicants being produced by HTPs that are not covered by commonly accepted lists should be evaluated. For the priority list of toxicants in combusted products, TobReg proposed a new approach requiring quantification of nicotine in smoke (previously only recommended as a measurand in tobacco) to accompany the levels of known harmful constituents, with the view that normalization of specific toxicants in relation to nicotine yield would enable measurement of toxicity of smoke generated in a standard regimen rather than in the quantity of smoke generated. Accordingly, nicotine has been added to a list of toxicants selected for testing and measuring, which additionally includes the nine toxicants proposed for mandated reduction, although nicotine does not fall under any requirement for mandated reduction. The expanded list of priority toxicants in mainstream cigarette smoke selected by

TobReg in 2015 has been reduced from 39 to 38 toxicants following a full review, which took into consideration any new analytical and/or toxicological information. This resulted in the removal of arsenic from the expanded priority list. Validated methods for mandated contents and emissions required by TobReg are now available.

4.4 US FDA LIST OF 93 HPHCS

The US FDA has established a list of 93 HPHCs in tobacco products and tobacco smoke (FDA, 2012a) and issued draft guidance on the reporting of an abbreviated list of 20 HPHCs in tobacco and mainstream cigarette smoke, for which analytical protocols are well established and widely available (FDA, 2012b). In mainstream cigarette smoke, 18 HPHCs are required to be reported, with 9 and 6 HPHCs required to be reported for smokeless tobacco products and cigarette filler (including roll-your-own), respectively. The protocols recommend machine smoking of cigarettes to be performed by using both the ISO 3308 and HCI regimens (Health Canada, 1999; ISO, 2012) and seven replicates to be used for determining all HPHCs, except nicotine and CO, for which 20 replicates are recommended. HPHC quantities should be expressed on a per-cigarette basis and reported by tobacco product manufacturers to the FDA. In addition, the FDA has encouraged tobacco product manufacturers to include HPHC data within new product applications.

4.5 PHILIP MORRIS INTERNATIONAL'S LIST OF 58 CONSTITUENTS

The list of constituents measured for evaluation of the mainstream aerosol composition of the Tobacco Heating System 2.2 (THS), an electrically heated tobacco product (EHTP) developed by Philip Morris International (PMI), is presented in Table 4.1 and compared with lists of priority smoke constituents proposed by TobReg (WHO, 2019a), Health Canada (Health Canada, 2000), and the FDA (FDA, 2012b, 2012a). PMI's list of 58 constituents (PMI 58 list) covers both smoke constituents and analytes determined by ISO standard methods (CO, nicotine, NFDPM, total particulate matter [TPM], and water) and representatives of all major toxicologically relevant chemical classes of compounds present in both the particulate and gas–vapor phases of cigarette smoke. The PMI 58 list was originally based on recommendations by the US Consumer Product Safety Commission on smoke constituents presenting toxicological concerns in low-ignition-propensity

cigarettes (U.S. Consumer Products Safety Commission, 1993) and compounds reported in cigarette smoke that have been classified as either known or probable human carcinogens by the International Agency for Research on Cancer (IARC, 2004). Additional HPHCs identified in mainstream cigarette smoke were considered and, if deemed relevant, included in the PMI 58 list of constituents requiring measurement for product evaluation. The PMI 58 list contains all constituents required for reporting by different regulatory authorities, including the 18 HPHCs that are subject to reporting in the FDA's abbreviated list (FDA, 2012b) and according to Health Canada (Health Canada, 2000) as well as all smoke constituents identified as priority toxicants and proposed for reporting by TobReg (WHO, 2019a).

4.6 HPHC EMISSIONS BY EHTPS

The underlying principle of the heated tobacco concept is that a number of the chemical processes occurring at the lit-end of a cigarette, linked to the high temperatures (>900°C) resulting from tobacco combustion (Baker, 2006, 2005, 1999, 1975), do not take place or are significantly reduced when tobacco is heated at a lower temperature (in the THS, the maximum temperature achieved within the tobacco substrate is approximately 320°C; Cozzani et al., 2020). These chemical processes are linked to the formation of a number of HPHCs that are not originally present in tobacco but are formed by pyrolysis. Moreover, the transfer of some HPHCs known to be present in cured tobacco leaves (such as TSNAs) to the aerosol is also reduced in EHTPs relative to cigarettes, because of the reduced operating temperature of the former. The lower operating temperature of an EHTP translates into a range of reductions in all measured HPHCs when comparing THS aerosol with the smoke of a reference cigarette (3R4F), either on a per-item basis or when normalized in relation to nicotine delivery.

4.6.1 Comparison of THS with the Reference Cigarette 3R4F

The mainstream emissions from both regular and mentholated THS tobacco sticks—referred to as THS Regular and THS Smooth Menthol, respectively—were compared with those from the 3R4F reference cigarette to demonstrate that heating rather than burning tobacco results in a reduction in HPHC formation. All experimental procedures for this comparison were conducted by Labstat International ULC (262 Manitou Drive, Kitchener, Ontario, N2C 1L3, Canada) in

TABLE 4.1
Lists of Priority Toxicants (HPHCs) Proposed by Regulatory Authorities, Alongside Those Measured by PMI for Quantification in the Mainstream Aerosol of Tobacco Products.

Mainstream aerosol Constituents	WHO 10 (2019)[a]	FDA 18 (2012b)[b]	WHO 38 (2019)[c]	HC 44 (2000)[d]	PMI 58[e]	FDA 93 (2012a)[f]
ISO PARAMETERS						
Nicotine	x	x	x	x	x	x
Carbon monoxide (CO)	x	x	x	x	x	x
Tar (NFDPM)					x	x
Total particulate matter (TPM)					x	
Water					x	
ALIPHATIC DIENES						
1,3-Butadiene	x	x	x	x	x	x
Isoprene		x	x	x	x	x
CARBONYLS						
Acetaldehyde	x	x	x	x	x	x
Acrolein	x	x	x	x	x	x
Formaldehyde	x	x	x	x	x	x
Crotonaldehyde		x	x	x	x	x
Acetone			x	x	x	x
Propionaldehyde			x	x	x	x
Butyraldehyde			x	x	x	
Methyl-ethyl-ketone (MEK)					x	x
MONOCYCLIC AROMATIC HYDROCARBONS						
Benzene	x	x	x	x	x	x
Toluene		x	x	x	x	x
Styrene				x	x	x
Ethylbenzene						x
N-NITROSAMINES						
4-(Methylnitrosamino)-1-(3-pyridyl)-1-butanone (NNK)	x	x	x	x	x	x
N-Nitrosonornicotine (NNN)	x	x	x	x	x	x
N-Nitrosoanabasine (NAB)			x	x	x	
N-Nitrosoanatabine (NAT)			x	x	x	
N-Nitrosodiethanolamine (NDELA)						x
N-Nitrosodiethylamine (NDEA)						x
N-Nitrosodimethylamine (NDMA)						x
N-Nitrosomethylethylamine (NEMA)						x
N-Nitrosomorpholine (NMOR)						x
N-Nitrosopiperidine (NPIP)						x
N-Nitrosopyrrolidine (NPYR)						x

POLYCYCLIC AROMATIC HYDROCARBONS						
Benzo[a]pyrene	x	x	x	x	x	x
Benz[a]anthracene					x	x
Dibenz[a,h]anthracene					x	x
Pyrene					x	
Benz[j]aceanthrylene						x
Benzo[b]fluoranthene						x
Benzo[k]fluoranthene						x
Benzo[b]furan						x
Benzo[c]phenanthrene						x
Chrysene						x
Cyclopenta[c,d]pyrene						x
Dibenzo[a,e]pyrene						x
Dibenzo[a,h]pyrene						x
Dibenzo[a,i]pyrene						x
Dibenzo[a,l]pyrene						x
Indeno[1,2,3-cd]pyrene						x
5-Methylchrysene						x
Naphthalene						x
ACID DERIVATIVES						
Acrylonitrile		x	x	x	x	x
Acetamide					x	x
Acrylamide					x	x
Caffeic acid						x
Ethyl carbamate (urethane)						x
Vinyl acetate						x
INORGANICS						
Ammonia		x	x	x	x	x
Hydrogen cyanide			x	x	x	x
Nitric oxide			x	x	x	
Nitrogen oxides			x	x	x	
Hydrazine						x
AROMATIC AMINES						
4-Aminobiphenyl		x	x	x	x	x
1-Aminonaphthalene		x	x	x	x	x
2-Aminonaphthalene		x	x	x	x	x
3-Aminobiphenyl			x	x	x	
o-Toluidine					x	x
o-Anisidine						x
A-α-C (2-Amino-9H-pyrido[2,3-b] indole)						x
2,6-Dimethylaniline						x
Glu-P-1 (2-Amino-6-methyldipyrido [1,2-a:3′,2′-d]imidazole)						x

Continued

TABLE 4.1
Lists of Priority Toxicants (HPHCs) Proposed by Regulatory Authorities, Alongside Those Measured by PMI for Quantification in the Mainstream Aerosol of Tobacco Products.—cont'd

Mainstream aerosol Constituents	WHO 10 (2019)[a]	FDA 18 (2012b)[b]	WHO 38 (2019)[c]	HC 44 (2000)[d]	PMI 58[e]	FDA 93 (2012a)[f]
Glu-P-2 (2-aminodipyrido[1,2-a:3′,2′-d]imidazole)						x
IQ (2-Amino-3-methylimidazo[4,5-f]quinoline)						x
MeA-α-C (2-Amino-3-methyl)-9H-pyrido[2,3-b]indole)						x
PhIP (2-Amino-1-methyl-6-phenylimidazo[4,5-b]pyridine)						x
Trp-P-1 (3-Amino-1,4-dimethyl-5H-pyrido[4,3-b]indole)						x
Trp-P-2 (1-Methyl-3-amino-5H-pyrido[4,3-b]indole)						x
PHENOLS						
m-Cresol			x	x	x	x
p-Cresol			x	x	x	x
o-Cresol			x	x	x	x
Catechol			x	x	x	x
Phenol			x	x	x	x
Hydroquinone			x	x	x	
Resorcinol			x	x	x	
HETEROCYCLIC AROMATIC HYDROCARBONS						
Furan						x
Quinoline			x	x	x	x
Pyridine			x	x	x	
Cadmium			x	x	x	x
METALS						
Lead			x	x	x	x
Mercury			x	x	x	x
Arsenic					x	x
Chromium					x	x
Nickel					x	x
Selenium					x	x
Beryllium						x
Cobalt						x
Polonium-210						x
Uranium-235						x
Uranium-238						x
EPOXIDES						
Ethylene oxide					x	x
Propylene oxide					x	x
HALOGENATED						
Vinyl chloride					x	x
Chlorinated dioxins (7)/furans (10)						x

NITRO COMPOUNDS		
Nitrobenzene	X	X
Nitromethane		X
2-Nitropropane		X
TOBACCO ALKALOIDS		
Anabasine		X
Nornicotine		X
PRODUCT SPECIFIC		
Glycerol	X	

[a] Priority toxicants selected by TobReg for testing and measuring, including the nine toxicants proposed for mandated reduction ("WHO"), plus nicotine.
[b] FDA abbreviated list of priority toxicants for tobacco products actually comprises 20 chemical constituents. However, measurements for cadmium and arsenic are required in tobacco substrate only.
[c] The previous extended list of 39 priority toxicants proposed by the WHO (2015) has been reduced to 38, with removal of the requirement for measuring arsenic following the release of the seventh report of the WHO study group on tobacco product regulation (WHO, 2019).
[d] Health Canada's Tobacco Reporting Regulations (SOR/2000−273) mandate the reporting of 40 aerosol constituents.
[e] The "PMI 58" list of analytes comprises 54 HPHCs, plus nicotine, TPM, NFDPM, and water. (Glycerol is a heated tobacco product-specific measurand.)
[f] The FDA list of 93 HPHCs requires measurement for more than 93 mainstream aerosol constituents, as multiple chlorinated dioxins and furans are represented as a single entry within this list. In addition, the *m*-, *o*-, and *p*-isomers of cresol are listed as a single constituent. Measurements for aflatoxin-B1, coumarin, and *N*-nitrosarcosine are required in tobacco substrate only. HPHCs, harmful and potentially harmful constituents; PMI, Philip Morris International.

accordance with their procedures and methods that were accredited according to ISO 17025 (ISO, 2017a). Prior to aerosol generation, all test items were conditioned in accordance with ISO 3402 conditions ($22°C \pm 1°C$ and $60\% \pm 3\%$ relative humidity (RH)), and the laboratory conditions during aerosol generation were maintained at $22°C \pm 2°C$ and $60\% \pm 5\%$ RH. All aerosol and smoke collections were performed in accordance with the HCI machine-smoking protocol (Health Canada, 1999) by using a linear smoking machine. For THS, vent blocking was not required, as the tobacco sticks are not ventilated (no perforation at the filter level). The butt length requirement did not apply either, as tobacco sticks are not consumed by combustion and remain the same size throughout use. Aerosol collection starts after the preheating period (30 s) and stops at 6 min, which is the end of the heating period. This results in exactly 12 puffs under HCI conditions. Tables 4.2 and 4.3 present the comparative yields for THS Regular versus 3R4F. Tables 4.4 and 4.5 present the comparative yields for THS Smooth Menthol versus 3R4F.

Fig. 4.1 is a graphical representation of the data in Table 4.3 and shows the proportion (%) of each HPHC relative to 3R4F (set at 100%) on a per-item basis.

Fig. 4.2 is a graphical representation of the data in Table 4.5 and shows the proportion (%) of each HPHC relative to 3R4F (set at 100%) on a per-item basis.

Comparison of deliveries between THS Regular and 3R4F on a per-item basis showed reductions in HPHCs in the former, ranging from 62.6% for mercury to more than 99% for aromatic amines, 1,3-butadiene, acrylonitrile, benzene, cadmium, ethylene oxide, hydrogen cyanide, isoprene, *m*-cresol, and *p*-cresol. For THS Smooth Menthol, comparison on a per-item basis with 3R4F showed reductions from 64.2% for mercury to more than 99% for aromatic amines, 1,3-butadiene, acrylonitrile, benzene, cadmium, ethylene oxide, hydrogen cyanide, isoprene, *m*-cresol, *o*-cresol, and *p*-cresol. The range of reductions achieved for the measured HPHCs is reflective of the different mechanisms involved in their formation, or volatility (for those already present in tobacco). Overall, relative to the 3R4F reference cigarette, the average reduction in the levels of HPHCs (upon applying analysis for the PMI 58 list of aerosol constituents) for THS was >92% for the regular tobacco stick and >93% for the mentholated tobacco stick, on a per-item basis. The reductions in the levels of HPHCs relative to nicotine delivery were slightly lower, as THS delivers less nicotine per stick than the reference cigarette, and the average reductions were >89% and >88% for the regular and mentholated tobacco stick variants, respectively.

TABLE 4.2
Main Aerosol Deliveries for THS Regular Tobacco Sticks and 3R4F Cigarettes.

Aerosol Deliveries Determined in Accordance with ISO 4387; 8454; 10315	Unit	3R4F			THS REGULAR		
		Mean	SD	N	Mean	SD	n
Glycerol[a]	mg/item	2.08	0.113	2	5.02	0.101	3
Nicotine	mg/item	1.74	0.039	2	1.29	0.047	3
Nicotine-free dry particulate matter (NFDPM)[b]	mg/item	25.0	1.14	2	19.4	1.62	3
Total particulate matter (TPM)	mg/item	41.4	3.28	2	50.9	2.90	3
Water[c]	mg/item	14.7	2.10	2	30.2	2.17	3

SD, standard deviation; n, number of items.

[a] Product-specific, not part of ISO parameters.

[b] ISO terminology NFDPM is used here to describe the aerosol-collected mass from THS. It should be noted that the NFDPM of THS has a very different constituent makeup than a cigarette. Glycerol, reported separately, is a part of NFDPM.

[c] The water value reported here was determined in accordance with ISO 4387 and is underestimated relative to the true value because of the significant water loss linked with the high water content of the THS aerosol. Accurate water measurements can only be obtained by using a modified procedure not available to Labstat (see (Ghosh and Jeannet, 2014)).

A later study, also performed by Labstat International ULC, compared the levels of HPHCs in the full FDA 93 list between THS Regular and Smooth Menthol and the 3R4F reference cigarette. The total reductions in HPHCs for THS Regular and Smooth Menthol relative to 3R4F (excluding nicotine) were found to be between 90.5% and 91.0% on a per-item basis and between 85.6% and 86.3% relative to nicotine delivery, respectively. These reductions are fully aligned with the calculated overall reductions in the 54 HPHCs contained in the PMI 58 list of aerosol constituents and demonstrate that measurement of these 54 HPHCs is sufficiently reliable for correctly estimating the overall reduction of HPHCs emitted by THS relative to cigarettes. In addition, the overall reduction in HPHCs remained consistent between the Regular and Smooth Menthol variants. The results from the analysis of the FDA list of 93 HPHCs are presented in Tables 4.6 and 4.7 for the Regular and Smooth Menthol product variants, respectively.

The analysis of the FDA 93 list of HPHCs required quantification of 108 chemical constituents (including nicotine). In the FDA 93 list, chlorinated dioxins and furans are listed as a single entry, and specific compounds are not defined. Labstat engaged an external laboratory (Maxxam Analytics International Corporation [now Bureau Veritas] o/a Maxxam Analytics, 6740 Campobello Road, Mississauga, Ontario, L5N 2L8) for analysis of these compounds and used Maxxam's standard list of 17 chlorinated dioxins/furans. Presumably a sum value would be required in order to report in accordance with the requirements of the FDA list. In addition, cresols are represented as a single entry in the FDA list, although the three isomeric forms (*ortho*-, *meta*-, and *para*-cresol) are generally determined independently. Three of the compounds in the FDA list are tobacco substrate specific and were not required to be measured in aerosol/smoke (aflatoxin B1, coumarin, and N-nitrososarcosine).

Beyond PMI's efforts to characterize the levels of recognized HPHCs in the aerosol of THS, several independent researchers have investigated, to a similar or lesser extent, the chemical composition of THS aerosol (Auer et al., 2017; Bekki et al., 2017; Farsalinos et al., 2018a, 2018b; Gasparyan et al., 2018; Ishizaki and Kataoka, 2019; Leigh et al., 2018; Li et al., 2019; Mallock et al., 2018; Salman et al., 2019; Uchiyama et al., 2018). The results published by independent researchers confirm the results reported by PMI, although the majority of these researchers only partially addressed the list of 54 HPHCs contained within the PMI 58 list of chemical constituents. Forster et al. (Forster et al., 2018) evaluated a list of constituents that contained all 54 HPHCs selected by PMI for evaluation of EHTPs. It should be noted that the analytical data reported by Forster et al. (2018) were also generated by Labstat International ULC and, therefore, with the same methods as those used for generating the data reported by PMI. Table 4.8 presents the results of the analysis of THS Regular aerosol (covering the PMI 58 list of constituents), which are currently available in the public domain.

TABLE 4.3

HPHCs Determined for Regular THS Tobacco Sticks and 3R4F Cigarettes (excluding the Main Aerosol Deliveries Reported in Table 4.2) and Percent Reductions Versus 3R4F Calculated on a Per-Item Basis.

PMI 58 HPHCs (Alphabetical Order)	Unit	3R4F			THS REGULAR			Reduction Relative to 3R4F (%)[a]
		Mean	SD	n	Mean	SD	n	
1-Aminonaphthalene	ng/item	20.9	0.145	2	0.0427	0.00513	3	99.8%
2-Aminonaphthalene	ng/item	17.5	0.497	2	0.0223	0.00321	3	99.9%
3-Aminobiphenyl	ng/item	4.60	0.137	2	0.0070	0.003	3	99.8%
4-Aminobiphenyl	ng/item	3.21	0.105	2	0.0087	0.0012	3	99.7%
Acetaldehyde	µg/item	1602	NA	1	192	11.6	3	88.0%
Acetamide	µg/item	13.0	0.501	2	2.96	0.134	3	77.3%
Acetone	µg/item	653	NA	1	30.7	1.86	3	95.3%
Acrolein	µg/item	158	NA	1	8.32	0.755	3	94.7%
Acrylamide	µg/item	4.50	0.294	2	1.58	0.0543	3	65.0%
Acrylonitrile	µg/item	21.2	1.44	2	0.145	0.0112	3	99.3%
Ammonia	µg/item	33.2	0.539	2	12.2	0.973	3	63.2%
Arsenic	ng/item	<7.49 (LOQ)	NA	2	<0.36 (LOD)	NA	3	NA
Benz[a]anthracene	ng/item	28.4	1.09	2	2.65	0.0647	3	90.7%
Benzene	µg/item	77.3	5.81	2	0.452	0.0395	3	99.4%
Benzo[a]pyrene	ng/item	13.3	0.660	2	0.736	0.0973	3	94.5%
1,3-Butadiene	µg/item	89.2	1.73	2	0.207	0.0160	3	99.8%
Butyraldehyde	µg/item	81.3	NA	1	20.7	1.52	3	74.5%
Cadmium	ng/item	89.2	9.31	2	<0.28 (LOQ)	NA	3	>99.7%
Carbon monoxide (CO)	mg/item	29.4	1.35	2	0.347	0.0462	3	98.8%
Catechol	µg/item	84.1	9.36	2	14.0	0.522	3	83.3%
Chromium	ng/item	<11.9 (LOD)	NA	2	<11.0 (LOQ)	NA	3	NA
m-Cresol	µg/item	4.24	0.461	2	0.0424	0.0045	3	99.0%
o-Cresol	µg/item	4.81	0.304	2	0.0779	0.0093	3	98.4%
p-Cresol	µg/item	9.60	0.929	2	0.0706	0.00816	3	99.3%
Crotonaldehyde	µg/item	49.3	NA	1	<3.29 (LOQ)	NA	3	>93.3%
Dibenz[a,h]anthracene	ng/item	<0.689 (LOQ)	NA	2	<0.124 (LOD)	NA	3	NA
Ethylene oxide	µg/item	16.0	1.18	2	<0.119 (LOQ)	NA	3	>99.3%
Formaldehyde	µg/item	79.4	NA	1	14.1	0.430	3	82.2%
Hydrogen cyanide	µg/item	329	16.2	2	<1.75 (LOQ)	NA	3	>99.5%
Hydroquinone	µg/item	94.5	10.3	2	6.55	0.461	3	93.1%
Isoprene	µg/item	891	35.8	2	1.51	0.129	3	99.8%

Continued

TABLE 4.3
HPHCs Determined for Regular THS Tobacco Sticks and 3R4F Cigarettes (excluding the Main Aerosol Deliveries Reported in Table 4.2) and Percent Reductions Versus 3R4F Calculated on a Per-Item Basis.—cont'd

PMI 58 HPHCs (Alphabetical Order)	Unit	3R4F			THS REGULAR			Reduction Relative to 3R4F (%)[a]
		Mean	SD	n	Mean	SD	n	
Lead	ng/item	31.2	2.78	2	2.23	0.351	3	92.8%
Mercury	ng/item	3.68	0.140	2	1.38	0.163	3	62.6%
Methyl-ethyl-ketone (MEK)	µg/item	183	NA	1	10.1	0.759	3	94.5%
Nickel	ng/item	<12.9 (LOD)	NA	2	<15.9 (LOD)	NA	3	NA
Nitric oxide (NO)	µg/item	484	7.20	2	12.6	0.418	3	97.4%
Nitrobenzene	µg/item	<0.038 (LOD)	NA	2	<0.011 (LOD)	NA	3	NA
Nitrogen oxides (NOx)	µg/item	538	8.78	2	14.2	0.413	3	97.4%
N-Nitrosoanabasine (NAB)	ng/item	29.0	1.08	2	2.35	0.0589	3	91.9%
N-Nitrosoanatabine (NAT)	ng/item	254	17.4	2	14.7	1.25	3	94.2%
4-(Methylnitrosamino)-1-(3-pyridyl)-1-butanone (NNK)	ng/item	244.7	7.54	2	7.80	0.423	3	96.8%
N-Nitrosonornicotine (NNN)	ng/item	271	8.49	2	10.1	0.205	3	96.3%
Phenol	µg/item	15.6	1.75	2	1.47	0.206	3	90.6%
Propionaldehyde	µg/item	109	NA	1	10.8	0.675	3	90.1%
Propylene oxide	ng/item	896	82.5	2	142.3	6.67	3	84.1%
Pyrene	ng/item	79.2	3.58	2	8.20	0.152	3	89.7%
Pyridine	µg/item	30.9	1.64	2	6.58	0.185	3	78.7%
Quinoline	µg/item	0.434	0.0246	2	<0.011 (LOQ)	NA	3	>97.5%
Resorcinol	µg/item	1.72	0.168	2	<0.055 (LOQ)	NA	3	>96.8%
Selenium[b]	ng/item	<4.42 (LOD)	NA	2	1.27	0.0577	3	NA
Styrene	µg/item	13.9	1.72	2	0.577	0.0916	3	95.8%
Toluene	µg/item	129	1.17	2	1.42	0.162	3	98.9%
o-Toluidine	ng/item	96.2	3.09	2	1.10	0.0243	3	98.9%
Vinyl chloride	ng/item	93.4	3.00	2	<0.657 (LOD)	NA	3	>99.3%

LOD, limit of detection, LOQ, limit of quantification, n, number of items; NA, not available; SD, standard deviation

[a] When HPHC values for both THS and 3R4F were below LOD or LOQ, no reduction could be calculated. For HPHC values found below LOD or LOQ for THS, with a corresponding value for 3R4F above the LOQ, the % reduction was calculated by using the LOD/LOQ value.

[b] In the case of selenium, the 3R4F value was below the LOD, while a value was reported for THS. However, the LOD for 3R4F was higher than the value reported for THS. In this case, a reduction could not be calculated.

TABLE 4.4

Main Aerosol Deliveries for Mentholated THS Tobacco Sticks and 3R4F Cigarettes.

Aerosol Deliveries Determined in Accordance with ISO 4387; 8454; 10315	Unit	3R4F			THS SMOOTH MENTHOL		
		Mean	SD	n	Mean	SD	n
Glycerol[a]	mg/item	2.15	0.11	2	4.41	0.10	3
Nicotine	mg/item	1.84	0.11	2	1.19	0.05	3
Nicotine-free dry particulate matter (NFDPM)[b]	mg/item	24.8	1.0	2	19.5	1.3	3
Total particulate matter (TPM)	mg/item	41.9	2.39	2	56.3	0.93	3
Water[c]	mg/item	15.3	1.55	2	35.6	0.59	3

[a–c] See legend to Table 4.2. *n*, number of items; *SD*, standard deviation

TABLE 4.5

HPHCs Determined for Mentholated THS Tobacco Sticks and 3R4F Cigarettes (excluding the Main Aerosol Deliveries Reported in Table 4.4) and Percent Reductions Versus 3R4F Calculated on a Per-Item Basis.

PMI 58 HPHCs (Alphabetical Order)	Unit	3R4F			THS SMOOTH MENTHOL			Reduction Relative to 3R4F (%)[a]
		Mean	SD	n	Mean	SD	n	
1-Aminonaphthalene	ng/item	20.9	0.8	2	0.043	0.012	3	99.8%
2-Aminonaphthalene	ng/item	17.3	0.5	2	0.022	0.007	3	99.9%
3-Aminobiphenyl	ng/item	4.61	0.24	2	0.008	0.001	3	99.8%
4-Aminobiphenyl	ng/item	3.21	0.22	2	0.009	0.002	3	99.7%
Acetaldehyde	µg/item	1612	NA	1	206	6	3	87.2%
Acetamide	µg/item	14.0	1.2	2	2.98	0.06	3	78.8%
Acetone	µg/item	648	NA	1	37.8	2.2	3	94.2%
Acrolein	µg/item	144	NA	1	9.79	1.66	3	93.2%
Acrylamide	µg/item	4.67	0.32	2	1.64	0.001	3	64.9%
Acrylonitrile	µg/item	22.1	0.3	2	0.127	0.017	3	99.4%
Ammonia	µg/item	32.2	1.3	2	11.1	1.1	3	65.4%
Arsenic	ng/item	<7.49 (LOQ)	NA	2	<1.2 (LOQ)	NA	3	NA
Benz[a]anthracene	ng/item	26.5	0.5	2	1.80	0.03	3	93.2%
Benzene	µg/item	79.7	2.9	2	0.453	0.046	3	99.4%
Benzo[a]pyrene	ng/item	12.5	0.3	2	0.539	0.081	3	95.7%
1,3-Butadiene	µg/item	92.8	3.1	2	0.223	0.030	3	99.8%
Butyraldehyde	µg/item	83.4	NA	1	21.1	0.4	3	74.7%
Cadmium	ng/item	89.2	9.3	2	<0.28 (LOQ)	NA	3	>99.7%
Carbon monoxide (CO)	mg/item	30.8	1.7	2	0.320	0.000	3	99.0%
Catechol	µg/item	92.8	6.8	2	11.5	1.0	3	87.6%
Chromium	ng/item	<11.9 (LOD)	NA	2	<3.31 (LOD)	NA	3	NA

Continued

TABLE 4.5

HPHCs Determined for Mentholated THS Tobacco Sticks and 3R4F Cigarettes (excluding the Main Aerosol Deliveries Reported in Table 4.4) and Percent Reductions Versus 3R4F Calculated on a Per-Item Basis.—cont'd

PMI 58 HPHCs (Alphabetical Order)	Unit	3R4F			THS SMOOTH MENTHOL			Reduction Relative to 3R4F (%)[a]
		Mean	SD	n	Mean	SD	n	
m-Cresol	µg/item	4.23	0.11	2	0.027	0.002	3	99.4%
o-Cresol	µg/item	4.58	0.30	2	0.048	0.005	3	99.0%
p-Cresol	µg/item	9.83	0.71	2	0.047	0.007	3	99.5%
Crotonaldehyde	µg/item	48.2	NA	1	<3.29 (LOQ)	NA	3	>93.2%
Dibenz[*a,h*]anthracene	ng/item	<0.689 (LOQ)	NA	2	<0.124 (LOD)	NA	3	NA
Ethylene oxide	µg/item	19.0	2.8	2	<0.119 (LOQ)	NA	3	>99.4%
Formaldehyde	µg/item	67.9	NA	1	15.2	0.0	3	77.7%
Hydrogen cyanide	µg/item	331	10	2	<1.75 (LOQ)	NA	3	>99.5%
Hydroquinone	µg/item	97.2	7.0	2	4.99	0.50	3	94.9%
Isoprene	µg/item	956	11	2	1.51	0.31	3	99.8%
Lead	ng/item	31.2	2.8	2	1.87	0.06	3	94.0%
Mercury	ng/item	3.70	0.32	2	1.32	0.09	3	64.2%
Methyl-ethyl-ketone (MEK)	µg/item	178	NA	1	13.9	0.2	3	92.2%
Nickel	ng/item	<43.1 (LOQ)	NA	2	<15.9 (LOD)	NA	3	NA
Nitric oxide (NO)	µg/item	500	9	2	13.0	0.4	3	97.4%
Nitrobenzene	µg/item	<0.038 (LOD)	NA	2	<0.011 (LOD)	NA	3	NA
Nitrogen oxides (NOx)	µg/item	554	11	2	14.5	0.5	3	97.4%
N-Nitrosoanabasine (NAB)	ng/item	31.1	2.5	2	2.29	0.21	3	92.6%
N-Nitrosoanatabine (NAT)	ng/item	248	15	2	12.8	1.4	3	94.9%
4-(Methylnitrosamino)-1-(3-pyridyl)-1-butanone (NNK)	ng/item	256	8	2	6.63	0.53	3	97.4%
N-Nitrosonornicotine (NNN)	ng/item	274	8	2	7.01	0.51	3	97.4%
Phenol	µg/item	17.1	0.9	2	0.953	0.045	3	94.4%
Propionaldehyde	µg/item	108	NA	1	12.0	0.6	3	88.9%
Propylene oxide	ng/item	1066	28	2	111	5	3	89.5%
Pyrene	ng/item	74.8	2.5	2	5.81	0.19	3	92.2%
Pyridine	µg/item	26.8	2.7	2	6.22	0.25	3	76.8%
Quinoline	µg/item	0.450	0.048	2	<0.011 (LOQ)	NA	3	>97.6%
Resorcinol	µg/item	1.86	0.23	2	<0.055 (LOQ)	NA	3	>97.0%

TABLE 4.5
HPHCs Determined for Mentholated THS Tobacco Sticks and 3R4F Cigarettes (excluding the Main Aerosol Deliveries Reported in Table 4.4) and Percent Reductions Versus 3R4F Calculated on a Per-Item Basis.—cont'd

PMI 58 HPHCs (Alphabetical Order)	Unit	3R4F			THS SMOOTH MENTHOL			Reduction Relative to 3R4F (%)[a]
		Mean	SD	n	Mean	SD	n	
Selenium[b]	ng/item	<4.42 (LOD)	NA	2	1.21	0.63	3	NA
Styrene	µg/item	12.3	2.3	2	0.457	0.070	3	96.3%
Toluene	µg/item	137	4	2	1.28	0.12	3	99.1%
o-Toluidine	ng/item	102	1	2	0.936	0.041	3	99.1%
Vinyl chloride	ng/item	92.5	7.7	2	<2.19 (LOQ)	NA	3	>97.6%

[a,b] See legend to Table 4.3. *LOD*, limit of detection, *LOQ*, limit of quantification, *n*, number of items; *NA*, not available; *SD*, standard deviation.

Amount relative to 3R4F value (%)

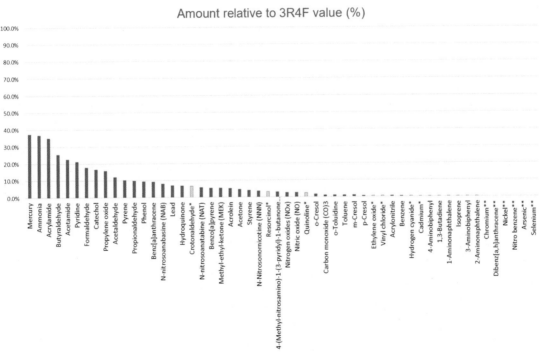

FIG. 4.1 Comparison of HPHC Emissions in the Aerosol Generated by Regular THS Tobacco Sticks With Those in 3R4F Smoke, Calculated on a Per-Item Basis. *HPHC*, harmful and potentially harmful constituent; *THS*, Tobacco Heating System 2.2. * Values determined for THS were below the LOQ or LOD, and, therefore, calculation of reduction relative to 3R4F was performed by using LOQ/LOD values. ** Values determined for both THS and 3R4F were below the LOQ or LOD, and, therefore, relative quantities were not calculable.

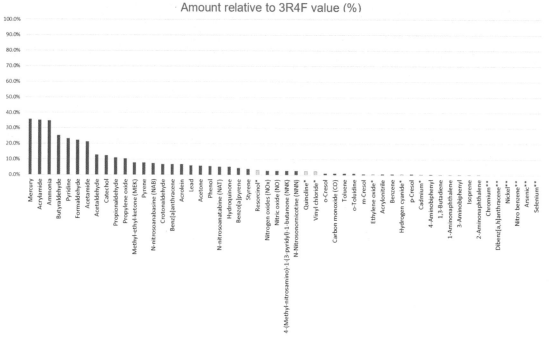

FIG. 4.2 Comparison of HPHC Emissions in the Aerosol Generated by Mentholated THS Tobacco Sticks With Those in 3R4F Smoke, Calculated on a Per-Item Basis. *HPHC*, harmful and potentially harmful constituent; *THS*, Tobacco Heating System 2.2. * Values determined for THS were below the LOQ or LOD, and, therefore, calculations of quantities relative to 3R4F were performed by using LOQ/LOD values. ** Values determined for both THS and 3R4F were below the LOQ or LOD, and, therefore, relative quantities were not calculable.

As can be seen in Table 4.8, the majority of the data are directly comparable among the investigations. It should be noted that, with the exception of the results reported by Schaller et al. (2016) (analysis performed at PMI), all data reported in this table were independently generated by Labstat International ULC. These data, together with the analytical data from other independent researchers (Bekki et al., 2017; Farsalinos et al., 2018a, 2018b; Gasparyan et al., 2018; Ishizaki and Kataoka, 2019; Leigh et al., 2018; Li et al., 2019; Mallock et al., 2018; Salman et al., 2019; Uchiyama et al., 2018), demonstrate that the methods used to quantify known HPHCs are well controlled and generate reliable results.

4.6.2 Comparison of THS with Cigarettes from the US Market

Although comparison of THS emissions with those of the 3R4F reference cigarette is a valid approach for assessing the reductions in HPHCs associated with EHTPs, it is recognized that such reference products are not entirely representative of the range of commercially available products in terms of tobacco blend or added humectants/flavoring (3R4F is an unflavored product). By using the data presented in Tables 4.2–4.5, the levels of the FDA abbreviated list of 18 HPHCs in THS aerosol can be compared with the median levels measured in smoke from cigarette brands commercially available in the US. The data for the commercial cigarettes were provided to PMI by Altria Client Services and included smoke chemistry data for the 31 brands shown in Table 4.9.

For the commercial cigarette brands, the yields of different constituents were measured by two different laboratories. In order to account for any potential interlaboratory difference, which might have led to systematic differences in reported yields, the yields were normalized to the laboratory-specific 3R4F research cigarette results prior to comparison. For the baseline comparator, the median of the mean yield for each of the 31 cigarette brands was calculated on a per-item basis (referred to as "US market map median"). The THS results were also normalized in relation to 3R4F values determined in parallel, in order to minimize

TABLE 4.6
FDA 93 List of HPHCs Determined for Regular THS Tobacco Sticks and 3R4F Cigarettes and Percent Reductions Versus 3R4F Calculated on a Per-Item Basis.

FDA 93 HPHCs (Alphabetical Order)	Unit	3R4F			THS REGULAR			Reduction Relative to 3R4F (%)[a]
		Mean	SD	n	Mean	SD	n	
Acetaldehyde	µg/item	1713	123	3	197	15.6	3	88.5
Acetamide	µg/item	12.3	0.354	3	3.28	0.116	3	73.3
Acetone	µg/item	697	47.8	3	31.5	4.92	3	95.5
Acrolein	µg/item	177	15.5	3	9.20	0.865	3	94.8
Acrylamide	µg/item	4.33	0.262	3	1.64	0.084	3	62.1
Acrylonitrile	µg/item	22.5	1.73	3	<0.107 (LOQ)	NA	3	>99.5
4-Aminobiphenyl	ng/item	2.81	0.238	3	0.008	0.0006	3	99.7
1-Aminonaphthalene	ng/item	18.4	0.423	3	<0.027 (LOQ)	NA	3	>99.9
2-Aminonaphthalene	ng/item	11.6	0.230	3	<0.012 (LOQ)	NA	3	>99.9
A-α-C (2-Amino-9*H*-pyrido [2,3-*b*]indole)	ng/item	206	4.82	3	1.49	0.244	3	99.3
Ammonia	µg/item	31.7	1.13	3	13.14	0.846	3	58.6
Anabasine	µg/item	1.15	0.143	3	0.952	0.040	3	16.9
o-Anisidine	ng/item	5.20	0.451	3	0.124	0.003	3	97.6
Arsenic	ng/item	8.23	0.180	3	<1.20 (LOQ)	NA	3	>85.4
Benz[*a*]anthracene	ng/item	31.6	2.27	3	2.75	0.353	3	91.3
Benz[*j*]aceanthrylene	ng/item	1.15	0.206	3	<0.104 (LOD)	NA	3	>90.9
Benzene	µg/item	83.1	3.02	3	0.483	0.023	3	99.4
Benzo[*a*]pyrene	ng/item	15.6	0.946	3	1.12	0.174	3	92.8
Benzo[*b*]fluoranthene	ng/item	13.9	0.816	3	1.20	0.133	3	91.4
Benzo[*b*]furan	µg/item	0.592	0.0243	3	0.027	0.003	3	95.4
Benzo[*c*]phenanthrene	ng/item	7.96	2.295	3	1.29	0.132	3	83.8
Benzo[*k*]fluoranthene	ng/item	4.86	0.379	3	0.607	0.061	3	87.5
Beryllium	pg/item	<11.9 (LOQ)	NA	3	<11.9 (LOQ)	NA	3	NA
1,3-Butadiene	µg/item	93.0	5.55	3	0.230	0.009	3	99.8
Cadmium	ng/item	99.4	4.84	3	<0.09 (LOD)	NA	3	>99.9
Caffeic acid	µg/item	<1.19 (LOD)	NA	3	<0.478 (LOD)	NA	3	NA
Carbon monoxide (CO)	mg/item	30.6	1.83	3	<0.067 (LOD)	NA	3	>99.8
Catechol	µg/item	98.1	7.34	3	12.9	0.941	3	86.8

Continued

TABLE 4.6
FDA 93 List of HPHCs Determined for Regular THS Tobacco Sticks and 3R4F Cigarettes and Percent Reductions Versus 3R4F Calculated on a Per-Item Basis.—cont'd

FDA 93 HPHCs (Alphabetical Order)	Unit	3R4F			THS REGULAR			Reduction Relative to 3R4F (%)[a]
		Mean	SD	n	Mean	SD	n	
CHLORINATED DIOXINS/FURANS								
2,3,7,8-Tetra CDD	pg/item	<3.9 (LOD)	NA	3	<3.7 (LOD)	NA	3	NA
1,2,3,7,8-Penta CDD	pg/item	<4.0 (LOD)	NA	3	<3.5 (LOD)	NA	3	NA
1,2,3,4,7,8-Hexa CDD	pg/item	<3.7 (LOD)	NA	3	<3.7 (LOD)	NA	3	NA
1,2,3,6,7,8-Hexa CDD	pg/item	<3.7 (LOD)	NA	3	<3.8 (LOD)	NA	3	NA
1,2,3,7,8,9-Hexa CDD	pg/item	<3.3 (LOD)	NA	3	<3.4 (LOD)	NA	3	NA
1,2,3,4,6,7,8-Hepta CDD	pg/item	<3.5 (LOD)	NA	3	<3.4 (LOD)	NA	3	NA
Octa CDD	pg/item	<200 (LOQ)	NA	3	<7.2 (LOD)	NA	3	NA
2,3,7,8-Tetra CDF	pg/item	<3.8 (LOD)	NA	3	<2.9 (LOD)	NA	3	NA
1,2,3,7,8-Penta CDF	pg/item	<3.8 (LOD)	NA	3	<3.5 (LOD)	NA	3	NA
2,3,4,7,8-Penta CDF	pg/item	<4.0 (LOD)	NA	3	<3.5 (LOD)	NA	3	NA
1,2,3,4,7,8-Hexa CDF	pg/item	<2.2 (LOD)	NA	3	<2.4 (LOD)	NA	3	NA
1,2,3,6,7,8-Hexa CDF	pg/item	<2.1 (LOD)	NA	3	<2.3 (LOD)	NA	3	NA
2,3,4,6,7,8-Hexa CDF	pg/item	<2.4 (LOD)	NA	3	<2.6 (LOD)	NA	3	NA
1,2,3,7,8,9-Hexa CDF	pg/item	<2.6 (LOD)	NA	3	<2.9 (LOD)	NA	3	NA
1,2,3,4,6,7,8-Hepta CDF	pg/item	<2.5 (LOD)	NA	3	<2.7 (LOD)	NA	3	NA
1,2,3,4,7,8,9-Hepta CDF	pg/item	<3.3 (LOD)	NA	3	<3.6 (LOD)	NA	3	NA
Octa CDF	pg/item	<4.4 (LOD)	NA	3	<5.4 (LOD)	NA	3	NA
Chromium	ng/item	<11.9 (LOD)	NA	3	<11.0 (LOQ)	NA	3	NA
Chrysene	ng/item	40.7	2.78	3	3.86	0.396	3	90.5
Cobalt	ng/item	<3.69 (LOD)	NA	3	<3.69 (LOD)	NA	3	NA
m-Cresol	µg/item	3.34	0.448	3	0.033	0.004	3	99.0

TABLE 4.6
FDA 93 List of HPHCs Determined for Regular THS Tobacco Sticks and 3R4F Cigarettes and Percent Reductions Versus 3R4F Calculated on a Per-Item Basis.—cont'd

FDA 93 HPHCs (Alphabetical Order)	Unit	3R4F			THS REGULAR			Reduction Relative to 3R4F (%)[a]
		Mean	SD	n	Mean	SD	n	
o-Cresol	µg/item	3.76	0.144	3	0.041	0.007	3	98.9
p-Cresol	µg/item	6.56	0.679	3	<0.034 (LOQ)	NA	3	>99.5
Crotonaldehyde	µg/item	55.2	4.40	3	<3.29 (LOQ)	NA	3	>94.0
Cyclopenta[c,d]pyrene	ng/item	6.00	0.392	3	1.96	0.260	3	67.3
Dibenz[a,h]anthracene	ng/item	0.797	0.102	3	<0.124 (LOD)	NA	3	>84.4
Dibenzo[a,e]pyrene	ng/item	<0.696 (LOQ)	NA	3	<0.125 (LOD)	NA	3	NA
Dibenzo[a,h]pyrene	ng/item	<0.236 (LOD)	NA	3	<0.141 (LOD)	NA	3	NA
Dibenzo[a,i]pyrene	ng/item	1.46	0.029	3	<0.132 (LOD)	NA	3	>91.0
Dibenzo[a,l]pyrene	ng/item	<0.423 (LOD)	NA	3	<0.254 (LOD)	NA	3	NA
2,6-Dimethylaniline	ng/item	8.01	0.417	3	0.316	0.019	3	96.1
Ethyl carbamate (urethane)	ng/item	<6.43 (LOD)	NA	3	<1.93 (LOD)	NA	3	NA
Ethylbenzene	µg/item	14.8	0.638	3	0.132	0.001	3	99.1
Ethylene oxide	µg/item	21.2	2.11	3	0.198	0.021	3	99.1
Formaldehyde	µg/item	70.2	6.17	3	7.10	0.607	3	89.9
Furan	µg/item	58.3	2.93	3	4.43	0.390	3	92.4
Glu-P-1 (2-Amino-6-methyldipyrido[1,2-a:3′,2′-d]imidazole)	ng/item	<0.239 (LOD)	NA	3	<0.095 (LOD)	NA	3	NA
Glu-P-2 (2-aminodipyrido[1,2-a:3′,2′-d]imidazole)	ng/item	<0.301 (LOD)	NA	3	<0.120 (LOD)	NA	3	NA
Hydrazine	ng/item	<6.79 (LOD)	NA	3	<2.04 (LOD)	NA	3	NA
Hydrogen cyanide	µg/item	433	5.50	3	2.06	0.040	3	99.5
Indeno[1,2,3-cd]pyrene	ng/item	5.36	0.196	3	<0.337 (LOQ)	NA	3	>93.7
IQ (2-Amino-3-methylimidazo[4,5-f]quinoline)	ng/item	6.73	0.757	3	<0.64 (LOD)	NA	3	>90.5
Isoprene	µg/item	812	11.8	3	1.33	0.077	3	99.8
Lead	ng/item	<25.7 (LOQ)	NA	3	<1.62 (LOQ)	NA	3	NA
MeA-α-C (2-Amino-3-methyl)-9H-pyrido[2,3-b]indole)	ng/item	26.6	0.872	3	<0.385 (LOQ)	NA	3	>98.6
Mercury	ng/item	4.36	0.360	3	2.11	0.071	3	51.6

Continued

TABLE 4.6
FDA 93 List of HPHCs Determined for Regular THS Tobacco Sticks and 3R4F Cigarettes and Percent Reductions Versus 3R4F Calculated on a Per-Item Basis.—cont'd

FDA 93 HPHCs (Alphabetical Order)	Unit	3R4F			THS REGULAR			Reduction Relative to 3R4F (%)[a]
		Mean	SD	n	Mean	SD	n	
5-Methylchrysene	ng/item	1.32	0.034	3	<0.094 (LOQ)	NA	3	>92.9
Methyl-ethyl-ketone (MEK)	µg/item	184	14.0	3	7.08	0.656	3	96.2
Naphthalene	ng/item	1197	83.1	3	7.34	1.18	3	99.4
Nickel	ng/item	<43.1 (LOQ)	NA	3	<15.9 (LOD)	NA	3	NA
Nicotine	mg/item	1.87	0.09	3	1.23	0.06	3	34.2
Nitrobenzene	µg/item	<0.038 (LOD)	NA	3	<0.011 (LOD)	NA	3	NA
Nitromethane	ng/item	809	85.6	3	51.2	3.43	3	93.7
2-Nitropropane	ng/item	36.5	6.69	3	8.40	0.553	3	77.0
N-Nitrosodiethanolamine (NDELA)	ng/item	<0.085 (LOD)	NA	3	<0.042 (LOD)	NA	3	NA
N-Nitrosodiethylamine (NDEA)	ng/item	<0.617 (LOD)	NA	3	<0.308 (LOD)	NA	3	NA
N-Nitrosodimethylamine (NDMA)	ng/item	6.43	0.219	3	2.79	0.209	3	56.6
N-Nitrosomethylethylamine (NEMA)	ng/item	<0.509 (LOD)	NA	3	<0.254 (LOD)	NA	3	NA
N-Nitrosomorpholine (NMOR)	ng/item	<0.550 (LOD)	NA	3	<0.275 (LOD)	NA	3	NA
4-(Methylnitrosamino)-1-(3-pyridyl)-1-butanone (NNK)	ng/item	232	7.31	3	9.00	0.485	3	96.1
N-Nitrosonornicotine (NNN)	ng/item	277	39.7	3	15.2	1.55	3	94.5
N-Nitrosopiperidine (NPIP)	ng/item	<0.172 (LOD)	NA	3	<0.086 (LOD)	NA	3	NA
N-Nitrosopyrrolidine (NPYR)	ng/item	36.8	6.41	3	<0.198 (LOD)	NA	3	>99.5
Nornicotine	µg/item	14.5	1.13	3	0.604	0.065	3	95.8
Phenol	µg/item	14.4	0.777	3	0.941	0.134	3	93.5
PhIP (2-Amino-1-methyl-6-phenylimidazo[4,5-b] pyridine)	ng/item	<0.365 (LOD)	NA	3	<0.486 (LOQ)	NA	3	NA
Polonium-210[b]	Bq/item	0.0062	0.0032	3	<0.005 (LOD)	NA	3	NA
Propionaldehyde	µg/item	125	8.97	3	12.2	1.16	3	90.2
Propylene oxide	ng/item	930	118	3	159	15.5	3	82.9
Quinoline	µg/item	0.409	0.019	3	<0.011 (LOQ)	NA	3	>97.3
Selenium	ng/item	<4.42 (LOD)	NA	3	<0.830 (LOQ)	NA	3	NA

TABLE 4.6
FDA 93 List of HPHCs Determined for Regular THS Tobacco Sticks and 3R4F Cigarettes and Percent Reductions Versus 3R4F Calculated on a Per-Item Basis.—cont'd

FDA 93 HPHCs (Alphabetical Order)	Unit	3R4F			THS REGULAR			Reduction Relative to 3R4F (%)[a]
		Mean	SD	n	Mean	SD	n	
Styrene	µg/item	13.0	1.53	3	0.328	0.036	3	97.5
Toluene	µg/item	143	6.74	3	1.40	0.054	3	99.0
o-Toluidine	ng/item	105	7.39	3	1.08	0.050	3	99.0
Trp-P-1 (3-Amino-1,4-dimethyl-5H-pyrido[4,3-b]indole)	ng/item	5.20	0.872	3	<0.098 (LOD)	NA	3	>98.1
Trp-P-2 (1-Methyl-3-amino-5H-pyrido[4,3-b]indole)	ng/item	6.37	0.751	3	<0.113 (LOD)	NA	3	>98.2
Uranium-235	Bq/item	<0.005 (LOD)	NA	3	<0.005 (LOD)	NA	3	NA
Uranium-238	Bq/item	<0.005 (LOD)	NA	3	<0.005 (LOD)	NA	3	NA
Vinyl acetate	ng/item	646	44.3	3	60.1	1.09	3	90.7
Vinyl chloride	ng/item	128	8.10	3	<0.657 (LOD)	NA	3	>99.5

LOD, limit of detection, LOQ, limit of quantification; n, number of items; NA, not available; SD, standard deviation.
[a] When HPHC values for both THS and 3R4F were below LOD or LOQ, no reduction could be calculated. For HPHC values found below LOD or LOQ for THS, with a corresponding value for 3R4F above the LOQ, the % reduction was calculated by using the LOD/LOQ value.
[b] Polonium-210 was not included in the average reduction calculation, as its presence is expressed in terms of Bq (becquerel, a unit of radioactivity) and not as a concentration (mass/stick). It is worth noting that the value determined for THS Regular was below the LOD. The same logic was applied for the mentholated product.

any interlaboratory and/or long-term analytical variability. The percent reductions in HPHC emissions for THS versus the US market map median was then calculated on a per-item basis and relative to nicotine delivery. The results are presented in Tables 4.10 and 4.11.

The percent reductions in HPHC levels determined for THS relative to the levels for the representative US commercial cigarettes, in terms of pattern and magnitude, were similar to those observed when comparing THS and 3R4F emissions. Overall, compared with the US market map cigarettes, the average reduction in 18 HPHCs from the FDA abbreviated list for THS was >94% on a per-item basis and >91% relative to nicotine delivery for the regular tobacco stick variant and >94% on a per-item basis and >91% relative to nicotine delivery for the mentholated tobacco stick variant. It is worth noting that the presence of menthol had no impact on the performance of the tobacco sticks, as similar levels of reduction in HPHCs for both the regular and mentholated variants, relative to 3R4F, were observed.

4.7 PRODUCT ROBUSTNESS
4.7.1 Influence of Smoking Regimen on Product Performance

The two most frequently employed smoking machine regimens for assessment of cigarette emissions are the ISO (ISO 3308) (ISO, 2012) and HCI (Health Canada, 1999), now ISO intense (ISO 20778) (ISO, 2018b), regimens. The ISO testing regimen (ISO 3308) (ISO, 2012) mandates a puff volume of 35 mL, a puff duration of 2 s, one puff per min frequency, and a bell-shaped puff profile. The HCI regimen prescribes a puff volume of 55 mL, a puff duration of 2 s, two puffs per min frequency, a bell-shaped puff profile, and an additional requirement that any ventilation holes present in the cigarettes are blocked. This is also the smoking regimen applied for assessment of EHTPs at PMI. The HCI smoking regimen was not developed to represent smoking behavior in humans, but was designed to generate emissions under a more intensive set of smoking parameters that would provide a "maximum" exposure limit that could be exceeded by very few smokers, thereby

TABLE 4.7
FDA 93 List of HPHCs Determined for Mentholated THS Tobacco Sticks and 3R4F Cigarettes and Percent Reductions Versus 3R4F Calculated on a Per-Item Basis.

FDA 93 HPHCs (Alphabetical Order)	Unit	3R4F			THS SMOOTH MENTHOL			Reduction Relative to 3R4F (%)[a]
		Mean	SD	N	Mean	SD	n	
Acetaldehyde	µg/item	1713	123	3	199	13.5	3	88.4
Acetamide	µg/item	12.3	0.354	3	3.21	0.067	3	73.9
Acetone	µg/item	697	47.8	3	32.5	3.02	3	95.3
Acrolein	µg/item	177	15.5	3	9.36	0.946	3	94.7
Acrylamide	µg/item	4.33	0.262	3	1.80	0.041	3	58.5
Acrylonitrile	µg/item	22.5	1.73	3	0.112	0.039	3	99.5
4-Aminobiphenyl	ng/item	2.81	0.238	3	0.010	0.001	3	99.6
1-Aminonaphthalene	ng/item	18.4	0.423	3	<0.027 (LOQ)	NA	3	>99.9
2-Aminonaphthalene	ng/item	11.6	0.230	3	<0.012 (LOQ)	NA	3	>99.9
A-α-C (2-Amino-9*H*-pyrido [2,3-*b*]indole)	ng/item	206	4.82	3	1.65	0.361	3	99.2
Ammonia	µg/item	31.7	1.13	3	13.4	0.780	3	57.9
Anabasine	µg/item	1.15	0.143	3	1.01	0.103	3	12.3
o-Anisidine	ng/item	5.20	0.451	3	0.131	0.010	3	97.5
Arsenic	ng/item	8.23	0.180	3	<1.20 (LOQ)	NA	3	>85.4
Benz[a]anthracene	ng/item	31.6	2.27	3	2.01	0.242	3	93.6
Benz[j]aceanthrylene	ng/item	1.15	0.206	3	<0.104 (LOD)	NA	3	>90.9
Benzene	µg/item	83.1	3.02	3	0.561	0.072	3	99.3
Benzo[a]pyrene	ng/item	15.6	0.946	3	0.740	0.065	3	95.2
Benzo[b]fluoranthene	ng/item	13.9	0.816	3	0.840	0.127	3	94.0
Benzo[b]furan	µg/item	0.592	0.0243	3	0.030	0.004	3	95.0
Benzo[c]phenanthrene	ng/item	7.96	2.295	3	0.860	0.051	3	89.2
Benzo[k]fluoranthene	ng/item	4.86	0.379	3	<0.395 (LOQ)	NA	3	>91.9
Beryllium	pg/item	<11.9 (LOQ)	NA	3	<11.9 (LOQ)	NA	3	NA
1,3-Butadiene	µg/item	93.0	5.55	3	0.273	0.028	3	99.7
Cadmium	ng/item	99.4	4.84	3	<0.28 (LOQ)	NA	3	>99.7
Caffeic acid	µg/item	<1.19 (LOD)	NA	3	<0.478 (LOD)	NA	3	NA
Carbon monoxide (CO)	mg/item	30.6	1.83	3	<0.067 (LOD)	NA	3	>99.8
Catechol	µg/item	98.1	7.34	3	12.7	0.949	3	87.1

CHLORINATED DIOXINS/FURANS

2,3,7,8-Tetra CDD	pg/item	<3.9 (LOD)	NA	3	<3.8 (LOD)	NA	3	NA
1,2,3,7,8-Penta CDD	pg/item	<4.0 (LOD)	NA	3	<3.9 (LOD)	NA	3	NA
1,2,3,4,7,8-Hexa CDD	pg/item	<3.7 (LOD)	NA	3	<3.2 (LOD)	NA	3	NA
1,2,3,6,7,8-Hexa CDD	pg/item	<3.7 (LOD)	NA	3	<3.1 (LOD)	NA	3	NA
1,2,3,7,8,9-Hexa CDD	pg/item	<3.3 (LOD)	NA	3	<2.8 (LOD)	NA	3	NA
1,2,3,4,6,7,8-Hepta CDD	pg/item	<3.5 (LOD)	NA	3	<20 (LOQ)	NA	3	NA
Octa CDD	pg/item	<200 (LOQ)	NA	3	<200 (LOQ)	NA	3	NA
2,3,7,8-Tetra CDF	pg/item	<3.8 (LOD)	NA	3	<3.1 (LOD)	NA	3	NA
1,2,3,7,8-Penta CDF	pg/item	<3.8 (LOD)	NA	3	<3.3 (LOD)	NA	3	NA
2,3,4,7,8-Penta CDF	pg/item	<4.0 (LOD)	NA	3	<3.2 (LOD)	NA	3	NA
1,2,3,4,7,8-Hexa CDF	pg/item	<2.2 (LOD)	NA	3	<2.8 (LOD)	NA	3	NA
1,2,3,6,7,8-Hexa CDF	pg/item	<2.1 (LOD)	NA	3	<2.7 (LOD)	NA	3	NA
2,3,4,6,7,8-Hexa CDF	pg/item	<2.4 (LOD)	NA	3	<20 (LOQ)	NA	3	NA
1,2,3,7,8,9-Hexa CDF	pg/item	<2.6 (LOD)	NA	3	<20 (LOQ)	NA	3	NA
1,2,3,4,6,7,8-Hepta CDF	pg/item	<2.5 (LOD)	NA	3	<20 (LOQ)	NA	3	NA
1,2,3,4,7,8,9-Hepta CDF	pg/item	<3.3 (LOD)	NA	3	<20 (LOQ)	NA	3	NA
Octa CDF	pg/item	<4.4 (LOD)	NA	3	<200 (LOQ)	NA	3	NA
Chromium	ng/item	<11.9 (LOD)	NA	3	<11.0 (LOQ)	NA	3	NA
Chrysene	ng/item	40.7	2.78	3	2.93	0.319	3	92.8
Cobalt	ng/item	<3.69 (LOD)	NA	3	<3.69 (LOD)	NA	3	NA
m-Cresol	µg/item	3.34	0.448	3	0.030	0.006	3	99.1
o-Cresol	µg/item	3.76	0.144	3	0.042	0.009	3	98.9
p-Cresol	µg/item	6.56	0.679	3	0.040	0.003	3	99.4
Crotonaldehyde	µg/item	55.2	4.40	3	<3.29 (LOQ)	NA	3	>94.0
Cyclopenta[c,d]pyrene	ng/item	6.00	0.392	3	1.12	0.149	3	81.3
Dibenz[a,h]anthracene	ng/item	0.797	0.102	3		NA	3	>84.4

Continued

TABLE 4.7
FDA 93 List of HPHCs Determined for Mentholated THS Tobacco Sticks and 3R4F Cigarettes and Percent Reductions Versus 3R4F Calculated on a Per-Item Basis.—cont'd

FDA 93 HPHCs (Alphabetical Order)	Unit	3R4F			THS SMOOTH MENTHOL			Reduction Relative to 3R4F (%)[a]
		Mean	SD	N	Mean	SD	n	
					<0.124 (LOD)			
Dibenzo[a,e]pyrene	ng/item	<0.696 (LOQ)	NA	3	<0.125 (LOD)	NA	3	NA
Dibenzo[a,h]pyrene	ng/item	<0.236 (LOD)	NA	3	<0.141 (LOD)	NA	3	NA
Dibenzo[a,i]pyrene	ng/item	1.46	0.029	3	<0.132 (LOD)	NA	3	>91.0
Dibenzo[a,l]pyrene	ng/item	<0.423 (LOD)	NA	3	<0.254 (LOD)	NA	3	NA
2,6-Dimethylaniline	ng/item	8.01	0.417	3	0.270	0.024	3	96.6
Ethyl carbamate (urethane)	ng/item	<6.43 (LOD)	NA	3	<1.93 (LOD)	NA	3	NA
Ethylbenzene	µg/item	14.8	0.638	3	0.151	0.017	3	99.0
Ethylene oxide	µg/item	21.2	2.11	3	0.234	0.068	3	98.9
Formaldehyde	µg/item	70.2	6.17	3	7.68	1.23	3	89.1
Furan	µg/item	58.3	2.93	3	4.49	0.437	3	92.3
Glu-P-1 (2-Amino-6-methyldipyrido[1,2-a:3',2'-d]imidazole)	ng/item	<0.239 (LOD)	NA	3	<0.095 (LOD)	NA	3	NA
Glu-P-2 (2-aminodipyrido[1,2-a:3',2'-d]imidazole)	ng/item	<0.301 (LOD)	NA	3	<0.120 (LOD)	NA	3	NA
Hydrazine	ng/item	<6.79 (LOD)	NA	3	<2.04 (LOD)	NA	3	NA
Hydrogen cyanide	µg/item	433	5.50	3	2.17	0.200	3	99.5
Indeno[1,2,3-cd]pyrene	ng/item	5.36	0.196	3	<0.337 (LOQ)	NA	3	>93.7
IQ (2-Amino-3-methylimidazo[4,5-f]quinoline)	ng/item	6.73	0.757	3	<0.640 (LOD)	NA	3	>90.5
Isoprene	µg/item	812	11.8	3	1.62	0.187	3	99.8
Lead	ng/item	<25.7 (LOQ)	NA	3	<0.490 (LOD)	NA	3	NA
MeA-α-C (2-Amino-3-methyl)-9H-pyrido[2,3-b]indole)	ng/item	26.6	0.872	3	<0.115 (LOD)	NA	3	>99.6
Mercury	ng/item	4.36	0.360	3	1.88	0.190	3	56.8
5-Methylchrysene	ng/item	1.32	0.034	3	<0.094 (LOQ)	NA	3	>92.9
Methyl-ethyl-ketone (MEK)	µg/item	184	14.0	3	7.10	0.710	3	96.1
Naphthalene	ng/item	1197	83.1	3	5.94	0.900	3	99.5

Nickel	ng/item	<43.1 (LOQ)	NA	3	<15.9 (LOD)	NA	3	NA
Nicotine	mg/item	1.87	0.09	3	1.23	0.13	3	34.2
Nitrobenzene	µg/item	<0.038 (LOD)	NA	3	<0.011 (LOD)	NA	3	NA
Nitromethane	ng/item	809	85.6	3	44.3	2.00	3	94.5
2-Nitropropane	ng/item	36.5	6.69	3	6.00	0.261	3	83.6
N-Nitrosodiethanolamine (NDELA)	ng/item	<0.085 (LOD)	NA	3	<0.042 (LOD)	NA	3	NA
N-Nitrosodiethylamine (NDEA)	ng/item	<0.617 (LOD)	NA	3	<0.308 (LOD)	NA	3	NA
N-Nitrosodimethylamine (NDMA)	ng/item	6.43	0.219	3	3.38	0.088	3	47.5
N-Nitrosomethylethylamine (NEMA)	ng/item	<0.509 (LOD)	NA	3	<0.254 (LOD)	NA	3	NA
N-Nitrosomorpholine (NMOR)	ng/item	<0.550 (LOD)	NA	3	<0.275 (LOD)	NA	3	NA
4-(Methylnitrosamino)-1-(3-pyridyl)-1-butanone (NNK)	ng/item	232	7.31	3	6.92	0.902	3	97.0
N-Nitrosonornicotine (NNN)	ng/item	277	39.7	3	9.50	1.62	3	96.6
N-Nitrosopiperidine (NPIP)	ng/item	<0.172 (LOD)	NA	3	<0.086 (LOD)	NA	3	NA
N-Nitrosopyrrolidine (NPYR)	ng/item	36.8	6.41	3	<0.198 (LOD)	NA	3	>99.5
Nornicotine	µg/item	14.5	1.134	3	0.521	0.012	3	96.4
Phenol	µg/item	14.4	0.777	3	0.812	0.088	3	94.4
PhIP (2-Amino-1-methyl-6-phenylimidazo[4,5-b] pyridine)	ng/item	<0.365 (LOD)	NA	3	<0.486 (LOQ)	NA	3	NA
Polonium-210[b]	Bq/item	0.0062	0.0032	3	<0.005 (LOD)	NA	3	NA
Propionaldehyde	µg/item	125	8.97	3	12.4	0.930	3	90.0
Propylene oxide	ng/item	930	118	3	158	25.1	3	83.0
Quinoline	µg/item	0.409	0.019	3	<0.011 (LOQ)	NA	3	>97.3
Selenium	ng/item	<4.42 (LOD)	NA	3	<0.830 (LOQ)	NA	3	NA
Styrene	µg/item	13.0	1.53	3	0.336	0.013	3	97.4
Toluene	µg/item	143	6.74	3	1.65	0.227	3	98.8
o-Toluidine	ng/item	105	7.39	3	1.08	0.089	3	99.0
Trp-P-1 (3-Amino-1,4-dimethyl-5H-pyrido[4,3-b]indole)	ng/item	5.20	0.872	3	<0.098 (LOD)	NA	3	>98.1
Trp-P-2 (1-Methyl-3-amino-5H-pyrido[4,3-b]indole)	ng/item	6.37	0.751	3	<0.113 (LOD)	NA	3	>98.2
Uranium-235	Bq/item	<0.005 (LOD)	NA	3	<0.005 (LOD)	NA	3	NA

Continued

TABLE 4.7
FDA 93 List of HPHCs Determined for Mentholated THS Tobacco Sticks and 3R4F Cigarettes and Percent Reductions Versus 3R4F Calculated on a Per-Item Basis.—cont'd

FDA 93 HPHCs (Alphabetical Order)	Unit	3R4F			THS SMOOTH MENTHOL			Reduction Relative to 3R4F (%)[a]
		Mean	SD	N	Mean	SD	n	
Uranium-238	Bq/item	<0.005 (LOD)	NA	3	<0.005 (LOD)	NA	3	NA
Vinyl acetate	ng/item	646	44.3	3	66.4	5.69	3	89.7
Vinyl chloride	ng/item	128	8.10	3	<0.657 (LOD)	NA	3	>99.5

[a,b] See legend to Table 4.6. *LOD*, limit of detection, *LOQ*, limit of quantification, *n*, number of items; *NA*, not available; *SD*, standard deviation.

TABLE 4.8
Comparison of Research Results for Regular THS Tobacco Sticks Across the Aerosol Constituents on the PMI 58 List.

PMI 58 HPHCs (Alphabetical Order)	Unit	MRTPA[a]	Schaller et al.[b]	FDA 93[c]	Forster et al.[d]	3R4F[e]
		Mean (SD)	Mean (SD)	Mean (SD)	Mean (SD)	Mean (SD)
1-Aminonaphthalene	ng/item	0.0427 (0.00513)	0.063 (0.003)	<0.027 (LOQ)	0.030 (0.013)	19.1 (1.5)
2-Aminonaphthalene	ng/item	0.0223 (0.00321)	<0.035 (LOQ)	<0.012 (LOQ)	0.016 (0.008)	14.4 (2.2)
3-Aminobiphenyl	ng/item	0.007 (0.003)	<0.013 (LOQ)	NA	0.005 (0.002)	3.96 (0.52)
4-Aminobiphenyl	ng/item	0.0087 (0.0012)	<0.021 (LOQ)	0.008 (0.0006)	<0.005 (LOQ)	2.83 (0.44)
Acetaldehyde	µg/item	192 (11.6)	213 (10)	197 (15.6)	327 (20)	1836 (295)
Acetamide	µg/item	2.96 (0.134)	4.13 (0.11)	3.28 (0.116)	3.07 (0.29)	12.8 (1.1)
Acetone	µg/item	30.7 (1.86)	33.8 (3.3)	31.5 (4.92)	30.2 (3.0)	686 (41)
Acrolein	µg/item	8.32 (0.755)	9.44 (0.44)	9.20 (0.865)	9.98 (1.13)	171 (20)
Acrylamide	µg/item	1.58 (0.0543)	2.27 (0.14)	1.64 (0.084)	1.35 (0.14)	4.53 (0.58)
Acrylonitrile	µg/item	0.145 (0.0112)	0.186 (0.014)	<0.107 (LOQ)	<0.107 (LOQ)	23.6 (5.0)
Ammonia	µg/item	12.2 (0.973)	15.6 (0.6)	13.14 (0.846)	10.6 (0.7)	34.1 (3.7)
Arsenic	ng/item	<0.36 (LOD)	<1.13 (LOQ)	<1.20 (LOQ)	0.822 (0.08)	6.62 (1.86)
Benz[a]anthracene	ng/item	2.65 (0.0647)	2.58 (0.09)	2.75 (0.353)	1.54 (0.04)	27.0 (3.1)
Benzene	µg/item	0.452 (0.0395)	0.575 (0.037)	0.483 (0.023)	0.457 (0.029)	84.9 (10.0)
Benzo[a]pyrene	ng/item	0.736 (0.0973)	1.19 (0.04)	1.12 (0.174)	0.582 (0.024)	13.6 (1.3)
1,3-Butadiene	µg/item	0.207 (0.016)	0.319 (0.037)	0.230 (0.009)	0.224 (0.016)	96.9 (8.8)

Butyraldehyde	µg/item	20.7 (1.52)	25.3 (1.4)	NA	1.20 (0.13)	59.7 (43.4)
Cadmium	ng/item	<0.28 (LOQ)	<0.350 (LOQ)	<0.09 (LOD)	<0.162 (LOD)	104 (13)
Carbon monoxide (CO)	mg/item	0.347 (0.0462)	0.598 (0.037)	<0.067 (LOD)	0.305 (0.017)	30.9 (1.5)
Catechol	µg/item	14.0 (0.522)	16.4 (0.3)	12.9 (0.941)	13.0 (0.2)	90.0 (6.4)
Chromium	ng/item	<11.0 (LOQ)	<0.170 (LOQ)	<11.0 (LOQ)	4.57 (0.71)	<LOQ
m-Cresol	µg/item	0.0424 (0.0045)	0.042 (0.003)	0.033 (0.004)	0.029 (0.002)	3.70 (0.42)
o-Cresol	µg/item	0.0779 (0.0093)	0.105 (0.009)	0.041 (0.007)	0.063 (0.004)	4.33 (0.51)
p-Cresol	µg/item	0.0706 (0.00816)	0.073 (0.005)	<0.034 (LOQ)	0.060 (0.005)	8.51 (1.18)
Crotonaldehyde	µg/item	<3.29 (LOQ)	3.75 (0.17)	<3.29 (LOQ)	2.00 (0.40)	60.1 (22.2)
Dibenz[a,h]anthracene	ng/item	<0.124 (LOD)	<1.00 (LOQ)	<0.124 (LOD)	<0.046 (LOD)	0.969 (0.545)
Ethylene oxide	µg/item	<0.119 (LOQ)	0.314 (0.006)	0.198 (0.021)	0.142 (0.020)	22.9 (7.1)
Formaldehyde	µg/item	14.1 (0.430)	5.22 (0.12)	7.10 (0.607)	5.93 (0.87)	64.5 (9.6)
Glycerol	mg/item	5.02 (0.101)	4.1 (0.55)	NA	4.28 (0.08)	2.29 (0.14)
Hydrogen cyanide	µg/item	<1.75 (LOQ)	3.78 (0.22)	2.06 (0.040)	3.21 (0.98)	384 (65)
Hydroquinone	µg/item	6.55 (0.461)	7.86 (0.32)	NA	5.40 (0.10)	87.8 (6.8)
Isoprene	µg/item	1.51 (0.129)	2.44 (0.26)	1.33 (0.077)	1.55 (0.20)	878 (51)
Lead	ng/item	2.23 (0.351)	<3.35 (LOQ)	<1.62 (LOQ)	42.9 (15.3)	25.5 (6.7)
Mercury	ng/item	1.38 (0.163)	1.02 (0.03)	2.11 (0.071)	1.99 (0.12)	4.11 (0.43)
Methyl-ethyl-ketone (MEK)	µg/item	10.1 (0.759)	7.94 (0.38)	7.08 (0.656)	6.80 (0.75)	203 (27)
Nickel	ng/item	<15.9 (LOD)	<0.550 (LOQ)	<15.9 (LOD)	1.22 (0.72)	<LOQ
Nicotine	mg/item	1.29 (0.047)	1.26 (0.12)	1.23 (0.06)	1.16 (0.03)	1.95 (0.143)
Nitric oxide (NO)	µg/item	12.6 (0.418)	21.0 (3.6)	NA	13.2 (1.1)	496 (13)
Nitrobenzene	µg/item	<0.011 (LOD)	0.092 (0.004)	<0.011 (LOD)	<0.011 (LOD)	<LOQ
Nitrogen oxides (NOx)	µg/item	14.2 (0.413)	22.6 (3.9)	NA	14.9 (1.2)	549 (20)
N-Nitrosoanabasine (NAB)	ng/item	2.35 (0.0589)	3.52 (0.24)	NA	3.14 (0.26)	29.0 (4.6)
N-Nitrosoanatabine (NAT)	ng/item	14.7 (1.25)	22.3 (0.8)	NA	21.0 (1.1)	273 (28)
4-(Methylnitrosamino)-1-(3-pyridyl)-1-butanone (NNK)	ng/item	7.80 (0.423)	10.1 (0.2)	9.00 (0.485)	10.6 (0.2)	258 (22)
N-Nitrosonornicotine (NNN)	ng/item	10.1 (0.205)	10.3 (0.2)	15.2 (1.55)	11.5 (0.8)	269 (20)
Phenol	µg/item	1.47 (0.206)	1.51 (0.12)	0.941 (0.134)	1.46 (0.08)	14.3 (1.5)
Propionaldehyde	µg/item	10.8 (0.675)	13.6 (0.8)	12.2 (1.16)	16.7 (1.3)	131 (14)
Propylene oxide	ng/item	142.3 (6.67)	175 (15)	159 (15.5)	134 (5)	1132 (393)

Continued

TABLE 4.8
Comparison of Research Results for Regular THS Tobacco Sticks Across the Aerosol Constituents on the PMI 58 List.—cont'd

PMI 58 HPHCs (Alphabetical Order)	Unit	MRTPA[a] Mean (SD)	Schaller et al.[b] Mean (SD)	FDA 93[c] Mean (SD)	Forster et al.[d] Mean (SD)	3R4F[e] Mean (SD)
Pyrene	ng/item	8.20 (0.152)	7.93 (0.40)	NA	5.88 (0.23)	81.1 (6.5)
Pyridine	µg/item	6.58 (0.185)	9.38 (0.48)	NA	4.05 (0.11)	35.8 (11.5)
Quinoline	µg/item	<0.011 (LOQ)	0.014 (0.001)	<0.011 (LOQ)	<0.011 (LOQ)	0.406 (0.039)
Resorcinol	µg/item	<0.055 (LOQ)	0.055 (0.007)	NA	<0.055 (LOQ)	1.75 (0.27)
Selenium	ng/item	1.27 (0.0577)	<0.550 (LOQ)	<0.830 (LOQ)	<0.219 (LOD)	<LOQ
Styrene	µg/item	0.577 (0.0916)	0.672 (0.032)	0.328 (0.036)	0.356 (0.039)	18.0 (6.8)
Tar (NFDPM)	mg/item	19.4 (1.62)	13.4 (1.4)	NA	22.3 (2.2)	28.6 (2.8)
Toluene	µg/item	1.42 (0.162)	1.61 (0.09)	1.40 (0.054)	1.33 (0.11)	151 (29)
o-Toluidine	ng/item	1.10 (0.0243)	1.204 (0.076)	1.08 (0.050)	0.938 (0.092)	93.1 (9.1)
Vinyl chloride	ng/item	<0.657 (LOD)	<3.47 (LOQ)	<0.657 (LOD)	<0.657 (LOD)	101 (15)
Water	mg/item	30.2 (2.17)	39.4 (2.3)	NA	25.4 (2.0)	14.5 (1.5)

LOD, limit of detection, *LOQ*, limit of quantification, *n*, number of items; *NA*, not available; *SD*, standard deviation.
[a] Analyses performed in support of PMI's Modified Risk Tobacco Product application, submitted to the FDA in November 2016: PMP S.A. Summaries of Research Findings on IQOS and HeatStick Products (.zip—75.4 MB, added May 24, 2017) https://www.fda.gov/tobacco-products/advertising-and-promotion/philip-morris-products-sa-modified-risk-tobacco-product-mrtp-applications#1.
[b] *Data from* Schaller et al. (2016) (Schaller et al., 2016).
[c] Supplementary data submitted to the FDA in support of PMI's Modified Risk Tobacco Product application in September 2018: Submission of an Amended Study Report as part of "P1 Characterization" and an Updated Clinical Study (.zip—376 MB) (added Nov 29, 2018), 93-FDA-HPHCs_THS-R-SM_Report_Release in Full.pdf, https://www.fda.gov/tobacco-products/advertising-and-promotion/philip-morris-products-sa-modified-risk-tobacco-product-mrtp-applications#1.
[d] Data from Forster et al. (2018).
[e] Mean values for 3R4F are overall means (standard deviations) calculated by using values reported for each of the HPHC datasets (<LOQ/<LOD values were treated as ½ LOQ or ½ LOD for calculation purposes, where all values were <LOQ or a combination of <LOQ and <LOD, a value of <LOQ was reported).

minimizing the likelihood that machine emissions would underestimate human exposure. However, it is widely recognized that even such an intensive regimen is not adequately representative of the extreme puffing behaviors exhibited by some smokers.

In order to assess the influence of smoking regimen on the performance of an EHTP, PMI performed a study (Goujon et al., 2020) to investigate the relative reductions in HPHC emissions achieved by THS versus the 3R4F reference cigarette over a range of machine-smoking conditions, including regimens more intense than HCI. In the absence of specific standards or recommendations for robustness testing, the alternative puffing regimens used for generating THS aerosol were selected on the basis of human puffing conditions observed in users (Poget et al., 2017), including a regimen representative of extreme-end usage conditions (110-mL puff volume, 4.5-s puff duration, and 22-s puff interval). The most extreme regimen for generating 3R4F mainstream smoke (80-mL puff volume, 2.4-s puff duration, and 25-s puff interval) was selected to exceed the extreme regimens used in other cigarette studies (CORESTA, 2016; Zenzen et al., 2012).

For this study, Labstat International ULC performed the aerosol generation for THS Regular and 3R4F, in accordance with the machine-smoking regimens described in Table 4.12, and quantified the 54 HPHCs contained in the PMI 58 list of aerosol constituents.

TABLE 4.9
List of the 31 Commercially Available Cigarette Brands Used for Comparison With THS Across the HPHCs on the FDA 18 List.

Basic Blue Pack Box	Marlboro Gold Pack Box	Marlboro Virginia Blend Box
Basic Box	Marlboro Menthol Blue Pack 100's Box	Merit Bronze Pack Box
Basic Gold Pack Box	Marlboro Menthol Blue Pack Box	Merit Gold Pack Box
Basic NonFilter Soft Pack	Marlboro Menthol Box	Parliament Menthol (Green Pack) Box
L&M Turkish Blend Box	Marlboro Menthol Gold Pack Box	Parliament Menthol (White Pack) 100's Box
Marlboro 100's Box	Marlboro Red Label Box	Parliament Menthol Silver Pack Box
Marlboro 72's Silver Pack Box	Marlboro Silver Pack 100's Box	Parliament Silver Pack Box
Marlboro Blend No. 27 Box	Marlboro Silver Pack Box	Virginia Slims 120s Gold Pack Box
Marlboro Box	Marlboro Skyline Box	Virginia Slims Silver Pack Box
Marlboro Craft Blend Reserve Box	Marlboro Special Blend (Gold Pack) 100's Box	Virginia Slims Superslims Box
Marlboro Gold Pack 100's Box		

For each regimen applied to 3R4F reference cigarettes (L, N, and H, described in Table 4.12) the use of both 50% and 100% ventilation occlusion was investigated. Standard ISO conditions (ISO 3308) were not represented (regimen L without ventilation blocking). However, an equivalent puffing regimen was employed with ventilation blocking, and HCI conditions were represented by regimen N with 100% ventilation blocking. The tobacco sticks used with THS do not have filter ventilation, and, therefore, ventilation blocking was not required/possible.

HPHC aerosol/smoke concentrations were calculated in terms of mass per item (tobacco stick/cigarette) and normalized with respect to nicotine delivery, which is commonly applied to estimate the level of toxicant exposure in cigarette smokers (Djordjevic et al., 2000; WHO, 2015). As a comparative approach, the data were also normalized in accordance with the total puff volume generated for each product, constituent, regimen, and replicate. Total puff volume was calculated as the product of the number of puffs and puff volume applied for each smoking regimen. The average number of puffs required to reach a predefined butt length for all items, per replicate, was used for the 3R4F cigarette, and the number of puffs predefined by the regimen was used for THS. Normalization in accordance with total puff volume is an approach that could be considered for comparison of performance for products that do not contain nicotine.

The reduction in HPHC concentrations observed for THS Regular aerosol relative to 3R4F was calculated as a percentage of the concentration in 3R4F cigarette mainstream smoke. Fig. 4.3 summarizes the average HPHC reductions calculated for each regimen combination, normalized on a nicotine basis, where the values ranged between 82.5% and 89.3%. Fig. 4.4 presents the average HPHC reductions calculated for each regimen combination by using absolute concentrations, where the values ranged between 88.1% and 95.9%. For the HCI regimen, the average reduction in absolute HPHC concentrations for THS aerosol relative to 3R4F cigarette smoke was 93.6%. This was in line with previously published results (Smith et al., 2016), where the majority of HPHCs measured in THS aerosol were reduced by more than 90%. For machine-smoking parameters that were more intense than the HCI regimen, the average HPHC reductions for THS relative to 3R4F were in the range of 93.1%–95.9%, regardless of the smoking regimen applied for the 3R4F reference cigarette. It should be noted that the numbers of HPHCs used to calculate the overall reductions varied because the values for some constituents were incalculable, as the majority (or all) of the measurements for these constituents were below the limits of detection or quantification, and only a maximum of 50 of the 54 quantified HPHCs were used for the calculations. These data demonstrate that the performance of THS, with respect to reducing the emissions of HPHCs relative to the 3R4F reference cigarette, is robust over a broad range of machine-smoking conditions and particularly so with the HCI and more intense regimens. This is an important factor, which ensures that a consistent reduction in exposure to HPHCs for users is maintained irrespective of how the product is used, because smoking and product use behavior are very individual processes.

TABLE 4.10
FDA Abbreviated List of 18 HPHCs Determined for Regular THS Tobacco Sticks and the US Market Map and Percent Reductions Versus 3R4F Calculated on a Per-Item and Nicotine Basis.

Aerosol Deliveries according to ISO 4387; ISO 8454; ISO 10315	Unit	US Market map Median	THS REGULAR			% Reduction relative to US market map on a per-item basis	% Reduction relative to US market map on a nicotine basis
			Mean	SD	n		
1-Aminonaphthalene	ng/item	32.1	0.0427	0.00513	3	99.8%	99.7%
2-Aminonaphthalene	ng/item	20.1	0.0223	0.00321	3	99.9%	99.8%
4-Aminobiphenyl	ng/item	3.43	0.0087	0.0012	3	99.7%	99.6%
Acetaldehyde	μg/item	1467	192	11.6	3	86.8%	79.6%
Acrolein	μg/item	159	8.32	0.755	3	94.3%	91.4%
Acrylonitrile	μg/item	23.6	0.145	0.0112	3	99.3%	98.9%
Ammonia	μg/item	31.0	12.2	0.973	3	69.3%	53.6%
Benzene	μg/item	87.0	0.452	0.0395	3	99.4%	99.1%
Benzo[a]pyrene	ng/item	15.3	0.736	0.0973	3	94.3%	91.0%
1,3-Butadiene	μg/item	117.0	0.207	0.0160	3	99.8%	99.7%
Carbon monoxide (CO)	mg/item	28.0	0.347	0.0462	3	98.8%	98.2%
Crotonaldehyde	μg/item	51.1	<3.29 (LOQ)	NA	3	>92.7%	>89.0%
Formaldehyde	μg/item	91.5	14.1	0.430	3	80.7%	71.0%
Isoprene	μg/item	1005	1.51	0.129	3	99.8%	99.8%
Nicotine	mg/item	2.00	1.29	0.047	3	NA	NA
4-(Methylnitrosamino) -1-(3-pyridyl)-1-butanone (NNK)	ng/item	128.0	7.80	0.423	3	94.3%	91.5%
N-Nitrosonornicotine (NNN)	ng/item	184	10.1	0.205	3	95.0%	92.8%
Toluene	μg/item	149	1.42	0.162	3	98.8%	98.2%

LOQ, limit of quantification; *n*, number of items; *NA*, not available; *SD*, standard deviation.

This was confirmed in clinical reduced—exposure studies in which smokers switched from cigarette smoking to THS use (Chapter 17).

4.7.2 Influence of Climatic Conditions on Product Performance

THS is a product designed to be available across all markets in the world where cigarettes are currently sold. Therefore, it is important to understand how the product behaves in different climatic conditions in terms of its ability to maintain the reductions in HPHC emissions. In order to address this, PMI investigated the levels of 54 HPHCs in THS aerosol when tobacco sticks were stored and aerosols were generated

under different climatic conditions and compared these with the emissions of the 3R4F reference cigarette. The investigated conditions were selected on the basis of a list of climatic zones defined by the International Conference on Harmonization and WHO for pharmaceutical stability testing to be representative of a hot/dry climate (30°C/35% RH; Zone III), a subtropical/Mediterranean climate (25°C/60% RH; Zone II), and a hot/higher humidity climate (30°C/75% RH; Zone IVb). In place of Zone II conditions, standard ISO conditions (ISO 3402) required for the conditioning and testing of tobacco and tobacco products were used (22°C/60% RH). For the purposes of this investigation, the climatic conditions were referred to as "dry,"

TABLE 4.11

FDA Abbreviated List of 18 HPHCs Determined for Mentholated THS Tobacco Sticks and the US Market Map and Percent Reductions Versus 3R4F Calculated on a Per-Item and Nicotine Basis.

Aerosol Deliveries according to ISO 4387; ISO 8454; ISO 10315	Unit	US Market map Median	THS SMOOTH MENTHOL			% Reduction relative to US market map on a per-item basis	% Reduction relative to US market map on a nicotine basis
			Mean	SD	n		
1-Aminonaphthalene	ng/item	32.1	0.043	0.012	3	99.8%	99.7%
2-Aminonaphthalene	ng/item	20.1	0.022	0.007	3	99.9%	99.8%
4-Aminobiphenyl	ng/item	3.43	0.009	0.002	3	99.7%	99.5%
Acetaldehyde	µg/item	1467	206	6	3	85.8%	76.2%
Acrolein	µg/item	159	9.79	1.66	3	93.2%	89.0%
Acrylonitrile	µg/item	23.6	0.127	0.017	3	99.4%	99.0%
Ammonia	µg/item	31.0	11.1	1.1	3	72.0%	54.2%
Benzene	µg/item	87.0	0.453	0.046	3	99.4%	99.0%
Benzo[a]pyrene	ng/item	15.3	0.539	0.081	3	95.8%	92.8%
1,3-Butadiene	µg/item	117.0	0.223	0.030	3	99.8%	99.6%
Carbon monoxide (CO)	mg/item	28.0	0.320	0.000	3	98.9%	98.2%
Crotonaldehyde	µg/item	51.1	<3.29 (LOQ)	NA	3	>92.7%	>88.1%
Formaldehyde	µg/item	91.5	15.2	0.035	3	79.3%	66.3%
Isoprene	µg/item	1005	1.51	0.31	3	99.8%	99.7%
Nicotine	mg/item	2.00	1.19	0.05	3	NA	NA
4-(Methylnitrosamino)-1-(3-pyridyl)-1-butanone (NNK)	ng/item	128.0	6.63	0.53	3	95.2%	92.2%
N-Nitrosonornicotine (NNN)	ng/item	184	7.01	0.51	3	96.5%	94.6%
Toluene	µg/item	149	1.28	0.12	3	98.9%	98.2%

LOQ, limit of quantification, n, number of items; NA, not available; SD, standard deviation;

TABLE 4.12

Smoking Parameters Applied for Assessment of Robustness of THS Performance.

Parameter	Unit	SMOKING PARAMETERS FOR THS					SMOKING PARAMETERS FOR 3R4F					
		L[a]	N[b]	A	H	E	L	L	N	N	H	H
Puff volume	mL	35	55	60	80	110	35	35	55	55	80	80
Puff interval	s	60	30	25	25	22	60	60	30	30	25	25
Puff duration	s	2	2	2.4	2.4	4.5	2	2	2	2	2.4	2.4
Puff count[c]	N	6	12	14	14	14	—	—	—	—	—	—
Ventilation blocking[d]	%	NA	NA	NA	NA	NA	50	100	50	100	50	100

[a] ISO 3308 machine-smoking regimen.
[b] HCI (Health Canada, 1999) machine-smoking regimen.
[c] For THS, the number of puffs is governed by the device, which operates for a maximum of 6 min or 14 puffs, whichever comes first. Puff counts for 3R4F were determined as the mean puff count for all items, per replicate, smoked to a predefined butt length.
[d] Ventilation blocking for THS was not applicable (NA), as tobacco sticks do not have filter ventilation perforations.

Goujon, C., Kleinhans, S., Maeder, S., Poget, L., & Schaller, J., 2020. Robustness of HPHC Reduction for THS 2.2 Aerosol Compared with 3R4F Reference Cigarette Smoke Under High Intensity Puffing Conditions. Beitr. Tab. Int. 29 (2), 66–83. https://doi.org/10.2478/cttr-2020-0008https://content.sciendo.com/configurable/contentpage/journals$002fcttr$002f29$002f2$002farticle-p66.xml.

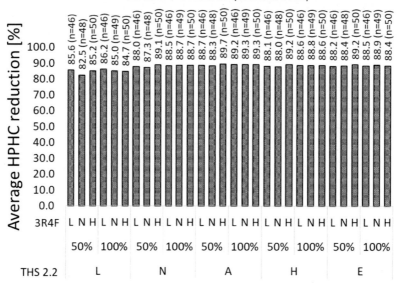

FIG. 4.3 Comparison of Average Reductions in HPHCs in THS Aerosol, Expressed as Percentage Relative to 3R4F Smoke Concentrations and Normalized by Nicotine Levels, Among Various Combinations of Smoking Regimens and Two Levels of Filter Ventilation Blocking (50% and 100%) for 3R4F. The Smoking Regimens L, N, A, H, and E are Defined in Table 4.12. *HPHC*, harmful and potentially harmful constituent; *THS*, Tobacco Heating System 2.2. (Goujon, C., Kleinhans, S., Maeder, S., Poget, L., & Schaller, J., 2020. Robustness of HPHC Reduction for THS 2.2 Aerosol Compared with 3R4F Reference Cigarette Smoke Under High Intensity Puffing Conditions. Beitr. Tab. Int. 29 (2), 66—83. https://doi.org/10.2478/cttr-2020-0008https://content.sciendo.com/configurable/contentpage/journals$002fcttr$002f29$002f2$002farticle-p66.xml.)

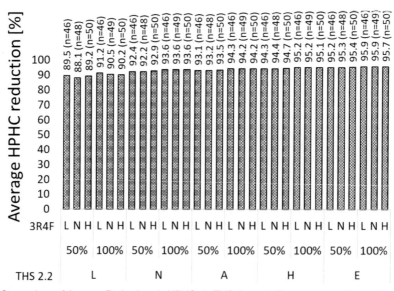

FIG. 4.4 Comparison of Average Reductions in HPHCs in THS Aerosol, Expressed as a Percentage Relative to 3R4F Smoke Concentrations, Among Various Combinations of Smoking Regimens and Two Levels of Filter Ventilation Blocking (50% and 100%) for 3R4F. The Smoking Regimens L, N, A, H, and E are defined in Table 4.12. *HPHC*, harmful and potentially harmful constituent; *THS*, Tobacco Heating System 2.2. (Goujon, C., Kleinhans, S., Maeder, S., Poget, L., & Schaller, J., 2020. Robustness of HPHC Reduction for THS 2.2 Aerosol Compared with 3R4F Reference Cigarette Smoke Under High Intensity Puffing Conditions. Beitr. Tab. Int. 29 (2), 66—83. https://doi.org/10.2478/cttr-2020-0008https://content.sciendo.com/configurable/contentpage/journals$002fcttr$002f29$002f2$002farticle-p66.xml.)

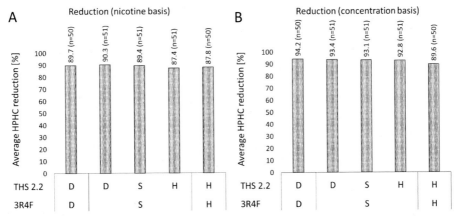

FIG. 4.5 Average Reductions in 51 HPHCs in THS Aerosol, Expressed as Percentage Relative to 3R4F Smoke with **(A)** and Without **(B)** Normalization for Nicotine Delivery, at Various Combinations of Ambient Temperature and Humidity Conditions (D, Dry 30°C/35% RH; S, Standard ISO 22°C/60% RH; H, Humid 30°C/75% RH).   *HPHC*, harmful and potentially harmful constituent; *RH*, relative humidity; *THS*, Tobacco Heating System 2.2.

"standard ISO," and "humid," respectively. The products were conditioned for at least 48 h under the same climatic conditions as those under which they were to be machine smoked.

As in the assessment performed for the effect of smoking regimen on product performance, the HPHC yields in aerosol/smoke were normalized in accordance with the total puff volume collected for each product, constituent, and replicate under the HCI smoking regimen. Fig. 4.5 presents the average reductions in all HPHCs quantified; the reduction values for some constituents (6 of 54) were not calculable because the determined concentrations were below the limits of detection or quantification.

Overall, the average reductions in HPHC concentrations for THS relative to 3R4F were in the range of 89.4%—94.2% (87.6%—89.7% on a nicotine basis), which is in line with previous findings (Goujon et al., 2020; Smith et al., 2016). Temperature and humidity had a marked impact on 3R4F smoke yields relative to THS aerosol yields; the effects of moisture on cigarette burn rate, puff number, retention in the tobacco rod and filter, and thermochemical reactions have been reported in several studies (Davis and George, 1965; Kobashi et al., 1959; Pang and Lewis, 2011; Zha and Moldoveanu, 2004). Comparison of the average reductions in HPHC concentrations for THS across all climatic conditions with the 3R4F values generated under standard ISO climatic conditions showed reductions in the range of 92.8%—93.4%, indicating that THS is less affected by moisture than

cigarettes. The results of this investigation support the continued use of standard ISO climatic conditions for assessment of EHTP performance relative to cigarettes smoked under the same conditions.

4.8 HPHC EMISSIONS BY EVPS AND HYBRID DEVICES

E-vapor products (EVPs) (Chapter 2), commonly referred to as "e-cigarettes," are available in a wide variety of forms (e.g., cigalikes, pens, tanks, pods, and mods), which comprise a battery-powered heater that is used to vaporize a liquid matrix (e-liquid) to deliver an aerosol (e-vapor) to the user. The e-liquid is usually a solution containing a mixture of propylene glycol (PG) and vegetable glycerin (VG), nicotine, flavorings, and other constituents, such as small quantities of water used to reduce the e-liquid viscosity. Hybrid devices are also available commercially, which operate by passing e-vapor through a tobacco matrix to provide flavor enhancement (Poynton et al., 2017) and, in products that operate with a nicotine-free e-liquid, deliver nicotine to the user (Takahashi et al., 2018). EVPs are currently sold worldwide (WHO, 2009) and, depending on location, may be subject to regulation as tobacco products, consumer products, or pharmaceutical products. However, some countries have banned EVPs, e-liquid refills that contain nicotine, and even EVPs that do not contain nicotine (Kennedy et al., 2017).

In most cases, EVP aerosols comprise water, nicotine, and the aerosol formers VG and PG, with the additional presence of flavor compounds. The emission of EVP toxicants is a function of a variety of factors, including device construction, device power, liquid constituents, and user behavior (WHO, 2019b). The use of low-quality ingredients is a potential source of unwanted impurities, in addition to the toxicants produced by thermal degradation of the aerosol formers (Beauval et al., 2017; Flora et al., 2016; Hutzler et al., 2014; Jensen et al., 2017), which are mainly aldehydes (Geiss et al., 2016; Gillman et al., 2016; Jensen et al., 2015; Kosmider et al., 2014; Sleiman et al., 2016). Flavoring compounds may also contribute to the generation of acetaldehyde, acrolein, formaldehyde, and other aldehydes in EVP aerosol (Guthery, 2016; Khlystov and Samburova, 2016). The nicotine used for preparation of e-liquids is extracted from tobacco; therefore, TSNAs might also be present in e-liquids as coextracted impurities or, in the case of hybrid devices, transferred from the tobacco matrix into the aerosol. In addition to known tobacco toxicants, e-cigarettes have been identified as containing potential toxicants such as glyoxal, methylglyoxal (Uchiyama et al., 2013), diacetyl and 2,3-pentanedione (Allen et al., 2016; Farsalinos et al., 2015), acetoin (Allen et al., 2016), and metals, such as copper (Lerner et al., 2015) and zinc (Williams et al., 2013). Because EVP devices may contain multiple metallic parts—including wiring, a heating element, solder connections, and structural components—there is a possibility for contamination of e-liquids with other elemental metals, such as chromium, nickel, aluminum, iron, lead, and tin. In addition, the contact between metals and e-liquids, specifically with heater filaments, has also been demonstrated to catalyze the formation of carbonyls at temperatures well below those expected during "dry wicking," which is a situation where insufficient e-liquid reaches the heater, resulting in significant overheating. This may be a contributing factor to the wide range of carbonyl values reported in the literature to date, suggesting that device materials may be an important variable for regulations designed for protecting public health (Saliba et al., 2018). Therefore, relevant measurements for assessment of EVP aerosols would include the main components of e-liquids (nicotine, water, VG, and PG), recognized thermal degradation products (including carbonyls such as formaldehyde, acetaldehyde, and acrolein), TSNAs, and metals, if their potential release by device elements cannot be excluded (Hess et al., 2017; Mishra et al., 2017).

Current regulations for e-cigarettes lag behind the existing controls that regulate tobacco and tobacco smoking, for which several regulatory bodies have compiled lists of potential toxicants (Burns et al., 2008; FDA, 2012a; Health Canada, 2000), and the FDA and WHO's TobReg have mandated the monitoring and reporting of selected toxicants (FDA, 2012b; WHO, 2019a). However, a revised version of the European Union Tobacco Products Directive (EUTPD; 2014/40/EU), which entered into force in May 2014, became applicable for EU Member States in May 2016, bringing the regulation of EVPs within its remit. Similarly, in the US, the FDA has deemed e-cigarettes subject to tobacco laws (FDA, 2016) and introduced regulations for new Premarket Tobacco Product Applications for EVPs (FDA, 2019). Within these guidelines, the FDA has recommended the analysis of 33 constituents in e-liquids and aerosols for new EVP applications: acetaldehyde, acetyl propionyl (also known as 2,3-pentanedione), acrolein, acrylonitrile, benzene, benzyl acetate, butyraldehyde, cadmium, chromium, crotonaldehyde, diacetyl, diethylene glycol, ethyl acetate, ethyl acetoacetate ethylene glycol, formaldehyde, furfural, glycerol, glycidol, isoamyl acetate, isobutyl acetate, lead, menthol, menthyl acetate, n-butanol, nickel, nicotine (any source, including total nicotine, unprotonated nicotine, and nicotine salts), NNK (4-(methylnitrosamino)-1-(3-pyridyl)-1-butanone), NNN (N-nitrosonornicotine), propionic acid, PG, propylene oxide, toluene, and any other constituents that may be considered appropriate for the product (e.g., flavorants considered to be respiratory irritants, such as benzaldehyde, vanillin, and cinnamaldehyde). Earlier documents issued by national standardization bodies in the United Kingdom (UK) and France (AFNOR, 2016; British Standards Institute (BSI), 2015) have recommended determination of nicotine, formaldehyde, acrolein, acetaldehyde, diacetyl, and some metals in e-cigarette aerosols. In the UK, this was later formalized into a list of aerosol constituents mandated by the Medicines and Healthcare products Regulatory Agency (MHRA, 2016), in accordance with the requirements of the EUTPD. Officially recognized analytical methods already exist for determining many of the aforementioned constituents in mainstream cigarette smoke. However, there are currently no standard analytical methods available for determining the concentrations of these constituents in e-liquids or their corresponding aerosols. The levels of constituents present in EVP aerosols can differ greatly from those present in cigarette smoke, sometimes being lower by several orders of magnitude, and the applicability of such methods for assessment of EVP aerosols remains to be evaluated with appropriate method validation and interlaboratory comparisons. Margham

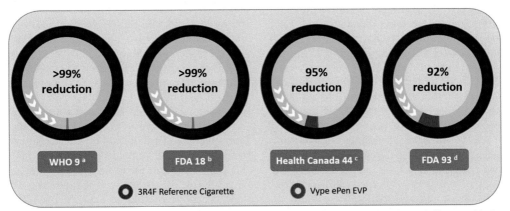

FIG. 4.6 Average Reductions in HPHC Emissions for an EVP Relative to the 3R4F Reference Cigarette Under the HCI Smoking Regimen.   Priority toxicants selected by TobReg for mandated reduction (WHO, 2019). FDA abbreviated list of priority toxicants for mainstream tobacco smoke (FDA, 2012b). Health Canada's mandated Tobacco Reporting Regulations (SOR/2000–273, Health Canada, 2000). FDA list of 93 HPHCs in mainstream tobacco smoke (FDA, 2012a). *EVP*, e-vapor product; *HCI*, Health Canada Intense; *HPHC*, harmful and potentially harmful constituent. (Data from Margham, J., McAdam, K., Forster, M., Liu, C., Wright, C., Mariner, D., Proctor, C., 2016. Chemical composition of aerosol from an E-cigarette: a quantitative comparison with cigarette smoke. Chem. Res. Toxicol. 29, 1662–1678. https://doi.org/10.1021/acs.chemrestox.6b00188.)

and colleagues (Margham et al., 2016) compared the emissions of an EVP (Vype ePen, operator-actuated heater) with those of the 3R4F reference cigarette by using the HCI smoking regimen (Health Canada, 1999). Analyses were performed to quantify the HPHCs listed by the WHO (nine toxicants mandated for lowering in cigarette smoke), Health Canada (Health Canada, 2000), and the FDA (FDA, 2012a; FDA, 2012b), although it should be noted that three HPHCs were omitted from the full FDA list of HPHCs owing to lack of available analytical methods. The average reductions in HPHC emissions observed for the EVP versus 3R4F, for each of the defined reporting lists, are presented in Fig. 4.6.

The choice of machine-smoking regimen used for generating EVP aerosol is as important as the selection of appropriate chemical markers for assessing EVP aerosol emissions. The use of smoking regimens developed for cigarettes for assessment of EVPs has been extensively deliberated by the Cooperation Centre for Scientific Research Relative to Tobacco (CORESTA). It was considered that neither of the regimens routinely applied for assessment of cigarette emissions—ISO (ISO 3308) or HCI (Health Canada, 1999)—were suitable for assessment of EVP aerosol, because many self-actuating devices (by detection of pressure drop) fail to activate fully and generate a representative aerosol. To overcome this issue, CORESTA released a recommended method, CRM 81 (CORESTA, 2015), which has since been adopted by ISO and issued as a standard

method (ISO 20768; ISO, 2018). It is broadly similar to the HCI machine-smoking regimen for cigarettes, but uses a square-shaped puff profile instead of a bell-shaped puff profile, with a 3-s puff duration, which ensures that the devices are fully activated and generate an aerosol during puffing. Similar specifications have also been adopted by Association Française de Normalisation (AFNOR) (AFNOR, 2016), and a meta-analysis of available data from smoking topography investigations in EVP users has shown that the machine-smoking regimen proposed by CORESTA (CORESTA, 2015) does represent the average consumers' puffing behavior for the EVP devices studied (Belushkin et al., 2018).

With the recent emergence of higher delivery "sub-ohm" EVP devices, many users are employing a direct-to-lung inhalation technique, where the inhaled volumes can be significantly higher than those in mouth-to-lung users. Accordingly, in their guidance for the evaluation of electronic nicotine delivery products (ENDPs), the FDA suggested evaluation of emissions by using a more intense aerosol generation regimen (FDA, 2019). A CORESTA technical guide (CORESTA, 2018) has also been published to address this need; it provides guidance on the criteria that should be considered when setting intense analytical aerosol generation parameters for EVPs. The main attributes are puff duration and, to a lesser extent, puff volume. Device settings, such as voltage setting, ventilation setting, and heating element age, are also identified as factors affecting aerosol generation and are recommended to be based on representative human usage (CORESTA, 2018). Furthermore, emissions may change depending on the level of e-liquid remaining in the device (Farsalinos and Gillman, 2017; Sleiman et al., 2016). While some studies have focused on start-of-use measurements (Flora et al., 2017) or the last puffs beyond the criteria specified by CORESTA in their recommended method CRM 81 (CORESTA, 2015) for end-of-life aerosol generation (Farsalinos and Gillman, 2017), it is important to assess the emissions from such products over their full life cycle and to consider the average levels of emissions. If properly designed and used, EVP devices should not overheat the e-liquid, as overheating is a significant source of toxicants related to EVP use. Therefore, it is imperative to define clear criteria for the end of aerosol generation, so that the results remain meaningful and, very importantly, comparable. Among others, these considerations have been addressed in CORESTA Technical Guide No. 25 (CORESTA, 2019a), and recommendations for stability assessments are addressed in CORESTA Technical Guide No. 26 (CORESTA, 2019b).

Because of the wide range of designs and materials used for construction of EVP devices, the multitude of possible user settings for some devices, and the vast array of e-liquid choices available to consumers, it is very challenging to establish standard conditions for assessing the performance of different types of product. With the proliferation of EVPs, new testing and product standards for this product category are being elaborated, and it is only recently that guidelines have been issued by the FDA to address the absence of requirements for manufacturers (FDA, 2019), although these are yet to be enforced for products that are already commercially available within the US. Such standards are an essential part of science-based regulations, serving to identify relevant analytes for quantification and ensuring that analytical methods are relevant considering the levels of such analytes in the aerosol of the products. The use of a standard EVP device for assessing e-liquids and the use of a standard e-liquid(s) for assessing the performance of different EVP devices are also approaches that are deliberated within the scientific community. Accordingly, UK authorities have recommend that e-liquid suppliers use a device that is most representative of their products' usage in the market (or which poses the highest potential risk to the consumer) for reporting aerosol constituent data (MHRA, 2016). This approach has been adopted in a recent study that investigated the levels of carbonyls (acetaldehyde, acrolein, and formaldehyde),

TSNAs (NNK and NNN), metals (arsenic, cadmium, chromium, lead, and nickel), benzene, 1,3-butadiene, and benzo[a]pyrene in a broad range of commercially available EVPs (Belushkin et al., 2020a, 2020b).

This study evaluated the levels of carbonyls emitted by a range of commercial devices in combination with a standard e-liquid, which is an approach that has been proposed by various standardization committees, including AFNOR (AFNOR, 2016) and the European Committee for Standardization. The levels of acetaldehyde, acrolein, and formaldehyde observed in the aerosols generated from the same e-liquid covered a wide range of concentrations, with a difference of almost three orders of magnitude between the highest and lowest concentrations of formaldehyde. This observation is most likely a reflection of the absolute temperatures to which the liquid was exposed in the different devices (Flora et al., 2017; Geiss et al., 2016; Hutzler et al., 2014), as the power and construction of EVP devices have been demonstrated to have a strong effect on carbonyl emissions (Geiss et al., 2016; Gillman et al., 2016; Kosmider et al., 2014; Sleiman et al., 2016), and dry wicking may have occurred in some of the devices (Farsalinos and Gillman, 2017). The study also used an arbitrary reference device (a widely available commercial open-tank system) to assess the carbonyl emissions associated with a number of commercially available e-liquids from different suppliers. In this setting, the ranges of carbonyl yields were much narrower, well within an order of magnitude, most likely because a single reference device was used to apply a more consistent temperature to each of the e-liquids. The differences among the e-liquids may have been due to compositional differences, either in terms of the PG and VG ratios used, which are known to result in different acetaldehyde, acrolein, and formaldehyde concentrations (Farsalinos and Gillman, 2017; Jensen et al., 2017; Laino et al., 2012, 2011; Wang et al., 2017), or in the use of certain flavor compounds that thermally decompose and add to the carbonyl load (Khlystov and Samburova, 2016). Table 4.13 presents comparative data for carbonyl emissions from a cigarette (represented by Marlboro Red), an EHTP (represented by THS with both regular and mentholated tobacco stick variants), and a variable-power EVP operated at two different power levels (10 and 14 W) by using a tobacco flavored e-liquid containing 18 mg/mL nicotine (Farsalinos et al., 2018b). Smoke and aerosols were generated in accordance with the HCI smoking regimen, and the data demonstrated that an EHTP, represented by THS, emits substantially lower levels of carbonyls than a commercial tobacco cigarette

TABLE 4.13
Comparative Carbonyl Emissions for Cigarettes, EHTPs, and EVPs, Normalized by Nicotine Delivery.

	Formaldehyde	Acetaldehyde	Acrolein	Propionaldehyde	Crotonaldehyde
Product	**MEAN YIELD (μG/MG NICOTINE)**				
Marlboro red	36.7 (7.6)	580.4 (88.3)	61.6 (7.8)	59.4 (9.8)	22.5 (8.0)
THS Regular	5.3 (1.5)	120.1 (19.4)	9.0 (3.3)	10.7 (3.1)	1.6 (0.4)
THS Menthol	4.1 (1.2)	147.3 (27.2)	8.6 (1.6)	9.2 (2.0)	1.6 (0.2)
EVP 10W	0.5 (0.2)	0.8 (0.3)	0.3 (0.1)	< LOD	< LOD
EVP 14W	0.6 (0.2)	0.9 (0.2)	0.3 (0.1)	< LOD	< LOD

Standard deviations for the means of five replicates are presented in parentheses. *EHTP*; electrically heated tobacco product; *EVPs*, e-vapor products.
Data from Farsalinos, K.E., Yannovits, N., Sarri, T., Voudris, V., Poulas, K., Leischow, S.J., 2018. Carbonyl emissions from a novel heated tobacco product (IQOS): comparison with an e-cigarette and a tobacco cigarette: carbonyl emissions in heated tobacco product. Addiction 113, 2099–2106. https://doi.org/10.1111/add.14365.

(Marlboro Red) and that an EVP emits even lower levels of carbonyls when operated correctly.

The EUTPD leaves the responsibility for adopting rules on flavors to the Member States, but requires that notifications for new products should include "a list of all ingredients contained in, and emissions resulting from the use of, the product, by brand name and type, including quantities thereof." The EUTPD also specifies a number of additives that cannot be used in EVPs, including vitamins, stimulants, and any additives that have known carcinogenic, mutagenic, or reproductive toxicological properties (EUTPD; 2014/40/EU). In the US, restrictions on the use of flavors in cartridge-based EVPs have been enforced, limiting the use of flavors to tobacco and menthol. However, e-liquids produced for use with refillable EVPs are not currently subject to such restrictions, and manufacturers are free to continue producing novel flavor variants. Flavor ingredients in tobacco and/or tobacco smoke were not included in the original priorities ascribed for tobacco and mainstream tobacco smoke in Articles 9 and 10 of the WHO FCTC, and, in 2017, the WHO reported that e-liquids were available in over 7500 unique flavors, with new flavors being introduced on a daily basis (WHO, 2017). Most of the e-liquid flavor ingredients used are "generally regarded as safe" (GRAS) when ingested. However, GRAS certification does not apply to chemicals that are inhaled, which includes flavor ingredients inhaled via EVP aerosols (Flavor and Extract Manufacturers Association (FEMA), 2013; Tierney et al., 2016). Although there is some evidence suggesting possible adverse health effects resulting from inhalation of EVP aerosols (Hwang et al., 2016; Yu et al., 2016), the role of flavors in this respect is largely unknown. However, some classes of flavor compounds reported in e-liquids pose potential health risks (Barrington-Trimis et al., 2014) and include the compound diacetyl, which has been directly linked to respiratory disease and has since been banned in many countries. In the absence of any formal requirements for quantification of flavors in e-liquids and their resulting aerosols, any analyses performed in relation to flavors will most likely focus on compounds that are known, or are suspected, to have a negative health impact for users.

4.9 CONCLUSION

The central tenet of tobacco harm reduction (Chapter 1) is that ENDPs emit substantially lower levels of toxicants than cigarettes (Chapter 3). It is, therefore, important to select a range of relevant HPHCs, measured by appropriate methods, to compare the emissions of ENDPs with those of cigarettes.

For HTPs, it is assumed that the HPHCs required for reporting by cigarette regulations may be directly relevant. On this basis, PMI assembled a list of 58 analytes to compare the emissions of THS with those of the 3R4F reference cigarette. This list includes the HPHCs listed by the WHO (WHO, 2019a) and Health Canada (Health Canada, 2000) and the abbreviated FDA list of 18 HPHCs (FDA, 2012b). A recent untargeted analysis of an EHTP aerosol showed that the substances emitted by THS are also present in cigarette smoke (Bentley et al., 2020) (Chapter 6). This confirms that the lists of priority HPHCs mandated for regulatory reporting of tobacco products remain applicable for assessment of EHTPs. On the basis of the PMI 58 list, a THS tobacco stick emits, on average, 92% less HPHCs than a 3R4F reference cigarette.

Although EVPs seem simpler than EHTPs, selecting a list of appropriate HPHCs for assessment is complex and should include substances that are not currently mandated for regulatory reporting of tobacco products. For instance, the FDA has recommended analysis of 33 constituents in e-liquids and aerosols for new EVP applications. Interestingly, this list includes only eight (1,3-butadiene, acetaldehyde, acrolein, benzene, CO, formaldehyde, NNK, and NNN) of the nine priority toxicants mandated by the WHO for lowering and regulation (WHO, 2008); benzo[*a*]pyrene is absent in the FDA list of 33.

Heating a nicotine-containing solution comprising PG, VG, and flavor ingredients to produce an aerosol would appear to be a simple process. However, devices constructed with poor materials, lacking appropriate electronic controls, and open to misuse can generate aerosols that may contain concentrations of specific toxicants equivalent to, or even greater than, those found in cigarette smoke (Belushkin et al., 2020a). The biggest issue with EVP emissions arises from e-liquid overheating, or dry wicking, leading to emission of high concentrations of carbonyls and epoxides from the thermal decomposition of PG, VG, and some chemical classes of flavor ingredients. Overheating can occur for a number of reasons, including the absence of electronic systems for detecting overheating, users applying excessive power with variable-power devices, and insufficient e-liquid reaching the heater because of liquid exhaustion (empty reservoir or very intense puffing by user) or higher liquid viscosity restricting the flow of e-liquid to the heater. However, this is not considered to be a danger to EVP users, because dry wicking events are aversive and hence avoided by the user (Farsalinos et al., 2017; McNeill et al., 2018, 2015). When EVPs operate within their intended parameters, the aerosol delivered contains significantly lower levels of toxicants than are present in cigarette smoke, and Public Health England has estimated that the use of EVPs is 95% less harmful than smoking cigarettes (McNeill et al., 2015), which is entirely supported by the data presented by Margham et al. (2016). However, assessment of EVP aerosols needs to take into account flavor ingredients to ensure that those not suitable for inhalation, or their potentially toxic degradation products, are minimized.

REFERENCES

AFNOR, 2016. XP D 90-300-3 Electronic Cigarettes and E-Liquids — Part 3. Requirements and Test Methods for Emissions. AFNOR, Paris, France.

Allen, J.G., Flanigan, S.S., LeBlanc, M., Vallarino, J., MacNaughton, P., Stewart, J.H., Christiani, D.C., 2016. Flavoring chemicals in E-cigarettes: diacetyl, 2,3-pentanedione, and acetoin in a sample of 51 products, including fruit-, candy-, and cocktail-flavored E-cigarettes. Environ. Health Perspect. 124, 733—739. https://doi.org/10.1289/ehp.1510185.

Auer, R., Concha-Lozano, N., Jacot-Sadowski, I., Cornuz, J., Berthet, A., 2017. Heat-not-burn tobacco cigarettes: smoke by any other name. JAMA Intern. Med. 177, 1050—1052. https://doi.org/10.1001/jamainternmed.2017.1419.

Baker, R.R., 2006. Smoke generation inside a burning cigarette: modifying combustion to develop cigarettes that may be less hazardous to health. Prog. Energy Combust. Sci. 32, 373—385. https://doi.org/10.1016/j.pecs.2006.01.001.

Baker, R.R., 2005. Smoke generation inside a burning cigarette. In: Presented at the 9th International Congress on Combustion By-Products and Their Health Effects, Tucson, Arizona, USA.

Baker, R.R., 1999. Smoke chemistry. In: Tobacco Production, Chemistry and Technology. Blackwell Science Ltd., Oxford, pp. 398—439.

Baker, R.R., 1975. Temperature variation within a cigarette combustion coal during the smoking cycle. High Temp. Sci. 7, 236—247.

Barrington-Trimis, J.L., Samet, J.M., McConnell, R., 2014. Flavorings in electronic cigarettes: an unrecognized respiratory health hazard? J. Am. Med. Assoc. 312, 2493—2494. https://doi.org/10.1001/jama.2014.14830.

Bartsch, H., Malaveille, C., Friesen, M., Kadlubar, F.F., Vineis, P., 1993. Black (air-cured) and blond (flue-cured) tobacco cancer risk. IV: molecular dosimetry studies implicate aromatic amines as bladder carcinogens. Eur. J. Canc. 29A, 1199—1207. https://doi.org/10.1016/s0959-8049(05)80315-6.

Beauval, N., Antherieu, S., Soyez, M., Gengler, N., Grova, N., Howsam, M., Hardy, E.M., Fischer, M., Appenzeller, B.M.R., Goossens, J.-F., Allorge, D., Garçon, G., Lo-Guidice, J.-M., Garat, A., 2017. Chemical evaluation of electronic cigarettes: multicomponent analysis of liquid refills and their corresponding aerosols. J. Anal. Toxicol. 41, 670—678. https://doi.org/10.1093/jat/bkx054.

Bekki, K., Inaba, Y., Uchiyama, S., Kunugita, N., 2017. Comparison of chemicals in mainstream smoke in heat-not-burn tobacco and combustion cigarettes. J. UOEH 39, 201—207. https://doi.org/10.7888/juoeh.39.201.

Belushkin, M., Esposito, M., Jaccard, G., Jeannet, C., Korneliou, A., Tafin Djoko, D., 2018. Role of testing standards in smoke-free product assessments. Regul. Toxicol. Pharmacol. 98, 1—8. https://doi.org/10.1016/j.yrtph.2018.06.021.

Belushkin, M., Tafin Djoko, D., Esposito, M., Korneliou, A., Jeannet, C., Lazzerini, M., Jaccard, G., 2020. Selected harmful and potentially harmful constituents levels in commercial e-cigarettes. Chem. Res. Toxicol. 33, 657—668. https://doi.org/10.1021/acs.chemrestox.9b00470.

Belushkin, M., Tafin Djoko, D., Esposito, M., Korneliou, A., Jeannet, C., Lazzerini, M., Jaccard, G., 2020. Quantification of Harmful and Potentially Harmful Constituents (HPHC)

Emission in Commercial E-Cigarettes. https://doi.org/10.26126/INTERVALS.2B85P7.1.

Bentley, M.C., Almstetter, M., Arndt, D., Knorr, A., Martin, E., Pospisil, P., Maeder, S., 2020. Comprehensive chemical characterization of the aerosol generated by a heated tobacco product by untargeted screening. Anal. Bioanal. Chem. 412, 2675–2685. https://doi.org/10.1007/s00216-020-02502-1.

British Standards Institute (BSI), 2015. PAS 54115:2015 Vaping Products, Including Electronic Cigarettes, E-Liquids, E-Shisha and Directly-Related Products - Manufacture, Importation, Testing and Labelling - Guide.

Burns, D.M., Dybing, E., Gray, N., Hecht, S., Anderson, C., Sanner, T., O'Connor, R., Djordjevic, M., Dresler, C., Hainaut, P., Jarvis, M., Opperhuizen, A., Straif, K., 2008. Mandated lowering of toxicants in cigarette smoke: a description of the World Health Organization TobReg proposal. Tobac. Contr. 17, 132–141. https://doi.org/10.1136/tc.2007.024158.

CORESTA, 2018. CORESTA Guide No. 22. Technical Guide for the Selection of Appropriate Intense Vaping Regimes for E-Vapour Devices.

CORESTA, 2016. CORESTA Recommended Method (CRM) N° 80. Use of the Part-Filter Method for the Estimation of Smokers' Exposure to Nicotine and Nicotine-free Dry Particulate Matter.

CORESTA, 2015. CORESTA Recommended Method (CRM) N° 81. Routine Analytical Machine for E-Cigarette Aerosol Generation and Collection - Definitions and Standard Conditions.

CORESTA, 2019. CORESTA Guide No. 25. Technical Guide for Aerosol Collection and Considerations when Testing E-Vapour Product Technologies.

CORESTA, 2019. CORESTA Guide No. 26. Technical Guide for Designing E-Vapour Product Stability Studies.

Costa, D.L., Kutzman, R.S., Lehmann, J.R., Drew, R.T., 1986. Altered lung function and structure in the rat after sub-chronic exposure to acrolein. Am. Rev. Respir. Dis. 133, 286–291. https://doi.org/10.1164/arrd.1986.133.2.286.

Cozzani, V., Barontini, F., McGrath, T., Mahler, B., Nordlund, M., Smith, M., Schaller, J.P., Zuber, G., 2020. An experimental investigation into the operation of an electrically heated tobacco system. Thermochim. Acta 684, 178475. https://doi.org/10.1016/j.tca.2019.178475.

Cunningham, F.H., Fiebelkorn, S., Johnson, M., Meredith, C., 2011. A novel application of the Margin of Exposure approach: segregation of tobacco smoke toxicants. Food Chem. Toxicol. 49, 2921–2933. https://doi.org/10.1016/j.fct.2011.07.019.

Davis, H., George, W., 1965. A dimensionless measure of filter selectivity: geometrical factors in cigaret construction which influence this measure. Beiträge Tabakforsch./Contrib. Tob. Res. 3 https://doi.org/10.2478/cttr-2013-0110.

Djordjevic, M.V., Stellman, S.D., Zang, E., 2000. Doses of nicotine and lung carcinogens delivered to cigarette smokers. J. Natl. Cancer Inst. 92, 106–111. https://doi.org/10.1093/jnci/92.2.106.

Farsalinos, K.E., Gillman, G., 2017. Carbonyl emissions in E-cigarette aerosol: a systematic review and methodological considerations. Front. Physiol. 8, 1119. https://doi.org/10.3389/fphys.2017.01119.

Farsalinos, K.E., Kistler, K.A., Gillman, G., Voudris, V., 2015. Evaluation of electronic cigarette liquids and aerosol for the presence of selected inhalation toxins. Nicotine Tob. Res. 17, 168–174. https://doi.org/10.1093/ntr/ntu176.

Farsalinos, K.E., Voudris, V., Spyrou, A., Poulas, K., 2017. E-cigarettes emit very high formaldehyde levels only in conditions that are aversive to users: a replication study under verified realistic use conditions. Food Chem. Toxicol. 109, 90–94. https://doi.org/10.1016/j.fct.2017.08.044.

Farsalinos, K.E., Yannovits, N., Sarri, T., Voudris, V., Poulas, K., 2018. Nicotine delivery to the aerosol of a heat-not-burn tobacco product: comparison with a tobacco cigarette and E-cigarettes. Nicotine Tob. Res. 20, 1004–1009. https://doi.org/10.1093/ntr/ntx138.

Farsalinos, K.E., Yannovits, N., Sarri, T., Voudris, V., Poulas, K., Leischow, S.J., 2018. Carbonyl emissions from a novel heated tobacco product (IQOS): comparison with an e-cigarette and a tobacco cigarette: carbonyl emissions in heated tobacco product. Addiction 113, 2099–2106. https://doi.org/10.1111/add.14365.

FDA, 2019. Premarket Tobacco Product Applications for Electronic Nicotine Delivery Systems. Guidance for Industry.

FDA, 2016. Deeming tobacco products to Be subject to the federal food, Drug, and cosmetic act, as amended by the family smoking prevention and tobacco control act; restrictions on the sale and distribution of tobacco products and required warning statements for tobacco products. Fed. Regist. 81, 28974–29106.

FDA, 2012. Harmful and potentially harmful constituents in tobacco products and tobacco smoke; established list. Fed. Regist. 77, 20034–20037.

FDA, 2012. Guidance for Industry - Reporting Harmful and Potentially Harmful Constituents in Tobacco Products and Tobacco Smoke under Section 904(a)(3) of the Federal Food, Drug, and Cosmetic Act - Draft Guidance. U.S. Department of Health and Human Services, Center for Tobacco Products (CTP).

Flavor and Extract Manufacturers Association (FEMA), 2013. Safety Assessment and Regulatory Authority to Use Flavors: Focus on E-Cigarettes.

Flora, J.W., Meruva, N., Huang, C.B., Wilkinson, C.T., Ballentine, R., Smith, D.C., Werley, M.S., McKinney, W.J., 2016. Characterization of potential impurities and degradation products in electronic cigarette formulations and aerosols. Regul. Toxicol. Pharmacol. 74, 1–11. https://doi.org/10.1016/j.yrtph.2015.11.009.

Flora, J.W., Wilkinson, C.T., Wilkinson, J.W., Lipowicz, P.J., Skapars, J.A., Anderson, A., Miller, J.H., 2017. Method for the determination of carbonyl compounds in E-cigarette aerosols. J. Chromatogr. Sci. 55, 142–148. https://doi.org/10.1093/chromsci/bmw157.

Forster, M., Fiebelkorn, S., Yurteri, C., Mariner, D., Liu, C., Wright, C., McAdam, K., Murphy, J., Proctor, C., 2018. Assessment of novel tobacco heating product THP1.0. Part 3: comprehensive chemical characterisation of harmful and potentially harmful aerosol emissions. Regul. Toxicol. Pharmacol. 93, 14–33. https://doi.org/10.1016/j.yrtph.2017.10.006.

Fowles, J., Dybing, E., 2003. Application of toxicological risk assessment principles to the chemical constituents of cigarette smoke. Tobac. Contr. 12, 424–430. https://doi.org/10.1136/tc.12.4.424.

FTC, 1967. Cigarettes: testing for tar and nicotine content. Federal Reg. Food Drug Admin. 32, 11178.

Gasparyan, H., Mariner, D., Wright, C., Nicol, J., Murphy, J., Liu, C., Proctor, C., 2018. Accurate measurement of main aerosol constituents from heated tobacco products (HTPs): implications for a fundamentally different aerosol. Regul. Toxicol. Pharmacol. 99, 131–141. https://doi.org/10.1016/j.yrtph.2018.09.016.

Geiss, O., Bianchi, I., Barrero-Moreno, J., 2016. Correlation of volatile carbonyl yields emitted by e-cigarettes with the temperature of the heating coil and the perceived sensorial quality of the generated vapours. Int. J. Hyg Environ. Health 219, 268–277. https://doi.org/10.1016/j.ijheh.2016.01.004.

Ghosh, D., Jeannet, C., 2014. An improved cambridge filter pad extraction methodology to obtain more accurate water and "tar" values: in situ cambridge filter pad extraction methodology. Beiträge zur Tabakforschung Int./Contribut. Tobacco Res. 26 https://doi.org/10.2478/cttr-2014-0008.

Gillman, I.G., Kistler, K.A., Stewart, E.W., Paolantonio, A.R., 2016. Effect of variable power levels on the yield of total aerosol mass and formation of aldehydes in e-cigarette aerosols. Regul. Toxicol. Pharmacol. 75, 58–65. https://doi.org/10.1016/j.yrtph.2015.12.019.

Goujon, C., Kleinhans, S., Maeder, S., Poget, L., Schaller, J.-P., 2020. Robustness of HPHC reduction for THS 2.2 aerosol compared with 3R4F reference cigarette smoke under high intensity puffing conditions. Beitr. Tab. Int. 29 (2), 66–83. https://doi.org/10.2478/cttr-2020-0008.

Guthery, W., 2016. Emissions of toxic carbonyls in an electronic cigarette. Beitr. Tabakforsch. Int. 27, 30–37.

Hammond, D., Wiebel, F., Kozlowski, L.T., Borland, R., Cummings, K.M., O'Connor, R.J., McNeill, A., Connolly, G.N., Arnott, D., Fong, G.T., 2007. Revising the machine smoking regime for cigarette emissions: implications for tobacco control policy. Tobac. Contr. 16, 8–14. https://doi.org/10.1136/tc.2005.015297.

Haussmann, H.-J., 2012. Use of hazard indices for a theoretical evaluation of cigarette smoke composition. Chem. Res. Toxicol. 25, 794–810. https://doi.org/10.1021/tx200536w.

Health Canada, 2000. Tobacco Reporting Regulations; SOR/200–273.

Health Canada, 1999. Health Canada Test Method T-115, Determination of "Tar", Nicotine and Carbon Monoxide in Mainstream Tobacco Smoke. http://healthycanadians.gc.ca/en/open-information/tobacco/t100/nicotine.

Hecht, S.S., 2006. Cigarette smoking: cancer risks, carcinogens, and mechanisms. Langenbeck's Arch. Surg. 391, 603–613. https://doi.org/10.1007/s00423-006-0111-z.

Hecht, S.S., 1999. Tobacco smoke carcinogens and lung cancer. J. Natl. Cancer Inst. 91, 1194–1210. https://doi.org/10.1093/jnci/91.14.1194.

Hecht, S.S., 1998. Biochemistry, biology, and carcinogenicity of tobacco-specific N-nitrosamines. Chem. Res. Toxicol. 11, 559–603. https://doi.org/10.1021/tx980005y.

Hess, C.A., Olmedo, P., Navas-Acien, A., Goessler, W., Cohen, J.E., Rule, A.M., 2017. E-cigarettes as a source of toxic and potentially carcinogenic metals. Environ. Res. 152, 221–225. https://doi.org/10.1016/j.envres.2016.09.026.

Hoffmann, D., Djordjevic, M.V., Hoffmann, I., 1997. The changing cigarette. Prev. Med. 26, 427–434. https://doi.org/10.1006/pmed.1997.0183.

Hoffmann, D., Hoffmann, I., 1998. Letters to the editor - tobacco smoke components. Beiträge zur Tabakforschung/Contribut. Tob. Res 18, 49–52. https://doi.org/10.2478/cttr-2013-0668.

Hutzler, C., Paschke, M., Kruschinski, S., Henkler, F., Hahn, J., Luch, A., 2014. Chemical hazards present in liquids and vapors of electronic cigarettes. Arch. Toxicol. 88, 1295–1308. https://doi.org/10.1007/s00204-014-1294-7.

Hwang, J.H., Lyes, M., Sladewski, K., Enany, S., McEachern, E., Mathew, D.P., Das, S., Moshensky, A., Bapat, S., Pride, D.T., Ongkeko, W.M., Crotty Alexander, L.E., 2016. Electronic cigarette inhalation alters innate immunity and airway cytokines while increasing the virulence of colonizing bacteria. J. Mol. Med. 94, 667–679. https://doi.org/10.1007/s00109-016-1378-3.

IARC (Ed.), 2004. IARC Monographs on the Evaluation of Carcinogenic Risks of Chemicals to Humans. Tobacco Smoke and Involuntary Smoking, vol. 83. IARC, Lyon.

Ishizaki, A., Kataoka, H., 2019. A sensitive method for the determination of tobacco-specific nitrosamines in mainstream and sidestream smokes of combustion cigarettes and heated tobacco products by online in-tube solid-phase microextraction coupled with liquid chromatography-tandem mass spectrometry. Anal. Chim. Acta 1075, 98–105. https://doi.org/10.1016/j.aca.2019.04.073.

ISO, 2018. ISO/DIS 20778 Cigarettes-Routine Analytical Cigarette Smoking Machine-Definitions and Standard Conditions with an Intense Smoking Regime.

ISO, 2018. ISO 20768:2018, Routine Analytical Vaping Machine - Definitions and Standard Conditions.

ISO, 2017. ISO 17025:2017, Last Rev 2018. General Requirements for the Competence of Testing and Calibration Laboratories.

ISO, 2013. ISO 8243:2013 Cigarettes - Sampling.

ISO, 2013. ISO 10315:2013, Cigarettes – Determination of Nicotine in Smoke Condensates – Gas-chromatographic Method.

ISO, 2012. ISO 3308: 2012, Routine Analytical Cigarette-Smoking Machine - Definitions and Standard Conditions. https://www.iso.org/standard/60404.html.

ISO, 2007. ISO 8454:2007, Last Rev: 2010. Cigarettes – Determination of Carbon Monoxide in the Vapour Phase of Cigarette Smoke – NDIR Method.

ISO, 1999. ISO 3402:1999 Tobacco and Tobacco Products - Atmosphere for Conditioning and Testing.

Jensen, R.P., Luo, W., Pankow, J.F., Strongin, R.M., Peyton, D.H., 2015. Hidden formaldehyde in e-cigarette aerosols. N. Engl. J. Med. 372, 392–394. https://doi.org/10.1056/NEJMc1413069.

Jensen, R.P., Strongin, R.M., Peyton, D.H., 2017. Solvent chemistry in the electronic cigarette reaction vessel. Sci. Rep. 7, 42549. https://doi.org/10.1038/srep42549.

Kennedy, R.D., Awopegba, A., De León, E., Cohen, J.E., 2017. Global approaches to regulating electronic cigarettes. Tobac. Contr. 26, 440–445. https://doi.org/10.1136/tobaccocontrol-2016-053179.

Khlystov, A., Samburova, V., 2016. Flavoring compounds dominate toxic aldehyde production during E-cigarette vaping. Environ. Sci. Technol. 50, 13080–13085. https://doi.org/10.1021/acs.est.6b05145.

Kobashi, Y., Sakaguchi, S., Izawa, M., 1959. On the influence of moisture content in cigarettes on combustion temperature and transferred amount of nicotine into cigarettes smoke. Bull. Agric. Chem. Soc. Jpn. 23, 532–535. https://doi.org/10.1080/03758397.1959.10857614.

Kosmider, L., Sobczak, A., Fik, M., Knysak, J., Zaciera, M., Kurek, J., Goniewicz, M.L., 2014. Carbonyl compounds in electronic cigarette vapors: effects of nicotine solvent and battery output voltage. Nicotine Tob. Res. 16, 1319–1326. https://doi.org/10.1093/ntr/ntu078.

Laino, T., Tuma, C., Curioni, A., Jochnowitz, E., Stolz, S., 2011. A revisited picture of the mechanism of glycerol dehydration. J. Phys. Chem. 115, 3592–3595. https://doi.org/10.1021/jp201078e.

Laino, T., Tuma, C., Moor, P., Martin, E., Stolz, S., Curioni, A., 2012. Mechanisms of propylene glycol and triacetin pyrolysis. J. Phys. Chem. 116, 4602–4609. https://doi.org/10.1021/jp300997d.

Leigh, N.J., Palumbo, M.N., Marino, A.M., O'Connor, R.J., Goniewicz, M.L., 2018. Tobacco-specific nitrosamines (TSNA) in heated tobacco product IQOS. Tobac. Contr. 27, s37–s38. https://doi.org/10.1136/tobaccocontrol-2018-054318.

Lerner, C.A., Sundar, I.K., Yao, H., Gerloff, J., Ossip, D.J., McIntosh, S., Robinson, R., Rahman, I., 2015. Vapors produced by electronic cigarettes and e-juices with flavorings induce toxicity, oxidative stress, and inflammatory response in lung epithelial cells and in mouse lung. PloS One 10, e0116732. https://doi.org/10.1371/journal.pone.0116732.

Li, X., Luo, Y., Jiang, X., Zhang, H., Zhu, F., Hu, S., Hou, H., Hu, Q., Pang, Y., 2019. Chemical analysis and simulated pyrolysis of tobacco heating system 2.2 compared to conventional cigarettes. Nicotine Tob. Res. 21, 111–118. https://doi.org/10.1093/ntr/nty005.

Mallock, N., Böss, L., Burk, R., Danziger, M., Welsch, T., Hahn, H., Trieu, H.-L., Hahn, J., Pieper, E., Henkler-Stephani, F., Hutzler, C., Luch, A., 2018. Levels of selected analytes in the emissions of "heat not burn" tobacco products that are relevant to assess human health risks. Arch. Toxicol. 92, 2145–2149. https://doi.org/10.1007/s00204-018-2215-y.

Margham, J., McAdam, K., Forster, M., Liu, C., Wright, C., Mariner, D., Proctor, C., 2016. Chemical composition of aerosol from an E-cigarette: a quantitative comparison with cigarette smoke. Chem. Res. Toxicol. 29, 1662–1678. https://doi.org/10.1021/acs.chemrestox.6b00188.

McNeill, A., Brose, L., Calder, R., Bauld, L., Robson, D., 2018. Evidence Review of E-Cigarettes and Heated Tobacco Products 2018. A Report Commissioned by Public Health England. Public Health England, London.

McNeill, A., Brose, L.S., Calder, R., Hitchman, S.C., Hajek, P., McRobbie, H., 2015. E-Cigarettes: An Evidence Update A Report Commissioned by Public Health England. Public Health England, London. https://assets.publishing.service.gov.uk/government/uploads/system/uploads/attachment_data/file/733022/Ecigarettes_an_evidence_update_A_report_commissioned_by_Public_Health_England_FINAL.pdf.

MHRA, 2016. E-cigarettes: Regulations for Consumer Products. Emissions Testing Guidance (updated April 2020).

Mishra, V.K., Kim, K.H., Samaddar, P., Kumar, S., Aggarwal, M.L., Chacko, K.M., 2017. Review on metallic components released due to the use of electronic cigarettes. Environ. Eng. Res. 22, 131–140.

Pang, X., Lewis, A.C., 2011. Carbonyl compounds in gas and particle phases of mainstream cigarette smoke. Sci. Total Environ. 409, 5000–5009. https://doi.org/10.1016/j.scitotenv.2011.07.065.

Pankow, J.F., Watanabe, K.H., Toccalino, P.L., Luo, W., Austin, D.F., 2007. Calculated cancer risks for conventional and "potentially reduced exposure product" cigarettes. Canc. Epidemiol. Biomarkers Prev.: Pub. Am. Associ. Canc. Res. Cospons. Am. Soci. Prevent. Oncol. 16, 584–592. https://doi.org/10.1158/1055-9965.EPI-06-0762.

Penn, A., Batastini, G., Soloman, J., Burns, F., Albert, R., 1981. Dose-dependent size increases of aortic lesions following chronic exposure to 7,12-dimethylbenz(a)anthracene. Canc. Res. 41, 588–592.

Penn, A., Snyder, C.A., 1996. Butadiene inhalation accelerates arteriosclerotic plaque development in cockerels. Toxicology 113, 351–354. https://doi.org/10.1016/0300-483X(96)03472-5.

Poget, L., Campelos, P., Jeannet, C., Maeder, S., 2017. Development of models for the estimation of mouth level exposure to aerosol constituents from a heat-not-burn tobacco product using mouthpiece analysis. Beiträge Tabakforsch./Contrib. Tob. Res. 27.

Poynton, S., Sutton, J., Goodall, S., Margham, J., Forster, M., Scott, K., Liu, C., McAdam, K., Murphy, J., Proctor, C., 2017. A novel hybrid tobacco product that delivers a tobacco flavour note with vapour aerosol (Part 1): product operation and preliminary aerosol chemistry assessment. Food Chem. Toxicol.: Int. J. Publish. Br. Indus. Biol. Res. Associ. 106, 522–532. https://doi.org/10.1016/j.fct.2017.05.022.

Pryor, W.A., 1997. Cigarette smoke radicals and the role of free radicals in chemical carcinogenicity. Environ. Health Perspect. 105, 875–882. https://doi.org/10.1289/ehp.97105s4875.

Rodgman, A., Green, C.R., 2003. Toxic chemicals in cigarette mainstream smoke — hazard and hoopla. Beitr. Tabakforsch. Int. 20, 481–545.

Rodgman, A., Perfetti, T.A., 2013. The Chemical Components of Tobacco and Tobacco Smoke, second ed. CRC Press, Taylor & Francis Inc (United States), Boca Raton, FL, USA.

Saliba, N.A., El Hellani, A., Honein, E., Salman, R., Talih, S., Zeaiter, J., Shihadeh, A., 2018. Surface chemistry of electronic cigarette electrical heating coils: effects of metal type on propylene glycol thermal decomposition. J. Anal. Appl. Pyrolysis 134, 520–525. https://doi.org/10.1016/j.jaap.2018.07.019.

Salman, R., Talih, S., El-Hage, R., Haddad, C., Karaoghlanian, N., El-Hellani, A., Saliba, N.A., Shihadeh, A., 2019. Free-base and total nicotine, reactive oxygen species, and carbonyl emissions from IQOS, a heated tobacco product. Nicotine Tob. Res. 21, 1285–1288. https://doi.org/10.1093/ntr/nty235.

Schaller, J.-P., Keller, D., Poget, L., Pratte, P., Kaelin, E., McHugh, D., Cudazzo, G., Smart, D., Tricker, A.R., Gautier, L., Yerly, M., Reis Pires, R., Le Bouhellec, S., Ghosh, D., Hofer, I., Garcia, E., Vanscheeuwijck, P., Maeder, S., 2016. Evaluation of the Tobacco Heating System 2.2. Part 2: chemical composition, genotoxicity, cytotoxicity, and physical properties of the aerosol. Regul. Toxicol. Pharmacol. 81 (Suppl. 2), S27–S47. https://doi.org/10.1016/j.yrtph.2016.10.001.

Sleiman, M., Logue, J.M., Montesinos, V.N., Russell, M.L., Litter, M.I., Gundel, L.A., Destaillats, H., 2016. Emissions from electronic cigarettes: key parameters affecting the release of harmful chemicals. Environ. Sci. Technol. 50, 9644–9651. https://doi.org/10.1021/acs.est.6b01741.

Smith, C.J., Hansch, C., 2000. The relative toxicity of compounds in mainstream cigarette smoke condensate. Food Chem. Toxicol. 38, 637–646. https://doi.org/10.1016/s0278-6915(00)00051-x.

Smith, M.R., Clark, B., Lüdicke, F., Schaller, J.-P., Vanscheeuwijck, P., Hoeng, J., Peitsch, M.C., 2016. Evaluation of the tobacco heating system 2.2. Part 1: description of the system and the scientific assessment program. Regul. Toxicol. Pharmacol. 81 (Suppl. 2), S17–S26. https://doi.org/10.1016/j.yrtph.2016.07.006.

Takahashi, Y., Kanemaru, Y., Fukushima, T., Eguchi, K., Yoshida, S., Miller-Holt, J., Jones, I., 2018. Chemical analysis and in vitro toxicological evaluation of aerosol from a novel tobacco vapor product: a comparison with cigarette smoke. Regul. Toxicol. Pharmacol. 92, 94–103. https://doi.org/10.1016/j.yrtph.2017.11.009.

Talhout, R., Schulz, T., Florek, E., van Benthem, J., Wester, P., Opperhuizen, A., 2011. Hazardous compounds in tobacco smoke. Int. J. Environ. Res. Publ. Health 8, 613–628. https://doi.org/10.3390/ijerph8020613.

Tierney, P.A., Karpinski, C.D., Brown, J.E., Luo, W., Pankow, J.F., 2016. Flavour chemicals in electronic cigarette fluids. Tobac. Contr. 25, e10–15. https://doi.org/10.1136/tobaccocontrol-2014-052175.

Uchiyama, S., Noguchi, M., Takagi, N., Hayashida, H., Inaba, Y., Ogura, H., Kunugita, N., 2018. Simple determination of gaseous and particulate compounds generated from heated tobacco products. Chem. Res. Toxicol. 31, 585–593. https://doi.org/10.1021/acs.chemrestox.8b00024.

Uchiyama, S., Ohta, K., Inaba, Y., Kunugita, N., 2013. Determination of carbonyl compounds generated from the E-cigarette using coupled silica cartridges impregnated with hydroquinone and 2,4-dinitrophenylhydrazine, followed by high-performance liquid chromatography. Anal. Sci. 29, 1219–1222. https://doi.org/10.2116/analsci.29.1219.

U.S. Consumer Products Safety Commission (US CPSC), 1993. Toxicity Testing Plan for Low Ignition-Potential Cigarettes, vol. 5. US CPS, Washington, DC.

Valavanidis, A., Vlachogianni, T., Fiotakis, K., 2009. Tobacco smoke: involvement of reactive oxygen species and stable free radicals in mechanisms of oxidative damage, carcinogenesis and synergistic effects with other respirable particles. Int. J. Environ. Res. Publ. Health 6, 445–462. https://doi.org/10.3390/ijerph6020445.

Vineis, P., Pirastu, R., 1997. Aromatic amines and cancer. Cancer Causes Control 8, 346–355. https://doi.org/10.1023/a:1018453104303.

Vorhees, D.J., Dodson, R.E., 1999. Estimation to Cigarette Smokers from Smoke Constituents in Proposed "Testing and Reporting of Constituents of Cigarette Smoke Regulations. Menzie-Cura & Associates, Inc.

Wang, P., Chen, W., Liao, J., Matsuo, T., Ito, K., Fowles, J., Shusterman, D., Mendell, M., Kumagai, K., 2017. A device-independent evaluation of carbonyl emissions from heated electronic cigarette solvents. PloS One 12, e0169811. https://doi.org/10.1371/journal.pone.0169811.

WHO, 2019. TobReg Scientific Recommendation: Updated Priority List of Toxicants in Combusted Tobacco Products.

WHO, 2019. TobReg Scientific Recommendation: Clinical Pharmacology of Nicotine in Electronic Nicotine Delivery Systems.

WHO, 2017. The Scientific Basis of Tobacco Product Regulation. Sixth report of a WHO study group (TobReg). WHOC Technical Report Series 1001.

WHO, 2015. WHO Study Group on Tobacco Product Regulation: Report on the Scientific Basis of Tobacco Product Regulations. Fifth Report of a WHO Study Group. Technical Report Series 989.

WHO, 2009. TobReg Scientific Recommendation: Devices Designed for the Purpose of Nicotine Delivery to the Respiratory System in Which Tobacco Is Not Necessary for Their Operation.

WHO, 2008. The Scientific Basis of Tobacco Product Regulation. Report of a WHO Study Group (TobReg). WHO Technical Report Series 951.

WHO, 2007. The Scientific Basis of Tobacco Product Regulation. Report of a WHO Study Group (TobReg). WHO Technical Report Series 945.

Williams, M., Villarreal, A., Bozhilov, K., Lin, S., Talbot, P., 2013. Metal and silicate particles including nanoparticles are present in electronic cigarette cartomizer fluid and aerosol. PLoS One 8, e57987. https://doi.org/10.1371/journal.pone.0057987.

Witschi, H., Espiritu, I., Maronpot, R.R., Pinkerton, K.E., Jones, A.D., 1997. The carcinogenic potential of the gas phase of environmental tobacco smoke. Carcinogenesis 18, 2035–2042. https://doi.org/10.1093/carcin/18.11.2035.

Wright, C., 2015. Standardized methods for the regulation of cigarette-smoke constituents. Trends Anal. Chem. 66, 118—127.

Xie, J., Marano, K.M., Wilson, C.L., Liu, H., Gan, H., Xie, F., Naufal, Z.S., 2012. A probabilistic risk assessment approach used to prioritize chemical constituents in mainstream smoke of cigarettes sold in China. Regul. Toxicol. Pharmacol. 62, 355—362. https://doi.org/10.1016/j.yrtph.2011.10.017.

Yu, V., Rahimy, M., Korrapati, A., Xuan, Y., Zou, A.E., Krishnan, A.R., Tsui, T., Aguilera, J.A., Advani, S., Crotty Alexander, L.E., Brumund, K.T., Wang-Rodriguez, J., Ongkeko, W.M., 2016. Electronic cigarettes induce DNA strand breaks and cell death independently of nicotine in cell lines. Oral Oncol. 52, 58—65. https://doi.org/10.1016/j.oraloncology.2015.10.018.

Zenzen, V., Diekmann, J., Gerstenberg, B., Weber, S., Wittke, S., Schorp, M.K., 2012. Reduced exposure evaluation of an Electrically Heated Cigarette Smoking System. Part 2: smoke chemistry and in vitro toxicological evaluation using smoking regimens reflecting human puffing behavior. Regul. Toxicol. Pharmacol. 64, S11—S34. https://doi.org/10.1016/j.yrtph.2012.08.004.

Zha, Q., Moldoveanu, S., 2004. The influence of cigarette moisture to the chemistry of particulate phase smoke of a common commercial cigarette. Beiträge zur Tabakforschung Int./Contribut. Tob. Res. 21, 184—191. https://doi.org/10.2478/cttr-2013-0779.

CHAPTER 5

Aerosol Physics and Dynamics

PASCAL PRATTE • JEAN-PIERRE SCHALLER • SERGE MAEDER

5.1 INTRODUCTION

In addition to their specific chemical compositions (Chapters 4, 6, and 7), aerosols have physical properties that may impact their respirability and volatility, two important parameters when evaluating their health effects through inhalation. In the context of electronic nicotine delivery product (ENDP) assessment, these are relevant parameters when assessing the impact of ENDP aerosols on nicotine delivery and health. Here, we present a brief overview of the key physical properties of aerosols and the techniques that are available for characterizing them. The aim is to provide general aerosol definitions, explain the working principles of instruments with their associated advantages/limitations, and describe some of their applications. Further details can be found in aerosol science textbooks. When not mentioned in the text, the statements introduced in this chapter refer to the *Aerosol Technology* textbook by W.C. Hinds (Hinds, 1999).

5.1.1 Aerosol Definition and Applications

A simple definition of an aerosol is that it is a collection of individual airborne physical objects of various sizes transported in a gas. These airborne physical objects may be in solid or liquid form (externally mixed) or both (internally mixed) and are characterized by a size ranging from 3 nm to a few hundred μm. At sizes larger than 1 mm, particles behave like macroscopic objects and are no longer an aerosol. At sizes smaller than 3 nm, the internal pressure of the particulate matter is so high that the structure often collapses and creates subnanometer molecular clusters. Many other alternative definitions of aerosol have become available in the literature since the term was first introduced in 1920 to refer to suspended particulate matter, aerocolloidal systems or dispersed systems (Hinds, 1999). This concept was first used to understand atmospheric processes such as cloud formation and was later extended to atmospheric pollution, strongly linked to

anthropogenic activities such as the use of combustion engines and natural occurrences such as volcanic eruptions or atmospheric photochemical reactions (Pandis et al., 1995). Aerosol emissions into the atmosphere generally impact the earth's radiative forcing and influence climate change (Kiehl and Trenberth, 1997). After 1980, industrial applications broadened and spread, leading to an increase in overall aerosol emissions. New technologies and manufacturing processes leading to emission of nanoparticles also raised concerns regarding human health and the risk of developing diseases (Bauer et al., 2010; Donaldson and Borm, 1998; Fariss et al., 2013; Klein et al., 2017; Rocha et al., 2010; You et al., 2015) and, consequently, increased mortality in the population (Pope et al., 2002). The risk of developing diseases is linked to physical and chemical aerosol properties taken together. Consequently, when studying how suspended particulate matter impacts health, it is imperative to consider the overall physicochemical properties of an aerosol, including its physical state, shape, and size-dependent chemical composition. In the next section, different aerosol emission sources will be described.

5.1.2 Aerosol Emission Sources and Size Classification

Aerosols released into the environment originate from numerous emission sources, are associated with different formation processes, and result in a range of suspended particulate matter with different physicochemical properties. Within this aerosol range, the two main families are defined as primary and secondary aerosols. Primary aerosols include, for instance, particles produced from erosion, grinding processes, ocean sprays, and biospore emissions. They are generally composed of suspended solid-like state or dust particulate matter characterized by an average size greater than 2.5 μm, the so-called coarse particle fraction or sedimentation mode. Given its large size, the coarse particle fraction is eliminated from the atmosphere within a few hours because of gravitational forces. In contrast, secondary aerosols are not formed mechanically but by indirect processes, such as vapor-to-droplet conversion or photochemical reactions and combustion (Hobbs, 2000). The resulting particulate matter can be in solid or liquid form or both physical states simultaneously. During their formation, secondary aerosols are often below a size of 100 nm and are categorized as the ultrafine particulate matter fraction. After a given aging time, coagulation starts while low volatile compounds condense on the existing seeds. These simultaneous processes allow secondary aerosols to reach an average size ranging from a few hundred nm to 1 μm. Consequently, aged secondary aerosols end up in the fine aerosol fraction also called the accumulation mode.

Different subcategories of aerosols are defined depending on the emission sources of secondary aerosols and the associated formation processes. To cite a few, mists are created mainly by the condensation of gas-phase water and organic acids, in particular, on to nanoscale dust particles when the dew point is reached. Fumes are generated during welding activities, in which a metal is exposed to plasma temperatures. In this case, a small amount of metal sublimates and results in a gas-phase metal, which condenses into droplets that rapidly solidify. In case a hot gas experiences a significant temperature drop, homogeneous nucleation may occur, and a secondary aerosol, categorized as a condensable aerosol, is released. The same process occurs during the formation of an aerosol from e-vapor products (EVPs) and electrically heated tobacco products (EHTPs). Another important aerosol category is smoke. In contrast to condensable aerosol, smoke is produced during the combustion process of a biomass and contains combustion-related nanoparticles in case the biomass is only partially thermally degraded (Butler and Mulholland, 2004). In fact, from incomplete combustion, organic residues aggregate and form a smoke containing combustion-related solid particles also called soot (Steiner et al., 2016). In this context, although smoke is an aerosol, an aerosol is not necessarily smoke. Because of their very different physicochemical properties, condensable aerosol or simply "aerosol" is the terminology associated with ENDPs, comprising EVPs and EHTPs, while "smoke" is used to describe combustion-related aerosols.

5.1.3 Aerosol Size and Time Evolution

When secondary aerosols are emitted into the environment, different mechanisms induce modifications to their physicochemical properties. These changes are attributed to, but not limited to, hygroscopic properties,

evaporation/condensation rates, transport mechanics, and coagulation/aggregation. Generally, the sources emit gases or vapors, which interact through chemical reactions or homogeneous and heterogeneous nucleation. Chemical reactions and high temperatures enable the formation of low volatile compounds and primary carbon particles, while homogeneous nucleation occurs in condensable aerosols. In the atmosphere, the more common process is heterogeneous nucleation where existing solid particles act as growing seeds for low volatile compounds to condense. In terms of energy, heterogeneous nucleation is favored over homogenous nucleation and explains phenomena such as fog and cloud formation (Mason, 1971). Homogenous nucleation needs to overcome a larger energy barrier to be initiated, where a sufficient amount of collisions in the gas phase is necessary to create stable nucleation seeds, while preventing them from evaporating during the time needed for the remaining gas phase to condense onto it. When the vapor pressure is in equilibrium with the liquid phase, the seeds reach a specific and relatively stable size. On a timescale of milliseconds to seconds, each suspended object is transported in random directions owing to Brownian motion, but at a slower pace than the gas phase. This random movement allows the particulate matter to collide and fuse via coagulation in case of droplets and aggregation in case of solid particles. As a result, the average aerosol particle size increases and, so, their number concentration decreases. In a timescale greater than minutes or hours, chemical reactions or reevaporation/condensation may occur. Generally, these phenomena are slow, and only marginally change the average particulate matter size before particles are removed from the carrier gas to surfaces by settling, diffusion, or rain.

5.1.4 Aerosol Size Distribution, Particulate Matter ("PMx"), Aerosol Deposition, and Size Definitions

As mentioned earlier, an aerosol is a collection of objects suspended in a carrier gas. In the case of an aerosol containing liquid droplets, the gas phase may be in thermodynamic equilibrium with the liquid (Beverley et al., 1998). This leads to a range of physicochemical properties that depend mainly on the emission sources. In order to characterize an aerosol, its chemical composition and associated physical properties are generally determined separately by using different techniques. While the chemical composition of an aerosol determines its biological effects, knowledge of its physical properties enables to determine how it is transported and delivered within a system such as the human lungs. Consequently, knowledge of an aerosol's physical properties is key both for estimating exposure to pollutants and optimizing therapeutic drug delivery via inhalation.

For characterizing the chemical composition of an aerosol, it is possible to collect samples by using filters and solvent traps and analyze their content by using analytical techniques such as liquid chromatography or gas chromatography coupled with mass spectrometric detection (Chapter 4). However, this does not provide information regarding the physical dimensions of the suspended particles or droplets. To do so, various techniques have been developed since the beginning of the 20th century by using different measurement principles. When analyzing an aerosol, the size distribution of its particles/droplets is measured. Because an aerosol generally contains particles/droplets with different sizes, the number or mass concentration of an aerosol is categorized into different size classes. Depending on how an aerosol evolves because of coagulation, condensation, evaporation, and chemical aging, the size distribution may increase or decrease around the average particle/droplet size value. Size distributions are often represented mathematically by using lognormal distributions instead of normal distributions, the rationale

being that a lognormal distribution cannot have negative values on the x-axis, which matches with the definition of diameter, which also cannot have a negative value (Hinds, 1999). Because lognormal distributions are skewed to the right-hand side, they are generally plotted to look like a normal distribution by using an x-axis with a logarithmic scale. From the fitted size distribution, two parameters are generally calculated. These are the count/mass median diameter (CMD/ MMD) and the geometric standard deviation (GSD), which are used to characterize the entire range of distribution properties. The lognormal distribution is a density function, implying that the area under the curve provides the total aerosol concentration linked to the dose fraction that can potentially be inhaled. Because each suspended object is assumed to be spherical, the associated mass depends on the third power of its diameter. Doubling the particle/droplet size increases the mass content by a factor of eight. However, because human lung geometry is complex, the associated deposition yield is not in a linear relationship with the particle/droplet size. In fact, competitive mechanisms, such as diffusion, settling, and impaction, result in a U-shaped deposition pattern, as shown in Fig. 5.1.

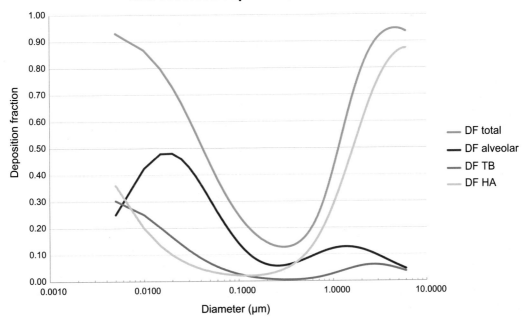

Size-resolved deposition fraction

FIG. 5.1 Size-dependent aerosol deposition fraction in human lungs for a person at rest. The green curve corresponds to the total deposition fraction (DF total), the *yellow curve* to the deposition fraction in the head airway fraction (DF HA), the *blue curve* to the deposition fraction in the tracheo–bronchial region fraction (DF TB), and the *red curve* to the deposition fraction in the alveolar region (DF alveolar). (Credit: W.C Hinds (Hinds, 1999).)

The larger the particle/droplet size, the higher the deposition in the head airways via settling and impaction mechanisms. If the aerosol particles/droplets are smaller than 300 nm, diffusion becomes increasingly dominant and leads to a relatively high fraction of deposition in the alveolar region. When an aerosol has an MMD of approximately 300 nm, diffusion, settling, and impaction are minimized, leading to a minimized aerosol deposition yield.

When considering aerosol inhalation into the human respiratory system, the aerosol particle/droplet size distribution provides an indirect but fair estimate of dose exposure. When solid water—insoluble particles are deposited in the lungs, dose exposure is evaluated by considering the particulate matter shape and its size-dependent chemical composition. For aerosols containing liquid droplets, the surrounding gas phase generally results in a higher chemical deposition yield than for suspended particulate matter alone. This is because gases diffuse faster than droplets, and, therefore, active compounds may be delivered more efficiently to the alveolar region if they are volatile enough. Consequently, aerosol size distribution taken alone is insufficient for estimating dose exposure in human lungs for liquid-/droplet-based aerosols. An alternative way to estimate the aerosol dose delivered in the lungs is to classify the droplets into larger size classes. For this purpose, coarse particulate matter was defined as PM_{10}, referring to the mass concentration of suspended particulate matter below or equal to 10 μm. This includes subcategories such as $PM_{4.0}$, referred to as respirable aerosol. $PM_{4.0}$ corresponds to a size below which at least 50% of the mass concentration can reach the alveolar region. This signifies that, out of the 50% of particulate matter passing through the trachea, only a fraction can deposit in the alveolar region, according to Fig. 5.1. Both PM_{10} and $PM_{4.0}$ are generally used to estimate the dose deposited in the upper part of the human respiratory system for aerosols containing particles with a large diameter, such as those for therapeutic drug delivery. Other categories are used to estimate the mass concentrations of aerosols that penetrate more deeply into the alveolar region. For instance, $PM_{2.5}$ is attributed to the fine particulate mass concentration fraction where at least 85% of suspended objects can reach the alveolar region. $PM_{1.0}$ corresponds to fine particulate matter equal to or smaller than 1 μm, in which at least 95% of the suspended objects can reach the alveolar region. Finally, $PM_{0.1}$ represents the ultrafine particles, or the so-called nanoparticles/nanodroplets, that penetrate at virtually 100% into the alveolar region. Owing to the simple definition for particulate matter, and the fact that direct gravimetric measurements can be achieved, regulatory bodies recommend determining PM_x gravimetrically for dose exposure estimation to pollutants or pharmaceutical aerosols (WHO Air Quality Guidelines, 2005).

5.1.4.1 Geometric diameter

In day-to-day life, the dimensions of macroscopic objects may be determined by using a ruler as a measuring tool, where the measurement is performed visually with a ruler exposed to the spectrum of natural or artificial white light. In this case, measurement is possible because the wavelengths present within white light are significantly smaller than common macroscopic objects. The same type of measurements is also possible when considering tiny objects magnified by using an optical microscope. When white light is used to perform an observation, it is said that geometric dimensions are measured (Hinds, 1999). However, the geometric diameter of spherical objects below 200 nm cannot be measured by using an optical microscope because white light wavelengths become equivalent to the dimensions of the object. However, it is still possible to observe nanoparticles by using wavelengths shorter than white light, such as the electron beams used in scanning electron microscopy techniques. A limitation to the measurement of geometric size diameter is that, for nonspherical particulate matter, the procedure for size measurement is not straightforward. One of the most popular techniques for determining the geometric diameter of tiny objects is to observe them by using an optical or a scanning electron microscope. To do so, the centroid of each particle is defined as the center of a circle that fits in the particle. This procedure is labor-intensive and, for obvious reasons, cannot be applied to needle-shaped particles or volatile liquid droplets, and it is not suitable for real-time measurements. Consequently, when the size distribution of an aerosol needs to be characterized, one solution is to introduce other size diameter definitions.

5.1.4.2 Aerodynamic diameter

One of the most important definitions of particle size involves indirect determination. The aerodynamic diameter is a measure of particulate matter behavior when accelerated in a flow. This parameter is defined as the equivalent sphere of unit density, having the same terminal velocity as a test aerosol for which the density and shape may be unknown. This definition has the advantage that particulate matter with different densities and shapes can be classified similarly, in accordance with their aerodynamic size diameter. In other words, aerodynamic diameter depicts how a given aerosol will be transported and deposited in a geometry such as the human lungs. The main application of the aerodynamic diameter is to estimate dose exposure in humans when exposed to indoor/outdoor particulate matter pollutants or therapeutic drugs. Although offline and real-time measurement techniques exist, aerodynamic aerosol sizing is generally limited to coarse and fine particulate matter and excludes the ultrafine fraction because of physical dynamic flow limitations.

5.1.4.3 Optical diameter

Optical diameter measurements are a good solution in certain cases where fast acquisition rates are needed to measure size distributions for aerosols as small as a couple of 100 nm in diameter. Similar to the definition for geometric diameter, optical size diameter is obtained by using light, although no visual observation is performed. In this case, the light beam interacts with the particulate matter, and the scattered light is collected to determine the physical properties of the aerosol, assuming that the particles are spherical. When all physical parameters of the suspended particles are known, the scattered light pattern can be used to determine the optical diameter of the suspended particulate matter. It is important to stress the fact that an optical diameter is a measure of how an incident light beam is scattered owing to the optical cross section of suspended objects. To do this, a high energy density monochromatic light wave is generally used to interact with particles. When a light source uses a wavelength close to the geometric size of individual particles, Mie scattering dominates the resultant scattering process (Hinds, 1999). In this case, the scattered light is a function of the observation angle, particle size/optical properties and light wavelength. When suspended objects in an aerosol pass individually through the light beam, Mie scattering provides a footprint for characterizing their optical diameter. For ultrafine particulate matter, where the light wavelength used is significantly larger than the particle geometric size, Rayleigh scattering dominates the scattering process. One of the major features of Rayleigh scattering is that it may be applied for the characterization of ultrafine particles/droplets or gases. In this case, forward and back scattering are more efficient, especially for shorter wavelengths (blue light), which explains why the sky looks blue on sunny days.

5.1.4.4 Mobility diameter

An alternative indirect measurement of aerosol physical properties is its mobility diameter. This is done by neutralizing or charging an aerosol and determining its trajectory when exposed to an electric field. In a case where an aerosol is neutralized in accordance with the Boltzmann charge equilibrium, only a small fraction of the charge remains on the suspended particulate matter. When subsequently applying an electric field in an engineered flow path containing the aerosol, only positively or negatively singly charged suspended particles can be deflected through a slit for further analysis according to their diameter-to-charge ratio. Alternatively, the suspended particulate matter can be charged to its maximum charging capacity and particle sizes are subsequently segregated into different size classes according to their aerosol electrical mobility. The mobility size diameter is generally used to characterize ultrafine particulate matter for high aerosol concentration sources. However, the main disadvantage of using the mobility size diameter definition is that the result depends on charging conditions that may differ from aerosol to aerosol.

5.1.5 Measurement Techniques and Challenges

Scientific instruments using these different sizing techniques can be purchased commercially for measuring suspended particulate matter size distributions. The selection of a methodology is generally made in consideration of the aerosol concentration and anticipated particle size distribution. Additional considerations may be the diameter type, how fast an aerosol is sized to avoid aging, and whether direct or indirect measurement is needed. Real-time techniques are preferred where a fast screening tool is required. This is typically the case for air pollution monitoring and clean room air control for fabrication processes or fundamental research. When an aerosol needs to be assessed for therapeutic applications, gravimetric methods are generally preferred for determining its aerodynamic diameter, although real-time techniques are also available for this purpose. This is because the gravimetric method allows direct size-segregated aerosol mass reading for evaluating dose exposure in human lungs. In general, instruments are unable to measure multiple parameters, and each measurement technique only allows measurement of a specific aerosol size parameter (i.e., geometric, aerodynamic, optical, or mobility diameter). Each method has advantages and limitations and is selected according to the required application. The next subsections provide a very brief and generic overview of available technologies.

5.1.5.1 Aerodynamic sizers

Aerodynamic sizers are used when aerosols with different particle densities and shapes need to be compared. In this case, the suspended objects' terminal velocities are measured and size-segregated according to their inertia. The test aerosol is generally diluted to ensure that individual suspended objects enter the inlet of the sizer. Downstream of the inlet, a dilution flow surrounding the aerosol allows it to accelerate and ensures that the suspended objects reach their terminal velocity. Further down the flow, a red-light laser is split into two parallel beams with a predefined distance in accordance with the instrument design. When a suspended object passes through the first and second beams, the scattered light is detected by a photomultiplier tube at different time intervals. On the basis of the interval between the first and second beam measurements, the time of flight of the suspended object is calculated, and the event is recorded. In accordance with the definition of aerodynamic diameter, the terminal velocity is used to calculate the aerodynamic diameter for each detected event. As a result, an aerodynamic size distribution can be obtained every second. This technique has the advantage of measuring the real-time physical properties of an aerosol and is useful for estimating dose exposure. The drawback of this technique is that dilution is needed to ensure that individual suspended objects enter one by one into the detection zone of the instrument. As a result, this dilution may affect the size distribution for volatile particles prior to their measurement, leading to underestimation of their original size. A second disadvantage is that the time-of-flight technique can only be applied for aerodynamic diameters above 500 nm. Below this size, all suspended objects match the air stream velocity, and size differentiation can no longer be achieved.

Alternatively, aerodynamic diameter can be determined by using offline techniques. One of the most popular methods is the use of a multistage cascade impactor, which enables collection of suspended particulate matter according to their inertia. An impactor consists of several stages, where each stage is a combination of nozzle and collection plate/surface. When an aerosol passes through a nozzle, the suspended particulate matter is accelerated, and particles larger than a critical size impact with the collection surface. Smaller particles flow around the collection surface and are transported to the next impactor stage and accelerated further so that smaller particle sizes are collected. To obtain a measurement for aerodynamic diameter, the different collection surfaces are weighed before and after aerosol collection. Because each impactor stage is characterized by a particle size range, the associated mass distribution can be plotted against the average particle size for each stage to obtain the aerosol aerodynamic diameter. The

main advantage of this technique is that the mass is measured directly and can be used to estimate dose exposure in human lungs (WHO Air Quality Guidelines, 2005). However, it has the disadvantage of being a very labor-intensive technique that is also not appropriate for the assessment of volatile aerosols.

5.1.5.2 Optical sizers
Optical sizers are often used in situations where rapid data acquisition is required, for example, when performing air quality monitoring. Different adapted laser wavelengths can be used depending on the instrument design and required working ranges for particle concentration and size. Currently, most optical sizers use Mie scattering to obtain optical size distributions ranging from a few hundred nm to several μm. This instrument type is commonly referred to as an optical particle counter (OPC), and it requires the suspended particles to enter into the laser beam section of the equipment one by one. The resulting scattered light for each suspended particle is detected by using a fixed wide-angle photodetector. The signal is interpreted to give the optical size of the suspended particulate matter on the basis of calibration performed with standard monodisperse spherical particles of known refractive indices. Calibration is an important step because the optical properties of an aerosol significantly affect the Mie scattering pattern and, hence, the data interpretation. Clearly, the closer the optical properties and geometrical shape of a test aerosol and the standard particles used for calibration are, the better will be the accuracy of measurement. Generally, the standard particles used for calibrating an OPC are nonabsorbing white monodisperse polystyrene sphere latex (PSL) particles. Consequently, an OPC cannot provide accurate data for the assessment of light-absorbing test aerosols, such as soot particles. Another simple way to characterize the physical properties of an aerosol is to use a photometer that measures scattered light at fixed narrow angles. In this case, the scattered light is less sensitive to the aerosol's refractive index, and it is possible to measure multiple suspended particles simultaneously and directly determine the aerosol mass concentration for large particle size classes, such as PM_x. Again, photometers need to be calibrated against gravimetric measurements in order to compensate for any physicochemical property differences between standard particles and those present in test aerosols.

5.1.5.3 Mobility diameter sizers
In cases where fine and ultrafine suspended particles need to be evaluated, measurement of electrical

mobility diameter is generally a good choice. When an aerosol is electrically neutralized, or charged, it can be sized by applying an electric field while measuring the movement of the suspended particulate matter. A frequently applied technique for measuring an aerosol's electrical mobility diameter uses a scanning mobility particle sizer. The aerosol is first neutralized and then introduced into a cylindrical column where a range of differential voltages are applied sequentially (scanned) to evaluate different particle size fractions, which are quantified by using a particle counter. The resulting data provide an electrical mobility size spectrum, ranging from approximately 10 to 1000 nm. A limitation of this technique is that a stable aerosol concentration is needed. This means that an aerosol cannot be measured when its concentration is transient, as is the case for cigarettes or ENDPs, where aerosol-generating puffs only last a few seconds. A second limitation is the fact that suspended particulate matter larger than 600 nm in size may carry multiple charges, which may introduce experimental artifacts even if mathematical corrections are applied.

An alternative type of instrument using corona discharge can also measure the electrical mobility diameter of an aerosol in real time. The corona discharge transfers the maximum possible electrical charge to the suspended particulate matter, and the applied voltage creates an electric field in a partial vacuum, which deflects the suspended particulate matter according to size. In other words, different particle sizes are characterized by different times of flight, which are collected at different positions on a segmented electrode rod coupled to an electrometer (or conductive impactor plates for some instruments). Each segment or impaction plate then measures the resulting electrical current, which is proportional to the particle number concentration. Although advantageous because measurements are performed in real time, this type of instrument is not suitable for evaluating volatile aerosols because of the evaporation in the low vacuum chamber and the fact that the electrometers are not sufficiently sensitive for measuring low particle number concentrations.

5.2 AEROSOL SIZE IN ENDPS
5.2.1 ENDP Aerosol and Cigarette Smoke Physical Assessment Strategy
As discussed earlier, a condensable aerosol is a secondary aerosol that is formed in the absence of combustion; it is simply referred to as "aerosol." By contrast, a combustion aerosol is commonly referred to as "smoke." Both

condensable aerosol and smoke are aerosols, but with substantially different physicochemical properties. A key point to consider when performing physical measurements of an aerosol is to define in what context the results will be used. Two approaches are used for assessing the physical properties of ENDP aerosols: real-time and offline measurements. Real-time tools are generally preferred for rapid screening and research purposes. These techniques enable direct comparison of different aerosols in terms of their physical properties while minimizing aerosol aging, which could bias the outcome of any comparison. Offline gravimetric methods are often used in cases where the aerodynamic diameter of an aerosol needs to be measured for estimating dose exposure or where size-segregated chemical analyses are required (WHO Air Quality Guidelines, 2005). In the next subsection, both approaches are addressed.

5.2.2 Aerosol Sizing Techniques for ENDPs
5.2.2.1 Laser scattering methodology and physical characterization of ENDP aerosols
As previously mentioned, real-time data acquisition can be used to characterize and compare ENDP aerosols and to verify whether or not an aerosol is respirable (mass median aerodynamic diameter [MMAD] <2.5 μm). Because EVPs and EHTPs produce condensable aerosols, the associated droplet sizes are generally in the submicron range. Aerodynamic sizers cannot measure particle/droplet sizes below 500 nm; therefore, it is not recommended to use such an instrument for physical characterization of ENDP aerosols. Optical and mobility sizers are generally considered to be good alternatives for measuring submicron droplet size distributions, although these techniques only provide an estimate of the actual size distribution. This is because the PSL particles used for calibrating these instruments have electrical potential and optical properties that generally differ from those of test aerosols. However, because the chemical composition of ENDP aerosols is much simpler than that of cigarette smoke, accurate estimates for ENDP aerosol size distributions may be achieved by using well-calibrated mobility or optical sizers. Owing to the inherent volatility of ENDP aerosols, droplet evaporation is the main issue associated with these measurements.

Since the beginning of the 21st century, many researchers have studied the particle/droplet size distributions in ENDP aerosols by using different techniques, but the size distribution results have been inconsistent from study to study. These studies used different equipment to obtain size distribution results for a range of

ENDPs, characterized by various cooling rates, applied power, liquid formulations, and tobacco substrate composition (Brown and Cheng, 2014). It is clear from this that accurate documentation regarding the testing conditions used when evaluating aerosol particle size distributions is required to ensure that consistent data are generated for comparative purposes.

For performing real-time measurements with ENDP aerosols, a TSI Laser Aerosol Spectrometer 3340 (LAS; TSI Incorporated, Shoreview, MN) was calibrated to measure optical size distributions and concentrations for spherical ENDP suspended droplets. The instrument monitored the scattering pattern of individual droplets by using a highly focused laser beam for optical sizes ranging from 0.090 to 7.500 μm in diameter. To determine whether the instrument calibration had been performed correctly by the supplier, four different standard PSL monodisperse particle sizes were selected to verify the accuracy and linearity of the instrument. This verification involved five repetitions per chosen PSL per day and was repeated over 3 days. The linearity of the size response for each day was determined together with the slope, intercept, and coefficient of determination (R^2), as shown in Table 5.1. For each testing day, the slopes ranged from 0.99 to 1.15, with an R^2 of 0.996−0.999, indicating excellent linearity, with a maximum slope variability of 15% when compared with the expected theoretical unit value. More details on the procedure and experimental setup have been published previously (Pratte et al., 2016).

To determine the impact of measuring an aerosol with a different refractive index than PSL particles (index of refraction, 1.59; see Table 5.3), di-ethyl-hexyl-sebacate (DEHS) monodisperse droplets (index of refraction, 1.45; see Table 5.3) of different sizes were produced by using a TSI Condensation Monodisperse Aerosol Generator.

The DEHS droplet size was determined by using a TSI particle aerosol monitor (PAM), which characterized the DEHS aerosols during the LAS measurements by measuring the light scattered at 90 degrees, assuming a monodisperse distribution and fixed refractive index. By using the PSL calibration, DEHS droplets were introduced into the instrument, and the size response was plotted as a function of the PAM output. When considering individual testing days, the linear fitting of the data was characterized by an R^2 value >0.993 (see Table 5.2). Although the LAS size response was found to be linear, DEHS droplet sizes were underestimated (the slope values were between 0.872 and 0.913, lower than the expected value of 1, over the three testing days). The black dots shown in Fig. 5.2 are the average measured size values for PSL particles; the dashed lines represent the boundaries for their likely distribution on the basis of the ±5% accuracy claimed by the instrument manufacturer. Clearly, the LAS response for PSL particles showed no bias when the PSL calibration curve was used. However, the triangle symbols in Fig. 5.2, representing DEHS droplets, reveal a clear bias, as the data points do not fall within the dashed lines. This demonstrates that a 9% variation in refractive index impacts the LAS size response and results in a negative bias of approximately 15%−20%. This 15%−20% bias does not account for any droplet evaporation, which may reduce droplet size prior to measurement. In practice, when droplets/particles with a refractive index similar to DEHS are tested, a correction factor of 1.20 should be applied to the particle size estimates.

5.2.2.2 Laser scattering methodology applied to ENDP aerosols

The aim of measuring the size response for selected DEHS droplets versus a PSL calibration was to verify whether adequate size distribution measurements can

---

TABLE 5.1
Fitting Parameters Calculated From Fitted LAS Linear Size Response Against PSL Supplier-Claimed Values.

Day	Slope	Intercept	R^2
1	0.99	−25.74	0.997
2	1.15	−57.97	0.996
3	0.96	10.33	0.999

LAS, laser aerosol spectrometer; PSL, polystyrene sphere latex.
Adapted from Pratte, P., Cosandey, S., Goujon-Ginglinger, C., 2016. A scattering methodology for droplet sizing of e-cigarette aerosols. Inhal. Toxicol. 28 (12), 537−545.

TABLE 5.2
Fitting Parameters Calculated From Fitted DEHS Linear Size Response Against DEHS Size Values Measured with PAM.

Day	Slope	Intercept	R^2
1	0.906	−78.610	0.995
2	0.913	−71.620	0.993
3	0.872	−17.495	0.999

DEHS, di-ethyl-hexyl-sebacate; PAM, particle Aerosol monitor.
Adapted from Pratte, P., Cosandey, S., Goujon-Ginglinger, C., 2016. A scattering methodology for droplet sizing of e-cigarette aerosols. Inhal. Toxicol. 28 (12), 537−545.

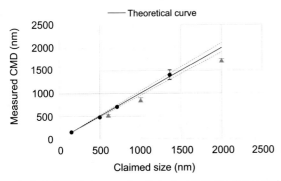

FIG. 5.2 LAS Response for Selected PSL Particles and DEHS Droplets as a Function of Expected or Claimed Values. *Circles* (●) and *triangles* (▲) represent the average count median diameters calculated for PSL and DEHS size distributions, respectively. *Error bars* represent the standard deviation of the data points. *Dashed straight lines* are upper and lower limits within which no bias is considered, taking instrument uncertainty into account. *CMD*, count median diameters; *DEHS*, di-ethyl-hexyl-sebacate; *LAS*, laser aerosol spectrometer; *PSL*, polystyrene sphere latex. (Adapted from Pratte, P., Cosandey, S., Goujon-Ginglinger, C., 2016. A scattering methodology for droplet sizing of e-cigarette aerosols. Inhal. Toxicol. 28 (12), 537–545.)

TABLE 5.3
Commercially Available e-Cigarettes Tested in the Study.

Sample	Formulation composition	Refractive index
PSL	N/A	1.59[b]
DEHS	N/A	1.45[b]
(A) e-cigarette Blu 18 mg[a]	75% glycerin, 25% water	1.436 ± 0.005
(B) e-cigarette Mark10 regular[a]	1.14% nicotine, 50.96% glycerin, 27.86% propylene glycol, 15.91% water, 4.13% others	1.436 ± 0.005
(C) e-cigarette Mark10 menthol[a]	1.18% nicotine, 2.29% menthol, 50.96% glycerin, 26.36% propylene glycol, 15.94% water, 3.27% others	1.429 ± 0.005
(D) e-cigarette Nicolite 16 mg[a]	20.20% glycerin, 74.13% propylene glycol, 5.96% water	1.433 ± 0.005

DEHS, di-ethyl-hexyl-sebacate; *PSL*, polystyrene latex spheres.
[a] Measured values via an Abbe refractometer;
[b] literature values (Eidhammer et al., 2008).
Adapted from Pratte, P., Cosandey, S., Goujon-Ginglinger, C., 2016. A scattering methodology for droplet sizing of e-cigarette aerosols. Inhal. Toxicol. 28 (12), 537–545.

be obtained for aerosols with refractive indices differing slightly from that of PSL. As demonstrated by the size response determined for selected DEHS droplets, the LAS produced a linear response, but the response has a systematic bias. EVPs produce an aerosol primarily composed of propylene glycol, glycerin, water, nicotine, and flavors. Consequently, prior to conducting e-vapor measurements, the refractive index of each tested liquid formulation was measured and compared with DEHS by using an Abbe refractometer. Data regarding the refractive index of each liquid tested are presented in Table 5.3. A relative difference smaller than 3% was observed between the refractive index values of DEHS and the liquid formulations, which was considered to be comparable. Therefore, the droplet size distributions for EVPs determined by using this methodology should be assumed to be linear and require correction for size underestimation of 15%–20%.

The EVPs identified in Table 5.3, with their associated e-liquid formulations, were used to produce puffs under the Health Canada Intense smoking regimen: 55-mL puff volume and 2-s puff duration (Canada, 1999). For conducting the tests, two different setups (Fig. 5.3) coupled to an LAS were used to obtain droplet size distributions, from which the count median diameter (CMD) and GSD were calculated as representative parameters. In the setup shown in Fig. 5.3A, aerosol was

produced by creating a negative pressure drop at the mouthpiece of the EVPs by pulling back the piston of a programmable dual syringe pump (PDSP). As a result, aerosol was drawn into the cylinder housing of the PDSP piston during a 2-s puff. The aerosol was then immediately exhausted from the PDSP housing by the return of the piston, pushing out the aerosol over a period of 1.4 s into two TSI aerosol diluters. A 1:10,000 dilution of the aerosol was made, ensuring that the droplets entered one by one into the LAS detector. Although the TSI diluters are designed to minimize droplet evaporation, e-vapor aerosols are generally considered to be highly volatile (Ingebrethsen et al., 2012; Schripp et al., 2013), and droplet sizes may change prior to measurement. The use of the PDSP pump in this setup increased the aerosol residence time by at least 3.4 s prior to measurement, which could have led to changes in aerosol size and concentration

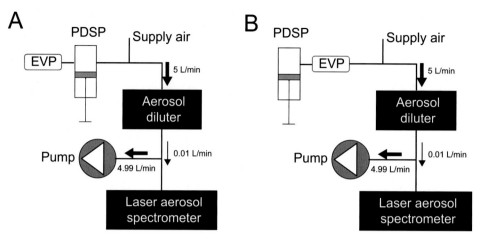

FIG. 5.3 **(A)** (standard setup) and **(B)** (monoport setup, represented by a rectangle between the PDSP and diluter), the two setups used to determine the size distributions of selected EVPs. *EVPs*, e-vapor products; *PDSP*, programmable dual syringe pump. (Adapted from Pratte, P., Cosandey, S., Goujon-Ginglinger, C., 2016. A scattering methodology for droplet sizing of e-cigarette aerosols. Inhal. Toxicol. 28 (12), 537–545.)

due to coagulation, wall deposition, and evaporation. In order to investigate the effects of this residence time prior to aerosol detection, an in-house monoport aerosol generator was developed, which forced air through the EVPs and transported aerosol directly into the measurement system, as shown in Fig. 5.3B.

The EVPs listed in Table 5.3 were evaluated by using the two experimental setups (Fig. 5.3A and B), and their relative aerosol size distributions were determined. Five replicates were evaluated by using the negative-pressure PDSP setup and three replicates by using the monoport (positive-pressure PDSP) aerosol generator. From the data generated, the CMD, GSD, and MMD parameters were calculated and reported in Table 5.4 (not corrected for bias). The use of the monoport aerosol generator led to droplet size distributions that partially exceeded the

LAS lower boundary working range. Consequently, the MMD parameters provided in Table 5.4 for the monoport aerosol generation setup should be interpreted as upper limit values. When comparing MMD data obtained for different EVPs tested by using the monoport aerosol generator, the values were found to be comparable, considering the uncertainties associated with the measurements. In the tests conducted with the PDSP setup, the MMD values differed for each e-cigarette, such that MMD(C) < MMD(A) ≈ MMD(D) < MMD(B) for samples C, A, D, and B, respectively. There were also significant differences between the MMD values obtained by using the two experimental setups. For all tested EVPs, the PDSP setup produced MMD values that were 17%–33% higher than the corresponding measurements made by using

TABLE 5.4
Calculated CMD, GSD, and MMD for Different Marketed EVPs.

Sample	MONOPORT CMD (nm)	GSD	MMD (nm)	PDSP CMD (nm)	GSD	MMD (nm)
(A)	138 ± 11	1.42	200 ± 26	166 ± 4	1.42	242 ± 19
(B)	136 ± 8	1.42	197 ± 25	191 ± 10	1.46	293 ± 19
(C)	130 ± 4	1.37	176 ± 10	158 ± 5	1.41	225 ± 9
(D)	136 ± 3	1.40	191 ± 8	163 ± 3	1.44	245 ± 6

CMD, count median diameter; *EVPs*, e-vapor products; *GSD*, Geometric standard deviation; *MMD*, mass median diameter.
Adapted from Pratte, P., Cosandey, S., Goujon-Ginglinger, C., 2016. A scattering methodology for droplet sizing of e-cigarette aerosols. Inhal. Toxicol. 28 (12), 537–545.

the monoport aerosol generator (see Table 5.4). This demonstrates the impact that aerosol residence time had on the resulting size distribution measurements. These differences in MMD can be attributed to thermal coagulation and gas-/vapor-phase condensation/evaporation processes occurring during the 3.4 s required to generate the aerosol and transfer it into the measurement system.

After this first evaluation, additional products were tested: two EVPs (same device but two different e-liquids) were compared with a reference cigarette (Kentucky 3R4F cigarette), the Tobacco Heating System 2.2 (THS), and a Carbon Heated Tobacco Product (CHTP). For the experiments, a PDSP was operated, as indicated in Fig. 5.3A, in accordance with the Health Canada Intense (55-mL puff volume and 2-s puff duration) and Cooperation Centre for Scientific Research Relative to Tobacco (2015) (55-mL puff volume, 3-s puff duration, and a square puff profile) regimens. The resulting MMD values, presented in Table 5.5, show that the largest MMD was attributable to the smoke produced from the 3R4F Kentucky reference cigarette. Compared with the MMDs of the aerosols generated by THS, CHTP, and the two EVPs (under the Health Canada regimen), the MMD of cigarette smoke was greater by a factor of approximately 1.3–2.0. Furthermore, the MMD values of the THS, CHTP, and EVP aerosols obtained under the Health Canada regimen generally overlapped in the range 256–391 nm.

In order to evaluate how the physical properties of an e-vapor aerosol were affected when its residence time in the PDSP was increased prior to droplet/particle

size measurement, the CORESTA regimen (CORESTA, 2015) was applied for assessing the aerosol of both EVPs. As presented in Table 5.5, the droplet size approximately doubled when the CORESTA regimen was applied instead of the Health Canada regimen. Overall, under both smoking regimens, both smoke and aerosols were found to contain particles/droplets in the respirable range (256–522 nm), with the total deposition yield in the airways calculated to be less than 20% (see Fig. 5.1).

5.2.2.3 ENDP aerosol physical properties compared with values in the literature

To evaluate the comparability of the results presented in the preceding subsections with those of other researchers, the data were compared with previously published values derived from a variety of experimental techniques. One research group applied the light extinction technique for different wavelengths to determine real-time aerosol size distributions, reporting average droplet size diameters in the range of 272–458 nm for undiluted EVP aerosols (Ingebrethsen et al., 2012). Another group used an electrical mobility instrument (FMPS 3091) to report droplet sizes in the range of 120–165 nm for EVPs containing different levels of nicotine (Fuoco et al., 2014). In indoor air quality assessments, the size distributions ranged from 20 to 300 nm (Geiss et al., 2015); in in vitro tests, the droplet sizes ranged from 120 to 180 nm (Zhang et al., 2013). In another study, light scattering was used to determine the volume median diameter for commercial EVPs, which approximated to 435 nm when no dilution was applied (Cabot et al., 2013). However, direct

TABLE 5.5
Aerosol Physical Parameters of Different Products (Health Canada and CORESTA Regimen).

Product type	Aerosol regimen	Number of replicates	CMD (nm)	GSD	MMD (nm)
Kentucky reference 3R4F cigarette	PDSP—health Canada	3	314 ± 13	1.51	522 ± 25
Tobacco heating system	PDSP—health Canada	3	168 ± 8	1.47	261 ± 14
Carbon heated tobacco product	PDSP—health Canada	3	213 ± 48	1.55	391 ± 146
EVP 1	PDSP—health Canada	1	212	1.50	345
EVP 2	PDSP—health Canada	1	162	1.48	256
EVP 1	PDSP—CORESTA	3	265 ± 30	1.57	492 ± 44
EVP 2	PDSP—CORESTA	3	263 ± 37	1.57	487 ± 65

comparison with previously published data has limited value, as the studies have used various techniques to measure different diameter types (e.g., aerodynamic, mobility, and optical) with different dilutions and sampling times. In this chapter, for the EVPs tested, the reported MMD values varied from 225 to 492 nm, which is in general agreement with the values reported by other external research groups (20–458 nm).

When measuring the particle/droplet size distribution of ENDP aerosols, it is of paramount importance to ensure that the chosen methodology provides linear results and that any measurement bias is understood. In addition, aerosol conditioning prior to measurement (dilution, temperature, and aging) should be equivalent when comparing different ENDP aerosols. The aim is not to obtain absolute size distribution measurements but to ensure direct comparability among the results generated from different ENDPs. However, one should ensure that ENDP aerosols are respirable and determine if they can be delivered to the alveolar region of the lungs. This requires ENDP droplet size distributions to be in the fine particulate matter fraction, with droplets smaller than 2.5 µm and preferably below 1 µm in diameter. In general, the larger the droplets, the greater their deposition in the upper airways of the lungs instead of penetration down to the alveolar region. However, in the case of ultrafine droplets, especially those below 20 nm in diameter, deposition is actually increased in the upper airways, which reduces the amount reaching the alveolar region. In general, the best compromise is to obtain ENDP droplet size distributions ranging between 100 nm and 1.0 µm, which enables aerosols to reach the alveolar region and minimizes upper airways deposition.

To summarize, when ENDP aerosols are tested under controlled conditions, an instrument must be well calibrated and capable of delivering repeatable size distribution measurements. The results, however, are dependent on exact experimental conditions (e.g., residence time), given the evolving nature of aerosols; therefore, the reported results should always be accompanied by a precise methodological description.

5.2.2.4 Gravimetric techniques for measuring ENDP aerosol size distribution

ENDPs can also be evaluated by using offline techniques for measuring the aerodynamic diameter of their aerosols. Generally, gravimetric methodologies are preferred because direct mass readings provide the aerosol mass distribution without any speculation on droplet density and enable accurate estimations of dose exposure to aerosol-borne substances (WHO Air Quality Guidelines,

2005). When wall losses attributable to specific measurement devices are well characterized, gravimetric methodologies have a good degree of accuracy, especially in the case of dry particulate matter, where only limited evaporation may occur during aerosol transport. In the case of droplets containing volatile compounds, aerosol mass size determination is challenging. If we consider impactor techniques, droplets are impacted on various collection substrates according to their aerodynamic size, and volatile substances will partially evaporate during the experiment, which may lead to an underestimation of the mass reading. Fortunately, this effect self-compensates across the range of size distributions when volatile substances are distributed evenly throughout the aerosol at the point of generation. By minimizing aerosol dilution, droplets coagulate and reach a quasi-steady-state equilibrium, which results in a larger, more stable median aerosol diameter than that obtained by real-time techniques. Consequently, impactor data should be used to evaluate the upper size distribution limit for ENDP aerosols in order to determine the aerosol fraction reaching the alveolar region and estimate the deposition yield of the suspended particulate matter in the lungs.

5.2.2.5 Comparing the physical properties of THS aerosol and cigarette smoke

Size distribution measurements of aerosol droplets were conducted by using a PIXE multistage cascade impactor (PIXE International Corp., Tallahassee, FL, USA). The test items were connected to the inlet of a PDSP (Burghart Messtechnik GmbH, Wedel, Germany), and the outlet of the PDSP was connected to a glass T-junction, which facilitated aerosol dilution before entry into the cascade impactor. The outlet of the PIXE cascade impactor was connected to a pump (Vacuubrand GmbH & CO KG, Wertheim, Germany) (see Fig. 5.4) (Boué et al., 2020).

The PIXE cascade impactor was composed of nine impactor stages, and the average MMAD and GSD values were estimated by using data from 10 aerosol sample replicates. The size distribution parameters for THS aerosol and 3R4F cigarette smoke are presented in Table 5.6 (Schaller et al., 2016). The MMAD values were similar for both 3R4F smoke and THS aerosol, with average values of 0.8 and 0.7 µm, respectively. However, the GSD was somewhat higher for THS aerosol than for 3R4F smoke. The most appropriate way to interpret such data is to determine the probability of finding the aerosol mass in a given droplet size range. In general, a 95% probability is applied, defined by lower and upper boundaries calculated as MMAD/

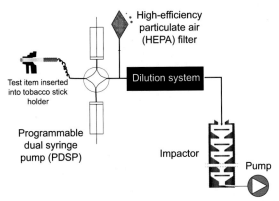

FIG. 5.4 Experimental setup for aerosol physical measurement. (Adapted from Boué, S., Goedertier, D., Hoeng, J., Kuczaj, A., Majeed, S., Mathis, C., et al., 2020. State-of-the-art methods and devices for the generation, exposure, and collection of aerosols from heat-not-burn tobacco products. Toxicol. Res. Appl. 4, 239784731989786.)

GSD^2 and MMAD × GSD^2, respectively. On the basis of these parameters, it was possible to determine whether 3R4F smoke and THS aerosol were respirable. To this end, the upper boundary values reported in Table 5.6 were compared with the maximum respirable aerosol size, which was 2.5 µm (for which at least 85% of the

aerosol reaches the alveolar region), and both smoke and aerosol were determined as being respirable.

When comparing these gravimetrically based MMAD measurements with the optical MMD values reported in Section 5.2, one can notice a substantial difference in the values, which deviate by more than 35%. As seen in Table 5.5, the MMD values for THS aerosol and 3R4F smoke were reported to be 261 ± 14 and 522 ± 25 nm, respectively. These values are significantly lower than the MMAD values obtained by using gravimetric measurements (0.7 and 0.8 µm for THS aerosol and 3R4F smoke, respectively) (Table 5.6), the difference being attributed to several factors. First, the MMD and MMAD measurements were determined by using different size diameter definitions. MMD is determined as the optical cross section of the aerosol/smoke particles, and MMAD is determined from their aerodynamic properties. Second, optical measurements require a relatively high dilution prior to the measurement, in contrast to the gravimetric approach, where the dilution is maintained as low as possible. As a result, droplet evaporation was enhanced in the optical measurements, resulting in the MMD values being lower compared with the gravimetrically determined MMAD values. Finally, the residence time of the aerosol/smoke prior to measurement was longer in the

TABLE 5.6
MMAD and GSD Results for 3R4F Smoke and THS Aerosol.

	3R4F SMOKE				THS AEROSOL			
Repetition	MMAD [µm]	GSD	LB [m]	UB [µm]	MMAD [µm]	GSD	LB [µm]	UB [µm]
1	0.9	2.1	0.4	1.8	0.8	2.6	0.3	2.1
2	0.8	1.9	0.4	1.5	0.7	2.3	0.3	1.7
3	0.8	1.9	0.4	1.5	0.7	2.1	0.3	1.4
4	0.9	1.7	0.5	1.5	0.7	1.9	0.4	1.3
5	0.9	1.6	0.5	1.4	0.7	2.0	0.3	1.3
6	0.8	1.9	0.4	1.5	0.7	2.2	0.3	1.6
7	0.9	1.9	0.5	1.6	0.8	2.5	0.3	1.9
8	0.6	1.4	0.5	0.9	0.6	2.3	0.3	1.3
9	0.8	1.8	0.5	1.5	0.6	2.3	0.3	1.5
10	0.7	1.8	0.4	1.3	0.7	3.2	0.2	2.3
Mean	0.8	1.8			0.7	2.3		
Mean GSD		1.3				1.5		

GSD, geometric standard deviation; LB, lower boundaries with a 95% confidence interval; MMAD, mass median aerodynamic diameter; UB, upper boundaries with a 95% confidence interval.
Adapted from Schaller, J.P., Keller, D., Poget, L., Pratte, P., Kaelin, E., Mchugh, D., et al., 2016. Evaluation of the tobacco heating system 2.2. Part 2: chemical composition, genotoxicity, cytotoxicity, and physical properties of the aerosol. Regul. Toxicol. Pharmacol. 81 Suppl. 2, S27—S47.

gravimetric method, resulting in larger MMAD values because of droplet coagulation. Although the different measurement approaches resulted in different size parameter values, it can be concluded that both THS aerosol and 3R4F cigarette smoke are respirable, as their determined MMD and MMAD values were less than 2.5 μm. The differences highlighted here show the importance of accurately reporting the testing approach, thereby allowing the observed differences to be rationalized by taking into account the evolving nature of such liquid droplet–based aerosols.

5.3 AEROSOL MASS CONCENTRATION RATE OF DECAY

As discussed throughout this chapter, aerosols generated by a heating process, as in case of the THS or EVPs, have different physicochemical properties than smoke, which is a result of biomass combustion. A qualitative sign of this fact is the longer visual persistence of smoke in comparison to an aerosol when released in an indoor environment: When smoke is released in an indoor environment, it can be visible for several minutes, as opposed to aerosol produced by an ENDP, which vanishes within seconds. This difference in the level of visual persistence may be explained by the chemical composition of ENDP aerosols, which is substantially different from that of cigarette smoke. The scientific evidence in Chapter 7 demonstrates that cigarette smoke contains combustion-related solid particles with a large amount of low volatile compounds, whereas THS aerosol contains lower amounts of low volatile compounds and no solid particles. The composition of smoke allows it greater stability upon dilution and over time compared with an aerosol generated by a heating process. In order to demonstrate this scientifically, cigarette smoke and aerosol from THS and an EVP were introduced, in separate experiments, into a designed and controlled indoor air quality environment as schematically described in Fig. 5.5 (Mitova et al., 2016). The smoke or aerosol $PM_{2.5}$ mass concentration was monitored by using a

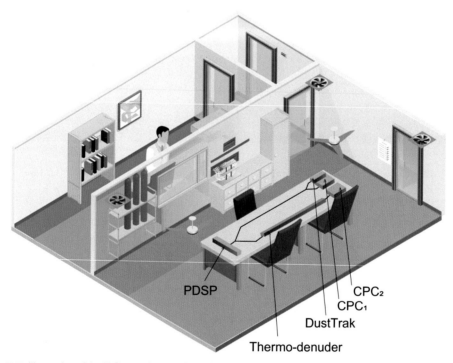

FIG. 5.5 Illustration of the IAQ room located in the facility of PMI R&D. The thermo-denuder and DustTrak unit measuring $PM_{2.5}$ for the less volatile and volatile fractions of the suspended particulate matter are identified in the figure. The condensation particle counter (CPC) units were used to measure the number concentration for the less volatile and volatile fractions of the suspended particulate matter. (Adapted from Mitova, M.I., Campelos, P.B., Goujon-Ginglinger, C.G., Maeder, S., Mottier, N., Rouget, E.G., et al., 2016. Comparison of the impact of the Tobacco Heating System 2.2 and a cigarette on indoor air quality. Regul. Toxicol. Pharmacol. 80, 91–101.)

real-time TSI DustTrak monitoring unit. The experiments were performed over a 5-day period by using a specially designed clean room with an applied ventilation rate of 0.5 h^{-1}. On each testing day, 1 h was dedicated to monitoring the background levels of PM$_{2.5}$, followed by a 2-h testing period where an aerosol, or smoke, was introduced into the room at the beginning of each hour (during the first 6−25 min). PM$_{2.5}$ data points were plotted as a function of time, as represented in Fig. 5.6 for cigarette smoke (commercially available brand, 0.5 mg nicotine) and THS aerosol and in Fig. 5.7 for EVP aerosol. For each hour of testing, the smoke or aerosol generation was stopped after 6−25 min, leading to a subsequent decay in aerosol mass concentration in the indoor air environment. The main reasons for the observed decline in PM$_{2.5}$ concentrations were the ventilation rate, wall deposition, and droplet evaporation.

In theory, if aerosol evaporation and wall deposition were assumed to be negligible, the time required to remove aerosol/smoke from the room would be driven

solely by the ventilation rate of decay (RD). This can be expressed in terms of the number of air changes per hour (h^{-1}) calculated by dividing the actual ventilation volumetric flow rate (m^3/h) by the volume (m^3) of the indoor air environment. Moreover, knowing the RD, the aerosol residence time (τ) can be calculated as $\tau = {}^1/_{RD}$, and, when three times τ is achieved, more than 95% of the aerosol will have been removed. In practice, aerosol wall deposition and evaporation effects are important, and τ should be measured rather than estimated from the ventilation rate. In order to calculate τ by using measured data, a natural logarithm conversion was applied to the aerosol mass concentration decay profile after aerosol generation was stopped. This produced a linear curve, from which the slope could be used to determine the actual RD and the related residence time τ. The inset in Fig. 5.6 shows a typical mathematical treatment applied to the smoke mass concentration profile of cigarettes, where the rates of decay were determined to vary between 0.80 and 0.83 h^{-1}, which were greater than the applied

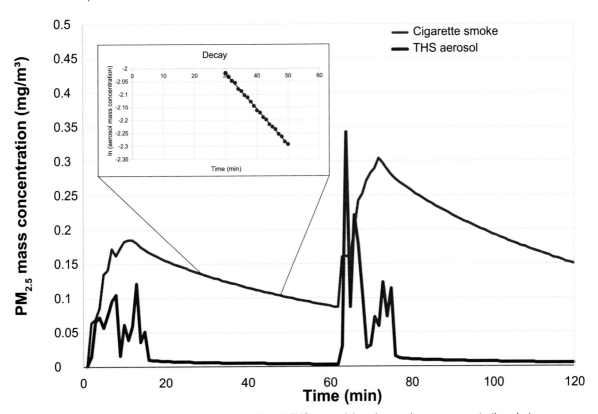

FIG. 5.6 Time-dependent smoke (*red curve*) and THS aerosol (*purple curve*) mass concentrations in two successive replicates. The inset in the figure shows the smoke mass concentration profile when the natural logarithm is applied. The slope of the straight line allows to calculate the effective rate of decay and the corresponding residence time.

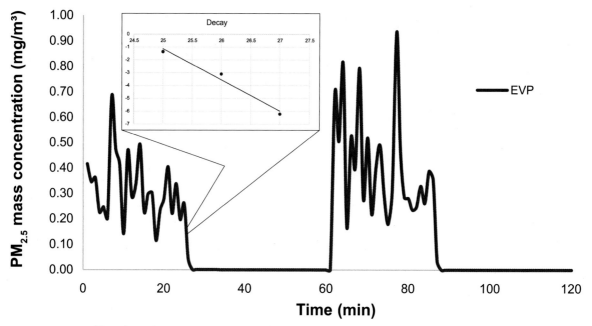

FIG. 5.7 Time-dependent e-vapor product (EVP) aerosol mass concentrations in two successive replicates. The inset in the figure shows the aerosol mass concentration profile when the natural logarithm is applied. The slope of the straight line allows to calculate the effective rate of decay and the corresponding residence time τ.

ventilation rate of $0.5\ h^{-1}$, excluding any consideration for wall losses or evaporation. In other words, the smoke mass concentration would be reduced by 95% after $3 \times \tau = 3 \times (1/0.8\ h^{-1}) = 3.75\ h$, as opposed to 6 h if the room ventilation rate alone was considered.

The same exercise was performed for the other tested products. For THS aerosol, it was only possible to estimate a RD, which equated to an aerosol lifetime of less than 1 min. This was because of the rapid evaporation of aerosol droplets occurring upon release into the indoor environment, which resulted in very few data points being generated (see Fig. 5.6). For the EVP aerosol, however, sufficient data points were obtained to achieve a reliable curve fit (see Fig. 5.7 inset). The calculated RD was found to be in the range $145{-}155\ h^{-1}$, which was considerably larger than the RD attributable to room ventilation alone ($0.5\ h^{-1}$). This means that the EVP aerosol mass concentration would be reduced by 95% after approximately 1 min, as opposed to 6 h if the room ventilation rate alone was considered. According to these results, EVP and THS aerosols dissipate approximately 225 times faster than cigarette smoke because of the higher volatility of ENDP aerosols compared with cigarette smoke.

5.4 SUMMARY

The intention of this chapter was to provide a general overview of aerosol definitions, aerosol physicochemical properties, and associated applications. An aerosol was defined as a collection of airborne objects of varying sizes suspended in a carrier gas. The concept of aerosol was discussed in light of its physical properties, including size distribution, which characterizes how the sizes of suspended particulate matter spread in the range of 3 nm to several 100 μm. Aerosols were categorized according to their formation process, with primary aerosols being produced mechanically and secondary aerosols being formed from vapor-to-droplet conversion, photochemical reactions, or combustion. Primary aerosols, often referred to as the coarse suspended particulate matter fraction (PM_{10} and $PM_{4.0}$), are rapidly eliminated from the atmosphere because of gravitational settling. In contrast, secondary aerosols are classified in the ultrafine or fine particulate matter fractions ($PM_{0.1}$ and $PM_{1.0}$ or $PM_{2.5}$), can persist in the atmosphere for hours or days, and are generally eliminated by diffusion mechanisms.

The importance of aerosol size distribution in relation to human dose exposure was also mentioned.

For coarse suspended particulate matter (PM_{10} and $PM_{4.0}$), the aerosol is mainly deposited in the upper part of the human respiratory tract. Smaller particulate fractions ($PM_{2.5}$ and $PM_{1.0}$) are considered to be the respirable fraction. In the context of evaluating the respirable fraction of an aerosol, different diameter definitions were introduced. Geometric diameter was defined as the size of an object determined by using light with wavelengths smaller than its relative size, by means of optical or scanning electron microscopy. However, real-time aerosol measurements are not possible with this technique. This chapter then introduced aerosol aerodynamic, optical, and mobility diameters. Aerosol aerodynamic diameter is derived from the measured terminal velocity of suspended objects with arbitrary density and shape, assuming an equivalent spherical diameter of unit density. It was also highlighted that the aerodynamic diameter could be obtained by both real-time and offline methodologies, and it was shown to be of key importance for estimating how an aerosol deposits in the human respiratory system. Optical and mobility diameters were also introduced, with particular attention paid to the optical diameter.

Physical property measurements for ENDP aerosols were separated into two complementary approaches. The first approach is used for fast screening and determining respirability; the second approach is used for estimating aerosol dose exposure. In the first case, an optical methodology was selected to evaluate ENDP aerosol physical properties for comparison with the values in the literature, and the mass median size diameters obtained by this method were found to be consistent with data in the public domain (20–458 nm). In this context, the size distribution values were considered to be comparable between different measurement devices, which can be used to assess aerosol respirability by considering the $PM_{2.5}$ definition. The gravimetric methodology is a labor-intensive approach, although essential for estimating the dose exposure in human lungs for a given aerosol. Here, a multistage cascade impactor (PIXE) was used to compare THS aerosol with smoke from the Kentucky reference 3R4F cigarette. The MMADs of 3R4F smoke and THS aerosol were found to be similar, with average values of 0.8 and 0.7 µm, respectively. When comparing gravimetrically based MMAD measurements with optical MMD measurements, a significant difference was observed in the reported values. This difference was attributed to various factors, such as the different size diameter definitions used, applied dilution, and aerosol residence time. Although the two different approaches resulted in different size parameter

values, it was concluded that both THS aerosol and 3R4F cigarette smoke comprise respirable suspended particulate matter, as their MMD and MMAD values were smaller than 2.5 µm.

Finally, this chapter addressed the major difference in volatility between ENDP aerosol and cigarette smoke, which is attributed to their different chemical and physical properties. To demonstrate this, cigarette smoke, THS aerosol, and an EVP aerosol were introduced, in separate experiments, into a specifically designed and controlled indoor air quality environment, where the $PM_{2.5}$ aerosol mass concentration was monitored by using a TSI DustTrak unit. After the smoke or aerosol emissions were stopped, the associated mass concentration decay rates of the ENDP aerosols were found to be higher than those of cigarette smoke by a factor of at least 225. This demonstrated that ENDP aerosols have higher volatility and substantially different physicochemical properties than cigarette smoke.

REFERENCES

Bauer, M., Moebus, S., Mohlenkamp, S., Dragano, N., Nonnemacher, M., Fuchsluger, M., et al., 2010. Urban particulate matter air pollution is associated with subclinical atherosclerosis: results from the HNR (Heinz Nixdorf Recall) study. J. Am. Coll. Cardiol. 56 (22), 1803–1808.

Beverley, K.J., Clint, J.H., Fletcher, P.D.I., 1998. Evaporation rates of pure liquids measured using a gravimetric technique. Phys. Chem. Chem. Phys. (1), 149–153.

Boué, S., Goedertier, D., Hoeng, J., Kuczaj, A., Majeed, S., Mathis, C., et al., 2020. State-of-the-art methods and devices for the generation, exposure, and collection of aerosols from heat-not-burn tobacco products. Toxicol. Res. Appl. 4, 239784731989786.

Brown, C.J., Cheng, J.M., 2014. Electronic cigarettes: product characterisation and design considerations. Tob. Control 23 (Suppl. 2), ii4–10.

Butller, K.M., Mulholland, G.W., 2004. Generation and transport of smoke components. Fire Technol. 40, 149–176.

Cabot, R., Koc, A., Yurteri, C.U., Mcaughey, J., 2013. Poster: aerosol measurement of e-cigarettes. In: 32nd Annual Conference, American Association for Aerosol Research, Portland, OR.

Canada, H., 1999. Test Method T-115, Determination of "Tar", Nicotine and Carbon Monoxide in Mainstream Tobacco Smoke.

CORESTA, 2015. 2014 Electronic Cigarette Aerosol Parameters Study. E-Cigarette Task Force, Technical report. https://www.coresta.org/sites/default/files/technical_documents/main/ECIG-CTR_ECigAerosolParameters-2014Study_March2015.pdf.

Donaldson, K., Borm, P.J., 1998. The quartz hazard: a variable entity. Ann. Occup. Hyg. 42 (5), 287–294.

Eidhammer, T., Montague, D.C., Deshler, T., 2008. Determination of index of refraction and size of supermicrometer particles from light scattering measurements at two angles. J. Geophys. Res. 113 (D16), D16206.

Fariss, M.W., Gilmour, M.I., Reilly, C.A., Liedtke, W., Ghio, A.J., 2013. Emerging mechanistic targets in lung injury induced by combustion-generated particles. Toxicol. Sci. 132 (2), 253–267.

Fuoco, F.C., Buonanno, G., Stabile, L., Vigo, P., 2014. Influential parameters on particle concentration and size distribution in the mainstream of e-cigarettes. Environ. Pollut. 184, 523–529.

Geiss, O., Bianchi, I., Barahona, F., Barrero-Moreno, J., 2015. Characterisation of mainstream and passive vapours emitted by selected electronic cigarettes. Int. J. Hyg. Environ. Health 218 (1), 169–180.

Hinds, W.C., 1999. Aerosol Technology, Properties, Behaviour, and Measurement of Airborne Particles, 2nd Edition. John Wiley & Sons Inc., New York.

Hobbs, P.V., 2000. Introduction to Atmospheric Chemistry. Cambridge University Press.

Ingebrethsen, B.J., Cole, S.K., Alderman, S.L., 2012. Electronic cigarette aerosol particle size distribution measurements. Inhal. Toxicol. 24 (14), 976–984.

Kiehl, J.T., Trenberth, K.E., 1997. Earth's annual global mean energy budget. Bull. Am. Meteorol. Soc. 78, 197–208.

Klein, S.G., Cambier, S., Hennen, J., Legay, S., Serchi, T., Nelissen, I., et al., 2017. Endothelial responses of the alveolar barrier in vitro in a dose-controlled exposure to diesel exhaust particulate matter. Part. Fibre Toxicol. 14 (1), 7.

Mason, B.J., 1971. The Physics of Clouds, second ed.

Mitova, M.I., Campelos, P.B., Goujon-Ginglinger, C.G., Maeder, S., Mottier, N., Rouget, E.G., et al., 2016. Comparison of the impact of the tobacco heating system 2.2 and a cigarette on indoor air quality. Regul. Toxicol. Pharmacol. 80, 91–101.

Pandis, S.N., Wexler, A.S., Seinfeld, J.H., 1995. Dynamic of tropospheric aerosols. J. Phys. Chem. (99), 9646–9659.

Pope 3rd, C.A., Burnett, R.T., Thun, M.J., Calle, E.E., Krewski, D., Ito, K., et al., 2002. Lung cancer, cardiopulmonary mortality, and long-term exposure to fine particulate air pollution. J. Am. Med. Assoc. 287 (9), 1132–1141.

Pratte, P., Cosandey, S., Goujon-Ginglinger, C., 2016. A scattering methodology for droplet sizing of e-cigarette aerosols. Inhal. Toxicol. 28 (12), 537–545.

Rocha, M., Apostolova, N., Hernandez-Mijares, A., Herance, R., Victor, V.M., 2010. Oxidative stress and endothelial dysfunction in cardiovascular disease: mitochondria-targeted therapeutics. Curr. Med. Chem. 17 (32), 3827–3841.

Schaller, J.P., Keller, D., Poget, L., Pratte, P., Kaelin, E., Mchugh, D., et al., 2016. Evaluation of the tobacco heating system 2.2. Part 2: chemical composition, genotoxicity, cytotoxicity, and physical properties of the aerosol. Regul. Toxicol. Pharmacol. 81 (Suppl. 2), S27–S47.

Schripp, T., Markewitz, D., Uhde, E., Salthammer, T., 2013. Does e-cigarette consumption cause passive vaping? Indoor Air 23 (1), 25–31.

Steiner, S., Bisig, C., Petri-Fink, A., Rothen-Rutishauser, B., 2016. Diesel exhaust: current knowledge of adverse effects and underlying cellular mechanisms. Arch. Toxicol. 90 (7), 1541–1553.

WHO Air Quality Guidelines, 2005. WHO Air Quality Guidelines for Particulate Matter, Ozone, Nitrogen Dioxide and Sulfur Dioxide. Summary of Risk Assessment.

You, R., Lu, W., Shan, M., Berlin, J.M., Samuel, E.L., Marcano, D.C., et al., 2015. Nanoparticulate carbon black in cigarette smoke induces DNA cleavage and Th17-mediated emphysema. Elife 4, e09623.

Zhang, Y., Sumner, W., Chen, D.R., 2013. In vitro particle size distributions in electronic and conventional cigarette aerosols suggest comparable deposition patterns. Nicotine Tob. Res. 15 (2), 501–508.

CHAPTER 6

Advanced Analytical Chemistry Methods to Characterize ENDP Aerosols

MARK BENTLEY • SERGE MAEDER

6.1 INTRODUCTION

Cigarette smoke contains more than 6000 constituents (Rodgman and Perfetti, 2013), which are distilled from tobacco or formed during pyrolysis and combustion reactions when tobacco is burned (Baker, 1987). Among these 6000+ chemicals, more than 100 are considered to be harmful and potentially harmful constituents (HPHCs). Their presence has been confirmed by various scientific and regulatory bodies (Burns et al., 2008; FDA, 2012a; IARC, 2004). In light of this knowledge, such regulatory bodies have compiled priority lists of smoke constituents (Burns et al., 2008; FDA, 2012a; Health Canada, 2000), and the US Food and Drug Administration (FDA) and World Health Organization's (WHO's) TobReg have mandated the monitoring and reporting of selected toxicants in cigarette emissions (FDA, 2012a; WHO, 2019). In the absence of information to the contrary, it is assumed that these HPHCs measured in cigarette smoke are also relevant for electrically heated tobacco products (EHTPs), which would include the Tobacco Heating System 2.2 (THS) developed by Philip Morris International (PMI).

In order to evidence the risk reduction potential of its electronic nicotine delivery product portfolio, PMI uses a structured scientific assessment program covering both nonclinical and clinical evaluations, which was applied for assessment of THS (Smith et al., 2016). The nonclinical assessment of THS involved targeted measurement of priority toxicants listed by the WHO (WHO, 2019) and Health Canada (Health Canada, 2000), and the FDA reduced panel of 18 constituents (FDA, 2012a), all of which are present in the list of 54 HPHCs routinely measured by PMI for development of EHTPs (Chapter 4). In addition, the list of 93 constituents identified as HPHCs by the FDA (2012b) were

also measured as a part of this nonclinical assessment (Chapter 4). Significant reductions were reported in the levels of all these priority toxicants in THS aerosol relative to the smoke of the 3R4F reference cigarette (University of Kentucky Center for Tobacco Reference Products, n.d.), with the majority of HPHCs being comparatively reduced by more than 90% (Schaller et al., 2016, Chapter 4).

However, despite these significant reductions in HPHCs in EHTP aerosols and an associated reduction in in vitro toxicity relative to 3R4F smoke (Schaller et al., 2016), the potential presence of toxicants beyond those highlighted by regulatory bodies—and those determined by using targeted methods—could not be discounted. Because lower temperatures are used for aerosol formation in heated tobacco products, where the absence of combustion has been confirmed (Cozzani et al., 2020), the question always arises as to whether a different set of toxicologically relevant compounds would be generated. To address this issue, PMI has applied a suite of untargeted analytical methods to more comprehensively characterize the aerosols delivered by EHTPs, represented by THS.

6.2 SCIENTIFIC APPROACH

In contrast to quantitative methods, which purely target chemical constituents (analytes) of interest to the exclusion of all others, untargeted methods are used to evaluate the chemical composition of a target chemical space by indiscriminate determination of all analytes relevant to that space. To that end, PMI has developed a portfolio of untargeted methods aimed at delivering maximum coverage of the chemical space related to tobacco-derived aerosols (Fig. 6.1). Because the chemical diversity of constituents within these aerosols is so

Toxicological Evaluation of Electronic Nicotine Delivery Products. https://doi.org/10.1016/B978-0-12-820490-0.00011-0

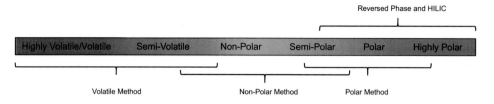

FIG. 6.1 Illustration of the suite of untargeted methods used to cover the anticipated chemical space of tobacco smoke and aerosol, indicating approximate overlaps between the methods. *HILIC*, hydrophilic interaction liquid chromatography. (Graphic from Bentley, M.C., Almstetter, M., Arndt, D., Knorr, A., Martin, E., Pospisil, P., Maeder, S., 2020. Comprehensive chemical characterization of the aerosol generated by a heated tobacco product by untargeted screening. Anal. Bioanal. Chem. 412, 2675–2685. https://doi.org/10.1007/s00216-020-02502-1.)

large, a number of overlapping methods using simplified sample collection and preparation techniques are required to ensure maximal analytical coverage. These methods are based on comprehensive two-dimensional gas chromatography with time-of-flight mass spectrometry (GCxGC–TOFMS) (Knorr et al., 2019) and liquid chromatography with high-resolution accurate mass spectrometry (LC–HRAM-MS) (Arndt et al., 2020). Although these methodologies were specifically developed to optimize analytical coverage, it is acknowledged that there will be some compromise associated with the application of nonspecific sample collection and preparation processes, and that some classes of chemicals will be less amenable to analysis than others. However, a range of different solvents suited to the different (overlapping) methods were used to minimize any shortfall, and only a small minority of constituents are considered to have been overlooked. For example, highly reactive compounds such as unstable radicals, which require specific analytical techniques for stabilization (or derivatization) prior to analysis, will be very short lived within the collection system. Mass spectrometric detection also has some limitations, such as its inability to detect compounds below the predefined scan range (such as carbon monoxide), metals, inorganic acids, ammonia, and compounds that do not easily ionize. There is also an upper mass range limitation of ca. 800 Da for the detection of chemical constituents. However, this was not expected to have had a significant impact, as compounds with a high molecular mass were not expected to have transferred substantially into the aerosol of THS, which relies on volatility for transfer. A number of other researchers have applied analytical screening techniques to investigate the composition of heated tobacco

aerosols in relation to cigarette smoke; however, the methods employed were only sufficient to characterize specific portions of the chemical space related to heated tobacco and cigarette aerosols (Savareear et al., 2019, 2018; Uchiyama et al., 2018).

Untargeted methods are semiquantitative, with the concentrations for large numbers of compounds being estimated versus a limited number of stable isotope–labeled reference materials of known concentration used as internal standards. For constituents amenable to gas chromatographic analysis, a comparison of quantitative values for recognized HPHCs determined by targeted methods with the corresponding semiquantified values from untargeted analysis demonstrated that, for analytes that were measurable by both techniques, untargeted analysis by GCxGC–TOFMS was able to semiquantify within a ±fourfold deviation from the true concentration (Knorr et al., 2019). A similar evaluation of the performance of liquid chromatography–based untargeted methods was not possible owing to the lack of comparative quantitative data, and semiquantification by this approach may only be described as being sufficient for estimating concentrations within a correct order of magnitude. Untargeted assessment is a time-consuming process, with the majority of the time being required for postanalysis data evaluation and the laboratory activities representing only a fraction of the overall effort. Each chromatographic peak for each individual chemical constituent requires in-depth evaluation for proposing a chemical name and providing a semiquantified concentration. Each experimentally determined mass spectrum is first compared with the mass spectra contained in both custom-built (Martin et al., 2012) and publicly/commercially available libraries; this produces a list of potential chemical (structural) proposals that can run into the hundreds. For each of these structural proposals, multiple prediction models are applied to predict parameters, such as boiling point, retention index, and fragmentation pattern, which are then compared with the experimentally determined values. Then, depending on the chemical structure identified for the chromatographic peak being evaluated, the most appropriate internal standard is used to provide a semiquantified estimate of abundance. In order to streamline this complex and highly time-consuming process, software platforms that automate the iterative steps required for accurately identifying each chemical constituent are used. For GCxGC–TOF methods, an in-house platform is used which interrogates mass spectral databases for spectral similarity and compares a number of predicted and measured parameters, including retention index and relative/absolute retention time in both chromatographic dimensions, in order to improve the confidence in identification (Knorr et al., 2019, 2013). For LC–HRAM-MS, a similar workflow is implemented by using the Progenesis QI software (Nonlinear Dynamics, Newcastle upon Tyne, UK), which also incorporates a modified MetFrag in silico fragmentation algorithm ("Nonlinear Dynamics web site. Progenesis QI theoretical fragmentation algorithm," n.d.; Wolf et al., 2010) to enable comparison of experimental and predicted first-order fragmentation spectra (Arndt et al., 2020).

The untargeted methodology developed at PMI may be applied in two different ways. When developing new platform concepts (such as EHTPs) or creating subsequent iterations of an existing platform, it is important to understand whether any new compounds are expressed in comparison to a reference product or a previous version. It is also important to identify whether any significant increases have occurred in the concentrations of constituents common to the "new" and "reference" product. To this end, untargeted differential screening is performed, whereby untargeted screening data from different products are statistically compared. Developed statistical models are used to filter compounds with significant differences, following which a ranking (RANK) procedure is used to consider the relative differences in abundance of each compound as well as the absolute abundance (Knorr et al., 2019). In this way, large differences between very low concentrations may be ranked as being less significant than smaller differences between very high concentrations. Because the ranking procedure is performed prior to extensive compound identification processes, it affords some reduction in the effort required for data processing. Where full characterization of a product's aerosol is required,

data processing for compound identification and semi-quantification is applied to all peaks identified. However, in this case, a reporting threshold of 100 ng/item (item = cigarette or tobacco stick) is applied, which serves to optimize the proportion of substances identified relative to a practicable amount of effort applied for their identification. It is estimated that less than 1% of the accumulated total mass estimated by untargeted analysis is represented by chemical constituents present in the aerosol at concentrations below this reporting threshold (Knorr et al., 2019). A concentration threshold is not applied for the untargeted differential screening process.

6.3 METHODS

A harmonized aerosol trapping approach was adopted for each of the analytical methods, because data from the different methods require combining to obtain final concentration values. Separate trapping is performed for the particulate phase and the gas–vapor phase (GVP), which together comprise the whole aerosol, thereby enabling individual chemical characterization of these two distinct phases. Aerosol from EHTPs and smoke from cigarettes are generated by using a linear smoking machine in accordance with the Health Canada Intense smoking regimen (Health Canada, 1999). The particulate phase, commonly referred to as total particulate matter (TPM), is collected by passing the smoke/aerosol through a Cambridge (glass fiber) filter pad. The GVP is trapped by using two microimpingers in series, which contain solvents maintained at subambient temperatures (Fig. 6.2).

For GCxGC–TOFMS analysis, internal standards for semiquantification are present within the solvents used to extract the Cambridge filter pads and within those used to trap the GVP. For LC–HRAM-MS, internal standards are added to the samples after aerosol collection but before chromatographic analysis. Aerosol samples are collected as an accumulation of smoke from up to three cigarettes or aerosol from up to five tobacco sticks for EHTPs. The number of accumulations is optimized to match the requirements for individual analytical methods, and replicate sample collection is performed for each required measurement (at least triplicate). The samples collected are then analyzed by GCxGC–TOFMS (Knorr et al., 2019) and LC–HRAM-MS (Arndt et al., 2020). Replicate injection of sample replicates for GCxGC–TOFMS analysis is not performed because of the highly complex nature of the sample extracts, particularly those for cigarettes, which reduces the effective lifetime of the chromatographic columns used and

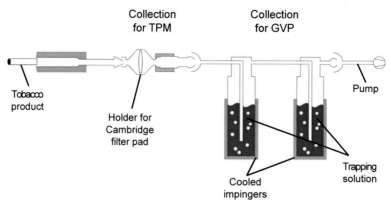

FIG. 6.2 General schematic for smoke/aerosol trapping. *GVP*, gas–vapor phase; *TPM*, total particulate matter. (Graphic from Bentley, M.C., Almstetter, M., Arndt, D., Knorr, A., Martin, E., Pospisil, P., Maeder, S., 2020. Comprehensive chemical characterization of the aerosol generated by a heated tobacco product by untargeted screening. Anal. Bioanal. Chem. 412, 2675–2685. https://doi.org/10.1007/s00216-020-02502-1.)

limits the number of injections that can be made per analytical run. For LC–HRAM-MS, each sample replicate for each method is injected 5 times for chromatographic analysis. The values reported for each method are the overall mean values for aerosol/smoke collections and any injection replicates, without the exclusion of any data.

6.4 UNTARGETED DIFFERENTIAL SCREENING

THS was shown to generate an aerosol that is significantly less complex than cigarette smoke and yields, on average, >90% lower levels of HPHCs than the 3R4F reference cigarette, as determined by using a number of quantitative (targeted) methods (Chapter 4). However, it remains unclear whether the HPHCs identified as requiring measurement in cigarette smoke are directly applicable for the assessment of EHTPs and whether the heating process generates other toxicants of concern that are not generated during combustion.

In order to investigate this possibility and to demonstrate that the THS aerosol does not present any new hazards beyond those associated with cigarette smoking, a number of investigative studies were designed and performed using untargeted differential screening. Untargeted differential screening was used to identify chemical constituents that were significantly higher in abundance in THS aerosol than in 3R4F smoke. By using a statistical approach, the chromatographic features (peaks, per method) of THS aerosol and 3R4F smoke were compared and those demonstrated to be significantly higher in abundance in THS were identified

and semiquantified in both THS and 3R4F. Features that were not of interest (i.e., abundance in THS ≤ 3R4F), which were approximately 10-fold higher in number than those for THS > 3R4F, were not taken through the identification and semiquantification process.

Table 6.1 presents a summary for the numbers of compounds determined to be present at higher concentrations in the three THS variants than in 3R4F by using both LC–HRAM-MS-based and GCxGC–TOFMS-based analyses.

Full details of the methodology and results for each analytical method and tobacco stick variant investigated can be found in the individual analytical reports, which were submitted to the FDA in support of PMI's MRTP application (Amendment to Philip Morris Products S.A. Modified Risk Tobacco Product Application, 2017: Response to August 4, 2017 FDA advice and information request letter including nontargeted differential screening, toxicological assessment, and peer review reports).

The total numbers of compounds observed in all three product variants combined are presented in the row entitled "All," which takes into account compounds that are common to the methods and/or product variants. For the 3 investigated product variants, 86 compounds in total were found at higher concentrations in (or were novel to) THS aerosols than in 3R4F smoke. To put this into context with cigarette smoke, approximately 4800 constituents (approximately 50 times more) were present at higher (or equivalent) concentrations in 3R4F smoke than in THS aerosols. This was determined by using the same untargeted

TABLE 6.1

Numbers of Compounds Determined to be at Higher Concentrations (or Uniquely Present) in THS Aerosol Compared With 3R4F Smoke by Using Untargeted Differential Screening

	LC–HRAM-MS ANALYSIS		GCXGC–TOFMS ANALYSIS			
Product	Number of compounds in THS > 3R4F	Number of unique compounds in THS	Number of compounds[a] in THS > 3R4F	Number of unique compounds in THS	Total number of compounds[a] in THS > 3R4F	Total number of unique compounds in THS
THSR	13	0	43	3	54	3
THSM	16	0	46	5	58	5
THSH	20	0	45	3	61	3
All	22	0	68	9	86	9

[a] The number of compounds identified accounts for the presence of both 1,2-propanediol and 1-hydroxy-2-propanone (both compounds were originally reported as a single entity in the reports sent to the FDA). *3R4F*, reference cigarettes; *GCxGC–TOFMS*, two-dimensional gas chromatography with time-of-flight mass spectrometry; *LC–HRAM-MS*, liquid chromatography with high-resolution accurate mass spectrometry; *THS*, Tobacco Heating System; *THSH*, THS Fresh Menthol; *THSM*, THS Smooth Menthol; *THSR*, THS Regular.

methodology. In addition, given that 3R4F is an unflavored reference cigarette, a proportion of the 86 compounds found at higher concentrations in THS aerosols would have been derived from the flavor systems applied to the tobacco stick variants.

Toxicological evaluation was performed for 80 of these compounds—those which were identified and subsequently assigned a Chemical Abstracts Service (CAS) number (toxicological evaluation was not performed for 1,2-propanediol). Of the 86 compounds, 5 were not present within the CAS registry system and were not subjected to any toxicological assessment. Of the 80 compounds evaluated for toxicological concern, 8 were reported as exhibiting structure–activity relationship alerts for potential genotoxicity or carcinogenicity that could not be ruled out through publicly available toxicological data. A further four compounds, namely furfural, 2-furanmethanol, 3-chloro-1,2-propanediol (3-MCPD), and glycidol, were classified as carcinogens and/or mutagens and were subjected to further in-depth toxicological evaluation (Amendment to Philip Morris Products S.A. Modified Risk Tobacco Product Application, 2017: Response to August 4, 2017 FDA advice and information request letter including nontargeted differential screening, toxicological assessment, and peer review reports). In response to these findings, presented to the FDA in May 2017 as part of PMI's Premarket Tobacco Product Application for the marketing of *IQOS* in the United States, the FDA summarized their review of these toxicological findings with the statement that "Although some of the chemicals are genotoxic or cytotoxic, these

chemicals are present in very low levels, and potential effects are outweighed by the substantial decrease in the number and levels of HPHCs found in combusted cigarettes" (FDA, 2019).

Because the data from this untargeted differential screening were only semiquantitative, it was considered necessary to perform additional targeted (quantitative) analysis for these four carcinogen/mutagens; to this end, replicate analyses were performed for comparing THS aerosol (regular product variant only; THSR) with 3R4F smoke. Table 6.2 presents the mean levels of furfural, 2-furanmethanol, 3-MCPD, and glycidol observed after replicate (x 4) determination of their comparative levels in THSR aerosol and 3R4F smoke. The levels of these compounds were also analyzed in a representative selection of commercially available cigarettes to understand the range of concentrations present in cigarette smoke. The resulting range of values for commercially available cigarettes is indicative of the fact that tobacco blend has an impact on the level of smoke constituents.

6.5 COMPREHENSIVE UNTARGETED SCREENING

In addition to the data generated by untargeted differential screening, and as a second step for evaluating the composition of THS aerosol, comprehensive characterization was performed by untargeted screening (Bentley et al., 2020). This investigation focused upon the regular product variant, whereby all constituents with a semiquantified abundance estimated to

TABLE 6.2
Targeted Analysis for Furfural, 2-Furanmethanol, 3-MCPD, and Glycidol (in THSR, 3R4F, and Representative Commercial Cigarettes)

Compound	Mean concentration 3R4F (μg/item)[a]	Mean concentration THSR (μg/item)[a]	Range of concentrations determined in commercial cigarettes (μg/item)
Furfural	25.9	31.1	26.1–54.1
2-Furanmethanol	7.00	39.2	6.53–12.9
3-MCPD	5.93	9.94	2.07–18.3
Glycidol	1.76	5.71	0.27–3.07

[a] Mean value of four aerosol replicates. *3-MCPD*, 3-chloro-1,2-propanediol; *3R4F*, reference cigarettes; *THS*, Tobacco Heating System; *THSR*, THS Regular.

be ≥ 100 ng/item were identified and reported. Smoke collected from the 3R4F reference cigarette was also analyzed in parallel in order to understand which of the constituents identified as being present in THS aerosol were also present in cigarette smoke. It is important to recognize that, during these investigations, 3R4F was used only as a comparator for constituents of interest identified in THS aerosol and that an effort to fully characterize the composition of 3R4F smoke was not planned or made. However, it was clear that the number of constituents estimated to be present in 3R4F smoke was approximately 10-fold higher than that observed in THS aerosol.

Being highly abundant in THS aerosol, water, nicotine, and glycerin were determined by separate quantitative methods and were not considered a part of this untargeted assessment. Excluding these constituents, a total of 529 compounds with concentrations ≥100 ng/item were identified as being present in THS aerosol by untargeted screening. By applying this nominal reporting threshold of ≥100 ng/item, it was estimated that close to 100% of the total aerosol mass determined by untargeted screening was evaluated (Knorr et al., 2019). Table 6.3 presents the information on all compounds present in THS aerosol above this reporting threshold as well as their corresponding concentrations in 3R4F smoke.

Three confidence categories were used for structural identification proposals (high, medium, and not identified) based on the combined scores calculated by using mass spectral similarity as well as by comparison of additional predicted and experimental parameters (Arndt et al., 2020; Knorr et al., 2019). The proposed structures were confirmed by comparative analysis using authentic analytical reference standards. This

approach confirmed 80% of the proposed structures, which corresponds to approximately 96% of the total aerosol mass determined by untargeted screening; only 0.2% of the total aerosol mass remained unidentified. Compounds identified with either "high" or "medium" confidence are yet to be confirmed by a reference standard, primarily owing to their lack of commercial availability.

Of these 529 compounds, 363 (68.6%) and 127 (24.0%) were exclusively found in the TPM and GVP, respectively, and 39 (7.4%) compounds were partitioned between the TPM and the GVP. The particulate phase comprised 81.3% of the total aerosol mass determined by untargeted screening, which was estimated to represent ca. 99% of the remaining collected aerosol mass after subtraction of the masses attributable to water, glycerin, and nicotine. Approximately 98% of the particulate phase mass estimated by untargeted screening comprised compounds that were either confirmed by using reference standards (95.4%) or identified with a high degree of confidence (2.5%). More than 80% of this estimated mass was represented by only 34 chemical constituents, with over 50% represented by just the four most abundant constituents (Fig. 6.3). Although the uncertainties associated with the experimental measurements should be acknowledged, the accumulated data (Bentley et al., 2020) represent the most comprehensive and technically achievable characterization of the TPM generated by an EHTP.

The GVP, which represented just under 20% of the total aerosol mass determined by untargeted screening, was represented by 166 compounds. More than 80% of the determined mass of the GVP present in THS aerosol was contributed by the 14 most abundant chemical constituents, with more than 50% represented by just

TABLE 6.3
The Most Abundant (≥100 ng/item) Chemical Constituents Present in the Aerosol of THS and Their Corresponding Concentrations in the Smoke of the 3R4F Reference Cigarette

Compound name	CAS number	Identification confidence	Aerosol fraction	Conc. in THS (µg/item)	Conc. in 3R4F (µg/item)
1-Hydroxy-2-propanone/ 1,2-propanediol[a]	116-09-6/7333-03-1	Confirmed	TPM	1135	502
Acetic acid	64-19-7	Confirmed	TPM	994[b]	2659
Propylene glycol	57-55-6	Confirmed	TPM	643	89.6
1-Monoacetin	106-61-6	Confirmed	TPM	409	434
Acetaldehyde	75-07-0	Confirmed	TPM/GVP	313	1253
Methanol	67-56-1	Confirmed	TPM/GVP	211	361
Solanesol	13190-97-1	Confirmed	TPM	179	3382
Isobutyraldehyde	78-84-2	Confirmed	GVP	116	259
Triacetin	102-76-1	Confirmed	TPM	112	194
Palmitic acid	57-10-3	Confirmed	TPM	105	266
3-(2-Hydroxymethoxy)-propane-1,2-diol	14641-24-8	Confirmed	TPM	100	267
Cembranoid degradation products (18 compounds)[c]	-	Confirmed	TPM	93.2	193
Isovaleraldehyde	590-86-3	Confirmed	TPM/GVP	88.7	245
13,14-Dihydroretinol	115797-14-3	Confirmed	TPM	79.1	152
Linolenic acid	463-40-1	Confirmed	TPM	57.9	157
Propanal	123-38-6	Confirmed	GVP	57.4	386
2-Methylbutyraldehyde	96-17-3	Confirmed	GVP	54.7	179
Propanoic acid	79-09-4	Confirmed	TPM	53.2	141
3-Pyridinol	109-00-2	Confirmed	TPM	52.8	218
β-Nicotyrine	487-19-4	Confirmed	TPM	52.4	100
Pyranone	28564-83-2	Confirmed	TPM	51.4	44.5
Oleic acid	112-80-1	Confirmed	TPM	50.2	107
Furfural	98-01-1	Confirmed	TPM/GVP	47.4	38.3
2-Monoacetin	100-78-7	Confirmed	TPM	46.8	30.0
Linoleic acid	60-33-3	Confirmed	TPM	43.0	123
2-Furanmethanol	98-00-0	Confirmed	TPM/GVP	37.5	9.47
Acetone	67-64-1	Confirmed	GVP	34.7	268
2,3-Butanedione	431-03-8	Confirmed	TPM/GVP	34.0	127
Anhydro sugar derivative	—	High	TPM	30.8	43.1
Octadecanoic acid	57-11-4	Confirmed	TPM	29.4	72.7
2-Methylfuran	534-22-5	Confirmed	GVP	28.2	175
Furan	110-00-9	Confirmed	GVP	24.3	214
Neophytadiene	504-96-1	Confirmed	TPM	23.8	43.0
1-Linolenoylglycerol	18465-99-1	Confirmed	TPM	23.5	42.8
5-Hydroxymethylfurfural	67-47-0	Confirmed	TPM	23.0	82.1

Continued

TABLE 6.3
The Most Abundant (≥100 ng/item) Chemical Constituents Present in the Aerosol of THS and Their Corresponding Concentrations in the Smoke of the 3R4F Reference Cigarette—cont'd

Compound name	CAS number	Identification confidence	Aerosol fraction	Conc. in THS (μg/item)	Conc. in 3R4F (μg/item)
α-Levantenolide	30987-48-5	Medium	TPM	22.8	74.8
2-Methyl-2-propenal	78-85-3	Confirmed	TPM/GVP	22.0	115
Pentadecanoic acid	1002-84-2	Confirmed	TPM	18.8	32.7
3-Chloro-1,2-propanediol	96-24-2	Confirmed	TPM	16.1	8.21
4,6-Dihydroxy-20-nor-2,7-cembradien-12-one	119613-98-8[d]	High	TPM	14.6	17.8
3-Methylpentanoic acid	105-43-1	Confirmed	TPM	14.5	12.8
5-Methylfurfural	620-02-0	Confirmed	TPM/GVP	14.2	5.25
1H-Pyrrole	109-97-7	Confirmed	TPM/GVP	14.0	24.8
Phytoene	540-04-5	Medium	TPM	13.8	247
Pyridine	110-86-1	Confirmed	TPM/GVP	13.7	68.4
6,10,14,18,22,26-Hexamethyl-5,9,13,17,21,25-heptacosahexaen-2-one	32304-17-9[d]	Medium	TPM	13.2	75.3
Butanoic acid	107-92-6	Confirmed	TPM	12.7	22.4
1-Acetyloxy-2-propanone	592-20-1	Confirmed	TPM/GVP	12.2	9.23
N-Octanoylnornicotine	38854-10-3	Confirmed	TPM	12.1	100
5,6-Dihydropyridin-2(1H)-one	6052-73-9	Confirmed	TPM	11.8	38.8
Methanethiol	74-93-1	Confirmed	GVP	11.7	22.9
Chloromethane	74-87-3	Confirmed	GVP	11.1	32.1
Heptacosane	593-49-7	Confirmed	TPM	10.2	8.41
α-Tocopherolquinone	7559-04-8	Confirmed	TPM	10.0	40.5
2-Butanone	78-93-3	Confirmed	GVP	10.0	128
3-Hydroxy-2-butanone	513-86-0	Confirmed	TPM/GVP	9.43	11.2
Arachidic acid	506-30-9	Confirmed	TPM	8.91	35.8
α-Cembratriene-diol	57605-80-8[d]	High	TPM	8.49	0.393
(9Z,12Z)-18-Hydroxy-9,12-octadecadienoic acid	4546-59-2	High	TPM	8.47	21.9
2-Cyclopentene-1,4-dione	930-60-9	Confirmed	TPM/GVP	8.40	2.01
2-Cyclopenten-1-one	930-30-3	Confirmed	TPM/GVP	8.20	46.9
2H-Pyran-2-one, tetrahydro-5-hydroxy	33691-73-5	Confirmed	TPM	8.16	4.13
2-Furancarboxylic acid, 3-methyl	4412-96-8	Confirmed	TPM	8.06	18.9
trans-Crotonaldehyde	123-73-9	Confirmed	TPM/GVP	7.87	210

TABLE 6.3
The Most Abundant (≥100 ng/item) Chemical Constituents Present in the Aerosol of THS and Their Corresponding Concentrations in the Smoke of the 3R4F Reference Cigarette—cont'd

Compound name	CAS number	Identification confidence	Aerosol fraction	Conc. in THS (μg/item)	Conc. in 3R4F (μg/item)
8,11-Epoxy-2,6,12-cembratrien-4-ol	75281-94-6[d]	Medium	TPM	7.79	19.6
Butanal	123-72-8	Confirmed	GVP	7.79	114
trans-Solanone	54868-48-3	Confirmed	TPM/GVP	7.75	12.7
Palmitoleic acid	373-49-9	Confirmed	TPM	7.46	22.0
Isoraimonol	82458-63-7	High	TPM	7.42	11.4
Scopoletin	92-61-5	Confirmed	TPM	7.21	42.3
Anatabine	581-49-7	Confirmed	TPM	7.15	11.8
Behenic acid	112-85-6	Confirmed	TPM	6.57	40.1
2,3-Pentanedione	600-14-6	Confirmed	GVP	6.43	17.0
Hexadecanoic acid, ethyl ester	628-97-7	Confirmed	TPM	6.43	< 0.100
2,5-Dimethylfuran	625-86-5	Confirmed	GVP	6.38	156
Dimethyldisulfide	624-92-0	Confirmed	GVP	6.34	74.1
2-Methyl-3-pyridinol	1121-25-1	Confirmed	TPM	6.23	41.0
5-Oxo-1-tetradecyl-3-pyrrolidinecarboxylic acid	10054-22-5	Medium	TPM	6.16	10.8
α-Tocopherol	10191-41-0	Confirmed	TPM	5.80	25.4
1,2-Benzenediol	120-80-9	Confirmed	TPM	5.73	56.5
Hydroquinone	123-31-9	Confirmed	TPM	5.71	80.6
2-Hydroxy-3-oxo-butanal	473-80-3	High	TPM/GVP	5.60	6.58
Andrograpanin	82209-74-3	Confirmed	TPM	5.57	61.7
N-Cyclohexylnicotinamide	10354-56-0	Medium	TPM	5.56	48.3
Lignoceric acid	557-59-5	Confirmed	TPM	5.47	30.1
2(5*H*)-Furanone	497-23-4	Confirmed	TPM	5.45	2.13
2-Methylbutanoic acid	116-53-0	Confirmed	TPM	5.28	8.08
Isoprene	78-79-5	Confirmed	GVP	5.24	49.1
Acrolein	107-02-8	Confirmed	GVP	5.20	463
3-Methylbutanoic acid	503-74-2	Confirmed	TPM	5.13	9.98
6-Methyl-3-pyridinol	1121-78-4	Confirmed	TPM	5.10	21.3
1,4,7,10-Cyclotetradecatetraene, 1,7,11-trimethyl-4(1-methyl ethenyl)	101159-07-3	High	TPM	4.93	11.9
Butyrolactone	96-48-0	Confirmed	TPM	4.80	1.08
Myristic acid	544-63-8	Confirmed	TPM	4.62	18.7
Stearidonic acid	20290-75-9	Confirmed	TPM	4.56	21.3
Hentriacontane	630-04-6	Confirmed	TPM	4.54	20.4
Benzene	71-43-2	Confirmed	GVP	4.41	106

Continued

TABLE 6.3
The Most Abundant (≥100 ng/item) Chemical Constituents Present in the Aerosol of THS and Their
Corresponding Concentrations in the Smoke of the 3R4F Reference Cigarette—cont'd

Compound name	CAS number	Identification confidence	Aerosol fraction	Conc. in THS (µg/item)	Conc. in 3R4F (µg/item)
Acetamide	60-35-5	Confirmed	TPM	4.30	38.7
3-Methylpalmitic acid	42172-35-0	Medium	TPM	4.27	11.7
3-Methylfuran	930-27-8	Confirmed	GVP	4.26	26.2
2-Cyclohexen-1-one, 2,4,4-trimethyl-3-(1,3-butadienyl)	84696-84-4	High	TPM	4.13	21.6
Harmaline	304-21-2	Confirmed	TPM	4.07	61.2
N-Formylnornicotine	3000-81-5	Confirmed	TPM	3.91	53.6
1,3,5,7,11-Cembrapentaene	420793-93-7[d]	High	TPM	3.89	8.60
Heptadecanoic acid	506-12-7	Confirmed	TPM	3.86	11.8
Octacosanoic acid	506-48-9	Confirmed	TPM	3.81	29.4
Tricosanoic acid	2433-96-7	Confirmed	TPM	3.80	18.3
Farnesylacetone	762-29-8	Confirmed	TPM	3.80	8.82
Toluene	108-88-3	Confirmed	GVP	3.80	77.5
Phenol	108-95-2	Confirmed	TPM	3.74	22.7
N'-Carbomethoxyanabasine	56078-09-2	High	TPM	3.71	53.2
Propanoic acid, 2-oxo-, methyl ester	600-22-6	Confirmed	TPM/GVP	3.70	19.5
2-Methyl-2-butene	513-35-9	Confirmed	GVP	3.60	92.6
1-(1-Oxohexyl)-2-(3-pyridinyl)-pyrrolidine	38854-09-0[d]	Confirmed	TPM	3.52	34.8
3-[1-(2-Furanylmethyl)-2-pyrrolidinyl]-pyridine	78210-85-2[d]	Confirmed	TPM	3.52	6.31
Retinol	68-26-8	Confirmed	TPM	3.48	6.82
Shikimic acid	138-59-0	Confirmed	TPM	3.41	23.5
3-Hydroxypalmitic acid	2398-34-7	Confirmed	TPM	3.38	26.9
Sclareolide	1216-84-8	Confirmed	TPM	3.31	4.50
Methylvinylketone	78-94-4	Confirmed	GVP	3.28	74.6
1-Hydroxy-2-butanone/ 1,2-butenediol	5077-67-8/ 50317-11-8	Confirmed	TPM	3.23	4.06
2-Methylpyrazine	109-08-0	Confirmed	TPM/GVP	3.20	27.7
2-Heptadecenoic acid, (2E)-	2825-78-7	Confirmed	TPM	3.20	11.9
Norharman	244-63-3	Confirmed	TPM	3.20	43.9
cis-4-Hydroxymethyl-2-methyl-1,3-dioxolane	3674-21-3	Confirmed	TPM	3.18	< 0.100
Nicoteine	366-18-7	Confirmed	TPM	3.18	23.6

TABLE 6.3
The Most Abundant (≥100 μg/item) Chemical Constituents Present in the Aerosol of THS and Their Corresponding Concentrations in the Smoke of the 3R4F Reference Cigarette—cont'd

Compound name	CAS number	Identification confidence	Aerosol fraction	Conc. in THS (μg/item)	Conc. in 3R4F (μg/item)
10-Nonadecenoic acid	67228-95-9	Medium	TPM	3.16	9.78
2,3-Dihydrofuran	1191-99-7	Confirmed	GVP	3.14	10.1
Cotinine	486-56-6	Confirmed	TPM	3.09	34.6
2-Hydroxy-γ-butyrolactone	19444-84-9	Confirmed	TPM	3.09	13.6
Methylformate	107-31-3	Confirmed	TPM/GVP	3.01	11.5
5-(Hydroxymethyl) dihydro-2(3H)-furanone	10374-51-3	Confirmed	TPM	2.85	18.9
1,4:3,6-Dianhydro-α-D-glucopyranose	4451-30-3	Confirmed	TPM	2.85	77.6
Acetonitrile	75-05-8	Confirmed	GVP	2.85	479
1-(1-Oxobutyl)-2-(3-pyridinyl)-pyrrolidine	69730-91-2[d]	Medium	TPM	2.81	5.46
2-Pyrrolidinone	616-45-5	Confirmed	TPM	2.81	20.9
2-Hydroxypyridine	72762-00-6	Confirmed	TPM	2.72	39.2
t-Phytol	253686-88-3	Confirmed	TPM	2.70	3.52
5,8,11-Eicosatriynoic acid	13488-22-7	Confirmed	TPM	2.70	4.63
3-Methoxybenzidine	3365-87-5	High	TPM	2.67	29.9
4-Dodecylphenol	104-43-8	Medium	TPM	2.60	7.10
2-Methyltriacontane	1560-72-1	High	TPM	2.56	12.8
Pentacosanoic acid	506-38-7	Confirmed	TPM	2.53	12.0
1-[4-Amino-2-methyl-5-(2-methylphenyl)-1H-pyrrol-3-yl] ethanone	56463-76-4	Medium	TPM	2.49	18.7
Cerotinic acid	506-46-7	Confirmed	TPM	2.48	14.2
Diacetin	102-62-5 or 25395-31-7	Confirmed	TPM	2.47	1.69
1-Keto-α-cyperone	38043-97-9	High	TPM	2.45	8.70
p-Xylene	106-42-3	Confirmed	GVP	2.39	47.8
3-Methylhentriacontane	4981-99-1	High	TPM	2.39	13.0
12-Isopropenyl-1,5,9-trimethyl-2,5,9-cyclotetradecatrien-1-ol	60026-11-1	High	TPM	2.37	30.4
Acrylic acid	79-10-7	Confirmed	TPM	2.36	35.9
2-Methyl-2-cyclopenten-1-one	1120-73-6	Confirmed	TPM/GVP	2.34	35.3
5-Methoxy-3-(2-pyridinylmethyl)-1H-indole	101832-06-8	High	TPM	2.33	33.2
2-Chloro-1,3-propanediol	497-04-1	Confirmed	TPM	2.32	2.30
Vernolic acid	503-07-1	Confirmed	TPM	2.31	14.7

Continued

TABLE 6.3
The Most Abundant (≥100 ng/item) Chemical Constituents Present in the Aerosol of THS and Their Corresponding Concentrations in the Smoke of the 3R4F Reference Cigarette—cont'd

Compound name	CAS number	Identification confidence	Aerosol fraction	Conc. in THS (μg/item)	Conc. in 3R4F (μg/item)
Heneicosanoic acid	2363-71-5	Confirmed	TPM	2.30	9.85
Myosmine	532-12-7	Confirmed	TPM	2.27	20.5
Dihydro-α-ionone	31499-72-6	Confirmed	TPM	2.24	2.89
3,4-Dimethyl-5-pentyl-2-furanundecanoic acid	57818-36-7	Medium	TPM	2.21	8.54
2-Hydroxytetracosanoic acid	544-57-0	Confirmed	TPM	2.19	21.8
Guaiacol	90-05-1	Confirmed	TPM/GVP	2.18	2.33
N-Ethylnorcotinine	359435-41-9	Confirmed	TPM	2.16	46.2
Retinal	116-31-4	Confirmed	TPM	2.13	4.33
3-Oxo-α-ionol	896107-70-3	Confirmed	TPM	2.11	9.64
Stigmasterol	83-48-7	Confirmed	TPM	2.08	21.9
β-Damascenone	23726-93-4	Confirmed	TPM	2.08	9.25
Phenylacetaldehyde	122-78-1	Confirmed	TPM/GVP	2.00	0.733
2-Acetylfuran	1192-62-7	Confirmed	TPM/GVP	1.99	2.38
2,5-Pyrrolidinedione	123-56-8	Confirmed	TPM	1.93	29.2
Triacontanoic acid	506-50-3	Confirmed	TPM	1.92	15.8
Geranylbenzoate	94-48-4	Medium	TPM	1.92	6.60
3-Methyl-pyridine	108-99-6	Confirmed	TPM	1.92	28.4
Furaneol	3658-77-3	Confirmed	TPM	1.92	2.89
2-[2-(4-Nonylphenoxy) ethoxy]ethyldecanoate	—	Medium	TPM	1.90	6.36
1-Butene	106-98-9	Confirmed	GVP	1.89	20.3
Pentacosane	629-99-2	Confirmed	TPM	1.88	1.08
Benzaldehyde	100-52-7	Confirmed	TPM/GVP	1.83	4.50
cis-2,6-Dimethyl-4-piperidinone	13200-35-6	Confirmed	TPM	1.82	1.22
1-(2,3,4,9-Tetrahydro-1H-β-carbolin-1-yl)acetone	69225-88-3	High	TPM	1.80	19.1
3-[1-(5-Ethyl-2-furanyl)-1H-pyrrol-2-yl] pyridine	78210-88-5	Medium	TPM	1.79	32.3
5-Methyl-2-pyridinol	1003-68-5	Confirmed	TPM	1.77	13.1
Nonacosane	630-03-5	Confirmed	TPM	1.77	7.65
3-Methyldotriacontane	20129-49-1	High	TPM	1.74	11.8
Cholest-7-en-3-ol	6036-58-4	Confirmed	TPM	1.71	8.55
(Z)-11-Eicosenoic acid	5561-99-9	Confirmed	TPM	1.68	4.07
2,6-Dimethylpyrazine	108-50-9	Confirmed	TPM/GVP	1.68	10.8

TABLE 6.3
The Most Abundant (≥100 μg/item) Chemical Constituents Present in the Aerosol of THS and Their Corresponding Concentrations in the Smoke of the 3R4F Reference Cigarette—cont'd

Compound name	CAS number	Identification confidence	Aerosol fraction	Conc. in THS (μg/item)	Conc. in 3R4F (μg/item)
1,4-Naphthalenedione, 2,3-dimethyl-6-(4,8,12-trimethyl tridecyl)-	68860-42-4[d]	Medium	TPM	1.67	9.33
2-Vinylfuran	1487-18-9	Confirmed	GVP	1.62	9.86
Campesterol	474-62-4	Confirmed	TPM	1.58	15.0
cis-2-Butene	590-18-1	Confirmed	GVP	1.53	50.4
1,3-Cyclopentadiene	542-92-7	Confirmed	GVP	1.51	82.8
β-Sitosterol	83-46-5	Confirmed	TPM	1.50	15.2
2-Methyl-2-butenal	497-03-0	Confirmed	GVP	1.49	9.20
2,4-Dimethylcyclopent-4-ene-1,3-dione	65656-90-8	High	TPM/GVP	1.49	2.73
3-Methyl-nonacosane	14167-67-0	High	TPM	1.48	6.39
Ethyl linolenate	1191-41-9	Confirmed	TPM	1.43	0.357
Ricinoleic acid	141-22-0	Confirmed	TPM	1.38	6.59
2-Methyl-3-phenyl-pyrazine	29444-53-9	Confirmed	TPM	1.37	32.8
Dihydrofuranone derivative	–	High	TPM	1.37	73.5
Acrylamide	79-06-1	Confirmed	TPM	1.34	5.81
2-Hydroxy-4,6-dimethylnicotinonitrile	769-28-8	Medium	TPM	1.32	5.92
Glycidol	556-52-5	Confirmed	TPM	1.31	0.439
3(2H)-Furanone, dihydro-2-methyl-	3188-00-9	Confirmed	TPM/GVP	1.30	0.561
Nicotelline	494-04-2	Confirmed	TPM	1.27	29.5
Pyridine, 3-[1-(5-propyl-2-furanyl)-1H-pyrrol-2-yl]	78210-89-6	Medium	TPM	1.27	30.3
cis-2-Pentene	627-20-3	Confirmed	GVP	1.26	40.0
2-Methyl-1-butene	563-46-2	Confirmed	GVP	1.25	44.9
1-(6-Hydroxy-1-oxooctyl)-2-(3-pyridinyl)-pyrrolidine	77829-17-5	Confirmed	TPM	1.24	38.7
(9Z,12Z,15Z)-18-Hydroxy-9,12,15-octadecatrienoic acid	51327-73-2	High	TPM	1.23	19.4
2,3′-Bipyridine	581-50-0	Confirmed	TPM	1.23	10.5
5-Methylcotinine	1076198-50-9	Confirmed	TPM	1.18	30.0
Heneicosane	629-94-7	Confirmed	TPM	1.17	0.495
cis-2-Methyl-1,3-pentadiene	1501-60-6	Confirmed	GVP	1.17	30.5

Continued

TABLE 6.3
The Most Abundant (≥100 ng/item) Chemical Constituents Present in the Aerosol of THS and Their Corresponding Concentrations in the Smoke of the 3R4F Reference Cigarette—cont'd

Compound name	CAS number	Identification confidence	Aerosol fraction	Conc. in THS (µg/item)	Conc. in 3R4F (µg/item)
4-(3-Hydroxy-2,6,6-trimethyl-1cyclohexen-1-yl)-3-buten-2-one	14398-34-6[d]	Confirmed	TPM	1.15	4.08
5,6-Dimethyl-3-pyridinol	61893-00-3	Confirmed	TPM	1.15	9.31
Nonadecanoic acid	646-30-0	Confirmed	TPM	1.15	3.90
Styrene	100-42-5	Confirmed	GVP	1.15	22.8
trans-2-Butene	624-64-6	Confirmed	GVP	1.14	30.4
Nicotine-N-oxide	2820-55-5	Confirmed	TPM	1.14	10.8
1H-Pyrrole, 1-methyl-	96-54-8	Confirmed	GVP	1.13	0.762
Methyl-pyroglutamate	4931-66-2	Confirmed	TPM	1.12	12.3
α-Acetylbutyrolactone	517-23-7	Confirmed	TPM	1.11	6.17
Hexadecanoic acid, methyl ester	112-39-0	Confirmed	TPM	1.10	5.67
Nonacosanoic acid	4250-38-8	Confirmed	TPM	1.07	8.85
6-(Heptyloxy)-3-pyridinamine	857219-70-6	High	TPM	1.07	28.7
2-Methyl-3-propyl-5,6-dihydropyrazine	15986-94-4	High	TPM	1.06	4.04
N-Formyl-anatabine	77264-87-0	Confirmed	TPM	1.06	14.0
2-Hydroxy-3-methyl-2-cyclopenten-1-one	80-71-7	Confirmed	TPM	1.06	8.33
2,3-Dimethyl-2-cyclopenten-1-one	1121-05-7	Confirmed	TPM/GVP	1.05	10.9
Ethyl linoleate	544-35-4	Confirmed	TPM	0.988	0.721
Nonanoic acid	112-05-0	Confirmed	TPM	0.968	1.97
Cyclopentanone	120-92-3	Confirmed	GVP	0.954	23.8
5-Hydroxymaltol	1073-96-7	Confirmed	TPM	0.938	0.491
5-Methyl-2(3H)-furanone	591-12-8	Confirmed	TPM/GVP	0.934	2.78
Pentane	109-66-0	Confirmed	GVP	0.922	36.4
cis-13-Docosenoamide	112-84-5	Confirmed	GVP	0.922	2.33
2-Methyldotriacontane	1720-11-2	High	TPM	0.917	6.33
17-Hydroxylinolenic acid	143343-97-9	Medium	TPM	0.905	4.23
Farnesylacetic acid	6040-06-8[d]	Confirmed	TPM	0.903	4.28
o-Toluic acid	118-90-1	Confirmed	TPM	0.900	14.3
Menthol	1490-04-6	Confirmed	TPM/GVP	0.894	1.16
24-Methylidenelophenol	1176-52-9	High	TPM	0.879	6.80
3-Methyl-2(1H)-pyridinone	1003-56-1	Confirmed	TPM	0.875	7.58
3,22,23-Trihydroxystigmastan-6-one	90524-90-6[d]	High	TPM	0.875	2.67

TABLE 6.3
The Most Abundant (≥100 μg/item) Chemical Constituents Present in the Aerosol of THS and Their Corresponding Concentrations in the Smoke of the 3R4F Reference Cigarette—cont'd

Compound name	CAS number	Identification confidence	Aerosol fraction	Conc. in THS (μg/item)	Conc. in 3R4F (μg/item)
Heptacosanoic acid	7138-40-1	Confirmed	TPM	0.874	5.88
Crotonic acid	3724-65-0	Confirmed	TPM	0.866	7.74
trans-4-hydroxymethyl-2-methyl-1,3-dioxolane	3674-22-4	Confirmed	TPM	0.857	< 0.100
cis-4-Methyl-2-pentene	691-38-3	Confirmed	GVP	0.855	37.8
3-Hydroxy-β-damascone	102488-09-5	High	TPM	0.803	3.59
Furancarboxylic acid, methyl ester	611-13-2	Confirmed	TPM/GVP	0.789	0.234
3-Furaldehyde	498-60-2	Confirmed	TPM/GVP	0.789	6.37
trans-3-Penten-2-one	3102-33-8	Confirmed	GVP	0.786	15.6
Loliolide	38274-00-9	Confirmed	TPM	0.782	5.44
α-Cyperone	473-08-5	Confirmed	TPM	0.782	4.35
3-(Furfuryloxy)-1,2-propanediol	20390-21-0	Medium	TPM	0.772	0.912
Vitamin K1	84-80-0	Confirmed	TPM	0.740	4.82
Megastigmatrienone (2 isomers)	5896-02-6	Confirmed	TPM	0.735	3.84
Cholesterol	57-88-5	Confirmed	TPM	0.732	6.90
trans-2-Pentenal	1576-87-0	Confirmed	GVP	0.718	4.75
1,3-Butadiene	106-99-0	Confirmed	GVP	0.716	75.4
3-Methyl-1-butene	563-45-1	Confirmed	GVP	0.706	34.8
Docosane	629-97-0	Confirmed	TPM	0.703	0.509
Dotriacontane	544-85-4	Confirmed	TPM	0.702	4.60
1-Methyl-1,4-cyclohexadiene	4313-57-9	Confirmed	GVP	0.698	7.46
3-Methyl-2-butanone	563-80-4	Confirmed	GVP	0.697	18.2
1-[4-(Dimethylamino)-2-butyn-1-yl]-5-methyl-2-pyrrolidinone	71970-74-6	Medium	TPM	0.686	20.7
4,8,13-Duvatriene-1,3-diol	7220-78-2	Confirmed	TPM	0.685	21.8
Limonene	138-86-3	Confirmed	GVP	0.684	3.49
3-Methyl-2-cyclopenten-1-one	2758-18-1	Confirmed	TPM	0.670	7.14
Thiirane	420-12-2	Confirmed	GVP	0.663	4.37
Cyclo(Pro-Leu)	5654-86-4	Confirmed	TPM	0.652	15.9
2-Ethylfuran	3208-16-0	Confirmed	GVP	0.647	13.3
Acetone cyanohydrin	75-86-5	Confirmed	GVP	0.647	20.2
2(3*H*)-Furanone, dihydro-5-(1-hydroxyethyl)	27610-27-1	Confirmed	TPM	0.641	0.336
16-Hydroxy-9-hexadecenoic acid	17278-80-7	Confirmed	TPM	0.636	27.1

Continued

TABLE 6.3
The Most Abundant (≥100 ng/item) Chemical Constituents Present in the Aerosol of THS and Their Corresponding Concentrations in the Smoke of the 3R4F Reference Cigarette—cont'd

Compound name	CAS number	Identification confidence	Aerosol fraction	Conc. in THS (μg/item)	Conc. in 3R4F (μg/item)
Pyrrole-2-carboxamide	4551-72-8	Confirmed	TPM	0.624	23.9
5-Methyl-1,3-cyclopentadiene	96-38-8	Confirmed	GVP	0.593	20.9
5-Methyl-2(5H)-furanone	591-11-7	Confirmed	TPM	0.590	0.417
2-Ethylpyrazine	13925-00-3	Confirmed	TPM/GVP	0.586	3.59
2,4-Dimethylfuran	3710-43-8	Confirmed	GVP	0.584	5.97
2-Methyl-butanenitrile	18936-17-9	Confirmed	GVP	0.580	45.9
2-Methyl-5-(prop-1-en-2-yl)-2-vinyltetrahydrofuran	54750-70-8	Confirmed	GVP	0.574	0.128
1-Methyl-3-(1-methylethyl)-2(1H)-pyrazinone	78210-68-1	Medium	TPM	0.570	8.57
Heptane	142-82-5	Confirmed	GVP	0.563	20.0
Phytuberol	56857-64-8	Medium	TPM	0.562	10.2
α-Amylcinnamyl alcohol	101-85-9	Confirmed	TPM	0.558	3.24
3-Hydroxysolavetivone	62623-88-5	High	TPM	0.553	4.22
trans-2-Pentene	646-04-8	Confirmed	GVP	0.552	42.0
6-Ethyl-5,6-dihydro-2H-pyran-2-one	19895-35-3	Confirmed	TPM	0.550	1.74
1-Chloro-2-propanone	78-95-5	Confirmed	GVP	0.546	4.89
Benzylalcohol	100-51-6	Confirmed	TPM	0.544	0.740
Phytone	502-69-2	Confirmed	TPM	0.543	5.70
3-Pyridinebutanol, d-amino	70898-36-1	Medium	TPM	0.541	16.6
Ethylvinylketone	1629-58-9	Confirmed	GVP	0.537	7.46
Triacontane	638-68-6	Confirmed	TPM	0.535	2.80
1-Methyl-1,3-cyclopentadiene	96-39-9	Confirmed	GVP	0.534	26.6
2-Methyl-heptane	592-27-8	Confirmed	GVP	0.529	7.39
Keto-ionone	27185-77-9	Medium	TPM	0.526	4.44
Solerone	29393-32-6	Confirmed	TPM	0.525	1.55
2-Farnesylethanol	67858-77-9[d]	High	TPM	0.522	10.8
Pentan-2-one	107-87-9	Confirmed	GVP	0.522	40.0
Geranyllinalool	1113-21-9	Confirmed	TPM	0.518	1.90
1-Acetyloxy-2-butanone	1575-57-1	Confirmed	TPM	0.516	0.752
(6E,10E,14E,18E)-2,6,10,15,19,23-Hexamethyl-1,6,10,14,18,22-tetracosahexaen-3-ol	97232-74-1	Medium	TPM	0.505	3.05

TABLE 6.3
The Most Abundant (≥100 μg/item) Chemical Constituents Present in the Aerosol of THS and Their Corresponding Concentrations in the Smoke of the 3R4F Reference Cigarette—cont'd

Compound name	CAS number	Identification confidence	Aerosol fraction	Conc. in THS (μg/item)	Conc. in 3R4F (μg/item)
6-Methyl-5-hepten-2-one	110-93-0	Confirmed	GVP	0.502	0.742
p-Menthene (Cyclohexene, 1-methyl-4-(1-methylethyl)-)	1195-31-9	Confirmed	GVP	0.492	7.73
1-Pentene	109-67-1	Confirmed	GVP	0.491	44.7
Phenylacetic acid	103-82-2	Medium	TPM	0.489	4.62
2,6,10,14,18-Pentamethyl-2,6,10,14,18-eicosapentaene	75581-03-2[d]	High	TPM	0.487	10.7
4-Methyl-1-pentene	691-37-2	Confirmed	GVP	0.487	18.0
2-Ethyl-3-pyridinol	61893-02-5	Confirmed	TPM	0.475	4.55
Pyrrolo[1,2-a]pyrazine-1,4-dione, hexahydro-3propyl-	26626-89-1[d]	Confirmed	TPM	0.474	16.8
3-Methyl-2-butenal	107-86-8	Confirmed	GVP	0.470	1.74
Propanenitrile	107-12-0	Confirmed	GVP	0.465	71.1
Dimethylsulfide	75-18-3	Confirmed	GVP	0.456	1.70
Dihydromaltol	38877-21-3	Confirmed	TPM	0.453	0.341
16-Hydroxy-hexadecanoic acid	506-13-8	Confirmed	TPM	0.447	5.72
3-Hydroxypropionaldehyde	2134-29-4	High	TPM	0.445	0.691
4-Methyl-2-pentanone	108-10-1	Confirmed	GVP	0.445	7.26
2-Methyloctacosane	1560-98-1	High	TPM	0.445	1.81
Methylacrylate	96-33-3	Confirmed	GVP	0.438	3.53
3-Hexene-2,5-dione	4436-75-3	Confirmed	GVP	0.437	3.92
2-Cyclohexen-1-one	930-68-7	Confirmed	TPM/GVP	0.436	1.55
13′-Hydroxy-γ-tocopherol	1215088-63-3	High	TPM	0.430	1.29
Squalene	111-02-4	Confirmed	TPM	0.429	2.54
2-Methyl-propanoic acid	79-31-2	Confirmed	TPM	0.425	2.45
12-Oxo-phytodienoic acid	67204-66-4	Medium	TPM	0.422	2.02
[1-Methyl-3-oxo-2-pentylidenecyclopentyl] acetic acid, (2E)-	958790-53-9	High	TPM	0.418	3.97
Tricosanal	72934-02-2	Confirmed	TPM	0.417	1.64
Stigmasta-5,7,22,25-tetraen-3-ol	119386-11-7	High	TPM	0.409	2.84
Higher molecular weight derivative of farnesylacetone (C22)	—	High	TPM	0.408	2.02

Continued

TABLE 6.3
The Most Abundant (≥100 ng/item) Chemical Constituents Present in the Aerosol of THS and Their Corresponding Concentrations in the Smoke of the 3R4F Reference Cigarette—cont'd

Compound name	CAS number	Identification confidence	Aerosol fraction	Conc. in THS (μg/item)	Conc. in 3R4F (μg/item)
2-Methyl-pyridine	109-06-8	Confirmed	TPM/GVP	0.407	14.3
β-Damascone	23726-91-2	Confirmed	TPM	0.402	1.37
2-Methylpentane	107-83-5	Confirmed	GVP	0.401	12.2
Higher molecular weight derivative of farnesylacetone (C26)	–	High	TPM	0.401	2.38
2,3-Dimethylfuran	14920-89-9	Confirmed	GVP	0.394	4.89
2-Hydroxycerotic acid	14176-13-7	Medium	TPM	0.387	4.35
1-Ethyl-9H-pyrido[3,4-β] indole	20127-61-1	Confirmed	TPM	0.378	12.1
2-Methylbutane	78-78-4	Confirmed	GVP	0.378	21.3
Glutarimide	1121-89-7	Confirmed	TPM	0.370	8.24
Plastoquinone 3	1168-52-1	High	TPM	0.365	1.00
3,4-Hexanedione	4437-51-8	Confirmed	GVP	0.362	1.39
2-Hydroxy-2-cyclopenten-1-one/1,2-cyclopentanedione	10493-98-8/ 3008-40-0	Confirmed	TPM	0.358	0.440
Scoparone	120-08-1	Confirmed	TPM	0.357	2.25
Cyclopentene	142-29-0	Confirmed	GVP	0.355	20.5
Ethylbenzene-	100-41-4	Confirmed	GVP	0.354	26.8
2,3-Dihydro-1,4-dioxin	543-75-9	Confirmed	GVP	0.346	2.32
Dihydro-4-hydroxy-2(3H)-furanone	7331-52-4	Confirmed	TPM	0.340	4.78
Cyclohexene, 3-(2-propenyl)- or Cyclohexene, 3-(1-methylethyl)-	5232-95-8 or 3983-08-2	Medium	GVP	0.333	4.95
trans-1,3-Pentadiene	2004-70-8	Confirmed	GVP	0.330	64.6
Pentan-3-one	96-22-0	Confirmed	GVP	0.328	14.1
Pyrazine	290-37-9	Confirmed	TPM/GVP	0.318	2.04
2-Methyl-2-propenoic acid	79-41-4	Confirmed	TPM	0.311	2.70
Cyclohexylphenylacetic acid	3894-09-5	Confirmed	TPM	0.309	3.68
Pentanal	110-62-3	Confirmed	GVP	0.308	3.08
3-Oxo-7,8-dihydro-a-ionol	60047-19-0	Confirmed	TPM	0.307	1.75
2,3-Dimethylpyrazine	5910-89-4	Confirmed	TPM/GVP	0.307	2.79
Geranylacetone	3796-70-1	Confirmed	TPM	0.294	1.39
3(2H)-Furanone	3511-31-7	Medium	TPM	0.294	< 0.100
2-Oxo-propionamide	631-66-3	Confirmed	TPM	0.291	4.95

TABLE 6.3
The Most Abundant (≥100 µg/item) Chemical Constituents Present in the Aerosol of THS and Their Corresponding Concentrations in the Smoke of the 3R4F Reference Cigarette—cont'd

Compound name	CAS number	Identification confidence	Aerosol fraction	Conc. in THS (µg/item)	Conc. in 3R4F (µg/item)
trans-2,6-Octadiene, 2,6-dimethyl-	2609-23-6	Confirmed	GVP	0.288	6.93
Glycidylacetate	6387-89-9	Confirmed	TPM	0.282	0.211
Cyclo(Phe-Pro)	3705-26-8	Confirmed	TPM	0.280	10.3
Harman	486-84-0	Confirmed	TPM	0.278	25.5
6,10,14,18-Tetramethyl-5,9,13,17-nonadecatetraen-2-one	6809-52-5	Confirmed	TPM	0.278	0.902
Squalene derivative (C28)	–	Medium	TPM	0.277	7.55
Norsolanadione	60619-46-7	High	TPM	0.275	3.14
2-Cyclopenten-1-one, dimethyl- (configurational isomer 1)	–	High	TPM/GVP	0.273	8.16
Higher molecular weight derivative of farnesylacetone (C30)	–	High	TPM	0.268	2.13
Norcotinine	5980-06-3	Confirmed	TPM	0.263	6.83
3-Hydroxy-4-methylbenzoic acid	586-30-1	High	TPM	0.260	2.09
1*H*-Pyrrole, 1-ethyl-	617-92-5	Confirmed	GVP	0.258	0.136
Benzene, 2-(1,3-butadienyl)-1,3,5-trimethyl-	5732-00-3	Confirmed	TPM	0.255	0.472
Isofucosterol	481-14-1	High	TPM	0.255	3.24
Octadecanoic acid, ethyl ester	111-61-5	Confirmed	TPM	0.253	< 0.100
1,2-Propadiene	463-49-0	Confirmed	GVP	0.249	19.5
Steroid derivative	–	High	TPM	0.247	2.06
trans-3-Methyl-2-pentene	616-12-6	Confirmed	GVP	0.246	24.7
Higher molecular weight derivative of α-longipinene or α-neoclovene	–	High	TPM	0.242	1.71
4-Ethenyl-2,6-dimethoxy-phenol	28343-22-8	Confirmed	TPM	0.241	5.75
3-Hexanone	589-38-8	Confirmed	GVP	0.240	1.60
N-Acetylanatabine	91565-91-2	Confirmed	TPM	0.239	14.6
p-Cresol	106-44-5	Confirmed	TPM	0.236	20.2
Formic acid	64-18-6	Confirmed	TPM	0.233	12.8
2-Ethyl-1-butene	760-21-4	Confirmed	GVP	0.233	5.11
Adenine	73-24-5	Confirmed	TPM	0.231	5.95
Caprolactone	502-44-3	Confirmed	TPM	0.229	< 0.100

Continued

TABLE 6.3
The Most Abundant (≥100 ng/item) Chemical Constituents Present in the Aerosol of THS and Their Corresponding Concentrations in the Smoke of the 3R4F Reference Cigarette—cont'd

Compound name	CAS number	Identification confidence	Aerosol fraction	Conc. in THS (µg/item)	Conc. in 3R4F (µg/item)
2-Heptanone	110-43-0	Confirmed	GVP	0.229	1.88
Octacosane	630-02-4	Confirmed	TPM	0.228	0.954
2-Acetylpyrrole	1072-83-9	Confirmed	TPM	0.225	0.371
N-Acetylanabasine	3350-86-5	Confirmed	TPM	0.221	7.26
Norfuraneol	19322-27-1	Confirmed	TPM	0.219	0.390
2-Heptanone, 6-methyl-	928-68-7	Confirmed	GVP	0.215	0.679
Benzoic acid, 2-hydroxy-4-methyl	50-85-1	Medium	TPM	0.214	1.74
N-acetyl-4(H)-pyridine	67402-83-9	High	TPM	0.213	< 0.100
Butyl-1H-imidazole	50790-93-7	Confirmed	TPM	0.213	6.18
4-Pentenal	2100-17-6	Confirmed	GVP	0.213	2.95
Phenol, 4-ethenyl-	2628-17-3	Confirmed	TPM	0.206	15.0
Methylpropionate	554-12-1	Confirmed	GVP	0.199	1.32
2,7,11-Trimethyl-1,6,10-dodecatriene	502723-87-7	High	TPM	0.198	6.147
2-Acetyl-2-hydroxy-γ-butyrolactone	135366-64-2	Confirmed	TPM	0.197	0.354
Labdanediol	10267-21-7[d]	High	TPM	0.196	< 0.100
Eicosane	112-95-8	Confirmed	TPM	0.194	0.247
2-Cyclopenten-1-one, 3-ethyl-2-hydroxy-	21835-01-8	Confirmed	TPM	0.194	1.66
Nicotinamide	98-92-0	Confirmed	TPM	0.192	4.32
Dimethyltrisulfide	3658-80-8	Confirmed	GVP	0.192	0.460
Hydrogen sulfide	7783-06-4	Confirmed	GVP	0.190	5.04
2,5-Hexanedione	110-13-4	Confirmed	TPM	0.190	0.515
2-Methyl-3-pentanone	565-69-5	Confirmed	GVP	0.189	1.21
2,3-Dimethyl-1-butene	563-78-0	Confirmed	GVP	0.188	16.9
Pentadecanal	2765-11-9	Confirmed	TPM	0.183	1.49
trans-2-Methyl-1,3-pentadiene	926-54-5	Confirmed	GVP	0.182	19.3
1-(4-Methylphenyl)-ethanone	122-00-9	Confirmed	TPM	0.182	0.754
cis-3-Methyl-2-pentene	922-62-3	Confirmed	GVP	0.179	21.2
3'-Hydroxycotinine	34834-67-8	Confirmed	TPM	0.178	7.22
4-Vinylguaiacol	7786-61-0	Confirmed	TPM	0.177	6.24
2,2,6-Trimethyl-1-(3-methylbuta-1,3-dienyl)-7-oxabicyclo[4.1.0]heptan-3-ol	1427305-74-5	Medium	TPM	0.177	3.48
Maltol	118-71-0	Confirmed	TPM	0.175	0.347

TABLE 6.3
The Most Abundant (≥100 μg/item) Chemical Constituents Present in the Aerosol of THS and Their Corresponding Concentrations in the Smoke of the 3R4F Reference Cigarette—cont'd

Compound name	CAS number	Identification confidence	Aerosol fraction	Conc. in THS (μg/item)	Conc. in 3R4F (μg/item)
3,4-Dimethyl-2,5-furandione	766-39-2	Confirmed	TPM	0.174	0.235
3-Methyl-2(5H)-furanone	22122-36-7	Confirmed	TPM	0.174	0.295
2H-Pyrrol-2-one, 4-ethyl-1,5-dihydro-3-methyl	766-45-0	High	TPM	0.173	12.4
(2-Isopropyl-1,3-dioxolan-4-yl)methanol	31192-94-6	High	TPM	0.171	< 0.100
α-Ionol	25312-34-9	Confirmed	GVP	0.169	< 0.100
10-Heneicosene	95008-11-0	Confirmed	TPM	0.167	0.442
2-Methylhydroquinone	95-71-6	Confirmed	TPM	0.166	4.86
1-Heptene	592-76-7	Confirmed	GVP	0.165	23.9
Isobutyronitrile	78-82-0	Confirmed	GVP	0.165	20.9
5-Methyl-2-furanmethanol	3857-25-8	Confirmed	TPM	0.164	< 0.100
5-Isopropyl-2,4-imidazolidinedione	16935-34-5	Confirmed	TPM	0.163	8.36
Pantolactone	79-50-5	Confirmed	TPM	0.163	0.278
cis-2,6-Octadiene, 2,6-dimethyl-	2492-22-0	Confirmed	GVP	0.160	4.44
1-Methylcyclopentene	693-89-0	Confirmed	GVP	0.160	19.4
Isocrotonic acid	503-64-0	Confirmed	TPM	0.159	1.53
2,5-Dihydro-3,5-dimethyl-2-furanone	5584-69-0	High	TPM	0.158	0.209
9-Eicosyne	71899-38-2	High	TPM	0.158	0.941
2-Methylphenol	95-48-7	Confirmed	TPM	0.158	6.73
Butyl-hydroxytoluene	128-37-0	Confirmed	TPM	0.155	< 0.100
cis-Phytol	854039-21-7	Confirmed	TPM	0.154	0.222
2-Vinyl-5-methylfuran	10504-13-9	Confirmed	GVP	0.153	0.330
trans-4-Methyl-2-pentene	674-76-0	Confirmed	GVP	0.151	7.43
cis-3-Hexene	7642-09-3	Confirmed	GVP	0.150	5.25
Cyclohexene	110-83-8	Confirmed	GVP	0.149	7.85
Diacetin monopropanoate	36600-62-1	Confirmed	TPM	0.149	1.69
1-Docosanol	661-19-8	Confirmed	TPM	0.149	0.534
4-Vinylpyridine	100-43-6	Confirmed	TPM	0.148	12.7
5-Cyanonicotine	42459-12-1	Confirmed	TPM	0.146	59.5
Thiophene	110-02-1	Confirmed	GVP	0.145	1.92
4-Vinylcatechol	6053-02-7	Confirmed	TPM	0.140	38.3
9-Nonadecene	31035-07-1	High	TPM	0.137	2.61

Continued

TABLE 6.3
The Most Abundant (≥100 ng/item) Chemical Constituents Present in the Aerosol of THS and Their Corresponding Concentrations in the Smoke of the 3R4F Reference Cigarette—cont'd

Compound name	CAS number	Identification confidence	Aerosol fraction	Conc. in THS (µg/item)	Conc. in 3R4F (µg/item)
4-Ethylguaiacol	2785-89-9	Confirmed	TPM	0.137	0.377
cis-Verbenol	18881-04-4	Confirmed	TPM	0.137	1.13
1-Hexadecanol	36653-82-4	Confirmed	TPM	0.136	0.833
2-Cyclopenten-1-one, dimethyl- (configurational isomer 2)	–	High	GVP	0.135	3.02
trans-Caryophyllene	87-44-5	Confirmed	TPM	0.135	1.22
7-Oxabicyclo[4.1.0] heptan-3-ol, 6-(3-hydroxy-1-butenyl)-1,5,5-trimethyl-)-	72777-88-9	Medium	TPM	0.135	1.31
1-Methylcyclohexene	591-49-1	Confirmed	GVP	0.134	2.78
Phenylethyl alcohol	60-12-8	Confirmed	TPM	0.133	0.381
Chloroethane	75-00-3	Confirmed	GVP	0.131	1.06
Cyclobutanone	1191-95-3	Confirmed	GVP	0.130	3.79
Linolenic acid, methyl ester	301-00-8	Confirmed	TPM	0.130	0.809
trans-2-Hexene	13269-52-8	Confirmed	GVP	0.130	17.4
Butanenitrile, 2-methylene	1647-11-6	Confirmed	GVP	0.130	12.3
2,4-Dimethyl pyridine	108-47-4	Confirmed	TPM	0.129	4.35
3-Acetoxypyridine	17747-43-2	Confirmed	TPM	0.128	8.17
Tridecane, 2,6,10-trimethyl-	3891-99-4	High	TPM	0.126	1.67
2-Methyl-2-hexene	2738-19-4	Confirmed	GVP	0.126	17.6
3,5-Dimethylcyclopentene	7459-71-4	High	GVP	0.126	7.18
2-Methylcyclopentanone	1120-72-5	Confirmed	GVP	0.125	6.85
3-(4,8,12-Trimethyltridecyl)furan	54869-11-3	Confirmed	TPM	0.125	0.260
N-Nitrosoanatabine	887407-16-1	Confirmed	TPM	0.125	0.955
4-Ethylcatechol	1124-39-6	Confirmed	TPM	0.124	5.84
Hexacosane	630-01-3	Confirmed	TPM	0.123	0.360
Bulnesol	22451-73-6	High	TPM	0.122	< 0.100
Nonane	111-84-2	Confirmed	GVP	0.121	3.34
Eicosane, 2-methyl-	1560-84-5	Confirmed	TPM	0.121	< 0.100
2-Furancarbonitrile	617-90-3	Confirmed	GVP	0.120	1.67
2-Methyl-1,4-pentadiene	763-30-4	Confirmed	GVP	0.119	9.84
1,2-Cyclohexanedione	765-87-7	Confirmed	TPM	0.119	< 0.100
trans,trans-2,4-Hexadiene	5194-51-4	Confirmed	GVP	0.119	16.3
2-Tritriacontanone	75207-55-5	High	TPM	0.118	2.00

TABLE 6.3
The Most Abundant (≥100 ng/item) Chemical Constituents Present in the Aerosol of THS and Their Corresponding Concentrations in the Smoke of the 3R4F Reference Cigarette—cont'd

Compound name	CAS number	Identification confidence	Aerosol fraction	Conc. in THS (μg/item)	Conc. in 3R4F (μg/item)
1,3-Cyclohexadiene	592-57-4	Confirmed	GVP	0.115	10.3
Docobosanal	57402-36-5	Confirmed	TPM	0.114	0.315
Sinapyl alcohol	537-33-7	Confirmed	TPM	0.114	7.95
Squalene oxide	7200-26-2	Confirmed	TPM	0.113	1.49
Octane, 3,3-dimethyl-	4110-44-5	Confirmed	GVP	0.111	0.610
N-Furfurylpyrrole	1438-94-4	Confirmed	TPM	0.108	0.103
3-Methyltritriacontane	14167-69-2	High	TPM	0.108	0.853
Octane	111-65-9	Confirmed	GVP	0.108	6.73
o-Cymene	527-84-4	Confirmed	GVP	0.106	0.323
9-Methyladenine	700-00-5	Confirmed	TPM	0.106	1.02
2-Methylnonadecane	1560-86-7	Confirmed	TPM	0.106	< 0.100
2(3*H*)-Furanone, dihydro-3-hydroxy-4,4-dimethyl-, (*R*)-	599-04-2	Confirmed	TPM	0.105	0.202
Nonadecane	629-92-5	Confirmed	TPM	0.105	0.194
2-Ethylpyridine	100-71-0	Confirmed	GVP	0.101	0.276
3-Methylcinnamic acid	3029-79-6	Medium	TPM	0.101	4.26
2,5-Dimethyl-3(2*H*)-furanone	14400-67-0	Confirmed	TPM	0.100	< 0.100
Not identified (GCxGC—TOFMS; 10 compounds)	–	Not identified	TPM	7.33	8.38
Not identified (GCxGC—TOFMS; 3 compounds)	–	Not identified	GVP	5.18	3.70

CAS, Chemical Abstracts Service; *GCxGC—TOFMS*, two-dimensional gas chromatography with time-of-flight mass spectrometry; *GVP*, gas—vapor phase; *THS*, Tobacco Heating System; *TPM*, total particulate matter.
[a] Semiquantified concentration represents the sum of concentrations of two tautomers, which interconvert inconsistently during analysis.
[b] Concentration determined quantitatively.
[c] Degradation experiments with suspected precursors confirmed the compound class proposal.
[d] CAS number corresponds to one of the isomeric forms of this compound.

4 compounds (Fig. 6.4). It was not possible to compare the analytically determined mass contribution of the GVP with any gravimetrically determined value, as it was not feasible to measure the mass of the GVP generated by using the trapping system, as described. Accordingly, no mass-based estimate for the achieved chemical coverage could be made. The major compound classes contributing to the GVP fraction were aldehydes, ketones, alcohols, and furanic compounds.

All 529 compounds found to be present in THS aerosol at concentrations above, or equivalent to, 100 ng/ item were also determined to be present in 3R4F smoke.

3R4F smoke was estimated to contain approximately 10 times the number of constituents as THS aerosol, with only a minority of the compounds being present in THS aerosol at concentrations exceeding those measured in 3R4F smoke.

6.6 CONCLUSION

In order to fully characterize the composition of the aerosol generated by an EHTP and evaluate the differences in its composition compared with cigarette smoke, a suite of complementary untargeted analytical methods was

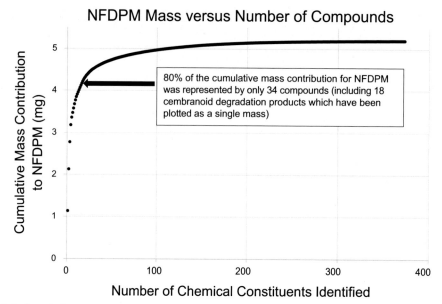

FIG. 6.3 Cumulative mass of individual chemical constituents contributing to THS 2.2 NFDPM (excluding glycerin) ranked in order from the highest (left) to the lowest (right) mass contribution.
NFDPM = TPM−[water + nicotine], nicotine-free dry particulate matter; *THS*, tobacco heating system.

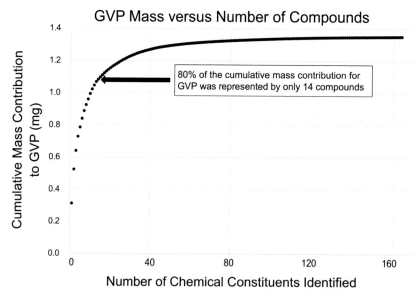

FIG. 6.4 Cumulative mass of individual chemical constituents contributing to THS GVP, ranked in order from the highest (left) to lowest (right) mass contribution. *GVP*, gas−vapor phase; *THS*, tobacco heating system. (Graphic from Bentley, M.C., Almstetter, M., Arndt, D., Knorr, A., Martin, E., Pospisil, P., Maeder, S., 2020. Comprehensive chemical characterization of the aerosol generated by a heated tobacco product by untargeted screening. Anal. Bioanal. Chem. 412, 2675−2685. https://doi.org/10.1007/s00216-020-02502-1.)

used, which was designed to cover the broadest possible range of chemical classes. With a 100-ng/item reporting threshold applied for untargeted screening, the chemical constituents found in THS aerosol were also confirmed to be present in cigarette smoke, with an apparent 10-fold reduction in the overall number of constituents present compared with cigarette smoke. It is, therefore, logical to assume that the priority toxicants currently selected for regulatory reporting of tobacco products by different authorities, including the FDA reduced list of 18 HPHCs for the United States (FDA, 2012a) and the Health Canada list of 44 HPHCs for Canada (Health Canada, 2000), will remain applicable for assessment of EHTPs. Of course, it is recognized that, with the application of such a reporting threshold, the presence of any compound representing a toxicological concern at concentrations below 100 ng/item would be overlooked. In order to address this shortfall, PMI has applied an untargeted differential screening approach that does not apply a concentration reporting threshold, in the context of "new hazard" identification. Evaluation of any potential "new hazard" should be made in context with the overall reductions in the numbers and quantities of chemical constituents, including known HPHCs, and in conjunction with the outcome of a range of biological assays that evaluate the aerosol as a whole (Chapters 13–15).

The comparative untargeted differential screening analyses identified three compounds unique to THS aerosol (*cis*-sesquisabinene hydrate, 61 ng/item; ethyl dodecanoate, 23 ng/item; and benzenemethanol, 4-hydroxy, 11 ng/item). All three compounds were present at concentrations below 100 ng/item, which demonstrated the ability of the methodology to identify differences at concentrations approximately one order of magnitude lower than the threshold applied for untargeted screening. Four additional compounds, not present within any list of priority toxicants currently used for regulatory reporting of tobacco products, were highlighted to be of toxicological concern, namely glycidol, 3-MCPD, 2-furanmethanol, and furfural. The range of values determined for these constituents in commercially available cigarettes was indicative of the fact that tobacco blend composition has an impact on smoke composition. However, the substantially decreased number and levels of HPHCs found in THS aerosol relative to cigarette smoke led to the conclusion that these reductions outweighed the potential detrimental effects presented by such compounds (FDA, 2019). The observed differences between THS aerosol and 3R4F smoke, particularly those for compounds determined to be unique to THS aerosol, are assumed to be due to added flavors (3R4F is an unflavored reference cigarette) and tobacco blend differences. Fig. 6.5 presents a graphical representation of the outcome of PMI's untargeted screening and untargeted differential screening activities regarding the composition of THS aerosol compared with 3R4F smoke.

Toxicants that are increased in, or specific to, EHTPs relative to cigarettes could be considered for inclusion in lists of HPHCs specific for such products. However, the small increase in the numbers of such specific HPHCs should be weighed and evaluated in the context of the overall reduction in the numbers and quantities

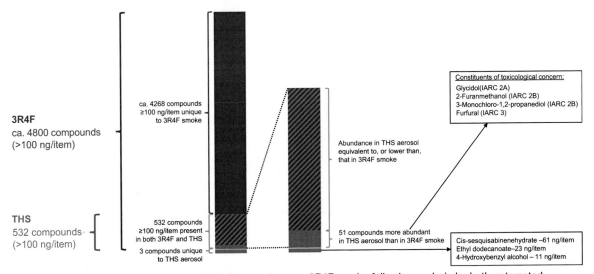

FIG. 6.5 Summary of findings for THS aerosol versus 3R4F smoke following analysis by both untargeted differential screening and untargeted screening. *THS*, tobacco heating system.

of chemical constituents, including known HPHCs (Schaller et al., 2016), and additionally assessed by biological assays that evaluate the aerosol as a whole (Chapters 13–15). To the best of our knowledge, this is the most comprehensive in-depth chemical characterization of an EHTP aerosol reported to date (Bentley et al., 2020).

It is not anticipated that such untargeted methodologies will be routinely applied for evaluation of e-vapor products (EVPs). The ingredients used for preparation of e-liquids should be of known identity and purity. The majority of toxicants related to EVP use are also known and can be measured by using targeted techniques. In addition, carbonyls, which are recognized as being the main chemical class of concern related to EVP use, require specific trapping techniques owing to their chemical reactivity and cannot be reliably measured by using the generic trapping techniques applied for untargeted screening.

REFERENCES

Amendment to Philip Morris Products S.A. Modified Risk Tobacco Product Application, 2017. Response to 4 August 2017 FDA Advice and Information Request Letter Including Non-targeted Differential Screening, Toxicological Assessment, and Peer Review Reports, 2017.

Arndt, D., Wachsmuth, C., Buchholz, C., Bentley, M., 2020. A complex matrix characterization approach, applied to cigarette smoke, that integrates multiple analytical methods and compound identification strategies for non-targeted liquid chromatography with high-resolution mass spectrometry. Rapid Commun. Mass Spectrom. 34 https://doi.org/10.1002/rcm.8571.

Baker, R.R., 1987. A review of pyrolysis studies to unravel reaction steps in burning tobacco. J. Anal. Appl. Pyrol. 11, 555–573. https://doi.org/10.1016/0165-2370(87)85054-4.

Bentley, M.C., Almstetter, M., Arndt, D., Knorr, A., Martin, E., Pospisil, P., Maeder, S., 2020. Comprehensive chemical characterization of the aerosol generated by a heated tobacco product by untargeted screening. Anal. Bioanal. Chem. 412, 2675–2685. https://doi.org/10.1007/s00216-020-02502-1.

Burns, D.M., Dybing, E., Gray, N., Hecht, S., Anderson, C., Sanner, T., O'Connor, R., Djordjevic, M., Dresler, C., Hainaut, P., Jarvis, M., Opperhuizen, A., Straif, K., 2008. Mandated lowering of toxicants in cigarette smoke: a description of the World Health Organization TobReg proposal. Tobac. Contr. 17, 132–141. https://doi.org/10.1136/tc.2007.024158.

Cozzani, V., Barontini, F., McGrath, T., Mahler, B., Nordlund, M., Smith, M., Schaller, J.P., Zuber, G., 2020. An experimental investigation into the operation of an electrically heated tobacco system. Thermochim. Acta 684, 178475. https://doi.org/10.1016/j.tca.2019.178475.

FDA, April 29, 2019. Premarket Tobacco Product Marketing Order TPL (Technical Project Lead Review) PM0000424-79. Section 6 - Summary of Toxicological Findings. https://www.fda.gov/media/124247/download (Accessed 16 May 20).

FDA, 2012a. Guidance for Industry - Reporting Harmful and Potentially Harmful Constituents in Tobacco Products and Tobacco Smoke under Section 904(a)(3) of the Federal Food, Drug, and Cosmetic Act - Draft Guidance.

FDA, 2012b. Harmful and potentially harmful constituents in tobacco products and tobacco smoke; established list. Fed. Regist. Food & Drug Adm. 77, 20034.

Health Canada, 2000. Tobacco Reporting Regulations. Part 3: Emissions from Designated Tobacco Products.

Health Canada, 1999. Health Canada Test Method T-115, Determination of "Tar", Nicotine and Carbon Monoxide in Mainstream Tobacco Smoke. http://healthycanadians.gc.ca/en/open-information/tobacco/t100/nicotine.

IARC monographs on the evaluation of carcinogenic risks of chemicals to humans. In: IARC (Ed.), 2004. Tobacco Smoke and Involuntary Smoking, vol. 83. IARC, Lyon.

Knorr, A., Almstetter, M., Martin, E., Castellon, A., Pospisil, P., Bentley, M.C., 2019. Performance evaluation of a nontargeted platform using two-dimensional gas chromatography time-of-flight mass spectrometry integrating computer-assisted structure identification and automated semiquantification for the comprehensive chemical characterization of a complex matrix. Anal. Chem. 91, 9129–9137. https://doi.org/10.1021/acs.analchem.9b01659.

Knorr, A., Monge, A., Stueber, M., Stratmann, A., Arndt, D., Martin, E., Pospisil, P., 2013. Computer-assisted structure identification (CASI)–an automated platform for high-throughput identification of small molecules by two-dimensional gas chromatography coupled to mass spectrometry. Anal. Chem. 85, 11216–11224. https://doi.org/10.1021/ac4011952.

Martin, E., Monge, A., Duret, J.-A., Gualandi, F., Peitsch, M.C., Pospisil, P., 2012. Building an R&D chemical registration system. J. Cheminf. 4, 11. https://doi.org/10.1186/1758-2946-4-11.

Nonlinear Dynamics web site, n.d. Progenesis QI Theoretical Fragmentation Algorithm. http://www.nonlinear.com/progenesis/qi/v2.4/faq/theoretical-fragmentation-algorithm.aspx. (Accessed 10 December 19).

Rodgman, A., Perfetti, T.A., 2013. The Chemical Components of Tobacco and Tobacco Smoke, second ed.

Savareear, B., Escobar-Arnanz, J., Brokl, M., Saxton, M.J., Wright, C., Liu, C., Focant, J.-F., 2019. Non-targeted analysis of the particulate phase of heated tobacco product aerosol and cigarette mainstream tobacco smoke by thermal desorption comprehensive two-dimensional gas chromatography with dual flame ionisation and mass spectrometric detection. J. Chromatogr. A 1603, 327–337. https://doi.org/10.1016/j.chroma.2019.06.057.

Savareear, B., Escobar-Arnanz, J., Brokl, M., Saxton, M.J., Wright, C., Liu, C., Focant, J.-F., 2018. Comprehensive comparative compositional study of the vapour phase of cigarette mainstream tobacco smoke and tobacco heating product aerosol. J. Chromatogr. A 1581–1582, 105–115. https://doi.org/10.1016/j.chroma.2018.10.035.

Schaller, J.-P., Keller, D., Poget, L., Pratte, P., Kaelin, E., McHugh, D., Cudazzo, G., Smart, D., Tricker, A.R., Gautier, L., 2016. Evaluation of the Tobacco Heating System 2.2. Part 2: chemical composition, genotoxicity, cytotoxicity, and physical properties of the aerosol. Regul. Toxicol. Pharmacol. 81, S27–S47.

Smith, M.R., Clark, B., Lüdicke, F., Schaller, J.-P., Vanscheeuwijck, P., Hoeng, J., Peitsch, M.C., 2016. Evaluation of the tobacco heating system 2.2. Part 1: description of the system and the scientific assessment program. Regul. Toxicol. Pharmacol. 81 (Suppl. 2), S17–S26. https://doi.org/10.1016/j.yrtph.2016.07.006.

Uchiyama, S., Noguchi, M., Takagi, N., Hayashida, H., Inaba, Y., Ogura, H., Kunugita, N., 2018. Simple determination of gaseous and particulate compounds generated from heated tobacco products. Chem. Res. Toxicol. 31, 585–593. https://doi.org/10.1021/acs.chemrestox.8b00024.

University of Kentucky Center for Tobacco Reference Products, n.d. 3R4F Preliminary Analysis.

WHO, 2019. TobReg Scientific Recommendation: Updated Priority List of Toxicants in Combusted Tobacco Products.

Wolf, S., Schmidt, S., Müller-Hannemann, M., Neumann, S., 2010. In silico fragmentation for computer assisted identification of metabolite mass spectra. BMC Bioinf. 11, 148. https://doi.org/10.1186/1471-2105-11-148.

CHAPTER 7

Other Species of Toxicological Concern not Classified as HPHCs

PASCAL PRATTE • MARK BENTLEY • JEAN-PIERRE SCHALLER • SERGE MAEDER

7.1 INTRODUCTION

Electronic nicotine delivery products (ENDPs) deliver nicotine and flavors at operating temperatures that are sufficient to release an aerosol from a solid- or liquid-based substrate. These operating temperatures are low enough to avoid combustion, which reduces thermal degradation of the evaporated molecules, thereby minimizing the levels of harmful and potentially harmful constituents (HPHCs) in ENDP aerosols (Chapters 4 and 6). Higher temperatures cause increased pyrolysis and initiate biomass combustion, which releases numerous toxicants into the generated smoke. Cigarette smoke contains highly reactive radicals and combustion-related carbon-based solid particles, which contribute to its toxicity. Comparing the levels of reactive radicals and combustion-related carbon-based particles in ENDP aerosols with those in cigarette smoke is important for evaluating the harm and disease risk reduction potential associated with switching from cigarette smoking to ENDP use.

7.2 RADICALS

Mainstream cigarette smoke has been shown to be highly complex comprising several thousand chemical substances distributed between the gas and particulate phases (Rodgman and Perfetti, 2013). It is composed of chemical constituents from a wide range of organic chemical classes, including saturated and unsaturated hydrocarbons, alcohols, aldehydes, ketones, carboxylic acids, esters, phenols, nitriles, terpenoids, and alkaloids (Baker, 1999; Dube and Green, 1982; Hoffmann et al., 2001). However, much of the research performed over the past decades has focused on a limited number of constituents, with more scrutiny applied to constituents in high abundance, with known pharmacological properties (Benowitz, 2009), and identified as harmful or potentially harmful for smokers (FDA, 2012; IARC, 2004). Constituents that cause oxidative stress in humans are perhaps some of the less scrutinized compounds present in tobacco smoke. A comprehensive review by Wooten and colleagues addressed the presence of chemical constituents in cigarette smoke that are related to oxidative stress, examining those that are known to increase the oxidant burden, decrease antioxidant protection, or result in the generation of reactive oxygen species and reactive nitrogen species (Wooten et al., 2006). In this chapter, we summarize the most recent information regarding the abundance of free radicals in ENDP aerosols relative to cigarette smoke.

Compared with cigarette smoke, aerosols from e-vapor products (EVPs) and electrically heated tobacco products (EHTPs) have been demonstrated to contain lower levels of all compounds in the list of HPHCs known to be present in tobacco and tobacco smoke (FDA, 2012) (Chapter 4). Free radicals, which also present potential health risks, are not routinely analyzed, and there is relatively little information available in the public domain regarding their emission from the increasing range of available ENDPs. In 2019, Shein and Jeschke compared the type and quantity of free radicals in the mainstream aerosol of 3R4F research cigarettes with those in two types of EVPs and one type of EHTP (Tobacco Heating System 2.2 [THS], developed by Philip Morris International [PMI]) (Shein and Jeschke, 2019). Free radicals and nitric oxide (NO) in the gas phase were spin trapped and quantified by electron paramagnetic resonance (EPR) spectroscopy, which employed a flow-through cell to enhance measurement reproducibility. Aerosol was generated in accordance with the Health Canada Intense (HCI) smoking regimen (Health Canada, 1999), and particulate matter was additionally collected by using a Cambridge filter pad (CFP). The authors reported at least a 99% reduction in the levels of spin-trapped organic radicals present in the EVP and EHTP aerosols relative to cigarette smoke,

Toxicological Evaluation of Electronic Nicotine Delivery Products. https://doi.org/10.1016/B978-0-12-820490-0.00015-8

with the radical levels in the aerosols being close to those observed in air blank samples. The radicals observed in cigarette smoke were identified as oxygen-centered, whereas those near the limit of detection in EVP and EHTP aerosols were found to be carbon-centered. Shein and Jeschke also reported reduced levels of NO (ca. 93% lower) in EHTP aerosol relative to cigarette smoke, with the levels in EVP aerosol falling below the limit of detection; persistent radicals in particulate matter trapped by using a CFP were only quantified in cigarette smoke (Shein and Jeschke, 2019).

A more recent publication (Bitzer et al., 2020) also confirmed a significantly reduced presence of gas vapor-phase (GVP) free radicals and an absence of persistent particulate-phase radicals in EVP and EHTP aerosols, in comparison with cigarette smoke. Aerosols generated by the EHTP, EVP, and a hybrid device were compared with smoke from the 1R6F reference cigarette (University of Kentucky, Lexington, KY, USA). This study showed that the GVP of 1R6F contained 568 ± 78.3 pmol radicals per puff (pmol/puff), whereas the GVP of the EHTP (12.6 ± 1.1 pmol/puff), hybrid device (12.1 ± 1.4 pmol/puff), and EVP (between 5.3 ± 0.5 and 47.8 ± 1.8 pmol/puff) contained significantly reduced levels of radicals.

While Shein and Jeschke noted the presence of oxygen-centered radicals in cigarette smoke (Shein and Jeschke, 2019) and carbon-centered radicals near the limit of detection in EVP and EHTP aerosols, Bitzer et al. investigated the differences in the polarity of free radicals by passing smoke/aerosol through polar and nonpolar solvents prior to spin trapping and EPR spectroscopy (Bitzer et al., 2020). The polarity of GVP radicals in the EVP aerosol was found to differ from that of GVP radicals in the EHTP aerosol and cigarette smoke, with the latter two producing more polar radicals than the EVP aerosol. These authors have also previously reported that the radical levels emitted by EVPs are influenced by device characteristics (e.g., voltage and coil resistance), e-liquid composition, and puffing behavior (Bitzer et al., 2018a,b, 2019; Goel et al., 2015; Reilly et al., 2019).

Exposure to inhaled free radicals presents a potentially significant health risk to smokers, as highly reactive chemical species can damage critical cellular pathways, leading to carcinogenesis and other disorders (CDC, 2010; Pryor, 1997). The reductions in radical emissions observed in EVP and EHTP aerosols relative to cigarette smoke are significant and exceed the reductions reported for recognized HPHCs (Chapter 4), lending further support to the view that EVPs and EHTPs are potentially less harmful than cigarettes.

7.3 COMBUSTION-RELATED SOLID PARTICLE ASSESSMENT

Chapter 5 makes a clear distinction between aerosols that are generated with and without combustion. When a biomass is heated without combustion, the resulting aerosol has substantially different properties than a combustion-related aerosol, which is defined as smoke. In addition to the fact that combustion-free aerosols and smoke may be differentiated by their different chemical composition, they also differ in the physical properties of their respective suspended particulate matter. Heating of biomass results in the formation of an aerosol that contains liquid droplets, whereas biomass combustion releases smoke that contains both liquid droplets and combustion-related solid particles, with the latter mainly comprising organic materials (Hildemann et al., 1991; Oha et al., 2011). These solid particles are generally insoluble in water and can persist in human lungs upon inhalation and may promote disease development (Bauer et al., 2010; Donaldson et al., 1998; Klein et al., 2017). In THS, the tobacco substrate is heated at temperatures below 320°C, where only distillation and low-temperature pyrolysis occur. Consequently, it is not expected that combustion-related solid particles will be released and transferred into the aerosol of THS (Cozzani et al., 2020). An experimental approach was established to demonstrate this with an EHTP and EVP by using cigarette smoke as a positive control.

7.3.1 Samples and Methodology

The approach described below has already been used (Pratte et al., 2017) to characterize aerosols from an EHTP (THS). This approach employed a Dekati thermo-denuder maintained at 300°C, close to the boiling point of glycerin (290°C), which is one of the main aerosol formers present in EHTP and EVP aerosols. The thermo-denuder consisted of two parts. The first comprised 1-m-long curved and straight tubing sections, which were insulated and heated to 300°C. The second part was a 0.60-m-long gas stripper, which captured volatiles by using a cartridge containing activated carbon, which was replaced after every 20 h of operation. To ensure that the gas stripper was operating efficiently, compressed air at room temperature was passed through the housing (70 L/min), ensuring that volatiles were trapped efficiently and potential recondensation was minimized. A schematic for the complete setup is presented in Fig. 7.1.

A programmable dual syringe pump (Burkhart Messtechnik GmbH, Wedel, Germany) was used for aerosol generation under the HCI smoking regimen (55-mL puff volume, 2-s puff, and 30-s puff interval). The aerosol, or

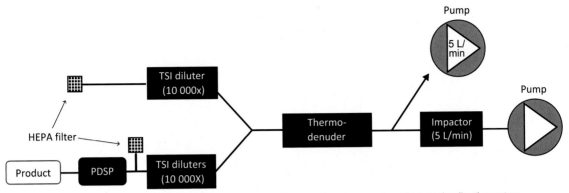

FIG. 7.1 Experimental design: Mainstream aerosol generation, thermo-denuding, and collection setup.

smoke, was then passed through two TSI dilution units in series, each operating with a dilution ratio of 100, resulting in an overall 10,000-fold dilution. The smoke/aerosol was passed through these serial diluters at a volumetric flow rate of 5 L/min; an additional dilution unit was used in parallel to provide makeup flow (5 L/min) with HEPA-filtered laboratory air, such that the total flow entering the thermo-denuder had a flow rate of 10 L/min. On the exit side, an equivalent vacuum flow rate of 10 L/min was applied, which ensured unrestricted gas flow through the thermo-denuder. This was achieved by using a TSI 3708 four-way splitter, which separated the flow equally between a filter-protected vacuum pump (5 L/min) and a two-stage impactor trap (5 L/min), which collected supermicron and submicron particles separately (Jalanti and Henchoz, 1990). The impactor traps were subsequently sent to Microscan (Microscan service SA [ISO/CEI 17025, STS n° 0472], Chavannes-près-Renens, Switzerland) to determine the presence of any residual particulate matter by scanning electron microscopy (SEM).

In order to ensure that the thermo-denuder was effectively removing liquid droplets from the introduced aerosol samples, model glycerin droplets were used to assess the efficiency of the thermo-denuder at 300°C. The droplet number concentration was measured upstream and downstream of the thermo-denuder, and the associated removal yield was estimated to be greater than 97% (Pratte et al., 2018). Therefore, the thermo-denuder was considered suitable for efficient separation of combustion-related particles from liquid droplets, facilitating their observation and elemental composition determination.

7.3.2 Results and Discussion

SEM with energy-dispersive X-ray (EDX) analysis showed that the impactor substrates used to trap thermo-denuded EHTP aerosol were very similar to blank samples (no

aerosol generation). Additionally, it was confirmed that both the blank and EHTP aerosol were free of combustion-related solid particles. Cigarette smoke was used as a positive control and compared with the blank and EHTP aerosol. It was essential to ensure that the technique could effectively isolate combustion-related particles on the impactor-collection substrates, in order to put the EHTP and blank results into context. The resulting SEM images are presented in Fig. 7.2.

A very low amount of particles, attributed to air and surface contamination from the experimental setup, can be observed in the images of the blank and thermo-denuded EHTP samples (Fig. 7.2B). This confirms that EHTP aerosol is entirely composed of liquid droplets and does not contain solid particles. In contrast, the images of smoke residue collected from the 3R4F cigarette clearly show a visible circle on the collection substrate (Fig. 7.2A). In-depth SEM analysis of the smoke residue revealed the presence of a myriad of agglomerated particle-forming clusters, whose surface number density was estimated to be greater than four million per square millimeter, as opposed to the blank and EHTP, for which less than a 1000 particles were observed. EDX analysis revealed that the smoke particles were composed mainly of organic materials, whereas the particles from the blank and EHTP aerosol samples were primarily composed of metallic oxides, attributed to suspended particles from the laboratory environment and released from the surfaces of the test bench. The size distribution of the particles collected from 3R4F smoke is presented in Fig. 7.3.

This shows that more than 80% of the smoke particles were smaller than 100 nm, which corresponds to the ultrafine or nanoparticle fraction, typically generated by an incomplete combustion process (Butler and Mulholland, 2004). Consequently, it can be concluded that the EHTP aerosol has substantially different physicochemical properties from cigarette smoke.

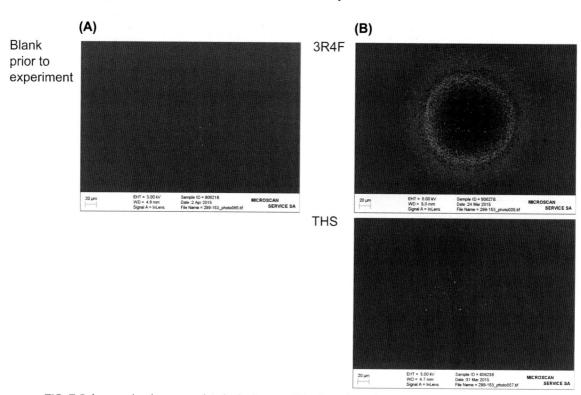

FIG. 7.2 Images showing accumulated submicron particles from the mainstream aerosol of (**A**) 3R4F and (**B**) EHTP (THS).The picture on the left side is the related blank prior to experiment.

7.3.3 Combustion-related Particles in Commercial Cigarettes and Evaluation of an EVP

To obtain more insights into the methodology, the smoke/aerosol of five commercial cigarette brands and an EVP were investigated for the presence and number of combustion particles. The total number of combustion-related solid particles released per cigarette was estimated by using the surface size distribution displayed in Fig. 7.3 (representative for smoke) and the concentration of particles measured downstream from the thermo-denuder. The data presented in Table 7.1 are corrected for aerosol dilution and thermo-denuder wall losses. For the tested commercial cigarettes, the number of solid particles released ranged from 5.9 to 7.3×10^{11}, in contrast to the $8.5-9.5 \times 10^{11}$ range for 3R4F. Overall, the associated combustion-related solid particle mass delivered per smoking run ranged from 683 to 1112 μg.

The EVP selected for evaluation was a product developed by PMI, which uses a mesh heater instead of the standard wick and coil system. The working principle is the same as that of a wick and coil system, where a liquid substrate is heated and the vapors generated

cool down to form an aerosol consisting of suspended liquid droplets, which are formed via homogeneous nucleation (Chapter 5). Given this aerosol-forming mechanism, the EVP aerosol was expected to contain only liquid droplets. For this experiment, 50 puffs were generated by using the CORESTA (Cooperation Centre for Scientific Research Relative to Tobacco) regimen (2015). The aerosol was thermo-denuded, collected on impactor-collection substrates, and compared with a blank sample. The associated SEM images are presented in Fig. 7.4 for the blank (left) and the thermo-denuded EVP aerosol (right). The two images are similar and confirm that the tested EVP generates an aerosol that contains only liquid droplets, in contrast to cigarette smoke, which contains combustion-related solid particles.

7.4 CONCLUSION

ENDPs emit significantly lower levels of recognized HPHCs than cigarettes (Chapter 4). In this chapter, we focused on other species of known toxicological concern, investigating the presence of highly reactive chemical radicals and combustion-related solid particles. External

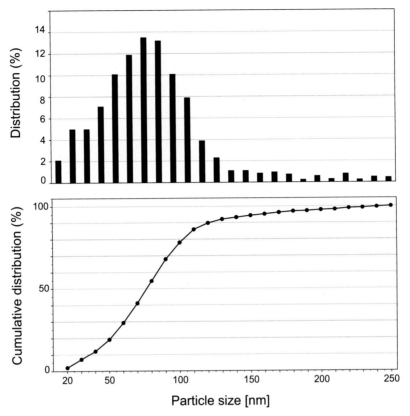

FIG. 7.3 Size distribution of deposited solid particles from 3R4F mainstream smoke, analyzed by SEM. The top panel shows the solid particle size distribution, and the bottom panel shows the cumulative size distribution. The x-axis represents the particle size in nanometers. *SEM*, scanning electron microscopy.

TABLE 7.1
Solid Particle Number Data (x10^{11}) per Test Item in Triplicates, Corrected for an Applied Aerosol Dilution of 20,000x.

Brand	Delicados	Karelia Tobacco Greece	Philip Morris Blue Caps	Camel CZ	MESKIE Filter	3R4F
Tar (mg)	1	6	7	10	10	10
Average, corrected for wall losses	6.6–7.3	5.9–6.4	6.6–7.3	6.3–6.9	6.3–6.9	8.5–9.5

research has shown that, in ENDP aerosols, gas-phase radicals are reduced by more than 99% relative to cigarette smoke, and persistent particulate-phase radicals are absent. In addition, NO levels were demonstrated to be approximately 93% lower in the EHTP aerosol (and undetected in EVP aerosol) than in cigarette smoke. Carbon-based solid particles, highly abundant in cigarette smoke, were not found in ENDP aerosols. These findings show that ENDPs emit not only lower levels of recognized HPHCs than cigarettes but also significantly lower levels of less studied, yet toxicologically relevant, cigarette smoke constituents.

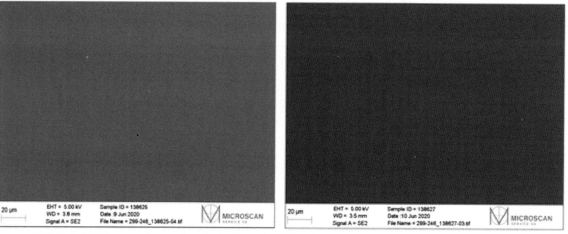

FIG. 7.4 SEM images of aerosols collected from the EVP with mesh heater that was not heated (left) and the same EVP but heated (right). The smoking regimen used was CORESTA, with 50 puffs.

REFERENCES

Baker, R.R., 1999. Smoke chemistry. In: Layten Davis, D., Nielsen, M.T. (Eds.), Tobacco Production, Chemistry and Technology. Blackwell Science Ltd., Oxford, pp. 308–439.

Bauer, M., Moebus, S., Mohlenkamp, S., Dragano, N., Nonnemacher, M., Fuchsluger, M., et al., 2010. Urban particulate matter air pollution is associated with subclinical atherosclerosis: results from the HNR (Heinz Nixdorf Recall) study. J. Am. Coll. Cardiol. 56 (22), 1803–1808.

Benowitz, N.L., 2009. Pharmacology of nicotine: addiction, smoking-induced disease, and therapeutics. Annu. Rev. Pharmacol. Toxicol. 49, 57–71.

Bitzer, Z.T., Goel, R., Reilly, S.M., Bhangu, G., Trushin, N., Foulds, J., et al., 2019. Emissions of free radicals, carbonyls, and nicotine from the NIDA standardized research electronic cigarette and comparison to similar commercial devices. Chem. Res. Toxicol. 32 (1), 130–138.

Bitzer, Z.T., Goel, R., Reilly, S.M., Elias, R.J., Silakov, A., Foulds, J., et al., 2018a. Effect of flavoring chemicals on free radical formation in electronic cigarette aerosols. Free Radic. Biol. Med. 120, 72–79.

Bitzer, Z.T., Goel, R., Reilly, S.M., Foulds, J., Muscat, J., Elias, R.J., et al., 2018b. Effects of solvent and temperature on free radical formation in electronic cigarette aerosols. Chem. Res. Toxicol. 31 (1), 4–12.

Bitzer, Z.T., Goel, R., Trushin, N., Muscat, J., Richie Jr., J.P., 2020. Free radical production and characterization of heat-not-burn cigarettes in comparison to conventional and electronic cigarettes. Chem. Res. Toxicol. 33 (7), 1882–1887.

Butler, K.M., Mulholland, G.W., 2004. Generation and transport of smoke components. Fire Technol. 40, 149–176.

CDC, 2010. How Tobacco Smoke Causes Disease: The Biology and Behavioral Basis for Smoking-Attributable Disease: A Report of the Surgeon General. Atlanta (GA).

Coresta E-Cigarette Task Force, 2015. Technical Report — Electronic Cigarette Aerosol Parameters Study.

Cozzani, V., Barontini, F., Mcgrath, T., Mahler, B., Nordlund, M., Smith, M., et al., 2020. An experimental investigation into the operation of an electrically heated tobacco system. Thermochim. Acta 684, 178475.

Donaldson, K., Li, X.Y., Macnee, W., 1998. Ultrafine (nanometre) particle mediated lung injury. J. Aerosol Sci. 29, 553–560.

Dube, M.F., Green, C.R., 1982. Methods of collection of smoke for analytical purposes. Rec. Adv. Tob. Sci. 8, 42–102.

FDA, 2012. Harmful and potentially harmful constituents in tobacco products and tobacco smoke; established list. Fed. Regist. 77 (64), 20034–20037.

Goel, R., Durand, E., Trushin, N., Prokopczyk, B., Foulds, J., Elias, R.J., et al., 2015. Highly reactive free radicals in electronic cigarette aerosols. Chem. Res. Toxicol. 28 (9), 1675–1677.

Health Canada, 1999. Health Canada Test Method T-115, Determination of "Tar", Nicotine and Carbon Monoxide in Mainstream Tobacco Smoke. http://healthycanadians.gc.ca/en/open-information/tobacco/t100/nicotine.

Hildemann, L.M., Markowsky, G.R., Jones, M.C., Cass, G.R., 1991. Submicrometer aerosol mass distributions of emissions from boilers, fireplaces, automobiles, diesel trucks, and meat-cooking operations. Aerosol Sci. Technol. 14, 138–152.

Hoffmann, D., Hoffmann, I., El-Bayoumy, K., 2001. The less harmful cigarette: a controversial issue. A tribute to Ernst L. Wynder. Chem. Res. Toxicol. 14 (7), 767–790.

IARC, 2004. IARC Monographs on the Evaluation of Carcinogenic Risks of Chemicals to Humans. In: Tobacco Smoke and Involuntary Smoking, vol. 83. IARC, Lyon.

Jalanti, T., Henchoz, P., 1990. Analytical scanning electron microscopy: a most important aid for solving microcontamination problems. Swiss Contam. Control 3 (4a), 428−432.

Klein, S.G., Cambier, S., Hennen, J., Legay, S., Serchi, T., Nelissen, I., et al., 2017. Endothelial responses of the alveolar barrier in vitro in a dose-controlled exposure to diesel exhaust particulate matter. Part. Fibre Toxicol. 14 (1), 7.

Oha, K.C., Leea, C.B., Leeb, E.J., 2011. Characteristics of soot particles formed by diesel pyrolysis. J. Anal. Appl. Pyrol. (92), 456−462.

Pratte, P., Cosandey, S., Goujon Ginglinger, C., 2017. Investigation of solid particles in the mainstream aerosol of the Tobacco Heating System THS2.2 and mainstream smoke of a 3R4F reference cigarette. Hum. Exp. Toxicol. 36 (11), 1115−1120.

Pratte, P., Cosandey, S., Goujon Ginglinger, C., 2018. Innovative methodology based on thermo-denuder principle for the detection of combustion related solid particles or high boiling point droplets: applications to cigarette and the Tobacco Heating System THS 2.2. J. Aerosol Sci. 120, 52−61.

Pryor, W.A., 1997. Cigarette smoke radicals and the role of free radicals in chemical carcinogenicity. Environ. Health Perspect. 105 (Suppl. 4), 875−882.

Reilly, S.M., Bitzer, Z.T., Goel, R., Trushin, N., Richie, J.P., 2019. Free radical, carbonyl, and nicotine levels produced by Juul electronic cigarettes. Nicotine Tob. Res. 21 (9), 1274−1278.

Rodgman, A., Perfetti, T.A., 2013. The Chemical Components of Tobacco and Tobacco Smoke, second ed. CRC Press, Boca Raton.

Shein, M., Jeschke, G., 2019. Comparison of free radical levels in the aerosol from conventional cigarettes, electronic cigarettes, and heat-not-burn tobacco products. Chem. Res. Toxicol. 32 (6), 1289−1298.

Wooten, J.B., Chouchane, S., Mc Grath, T.E., 2006. Ch 2 − tobacco smoke constituents affecting oxidative stress. In: Halliwell, B.B., Poulsen, H.E. (Eds.), Cigarette Smoke and Oxidative Stress. Springer, Heidelberg.

CHAPTER 8

Environmental Impact: Influence of ENDPs on Indoor Air Quality

CATHERINE GOUJON-GINGLINGER • MAYA I. MITOVA

8.1 INTRODUCTION

It is well established that environmental tobacco smoke (ETS) is a contributor to indoor air pollution and negatively affects indoor air quality (IAQ) (de Blas et al., 2012; Rösch et al., 2014). Therefore, in the context of tobacco harm reduction (Chapter 1), it is important to understand to what extent indoor use of electronic nicotine delivery products (ENDPs) (Chapter 2) impacts IAQ. ENDPs have been shown to emit significantly lower levels of toxicants than cigarettes (Chapters 4, 6 and 7), which is expected to translate into a lower impact on IAQ. The objective of IAQ studies is to evaluate whether reduced toxicant emissions translate into reduced impact on air quality when ENDPs are used indoors. This chapter provides an overview of air quality and summarizes different studies that have evaluated the impact of ENDPs on IAQ.

8.2 WHAT IS INDOOR AIR QUALITY?

Common terms and definitions used in the context of IAQ are listed below in alphabetic order.

Acceptable IAQ:

- Air in which there are no known contaminants at harmful concentrations as determined by cognizant authorities and with which a substantial majority (80% or more) of people exposed do not express dissatisfaction (ASHRAE, 2016a)
- Air toward which a substantial majority of occupants express no dissatisfaction with respect to odor or sensory irritation and in which there are not likely to be contaminants at concentrations that are known to pose a health risk (ASHRAE, 2016b)
- Air in an occupied space toward which a substantial majority of occupants express no dissatisfaction and that is not likely to contain contaminants at concentrations leading to exposures that pose a significant health risk (ISO 16814, 2008).

Acceptable perceived IAQ: Air in an occupied space toward which a substantial majority of occupants express no dissatisfaction on the basis of odor or sensory irritation (ISO 16814, 2008).

Airborne particulate matter/suspended particulate matter: A complex mixture of organic and inorganic substances contained in solid or liquid form or as a mixture of solid and liquid particles suspended in air. On the basis of their respective aerodynamic diameters, the particulates are separated into (DFG, 2014; WHO, 2000)

- Coarse fraction (mode): The fraction of particles with an aerodynamic diameter >2.5 µm, commonly reported in µg/m^3. This fractions includes
  - PM_{10}: Particulate matter with an aerodynamic diameter ≤10 µm
  - Respirable suspended particles (RSP): Particles with an aerodynamic diameter ≤4 µm (PM_4), which can penetrate into and be at least 50% deposited in the nonciliated portion of the lungs.
- Fine fraction (mode): The fraction of particles with an aerodynamic diameter <2.5 µm. This faction includes
  - $PM_{2.5}$: Particulate matter with an aerodynamic diameter ≤2.5 µm; commonly reported in µg/m^3
  - PM_1: Particulate matter with an aerodynamic diameter ≤1 µm (submicron PM); commonly reported in µg/m^3 and in particles/cm^3 (particle number concentration, PNC)
  - Ultrafine particles (UFP; nanoparticles/nanodroplets): Often refers to $PM_{0.1}$, which is particulate matter with an aerodynamic diameter ≤0.1 µm. In this chapter, we use this term for PM with particle diameter below 500 nm (Baldauf et al., 2016), commonly reported in particles/cm^3 (PNC).

Ambient air: The air surrounding a building; the source of outdoor air brought into a building (ASHRAE, 2016a,b).

Breathing zone: The region within an occupied space between planes 75 and 1800 mm above the floor and

Toxicological Evaluation of Electronic Nicotine Delivery Products. https://doi.org/10.1016/B978-0-12-820490-0.00006-7

more than 600 mm from the walls or fixed air-conditioning equipment (ASHRAE, 2016a,b).

Cognizant authority: An agency or organization that has the expertise and jurisdiction to establish and regulate concentration limits for airborne contaminants or an agency or organization that is recognized as authoritative and has the scope and expertise to establish guidelines, limit values, or concentration levels for airborne contaminants (ASHRAE, 2016a,b).

Environmental aerosol: Multiphase systems of particulate solids or liquids dispersed in gases and, in particular, in air. Aerosols include dusts, fumes, and mists (DFG, 2014):

- Dusts: Consist of particles of solid matter that have been produced mostly by mechanical processes or have been stirred up and dispersed in gases, in particular, in air. Airborne particles can not only be composed of compact, fine particles and free ultra-fine primary particles but can also consist of their aggregates or agglomerates.
- Fumes are dispersions of very finely divided solid matter in gases, in particular, in air. They arise in thermal processes (e.g., welding fumes, metal oxide fumes, soot, and flue ash) or chemical processes (e.g., the reaction of ammonia with hydrogen chloride).
- Mists are dispersions of particulate liquids (droplets) in gases, in particular, in air. They arise during nebulization of liquids, during condensation from the vapor phase, and during chemical processes (e.g., oil mist, hydrogen chloride in damp air, and artificial fog).

ETS: The "aged" and diluted combination of both sidestream smoke (smoke from the lit end of a cigarette or other tobacco product) and exhaled mainstream smoke (smoke that is exhaled by a smoker). ETS is commonly referred to as secondhand smoke (Baker and Proctor, 1990; FCTC, 2015; Jenkins et al., 2000).

Guideline value: Concentration of a pollutant in the air below which the risk for occurrence of adverse health effects is negligibly low (ISO 16814, 2008). It is derived on the basis of toxicological or precautionary considerations by using corresponding base values such as no observed adverse effect level, lowest observed adverse effect level, bench mark dose, etc. (Salthammer, 2011).

Indoor air: The air in an enclosed occupiable space (e.g., a dwelling or public building) (ISO 16814, 2008; ASHRAE, 2016a).

Occupational exposure limit/occupational exposure standard value (OEL): Values set by competent national authorities or other relevant national institutions as limits for concentrations of hazardous compounds in workplace air to prevent adverse health effects on healthy adult workers (ISO 16814, 2008).

Occupational exposure time–weighted average values: Airborne concentration standard values set by competent national authorities as limits for time-weighted average (TWA) concentrations of hazardous compounds over an 8-h working day, for a 5-day work week (ISO 16814, 2008).

Outdoor air: Ambient air and ambient air that enters a building through a ventilation system through intentional openings for natural ventilation (door or window) or by infiltration (ASHRAE, 2016a,b).

Particulate matter (PM): Solid or liquid particles in air, typically in the size range 0.01–100 μm in aerodynamic diameter.

Perceived air quality: Quality of air perceived by the occupants and expressed by the percentage of persons that perceive the air quality as unacceptable (percent dissatisfied) (ISO 16814, 2008).

Reference value: Value for a chemical substance in an environmental medium is a value that has been derived from a series of corresponding measured values of a random sample from a population on the basis of a specified procedure (c.f. discussion in review (Salthammer, 2011).

Public place: All places accessible to the general public or places for collective use, regardless of ownership or right of access (FCTC, 2007, 2015).

Total volatile organic compounds (TVOCs): The sum of all peaks (identified and unidentified) eluting between and including hexane (C_6) and hexadecane (C_{16}) on a nonpolar column. It considers the contributions of individual peaks (identified and unidentified), quantified in toluene equivalents, when present at concentration levels above the lowest calibration standard (0.0070 μg/tube, corresponding to approximately 2 μg/m^3) (EN 16516, 2017; International Organization for Standardization ISO ISO 16000-6, 2011).

8.3 INDOOR AIR AND INDOOR POLLUTION SOURCES

Indoor air naturally contains a mixture of different physical, biological, and chemical airborne pollutants. Some of these are released from indoor sources, while others result from entry of polluted outdoor air, or they have a mixed origin (Jones, 1999; Kelly and Fussell, 2019). More particularly, it is known that many building, construction, and interior materials are major sources of airborne pollutants; however, in cases where such materials are made of minerals (e.g., concrete, glass, mineral fibers, and gypsum) or stainless steel, the emissions of volatile organic compounds (VOCs) are considerably lower or nonexistent (Kotzias and

Pilidis, 2017; Niu and Burnett, 2001). It is also known that some mineral earth—derived materials such as brick, concrete, and tiles are classified as low VOC-emitting materials, but they might be sources of radon (Niu and Burnett, 2001). Furthermore, it has long been recognized that indoor air pollution may arise from biological sources, such as pets, ornamental plants, molds, microorganisms, and viruses (Kelly and Fussell, 2019). Besides, the presence of contaminants can be attributed to various human activities such as cooking and cleaning, smoking, or the use of personal care products (Kelly and Fussell, 2019; Weschler, 2009).

It is interesting to note that several airborne indoor constituents, including PM, carbon monoxide (CO), and nitrogen dioxide (NO_2), infiltrate from outdoors, and their indoor levels are influenced not only by indoor sources but also by the level of ambient pollution in building surroundings (e.g., proximity to intense road traffic or industry) (Jones, 1999; Kelly and Fussell, 2019). Other airborne constituents, such as formaldehyde, are considered to be specific indoor pollutants. This is because, even if they are emitted by numerous outdoor natural sources and during anthropogenic activities (biomass combustion, volcanic activity, decomposition, and industrial and traffic emissions), outdoor air either does not contribute to indoor pollution or the contribution is minor, except in highly polluted urban areas (Salthammer et al., 2010; WHO, 2010). The reasons for the low formaldehyde concentrations in ambient air—typically around $1-4\ \mu g/m^3$—are, first, the fast oxidation of formaldehyde to carbon dioxide in sunlight, and, second, its reaction with hydroxyl radicals to produce formic acid (WHO, 2010). The estimated half-life for these reactions is about 1 h, depending on the environmental conditions (WHO, 2010).

During the last decades, continuous sources of indoor pollutants, such as VOCs and formaldehyde emissions from building products, have been assessed comprehensively (Logue et al., 2011; Niu and Burnett, 2001; Salthammer et al., 2010; Weschler, 2009). A review has been published which summarizes the results of various studies on indoor pollution sources and the changes in their emanation profiles since the 1950s (Weschler, 2009).

More recently, studies have focused on the effect of different everyday life and recreational activities on air quality. There is increasing evidence that, when such activities take place in areas with limited ventilation, numerous airborne pollutants are released at harmful concentrations. Indeed, it has been shown that not only cigarette smoking (U.S. Department of Health and Human Services, 2014; Zhang and Smith, 2003) but

also, as mentioned above, cooking (Abdullahi et al., 2013; Bekö et al., 2013; Seaman et al., 2007), cleaning (Nazaroff and Weschler, 2004), and even activities associated with perception of wellness, such as using personal care products and perfume (Höllbacher et al., 2017; Mitova et al., 2019b; Steinemann, 2015) and playing sports (Alves et al., 2013; Andrade and Dominski, 2018; Mitova et al., 2019b; Ramos et al., 2014, 2015; Stathopoulou et al., 2008), could be substantial sources of different harmful airborne constituents.

Furthermore, what has become clear from the different studies conducted is that the very presence of human beings in a confined space influences the indoor air chemistry. In fact, not only bioeffluents such as carbon dioxide and odors but also CO (Cunnington and Hormbrey, 2002; Maga et al., 2017), NO (Travers et al., 2007), NH_3 (Giannoukos et al., 2014), and some VOCs originating from exhaled breath, sweat, skin, and other biological excretes are released into air (de Lacy Costello et al., 2014; Giannoukos et al., 2014; Mochalski et al., 2013; Perbellini et al., 2003; Sun et al., 2017; Turner et al., 2006). Several of these compounds are indicative of human residence as described for public environments (Kwak et al., 2015; Tang et al., 2016; Veres et al., 2013; Williams et al., 2016) and simulated residential environments (Mitova et al., 2019b). A review of studies on the effects of human emissions on chemical reactions occurring indoors showed (Weschler, 2016) that, under typical conditions, the occupant residues scavenge oxidants from indoor air and produce different by-products.

Thus, it can be clearly seen that IAQ is influenced by a huge variety of factors, and what is particularly noteworthy is that, simply through their presence, humans also have a polluting effect.

8.4 IAQ GUIDELINES

The primary goal of air quality legislation is to guarantee the best possible air quality in all types of environments (EU, 2004, 2008; Kuklinska et al., 2015). There are two main characteristics that are assessed in relation to IAQ:

- the indoor presence of chemical, physical, and biological airborne contaminants causing adverse health effects and
- the so-called comfort parameters such as climatic parameters (temperature, humidity, and air velocity) and odor.

The use of ENDPs has no influence on climatic parameters, nor does it cause biological contamination of the indoor environment. For these reasons, the legislation on these parameters is not further discussed in this text. Instead, this overview will concentrate on the basis considered by different countries and authorities to establish regulations concerning chemical and physical indoor pollutants.

Although indoor air pollution is a global problem, air quality policies are at varying stages of development in different countries. In general, the most economically developed countries have established standards and strategies to reduce air pollution, and ambient air quality is regulated in the vast majority of these countries. However, the list of airborne pollutants, their maximum permitted levels, and pollution management strategies can differ from country to country (Japan's regulations and environmental law, 2020; Russian Standard ГН 2.1.6.3492-17, 2018; AAQS, 2020; AQS, 2020; de Leeuw et al., 2016; de Leeuw and Ryssenaars, 2011; Harashima and Morita, 1998; Huang et al., 2018; Kuklinska et al., 2015; Marco and Bo, 2013; Riojas-Rodríguez et al., 2016). The regulatory landscape with regard to ambient air quality has been the subject of several reviews. For example, a review of the development of United States (US) and European Union (EU) ambient air quality policies, together with their comparative assessment, was published by Kuklinska and co-workers (Kuklinska et al., 2015). Additionally, the ambient air quality standards in the EU, EU member states, Australia, Canada, China, India, Japan, New Zealand, Switzerland, and the US and those set forth by the World Health Organization (WHO) were comparatively evaluated by the European Topic Center on Air Pollution and Climate Change Mitigation (de Leeuw et al., 2016; de Leeuw and Ryssenaars, 2011). The legal framework for ambient air quality control in the countries of South America and the Caribbean, together with the mean pollutant levels in all capitals and large cities, was also reviewed (Riojas-Rodríguez et al., 2016).

When specifically considering IAQ standards, it is crucial to keep in mind that determining indoor contaminant concentration limits is a particularly complex task. This is because only limited data are available on the health effects of different airborne pollutants and their mixtures and for different human populations, including sensitive individuals (the elderly, children, pregnant women, the sick, people suffering from allergies, etc.). Moreover, in contrast to the ambient air quality standards, the implementation of which is based on extensive monitoring networks, comparable monitoring for the vast majority of indoor environments is very difficult if not impossible (Kotzias, 2005; Salthammer, 2011). In addition, occupants are exposed indoors to mixtures of airborne constituents

that have significant local and temporal variations in their patterns (Salthammer, 2011). What further complicates matters is that all residential environments, which account for the vast majority of indoor environments, can only be partially regulated, as they belong to the private sphere of the occupants (Kotzias et al., 2005; Salthammer, 2011).

Consequently, in many countries, the regulation at working places (an umbrella term referring to both industrial and nonindustrial environments) has become, by far, the most well-established policy for IAQ. Table 8.1 summarizes information from different authorities in several countries that have set OELs for airborne pollutants. These exposure limits are based on values intended to protect healthy adult workers from health effects that might result from exposure over an 8 h workday for a 40- to 42 h workweek. The background, approaches, and recent trends for setting OELs on the basis of toxicological data from animal and human studies were reviewed (Nielsen and Ovrebo, 2008). OELs are developed and set by competent national authorities or adopted from international sources (Nielsen and Ovrebo, 2008; Schenk et al., 2008; Schmitz-Felten and Lissner, 2008). OELs established by 18 different entities were reviewed (Schenk et al., 2008). All these institutions had developed OELs for a total of 1341 substances; but, only 25 were common to all of the institutions, and more than one-third of the substances were regulated by a single organization (Schenk et al., 2008). In another review, comparison of OELs in 25 member states of the EU showed that there is a tendency toward harmonization in the limit values for common substances, but no harmonization exists in the number of substances in the different national lists or in the legal character of the OELs, where we can observe broad variations from "binding" to "orienting" (Schmitz-Felten and Lissner, 2008).

More specific IAQ standards for nonindustrial environments (offices and educational facilities) have been implemented in several countries; however, far fewer standards which consider heterogeneous populations, including protection of sensitive individuals, have been established for residential settings (Abdul-Wahab et al., 2015). The WHO has developed specific IAQ guidelines to protect the public from the risk of ill effects that might result from exposure to several airborne compounds commonly present in indoor air and in concentrations of health concern (WHO, 2010). The WHO guideline values aim to provide a uniform basis for protecting the public from the adverse effects of exposure to indoor air pollution. These values generally have the character of recommendations and

TABLE 8.1
Summary of Representative National and International Organizations that have Set Occupational Exposure Limits.

Occupational Exposure Limit	Abbreviation	Agency	Legal Character	Country
Workplace Exposure Standards	WES	Safe Work Australia	Indicative[a]	Australia
Canadian Occupational Safety and Health Regulations	COSHR	Canadian federal government	Requirements	Canada
Occupational exposure limits	OEL	EU Occupational Health and Safety administration (EU-OSHA)	Binding and indicative	European Union
Valeurs Limites d'Exposition Professionelle	VLEP	Insititut National de Recherche et de Sécurité (INRS)	Binding and indicative	France
Maximum concentrations in the workplace air (Maximale arbeitsplatz-Konzentration)	MAK	Deutsche Forschungs-gemeinschaft (DFG)	Enforceable standard	Germany
Occupational exposure limit	OEL	Japan Society for Occupational Health	Reference[a]	Japan
Maximum concentrations in the workplace air (Maximale arbeitsplatz-Konzentration)	MAK	Schweizerische Unfallversicherungsanstalt (SUVA)	Enforceable standard	Switzerland
Permissible exposure limit	PEL	US Occupational Health and Safety administration (OSHA)	Enforceable standard	United States
Threshold limit values	TLV	American Conference of Governmental Industrial Hygienists (ACGIH)	Guidelines	United States
Recommended exposure limits	REL	US National Institute for Occupational Safety and Health (NIOSH)	Recommended	United States

[a] Australia and Japan point out that the threshold values do not represent a definitive borderline between safe and hazardous conditions.

are intended to be used as a scientific basis for legally enforceable standards. Several other organizations have developed guideline values for nonindustrial environments. Nevertheless, there is currently no single institution developing guidelines or establishing regulatory levels for *all* indoor air pollutants, nor are values available for *all* contaminants of potential concern. Indeed, the situation today is that a number of organizations offer guideline values, but only for *selected* indoor air contaminants. A summary of representative guidelines for nonindustrial environments is given in Table 8.2. Basically, in cases where no IAQ guidelines are available for certain airborne constituents, ambient air quality standards are applied instead, as was the practice for many countries before specific IAQ guidelines were developed. In such cases, 24 h thresholds for indoor pollutants are adopted, and these thresholds are based on the annual guideline values for outdoor air (Kotzias et al., 2005). It is important to highlight that,

although the OELs are specifically developed for indoor environments, they do not take into consideration exposure of sensitive populations; therefore, they are commonly well above the thresholds for odor, sensory irritation, and even health effects defined for the general population and cannot be applied as such to residential environments (Kotzias et al., 2005; Oppl and Neuhaus, 2008; Persily, 2015). Sometimes the OELs are divided by a factor of 10 to take into account more sensitive populations in indoor settings (Oppl and Neuhaus, 2008; Persily, 2015), and these OELs are applied together with proposals for additional safety factors of 10 for all substances with dose-dependent effects (Oppl and Neuhaus, 2008). Thus, it can be seen that standards vary considerably worldwide, and much caution must be observed when making comparisons.

Two approaches have been defined for expressing IAQ with regard to health risk to occupants and/or occupants' perception (ISO 16814, 2008):

TABLE 8.2
Summary of Representative National and International Organizations that have Set Exposure Limits for Nonindustrial Environments.

Exposure Limit, General Population	Abbreviation	Agency	Legal Character	Country
Recommended exposure limit and indoor air reference levels		Canadian federal government, Health Canada (HC)	Recommended	Canada
Indoor exposure Limits in EU		European Commission	Recommended	EU
Guide value I and guide value II (Richtwerte I and II)	RW I and RW II	Umweltbundesamt	Guidelines	Germany
IAQ levels of Hong Kong (Excellent and Good Class IAQ)		Government of the Hong Kong Special administrative Region	Guidelines	Hong Kong
IAQ guideline for sick house syndrome prevention		Ministry of Health, Labour and Welfare of Japan	Guidelines	Japan
Reference exposure level	REL	Office of Environmental Health Hazard Assessment (OEHHA)	Guidelines	United States
Minimal Risk Levels	MRL	Agency for Toxic Substances and Disease Registry (ATSDR)	Guidelines	United States
WHO guidelines for IAQ		World Health Organization (WHO)	Guidelines	Worldwide

- In terms of health, airborne pollutant concentrations are compared with guideline or reference values established by cognizant authorities. Frequently, airflow rates for hygiene are imposed.
- In terms of acceptability, the percentage of dissatisfied persons (persons who perceive that the air quality is unacceptable) is an expression of the quality of air from a comfort point of view. However, this criterion varies depending on if it is based on unadapted (people entering indoor space) or adapted people (habituated to an indoor space) (Olesen, 2012; Persily, 2015).

Despite the fact that definitions for acceptable IAQ exist (ISO 16814, 2008; ASHRAE, 2016a,b), at present, there is no scientific agreement on their quantitative characterization. As stated in ASHRAE 62.1-2016: "Meeting one, some, or all of the listed (airborne constituents concentration) values does not ensure that acceptable IAQ (as defined in ASHRAE 62.1) will be achieved" (ASHRAE, 2016a). Nevertheless, it is generally accepted that the introduction and application of guideline values for certain compounds is, for all intents and purposes, a step forward toward better IAQ (Salthammer, 2011).

The most efficient strategies for improvement of IAQ are, first, source control, and second, dilution of airborne constituents (Kotzias and Pilidis, 2017; Niu and Burnett, 2001). Source control includes either elimination of the pollution source or substitution with materials or

equipment that contaminate at a lower rate. In contrast, dilution is commonly linked to ventilation, which allows the indoor concentrations of pollutants to be reduced to acceptable levels (ISO 16814, 2008). The US and EU ventilation standards set forth the required ventilation rates for different types of indoor environments on the basis of human occupancy and floor area (EN 13779, 2007; EN 15251, 2007; ASHRAE, 2016a,b). The ventilation measures put in place for human occupancy aim to remove bioeffluents and pollution resulting from activities, while those for the floor area are intended to reduce pollution emanating from the building materials and interior items (EN 13779, 2007; EN 15251, 2007; ASHRAE, 2016a,b). The two EU norms also provide additional ventilation rates for areas where cigarette smoking is permitted (EN 13779, 2007; EN 15251, 2007).

8.5 REQUIREMENTS FOR DESIGN OF STUDIES ON ENVIRONMENTAL AEROSOLS OF ENDPS

Typically, the indoor concentration of an airborne pollutant in an enclosed environment depends on its rate of emission from the pollution source, volume of air contained in the indoor space into which the contaminant is dispersed, rate of removal of the pollutant from the air via reaction or settling,

TABLE 8.3

Summary of Indoor Air Constituents Measured during Simulation with Combustion Products (Candles [Tealights], Incense Sticks, and Cigarettes) Compared With the Background Levels in an Empty IAQ Room, Background Levels with Panelists, and Simulation with THS. Simulated Environment, "Residential Category III" (0.5

Items for a 2 h Session	BKG for Tealights[c]	Tealights	BKG for Incense Stick[c]		Incense Stick		Cigarette-1[D]		Cigarette-2[D]		BKG for THS[E]		THS[F]	
	0	3	0		1		12		2		0		12	
Airborne Constituent[a,b]	Mean (µg/m³)	Mean (µg/m³)	Mean (µg/m³)	SD (µg/m³)	Mean (µg/m³)	SD (µg/m³)	Mean (µg/m³)	SD (µg/m³)	Mean (µg/m³)	SD (µg/m³)	Mean (µg/m³)	SD (µg/m³)	Mean (µg/m³)	SD (µg/m³)
RSP-gravimetry	NM	NM	9.01	2.13	171	10.1	643	23.6	127	4.72	11.3	8.8	18.9	14.8
UVPM-THBP	NM	NM	<1.61	NA	13.9	0.698	92.9	2.40	17.7	0.212	<1.61	NA	<1.61	NA
FPM-scopoletin	NM	NM	<0.132	NA	3.62	0.128	20.4	0.543	4.20	0.048	<0.132	NA	<0.132	NA
Acetaldehyde	NM	NM	3.61	0.082	25.8	0.602	126	7.74	30.0	1.12	3.32	0.280	6.76	0.760
Acrolein	NM	NM	<0.199	NA	5.31	0.173	12.4	1.96	2.75	0.120	<0.199	NA	<0.199	NA
Crotonaldehyde	NM	NM	<0.116	NA	0.862	0.026	3.57	0.207	0.802	0.028	<0.116	NA	<0.116	NA
Formaldehyde	NM	NM	12.5	0.217	41.5	0.721	74.9	4.44	24.4	1.32	13.0	2.24	10.8	1.05
Acrylonitrile	NM	NM	<0.652	NA	0.675	0.047	5.28	0.309	1.23	0.050	<0.652	NA	<0.652	NA
Benzene	NM	NM	0.608	0.074	75.8	1.85	14.9	0.964	4.47	0.301	1.00	0.127	0.943	0.119
1,3-Butadiene	NM	NM	<2.57	NA	11.6	0.211	17.6	0.783	4.17	0.199	<2.57	NA	<2.57	NA
Isoprene	NM	NM	3.83	0.689	12.9	0.546	173	8.53	50.0	1.98	8.65	0.61	9.85	1.32
Toluene	NM	NM	<1.48	NA	11.6	0.222	26.7	2.07	8.87	0.437	2.68	0.280	2.32	0.306
TVOC	NM	NM	14.5	1.79	338	9.24	479	19.4	63.4	0.730	20.4	0.632	22.2	0.933
CO	224	534	273	NA	1769	NA	3295	125	1402	NA	543	11.3	503	29.0
NO	4.73	75.5	17.6	NA	31.2	NA	82.5	7.94	72.2	NA	35.2	1.18	26.1	6.39
NOx	20.0	147	32.0	NA	53.0	NA	117	8.29	102	NA	53.7	1.53	41.6	8.97

Abbreviations: BKG, background; FPM, fluorescent particulate matter; NA, not applicable; NM, not measured; RSP, respirable suspended particles; SD, standard deviation; TVOC, total volatile organic compounds; UVPM-THBP, ultraviolet particulate matter-2,2',4,4'-tetrahydroxybenzophenone.

[a] Standard deviation is not reported for online measurements if they are performed only on 1 day (CO, NH_3, NO, and NO_x).

[b] Background of an unoccupied IAQ room.

[c] Background of an unoccupied IAQ room.

[d] Data for Cigarette-1 (total of 12 cigarettes/2 h; one cigarette lighted every 10 min; time to smoke one cigarette, 5–7 min) (Mitova et al., 2019a), Cigarette-2 (total of 2 cigarettes/2 h; one cigarette lighted every 60 min; time to smoke one cigarette, 5–7 min).

[e] Background with 3 people remaining in the IAQ room for 2 h (Mitova et al., 2019a).

[f] Data for THS (total of 12 tobacco sticks/2 h; one tobacco stick consumed every 10 min, time to use one tobacco stick, 5–7 min) were acquired during a study performed in 2016 (Mitova et al., 2019a).

TABLE 8.4.

Summary of Indoor Air Constituents Measured ($\mu g/m^3$) in a Surrogate Environmental Aerosol of P2V2 Generated by Machine Puffing (12 Sticks for 2 h) of the Experiment Under a Simulated "Residential Category III" Environment (0.5 h⁻¹)

Airborne Constituent[a,b]	BKG DAY 1		BKG DAY 2		BKG DAY 3		BKG DAY 4		P2V2 DAY 1		P2V2 DAY 2		P2V2 DAY 3		P2V2 DAY 4	
	Mean	SD	Mean	SD	Mean	SD	Mean	SD	Mean	SD	Mean	SD	Mean	SD	Mean	SD
RSP-gravimetry	<8.11	NA	<8.11	NA	<8.54	1.06	<8.11	NA	95.8	11.1	77.6	4.88	85.9	4.92	77.8	1.96
UVPM-THBP	<0.39	NA	<0.39	NA	<0.39	NA	<0.39	NA	4.11	0.11	4.10	0.22	4.08	0.13	3.88	0.16
FPM-scopoletin	<0.01	NA	<0.01	NA	<0.01	NA	<0.01	NA	0.58	0.01	0.58	0.02	0.58	0.01	0.55	0.01
Solanesol	<0.01	NA	<0.01	NA	<0.01	NA	<0.01	NA	1.45	0.08	1.30	0.06	1.52	0.06	1.03	0.09
3-Ethenylpyridine	<0.02	NA	<0.02	NA	<0.02	NA	<0.02	NA	0.12	0.00	0.11	0.00	0.12	0.00	0.12	0.01
Nicotine	<0.25	NA	0.68	0.04	0.80	0.03	0.96	0.02	24.4	0.36	26.6	0.50	27.7	1.58	28.7	1.50
Acetaldehyde	1.83	0.04	2.34	0.09	1.85	0.04	1.81	0.03	45.5	0.53	49.2	0.96	48.9	1.07	48.1	1.04
Acrolein	<0.06	NA	<0.06	NA	<0.06	NA	<0.06	NA	3.27	0.07	3.55	0.12	3.27	0.12	3.81	0.15
Crotonaldehyde	<0.07	NA	<0.07	NA	<0.07	NA	<0.07	NA	1.47	0.02	1.67	0.03	1.59	0.04	1.73	0.05
Formaldehyde	<6.01	0.13	<7.32	0.26	<6.10	0.10	<6.19	0.13	20.9	0.39	22.5	0.47	21.3	0.57	21.5	0.31
Acrylonitrile	<0.14	NA	<0.14	NA	<0.14	NA	<0.14	NA	<0.14	NA	<0.28	NA	<0.28	NA	<0.14	NA
Benzene	0.38	0.02	0.67	0.03	0.41	0.03	0.38	0.01	4.78	0.06	5.24	0.37	4.91	0.15	4.79	0.15
1,3-Butadiene	<0.67	NA	<0.67	NA	<0.67	NA	<0.67	NA	<1.66	NA	<2.65	NA	<2.16	NA	<2.65	NA
Isoprene	1.37	0.06	1.82	0.07	1.13	0.07	1.38	0.04	3.24	0.17	3.60	0.12	3.30	0.11	2.82	0.13

Toluene	0.55	0.05	1.50	0.07	0.95	0.05	0.78	0.02	1.36	0.04	1.89	0.13	1.93	0.05	1.38	0.05
TVOC	4.32	0.10	9.50	1.22	6.79	0.24	6.97	0.05	39.5	3.26	47.2	2.78	56.6	1.82	54.0	5.93
Glycerin	<3.08	NA	<3.08	NA	<3.08	NA	<3.65	0.80	85.6	6.77	78.7	5.58	88.9	2.00	82.6	4.29
Propylene glycol	<15.5	NA	<15.5	NA	<15.5	NA	<15.5	NA	18.6	1.56	17.8	0.71	17.0	0.80	15.7	0.21
NNK	<2.6e-05	NA	<2.6e-05	NA	<2.6e-05	NA	<2.6e-05	NA	9.0e-04	2.8e-05	9.3e-04	6.0e-05	1.1e-03	7.2e-05	1.1e-03	9.5e-05
NNN	<6.4e-05	NA	<6.4e-05	NA	1.07e-04	0e+00	<6.4e-05	NA	1.5e-03	2.5e-05	1.5e-03	5.6e-05	1.5e-03	4.7e-05	1.5e-03	4.0e-05
PM$_1$	<5.00		<5.00		<5.00		<5.00		55.4		53.4		58.8		55.2	
PM$_{2.5}$	<5.00		<5.00		<5.00		<5.00		60.1		56.6		63.0		59.4	
UFP count/cm^3	NM		NM		1075		1010		NM		108402		101504		106734	
UFP size	NM		NM		51		36		NM		63		65		64	
CO	287		447		252		248		2193		2371		2299		2217	
NH$_3$	8.3		11.5		8.9		10.7		19.6		22.8		20.6		21.0	
NO	11.2		49.9		14.1		10.7		29.8		43.9		27.0		29.7	
NO$_x$	14.7		55.3		22.6		20.1		37.3		53.9		40.0		42.6	

[a] Abbreviations: BKG, background; FPM, fluorescent particulate matter; NA, not applicable; NNK, nicotine-derived nitrosamine ketone; NM, not measured; NNN, N-nitrosonornicotine; P2V2, platform 2 version 2, a carbon heated tobacco product; RSP, respirable suspended particles; SD, standard deviation; TVOC, total volatile organic compounds; UFP, ultrafine particles; UVPM, ultraviolet particulate matter–2,2′,4,4′-tetrahydroxybenzophenone.

[b] Standard deviation is not reported for online measurements (PM$_1$, PM$_{2.5}$, UFP, CO, NH$_3$, NO, and NO$_x$).

reemission rates from indoor surfaces, rate of air exchange with the outside atmosphere, and outdoor pollutant concentration (ISO 16000-1, 2004; Jones, 1999; Kelly and Fussell, 2019). Thus, it is crucial that the experimental design for emission assessment of a consumer product takes all these variables into account and considers of equal importance the experimental location for performing the measurements, protocol for conducting sampling, and markers to be measured.

The experimental protocols for evaluation of environmental aerosols of ENDPs are based on the general requirements for assessment of common indoor pollution sources such as building materials and consumer products. Customarily, exposure of the general population to indoor pollution is evaluated via large monitoring studies with statistical assessment of the source of variance of airborne constituent concentrations in relation to the different indoor microenvironments (Edwards et al., 2001; Hoffmann et al., 2000). The goal of these studies is to reveal typical pollutant sources for the different microenvironments in order to subsequently study them in more detail either in real-life environments (field or real-world studies) or in controlled experimental conditions in exposure chambers (model environments). Although measuring airborne constituent concentrations in real-life environments has the obvious advantage of providing data for existing enclosed settings, it is apparent that confounding indoor emission sources cannot be discriminated and that both outdoor air and varying environmental parameters could impact the results when such an experimental setup is used.

Assessment of the indoor emissions of building and interior materials and items, which are continuous sources of pollution, is typically standardized and conducted in exposure chambers. For example, the requirements for evaluation of VOC emissions of construction products are described in the European norm EN 16516 (EN 16516, 2017) and an ISO standard (ISO 16000-9, 2006). Such standards are applied, for example, for assessment of products for compliance with "Conformité Européenne" marking and voluntary low VOC emissions labeling (e.g., different eco-labels) (Oppl, 2014). However, many consumer products, such as cleaning agents and personal care products, are sources of emissions with temporary (short-term or intermittent) patterns, and, therefore, different experimental setups are required to evaluate them properly. Standardization for assessment of this kind of emissions is currently under development (Bartzis et al., 2015).

Standardized assessment procedures for building and interior materials and items as well as consumer products allow evaluation of compliance with requirements for low-polluting materials and/or proper comparison of emissions of products and materials from different suppliers in predefined experimental conditions. Nonetheless, the applicability of the measured emissions to real-room situations is somewhat limited because the exposure chambers do not resemble real rooms in size or configuration, and they customarily lack furniture. Indeed, as mentioned above, experiments for evaluating emissions in real indoor settings can neither exclude nor control the influence of outdoor pollution or climatic parameters. Consequently, the use of model rooms that simulate a real room in size, configuration, and furnishings but are equipped with a supply of filtered air and have controlled environmental parameters is becoming increasingly popular (Höllbacher et al., 2017; Licina et al., 2017). A European standard describes the standard parameters for such a model room (environmentally controlled room)—the so-called "European reference room" (EN 16516, 2017)—that might be used to either build a model room or recalculate the measured emissions of an existing model room to those of the reference room.

ENDPs are consumer products with temporary emission patterns that arise when the products are used. As mentioned previously, currently, as for other consumer products with intermittent emanations, there are no officially standardized procedures for assessment of ENDPs. For that reason, different research groups assess the environmental aerosols emitted during consumption of ENDPs in different settings, including exposure chambers, model rooms, and real-world environments (Cancelada et al., 2019; Meišutovič-Akhtarieva et al., 2019; Mitova et al., 2016, 2019a; Protano et al., 2016, 2017; Zainol Abidin et al., 2017). In view of our experience with these products and on the basis of a critical review of the literature, we can propose several recommendations for the design of ENDP assessment studies.

The mainstream aerosols released during consumption of ENDPs are intended to be inhaled by the consumers, and, considering the concentrations of the mainstream aerosol constituents and their retention rates in the human body, low levels of airborne constituents in the environmental aerosol can be predicted. Because of this expected low level of environmental pollution, during the initial stages of evaluation of ENDPs, it is reasonable to evaluate their environmental aerosols via simulation in an environmentally controlled room fitted with an air filtration unit to remove or reduce potential contamination by polluted outdoor air and having controlled environmental parameters for reducing measurement variability. In such an experimental approach, the evaluations could be conducted with either aerosolization machines or human users. Studies with machine-puffing regimens have the advantage of being less variable and are, therefore, commonly applied for method development and validation purposes (Gómez Lueso et al., 2018; Mottier et al., 2016). However, they provide a nonrealistic scenario for assessment of actual indoor exposure to the environmental aerosols of ENDPs, because surrogate environmental aerosols are generated in such scenarios, (e.g., aged and diluted mainstream aerosol of ENDPs), and, therefore, the actual levels of airborne constituents emitted during the use of ENDPs are overestimated. In contrast, studies with consumption of ENDPs by human users allow assessment of the products with both a genuine puffing regimen and realistic retention of mainstream aerosol constituents after inhalation. In addition, such experimental designs take into account certain consumption issues such as mouth spill of the aerosol. Still, it is important to underline that, in such an experimental setup, it is crucial to evaluate and take into account the emissions resulting from human presence. In fact, as discussed in the Introduction and investigated in more detail in a study (Mitova et al., 2019b), during human residence in a confined space, several airborne constituents reach quantifiable levels in room air. Accordingly, the following implications for experimental design need to be considered. First, measurement of a proper background. It is essential to remember that empty room air is an appropriate background only for experiments with aerosolization machines. In contrast, an appropriate background for experiments with human users is the "room air" obtained in the presence of the same number of panelists as are present during sessions where ENDPs are consumed. Second, it is also important to consider the schedule of the experiments; indeed, if the experiments are conducted in a sequence, a compulsory purge of the experimental room is required between the experiments in order to ensure that human-related emanations are removed and that airborne constituents return to their initial levels. Third, when carrying out evaluations of environmental aerosols of ENDPs, it is crucial that the experiments be replicated several times in order to properly capture the variations in the background and in the environmental aerosols of ENDPs. Even with aerosolization machines, despite the overall good reproducibility of the experiments, some variability related to normal experimental uncertainty is observed. When human users consume the product, this variability naturally increases, and this variation needs to be incorporated into the experimental design to ensure that differences in consumption behavior are properly captured. Finally, every effort should be made to reduce as much as reasonably possible the background levels of the measured airborne constituents. As discussed in the Introduction, this means that all sources of contamination, such as use of personal care products and perfumes and consumption of food and drinks, must be controlled or avoided. Concretely, this entails introducing restrictions on the use of personal care products (including but not limited to the use of standardized nonscented toiletries and prohibition of the use of perfume and aftershave) by both the persons participating in the experiments and the staff entering the environmentally controlled room. Equally importantly, consumption of food and drinks in the environmentally controlled room is strictly prohibited.

Conducting experiments on evaluation of environmental aerosols of ENDPs in real-life environments is, in principal, more challenging, as it is difficult to implement many requirements that can be applied straightforwardly in the study design in a model room (e.g., control over the number of persons, requirements for the use of personal care products, and restrictions on the consumption of food and drinks). An important recommendation in such cases is to closely monitor all these parameters during the experiments, including counting the number of persons present and keeping records, whenever possible, on the food and drinks served in addition to the consumed ENDPs. Moreover, because it is often not possible to use filtered air in field studies, it is of critical importance to include additional background measurements (e.g., of the unoccupied experimental location) or perform outdoor air measurements in parallel, whenever feasible.

Concerning the sampling protocol to be applied for evaluation of environmental aerosols of ENDPs, general recommendations as described in international standards are to be followed, in particular, those for intermittent emission sources (for more details c. f. ISO 16000-1 and ISO 16000-5 (ISO 16000-1, 2004; ISO 16000-5, 2007)). Most standards set forth the measurements to be performed at breathing height (ISO 16000-1, 2004; EN 13779, 2007; EN 15251, 2007; ASHRAE, 2016a,b). To implement this requirement, the typical position of the persons in the enclosed environments (e.g., sitting or standing) is to be taken into account. Several norms stipulate that, whenever measurements are taken in real-life environments, the environment must be the place where residents spend most of their time, and the measurements must be conducted during typical high-load conditions (ISO 16000-1, 2004; EN 15251, 2007; ISO 16000-5, 2007).

Similarly to cases of other intermittent emissions sources, it is important to consider the setting of the distance between the source of emission (puffing on ENDPs and exhaling) and the sampling equipment. International standards do not stipulate any fixed distance for evaluation of intermittent emission sources and simply recommend considering the scope of the measurements when deciding on the sampling location (ISO 16000-1, 2004; ISO 16000-5, 2007). As shown for electrically heated tobacco products (EHTPs) and e-vapor products (EVPs), the measured emissions of PM, and probably other PM markers not evaluated in these studies, decrease with increasing distance to the measurement equipment (Martuzevicius et al., 2019; Meišutovič-Akhtarieva et al., 2019). Accordingly, the exposure of potential bystanders to emissions of ENDPs will vary in different social situations. Thus, for studies in model rooms, it is recommended to define the distances between the points of emission (puffing on ENDPs and exhaling) and the measurement equipment according to the situation intended to be simulated and the related interpersonal distances. Nowadays, the four most important interpersonal distances are described as follows: intimate distance (up to 46 cm, used for embracing, touching, or whispering), personal distance for interactions among good friends or family (46–122 cm), social distance for interactions among acquaintances (1.2–3.7 m), and public distance used for public speaking (3.7–7.6 m and more) (Hall, 1966). Concerning studies in real-life environments with multiple users of ENDPs who do not typically remain fixed at one place, the general recommendation for collecting and determining the average concentrations of airborne constituents is to be applied. More specifically, this means that the center of the room is considered as the most suitable sampling location, and, in cases where this is not possible, the samplers are to be located no closer than 1 m to any wall (ISO 16000-1, 2004; ISO 16000-5, 2007). In both sampling positions, places in the sun, nearby heating systems, or with noticeable draught or nearby ventilation channels are to be avoided, because this might influence the measurement results (ISO 16000-1, 2004; ISO 16000-5, 2007).

Measurement of a representative set of markers (or tracers) allows proper characterization of the environmental aerosols of ENDPs. Depending on their compartmentalization, the markers are classified as particulate-phase or gas-phase markers and, depending on their specificity to the source, as specific or nonspecific tracers. Many constituents have been evaluated in studies on the environmental aerosols of ENDPs (Tables 8.5 and 8.6). Several of these constituents were measured for general characterization of IAQ or to verify if there is any similarity

between ENDP environmental aerosols and the ETS from cigarettes and other emissions from combustible sources. Therefore, these constituents are not to be considered as tracers of environmental aerosols of ENDPs but rather as general markers for indoor pollution. Indeed, to fulfill the requirements for specificity, a tracer must be a unique compound contained in the aerosol of ENDPs and absent in background air. As a matter of fact, there are very few markers specific to the environmental aerosols of ENDPs, such as nicotine, glycerin, and propylene glycol. These are major compounds in the mainstream aerosols of ENDPs (Chapters 4 and 6), and they occur in the exhaled breath of the users. Nicotine is a component of many solaneceous plants, such as eggplants and tomatoes, but in quantities significantly below those present in tobacco or e-liquids (Domino et al., 1991). Thus, most indoor environments are usually free of this compound, and its occurrence in such environments is typically related to smoking cigarettes, cigars, and pipes or using ENDPs. Similarly, glycerin and propylene glycol are contained in many personal care and cleaning products, and, therefore, some real-life indoor environments might contain low levels of these constituents. Nevertheless, the indoor use of ENDPs is characteristically coupled with an increase in the indoor concentrations of glycerin and propylene glycol above the background levels.

In addition, solanesol is considered a specific tracer for all heated tobacco products (HTPs); but, it is present in their environmental aerosols at very low concentrations, probably because of its low volatility and retention in the human body (Armitage et al., 2004). Moreover, nicotine-derived nitrosamine ketone (NNK) and N-nitrosonornicotine (NNN), two tobacco-specific nitrosamines (TSNAs) present in the low nanogram-per-stick range in EHTP aerosols (Schaller et al., 2016), might possibly be good candidates to serve as specific tracers, because they are not common airborne constituents. However, their very low concentrations in ENDP aerosols and high retention rates in the users' bodies will complicate their use as tracers. It is important to highlight that none of the above listed compounds is an air quality marker.

Studies evaluating the impact of environmental aerosols of ENDPs on IAQ commonly measure airborne PM, UFPs, carbonyls, and TVOCs. Although none of these constituents is, per se, unique for any product, if used in combination, they are valuable tracers of ENDP environmental aerosols given that their concentrations in the background are taken into consideration in the evaluations. UFPs and PM_1 are nonspecific tracers of EHTPs (Forster et al., 2018; Meišutovič-Akhtarieva et al., 2019;

TABLE 8.5
Summary of Representative IAQ Studies on EHTPs Conducted in Model Environments.

Publication	Product	Constituents[a]	Control on Environmental Parameters	Air Changes/h (h^{-1})	Volume (m^3)	No. of Persons	Sampling Duration (min)	No. of Products
Cancelada et al. (2019)	THS	Nicotine, pyridine, 3-ethenylpyridine, pyrrole, N-methylformamide, acrylonitrile, 3-ethylpyridine, 2,3-dimethylpyridine, acetaldehyde, diacetyl, butanal, acetone, propanal, benzaldehyde, methacrolein, acrolein, crotonaldehyde, formaldehyde, 2-butanone, m-tolualdehyde, hexaldehyde, acetol, furfural, glycidol, 2-furanmethanol, isoprene, menthol, phenol, p-cresol, m-cresol, o-cresol, benzene, quinolone, naphtalene	Yes	0.3	0.2	0^b	180^f	1 (12 puffs)
Caponnetto et al. (2018)	THS, THP, cigarette	CO	–	–	–	1^c	45	1

Continued

TABLE 8.5
Summary of Representative IAQ Studies on EHTPs Conducted in Model Environments.—cont'd

Publication	Product	Constituents[a]	Control on Environmental Parameters	Air Changes/h (h^{-1})	Volume (m^3)	No. of Persons	Sampling Duration (min)	No. of Products
Forster et al. (2018)	THP, cigarette	PNC, PM (1–10 μm), MMD, RSP-gravimetry, nicotine, 3-ethenylpyridine, acetaldehyde, acrolein, crotonaldehyde, formaldehyde, acrylonitrile, benzene, 1,3-butadiene, isoprene, toluene, acrylamide, TVOCs, glycerin, propylene glycol, TSNAs, PAHs, CO, NO, NO_2, NO_x	Yes	1.2, 2.2, 7.7	37.8	4	240	20–32 tobacco sticks versus 20–32 cigarettes
Ichitsubo and Kotaki (2018)	NTV	PM, RSP-gravimetry, UVPM, FPM, solanesol, nicotine, 3-ethenylpyridine, acetaldehyde, acetone, formaldehyde, toluene, TVOCs, glycerin, propylene glycol, triacetin, CO, CO_2, NH_3	Yes	6.9, 12.2, 40	16.6	1–6	60	32–288 puffs versus 2–18 cigarettes
Meišutovič-Akhtarieva et al. (2019)	THS, cigarette	PNC (10–420 nm), PM (0.006–10 μm, 3-ethenylpyridine, nicotine, acetaldehyde, formaldehyde, CO, CO_2	Yes	0.2, 0.5, 1.0	35.8	1–5	30	1–5 tobacco sticks versus 1 cigarette

Mitova et al. (2016)	THS, cigarette	RSP-gravimetry, UVPM, FPM, solanesol, nicotine, 3-ethenylpyridine, acetaldehyde, acrolein, crotonaldehyde, formaldehyde, acrylonitrile, benzene, 1,3-butadiene, isoprene, toluene, CO, NO, NO$_x$	Yes	1.2, 2.2, 7.7	72.3	3–5[d]	240	12–24 tobacco sticks versus 12–24 cigarettes
Mitova et al. (2019a)	THS, cigarette	PM$_{1-2.5}$, UVPM, FPM, solanesol, nicotine, 3-ethenylpyridine, acetaldehyde, acrolein, crotonaldehyde, formaldehyde, acrylonitrile, benzene, 1,3-butadiene, isoprene, toluene, TVOCs, glycerin, propylene glycol, NNK, NNN, CO, NO, NO$_x$	Yes	0.5	72.3	3[d]	120	12
PMI, 2018	THS, THP, NTV	PM$_{1-10}$, solanesol, nicotine, 3-ethenylpyridine, acetaldehyde, acrolein, crotonaldehyde, formaldehyde, acrylonitrile, benzene, 1,3-butadiene, isoprene, toluene, TVOCs, glycerin, propylene glycol, NNK, NNN, CO, NO, NO$_x$, NH$_3$	Yes	4.3	72.3	4–16[e]	120	8 or 39 tobacco sticks of THS; 39 tobacco sticks of THP; 39 vaping sessions with NTV

Continued

TABLE 8.5
Summary of Representative IAQ Studies on EHTPs Conducted in Model Environments.—cont'd

Publication	Product	Constituents[a]	Control on Environmental Parameters	Air Changes/h (h⁻¹)	Volume (m³)	No. of Persons	Sampling Duration (min)	No. of Products
PMI, 2018	THS, THP, NTV, cigarette	PM_{1-10}, UFPs, solanesol, nicotine, 3-ethenylpyridine, acetaldehyde, acrolein, crotonaldehyde, formaldehyde, glycerin, propylene glycol, CO, NO, NO_x, NH_3	Yes	9.6	72.3	13[d]	15	24 tobacco sticks for THS and THP, 12 vaping sessions of NTV; 24 cigarettes
PMI, 2020	THS	UFPs, $PM_{1-2.5}$	Yes	0.5	72.3	4[d]	120	12
Protano et al. (2016)	THS, EVP, cigarette, hand-rolled cigarette	Particle size distribution (5.6–560 nm)	No	0.7	52.7	1	60	1
Protano et al. (2017)	THS, EVP, cigarette, hand-rolled cigarette, cigar, pipe	Particle size distribution (5.6–560 nm)	No	0.7	52.7	1	60	1
Ruprecht et al. (2017)	THS, EVP, cigarette	BC (880 nm), BC (370 nm), PNC (>0.3 μm, >1 μm, nm), PM_{1-10}, carbonyls (acetaldehyde, acrolein, formaldehyde), metals and trace organic compounds in suspended PM	No	1.5	48	2–3	120–180	13 vaping session for EVP, 10–14 tobacco sticks, 9 cigarettes

Abbreviations: *BC*, black carbon; *EVP*, e-vapor product; *FPM*, fluorescent particulate matter; *MMD*, mass median diameter; *NNK*, nicotine-derived nitrosamine ketone; *NNN*, N-nitrosonornicotine; *NTV*, Novel Tobacco Vapor product; *PAH*, polycyclic aromatic hydrocarbon; *PM*, particulate matter; *PNC*, particle number concentration; *PSD*, particle size distribution; *RSP*, respirable suspended particle; *THP*, Tobacco Heating Product 1.0; *THS*, Tobacco Heating System 2.2; *TSNA*, tobacco-specific nitrosamine; *TVOC*, total volatile organic compound; *UFP*, ultrafine particle; *UVPM*, ultraviolet particulate matter.

a Assessment of exposure based on calculated exhaled mainstream and sidestream emissions in experiments with machine puffing.
b Assessment of exposure based on calculated exhaled mainstream and sidestream emissions in experiments with machine puffing.
c Study on exhaled breath.
d Of the total number of persons in these experiments, 1 was a bystander.
e n these experiments, 1 person was a bystander in sessions with 4–12 participants, while 2 persons were bystanders in the sessions with 16 participants.
f Sampling for sidestream emission assessment.

TABLE 8.6
Summary of Representative IAQ Studies on EVPs Conducted in Model Environments with Human Users.

Publication	EVP	Constituents[a]	Control on Environmental Parameters	Air Changes/ h (h^{-1})	Volume (m^3)	No. of Persons/ No. of Vapers	Sampling Duration (min)	No. of Products
Avino et al. (2018)	Open tank	PNC (>4 nm), PM$_{1-10}$, BC, PSD (14–700 nm)	NI	0.2	40	NI	60	Ad libitum for 5 min
Czogala et al. (2014)	Cigalike	PM$_{2.5}$, nicotine, VOCs, CO	No	1.4–4.4	39	1/1	60	2x ad libitum for 5 min, with a 30-min interval
Liu et al. (2017)	Cigalike and open tank	Nicotine, carbonyls (acetaldehyde, acetone, acrolein, benzaldehyde, butanal, 2-butanone, crotonaldehyde, 2,5-dimethylbenzaldehyde, formaldehyde, hexaldehyde, isovaleraldehyde, o-/m-/p-tolualdehyde, propanal, valeraldehyde), benzene, 1,3-butadiene, furan, isoprene, toluene, ethylene oxide, vinyl chloride, propylene oxide, nitromethane, 2-nitropropane, vinyl acetate, ethylbenzene, glycerin, propylene glycol, trace metals (Ar, Cr, Ni, Cd)	Yes	2.2	114	10/9	240	720 puffs, ad libitum: 747 –1649 puffs
Martuzevicius et al. (2019)	Disposable cigalike, cigalike cartomizer, and open tank	PNC, PM (0.006–10 μm)	Yes	0, 1.0, 2.0	35.8	1/1	5	Ad libitum 5 puffs

Continued

TABLE 8.6
Summary of Representative IAQ Studies on EVPs Conducted in Model Environments with Human Users.—cont'd

Publication	EVP	Constituents[a]	Control on Environmental Parameters	Air Changes/h (h^{-1})	Volume (m^3)	No. of Persons/No. of Vapers	Sampling Duration (min)	No. of Products
Melstrom et al. (2017)	Disposable cigalike and open tank	PNC, PM$_{2.5}$, nicotine	NI	5	52.6	9/3	120	Ad libitum
O'Connell et al. (2015)	Disposable cigalike	Nicotine, carbonyls (acetaldehyde, acrolein, formaldehyde), TVOCs, PAHs (acenaphthene, acenaphthylene, anthracene, benz[a]anthracene, benzo[b]fluoranthene, benzo[k]fluoranthene, benzo[ghi]perylene, benzo[a]pyrene, chrysene, dibenz[a,h]anthracene, fluoranthene, fluorine, indeno[1,2,3-cd]pyrene, naphthalene, phenanthrene, pyrene), glycerin, propylene glycol, TSNAs (NNK, NNN, NAT, NAB), CO$_2$, CO, NO, NO$_2$, O$_3$, trace metals (Ag, Al, As, Ba, Be, Cd, Co, Cr, Cu, Hg, Mn, Ni, P, Pb, Sb, Se, Tl, Zn)	No	0.8	38.5	5/3	165	Ad libitum
PMI, 2015	Cigalike, open tank	Nicotine, 3-ethenylpyridine, acetaldehyde, formaldehyde, TVOCs, glycerin, propylene glycol	Yes	1.2	72.3	3/2	240	12 vaping sessions

Protano et al. (2016)	Open tank	PNC and PSD (5.6–560 nm)	No	0.7	52.7	1/1	60	12 puffs
Protano et al. (2017)	Open tank	PNC and PSD (5.6–560 nm)	No	0.7	52.7	1/1	60	12 puffs
Protano et al. (2018)	Different models, open tank	PM_1, $PM_{2.5}$, PM_4, PM_{10}	No	0.7	52.7	1/1	60	12 puffs
Ruprecht et al. (2017)	Open tank	BC (880 nm), BC (370 nm), PNC (>0.3 μm, >1 μm, nm), $PM_{1–10}$, carbonyls (acetaldehyde, acrolein, formaldehyde), metals, and trace organic compounds in suspended PM	No	1.5	48	2–3/2–3	120–180	13 vaping sessions of 7 puffs
Saffari et al. (2014)	Open tank	BC (370–950 nm), VOCs in PM (n-alkane: n-C20, n-C22, n-C24, n-C25, n-C26, n-C30, n-C31, n-C32, n-C33, n-C34, n-C35, n-C36, n-C37, n-C38, fatty acids: 10:0, 12:0, 14:0, 15:0, 16:0, 17:0, 16:1, 18:2, 20:0, 22:0, 23:0, 24:0, 25:0, 26:0, 28:0, 30:0, suberic acid, azelaic acid, PAHs: benzo[a]pyrene, benzo[b]fluoranthene, benzo[k]fluoranthene, benzo[e]pyrene, benzo[ghi]perylene, chrysene, indeno[1,2,3-cd]pyrene), trace inorganics in PM (Al, B, Ca, Co, Cr, Fe, K, Mg, Mn, Ni, S, Ti, V), CO	No	1.1	48	2/1	ND	2 vaping sessions of 7 puffs

Continued

TABLE 8.6
Summary of Representative IAQ Studies on EVPs Conducted in Model Environments with Human Users.—cont'd

Publication	EVP	Constituents[a]	Control on Environmental Parameters	Air Changes/h (h^{-1})	Volume (m^3)	No. of Persons/ No. of Vapers	Sampling Duration (min)	No. of Products
Schober et al. (2014)	Open tank	PNC, PM, PM_1, $PM_{2.5}$, PM_{10}, nicotine, carbonyls (acetaldehyde, acrolein, aceton, benzaldehyde, butyraldehyde, formaldehyde), VOC (benzene, benzyl alcohol, benzylbenzoate, 2,5–dimethylfuran, 3-ethenylpyridine, L-limonene, menthol, vanillin), glycerin, propylene glycol, PAHs(acenaphthene, acenaphthylene, anthracene, benz[a] anthracene, benzo[b] fluoranthene, benzo[ghi] perylene, benzo[a] pyrene, chrysene, dibenz [ah]anthracene, fluoranthene, fluorene, indeno[1,2,3-cd]pyrene, naphthalene, phenanthrene, pyrene), metals (Al, As, Bi, Ca, Cd, Ce, Co, Cr, Cu, Fe, K, La, Mg, Mn, Mo, Na, Ni, Pb, Sb, Sn, Ti, Tl, V, Zn), Co, CO_2	No	0.6	45	3	120	Ad libitum
Schripp et al. (2013)	Open tank	PNC (5.6–560 nm), nicotine, carbonyls (acetaldehyde, aceton, formaldehyde, propanal), glycerin, propylene glycol, TVOCs	Yes	0.3	8	1/1	15	6 puffs

Volesky et al. (2018)	Cigalike, open tank, and open tank with adjustable voltage	PNC, PM$_{2.5}$	Yes (t°)	NI	38	2/1	22	7 puffs
van Drooge et al. (2018)	NI	PNC, PSD, PM$_1$, PM$_{2.5}$, PM$_{10}$, BC, nicotine, carbonyls (acetone, formaldehyde), VOCs (benzene, ethylbenzene, naphthalene, o-/m-/p-xylene, toluene), TVOCs, trace organic compounds in PM (nicotine, glycerin, levoglucosan, PAHs (benz[a]anthracene, benzo[b+j+k]fluoranthene, benzo[ghi]perylene, benzo[a]pyrene, benzo[e]pyrene, chrysene, fluoranthene, indeno[1,2,3-cd]pyrene, phenanthrene, pyrene)	No	NM	146	10/5	720	NI

[a] Abbreviations: *BC*, black carbon; *EVP*, e-vapor product; *NAB*, N-nitrosoanabasine; *NAT*, N-nitrosoanatabine; *NI*, not indicated; *NNK*, nicotine-derived nitrosamine ketone; *NNN*, N-nitrosonornicotine; *PAH*, polycyclic aromatic hydrocarbon; *PM*, particulate matter; *PNC*, particle number concentration; *PSD*, particle size distribution; *TSNA*, tobacco-specific nitrosamine; *TVOC*, total volatile organic compound; *VOC*, volatile organic compound.

Mitova et al., 2019a; Protano et al., 2016, 2017; Schober et al., 2019) and EVPs (Fromme and Schober, 2015; Martuzevicius et al., 2019; Protano et al., 2016, 2017; Schober et al., 2014, 2019). Concerning carbonyls, acetaldehyde is a good nonspecific tracer of EHTPs and is, therefore, applied in studies in controlled experimental conditions; nevertheless, it has somewhat limited application in real-life environments because of its many other potential sources (Höllbacher et al., 2017; Mitova et al., 2019b). Formaldehyde in EHTPs and formaldehyde and acetaldehyde in EVPs are emitted at very low levels during the use of the products and, as a result, are "immersed" in the typical indoor background even in experiments in model rooms with filtered air (Forster et al., 2018; Meišutovič-Akhtarieva et al., 2019; Mitova et al., 2016, 2019a; Schober et al., 2014, 2019).Therefore, these compounds are not useful tracers of the respective environmental aerosols of ENDPs. Acrolein, a minor airborne carbonyl related to thermal degradation of glycerin (Barker-Hemings et al., 2011), has the potential to be a good nonspecific tracer in controlled experimental conditions in model rooms and experimental chambers. However, in real-life environments, the applicability of acrolein as a tracer of environmental aerosols of ENDPs is inadequate for locations where food is prepared or served, because acrolein is a known thermal degradation product of fats (Gomes et al., 2002; Seaman et al., 2007). More importantly, the most serious drawback today of using airborne acrolein as a tracer for ENDPs is the trapping method (a 2,4-dinitrophenylhydrazine cartridge) generally used for this assessment, which causes the formation of artifacts leading to variability in the measurements (Schulte-Ladbeck et al., 2001). In fact, due to interferences in the determination of acrolein inherent with this classical method contradictory data are found in the literature and serious problems have been observed in interlaboratory comparisons (Schulte-Ladbeck et al., 2001).

Concerning the compounds measured in the TVOC window (International Organization for Standardization ISO ISO 16000-6, 2011), once again, very few can be regarded as candidate tracers. Thus, for mentholated EHTPs, the flavor compound menthol (mentholated products only) and for both mentholated and nonmentholated EHTPs acetol partially fulfill the requirement for uniqueness because they are also emitted from other indoor sources and, accordingly, could serve as tracers for measurements under controlled experimental conditions in model rooms. Great caution must be taken when using these compounds for measurements in real-life environments,

and their background levels must be carefully monitored. Moreover, some minor compounds (Chapter 6) such as glycidol, 2-furanmethanol, 3-chloro-1,2-propanediol, and furfural could be candidates for tracing EHTP environmental aerosols; but, their very low levels in the mainstream aerosols of EHTPs (Bentley et al., 2020) might significantly limit their applicability. Once again, great caution must be taken when using these compounds as tracers, and the background levels must be carefully monitored.

Studies aiming to discriminate the consumption of cigarettes and ENDPs commonly apply measurement of compounds attributed to combustion or high-temperature pyrolysis, such as ultraviolet particulate matter (UVPM), fluorescent particulate matter (FPM), 3-ethenylpyridine, acrylonitrile, benzene, 1,3-butadiene, isoprene, toluene, CO, nitrogen oxide (NO), and combined oxides of nitrogen (NO_x). Of these compounds, only 3-ethenylpyridine is a specific pyrolysis product related to thermal degradation of nicotine in tobacco products (Vainiotalo et al., 2001). However, the operating temperature of ENDPs is below that required for its generation (Smith et al., 2016). It is important to remember that benzene, toluene, CO, NO, and NO_x are common traffic emissions (Edwards et al., 2001; WHO, 2010), while isoprene is a human presence–related marker (Kwak et al., 2015; Mitova et al., 2019b). Consequently, all these compounds are commonly quantified in all indoor environments and, as mentioned previously, their concentrations in the background must always be considered.

In summary, airborne acetaldehyde, nicotine, glycerin, PM_1, and UFP are suitable tracers for the use of EHTPs, especially when used in combination. Similarly, airborne nicotine, glycerin, propylene glycol, UFP, and PM_1 are useful markers for indoor consumption of EVPs. Except nicotine, these compounds could be emitted by several other indoor sources, and, therefore, it is crucial to carefully monitor their concentrations in the background air in the same experimental conditions. To ensure proper evaluation of the environmental aerosols of ENDPs, it is recommended to conduct the experiments in model rooms with filtered air that allow control of environmental parameters. Assessments of ENDPs in real-life environments must take into careful consideration possible confounding sources of pollution. Finally, all recommendations of international norms for measurement of intermittent pollution sources in terms of sampling protocol must be implemented with due regard to the monitoring objectives of the study.

8.6 STUDIES IN MODEL ENVIRONMENTS

To enhance our understanding of the characteristics of environmental aerosols of ENDPs, this section will start with an overview of experimental data on emissions of consumer products based on combustion as well as data on environmental aerosols of some other alternative nicotine delivery products, such as carbon heated tobacco products (CHTPs). Experimental data on environmental aerosols of EHTPs and EVPs will be summarized in the subsequent subsections.

8.6.1 IAQ During Indoor Use of Combustion Sources

ENDPs are products intended as an alternative source of nicotine for adult smokers who would otherwise continue to smoke. For that reason, the impact of ENDPs, including that on IAQ, is commonly compared with that of cigarettes. Cigarette smoking is recognized as a substantial indoor pollution source leading to emission of numerous airborne pollutants (U.S. Department of Health and Human Services, 2014). Generally, it is important to make a clear distinction between the impact on IAQ of consumer products based on combustion and high-temperature pyrolysis and the types of impact that imply different mechanisms for aerosolization. In fact, the great majority of airborne constituents released during smoking are also found in the emissions of other common combustion-based products, such as candles and incense. Although the general public is aware of the detrimental health impact of indoor smoking, there is very low awareness outside expert circles of the harmful impact of other combustible products that are commonly used indoors. Table 8.3 summarizes comparative data on smoking 2 or 12 cigarettes, burning three tealights or one incense stick, and using a representative ENDP, the tobacco heating system 2.2 (THS), in an environmentally controlled room—the so-called IAQ room—in Philip Morris International (PMI). All experiments were performed with ventilation representative of simulated residential environments ($0.5 \ h^{-1}$) (EN 15251, 2007). Under the experimental conditions, burning three tealights and one incense stick indoors led to an increase above the room background levels of the noxious gases CO, NO, and NO_x. Furthermore, measurements demonstrated that burning one incense stick caused an increase above the room background level of all off-line markers (RSP by gravimetry, UVPM, FPM, acrylonitrile, benzene, 1,3-butadiene, isoprene, toluene, acetaldehyde, acrolein, crotonaldehyde, and formaldehyde). Burning three tealights generated comparable levels of NO and higher concentrations of NO_x than smoking 12 cigarettes[1] (Figs. 8.1 and 8.2). Likewise, burning one incense stick led to comparable levels of TVOCs and higher concentrations of the carcinogenic compound benzene than smoking 12 cigarettes. Furthermore, burning one incense stick resulted in a greater increase in the concentrations of benzene (17-fold increase), acrolein, formaldehyde, 1,3-butadiene, and TVOCs than smoking two cigarettes. In contrast, in this experimental setup, consumption of THS (12 tobacco sticks/2 h) had a completely different influence on the indoor environment: Only acetaldehyde increased above the background levels, and only very slightly, while all the other constituents measured in this comparison remained at background levels. Consistent with these results are the conclusions of a review that compared the environmental aerosols of THS and EVPs with the emissions of candles, incense, and mosquito coils (Kauneliene et al., 2018). Indeed, on the basis of analyses of published data, this review highlighted that incense and mosquito coils generated higher levels of aldehydes, VOCs, and $PM_{2.5}$, while candles generated higher $PM_{2.5}$ and had no influence on formaldehyde concentrations in comparison to THS and EVPs indoors. Consequently, the authors of the review concluded that persons in proximity to such non-nicotine combustion products might be exposed to greater levels of pollutants than persons standing near an ENDP user (Kauneliene et al., 2018).

In short, rigorous scientific data have clearly demonstrated that all consumer products that are based on combustion and high-temperature pyrolysis generate substantial emissions of PM, carbonyls, VOCs, and noxious gases.

8.6.2 IAQ During Indoor Use of CHTPs

CHTPs are a distinct category of HTPs that use a glowing carbon tip to generate aerosol from processed tobacco instead of the electronically controlled heating mechanism such as used in THS. The design of CHTPs reduces the amount of sidestream emissions because the combustion and high-temperature pyrolysis occur only in the carbon heat source, which decreases the generation of harmful and potentially harmful constituents (HPHCs) in the mainstream aerosol (Bombick et al., 1998). The assessments of Bombick et al. and Nelson et al. (Bombick et al., 1998; Nelson et al., 1998) on the indoor use of CHTPs showed that the ETS marker levels after CHTP use were reduced by at least 80% relative to those after smoking commercial cigarettes, with the exception of CO, which was reduced by 11%—30%.

---

[1]Commercially available brand (0.5 mg nicotine).

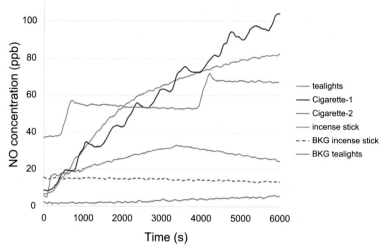

FIG. 8.1 Online measurements of NO under "Residential category III" environment (0.5 h^{-1}) for simulation with combustible products—tealights, incense stick, and cigarettes (Cigarette-1, 12 cigarettes (Mitova et al., 2019a); Cigarette-2, 2 cigarettes)—relative to the background levels in an empty IAQ room (BKG).

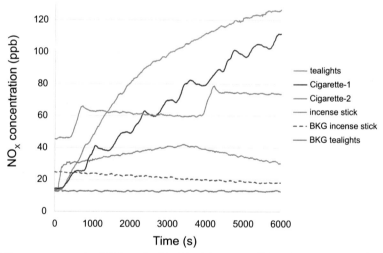

FIG. 8.2 Online measurements of NO$_x$ under "Residential category III" environment (0.5 h^{-1}) for simulation with combustible products—tealights, incense stick, and cigarettes (Cigarette-1, 12 cigarettes (Mitova et al., 2019a); Cigarette-2, 2 cigarettes)—relative to the background levels in an empty IAQ room (BKG).

The impact on IAQ of another CHTP prototype, termed P2V2, was evaluated in the IAQ room in PMI under the ventilation conditions (0.5 h^{-1}) recommended for simulating a residential environment (EN 15251, 2007). The indoor air concentrations of 27 constituents were determined (Table 8.4) in experiments that used a model with a machine-puffing regimen (surrogate environmental aerosol; 6 sticks/h; 2 h sessions). In general, relative to a reference cigarette, the mainstream aerosol of P2V2 shows a similar reduction in HPHC concentrations as the mainstream aerosol of THS. However, in contrast to THS, P2V2 shows a quantifiable release of several HPHCs in sidestream emissions (e.g., acrolein at 77.9 μg/stick and benzene at 52.4 μg/stick). For this reason, under a high-load environment (0.5 h^{-1}; 12 sticks in 2 h), we expected to observe an increase in the concentrations of several constituents above the levels in background air. As a matter of fact, of the 27 airborne constituents measured in experiments with a surrogate environmental aerosol of P2V2, only acrylonitrile and 1,3-butadiene did not increase above the background (below the lower limit of quantification) level. Furthermore, there was only a slight increase in isoprene and toluene levels; it was, therefore, concluded that, in experiments with panelists, the isoprene and toluene emissions resulting from P2V2 consumption would probably be immersed in the background air levels.

The indoor concentrations of markers of combustion (CO, NO, NO_x, UVPM, and FPM) and high-temperature pyrolysis (3-ethenylpyridine for pyrolysis of nicotine and acetaldehyde, acrolein, and formaldehyde for pyrolysis of glycerin and other constituents of the tobacco matrix) in the surrogate environmental aerosol of P2V2 were all increased above the levels in the background air, although they were below the levels in experiments with the same amounts of cigarettes. The levels of airborne acetaldehyde, acrolein, and CO during indoor consumption of P2V2 reached those typical in the ETS generated during smoking of two cigarettes. Conversely, the concentrations of formaldehyde in the environmental aerosol of P2V2 were slightly below those in the ETS of two cigarettes, while the concentrations of NO and NO_x were reduced by at least 50% and those of the rest of the constituents by more than 70%.

Furthermore, compounds typical to the mainstream aerosol of P2V2 were identified in the TVOC trace (Fig. 8.3).

The carcinogenic compounds benzene, NNK, and NNN were quantified at concentrations similar to those in the ETS of 2 cigarettes and, in the case of NNN, even at levels similar to those in the ETS of 12 cigarettes. This result was quite unexpected considering the levels of NNN in the mainstream aerosol of P2V2 (13.8 ng/stick, similar to that in the mainstream aerosol of THS). This observation strongly suggests the occurrence of an artifact formation during sampling—for example, from the nornicotine and NO_x generated during consumption of P2V2—and merits further investigation.

The results for the surrogate environmental aerosols of P2V2 are consistent with data published for other CHTP prototypes (Bombick et al., 1998; Nelson et al., 1998).

It is important to underline that the data for surrogate environmental aerosols of EHTPs and EVPs in the same experimental conditions (0.5 h^{-1}; machine aerosolization; THS with 12 tobacco sticks under the Health Canada puffing regimen; EVP Platform 4, P4 with 100 puffs under the CORESTA puffing regimen) are different from those of P2V2. Thus, 3-ethenylpyridine, a marker of nicotine pyrolysis, was never quantified within the method working range in experiments with

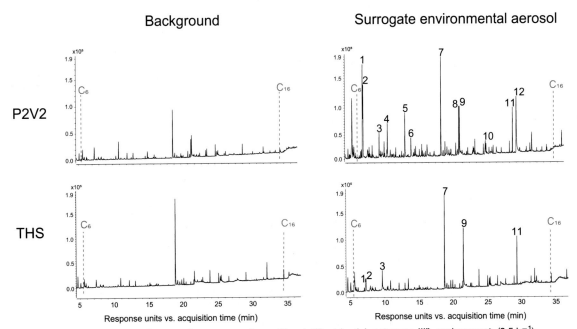

FIG. 8.3 Total volatile organic compounds profile at "Residential category III" environment (0.5 h^{-1}).
Compounds: Acetol (1), benzene (2), propylene glycol (3), toluene (4), furfural (5), 2-furanmethanol (6), benzaldehyde (7), ᴅ-limonene (8), benzyl alcohol (9), benzoic acid (10), triacetin (11), and nicotine (12).

THS and P4. Furthermore, formaldehyde, NO, and NO_x levels never exceeded the background levels in the surrogate environmental aerosols of THS and P4, while acrolein, crotonaldehyde, NNK, and NNN were measured below their reporting limits. Quite interestingly, the TVOC traces for THS and P2V2 were also different. Indeed, compounds such as furfural and 2-furanmethanol appeared in the TVOC trace of the surrogate environmental aerosol of P2V2 (Fig. 8.3) but not in that of THS, despite the fact that these compounds were quantified in THS mainstream aerosol (Bentley et al., 2020).

In the surrogate environmental aerosol of P2V2, the concentrations of the following constituents were above the guideline values:
- RSP (air quality marker): 84.3 µg/m³; guideline values, 10 µg/m³ (WHO, 2005) and 25 µg/m³ (Air Quality Standards EU, 2020)
- Acrolein (respiratory toxicant): 3.47 µg/m³; guideline value, 0.35 µg/m³ (California Office of Environmental Health Hazard Assessment, 2018)
- Benzene (carcinogen): 4.93 µg/m³; guideline values, 3 µg/m³ (California Office of Environmental Health Hazard Assessment, 2018) and 5 µg/m³ (Air Quality Standards EU, 2020)
- Airborne NNN and NNK at quantifiable levels; note that both NNN and NNK are carcinogens of group 1 (International Agency for Research on Cancer IARC, 2012)

On the basis of these findings, it is reasonable to conclude that the effect of CHTPs on the direct user, who is the person closest to the pollution source, will be lower than the effect of indoor exposure to the same amount of cigarettes. However, considering the similarity between the surrogate environmental aerosol of CHTPs and diluted ETS, and taking into account that the former surpasses the indoor guideline values of several constituents, it can be seen that CHTP consumption has an adverse effect on the overall IAQ in environments with the ventilation typically observed in residential buildings. Accordingly, CHTPs are not for indoor use, and their usage must be governed by the regulations for protection of bystanders implemented for cigarettes. It is also interesting to note that the indoor emissions of CHTPs are markedly different from those in the environmental aerosols generated during indoor use of EHTPs and EVPs.

8.6.3 IAQ During Indoor Use of EHTPs
Experimental evidence from studies conducted in exposure chambers has clearly indicated that the environmental aerosols emitted by EHTPs have a significantly

lower impact on an indoor environment than ETS generated by smoking cigarettes (Cancelada et al., 2019; Forster et al., 2018; Frost-Pineda et al., 2008; Ichitsubo and Kotaki, 2018; Meišutovič-Akhtarieva et al., 2019; Mitova et al., 2016, 2019a; Oey et al., 2008; Protano et al., 2016, 2017; Roethig et al., 2005; Ruprecht et al., 2017; Tricker et al., 2009). This is predictable because the aerosol formation from EHTPs does not entail tobacco combustion or high-temperature pyrolysis, which results in a substantial decrease in HPHCs emissions (Chapter 4). Furthermore, by design, EHTPs have no smoldering tip discharging sidestream smoke. Consequently, the main contributors to the indoor pollution caused by cigarettes are absent in EHTPs.

Studies investigating early prototypes, the so-called Electrically Heated Cigarette Smoking Systems (EHCSS), showed significant reductions in most ETS markers relative to cigarette smoking (Frost-Pineda et al., 2008; Oey et al., 2008; Roethig et al., 2005; Tricker et al., 2009). Environmental aerosol assessments of the first three generations of EHCSS demonstrated that the levels of gas-phase markers—including CO, TVOC, and 3-ethenylpyridine—were similar to nonsmoking levels, while ammonia concentrations were reduced by 40% (Frost-Pineda et al., 2008; Oey et al., 2008; Roethig et al., 2005). The concentrations of airborne particulate–phase markers, such as RSP-gravimetry, UVPM, FPM, and solanesol, in aerosols of the first two generation prototypes were 44%–98% below those in cigarette smoke (Oey et al., 2008; Roethig et al., 2005), while they all showed more than 93% reductions in the third-generation prototype aerosol (Frost-Pineda et al., 2008). A study conducted under a simulated "Office" environment with three levels of ventilation and a simulated "Hospitality" environment with low ventilation revealed that 24 out of 29 measured ETS markers in EHCSS aerosol had mean reductions greater than 90%, and that 5 of the measured airborne constituents had mean reductions between 80% and 90% in comparative experiments with cigarettes (Tricker et al., 2009).

While these early EHTP prototypes were not commercially successful, new EHTPs and hybrid products (Chapter 2) are now available, and their respective impact on air quality during indoor use has been evaluated (Forster et al., 2018; Ichitsubo and Kotaki, 2018; Mitova et al., 2016, 2019a). Summarized below are representative studies on IAQ of EHTPs published until the end of 2019 (Table 8.5).

The environmental aerosol generated during indoor use of THS is by far the most extensively studied (Mitova et al., 2016, 2019a). The design of these studies under simulated environmental conditions in the IAQ room was based on the European ventilation performance standard EN 15251 (EN 15251, 2007). A few other studies have been performed externally with different designs in an exposure chamber (Meišutović-Akhtarieva et al., 2019) and in environments with limited control on environmental parameters (Protano et al., 2016, 2017; Ruprecht et al., 2017). Another external study used sidestream and exhaled mainstream emissions of THS to predict their impact on IAQ in commonly encountered scenarios (Cancelada et al., 2019).

Protano et al. (Protano et al., 2016) comparatively evaluated particle size distribution in the range 5.6−560 nm during consumption of one tobacco stick of THS, 12 puffs of an EVP, and smoking of one cigarette (either classical or hand-rolled cigarette) at $0.7 \, h^{-1}$. The experiments were conducted with a Fast Mobility Particle Sizer spectrometer positioned 2 m away from the consumer and 1.5 m above the floor in a $52.7 \, m^3$ room, with no control of environmental parameters. The submicron particles generated during THS consumption were 4-times lower in quantity compared with the emissions generated by smoking cigarettes and at similar levels to those of EVPs. Most importantly, the emissions of submicron particles from both THS and EVPs immediately returned to the levels typical for background air, in sharp contrast to those from cigarettes, which persisted at elevated concentrations till the end of the experiments. The outcome of this study demonstrated that exposure to submicron particles occurred only during consumption of THS and EVPs, and it became negligible when the devices were turned off.

This initial experiment was extended with two additional products to allow comparative evaluation of the impact of four different types of combustion-based smoking products (cigarette, hand-rolled cigarette, cigar, and pipe) versus THS and a representative EVP (Protano et al., 2017). The experimental settings were equivalent to the ones described above (Protano et al., 2016) except for the replicate sessions conducted consecutively in the latter study. Similar to the previous study, the submicron particle emissions from THS and the EVP were significantly below those from all of the evaluated combustion-based smoking products. Assessment of temporal trends in the submicron particle traces revealed that the average emissions during the entire EVP session were lower than those of THS, even if the maximum values during consumption itself were higher for EVPs. In direct contrast to the outcome of the earlier study (Protano et al., 2016), this additional evaluation showed that particle number concentrations followed a slightly increasing trend for THS, while those for EVPs returned to the background levels (Protano et al., 2017).

Caponetto et al. investigated the CO exposure incurred with two commercially available EHTPs by comparatively assessing CO concentrations in the exhaled breath of smokers puffing the two EHTPs and cigarettes (Caponnetto et al., 2018). No increase in exhaled CO was observed in any of the study participants during experiments with the tested EHTPs. In contrast, smoking cigarettes resulted in elevated levels of exhaled CO. Because the constituents of exhaled breath are an important contributor to the environmental aerosols of EHTPs, these findings might be extrapolated to conclude that indoor use of the tested EHTPs had a very low impact, if any, on CO concentrations.

Ruprecht et al. (Ruprecht et al., 2017) described the analysis of 11 airborne constituents (black carbon [hereafter BC] at 880 nm; BC at 370 nm; particle counts >0.3 μm and >1.0 μm; nanoparticles; PM_1; $PM_{2.5}$; PM_{10}; acrolein; acetaldehyde; and formaldehyde) together with metals and trace organic compounds in total suspended PM in experiments that comparatively evaluated the environmental aerosols generated during indoor consumption of THS, an EVP, and a cigarette. The sampling site was a room in an apartment with no control on environmental parameters ($48 \, m^3$; $1.5 \, h^{-1}$). The sampling equipment was placed 2 m from the panelists, and, over a period of 3 h, 13 vaping sessions were conducted with the EVP, 10−14 tobacco sticks of THS were used, or 9 cigarettes smoked. The background concentrations of airborne constituents were monitored before the consumption sessions with the three different products for BC and the different PM measurements; the background levels of the three carbonyls were determined from outdoor air at the same time as the experimental measurements. Consequently, the analyses of carbonyls in this study lacked the required baseline controls of the indoor levels, which would have required human presence but without any product use (see Section 8.5). During the experiments with indoor consumption of THS, negligible levels of organic compounds with absorption at 370 nm were measured ($0.57 \, \mu g/m^3$ with 46% relative standard deviation [RSD]; <1% vs. measurement for cigarette smoke), while no soot whatsoever was detected in the BC measurements at 880 nm. A temporary increase related to THS consumption was observed in >0.3 μm particle counts as well as in nanoparticles. In agreement with published data, an increase in acetaldehyde concentrations attributable to THS was seen (Meišutović-Akhtarieva et al., 2019; Mitova et al., 2016, 2019a). Moreover, the study showed that there was no increase in the levels of metals in suspended PM, polycyclic aromatic hydrocarbons (PAH), hopanes, or steranes during THS consumption, relative to the control. Conversely, residues of n-alkanes, organic acids, and levoglucosan were detected in suspended PM. The most abundant of the n-alkanes (hentriacontane and heptacosane) and fatty acids (palmitic and linoleic acids) are common plant metabolites, which were identified in the PM of the mainstream aerosol of THS (Bentley et al., 2020) (Chapter 6); thus, their presence at low to negligible levels in the indoor environment during THS use is plausible. However, in this study PM_1-PM_{10}, acrolein, and formaldehyde levels during indoor THS use were reported to slightly exceed the background levels. However, these results were not supported by other studies (Meišutovič-Akhtarieva et al., 2019; Mitova et al., 2016, 2019a; Schober et al., 2019).

Meisutovic-Akhtarieva et al. conducted a study of the impact of THS on IAQ in an exposure chamber (35.8 m³; filtered air; controlled environmental parameters) with sample collection/monitoring in the breathing zone of a heated "dummy" (Meišutovič-Akhtarieva et al., 2019). The concentrations of nine airborne constituents (PNC, 10−420 nm; size-segregated PM concentrations, 0.006−10 µm; nicotine, 3-ethenylpyridine, acetaldehyde, formaldehyde, CO, and CO_2) were evaluated in a series of experiments in which the following conditions were varied: number of parallel users (1, 3, or 5), distance to the bystander (0.5, 1, or 2 m), ventilation rate (0.2, 0.5, or 1 h⁻¹), and relative humidity (RH: 30%, 50%, or 70%). The indoor concentrations of the nine analytes were measured during and after THS use. Cigarette smoking (1 cigarette; 2 m distance; 0.5 h⁻¹; 50% RH) was used as a positive control. In good agreement with published data (Mitova et al., 2016, 2019a; Protano et al., 2016, 2017), the experiments with THS showed an increase above the background in the indoor concentrations of nicotine, acetaldehyde, PNC, and PM; the rest of the analytes remained at background levels. Likewise, the indoor concentrations of all nine airborne constituents, except that of the human bioeffluent CO_2, during cigarette smoking exceeded those in the background and during THS sessions, even when the lowest number of products and furthest distance to the collection point were applied. An overall increase in PM was attributable to THS use, as analysis of particle size distribution revealed a mode at the smallest particle diameter. Overall, during THS use in these experiments, PM > 1 µm was measurable during exhalation at close distance and with five simultaneous users. Similarly, a distinct sawtooth pattern was apparent in the online trace of PM during THS consumption at a distance of 0.5 m, while progressively longer distances resulted in lower intensity or absence of peaks. "Masking" of the peaks in the online PM trace was also observed with an increase in ambient humidity together with a correlated rise in the measured aerodynamic diameter, probably related to particle growth. In addition, dry air conditions (30% RH) led to a decrease in the PNC after THS consumption. As stated by the authors, all these observations were explainable by the high volatility of the liquid droplets generated during THS use, their dispersion in approximately 6−8 s, and, consequently, their lower probability of reaching a "bystander" at distances greater than 0.5 m at low usage intensity and ambient humidity. Similar conclusions were drawn about the other constituents attributable to THS consumption. Thus, the concentrations of airborne nicotine and acetaldehyde showed a slight upward trend with increasing numbers of simultaneous users; with regard to nicotine levels, the distance between the user and bystander also played a role, with a significant drop in the indoor concentrations of nicotine with increasing distance. Concerning acetaldehyde, the authors emphasized that the measured concentrations fell within the range of mean concentrations observed in residential and public environments.

Cancelada et al. analyzed VOCs in the mainstream and sidestream emissions of three commercial brands of THS in a small exposure chamber (0.2 m³; filtered air; 0.3 h⁻¹) by using smoking machines operated under the Health Canada regimen (1 tobacco stick with 12 puffs) (Cancelada et al., 2019). The mainstream emissions were collected during consumption of the tobacco sticks, while putative sidestream[2] emissions were collected for the following 3 h to maximize the collected air volumes. The results were used to compare THS emission profiles with those of cigarettes and EVPs. In addition, the contributions from the sidestream and calculated exhaled mainstream emissions of THS were used to predict the indoor air concentrations of acrolein

---

[2]The authors of this study consider that "once the [THS] device is activated, the tobacco stick is heated independently of the frequency and intensity of puffing, generating sidestream emissions that contribute to increasing indoor pollutant levels, as do exhaled mainstream emissions." Of the 33 identified and quantified compounds in the three investigated THS flavors, 9−10 compounds were reported "<reporting limit," 7−8 compounds with RSDs exceeding 50%, and 12−13 compounds with RSDs exceeding 30%. It is important to underline that, of the nitrogenated compounds mentioned as tobacco smoke markers, only 2 (pyridine and pyrrole) were reported with sufficient analytical precision (<15%), while the rest were either below reporting limit or with RSDs above 100% (3-ethenylpyridine). Nicotine was not quantified because of an issue either with trapping or with experimental conditions (high surface-to-volume ratio of the chamber combined with low ventilation).

in two scenarios: a residential space with a nonuser living with a user and a bar to serve as an example of a public space with multiple users. This study is the first report of qualitative and quantitative analyses of sidestream emissions of THS. It is of overall good quality, although a few limitations of the data analyses and the insufficient analytical precision[2] need to be mentioned. For example, the concentrations of 3-ethenylpyridine and glycidol in sidestream emissions were reported with 100% RSD, leaving the reader with the puzzling question as to whether these compounds were present at all even after significant concentration of the putative emissions and long sampling times or whether insufficient method sensitivity and precision combined with an inadequate number of replicates (two) was responsible for the results. Furthermore, the findings on modeling of exposure to acrolein in residential and bar environments were incorrectly generalized as shown in this extract: *"Pollutant levels were predicted for a variety of scenarios, contributing to establishing the impacts of IQOS on indoor air quality."*

The IAQ during indoor use of the Tobacco Heating Product 1.0 (THP) was evaluated in comparison to cigarette smoking and background air with human presence (Forster et al., 2018). The experiments were conducted in a furnished room with filtered air (37.8 m^3) under simulated "Residential" (1.2 h^{-1}), "Office" (2.2 h^{-1}), and "Hospitality" (7.7 h^{-1}) conditions similar to those in the study on THS (Mitova et al., 2016); but, unlike in the former study, the number of users was kept the same during all sessions (four users), and the total number of tobacco sticks used was higher (Residential, 20 tobacco sticks; Office, 32 tobacco sticks; and Hospitality, 32 tobacco sticks). Most of the 40 airborne constituents analyzed were below detectable levels or at baseline levels. Consistent with published data for THS (Meišutović-Akhtarieva et al., 2019; Mitova et al., 2016, 2019a; Protano et al., 2016, 2017), indoor use of THP increased the concentrations of nicotine, acetaldehyde, and PNC above the background levels. However, in this investigation, PM$_1$–PM$_{10}$[3] levels were reported to exceed the background levels in "Office" and "Hospitality" conditions but not in the "Residential" condition, while an almost negligible increase was observed in formaldehyde levels in "Residential" and "Office" environments. The levels of all airborne constituents attributable to THP were typically more than 90% lower than those in cigarette smoke.

Ichitsubo and Kotaki (Ichitsubo and Kotaki, 2018) examined the impact of using the Novel Tobacco Vapor

product (NTV) on IAQ in a walk-in exposure chamber (16.6 m^3; filtered air; controlled environmental parameters) in comparison to empty chamber air, background air with human presence, and cigarette smoking. Simulated nonsmoking environments ("Conference Room": 6.9^{-h}, 32 puffs of NTVs vs. 2 cigarettes; "Dining Room": 12.2^{-h}, 48 puffs of NTVs vs. 3 cigarettes) and one ventilated smoking environment ("Smoking Lounge": 40^{-h}, 288 puffs of NTVs vs. 18 cigarettes) were used, and the ventilation rate, design occupancy, and number of sticks were based on US (ASHRAE, 2001; Glantz and Schick, 2004) and EU standards (EN 15251, 2007). Therefore, the experimental design of this particular investigation was somewhat different from those for THS and THP (Forster et al., 2018; Mitova et al., 2016, 2019a). All 18 airborne markers analyzed during NTV use were either below the quantification limits of the methods or at background levels, leading to the conclusion that, under the simulations tested, the NTV product had no measurable effect on IAQ in nonsmoking or smoking areas.

In 2014, PMI investigated the concentrations of 18 airborne markers during indoor use of the nonmentholated version of THS in simulations of two public environments ("Office": 2.2 h^{-1}, 16 tobacco sticks; "Hospitality": 7.7 h^{-1}, 24 tobacco sticks) and a residential setting ("Residential category II": 1.2 h^{-1}, 12 tobacco sticks) in an IAQ room (Mitova et al., 2016). A later study examined the levels of 24 airborne constituents under a simulated high-load residential environment with low ventilation ("Residential category III," 0.5^{-h}) combined with a high consumption rate of THS (6 tobacco sticks/h; total of 12 tobacco sticks) (Mitova et al., 2019a). These studies showed that indoor use of THS led to an increase in the concentrations of acetaldehyde, glycerin, and nicotine—the three major compounds in THS mainstream aerosol (Schaller et al., 2016)—to above their background levels, while the rest of the measured airborne constituents remained below the reporting limits or at background levels. The data were consistent with external results (Meišutović-Akhtarieva et al., 2019; Schober et al., 2019). Some discrepancies in the reporting of airborne PM between the PMI studies on THS (Mitova et al., 2016, 2019a) and those conducted externally (Protano et al., 2016, 2017; Ruprecht et al., 2017) were noted and criticized (Simonavicius et al., 2018). One of the PMI studies used RSP-gravimetric measurement to compare PM generated by cigarettes and THS (Mitova et al., 2016). This gravimetric measurement is a reference ISO method (ISO 15593, 2001), with broad application (Sousan et al., 2016) and is suitable for demonstrating the differences in PM between the ETS of

---

[3]The LOQ of the DustTrak used for monitoring PM$_1$–PM$_{10}$ was reported to be 1 μg/m^3 for each mass fraction.

cigarettes and environmental aerosol of THS. In fact, for airborne solid particles or low-volatility droplets (which would be the case for ETS), the methodology would allow sufficient residues to be collected on the filter for performing measurements; in contrast, very low amount of residue would be collected on the filter if the environmental aerosols were based only on volatile liquid droplets. A later study applied light-scattering detection to monitor PM in the environmental aerosols of THS and reported mean values below the limit of detection (LOD) (Mitova et al., 2019a). Investigations on THS consumption conducted by varying several experimental parameters (distance to the measurement equipment, number of users, ventilation rate, and humidity) revealed that distance to the measurement equipment and intensity of THS use significantly influenced the measurement of PM (Meišutovič-Akhtarieva et al., 2019). Indeed, a distinct sawtooth pattern attributable to THS use was observed in the PNC trace at a close distance, while, with increasing distance, the peaks decreased in size and, in some cases, disappeared entirely. Likewise, higher numbers of simultaneously consumed tobacco sticks led to more intense signals. Interestingly, this study also showed that particle size distribution has a mode at the smallest particle

diameter of the measurement equipment (Meišutovič-Akhtarieva et al., 2019). As a matter of fact, as reported in a study in a passenger car, UFP generation was attributable to THS use, while no increase in $PM_{2.5}$ was measured in the same experiment (Schober et al., 2019). To verify these findings, a series of experiments were conducted under low ventilation ("Residential category III"; 0.5^{-h}), with three users consuming THS ad libitum; UFP and PM_1-PM_{10} levels were measured simultaneously online. Indeed, consumption of one tobacco stick was not registered in the online trace of any of the monitors, whereas two or three tobacco sticks consumed simultaneously or with short delay were easily detected (Fig. 8.4). Likewise, all size-segregated channels of the DustTrak monitor were activated and gave similar responses within the typical method uncertainties following simultaneous use of two or three tobacco sticks. Such responses indicated that PM with an aerodynamic diameter below 1 μm was generated during THS use. In line with the results of external studies (Meišutovič-Akhtarieva et al., 2019; Protano et al., 2016, 2017), a temporary increase in UFP and PM was observed, but, in both cases, the concentrations returned to close to background levels almost immediately. As discussed in detail by Meišutovič et al.

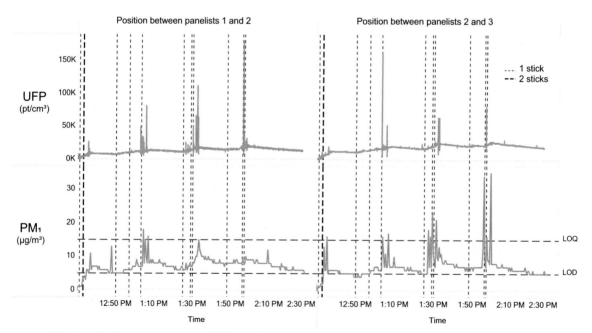

FIG. 8.4 Online measurements of UFP and PM_1 under simulated "Residential category III" environment (0.5 h^{-1}) in sessions with ad libitum consumption of THS. A total of 12 tobacco sticks were consumed by 3 panelists and measured simultaneously by UFP and PM analyzers placed at a 1.0 m distance from the panelists. One set of analyzers was positioned between Panelists 1 and 2 and a second set between Panelists 2 and 3.

(Meišutovič-Akhtarieva et al., 2019), this can be explained by the generation of an aerosol of liquid droplets consisting of highly volatile ingredients, which evaporated within seconds. Indeed, in additional experiments performed in PMI, the mean PM_1 (as well as $PM_{2.5}$) levels during indoor use of THS were below the limits of quantification (LOQ) of the method, even if several peaks were monitored in the online trace.

Following an initial study in 2014 (Mitova et al., 2016), an additional evaluation in a simulated "Hospitality" environment was conducted in 2018. However, in contrast to the former investigation, the second study did not include additional ventilation for smoking in the calculations (EN 15251, 2007). Consequently, the defined ventilation (existing buildings: non−low-polluted building and category III indoor environment) represents the lowest ventilation for restaurants according to the EU norm (EN 15251, 2007) and matches the ventilation given by the US norm for restaurant dining rooms (ASHRAE, 2016a) ($312 \, m^3/h$ and 4.3^{-1} vs. $309 \, m^3/h$ and 4.3^{-1}, respectively). Two sets of experiments were conducted with THS.[4] In the first set (simulation "Restaurant 20% HTP users"), 8 tobacco sticks of THS were used, with 4 tobacco sticks being consumed simultaneously at the beginning of the first hour and 4 tobacco sticks at the beginning of the second hour of the experiment. In the second set (simulation "Restaurant 100% HTP users"), 39 tobacco sticks of THS in total were consumed throughout the session, with two to three simultaneous consumptions. Furthermore, separate experiments with NTV and THP were conducted, with 39 vaping sessions of 10 min for NTV (no control on the number of puffs) and 39 tobacco sticks for THP, respectively, following the same consumption rate as that used for THS. The panelists could freely choose among three different flavors of THS and THP, and five different flavors of NTV. Before each THS, NTV, and THP session, a background session was performed with the same volunteers as those in the product-use session. The indoor air concentrations of 24 constituents were determined, including those of a particulate-phase tobacco-specific marker (solanesol), gas-phase tobacco-specific markers (3-ethenylpyridine

and nicotine), VOCs (acrylonitrile, benzene, 1,3-butadiene, isoprene, and toluene), low-molecular-weight carbonyls (acetaldehyde, acrolein, crotonaldehyde, and formaldehyde), aerosol formers (glycerin and propylene glycol), TSNAs (NNN and NNK), TVOC (expressed as toluene equivalents), gases (online measurement; CO, NO, NO_x, and NH_3), and PM (PM_1, $PM_{2.5}$, and PM_{10}).

Most of the constituents measured in the environmental aerosols of THS were below the reporting limits or at background levels. In accordance with the results of previously conducted studies (Mitova et al., 2016, 2019a), THS use led to an increase above background levels in the concentrations of nicotine, acetaldehyde, and glycerin in both "Restaurant 20% HTP users" and "Restaurant 100% HTP users" simulations. Moreover, owing to consumption of mentholated flavors, with a corresponding appearance of menthol peaks in the TVOC trace, the TVOC values exceeded the background concentrations. The real-time measurements of PM were below the LOQ, with a slight pattern in the online trace attributable to THS consumption (Fig. 8.5). The environmental aerosol of THP had a similar impact on IAQ as that of THS. However, the indoor concentrations of nicotine and acetaldehyde after THP use were somewhat lower than those after THS use (mean [standard deviation]: nicotine, 1.93 [0.04] vs. 4.22 [0.44] µg/m^3; acetaldehyde, 5.29 [0.10] vs. 7.10 [0.36] µg/m^3) (Fig. 8.6). The environmental aerosol of NTV had a relatively close resemblance to that of the EVP. Indeed, acetaldehyde showed no increase above the background level, while nicotine, glycerin, and propylene glycol showed an increase, and the concentrations of glycerin and, in particular, propylene glycol in the NTV aerosol exceeded those in the environmental aerosols of THS and THP (Fig. 8.6).

Another comparative assessment of environmental aerosols during indoor use of THS, THP, and NTV versus background and cigarette smoking (positive control) was conducted under a simulated "Smoking lounge" environment ($694 \, m^3/h$; $9.6 \, h^{-1}$; occupant density, $1.9 \, m^2$/person; 12 volunteer panelists and 1 PMI staff member; sessions, 15 min). In accordance with the established protocol, background measurement was performed with people present in the IAQ room but not using any tobacco product. All product-use sessions were conducted with 24 tobacco sticks in total for THS and THP (12 tobacco sticks consumed simultaneously, followed by simultaneous consumption of 12 more tobacco sticks), 12 vaping sessions of 10 min for NTV (no control on the number of puffs), and 24 cigarettes for the positive control. The panelists freely chose from among three different flavors of each

---

[4]The design occupancy for restaurant set forth in EN 15251 is of $1.5 \, m^2$/person corresponding to 16 persons for the IAQ room ($24.1 \, m^2$). Considering the consumption rate given in EN 15251 (20% users, consuming 1.5 sticks/h) at design occupancy of 16 persons (i) total of 8 tobacco sticks will correspond to 20% EHTP users: 16 persons x 0.2 × 1.5 sticks/h x 2h = 7.68 sticks rounded to 8 sticks; (ii) 39 tobacco sticks will correspond to 100% EHTP users: 16 persons x 1 × 1.5 sticks/h x 2h = 38.4 sticks rounded to 39 sticks.

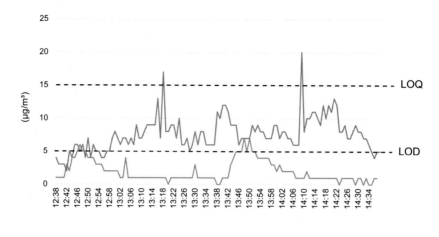

—8 Tobacco sticks   —39 Tobacco sticks

FIG. 8.5 Comparison of online measurements of PM$_1$ in sessions with 8 tobacco sticks versus 39 tobacco sticks consumed under a simulated "Hospitality" environment (4.3 h^{-1}).

of the EHTPs and two different brands of cigarettes. The indoor air concentrations of 16 constituents were determined, including offline measurement of 3-ethenylpyridine, nicotine, acetaldehyde, acrolein, crotonaldehyde, formaldehyde, and glycerin, propylene glycol, and online measurement of gases (CO, NH$_3$, NO, and NO$_x$), PM (PM$_1$, PM$_{2.5}$, and PM$_{10}$), and UFPs. The results obtained were concordant with those in the other simulated environments. Indeed, a significant increase in all airborne constituents except propylene glycol was observed with cigarette smoking (positive control). Furthermore, for all three EHTPs, the indoor concentrations of formaldehyde, CO, NH$_3$, NO, and NO$_x$ remained at background levels during consumption and those of 3-ethenylpyridine, acrolein, crotonaldehyde, and propylene glycol were below the reporting limits of the methods. In agreement with the results obtained in the simulated "Hospitality" condition, all three EHTPs caused an increase above background levels in nicotine and glycerin upon consumption, while acetaldehyde exceeded the background levels only in the THS and THP sessions. An increase in PM and UFPs was observed in these experiments. The mean levels of PM$_1$–PM$_{10}$ were somewhat similar with the three EHTPs. The mean levels for UFPs were similar with THS and NTV use, while they were lower with THP use. In the sessions with cigarettes, the measured PM$_1$–PM$_{10}$ and UFP levels were more than one order of magnitude above those in the sessions with the EHTPs.

To sum up, the studies on environmental aerosols of EHTPs demonstrated low levels of contamination of the

indoor environment irrespective of the ventilation rate applied. As a matter of fact, the available data demonstrated that most of the markers typical of ETS are not measurable during indoor use of EHTPs. This includes not only cigarette smoking–related markers such as 3-ethenylpyridine but also characteristic IAQ markers such as formaldehyde, benzene, toluene, CO, NO, and NO$_x$. Indoor consumption of EHTPs increases the concentrations of airborne nicotine, acetaldehyde, glycerin, and—in cases where mentholated products are consumed—menthol, with a corresponding increase in TVOC values. All these constituents are measured in the low parts per billion range, and their concentrations increase with the number of tobacco sticks consumed and, accordingly, decrease with increased ventilation rate. However, their levels, by no means, surpass the defined guideline values[5] (California Office of Environmental Health Hazard Assessment, 2018; US Occupational Safety and Health Administration US OSHA, 2020; ACGIH, 2001; EU OSHA, 2006). Moreover, the measured acetaldehyde concentrations fell within the typical range of the mean concentrations observed in residential and public environments (Kauneliene et al., 2018; Meišutovič-Akhtarieva et al., 2019; Mitova et al., 2019a). Some external research showed that acrolein concentrations are above the background levels in environmental aerosols of EHTPs

---

[5] Acetaldehyde, 140 μg/m^3 (chronic reference exposure level of OEHHA); glycerin, 10,000 μg/m^3 (occupational exposure limit, threshold limit value of ACGIH); and nicotine, 500 μg/m^3 (occupational exposure limit for US OSHA and EU OSHA).

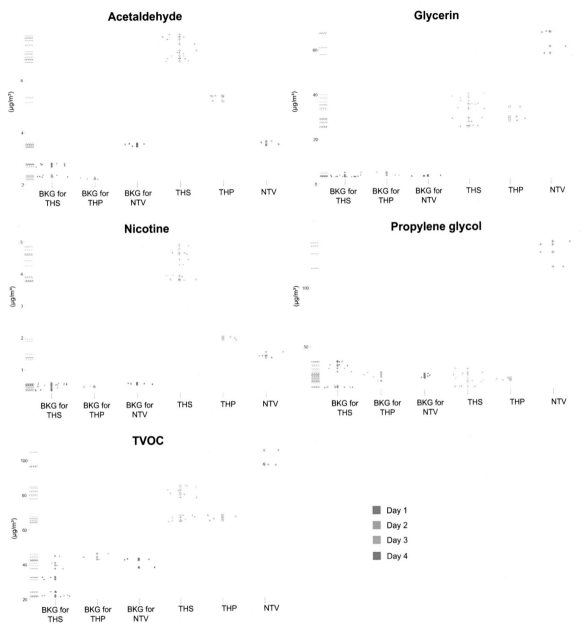

FIG. 8.6 Comparison of the measured concentrations of airborne acetaldehyde, glycerin, nicotine, propylene glycol, and TVOCs in sessions involving THS, THP, and NTV use in a simulated "Hospitality" environment (4.3 h⁻¹). THS (4 replicates) and THP (1 replicate) 39 tobacco sticks consumed; NTV (1 replicate), 39 vaping sessions.

(Ruprecht et al., 2017) or that the predicted concentrations might exceed the chronic exposure levels in small places with poor ventilation (Cancelada et al., 2019). There is no doubt that air is low quality in small places with poor ventilation. Nevertheless, our current experimental data, obtained with a validated and accredited method, do not support the presumption that an increase in airborne acrolein attributable to EHTP use occurs at the ventilation and consumption rates studied. Indoor use of hybrid products such as

NTV does not lead to an increase in the indoor levels of acetaldehyde, but it causes an increase in propylene glycol levels. In contrast, propylene glycol levels are very low in the environmental aerosol of classical EHTPs such as THS and THP. Concerning PM, the available data showed that the exposure varies depending on the intensity of use and distance to the user. Thus, PM_{1-10} is quantifiable in cases where all of the following conditions are fulfilled: (i) The equipment measures PM below 1 µm; (ii) more than 2 tobacco sticks are consumed simultaneously; and (iii) the distance between the user and measurement equipment is below 1.5 m. All in all, UFPs seem a more reliable tracer for the environmental aerosols of EHTPs than the conventional PM_{1-10}. Finally, the impact on the bystander significantly decreases with increasing distance to the EHTP user, and it occurs over short period of time, with a rapid decrease after consumption.

8.6.4 IAQ During Indoor Use of EVPs

EVP aerosol is generated when a user draws a puff. The only environmental aerosol to which a bystander is exposed is the *exhaled* aerosol—that is, the mainstream aerosol constituents that are not retained in the respiratory tract of the EVP user (Hess et al., 2016). Considering the high level of retention of the major constituents of the mainstream aerosols of EVPs (>90% for nicotine and propylene glycol; >80% for glycerin) (St Helen et al., 2016), it can safely be assumed that the levels of constituents in indoor air will, accordingly, be low. In fact, there is scientific agreement that the risk of bystanders being passively exposed to environmental aerosols is likely to be far lower in environments where EVPs are used than would be the case in the presence of ETS (PHE, 2016a; PHE, 2016b; FCTC, 2014, 2016; Hess et al., 2016).

Several studies have evaluated the impact of EVPs on IAQ by using a machine-puffing model (Czogala et al., 2014; Geiss et al., 2015; Lampos et al., 2019; McAuley et al., 2012). As mentioned previously, in general, such types of studies overestimate the concentrations of airborne constituents, because they do not take into account the retention of constituents in the body of the users. Geiss et al. assessed the surrogate environmental aerosols of representative EVPs in a walk-in exposure chamber with controlled environmental parameters (30 m³; filtered air, 0.5 h⁻¹; 6 series of 13 puffs with 5 min intervals) (Geiss et al., 2015). In these experiments, PM in the range of 20−300 nm, nicotine, glycerin, and propylene glycol increased above the background levels, while all carbonyls measured were below the detection limits. Furthermore, the

concentrations of PM larger than 300 nm immediately dropped to the baseline levels after each vaping session. In a further study, McAuley et al. predicted the concentrations of 11 airborne analytes in a 40 m³ room on the basis of assessment of the surrogate environmental aerosols of four EVPs and concluded that there was no significant risk of harm in their noncancer or cancer risk analyses (McAuley et al., 2012). A study by Czogala et al. investigated the indoor concentrations of $PM_{2.5}$, nicotine, CO, and VOCs in a room with limited control of environmental parameters (39 m³; 2 vaping sessions of 7 or 15 puffs) and with varying ventilation rates (4−12 h⁻¹); in good agreement with the results of similar studies, CO and VOCs remained at background levels, while nicotine exceeded its background levels (Czogala et al., 2014). An increase in $PM_{2.5}$ concentrations was measured during vaping, and the levels returned to the background values after the consumption was stopped. In a study by Lampos et al. the PNC and PM_1 values of five different EVPs were determined during machine puffing in a room with low ventilation conditions (35 m³; 0.2 h⁻¹; no air filtration) (Lampos et al., 2019). Consistent with the findings of similar studies, the aerosol mass concentrations rose very rapidly immediately on drawing the initial puff, and they subsequently dropped sharply back to the baseline levels as a result of fast dissipation of the generated liquid droplets; consequently, overall, the average particle levels were low. Indeed, it is interesting to note that, although all these studies used machine puffing of EVPs—which meant there was a related overestimation of airborne constituents in the environmental aerosols (Czogala et al., 2014; Geiss et al., 2015; Lampos et al., 2019; McAuley et al., 2012)—the results systematically showed that only nicotine, glycerin, and propylene glycol increased above the background levels, while PM reached high concentrations during machine puffing and then dropped rapidly to baseline levels when the puffing stopped.

In the last decade, a number of IAQ studies have been published on EVP use by human vapers in model environments with limited control of environmental parameters (Avino et al., 2018; Czogala et al., 2014; Melstrom et al., 2017; O'Connell et al., 2015; Protano et al., 2018; Protano et al., 2016; Protano et al., 2017; Ruprecht et al., 2017; Saffari et al., 2014; van Drooge et al., 2018; Volesky et al., 2018) and in exposure chambers with controlled environmental parameters (Liu et al., 2017; Martuzevicius et al., 2019; Schripp et al., 2013). Varying experimental conditions were applied in these studies, with wide variation in room volume, ventilation rate, number of simultaneous users, vaping rate, and session duration (Table 8.6). Some of these studies were recently reviewed (Fernández et al., 2015; Fromme and Schober, 2015; Hess et al., 2016; Kauneliene et al., 2018; Zainol Abidin et al., 2017).

In particular, a number of these studies investigated the indoor concentrations of $PM_{2.5}$ during indoor use of EVPs (Avino et al., 2018; Czogala et al., 2014; Martuzevicius et al., 2019; Melstrom et al., 2017; Ruprecht et al., 2017; Schober et al., 2014; van Drooge et al., 2018; Volesky et al., 2018). Several of these investigations also included measurement of PM_1 and PM_{10} (Avino et al., 2018; Martuzevicius et al., 2019; Protano et al., 2018; Ruprecht et al., 2017; Schober et al., 2014; van Drooge et al., 2018). The findings of these assessments differed, and the overall mean concentrations of $PM_{2.5}$ during EVP consumption varied over a broad range. This can be partially explained by the different experimental setups used in these studies (Table 8.6). Furthermore, some studies reported extreme values (Melstrom et al., 2017; Protano et al., 2018; Volesky et al., 2018); indeed, Melstrom et al. recorded mean $PM_{2.5}$ levels as high as 1.45 mg/m^3 during EVP use (3 vapers; 5 h^{-1}). The authors explained in their "Methods" section that the real-time monitor used has no accepted calibration factor, and, therefore, the values were reported as unadjusted numbers (Melstrom et al., 2017). In a further study, Volesky et al. reported cumulative mean $PM_{2.5}$ concentrations during vaping of three different types of EVPs in the range of 21.8−67.0 mg/m^3 at 0.5 m and 14.1−71.6 mg/m^3 at a 1 m distance (Volesky et al., 2018). The authors provided detailed information in their "Materials and Methods" section, explaining the overestimation: The real-time monitor was calibrated by using Arizona Road Dust, a calibrator not suitable for ambient aerosols, as is well described in the literature (Wallace et al., 2010). They reported two types of average values as "cumulative mean concentrations" and "mean" values (Volesky et al., 2018). In fact, the $PM_{2.5}$ mean values were in the range of 364−1117 µg/m^3 at 0.5 m and 168−1193 µg/m^3 at 1 m; although these values were still rather on the high end of the reported $PM_{2.5}$ range, overall, they concurred better with the results of similar studies than the cumulative mean concentrations did (Avino et al., 2018; Martuzevicius et al., 2019; Ruprecht et al., 2017; Schober et al., 2014; van Drooge et al., 2018). In a study by Protano et al. the authors reported median and mean PM_1 levels of 3.48 and 14.9 mg/m^3, respectively, for some sessions with fourth-generation open-tank EVPs (Protano et al., 2018). The authors (Protano et al., 2018) gave no details on the validation of the real-time monitor used or the calibration factor;

however, it is plausible that this study—similar to the other two studies (Melstrom et al., 2017; Volesky et al., 2018)—either reported unadjusted numbers or followed an unsuitable calibration procedure.

It is important to highlight that not all online sensors and methods for measuring $PM_{2.5}$ are suitable for assessment of EVP environmental aerosols. Indeed, the environmental aerosols of EVPs consist of liquid droplets with aerodynamic diameters in the submicron range, which dissipate fast. As emphasized by Martuzevicius et al. PM emissions during EVP use may only be recorded by instruments with high temporal resolution and the capability to measure particles smaller than 300 nm in aerodynamic diameter (Martuzevicius et al., 2019). It is also interesting to note that the same authors mentioned that, because of droplet evaporation over the collection period, it is difficult to determine particle concentrations with filter-based methods by using gravimetric measurements (Martuzevicius et al., 2019).

Overall, despite the differences in the reported values of PM inherent to the different experimental setups (Table 8.6) used in these published studies, the plots of the online traces of PM were very similar among the studies (Martuzevicius et al., 2019; Melstrom et al., 2017). Indeed, all experiments showed peaks of PM concurrent with the puffing schedule, with a substantial increase in particle concentration following exhalation and a rapid decrease after puffing.

Furthermore, in agreement with the PM measurements, EVP puffing led to a rapid increase in PNC by several orders of magnitude over background levels, followed by a very fast decrease to almost background levels within seconds (Volesky et al., 2018). However, an investigation reported UFP values that were slightly above baseline levels 10 min after stopping vaping, in contrast to the simultaneously measured $PM_{2.5}$, which returned to baseline levels (Volesky et al., 2018). Contrarily, in another study with real-time measurements made over a 12 h period, the PNC levels in the background session with human presence were higher than those detected during the vaping sessions (van Drooge et al., 2018). Indeed, a typical sawtooth pattern in the online traces of PNC was evident at close distances to the bystander (0.5 and 1 m), while the impact of the exhaled puffs was not detectable at 2 m (Martuzevicius et al., 2019). The authors put forward an explanation for this phenomenon that the liquid droplets likely dissipated and, therefore, did not reach the measuring equipment located at the bystander position.

The particle size distributions of EVP environmental aerosols reported in previous studies were in the submicron range but varied in absolute number. Martuzevicius et al. reported two modes—at 150 and 20–30 nm—at a close distance to the bystander, with a clear shift to the smaller mode with aging of the aerosol and increasing distance (Martuzevicius et al., 2019). Similarly, the presence of bimodal aerosols during EVP use was reported for an 8 m³ chamber, with one maximum in the range of 30 nm and another in the range of 100 nm (Schripp et al., 2013). Other studies reported the aerodynamic diameters of EVP environmental aerosol particles to be either 30 nm (Avino et al., 2018) or 24–36 nm (Schober et al., 2014).

A number of studies have investigated the concentrations of airborne nicotine in environmental aerosols of EVPs (Czogala et al., 2014; Liu et al., 2017; Melstrom et al., 2017; Schober et al., 2014; van Drooge et al., 2018). Similar to the findings on PM and PNC, the absolute numbers varied among the studies, although most investigations reported an increase in nicotine levels above the background, with values in the low μg/m³ range (Czogala et al., 2014; Liu et al., 2017; Melstrom et al., 2017; Schober et al., 2014; van Drooge et al., 2018). All the above-mentioned studies measured gas-phase nicotine; but, in one study (van Drooge et al., 2018), nicotine was also found in the ng/m³ range in the PM of environmental aerosols of EVPs.

A relatively small number of studies have assessed the concentrations of the two aerosol formers glycerin and propylene glycol during indoor use of EVPs (Liu et al., 2017; O'Connell et al., 2015; Schober et al., 2014; Schripp et al., 2013). All but two investigations found an increase in these two aerosol formers above background levels, attributable to EVP consumption: O'Connell et al. reported glycerin levels below quantification limits (O'Connell et al., 2015), while Schripp et al. reported concentrations of propylene glycol between LOD and LOQ (Schripp et al., 2013).

The indoor concentrations of carbonyls during vaping were evaluated in several studies (Liu et al., 2017; O'Connell et al., 2015; Ruprecht et al., 2017; Schober et al., 2014; van Drooge et al., 2018). The levels of the carbonyls measured were within the range of background variation in some studies (Liu et al., 2017; Schober et al., 2014; Schripp et al., 2013), whereas, in others, formaldehyde (van Drooge et al., 2018) or both formaldehyde and acetaldehyde (O'Connell et al., 2015; Ruprecht et al., 2017) were slightly increased above background levels.

A few studies have assessed the indoor concentrations of several VOCs (Czogala et al., 2014; Liu et al., 2017; O'Connell et al., 2015; Schober et al., 2014; Schripp et al., 2013; van Drooge et al., 2018). The

VOC values were reported to be within the range of background variation for the EVP sessions in most studies. Only a few VOCs were found to have slightly increased above the background levels in some studies, but the compounds listed differed from one study to another (Liu et al., 2017; van Drooge et al., 2018).

The concentrations of PAHs during EVP sessions were investigated in three studies; interestingly, the findings differed significantly among the studies (O'Connell et al., 2015; Schober et al., 2014; van Drooge et al., 2018). One study reported no increase in PAHs above the background levels (O'Connell et al., 2015), while another mentioned an increase of 20% in the concentrations of several PAHs (Schober et al., 2014); the third study reported an increase in different PAHs, but emphasized that the scale of increase was very small compared with those described in other indoor studies in urban zones (van Drooge et al., 2018). In addition, Saffari et al. evaluated the concentrations of VOCs and PAHs in suspended PM and concluded that particle-phase hopanes, steranes, and PAHs were not attributable to vaping (Saffari et al., 2014).

The concentrations of inorganic elements and metals were assessed by several research groups (Liu et al., 2017; O'Connell et al., 2015; Ruprecht et al., 2017; Saffari et al., 2014; Schober et al., 2014). Some studies found the concentrations of all evaluated metals to be either below the reporting limits or within background variations (Liu et al., 2017; O'Connell et al., 2015). This was in direct contrast with other studies that reported an increase in a few inorganics above background levels (Ruprecht et al., 2017; Saffari et al., 2014; Schober et al., 2014).

A very small number of studies have investigated the indoor concentrations of some other airborne constituents (Table 8.6). All these studies concurred that there was no increase whatsoever in BC concentrations during vaping (Avino et al., 2018; Ruprecht et al., 2017; Saffari et al., 2014; van Drooge et al., 2018). Likewise, there was agreement that indoor vaping did not influence the concentrations of gases (CO, CO_2, NO, NO_2, and O_3) (Czogala et al., 2014; O'Connell et al., 2015; Saffari et al., 2014; Schober et al., 2014). A further investigation (O'Connell et al., 2015) reported no increase in the concentrations of airborne TSNAs above background levels.

In 2015, PMI investigated the concentrations of seven airborne markers (3-ethenylpyridine, nicotine, glycerin, propylene glycol, acetaldehyde, formaldehyde, and TVOCs) during indoor use of two representative cigalike products and one refillable open-tank EVP. All products were PMI brands, and the experiments were performed in a simulated residential setting ("Residential category II": 1.2 h^{-1}; 12 vaping sessions) in a dedicated IAQ room, with a protocol similar to that used in the first set of experiments with THS (Mitova et al., 2016). Each session of 5 h was conducted on a separate day, starting with background (Monday, three persons present, not using any product), followed by vaping of the three EVPs on 3 consecutive days (Tuesday–Thursday, two vapers, one bystander). The study was conducted with three repetitions of each session in 3 separate weeks. The results showed that the concentrations of three analytes (acetaldehyde, formaldehyde, and TVOCs) were not increased in the environmental aerosol of any of the evaluated EVPs relative to the background levels, while 3-ethenylpyridine was below the reporting limits in both the background and vaping sessions. The nicotine, glycerin, and propylene glycol levels in the environmental aerosols of all three EVP brands were higher than their background levels. These results were, overall, in good agreement with the published data of two other research groups (Liu et al., 2017; Schober et al., 2014). Moreover, the increase in nicotine above background levels corroborated the findings of several studies (Czogala et al., 2014; Liu et al., 2017; Melstrom et al., 2017; Schober et al., 2014; van Drooge et al., 2018).

To conclude, similar to the IAQ studies on EHTPs, studies on environmental aerosols of EVPs have systematically demonstrated that contamination of the indoor environment following EVP use is very low, irrespective of the ventilation rate applied. Published external data and our internal results have shown that, although indoor vaping increases the concentrations of airborne nicotine, glycerin, propylene glycol, and submicron PM, the measured levels by no means exceed the exposure limits defined for nicotine, glycerin, and propylene glycol (US Occupational Safety and Health Administration US OSHA, 2020; ACGIH, 2001; EU OSHA, 2006; AIHA, 2011). Moreover, there is consensus that the PM emitted during EVP use consists of highly volatile liquid droplets that evaporate within seconds following exhalation. Thus, exposure to PM during vaping is limited to a very short period of time and is further restricted by distance, with bystanders being exposed only when in close proximity to the EVP user.

When comparing the results of the different studies reported here, we observed cases of both agreement and disagreement in the experimental findings, particularly concerning the huge variation in the concentrations of several constituents. Indeed, as highlighted in a review (Zainol Abidin et al., 2017), considering the broad range of reported values (including those for

nicotine, glycerin, propylene glycol, and submicron PM) and taking into account the variety of experimental settings, it is clear that there is a strong need for standardizing experimental protocols for measurement of environmental aerosols of EVPs.

At the same time, aside from the question of standardization, it is important to highlight that there is overall agreement in the scientific community that, compared with cigarettes, exhaled EVP aerosols release much lower levels of chemicals indoors and, considering the current exposure limits, are unlikely to pose an issue to bystanders.

8.7 STUDIES IN REAL-LIFE ENVIRONMENTS

As mentioned previously, existing studies have strictly used relevant norms, defined protocols, and controlled conditions for evaluating the specific impact of EHTPs and EVPs on IAQ in model environments and comparing this impact with that of ETS from cigarettes. Such scientific rigor minimizes the risk of potentially misinterpreting data and drawing erroneous conclusions regarding the impact of a product on air quality. However, only by conducting assessments in existing enclosed settings where typical real-life activities take place (such as cooking, wearing cosmetics, or simply use of the product in the presence of other people) and the product can be consumed without any restraint is it possible to gain a clear understanding of the actual impact of EHTPs and EVPs. Here, it is crucial to keep in mind the importance of measuring a proper background, as discussed in detail in Section 8.5.

Over the last decade, several studies have assessed the impact of usage of EHTPs, as well as certain EVPs, in indoor environments representative of residential and public places. Most of these studies compared the environmental aerosols from such products with those from combustion sources such as cigarettes and waterpipes or some common sources of indoor pollution (incense and mosquito coils) (Kauneliene et al., 2018). Depending on the regulatory framework considered (public places allowing or prohibiting ENDP use and/ or cigarette smoking) and the purpose of the study (evaluating the impact of ETS related to passive exposure), certain studies also considered comparisons with background air (no use of any product) and air quality guidelines. It is important to note that these studies differed not only in the residential and public environments used but also in the list of constituents measured in the air, even if most of them measured formaldehyde, benzene, toluene, and PM$_{2.5}$. Thus, it is somewhat difficult to draw conclusions on the basis of the reported overall findings. An additional point of concern is that most of these studies simply assumed that the regulatory norms for occupational exposure in terms of adequate ventilation were respected and did not systematically verify the ventilation rates.

This subchapter presents various studies published until the end of 2019 (listed in Table 8.7) which are considered representative for this topic and highlights their main outcomes and limitations. As mentioned above, there is a degree of inconsistency among the various studies, and, with regard to EVPs in particular, a review of studies involving human volunteers under natural settings (Zainol Abidin et al., 2017) highlighted that the inconsistency could mainly be attributed to a lack of standardization.

Case study—Residential, public, or transport environments. Kaunelienė et al. (Kauneliene et al., 2018) performed a comprehensive comparative analysis of the

changes in air quality resulting from EHTP and EVP use, cigarette smoking, waterpipe use, and burning of incense and mosquito coils in various environments, especially with combustion-based pollution sources present. Compared with the concentrations measured during EHTP and EVP use, real-life public and transport environments had equivalent or significantly higher levels of formaldehyde, acetaldehyde, benzene, and toluene.

Case study—Residential environment. Ballbè et al. (Ballbè et al., 2014) conducted the first passive exposure study that combined air collection and biological tests on saliva and urine for EVPs versus cigarettes and background levels. The study included 54 volunteer nonsmokers exposed at home to second-hand smoke, environmental aerosol of EVPs, or neither. The product consumption varied from one to above seven per day, whereas the duration of exposure per day was quite

TABLE 8.7
Summary of Representative IAQ Studies on EHTPs and EVPs Conducted in Real-Life Environments.

Real-life environment	Product	Constituents[a]	Initiator/author (year)
Residential, public, transport	THS, EVPs, cigarette, waterpipe, incense, mosquito coils	PM ($PM_{2.5}$, UFPs), carbonyls (acetaldehyde, formaldehyde), VOCs (benzene, toluene), propylene glycol	Kauneliene et al. (2018)
Residential	EVP, cigarette	Nicotine Cotinine in saliva and urine	Ballbè et al. (2014)
Vaping convention	EVP	PM ($PM_{2.5}$)	Soule et al. (2017)
Vaping convention	EVP	PM (PM_{10}), CO_2, NO_2, TVOCs	Chen et al. (2017)
Vaping convention	EVP	PM ($PM_{2.5}$), VOCs	Kaufman et al. (2018)
Catering and entertainment	THS	CO, CO_2, NH_3, formaldehyde, benzo[a]pyrene, nicotine	Prodanchuk et al. (2017)
Nightclub	THS	PNC, PSD, $PM_{2.5}$, PM_{10}, acetaldehyde, formaldehyde, nicotine, 3-ethenylpyridine, CO_2	Kaunelienė et al. (2019)
Transport	THS	PM ($PM_{2.5}$, UFPs), carbonyls (acetone, acrolein, acetaldehyde, benzaldehyde, 2-butanon, butyraldehyde, formaldehyde, propionaldehyde), 19 VOCs, CO, CO_2	Schober et al. (2019)
Restaurant	THS	PM ($PM_{2.5}$), carbonyls (acetaldehyde, acrolein, crotonaldehyde, formaldehyde), nicotine, TSNA (NNN, NNK)	PMI, 2018

[a] Abbreviations: *EHTP*, electrically heated tobacco product; *EVP*, e-vapor product; *NNK*, nicotine-derived nitrosamine ketone; *NNN*, N-nitrosonornicotine; *PM*, particulate matter; *PNC*, particle number concentration; *PSD*, particle size distribution; *THS*, Tobacco Heating System 2.2; *TSNA*, tobacco-specific nitrosamine; *TVOC*, total volatile organic compound; *UFP*, ultrafine particle; *VOC*, volatile organic compound.

stable, with a range of 1–2 h for 74% of the subjects. Nicotine present in the air was collected over 1 week, and its associated biomarker, cotinine, was measured at the end of the week. The results showed a clear correlation between airborne nicotine and salivary and urinary cotinine levels. Overall, the biological test revealed no statistically significant difference, particularly in urine levels, between nonsmokers exposed to cigarettes and EVPs. This is especially interesting given that the nicotine levels in these two environments were very different, with the concentrations being approximately 5.7 times higher in homes with smokers than in homes with EVP users. Such a difference in airborne nicotine concentrations was anticipated, as cigarettes produced sidestream smoke containing significant levels of nicotine, whereas EVPs do not produce sidestream smoke. The study demonstrated the clear benefit of combining air collection and measurement of biomarkers of exposure, particularly for nicotine. However, the conditions of exposure in this test varied considerably, and the distribution of volunteers was not spread appropriately, as only 5 persons were exposed to EVP emissions versus 25 who were exposed to ETS and 24 who were in control homes. Taking into consideration this uneven distribution in the study groups, it would have been highly beneficial to repeat the experiment to provide a more robust basis on which to draw conclusions.

Case study—Public environment (vaping convention). Soule et al. (Soule et al., 2017) designed a study to assess air quality before, during, and after EVP use in a natural public setting. For this purpose, they conducted measurements during a 2-day event in a large hotel meeting room, involving 59–87 EVP users (1.47–2.14 active EVP use density per 100 m^3). PM$_{2.5}$ measurements taken before, during, and after the event showed that the particle concentrations increased significantly during the event, with median levels of 311.68–818.88 μg/m^3 (average of values recorded at six time points) versus a baseline of 1.92–3.20 μg/m^3. The interest of this study, in addition to the robust approach for PM$_{2.5}$ measurement, was investigation of aerosol evolution in the room after EVP use. Indeed, PM$_{2.5}$ median levels measured 17 h after the EVP session varied from 12.80 to 15.52 μg/m^3. These results were expected, as environmental aerosol from EVPs is known to be composed of liquid droplets in suspension that have a tendency to evaporate quickly. However, the authors did not investigate the composition of the EVP environmental aerosol; consequently, it was not possible to demonstrate differences in chemical composition between the environmental aerosol of EVP and

ETS. Moreover, the authors acknowledged that there was a clear need to validate the equipment—in this case a Sidepak AM510 online sensor—for measuring purposes and further recognized that the limited knowledge of environmental aerosol composition meant that it was not possible to set an accepted calibration factor for EVP aerosol. Lastly, the excessively large size of the room unfortunately prevented exploration of aerosol dispersion and kinetics of the particles, which would have merited further study.

Case study—Public environment (vaping convention). Chen et al. (2017) conducted a similar study to that of Soule et al. (assessment of EVPs; large room; high number of attendees) (Soule et al., 2017) but extended the range of constituents screened in the air and focused on extreme conditions. This study aimed to assess the conditions in vaping conventions where vapers compete against each other to produce the largest exhaled aerosol plumes. The study considered both real-time measurements of PM$_{10}$, TVOC, CO$_2$, and NO$_2$ and offline measurement of nicotine based on air collected over a period of 7 h, with the purpose of identifying potential correlations between the constituents. Moreover, information on smell and visibility perception was recorded, and, for the latter point, pictures were taken throughout the event for visualizing the aerosol density. The authors made several observations which should be commented upon. First, a very high concentration of nicotine (124.7 μg/m^3 on average) was measured, which not only was clearly attributable to EVP usage but also, more importantly, probably reflected the unusual vaping behavior of the attendees: The aerosol was most likely not inhaled, and nicotine uptake was, therefore, extremely low. As a consequence, although the data collected fell within the same range as the historical data for ETS in nightclubs, it is important to note that the number of attendees (75–600 including, presumably, a significant percentage of EVP users) and the high consumption of EVPs reported by the assessor meant that the setting was very particular. Therefore, the findings cannot be reasonably considered as a reflection of a more generalized setting. Indeed, it would have been preferable to have additional points of measurement, not only during the event but also afterward, in order to track the evolution of nicotine in the air. In fact, the authors recognized this point and suggested such an investigation for assessing third-hand aerosols. Second, the findings highlighted a clear correlation among PM$_{10}$, TVOCs, and CO$_2$ levels, whereas NO$_2$ levels did not vary throughout the event. The fact that NO$_2$, which is a known combustion marker, was stable throughout the experiment corroborated the findings of a large body of studies that have reported differences in aerosol composition between combustion products and nicotine-containing products such as EVPs. Interestingly, the results for CO_2, a typical bioeffluent considered a nonspecific human-presence marker, showed that the number of attendees had a clear impact on the measurements. This was also demonstrated by the high concentrations of PM_{10} and TVOCs, attributed to a combination of several factors: human presence, product consumption, and ventilation. Unfortunately, because the study did not report detailed information, it was not possible to clearly determine the influence of human presence versus ventilation versus EVP use. Nevertheless, relative to similar events held inside the venue but not involving EVP use, the EVP event registered a significant increase in the three correlated markers. However, it should be highlighted that the authors interpreted the results for TVOCs with great caution because they suspected some problems related to sensitivity of the sensors. TVOC sensors are known to be nonspecific and sensitive to cross-contamination; hence, it is highly probable that the extreme conditions of the study setting led to interference in the measurements. This factor might also explain issues that were encountered with the PM_{10} sensor. A further point related to the study design is that it would have been helpful to perform offline measurements of glycerin and propylene glycol at different time points and correlate these with the TVOC and PM_{10} online values. Such additional measurements would have provided valuable information, allowing greater insight into the possible correlations among the different constituents. Finally, the assessors characterized the smell as strong and reported very low visibility values during the EVP event; but, unfortunately, these interesting observations were not investigated further. To sum up, although overall the study is of interest in that it assessed EVPs under extreme consumption conditions, these conditions are not representative of common EVP use and, therefore, the findings cannot be extrapolated to more general, or typical, usage of such products.

Case study—Public environment (vaping convention). Kaufman et al. (Kaufman et al., 2018) conducted an interesting study—complementing the investigation of Soule et al. (Soule et al., 2017)—to characterize the chemical composition of the environmental aerosol during EVP use at a vape festival. For this purpose, they performed online measurement of $PM_{2.5}$ and trapped VOCs on thermal desorption tubes during an EVP event involving 158 to 223 people, including 20 to 34

active users. The online measurement showed an increase in $PM_{2.5}$ levels during the EVP sessions, with an average concentration of 100.15 µg/m^3 measured during the event, compared to <10 µg/m^3 at baseline. Total VOC levels, based on 28 detected compounds, increased to 330.0 µg/m^3 during the EVP sessions, compared to 220.0 µg/m^3 at baseline. Unsurprisingly, the compounds that presented a significant difference in average levels between the EVP sessions and baseline were glycerin and propylene glycol, with differences of 35 and 107 µg/m^3 from baseline, respectively. Most importantly, under the trapping conditions applied during the EVP event, no new VOCs were detected, and no increases in carbonyls such as acetaldehyde and acrolein were noted. It would have been beneficial to measure nicotine in addition to VOCs and bridge the glycerin and propylene glycol concentrations in air with the e-liquid consumption during the EVP event.

Case study—Public environment (catering and entertainment). A study conducted in 2015 (Prodanchuk et al., 2017) aimed at measuring the pollution level of indoor air before, during, and after EHTP use and cigarette smoking at a catering and entertainment venue, without any air renewal during the experiments. While 10 participants either used EHTPs or smoked cigarettes, 60 participants (bystanders) did not use any tobacco product during the experiments. The measurements were taken over four consecutive 1 h sessions: (1) empty room background session (no human presence); (2) background session with participants (recreational activities without use of any tobacco product); (3) sessions with EHTP use or cigarette smoking; and (4) background session with participants after use of tobacco products (recreational activities without use of any tobacco product). The concentrations of six compounds were evaluated: CO, CO_2, nicotine, benzo[a]pyrene, formaldehyde, and ammonia. Benzo[a]pyrene, nicotine, and ammonia were not detected in the indoor air collected during or after the EHTP session (where 80 EHTPs were consumed), although slight increases in CO, CO_2, and formaldehyde concentrations were observed. The authors inferred that these increases were not caused by EHTP use but resulted from the intensified breathing of participants during their activities, a phenomenon reported in the literature (Schober et al., 2019; Schripp et al., 2013). Moreover, this outcome could be explained by the experimental settings (i.e., no air renewal between the background session with participants and the EHTP session), as described in the literature for formaldehyde (Mitova et al., 2019b). In addition to the similarity in the results of chemical analysis before and after usage, the participants reported that they subjectively perceived the indoor air during and after EHTP use as being practically the same as that before EHTP use. In the smoking session, the levels of all measured compounds increased in the indoor air during and after smoking of 80 cigarettes, in contrast to the trends observed in the EHTP sessions. Furthermore, all participants, both smokers and bystanders, described the indoor air as smoke-laden, suffocating, and of a nature that caused choking and, sometimes, mild eye irritation. This study is of particular interest because it considered intensive conditions of EHTP use (80 EHTPs in 1 h without ventilation). It also substantiates the conclusions on the significant and unambiguous qualitative and quantitative differences in air quality during cigarette smoking and ETHP use.

Case study—Public environment (nightclub). Kauneliene et al. performed a study aimed at assessing the impact of EHTP use in the real-life situation of a nightclub environment in two sets of experiments (Kaunelienė et al., 2019). In the first set, THS-generated emissions were evaluated at $0.5 \, h^{-1}$ in five sessions during nonoperating hours of the club: empty room air background, background with 10 persons not using any tobacco product, 10 persons using THS simultaneously, background with 30 persons not using any tobacco product, and finally 30 persons scattered throughout the main club area and using THS simultaneously. In the second set, IAQ was assessed before club opening (background) and throughout normal nightclub operation, and due consideration was given to the fact that the ventilation was adjusted between 2.6 and $10 \, h^{-1}$ depending on occupancy levels. In compliance with local regulations, during normal nightclub operation, cigarette smoking was only allowed in a designated smoking room. PNC, PM_{10}, $PM_{2.5}$, CO_2, formaldehyde, acetaldehyde, nicotine, and 3-ethenylpyridine were measured in both sets of experiments. THS use in the first set of experiments led to an increase in PNC levels above the background, especially when 30 persons used THS simultaneously. However, it is important to highlight that, when put in the context of a nightclub in full operation, these median PNC levels were within a similar range of, or even slightly below, the median background levels before club opening. Furthermore, the values recorded for PNC while the nightclub was in operation were one order of magnitude higher than those recorded during THS use. This clear difference in PNC levels was attributed to other sources of emission such as a fog machine, commonly used in such an environment, and possibly cross-contamination from the adjacent smoking area. Moreover, THS use resulted in only a slight increase in the indoor concentrations of $PM_{2.5}$ and PM_{10}, and—similar to that in case of PNC—this increase was in the range of background variations before club opening and substantially below the levels measured during normal night-club operation. Assessment of particle size distribution in all measurement scenarios indicated an ultrafine mode, with the major portion of particles being within the nucleation size range. These data are consistent with those found in an earlier investigation of environmental aerosols of THS in an exposure chamber (Meišutovič-Akhtarieva et al., 2019) and were attributed to rapid evaporation of the liquid droplets generated during THS use. Concerning formaldehyde and acetaldehyde, overall, the indoor concentrations of these compounds during THS use remained within the range of background variations, with the exception of a slight increase in one of the measurement zones during simultaneous use of 30 tobacco sticks of THS. The mean airborne acetaldehyde levels recorded during club operation were above those obtained in all other experiments, and these results can potentially be attributed to the consumption of alcohol-containing beverages. Airborne nicotine levels increased above the background during both sessions with THS use, while 3-ethenylpyridine remained at background levels. It is noteworthy that, although the club is officially considered a nonsmoking environment, the indoor concentrations of nicotine and 3-ethenylpyridine during normal operating hours were either in a similar range to those in the experiments with THS or even increased in one of the collection zones. These results were attributed to cross-contamination with pollutants from the adjacent smoking area. This, in turn, raised the concern that cigarette smoking remained a very important pollution factor even though the club was officially defined as a nonsmoking environment. On the basis of the results, the authors concluded that, relative to other thermal aerosol sources and unlike cigarette smoking, THS might not be a distinguishable source of particles or gaseous pollutants in crowded real-life environments even when used indoors.

Case study—Transport environment (car). Schober et al. (Schober et al., 2019) made a significant contribution to our understanding of the effects on IAQ of ENDP use by assessing the indoor use of representative EHTPs and EVPs in seven cars in comparison with cigarette smoking. Indeed, because a car environment is smaller and less ventilated than a normal indoor setting, it would be reasonable to assume that passengers in a car could be exposed to higher levels of emissions than occupants in a less confined environment (such as an apartment setting, for instance). Moreover, private venues such as homes and cars are important sources of secondhand smoke exposure, as smoke-free legislation in many countries bans smoking in indoor public and work places. Schober et al. measured the IAQ in the cars with no persons present, in order to obtain background levels; subsequently, they measured the IAQ in the cars separately after use of THS, a representative refillable EVP, or cigarettes.

The results showed that, following THS use, 18 of the 19 measured VOCs remained at levels similar to the background, and only nicotine levels increased, with concentrations between 4 and 12 µg/m^3 (in three of the seven cars). Upon EVP use, the levels of nicotine increased in the range of 4−10 µg/m^3 in four of the seven cars, and higher concentrations of the aerosol former propylene glycol were found in five cars (50−762 µg/m^3). In contrast, cigarette smoking led to not only an increase in nicotine levels (8−140 µg/m^3) but also higher concentrations of 3-ethenylpyridine, benzene, toluene, and furfural. Neither THS nor EVP use had an impact on the concentrations of CO, any of the six carbonyls investigated (benzaldehyde, butyraldehyde, acrolein, formaldehyde, acetaldehyde, and propionaldehyde), or either of the two ketones (acetone and 2-butanon). The concentrations of all these compounds remained either below the LOD or within the range of background levels (i.e., no product use). Conversely, cigarette smoking led to increased concentrations of formaldehyde, acetaldehyde, and acetone in the interior air.

THS use had almost no impact on the mean number concentrations of PM$_{>300\ nm}$ or concentrations of PM$_{2.5}$ inside the cars, although it caused an increase in UFP levels (range, 25−300 nm) in all the vehicles. Compared with THS use, EVP consumption led to emission of larger particles (>300 nm) and higher concentrations of PM$_{2.5}$, although the mean number concentration of UFPs (25−300 nm) tended to be higher upon THS use. In five of the seven cars, there was a steep increase in PM$_{2.5}$ concentrations (75−490 µg/m^3) upon EVP use, relative to the background (6−11 µg/m^3). However, the highest load of PM was detected following cigarette smoking, with mean PM$_{2.5}$ concentrations of 64−1988 µg/m^3 and 1.3- to 17-fold higher counts of UFPs compared with the control. It is important to highlight that, although THS use also resulted in higher concentrations of nanoparticles (25−300 nm in diameter, 9%−232% increase above the background) than no smoking activity in the cars, the concentrations were far lower than those in case of cigarette smoking. EVP consumption led to lower concentrations of UFPs than THS use.

Although the authors attempted to factor in many variables in their assessment, the results showed significant variability, which might have been due to differences among the cars, ventilation efficiencies of the cars, and product consumption patterns.

The authors concluded that, although the impact of THS use on air quality inside the car was clearly much lower than the detrimental effects of cigarette smoking, it remained problematic, as the levels of nicotine and UFPs in the 25−300 nm range were higher than background levels. They reached a similar conclusion on EVP use on the basis of the increase in nicotine, propylene glycol, UFPs, and PM$_{2.5}$ above background levels. This work provides interesting insights into the impact of ENDPs on air quality in a small-volume space. Nevertheless, as was the case in the other studies described above (Chen et al., 2017; Kaufman et al., 2018; Soule et al., 2017), the conclusions on the impact of EHTP and EVP use on IAQ overemphasized the emission of UFPs and PM and did not provide any additional information to substantiate the actual presence or absence of toxic properties. It is important to stress that, as intensively discussed among experts in the field, it is not the mere presence of PM and UFPs, per se, that causes adverse health effects; rather, it is their physicochemical properties—such as chemical composition as well as the volatility and solubility of the particles' components—that are responsible (Baldauf et al., 2016; Cassee et al., 2013; Notter, 2015).

Case study—Public environment (restaurant). In addition to the air quality studies (presented above) performed in residential and public environments, PMI conducted a study in a restaurant in Japan in 2018. The aim was to assess whether passive exposure to the environmental aerosol emitted by THS use during dinner events, where food and alcohol were served, had a negative impact on air quality and led to increased exposure of nonsmoking bystanders. It is important to emphasize that, at the time of the study, the use of tobacco- and nicotine-containing products in restaurants and bars in Japan was permitted at the discretion of the venue owner. Six dining events, each of approximately 4 h' duration, were organized over a period of 2 weeks: two events, where no tobacco- or nicotine-containing product use was allowed (nonexposure events) and four events where only THS use was allowed (exposure events). Cigarette smoking was not permitted in the restaurant throughout the study. Approximately 139 persons participated in the two nonexposure events, and 260 persons participated in the four exposure events. The former group was composed of nonsmokers, THS users, and cigarette smokers. During the exposure events, a group of THS users who were allowed to use THS during the events was added. More details on the study design are provided in Chapter 19.

Air quality during the events was assessed by measuring the concentrations of selected environmental aerosol constituents in the air; additionally, the urinary levels of biomarkers of exposure to selected HPHCs were measured in all groups prior to and after the events. The environmental aerosol constituents were PM ($PM_{2.5}$), carbonyls (acetaldehyde, acrolein, crotonaldehyde, and formaldehyde), nicotine, and TSNAs (NNN and NNK). The main observations in terms of IAQ are discussed below.

The nicotine levels during the nonexposure events were between 0.10 and 0.18 $\mu g/m^3$, whereas the highest average nicotine concentration recorded in the air during any of the exposure events was about 1.5 $\mu g/m^3$ (maximum, 2.26 $\mu g/m^3$). These results were in line with those reported in a nightclub (Kaunelienė et al., 2019). Furthermore, no quantifiable levels of TSNAs (NNN and NNK) were found in the air during the nonexposure events or, more importantly, exposure events. The biomarkers of exposure results are described in Chapter 19.

The airborne carbonyls measured as part of the air quality assessment (acrolein, formaldehyde, crotonaldehyde, and acetaldehyde) are not specific to EHTPs, and many other emission sources of these compounds exist in everyday life (Höllbacher et al., 2017; Mitova et al., 2019b; Salthammer et al., 2010). Extensive analyses and cross-correlations between various sources (including the number of THS used and food and alcohol consumption) present during the events indicate that, in a real-life setting, THS use was not a major source of any of the carbonyls measured in the air. On the basis of the results of previous studies, a minor contribution of THS to the concentrations of acetaldehyde in the indoor air of a restaurant could be assumed (Meišutovič-Akhtarieva et al., 2019; Mitova et al., 2016, 2019a). However, as discussed by Kaunelienė et al. these levels are negligible considering the exposure to these compounds that already exists in today's real-life environment (Kauneliene et al., 2018).

To sum up, this study showed the relevance of combining air quality assessment and measurements of urinary levels of biomarkers of exposure in participants during such events and helped understand and characterize potential sources of exposure, in particular, EHTP use versus background exposure in the building, study participants, food, and beverages.

Other. So far, no study has been published on assessing emissions from surfaces after EHTP use or on the reactivity/aging of the aerosol in real-life settings. Regarding EVPs, Bush and Goniewicz published the outcomes of a pilot study that assessed nicotine deposition on windows, walls, and floors in houses (nonsmoker, smoker, and e-cigarette user) (Bush and Goniewicz, 2015). The authors noted a clear difference between EVP (7.7 ± 17.2 $\mu g/m^3$) and cigarette (1303 ± 2676 $\mu g/m^3$) households even though they observed a large variation.

To summarize, existing scientific evidence has demonstrated that ENDP use in real-life public, residential, and transport environments has a significantly lower impact on IAQ than cigarette smoking. In good agreement with the studies in model environments, studies in these settings showed that the levels of conventional airborne pollutants such as benzene, toluene, carbonyls, CO, and NO_x were in the range of background variations during ENDP use. Interestingly, acetaldehyde—which commonly increased above the background level in studies on EHTPs in model environments—did not systematically exceed the background levels in these real-life investigations. Furthermore, most of the studies reported very low-level increases in nicotine concentrations above the background during EHTP and EVP consumption. Notably, the nicotine concentrations measured were in the range of cross-contamination values from an adjacent smoking area, as demonstrated in one of the studies in a night club. However, assessment of nicotine concentrations during vaping festivals with intentional excessive EVP use and no inhalation (e.g., competitions for producing the largest exhalation plume) showed elevated nicotine levels. Moreover, one particular study showed an increase in UFPs levels above the background during EHTP use in cars, while another study in a nightclub demonstrated that the UFP levels following simultaneous use of the product by multiple users were within the range measured during normal club operation. Similarly, an observation attributable to EVP use was an increase in UFP and PM concentrations in small-volume venues (cars) and during intentional excessive product use, such as that occurring at vaping festivals. Finally, a single study evaluated the residual levels of PM pollution following a vaping festival and showed concentrations similar to the background. This is in agreement with the findings of studies in model environments, which showed a temporary increase in PM levels only during product consumption.

8.8 CONCLUSION

The literature overview presented in this chapter confirms that the impact of indoor use of ENDPs on air quality is substantially lower than that of cigarette smoking. This is further supported by the outcomes of several studies on other combustion-based tobacco products such as cigars and pipes. Most importantly, the composition and qualitative and quantitative characteristics of the environmental aerosols of ENDPs differ considerably from those of ETS. Indeed, ENDP consumption generates submicron liquid droplets consisting of highly volatile ingredients. Depending on the ventilation rate, volume of the enclosed environment, and intensity of use, studies have reported some differences in the aerodynamic diameter of the liquid droplets. These droplets dissipate within seconds; accordingly, exposure to UFPs is restricted to a very short period of time and only to persons located at close proximity to the ENDP users. This is in sharp contrast to the PM of ETS, which is far more stable, lingers in enclosed environments (Chapter 5), and leads to substantial build-up of indoor pollution, particularly at high smoking rates and low ventilation levels.

There are certain differences in the qualitative patterns of the environmental aerosols of EHTPs and EVPs. Indeed, in simulations in model indoor environments, nicotine, acetaldehyde, glycerin, and—in cases where mentholated products are consumed—menthol, together with UFPs, were found to be increased above background levels in the environmental aerosols of EHTPs. In real-life environments, depending on the overall level of background pollution, these low-level increases were either measurable or within the background variation, particularly in case of acetaldehyde and UFPs, which are emitted from multiple indoor sources. Concerning the environmental aerosols of EVPs, most of the studies agree that, during indoor vaping, the concentrations of nicotine, the aerosol formers glycerin and propylene glycol, UFPs, and—in some studies—$PM_{2.5}$ are increased above background levels.

A number of discrepancies were noted among the studies in the values reported for different airborne constituents in the environmental aerosols of EHTPs and EVPs, particularly in the case of EVPs. These discrepancies can be partially explained by the differences in study design, including volume of the indoor space, air changes per hour, and consumption rate. The existence of these discrepancies clearly highlights the need for standardization of IAQ assessment of EHTPs and EVPs.

To conclude, the scientific evidence shows that ENDP use in environments where regulatory norms for adequate ventilation are respected has no adverse effect on air quality according to the guideline values set forth in air quality guidelines. Furthermore, to contextualize the actual impact of ENDPs, it is important to take into account the airborne pollutants levels in current real-life environments. These points merit full consideration in the ongoing debate on the health impact on bystanders exposed to ENDPs. Lastly, ENDPs should be used with caution and courtesy around other adults and only where local regulations permit use. Furthermore, as a general precaution, users should refrain from consuming such products in the presence of pregnant women or children.

REFERENCES

AAQS, 2020. China Releases New Ambient Air Quality Standards, Ambient Air Quality Standards (AAQS) (GB 3095-2012). Clean Air Asia. Available from: https://cleanairasia.org/node8163/. Accessed 24 January 2020.

Abdul-Wahab, S.A., Chin Fah En, S., Elkamel, A., Ahmadi, L., Yetilmezsoy, K., 2015. A review of standards and guidelines set by international bodies for the parameters of indoor air quality. Atmos. Pollut. Res. 6, 751–767. https://doi.org/10.5094/apr.2015.084.

Abdullahi, K.L., Delgado-Saborit, J.M., Harrison, R.M., 2013. Emissions and indoor concentrations of particulate matter and its specific chemical components from cooking: a review. Atmos. Environ. 71, 260–294. https://doi.org/10.1016/j.atmosenv.2013.01.061.

Air Quality Standards EU, 2020. Environment. Air. Air Quality Standards (AQS). European Commission. Available from: https://ec.europa.eu/environment/air/quality/standards.htm. Accessed 27 September 2020.

Alves, C.A., Calvo, A.I., Castro, A., Fraile, R., Evtyugina, M., Bate-Epey, E.F., 2013. Indoor air quality in two university sports facilities. Aeros. Air Qual. Res. 13, 1723–1730. https://doi.org/10.4209/aaqr.2013.02.0045.

American Conference of Governmental Industrial Hygienists (ACGIH), 2001. Threshold Limit Value for Glycerin Mist. American Conference of Governmental Industrial Hygienists.

American Industrial Hygiene Association (AIHA), 2011. Workplace Environmental Exposure Level (WEEL) Values. AIHA Guidline Foundation.

American Society of Heating, Refrigerating and Air-Conditioning Engineers (ASHRAE) ANSI/ASHRAE Standard 62-2001, 2001. Ventilation for Acceptable Indoor Air Quality. American Society of Heating, Refrigerating and Air-Conditioning Engineers, Inc., Atlanta, GA.

American Society of Heating, Refrigerating and Air-Conditioning Engineers (ASHRAE) ANSI/ASHRAE Standard 62.1-2016, 2016a. Ventilation for Acceptable Indoor Air Quality. American Society of Heating, Refrigerating and Air-Conditioning Engineers, Inc., Atlanta, GA.

American Society of Heating, Refrigerating and Air-Conditioning Engineers (ASHRAE) ANSI/ASHRAE Standard 62.2-2016, 2016b. Ventilation for Acceptable Indoor

Air Quality in Residential Buildings. American Society of Heating, Refrigerating and Air-Conditioning Engineers Inc., Atlanta, GA.

Andrade, A., Dominski, F.H., 2018. Indoor air quality of environments used for physical exercise and sports practice: systematic review. J. Environ. Manag. 206, 577–586. https://doi.org/10.1016/j.jenvman.2017.11.001.

Armitage, A.K., Dixon, M., Frost, B.E., Mariner, D.C., Sinclair, N.M., 2004. The effect of inhalation volume and breath-hold duration on the retention of nicotine and solanesol in the human respiratory tract and on subsequent plasma nicotine concentrations during cigarette smoking. Beitr. Tabakforsch. Int. 21, 240–249. https://doi.org/10.2478/cttr-2013-0786.

Avino, P., Scungio, M., Stabile, L., Cortellessa, G., Buonanno, G., Manigrasso, M., 2018. Second-hand aerosol from tobacco and electronic cigarettes: evaluation of the smoker emission rates and doses and lung cancer risk of passive smokers and vapers. Sci. Total Environ. 642, 137–147. https://doi.org/10.1016/j.scitotenv.2018.06.059.

AQS, 2020. Environmental Quality Standards in Japan – Air Quality. Air & Transportation. Ministry of the Environment, Government of Japan. Available from: http://www.env.go.jp/en/air/aq/aq.html. Accessed 24 January 2020.

Baker, R.R., Proctor, C.J., 1990. The origins and properties of environmental tobacco smoke. Environ. Int. 16, 231–245. https://doi.org/10.1016/0160-4120(90)90117-o.

Baldauf, R., Devlin, R., Gehr, P., Giannelli, R., Hassett-Sipple, B., Jung, H., Martini, G., McDonald, J., Sacks, J., Walker, K., 2016. Ultrafine particle metrics and research considerations: review of the 2015 UFP workshop. Int. J. Environ. Res. Publ. Health 13, 1054. https://doi.org/10.3390/ijerph13111054.

Ballbè, M., Martínez-Sánchez, J.M., Sureda, X., Fu, M., Pérez-Ortuño, R., Pascual, J.A., Saltó, E., Fernández, E., 2014. Cigarettes vs. e-cigarettes: passive exposure at home measured by means of airborne marker and biomarkers. Environ. Res. 135, 76–80. https://doi.org/10.1016/j.envres.2014.09.005.

Barker-Hemings, E., Cavallotti, C., Cuoci, A., Faravelli, T., Ranzi, E., 2011. A Detailed Kinetic Study of Pyrolysis and Oxidation of Glycerol (Propoane-1,2,3-Triol). MCS 7, Cagliari, Sardinia, Italy.

Bartzis, J., Wolkoff, P., Stranger, M., Efthimiou, G., Tolis, E.I., Maes, F., Nørgaard, A.W., Ventura, G., Kalimeri, K.K., Goelen, E., Fernandes, O., 2015. On organic emissions testing from indoor consumer products' use. J. Hazard. Mater. 285, 37–45. https://doi.org/10.1016/j.jhazmat.2014.11.024.

Bekö, G., Weschler, C.J., Wierzbicka, A., Karottki, D.G., Toftum, J., Loft, S., Clausen, G., 2013. Ultrafine particles: exposure and source apportionment in 56 Danish homes. Environ. Sci. Technol. 47, 10240–10248. https://doi.org/10.1021/es402429h.

Bentley, M.C., Almstetter, M., Arndt, D., Knorr, A., Martin, E., Pospisil, P., Maeder, S., 2020. Comprehensive chemical characterization of the aerosol generated by a heated tobacco product by untargeted screening. Anal. Bioanal. Chem. https://doi.org/10.1007/s00216-020-02502-1.

Bombick, B.R., Avalos, J.T., Nelson, P.R., Conrad, F.W., Doolittle, D.J., 1998. Comparative studies of the mutagenicity of environmental tobacco smoke from cigarettes that burn or primarily heat tobacco. Environ. Mol. Mutagen. 31, 169–175. https://doi.org/10.1002/(sici)1098-2280(1998)31:2. <169::aid-em9>3.0.co;2-h.

Bush, D., Goniewicz, M.L., 2015. A pilot study on nicotine residues in houses of electronic cigarette users, tobacco smokers, and non-users of nicotine-containing products. Int. J. Drug Pol. 26, 609–611. https://doi.org/10.1016/j.drugpo.2015.03.003.

California Office of Environmental Health Hazard Assessment (OEHHA), December 21, 2018. Acute, 8-Hour and Chronic Reference Exposure Level (REL) Summary. Available from: https://oehha.ca.gov/air/general-info/oehha-acute-8-hour-and-chronic-reference-exposure-level-rel-summary.

Cancelada, L., Sleiman, M., Tang, X., Russell, M.L., Montesinos, V.N., Litter, M.I., Gundel, L.A., Destaillats, H., 2019. Heated tobacco products: volatile emissions and their predicted impact on indoor air quality. Environ. Sci. Technol. 53, 7866–7876. https://doi.org/10.1021/acs.est.9b02544.

Caponnetto, P., Maglia, M., Prosperini, G., Busà, B., Polosa, R., 2018. Carbon monoxide levels after inhalation from new generation heated tobacco products. Respir. Res. 19, 164. https://doi.org/10.1186/s12931-018-0867-z.

Cassee, F.R., Héroux, M.-E., Gerlofs-Nijland, M.E., Kelly, F.J., 2013. Particulate matter beyond mass: recent health evidence on the role of fractions, chemical constituents and sources of emission. Inhal. Toxicol. 25, 802–812. https://doi.org/10.3109/08958378.2013.850127.

Chen, R., Aherrera, A., Isichei, C., Olmedo, P., Jarmul, S., Cohen, J.E., Navas-Acien, A., Rule, A.M., 2017. Assessment of indoor air quality at an electronic cigarette (vaping) convention. J. Expo. Sci. Environ. Epidemiol. 28, 522–529. https://doi.org/10.1038/s41370-017-0005-x.

Cunnington, A.J., Hormbrey, P., 2002. Breath analysis to detect recent exposure to carbon monoxide. Postgrad. Med. 233–237.

Czogala, J., Goniewicz, M.L., Fidelus, B., Zielinska-Danch, W., Travers, M.J., Sobczak, A., 2014. Secondhand exposure to vapors from electronic cigarettes. Nicotine Tob. Res. 16, 655–662. https://doi.org/10.1093/ntr/ntt203.

de Blas, M., Navazo, M., Alonso, L., Durana, N., Gomez, M.C., Iza, J., 2012. Simultaneous indoor and outdoor on-line hourly monitoring of atmospheric volatile organic compounds in an urban building. The role of inside and outside sources. Sci. Total Environ. 426, 327–335. https://doi.org/10.1016/j.scitotenv.2012.04.003.

de Lacy Costello, B., Amann, A., Al-Kateb, H., Flynn, C., Filipiak, W., Khalid, T., Osborne, D., Ratcliffe, N.M., 2014. A review of the volatiles from the healthy human body. J. Breath Res. 8, 014001. https://doi.org/10.1088/1752-7155/8/1/014001.

de Leeuw, F., Benešová, N., Horálek, J., 2016. Evaluation of International Air Quality Standards. ETC/ACM Technical Paper 2016/10. European Topic Centre on Air Pollution and Climate Change Mitigation, Bilthoven, The Netherlands.

de Leeuw, F., Ruyssenaars, P., 2011. Evaluation of Current Limit and Target Values as Set in the EU Air Quality Directive. ETC/ACM Technical Paper 2011/3. European Topic Centre on Air Pollution and Climate Change Mitigation, Bilthoven, The Netherlands.

Deutsche Forschungsgemeinschaft (DFG) DFG, 2014. List of MAK and BAT values 2014. Maximum concentrations and biological tolerance values at the workplace, Report No 50. In: Hartwig, A. (Ed.), Report of the Commission for the Investigation of Health Hazards of Chemical Compounds in the Work Area. Deutsche Forschungsgemeinschaft. Commission for the Investigation of Health Hazards of Chemical Compounds in the Work Area, Weinheim, Germany.

Domino, E.F., Hornbach, E., Demana, T., 1991. The Nicotine Content of Common Vegetables. University of Michigan, Wilmington, NC USA.

Edwards, R.D., Jurvelin, J., Koistinen, K., Saarela, K., Jantunen, M., 2001. VOC source identification from personal and residential indoor, outdoor and workplace microenvironment samples in EXPOLIS-Helsinki, Finland. Atmos. Environ. 35, 4829−4841. https://doi.org/10.1016/s1352-2310(01)00271-0.

EU, 2004. Comparison of the EU and US Air Quality Standards and Planning Requirements.

EU, 2008. Directive 2008/50/EC of the European parliament and of the council of 21 May 2008 on ambient air quality and cleaner air for Europe. Off. J. Eur. Union 152, 1−44.

European Agency for Safety and Health at Work (EU OSHA), 2006. Directive 2006/15/EC - Indicative Occupational Exposure Limit Values [2018 21 December]; Available from: https://osha.europa.eu/en/legislation/directives/commission-directive-2006-15-ec.

European Committee for Standardization European Standard EN 13779, 2007. Ventilation for Non-residential Buildings − Performance Requirements for Ventilation and Room-Conditioning Systems. European Committee for Standardization; CEN Comité Européen de Normalisation, Brussels.

European Committee for Standardization European Standard EN 15251, 2007. Indoor Environmental Input Parameters for Design and Assessment of Energy Performance of Buildings Addressing Indoor Air Quality, Thermal Environment, Lighting and Acoustics. European Committee for Standardization; CEN Comité Européen de Normalisation, Brussels.

European Committee for Standardization European Standard EN 16516, 2017. Construction Products: Assessment of Release of Dangerous Substances - Determination of Emissions into Indoor Air. European Committee for Standardization; CEN Comité Européen de Normalisation.

FCTC, 2007. Guidelines for Implementation of Article 8 of the WHO FCTC. Guidelines on Protection from Exposure to Tobacco Smoke. Framework Convention on Tobacco Control (FCTC). World Health Organization (WHO) [2020 10 February]; Available from: https://www.who.int/fctc/guidelines/adopted/article_8/en/.

FCTC, 2014. Electronic Nicotine Delivery Systems. Framework Convention on Tobacco Control (FCTC). World Health Organization (WHO). Report by WHO, 2014; Sixth session.

FCTC, 2015. Glossary of Terms Used in the WHO FCTC and its Intruments_2nd Version. Framework Convention on Tobacco Control (FCTC). World Health Organization (WHO) [2020 10 February]; Available from: https://www.who.int/fctc/reporting/glossary_fctc/en/.

FCTC, 2016. Electronic Nicotine Delivery Systems and Electronic Non-nicotine Delivery Systems. Framework Convention on Tobacco Control (FCTC). World Health Organization (WHO). Report by WHO. 2016 [10 February 2020].

Fernández, E., Ballbè, M., Sureda, X., Fu, M., Saltó, E., Martínez-Sánchez, J.M., 2015. Particulate matter from electronic cigarettes and conventional cigarettes: a systematic review and observational study. Curr. Environ. Health Rep. 2, 423−429. https://doi.org/10.1007/s40572-015-0072-x.

Forster, M., McAughey, J., Prasad, K., Mavropoulou, E., Proctor, C., 2018. Assessment of tobacco heating product THP1.0. Part 4: characterisation of indoor air quality and odour. Regul. Toxicol. Pharmacol. 93, 34−51. https://doi.org/10.1016/j.yrtph.2017.09.017.

Fromme, H., Schober, W., 2015. Waterpipes and e-cigarettes: impact of alternative smoking techniques on indoor air quality and health. Atmos. Environ. 106, 429−441. https://doi.org/10.1016/j.atmosenv.2014.08.030.

Frost-Pineda, K., Zedler, B.K., Liang, Q., Roethig, H.J., 2008. Environmental tobacco smoke (ETS) evaluation of a third-generation electrically heated cigarette smoking system (EHCSS). Regul. Toxicol. Pharmacol. 52, 118−121. https://doi.org/10.1016/j.yrtph.2008.06.007.

Geiss, O., Bianchi, I., Barahona, F., Barrero-Moreno, J., 2015. Characterisation of mainstream and passive vapours emitted by selected electronic cigarettes. Int. J. Hyg. Environ. Health 218, 169−180. https://doi.org/10.1016/j.ijheh.2014.10.001.

Giannoukos, S., Brkic, B., Taylor, S., France, N., 2014. Monitoring of human chemical signatures using membrane inlet mass spectrometry. Anal. Chem. 86, 1106−1114. https://doi.org/10.1021/ac403621c.

Glantz, S., Schick, S., 2004. Implications of ASHRAE'S guidance on ventilation for smoking-permitted areas. ASHRAE J. 46, 54−59.

Gomes, R., Meek, M.E., Eggleton, M., 2002. Acrolein. Concise International Chemical Assessment Document 43. 2002 [2019 12 March 2019]; Available from: http://inchem.org/documents/cicads/cicads/cicad43.htm.

Gómez Lueso, M., Mitova, M.I., Mottier, N., Schaller, M., Rotach, M., Goujon-Ginglinger, C.G., 2018. Development and validation of a method for quantification of two tobacco-specific nitrosamines in indoor air. J. Chromatogr. A 1580, 90−99. https://doi.org/10.1016/j.chroma.2018.10.037.

Hall E.T., 1966. The Hidden Dimension. Anchor, USA.

Harashima, Y., Morita, T., 1998. A comparative study on environmental policy development processes in the three East Asian countries: Japan, Korea, and China. Environ. Econ. Pol. Stud. 1, 39−67. https://doi.org/10.1007/bf03353894.

Hess, I., Lachireddy, K., Capon, A., 2016. A systematic review of the health risks from passive exposure to electronic cigarette vapour. Public Health Res. Pract. 26 https://doi.org/10.17061/phrp2621617.

Hoffmann, K., Krause, C., Seifert, B., Ullrich, D., 2000. The German Environmental Survey 1990/92 (GerES II): sources of personal exposure to volatile organic compounds. J. Expo. Anal. Environ. Epidemiol. 10, 115. https://doi.org/10.1038/sj.jea.7500084.

Höllbacher, E., Ters, T., Rieder-Gradinger, C., Srebotnik, E., 2017. Emissions of indoor air pollutants from six user scenarios in a model room. Atmos. Environ. 150, 389−394. https://doi.org/10.1016/j.atmosenv.2016.11.033.

Huang, J., Pan, X., Guo, X., Li, G., 2018. Health impact of China's Air Pollution Prevention and Control Action Plan: an analysis of national air quality monitoring and mortality data. Lancet Planet. Health 2, e313−e323. https://doi.org/10.1016/s2542-5196(18)30141-4.

Hygienic standard ГН 2.1.6.3492-17, 2018. Maximum Permissible Concentration of Pollutants in the Air of Urban and Rural Settlements (Предельно ДоЦустимые концентрации ЪЩДКЦ заГрязняющич Веществ В атмосферном Воздуче Городскич и сельскич ПоселенийЦ. ГиГиенические нормативы ГН ЫҺЪҺЯҺЪЭыЫкЪщ.

Ichitsubo, H., Kotaki, M., 2018. Indoor air quality (IAQ) evaluation of a Novel Tobacco Vapor (NTV) product. Regul. Toxicol. Pharmacol. 92, 278−294. https://doi.org/10.1016/j.yrtph.2017.12.017.

International Agency for Research on Cancer (IARC), 2012. Agents Classified by the IARC Monographs, Volumes 1−127. IARC Monogaphs on the Identification of Carcinogenic Hazards to Humans. International Agency for Research on Cancer. Available from: https://monographs.iarc.fr/agents-classified-by-the-iarc/. Accessed 27 September 2020.

International Organization for Standardization (ISO) ISO 15593, 2001. Environmental Tobacco Smoke − Estimation of its Contribution to Respirable Suspended Particles − Determination of Particulate Matter by Ultraviolet Absorbance and by Fluorescence. International Organization for Standardization (ISO), Geneva, Switzerland.

International Organization for Standardization (ISO) ISO 16000-1, 2004. Indoor Air Part 1: General Aspects of Sampling Strategy. International Organization for Standardization (ISO), Geneva, Switzerland.

International Organization for Standardization (ISO) ISO 16000-5, 2007. Indoor Air Part 5: Sampling Strategy for Volatile Organic Compounds (VOCs). International Organization for Standardization (ISO), Geneva, Switzerland.

International Organization for Standardization (ISO) ISO 16000-6, 2011. Indoor Air Part 6: Determination of Volatile Organic Compounds in Indoor and Test Chamber Air by Active Sampling on Tenax TA Sorbent, Thermal Desorption and Gas Chromatography Using MS or MS-FID. International Organization for Standardization (ISO), Geneva, Switzerland.

International Organization for Standardization (ISO) ISO 16000-9, 2006. Indoor Air Part 9: Determination of the Emission of Volatile Organic Compounds from Building Products and Furnishing − Emission Test Chamber Method. International Organization for Standardization (ISO), Geneva, Switzerland.

International Organization for Standartization (ISO) ISO 16814, 2008. Building Environment Design. Indoor Air Quality. Methods of Expressing the Quality of Indoor Air for Human Occupancy. International Organization for Standartization.

Japan's regulations and environmental law, 2020. Air Pollution. Environmental Policy, Ministry of the Environment, Japan. Ministry of the Environment. Available from: http://www.env.go.jp/en/coop/pollution.html. Accessed 24 January 2020.

Jenkins, R.A., Guerin, M.R., Tomkins, B.A., 2000. The Chemistry of Environmental Tobacco Smoke: Composition and Measurement, second ed. CRC Press, Boca Raton, Florida, USA.

Jones, A.P., 1999. Indoor air quality and health. Atmos. Environ. 33, 4535−4564. https://doi.org/10.1016/s1352-2310(99)00272-1.

Kaufman, P., Dubray, J., Soule, E.K., Cobb, C.O., Zarins, S., Schwartz, R., 2018. Analysis of secondhand E-cigarette aerosol compounds in an indoor setting. Tob. Regul. Sci. 4, 29−37. https://doi.org/10.18001/trs.4.3.3.

Kauneliene, V., Meisutovic-Akhtarieva, M., Martuzevicius, D., 2018. A review of the impacts of tobacco heating system on indoor air quality versus conventional pollution sources. Chemosphere 206, 568−578. https://doi.org/10.1016/j.chemosphere.2018.05.039.

Kaunelienė, V., Meišutovič-Akhtarieva, M., Prasauskas, T., Čiužas, D., Krugly, E., Keraitytė, K., Martuzevičius, D., 2019. Impact of using a tobacco heating system (THS) on indoor air quality in a nightclub. Aeros. Air Qual. Res. 19, 1961−1968. https://doi.org/10.4209/aaqr.2019.04.0211.

Kelly, F.J., Fussell, J.C., 2019. Improving indoor air quality, health and performance within environments where people live, travel, learn and work. Atmos. Environ. 200, 90−109. https://doi.org/10.1016/j.atmosenv.2018.11.058.

Kotzias, D., 2005. Critical Appraisal of the Setting and Implementation of Indoor Exposure Limits in the EU. Institute for Health and Consumer Protection Physical and Chemical Exposure Unit, Ispra, Italy.

Kotzias, D., Koistinen, K., Kephalopoulos, S., Carrer, P., Maroni, M., Schlitt, C., Jantunen, M., Cochet, C., Kirchner, S., Lindvall, T., McLaughlin, J., Molhave, L., 2005. The INDEX Project − Critical Appraisal of the Setting and Implementation of Indoor Exposure Limits in the EU.

Kotzias, D., Pilidis, G., 2017. Building design and indoor air quality − experience and prospects. Fresenius Environ. Bull. 26, 323−326.

Kuklinska, K., Wolska, L., Namiesnik, J., 2015. Air quality policy in the U.S. and the EU − a review. Atmos. Pollut. Res. 6, 129−137. https://doi.org/10.5094/apr.2015.015.

Kwak, J., Geier, B.A., Fan, M., Gogate, S.A., Rinehardt, S.A., Watts, B.S., Grigsby, C.C., Ott, D.K., 2015. Detection of volatile organic compounds indicative of human presence in the air. J. Separ. Sci. 38, 2463−2469. https://doi.org/10.1002/jssc.201500261.

Lampos, S., Kostenidou, E., Farsalinos, K., Zagoriti, Z., Ntoukas, A., Dalamarinis, K., Savranakis, P., Lagoumintzis, G., Poulas, K., 2019. Real-time assessment of E-cigarettes and conventional cigarettes emissions: aerosol size distributions, mass and number concentrations. Toxics 7, 45. https://doi.org/10.3390/toxics7030045.

Licina, D., Tian, Y., Nazaroff, W.W., 2017. Emission rates and the personal cloud effect associated with particle release from the perihuman environment. Indoor Air 27, 791–802. https://doi.org/10.1111/ina.12365.

Liu, J., Liang, Q., Oldham, M., Rostami, A., Wagner, K., Gillman, I., Patel, P., Savioz, R., Sarkar, M., 2017. Determination of selected chemical levels in room air and on surfaces after the use of cartridge- and tank-based E-vapor products or conventional cigarettes. Int. J. Environ. Res. Publ. Health 14, 969. https://doi.org/10.3390/ijerph14090969.

Logue, J.M., McKone, T.E., Sherman, M.H., Singer, B.C., 2011. Hazard assessment of chemical air contaminants measured in residences. Indoor Air 21, 92–109. https://doi.org/10.1111/j.1600-0668.2010.00683.x.

Maga, M., Janik, M.K., Wachsmann, A., Chrząstek-Janik, O., Koziej, M., Bajkowski, M., Maga, P., Tyrak, K., Wójcik, K., Gregorczyk-Maga, I., Niżankowski, R., 2017. Influence of air pollution on exhaled carbon monoxide levels in smokers and non-smokers. A prospective cross-sectional study. Environ. Res. 152, 496–502. https://doi.org/10.1016/j.envres.2016.09.004.

Marco, G., Bo, X., 2013. Air quality legislation and standards in the European union: background, status and public participation. Adv. Clim. Change Res. 4, 50–59. https://doi.org/10.3724/sp.J.1248.2013.050.

Martuzevicius, D., Prasauskas, T., Setyan, A., O'Connell, G., Cahours, X., Julien, R., Colard, S., 2019. Characterization of the spatial and temporal dispersion differences between exhaled E-cigarette mist and cigarette smoke. Nicotine Tob. Res. 21, 1371–1377. https://doi.org/10.1093/ntr/nty121.

McAuley, T.R., Hopke, P.K., Zhao, J., Babaian, S., 2012. Comparison of the effects of e-cigarette vapor and cigarette smoke on indoor air quality. Inhal. Toxicol. 24, 850–857. https://doi.org/10.3109/08958378.2012.724728.

Meišutovič-Akhtarieva, M., Prasauskas, T., Čiužas, D., Krugly, E., Keraitytė, K., Martuzevičius, D., Kaunelienė, V., 2019. Impacts of exhaled aerosol from the usage of the tobacco heating system to indoor air quality: a chamber study. Chemosphere 223, 474–482. https://doi.org/10.1016/j.chemosphere.2019.02.095.

Melstrom, P., Koszowski, B., Thanner, M.H., Hoh, E., King, B., Bunnell, R., McAfee, T., 2017. Measuring PM2.5, ultrafine particles, nicotine air and wipe samples following the use of electronic cigarettes. Nicotine Tob. Res. 19, 1055–1061. https://doi.org/10.1093/ntr/ntx058.

Mitova, M.I., Bielik, N., Campelos, P.B., Cluse, C., Goujon-Ginglinger, C.G., Jaquier, A., Gomez Lueso, M., Maeder, S., Pitton, C., Poget, L., Polier-Calame, J., Rotach, M., Rouget, E.G.R., Schaller, M., Tharin, M., Zaugg, V., 2019a. Air quality assessment of the tobacco heating system 2.2 under simulated residential conditions. Air Qual. Atmos. Health 12, 807–823. https://doi.org/10.1007/s11869-019-00697-6.

Mitova, M.I., Campelos, P.B., Goujon-Ginglinger, C.G., Maeder, S., Mottier, N., Rouget, E.G., Tharin, M., Tricker, A.R., 2016. Comparison of the impact of the tobacco heating system 2.2 and a cigarette on indoor air quality. Regul. Toxicol. Pharmacol. 80, 91–101. https://doi.org/10.1016/j.yrtph.2016.06.005.

Mitova, M.I., Cluse, C., Goujon-Ginglinger, C.G., Kleinhans, S., Rotach, M., Tharin, M., 2019b. Human chemical signature: investigation on the influence of human presence and selected activities on concentrations of airborne constituents. Environ. Pollut. 257, 113518. https://doi.org/10.1016/j.envpol.2019.113518.

Mochalski, P., King, J., Klieber, M., Unterkofler, K., Hinterhuber, H., Baumann, M., Amann, A., 2013. Blood and breath levels of selected volatile organic compounds in healthy volunteers. Analyst 138. https://doi.org/10.1039/c3an36756h.

Mottier, N., Tharin, M., Cluse, C., Crudo, J.R., Lueso, M.G., Goujon-Ginglinger, C.G., Jaquier, A., Mitova, M.I., Rouget, E.G.R., Schaller, M., Solioz, J., 2016. Validation of selected analytical methods using accuracy profiles to assess the impact of a tobacco heating system on indoor air quality. Talanta 158, 165–178. https://doi.org/10.1016/j.talanta.2016.05.022.

Nazaroff, W.W., Weschler, C.J., 2004. Cleaning products and air fresheners: exposure to primary and secondary air pollutants. Atmos. Environ. 38, 2841–2865. https://doi.org/10.1016/j.atmosenv.2004.02.040.

Nelson, P.R., Kelly, S.P., Conrad, F.W., 1998. Studies of environmental tobacco smoke generated by different cigarettes. J. Air Waste Manag. Assoc. 48, 336–344. https://doi.org/10.1080/10473289.1998.10463685.

Nielsen, G.D., Ovrebo, S., 2008. Background, approaches and recent trends for setting health-based occupational exposure limits: a minireview. Regul. Toxicol. Pharmacol. 51, 253–269. https://doi.org/10.1016/j.yrtph.2008.04.002.

Niu, J.L., Burnett, J., 2001. Setting up the criteria and credit-awarding scheme for building interior material selection to achieve better indoor air quality. Environ. Int. 26, 573–580. https://doi.org/10.1016/s0160-4120(01)00043-5.

Notter, D.A., 2015. Life cycle impact assessment modeling for particulate matter: a new approach based on physico-chemical particle properties. Environ. Int. 82, 10–20. https://doi.org/10.1016/j.envint.2015.05.002.

O'Connell, G., Colard, S., Cahours, X., Pritchard, J., 2015. An assessment of indoor air quality before, during and after unrestricted use of E-cigarettes in a small room. Int. J. Environ. Res. Publ. Health 12, 4889–4907. https://doi.org/10.3390/ijerph120504889.

Oey, J., Lau, R.W., Roethig, H.J., 2008. Determination of environmental tobacco smoke from a second-generation electrically heated cigarette smoking system and conventional cigarettes. Beiträge zur Tabakforschung Int./Contrib. Tob. Res. 23, 1–7. https://doi.org/10.2478/cttr-2013-0843.

Olesen, B.W., 2012. Revision of EN 15251: indoor environmental criteria. REHVA J. 49 (4), 6–13.

Oppl, R., 2014. New European VOC emissions testing method CEN/TS 16516 and CE marking of construction products. Innenraumluft 3, 62–68.

Oppl, R., Neuhaus, T.R., 2008. Emission Specifications in Europe and the US – Limit Values (TVOC, LCI, CREL) in Critical Discussion, Indoor Air 2008, Copenhagen, Denmark.

Perbellini, L., Princivalle, A., Cerpelloni, M., Pasini, F., Brugnone, F., 2003. Comparison of breath, blood and urine concentrations in the biomonitoring of environmental exposure to 1,3-butadiene, 2,5-dimethylfuran, and benzene. Int. Arch. Occup. Environ. Health 76, 461–466. https://doi.org/10.1007/s00420-003-0436-7.

Persily, A., 2015. Challenges in developing ventilation and indoor air quality standards: the story of ASHRAE standard 62. Build. Environ. 91, 61–69. https://doi.org/10.1016/j.buildenv.2015.02.026.

Prodanchuk, M.G., Podrushnyak, A.E., Malysheva, O.E., Stroy, A.M., Zaval'na, V.V., Moroz, T.I., Kruk, V.I., Shutova, T.V., 2017. Potential Risk Assessment of the Electrically Heated Tobacco System (EHTS) Use. Problem articles 1-2 5-14.

Protano, C., Avino, P., Manigrasso, M., Vivaldi, V., Perna, F., Valeriani, F., Vitali, M., 2018. Environmental electronic vape exposure from four different generations of electronic cigarettes: airborne particulate matter levels. Int. J. Environ. Res. Publ. Health 15, 2172. https://doi.org/10.3390/ijerph15102172.

Protano, C., Manigrasso, M., Avino, P., Sernia, S., Vitali, M., 2016. Second-hand smoke exposure generated by new electronic devices (IQOS(R) and e-cigs) and traditional cigarettes: submicron particle behaviour in human respiratory system. Ann. Ig. 28, 109–112. https://doi.org/10.7416/ai.2016.2089.

Protano, C., Manigrasso, M., Avino, P., Vitali, M., 2017. Secondhand smoke generated by combustion and electronic smoking devices used in real scenarios: ultrafine particle pollution and age-related dose assessment. Environ. Int. 107, 190–195. https://doi.org/10.1016/j.envint.2017.07.014.

Public Health England (PHE), 2016a. Report of PHE Stakeholder 'Conversation' on Use of E-Cigarettes in Enclosed Public Places and workplaces. Public Health England, London.

Public Health England (PHE), 2016b. Use of E-Cigarettes in Public Places and Workplaces: Advice to Inform Evidence-Based Policy Making. Public Health England, London.

Ramos, C.A., Reis, J.F., Almeida, T., Alves, F., Wolterbeek, H.T., Almeida, S.M., 2015. Estimating the inhaled dose of pollutants during indoor physical activity. Sci. Total Environ. 527–528, 111–118. https://doi.org/10.1016/j.scitotenv.2015.04.120.

Ramos, C.A., Wolterbeek, H.T., Almeida, S.M., 2014. Exposure to indoor air pollutants during physical activity in fitness centers. Build. Environ. 82, 349–360. https://doi.org/10.1016/j.buildenv.2014.08.026.

Riojas-Rodríguez, H., Silva, A.S.D., Texcalac-Sangrador, J., Moreno-Banda, G., 2016. Air pollution management and control in Latin America and the Caribbean: implications for climate change. Rev. Panam. Salud Pública 40, 150–159.

Roethig, H.J., Kinser, R.D., Lau, R.W., Walk, R.A., Wang, N., 2005. Short-term exposure evaluation of adult smokers switching from conventional to first-generation electrically heated cigarettes during controlled smoking. J. Clin. Pharmacol. 45, 133–145. https://doi.org/10.1177/0091270004271253.

Rösch, C., Kohajda, T., Röder, S., Bergen, M.v., Schlink, U., 2014. Relationship between sources and patterns of VOCs in indoor air. Atmos. Pollut. Res. 5, 129–137. https://doi.org/10.5094/apr.2014.016.

Ruprecht, A.A., De Marco, C., Saffari, A., Pozzi, P., Mazza, R., Veronese, C., Angellotti, G., Munarini, E., Ogliari, A.C., Westerdahl, D., Hasheminassab, S., Shafer, M.M., Schauer, J.J., Repace, J., Sioutas, C., Boffi, R., 2017. Environmental pollution and emission factors of electronic cigarettes, heat-not-burn tobacco products, and conventional cigarettes. Aerosol. Sci. Technol. 51, 674–684. https://doi.org/10.1080/02786826.2017.1300231.

Saffari, A., Daher, N., Ruprecht, A., De Marco, C., Pozzi, P., Boffi, R., Hamad, S.H., Shafer, M.M., Schauer, J.J., Westerdahl, D., Sioutas, C., 2014. Particulate metals and organic compounds from electronic and tobacco-containing cigarettes: comparison of emission rates and secondhand exposure. Environ. Sci. 16, 2259–2267. https://doi.org/10.1039/c4em00415a.

Salthammer, T., 2011. Critical evaluation of approaches in setting indoor air quality guidelines and reference values. Chemosphere 82, 1507–1517. https://doi.org/10.1016/j.chemosphere.2010.11.023.

Salthammer, T., Mentese, S., Marutzky, R., 2010. Formaldehyde in the indoor environment. Chem. Rev. 110, 2536–2572. https://doi.org/10.1021/cr800399g.

Schaller, J.P., Keller, D., Poget, L., Pratte, P., Kaelin, E., McHugh, D., Cudazzo, G., Smart, D., Tricker, A.R., Gautier, L., Yerly, M., Reis Pires, R., Le Bouhellec, S., Ghosh, D., Hofer, I., Garcia, E., Vanscheeuwijck, P., Maeder, S., 2016. Evaluation of the tobacco heating system 2.2. Part 2: chemical composition, genotoxicity, cytotoxicity, and physical properties of the aerosol. Regul. Toxicol. Pharmacol. 81 (Suppl. 2), S27–S47. https://doi.org/10.1016/j.yrtph.2016.10.001.

Schenk, L., Hansson, S.O., Rudén, C., Gilek, M., 2008. Occupational exposure limits: a comparative study. Regul. Toxicol. Pharmacol. 50, 261–270. https://doi.org/10.1016/j.yrtph.2007.12.004.

Schmitz-Felten, E., Lissner, L., 2008. Occupational exposure limits in 25 member states of the EU. Gefahrst. Reinhalt. Luft 68, 257–269.

Schober, W., Fembacher, L., Frenzen, A., Fromme, H., 2019. Passive exposure to pollutants from conventional cigarettes and new electronic smoking devices (IQOS, e-cigarette) in passenger cars. Int. J. Hyg. Environ. Health 222, 486–493. https://doi.org/10.1016/j.ijheh.2019.01.003.

Schober, W., Szendrei, K., Matzen, W., Osiander-Fuchs, H., Heitmann, D., Schettgen, T., Jorres, R.A., Fromme, H., 2014. Use of electronic cigarettes (e-cigarettes) impairs indoor air quality and increases FeNO levels of e-cigarette consumers. Int. J. Hyg. Environ. Health 217, 628–637. https://doi.org/10.1016/j.ijheh.2013.11.003.

Schripp, T., Markewitz, D., Uhde, E., Salthammer, T., 2013. Does e-cigarette consumption cause passive vaping? Indoor Air 23, 25–31. https://doi.org/10.1111/j.1600-0668.2012.00792.x.

Schulte-Ladbeck, R., Lindahl, R., Levin, J.O., Karst, U., 2001. Characterization of chemical interferences in the determination of unsaturated aldehydes using aromatic hydrazine reagents and liquid chromatography. J. Environ. Monit. 3, 306–310. https://doi.org/10.1039/b101354h.

Seaman, V.Y., Bennett, D.H., Cahill, T.M., 2007. Origin, occurrence, and source emission rate of acrolein in residential indoor air. Environ. Sci. Technol. 41, 6940–6946. https://doi.org/10.1021/es0707299.

Simonavicius, E., McNeill, A., Shahab, L., Brose, L.S., 2018. Heat-not-burn tobacco products: a systematic literature review. Tobac. Contr. https://doi.org/10.1136/tobaccocontrol-2018-054419.

Smith, M.R., Clark, B., Ludicke, F., Schaller, J.P., Vanscheeuwijck, P., Hoeng, J., Peitsch, M.C., 2016. Evaluation of the tobacco heating system 2.2. Part 1: description of the system and the scientific assessment program. Regul. Toxicol. Pharmacol. 81 (Suppl. 2), S17–S26. https://doi.org/10.1016/j.yrtph.2016.07.006.

Soule, E.K., Maloney, S.F., Spindle, T.R., Rudy, A.K., Hiler, M.M., Cobb, C.O., 2017. Electronic cigarette use and indoor air quality in a natural setting. Tobac. Contr. 26, 109–112. https://doi.org/10.1136/tobaccocontrol-2015-052772.

Sousan, S., Koehler, K., Thomas, G., Park, J.H., Hillman, M., Halterman, A., Peters, T.M., 2016. Inter-comparison of low-cost sensors for measuring the mass concentration of occupational aerosols. Aerosol. Sci. Technol. 50, 462–473. https://doi.org/10.1080/02786826.2016.1162901.

St Helen, G., Havel, C., Dempsey, D.A., Jacob 3rd, P., Benowitz, N.L., 2016. Nicotine delivery, retention and pharmacokinetics from various electronic cigarettes. Addiction 111, 535–544. https://doi.org/10.1111/add.13183.

Stathopoulou, O.I., Assimakopoulos, V.D., Flocas, H.A., Helmis, C.G., 2008. An experimental study of air quality inside large athletic halls. Build. Environ. 43, 834–848. https://doi.org/10.1016/j.buildenv.2007.01.026.

Steinemann, A., 2015. Volatile emissions from common consumer products. Air Qual. Atmos. Health 8, 273–281. https://doi.org/10.1007/s11869-015-0327-6.

Sun, X., He, J., Yang, X., 2017. Human breath as a source of VOCs in the built environment, Part II: concentration levels, emission rates and factor analysis. Build. Environ. 123, 437–445. https://doi.org/10.1016/j.buildenv.2017.07.009.

Tang, X., Misztal, P.K., Nazaroff, W.W., Goldstein, A.H., 2016. Volatile organic compound emissions from humans indoors. Environ. Sci. Technol. 50, 12686–12694. https://doi.org/10.1021/acs.est.6b04415.

Travers, J., Marsh, S., Aldington, S., Williams, M., Shirtcliffe, P., Pritchard, A., Weatherall, M., Beasley, R., 2007. Reference ranges for exhaled nitric oxide derived from a random community survey of adults. Am. J. Respir. Crit. Care Med. 176, 238–242. https://doi.org/10.1164/rccm.200609-1346OC.

Tricker, A.R., Schorp, M.K., Urban, H.J., Leyden, D., Hagedorn, H.W., Engl, J., Urban, M., Riedel, K., Gilch, G., Janket, D., Scherer, G., 2009. Comparison of environmental tobacco smoke (ETS) concentrations generated by an electrically heated cigarette smoking system and a conventional cigarette. Inhal. Toxicol. 21, 62–77. https://doi.org/10.1080/08958370802207334.

Turner, C., Španĕl, P., Smith, D., 2006. A longitudinal study of ethanol and acetaldehyde in the exhaled breath of healthy volunteers using selected-ion flow-tube mass spectrometry. Rapid Commun. Mass Spectrom. 20, 61–68. https://doi.org/10.1002/rcm.2275.

US Occupational Safety and Health Administration (US OSHA), April 14, 2020. Permissible Exposure Limits (PEL). OSHA Annotated Table Z-1. Available from: https://www.osha.gov/dsg/annotated-pels/tablez-1.html.

U.S. Department of Health and Human Services (DHHS), 2014. The Health Consequences of Smoking: 50 Years of Progress. A Report of the Surgeon General. U.S. Department of Health and Human Services, Centers for Disease Control and Prevention, National Center for Chronic Disease Prevention and Health Promotion, Office on Smoking and Health, Atlanta, GA.

Vainiotalo, S., Vaaranrinta, R., Tornaeus, J., Aremo, N., Hase, T., Peltonen, K., 2001. Passive monitoring method for 3-ethenylpyridine: a marker for environmental tobacco smoke. Environ. Sci. Technol. 35, 1818–1822. https://doi.org/10.1021/es0002058.

van Drooge, B.L., Marco, E., Perez, N., Grimalt, J.O., 2018. Influence of electronic cigarette vaping on the composition of indoor organic pollutants, particles, and exhaled breath of bystanders. Environ. Sci. Pollut. Control Ser. 26, 4654–4666. https://doi.org/10.1007/s11356-018-3975-x.

Veres, P.R., Faber, P., Drewnick, F., Lelieveld, J., Williams, J., 2013. Anthropogenic sources of VOC in a football stadium: assessing human emissions in the atmosphere. Atmos. Environ. 77, 1052–1059. https://doi.org/10.1016/j.atmosenv.2013.05.076.

Volesky, K.D., Maki, A., Scherf, C., Watson, L., Van Ryswyk, K., Fraser, B., Weichenthal, S.A., Cassol, E., Villeneuve, P.J., 2018. The influence of three e-cigarette models on indoor fine and ultrafine particulate matter concentrations under real-world conditions. Environ. Pollut. 243, 882–889. https://doi.org/10.1016/j.envpol.2018.08.069.

Wallace, L.A., Wheeler, A.J., Kearney, J., Van Ryswyk, K., You, H., Kulka, R.H., Rasmussen, P.E., Brook, J.R., Xu, X., 2010. Validation of continuous particle monitors for personal, indoor, and outdoor exposures. J. Expo. Sci. Environ. Epidemiol. 21, 49–64. https://doi.org/10.1038/jes.2010.15.

Weschler, C.J., 2009. Changes in indoor pollutants since the 1950s. Atmos. Environ. 43, 153–169. https://doi.org/10.1016/j.atmosenv.2008.09.044.

Weschler, C.J., 2016. Roles of the human occupant in indoor chemistry. Indoor Air 26, 6–24. https://doi.org/10.1111/ina.12185.

WHO, World Health Organization (WHO), 2000. Chapter 7.3 Particulate Matter. WHO Regional Office for Europe [2019 1 July].

WHO, World Health Organization (WHO), 2010. WHO Guidelines for Indoor Air Quality: Selected Pollutants [2018 21 December 2018]; Available from: https://www.ncbi.nlm.nih.gov/pubmed/23741784.

Williams, J., Stönner, C., Wicker, J., Krauter, N., Derstroff, B., Bourtsoukidis, E., Klüpfel, T., Kramer, S., 2016. Cinema audiences reproducibly vary the chemical composition of air during films, by broadcasting scene specific emissions on breath. Sci. Rep. 6 https://doi.org/10.1038/srep25464.

World Health Organization (WHO), 2005. WHO Air Quality Guidelines for Particulate Matter, Ozone, Nitrogen Dioxide and Sulfur Dioxide. Global Update 2005. Summary of Risk Assessment [2018 21 December]; Available from: https://apps.who.int/iris/bitstream/handle/10665/69477/WHO_SDE_PHE_OEH_06.02_eng.pdf;jsessionid=B9E6E04C7D88C16E4033585544FE4853?sequence=1.

Zainol Abidin, N., Zainal Abidin, E., Zulkifli, A., Karuppiah, K., Syed Ismail, S.N., Amer Nordin, A.S., 2017. Electronic cigarettes and indoor air quality: a review of studies using human volunteers. Rev. Environ. Health 32, 235−244. https://doi.org/10.1515/reveh-2016-0059.

Zhang, J., Smith, K.R., 2003. Indoor air pollution: a global health concern. Br. Med. Bull. 68, 209−225. https://doi.org/10.1093/bmb/ldg029.

CHAPTER 9

A Systems-Based Approach to Toxicity Testing

JULIA HOENG • MARJA TALIKKA • BJOERN TITZ • AMIN CHOUKRALLAH •
STÉPHANIE BOUÉ • NIKOLAI V. IVANOV • DIEGO MARESCOTTI • FLORIAN MARTIN •
MANUEL C. PEITSCH

9.1 INTRODUCTION TO SYSTEMS TOXICOLOGY

Toxicity testing is essential to drug development, food safety, ecotoxicology, and other areas where human activity might impact biological systems and organisms. Toxicity testing is particularly crucial when assessing the risk of substances or products that might impact human health, and it, therefore, relies heavily on robust regulatory frameworks, guidelines, and bioassays. However, the demand for more informed risk assessment and better decisions has fostered the development of more comprehensive and integrative testing strategies that go beyond the scope of a fixed battery of tests (Rovida et al., 2015b). Such strategies leverage the most recent developments in measurement technologies to generate detailed systems-wide molecular data and integrate them with traditional toxicity data by using computational approaches (Committee on Toxicity Testing and Assessment of Environmental Agents, 2007; Hartung, 2010; Hartung et al., 2017; Rovida et al., 2015b; Sauer et al., 2016; Sturla et al., 2014). Indeed, it has been postulated that there will be a shift from traditional toxicity testing toward efforts focused on exploring and improving our understanding of the signaling pathways that are perturbed by biologically active substances or their metabolites (Krewski et al., 2010; Hartung, 2010). To this end, adverse outcome pathways (AOPs) have been suggested as a means to reduce the uncertainty in extrapolating in vitro data in a causal chain of events by leveraging validated high-confidence links between assay endpoints and disease mechanisms (Clippinger et al., 2018; Lowe et al., 2017; Rovida et al., 2015a).

Systems toxicology approaches combine several omics platforms, various structural and functional "apical" measurements with preexisting knowledge, and computational modeling to gain mechanistic and quantitative insights into the biological effects of substance exposure (Hartung et al., 2017; Sturla et al., 2014). Therefore, the objective of systems toxicology is to understand and quantify the effects of toxicant exposure along the causal chain of events linking smoking to disease (CELSD) by combining biological network models (descriptions of biological process knowledge) with quantitative measurements at all levels of biological organization (Hoeng et al., 2012; Sturla et al., 2014) (Chapter 3) (Fig. 9.1). Thereby, systems toxicology augments the predictive power of toxicity testing (Chapter 3) and enables better-informed risk assessments (Sturla et al., 2014). In particular, systems toxicology enables mechanism-by-mechanism comparison of the biological effects of different exposures.

The advantages of systems toxicology approaches have recently been recognized in regulatory toxicology and pharmacology and are being leveraged in various applications. For instance, multiomics studies have been conducted to provide nonbiased insights into the toxic mode of action of pesticides (Simoes et al., 2019), metals (Chai et al., 2019), and nanomaterials (Wang et al., 2019); the hormetic actions of fullerene crystals on *Daphnia* (Wang et al., 2019); the benefits of trace elements against chemical toxicity (Chauhan et al., 2020); and the effects of climate change on the environment (Hennon and Dyhrman, 2020). These are only a few examples of the recently emerging spectrum of systems toxicology applications in science and applied research (Fig. 9.2).

From a regulatory perspective, there have been demands emerging for standardization and validation of systems toxicology approaches, and high-level frameworks are being developed to this end. For example, the United States (US) National Research Council,

Toxicological Evaluation of Electronic Nicotine Delivery Products. https://doi.org/10.1016/B978-0-12-820490-0.00009-2

189

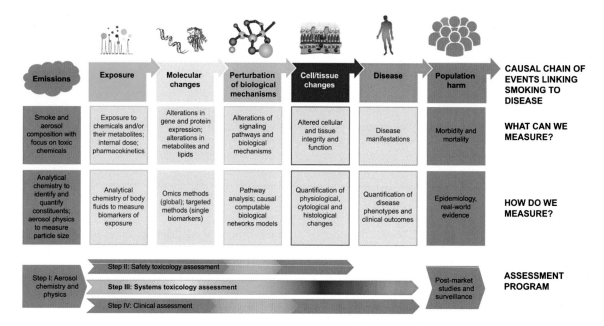

FIG. 9.1 Application of systems toxicology assessment to the CELSD. CELSD, causal chain of events linking smoking to disease. (Adapted from Sturla, S.J., Boobis, A.R., Fitzgerald, R.E., Hoeng, J., Kavlock, R.J., Schirmer, K., Whelan, M., Wilks, M.F., Peitsch, M.C., 2014. Systems toxicology: from basic research to risk assessment. Chem. Res. Toxicol. 27, 314–329. https://pubs.acs.org/doi/10.1021/tx400410s. Further permissions related to the material should be directed to the ACS.)

commissioned by the US Environmental Protection Agency, developed a vision for toxicity testing in the 21st century (called Tox 21-c) (Committee on Toxicity Testing and Assessment of Environmental Agents, 2007). More recently, the "Frank R. Lautenberg Chemical Safety for the 21st Century Act" provided an update of the Toxic Substances Control Act, aiming at reducing and replacing vertebrate animal studies and improving the relevance and quality of risk assessment by leveraging computational toxicology and bioinformatics, high-throughput screening (HTS) methods, in vitro studies, systems biology, and other elements of systems toxicology (U.S.Congress, 2016).

In the field of electronic nicotine delivery product (ENDP) testing, advanced nonclinical systems toxicological assessment enables detailed comparison of the effects of cigarette smoke (CS) and ENDP aerosols on biological mechanisms causally associated with smoking-related diseases. Such studies employ computational methods to analyze a broad array of comprehensive molecular measurements (transcriptomics, proteomics, genomics, and lipidomics endpoints) in addition to the standard measurements used in toxicity studies and the disease endpoints evaluated in animal

models of disease (e.g., emphysema, lung function, atherosclerotic plaque size, and lung tumor incidence).

Several human-derived in vitro model systems have been developed by following a systems toxicology–based approach, thus enabling—for example—comparative assessment of the effects of Tobacco Heating System (THS; an ENDP described in Chapter 2) aerosol and CS on vascular inflammation, endothelial dysfunction, and airway epithelium toxicity (Chapter 13). These studies have shown that THS aerosol exposure leads to significantly and consistently reduced perturbations of the biological mechanisms affected by CS. These mechanisms include oxidative stress, inflammation, DNA damage, xenobiotic metabolism, and cell death. Furthermore, systems toxicology–based approaches can augment in vivo safety toxicology studies (Chapter 14), studies in animal models of disease (Chapter 15), as well as clinical studies.

9.2 DESIGN OF SYSTEMS TOXICOLOGY EXPERIMENTS

Scientific questions should always drive the experimental design as well as the choice of methods and

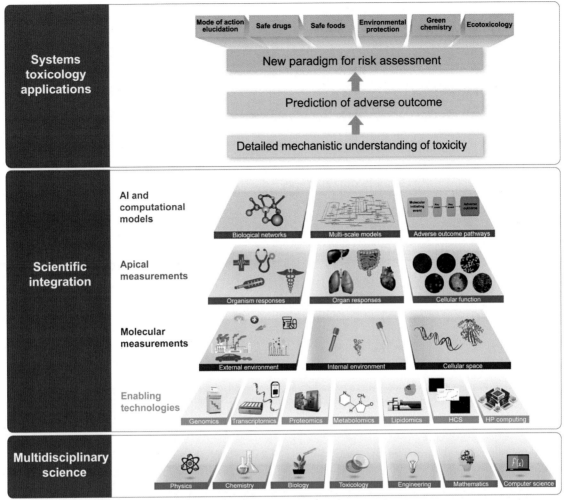

FIG. 9.2 Systems toxicology applications. (Adapted from Sturla, S.J., Boobis, A.R., Fitzgerald, R.E., Hoeng, J., Kavlock, R.J., Schirmer, K., Whelan, M., Wilks, M.F., Peitsch, M.C., 2014. Systems toxicology: from basic research to risk assessment. Chem. Res. Toxicol. 27, 314–329. https://pubs.acs.org/doi/10.1021/tx400410s. Further permissions related to the material should be directed to the ACS.)

analyses that will be conducted on the study samples. When the scientific questions are clear, it is feasible to assign adequate exposure modalities and choose the appropriate biological test systems. Ideally, the study should capture the toxicity and mechanisms of toxicity to discriminate stimuli that are likely to cause harm in humans. The experimental design defines the experimental system that is subjected to a standardized time- and dose-dependent exposure regimen with the aim of answering the scientific questions set beforehand (Hoeng et al., 2014).

A well-thought-out statistical design, such as using an adequate number of biological replicates, ensures that neither experimental errors nor external variables drive the study conclusions over the true biological effects. Sample randomization is particularly important to avoid any effects that might be introduced by batch variation of supply or variations in the treatment, sample collection, extraction, or isolation steps. Any known source of variability should be controlled (Hoeng et al., 2014) (Fig. 9.3).

The design of a systems biology experiment also needs to account for the fact that a priori knowledge is limited, considering the large amount of information obtained through high-density molecular measurements. This sets unique requirements for the design to enable

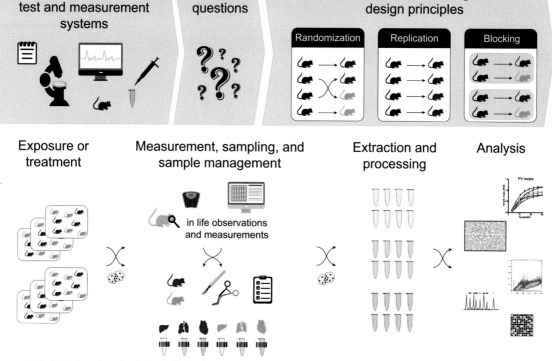

FIG. 9.3 A major step in toxicological assessment entails analysis of the exposure—response relationship. Together with selection of an appropriate model organism and a sufficient number of replicates, doses and time points always require careful consideration prior to the experiment.

robust insights unaffected by too many assumptions (Kreutz and Timmer, 2009). Moreover, it will be important that toxicologists, biologists, computational scientists, and other experts in the field continue to work with regulatory agencies on efficient strategies for describing unified and consistent experimental setups and designs, exposure conditions, and computational data analyses to achieve harmonized methodologies for robust toxicology assessment. Outside the field of tobacco harm reduction, the Chemical Effects in Biological Systems database compiled by the National Center for Toxicogenomics within the National Institute of Environmental Health Science encompasses over 8,000 studies, including carcinogenicity, short-term toxicity, and genetic toxicity studies. The database also includes study designs, clinical chemistry and histopathological findings, and a wealth of microarray and proteomics data from in vivo and in vitro exposure studies for over 11,000 test articles (exposure agents) (Lea et al., 2017).

9.3 TECHNOLOGY PLATFORMS FOR MEASURING A LARGE NUMBER OF BIOLOGICAL CHANGES SIMULTANEOUSLY

9.3.1 High-content Screening

The 3R principles (Replacement, Reduction, and Refinement of animal testing) have prompted the development of rapid and cost-effective methods for prescreening and classifying compounds that are suspected to cause adverse effects in humans. The National Toxicology Program is responsible for the remarkable initiative for developing an HTS program that aims to narrow down the number of compounds that go further to animal testing (Tice et al., 2007; National Toxicology Program NTP, 2004). The assays use several cell types in cell viability and cytotoxicity assays, and compound profiles are assessed across several cell types with structure—activity relationship kinetic signatures (Xia et al., 2008). Hence, HTS can be used to classify compounds into groups that possess similar activity as well as develop predictive models to limit and maximally benefit from in vivo testing.

High-content screening (HCS) is an image-based tool for rapid screening of compounds. It allows quantitative analysis of images derived from high-throughput microscopy, which can process thousands of samples. With sophistication come multiple considerations: In addition to assay design, it is necessary to consider selection of fluorophore markers, sample handling, and image acquisition, transfer, storage, and processing. Additionally, feature extraction and data preprocessing must be performed prior to final data analysis (Usaj et al., 2016; Zingler and Heyse, 2008).

Efforts in including HCS assays as part of the assessment of harmful and potentially harmful constituents of tobacco smoke have proven that the combination of cell impedance—based technologies with HCS allows rapid and cost-effective toxicological screening of multiple constituents at the same time (Marescotti et al., 2016).

For ENDP assessment, phenotypic HCS assays can be combined with real-time cellular analysis (impedance-based) and gene expression profiling to evaluate the toxicity of e-liquids. In addition to its utility in e-liquid assessment (Gonzalez-Suarez et al., 2017), such an assay toolbox is valuable for filtering out potentially hazardous flavor ingredients before testing them in more complex and expensive experiential systems such as organotypic cultures or rodents (Marescotti et al., 2020; Iskandar et al., 2016).

9.3.2 Omics Technologies
9.3.2.1 Genomics and Transcriptomics
Genomics is the study of the function, structure, regulation, and evolution of genomes and their associated biological processes. With the advent of high-throughput sequencing (HTseq) and microarray technologies, genomics investigations have rapidly evolved from simple analysis of gene sequences to a holistic approach aiming to dissect all biological processes associated with the genomes. The cost of genomic sequencing has decreased tremendously, making it accessible also to areas outside toxicological or clinical research, leading to the development of direct-to-consumer genomic profiling (Roberts and Ostergren, 2013).

In addition to DNA sequence analysis, genomics encompasses the study of transcription, replication, chromatin organization, and DNA damage and repair, to name a few. Alterations in any of these processes by endogenous or external factors might cause cellular dysfunction and eventually lead to a disease state.

Genomics investigations are an important part of risk assessment protocols for various products, including food, drugs, cosmetics, and ENDPs.

Exposure to CS induces various genomic perturbations, including DNA adduct formation (Ma et al., 2019), mutations, epigenetic changes, and perturbations in gene transcription (reviewed in Choukrallah et al., 2018). Given the central role of these biological processes in smoking-related disease onset and progression, it is crucial to investigate the genomic impact of alternative tobacco and nicotine-containing products in order to support their reduced-risk claims.

This section will briefly summarize current genomics techniques and their use in the context of risk assessment with emphasis on comparing the effects of ENDP aerosols and CS.

9.3.2.1.1 Analysis of DNA sequences. DNA sequencing by HTseq can be used to discover single-nucleotide polymorphisms (SNPs) and localize mutations (Leshchiner et al., 2012). The two main HTseq approaches include whole-genome sequencing (WGS) and whole-exome sequencing (WES); the latter only targets exons and, therefore, reduces the sequencing burden.

Both WGS and WES are massively used in the context of genome-wide association studies that aim to identify possible associations between genetic loci and traits including disease risk, susceptibility to environmental factors including smoking (Gage et al., 2016; Cai et al., 2017), and response to drugs (Kogelman et al., 2019; Gormley et al., 2016).

Smoking is associated with elevated mutation burdens in various tissues (Alexandrov et al., 2016), which might increase the risk of cancer. In this context, WGS is a powerful tool for comparing the mutational profiles induced by CS and ENDP aerosol exposure in humans and model organisms.

HTseq is also used to study microbiome diversity, a field known as metagenomics. The microbiome is impacted by environmental factors and is associated with a number of diseases (Shreiner et al., 2015). Microbiome research is rapidly expanding, as increasing numbers of microbial genomes are being sequenced and annotated. Given that CS exposure is associated with microbiome alterations in various tissues (Lee et al., 2018), it is important to investigate how ENDPs affect the microbiome in comparison with CS.

9.3.2.1.2 Analysis of natural DNA modifications and DNA adducts. DNA molecules can naturally undergo a number of chemical modifications that play an important role in genome regulation. DNA methylation—which most commonly results in methylation of cytosine to 5-methylcytosine (5 mC)—is the best characterized DNA modification. It occurs mainly at CpG dinucleotides and is considered a repressive epigenetic mark (Lei et al., 1996). Whole-genome bisulfite sequencing (WGBS) is currently the gold standard technique for assessing DNA methylation at base-resolution scale. Bisulfite treatment allows us to distinguish methylated and unmethylated cytosines, because the latter are converted to uracil and read as thymine, whereas methylated cytosines remain unchanged (Frommer et al., 1992). Subsequent bioinformatics analyses allow us to compute the methylation status of all cytosines in the genome. DNA methylation can also be assessed by microarrays but for a limited set of loci. CS has been shown to alter DNA methylation profiles in human tissues (Joehanes et al., 2016). In mice, WGBS investigations of the lungs have shown that CS-associated perturbations of DNA methylation are reduced upon cessation or switching to ENDPs (Choukrallah et al., 2019).

Exposure to certain carcinogens induces aberrant covalent modifications termed DNA adducts, which lead to alterations in many genomics processes (Rajalakshmi et al., 2015). For example, metabolic activation of benzo[*a*]pyrene (BaP), a polycyclic aromatic hydrocarbon found in CS, can lead to formation of DNA adducts, which, in turn, can lead to mutations (Iskandar et al., 2016).Therefore, BaP is considered as one of the major causes of CS-associated cancers (Pfeifer et al., 2002). Recently, a number of methods have been developed that combine immunoprecipitation and HTseq to localize DNA adducts and DNA-damage repair at a genome-wide level (Li et al., 2017; Vaughn et al., 2020).

9.3.2.1.3 Analysis of chromatin properties. Chromatin is a DNA–histone complex which packages DNA in a compact form to fit into the nucleus. Several histone residues carry covalent posttranslational modifications (PTMs), including acetylation, phosphorylation, and methylation. Histone PTMs are controlled by many epigenetic enzymes and play a central role in transcription, DNA-damage repair, and DNA replication. A number of epigenetic enzymes and their associated substrates are sensitive to environmental exposures and directly linked to many human diseases (Araki and Mimura, 2017). Genome-wide mapping of PTMs provides information about chromatin structure and its transcriptional competency. The gold standard technique for mapping

PTMs and other DNA-binding proteins is chromatin immunoprecipitation (ChIP) followed by HTseq (ChIP-seq). ChIP-seq involves an immunoprecipitation step that uses antibodies directed against the target protein. The reads resulting from sequencing of the captured DNA are mapped to the reference genome to identify the binding sites of target proteins (Schmidt et al., 2009).

Chromatin accessibility can also be assessed by ATAC-seq (assay for transposase-accessible chromatin using sequencing). ATAC-seq involves simultaneous fragmentation and adapter ligation by using Tn5 transposase, which inserts sequencing adapters into open chromatin regions, which are further amplified by HTseq (Buenrostro et al., 2015). After read mapping to the reference genome, the open chromatin regions are identified by using peak-calling algorithms. Recently, ATAC-seq has been used to show that, in retinal pigmented epithelium cells, CS exposure recapitulates the chromatin accessibility alterations observed in age-related macular degeneration (Wang et al., 2018).

9.3.2.1.4 Transcriptomics analysis. Thanks to rapid advances in microarrays and RNA sequencing (RNA-Seq), transcriptomics analysis has become a fast and affordable endpoint. Microarrays now cover the majority of known transcripts, including protein-coding RNAs and noncoding RNAs (ncRNA). Microarray data processing is now a well-standardized process, which makes this technology suitable for large-scale clinical and nonclinical studies. While microarrays enable standardized comparison of transcript abundance across studies, they are also limited by design and cannot cover the complete genome or help discover new transcripts. RNA-Seq allows measurement of transcript abundance for any RNA family, including messenger RNAs (mRNA), microRNAs (miRNA), and long ncRNAs. Moreover, RNA-seq raw data are reported in a simple and standard text-based format (fastq format), thus allowing platform-independent comparison of datasets generated in different laboratories.

9.3.2.2 Proteomics

Proteomics leverages highly multiplexed measurement technologies to study the function, structure, regulation, and biological networks of proteins. Proteins are structural and functional core elements of biological networks: They form biological structures, mediate biological activities, and compute and transmit information. Analysis of proteins plays an important role in toxicological assessment studies. For example, toxicants trigger the release of cytokines and chemokines as a part of inflammatory processes (Phillips et al., 2016a), induce cellular stress and xenobiotic metabolism programs (Titz et al., 2020), and cause cellular and tissue damage, which is revealed by marker proteins (Ramaiah, 2007).

The diversity of proteomics approaches reflects the structural and functional diversity of proteins. These approaches are optimized for identification and quantification of many proteins simultaneously.

9.3.2.2.1 Antibody-based approaches.
Generally, proteins are identified and quantified either by affinity-reagent—based methods or, more directly, by mass spectrometry (MS)-based methods. For the first category, antibodies are the most commonly employed affinity reagents for detecting and quantifying proteins. However, there exist alternative affinity reagents, such as aptamers, which are DNA or RNA molecules selected for their high binding affinity to a protein of interest (Dunn et al., 2017).

While Western blotting is not commonly considered a proteomics method, miniaturized versions of this technique have been developed that support multiplexed and higher-throughput protein analyses (Ciaccio et al., 2010). The advantage of Western blots is that they provide an estimate of the molecular weight of the detected protein(s), but—even with recent adaptations—this measurement format is not suited for accurate protein quantitation and higher throughput.

Traditionally, enzyme-linked immunosorbent assays (ELISA) have supported high-throughput quantification of proteins. In this assay format, the binding of antibodies to a protein of interest is more directly coupled to a quantitative readout (e.g., chromogenic, fluorogenic, or electrochemiluminescent readout). Importantly, several multiplexed methods based on the general ELISA principle have been developed, often with improved measurement characteristics. Antibody protein arrays allow highly multiplexed quantification (Sutandy et al., 2013): Antibodies are spotted at defined positions on a miniaturized solid support; this array is then incubated with the sample, and pools of detection antibodies are used to determine the protein levels. Reverse-phase protein arrays can also be constructed by spotting the protein samples of interest onto a solid support and subsequently probing these sample arrays with antibodies against the targets of interest (Sutandy et al., 2013). Multiplexed ELISA-type assays that use a bead-based format, rather than leverage a solid support, have

also been implemented. For example, the xMAP platform (Luminex, Austin, TX, USA) is based on antibody-coupled microspheres that can be distinguished in a multiplexed format by their specific fluorescence signal (Dunbar and Hoffmeyer, 2013). By simultaneously identifying the microsphere as well as the binding of a fluorophore-conjugated detection antibody, it is possible to quantify up to 100 proteins in a single assay.

The majority of protein assays conducted today rely on affinity reagents, which makes them critically dependent on the availability of high-quality affinity reagents (Vicari, 2013; Aebersold et al., 2013; Baker, 2015). Stringent antibody validation approaches are, therefore, essential (Edfors et al., 2018). For example, a previous study found that a quarter of 246 evaluated antibodies used in epigenetic studies lacked specificity (Egelhofer et al., 2011).

9.3.2.2.2 MS-based methods.
MS-based approaches allow direct identification and quantification of proteins. Progress in MS instrumentation and methods has allowed continuous improvements in the sensitivity and coverage of proteome analyses (e.g., Lesur and Domon, 2015; Bruderer et al., 2015; Eliuk and Makarov, 2015). The most common approach to MS-based proteomics uses a "bottom—up" strategy, whereby isolated proteins are first cleaved into peptides with a specific protease (most commonly, trypsin and Lys-C); these peptides are subsequently (chromatographically) separated and identified and quantified with a mass spectrometer (Titz et al., 2014).

Depending on the available MS instrumentation and experimental needs, proteomics scientists can choose from a variety of quantification methods. There are two distinct quantification approaches: label-based methods, which use modified proteins/peptides, and label-free methods, which directly quantify native peptides.

A commonly used label-based quantification approach employs isobaric tags (e.g., iTRAQ and TMT labeling) (Titz et al., 2015; Wiese et al., 2007; Thompson et al., 2003). In these methods, quantification relies on chemical modification (tagging) of the peptides in a sample: Different samples labeled with different tags are pooled, and the relative MS intensities of the ions derived from these tags are taken to represent the relative peptide abundances in the analyzed samples.

In the popular MS-based label-free quantification approach, the mass spectrometer is programmed to identify as many peptides during a run as possible, and each of the identified peptides is (relatively) quantified as the area under its chromatographic elution peak (Tyanova et al., 2016). For robust quantification, additional features have been added to this basic concept; for example, the number of missing values is reduced by including chromatographic run-to-run alignment.

While these "shotgun" methods broadly capture protein profiles, the so-called "targeted" proteomics methods can be beneficial owing to their greater robustness and quantitative accuracy, which is especially relevant for clinical applications or for establishing quantitative models (Gillette and Carr, 2013; Carr et al., 2014). These methods aim to accurately quantify a predefined protein panel and include matched heavy-isotope–labeled standard peptides to facilitate robust quantification and consistency, even across different laboratories (Addona et al., 2009).

Data-independent acquisition methods combine systematic, untargeted MS acquisition with targeted computational analysis and are gaining popularity (Gillet et al., 2012). These methods provide high quantification accuracy for a consistently sampled large part of the proteome, which enables comparisons across large sets of MS runs (Gillet et al., 2012; Bruderer et al., 2015).

9.3.2.3 Lipidomics

Lipidomics investigates the structure, function, and interactions of the broad chemical class of lipids. Lipids have diverse biological roles: They form structures (e.g., membranes), act as signaling mediators (e.g., eicosanoids), and serve as energy storage molecules as well as precursors of other metabolites (van Meer et al., 2008). Owing to their important physiological roles, lipid alterations also importantly contribute to disease processes such as those in cardiovascular diseases, chronic obstructive pulmonary disease (Ekroos et al., 2020), infectious diseases (Morita et al., 2013; Wenk, 2006), and diabetes (Gross and Han, 2007). In toxicology, lipid alterations are, for example, induced by hepatotoxic compounds in the liver (Xu et al., 2019) as well as by CS exposure in the lungs (Titz et al., 2016a; Kogel et al., 2016).

The chemical space of lipid molecules is especially large. Indeed, the lipidome of eukaryotic cells consists of thousands of individual lipid species (van Meer, 2005). Thus, lipidome analysis requires sophisticated measurement approaches, such as those enabled by MS-based methods for lipid identification and quantification (Jung et al., 2011).

In shotgun lipidomics approaches, lipid extracts from a sample are directly injected into the mass spectrometer. This simple setup, which allows identification and quantification of hundreds of lipid species, includes select internal standards for improving quantitative accuracy (Heiskanen et al., 2013; Ekroos, 2012). As in proteomics, targeted lipidomics methods are commonly employed that combine chromatographic separation of lipids and their targeted identification and quantification in a mass spectrometer (Weir et al., 2013). This allows analysis of low abundance lipid species and complex lipid mixtures that are not amenable to shotgun analysis. Ideally, for each targeted analyte, a corresponding internal standard is included to achieve high analytical sensitivity and selectivity, even for less-abundant lipids.

9.3 PROCESSING HIGH-DENSITY DATA

Systems toxicology approaches generate massive amounts of data, which require a high-performance computing environment. This environment provides users with the infrastructure, software, and services required for storing and analyzing data as well as archiving them for future use.

Like in experimental science, where new in vitro and in vivo model systems are often needed to complement standard cell lines and animal models, computational systems toxicology (Hoeng and Peitsch, 2015) often requires specific algorithms and simulation software tailored to address specific scientific questions that cannot be answered with the available ready-to-use solutions.

By definition, high-throughput technologies produce large amounts of data that require considerable efforts to process and analyze. For example, the ToxCAst pipeline (tcpl) provides tools for data storage and normalization as well as solutions for visualization and dose–response modeling (Filer et al., 2017). Multiple other solutions exist for HCS data analysis, ranging from commercial packages to open-source solutions. Similar to tcpl and with additional capabilities, the GLobal Assessment of Dose-IndicAtor in TOXicology (GladiaTOX) operates as a flexible web service that allows users to fetch images from their proprietary sources, process data, and export reports in pdf format (Belcastro et al., 2019).

Raw omics data are generally converted into a systems response profile (SRP), which describes the degree to which the measured molecules are changed in treated samples relative to control samples. The steps leading up to SRPs include quality control of the raw data and data normalization (Hoeng et al., 2014). For example, Affymetrix GeneChip analysis delivers intensity measurements per probe, which need to be converted to values that correspond to genes (i.e., mRNA-based intensities). The robust multiarray analysis (RMA) algorithm for Affymetrix gene expression microarrays performs background correction, normalization, and summarization in a modular way. Ideally, all data are normalized as a single batch, but, when this is not possible, the frozen RMA estimates probe-specific effects and precomputes and freezes them on the basis of information from large publicly available microarray databases (McCall et al., 2010).

A volcano plot is a graphical presentation of statistical significance (p value) versus magnitude of change (fold change) and is commonly used to illustrate statistically significant and large molecular changes in the treated samples relative to control samples (Cui and Churchill, 2003) (Fig. 9.4).

While an individual, molecule-by-molecule investigation of the regulated molecules might provide some early insights into the biological meaning of the data, additional tools are required to interpret the data in the context of biological pathways. The Database for Annotation, Visualization and Integrated Discovery bioinformatics database (Huang et al., 2009) and the Protein Analysis Through Evolutionary Relationships (Mi et al., 2019) system use overrepresentation analysis to statistically map regulated molecules onto biological pathways. The biological pathways used by these tools are taken from databases such as the Kyoto Encyclopedia of Gene and Genomes (Kanehisa, 2000), BioCarta (Nishimura, 2001), and Reactome (Joshi-Tope et al., 2005). The different pathways tools and databases have been discussed and compared previously (Talikka et al., 2015).

When the number of regulated molecules is small, the statistical thresholds can be relaxed, and, instead, fold changes should be used as determinants of importance. Gene set enrichment analysis gathers molecules with the highest fold changes in the data and maps them to a priori-defined gene sets assigned to diverse biological functions (Subramanian et al., 2005).

Finally, there are more advanced computational approaches that are not only based on the abundance of

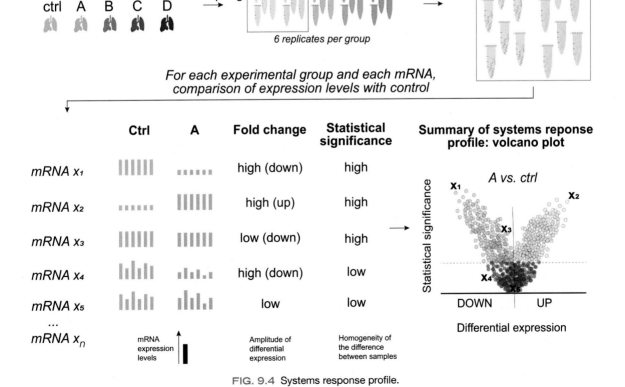

FIG. 9.4 Systems response profile.

the molecules involved in a given pathway or process but also take into account the way the molecules interact with each other to carry out their biological functions (Khatri et al., 2012; Shojaie and Michailidis, 2009). In Section 9.6, we describe a comprehensive approach that employs causal biological network (CBN) models and specific algorithm to analyze molecular data.

9.4 MULTIOMICS ANALYSIS

As outlined above, the rapid advances in high-throughput "omics" technologies have led to the development of different types of omics data, including gene expression, miRNA expression, SNP, metabolomics/lipidomics, and protein expression data. Each of these experimental data types potentially provides complementary information about the study organism as a whole and its response to a toxicological challenge. While computational analyses of individual data modalities provide relevant insights, multiomics data integration can provide deeper insights and more robust conclusions. Such integrative views are especially relevant, as toxicological effects involve multiple molecular layers. For example, CS exposure causes changes in proteins (Kenche et al., 2016), lipids (Rahman et al., 2002; Morissette et al., 2015), metabolites (Vulimiri et al., 2009; Zanetti et al., 2017), and transcriptional programs (Phillips et al., 2016b; Faner et al., 2016) in the lungs.

The potential benefits of such integrative multiomics analyses have been summarized in recent review articles (Hartung et al., 2017; Dellafiora and Dall'Asta, 2017). Previous multiomics toxicology studies have investigated, for example, doxorubicin cardiotoxicity (Holmgren et al., 2018), renal cisplatin toxicity (Wilmes et al., 2015), and lung nanoparticle toxicity (Dekkers et al., 2018). In the context of ENDP assessment, multiomics data have enabled evaluation of the diverse molecular effects (on lipid metabolism, oxidative stress responses, immune responses, etc.) in the lungs of mice and rats exposed to CS and ENDP aerosols (Titz et al., 2016b; Kogel et al., 2016).

While these two previous studies performed multiomics integration at the data interpretation stage, we recently employed Multi-Omics Factor Analysis and multimodality functional network interpretation for a more direct joint analysis of lung exposure responses across five omics data modalities (Titz et al., 2020). In a 6-month systems toxicology study in *Apoe*$^{-/-}$ mice, we measured how exposure to aerosols from the ENDP THS and a Carbon Heated Tobacco Product (CHTP) prototype affected lung proteins, mRNAs, miRNAs, lipids, and metabolites in comparison with CS. In total, these measurements captured approximately 17,500 mRNAs, 5,000 proteins, 670 metabolites, 400 lipids, and 360 miRNAs. Across all five omics data types, CS exposure was associated with increased inflammatory and oxidative stress response as well as lipid/surfactant alterations. In contrast, THS and CHTP aerosol exposure had much more limited or no effects. Of note, this integrated analysis also revealed the complex immunoregulatory interactions triggered by CS exposure in the lungs.

Taken together, our work and the work of others demonstrate the benefits of integrative multiomics analysis in toxicology studies for both gaining additional molecular insights and supporting more robust conclusions.

9.5 CBN MODELS

To get the most value out of systems biology and toxicology studies, it is beneficial if the biochemical mechanisms affected by the exposures are known a priori. While several pathway databases can help understand how the observed molecular changes impact biological processes as a whole (Khatri et al., 2012), they are often very generalized and not built for a specific context (e.g., organ system and disease). Network science, the applications of which are well developed in system biology, offers a platform for systematically exploring the mechanistic effects of chemical exposures and their impact on human health (Barabasi and Oltvai, 2004; Santolini and Barabási, 2018). The objective of systems biology and toxicology research is to discover the mechanisms affected by a specific exposure and represent this knowledge as well-documented and annotated biological network models that are specific for both the active substance or mixture and the exposed biological system.

For assessment of ENDPs—the aerosols of which are inhaled—it is of utmost importance to evaluate their biological effects in the context of lung biology. To this end, CBN models have been developed that contain large amounts of molecular and pathway information about lung-specific biological processes. These models enable analysis of high-density data in the context of lung biology. A dedicated website, http://causalbionet.com/, hosts a database of available and downloadable network models (Talikka et al., 2015; Boué et al., 2015).

9.5.1 Network Model Building

While comprehensive representation of biological networks as intertwined molecular pathways is an important attribute of CBN models, their true value comes from the fact that they are computable. The biological network models are encoded by using a special syntax embedded in the biological expression language (BEL) (Fluck et al., 2016). BEL allows biologists to represent facts written in scientific publications as cause and effect relationships between molecules by using a controlled vocabulary that allows computational linking of statements into a network representation (Fig. 9.5).

Building CBN models requires not only a computable language but also certain rules. First, these rules should define the model boundaries on the basis of the modeled biological process as well as the tissue or organ that is relevant to the study objective and associated data. Second, as signaling pathways might contribute to several different cellular processes, one should take care to include all signaling elements that are essential to the model. However, the specificity of the signaling elements to the modeled process must be retained in order to avoid too much overlap with other processes that use the same pathways (Talikka et al., 2015). Furthermore, there can be differences among the approaches taken by individual biocurators, and, hence, additional rules can be set to ensure consistency.

The model building begins with selection of articles that are pertinent to the modeled biological process. These articles are then subjected to biocuration with the aim of covering all known signaling pathways involved in the biological process to be modeled. In addition to providing the syntax, BEL also allows extensive annotation of the context of an observation, such as tissue, cell line, disease state, and species. During curation, as much of this information as possible is captured in order to gather rich metadata around each cause and effect statement. Once a sufficient number or articles have been curated, all curated statements can be compiled into a network representation (typically a graph) that can be viewed by using network visualization software such as Cytoscape (Lopes et al., 2010). In these graphs, the nodes represent biological entities (i.e., molecules), and the edges represent the relationships between the biological entities. Using the visualization software (for example, with Cytoscape), one can review the network models and further improve them by refining their structure and boundaries on the basis of additional literature-derived information or experimental data.

9.5.2 Quantifying the Effects on Biological Processes

A major benefit of computable biological network models is that they enable network-specific scoring of omics data and, thereby, extraction of biological process—relevant insights from the thousands of data points in the SRPs. The use of a network perturbation amplitude (NPA)

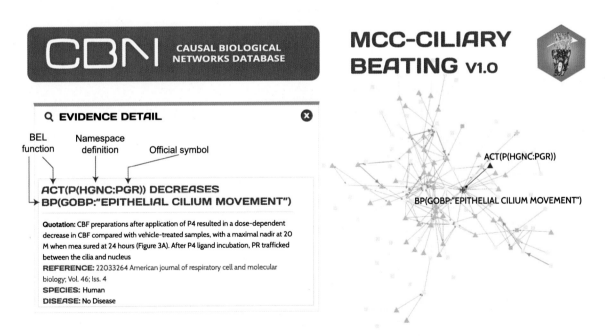

FIG. 9.5 BEL and the CBN model database. Left: Scientific facts written in natural language can be represented in BEL. Right: A typical graphic representation of a biological network. *BEL*, biological expression language; *CBN*, causal biological networks.

algorithm, developed for computing a single quantitative value for each CBN model (Martin et al., 2014; Hoeng et al., 2014), allows quantitative mechanism-by-mechanism comparison of different exposures or treatments. The NPA algorithm takes into account the molecular entities in the CBN, the structure of the CBN (edges between nodes), as well as experimental variability (Fig. 9.6).

Finally, the overall biological effect of an active substance or mixture on a biological system is estimated by aggregating the quantitative NPA values from several CBN models into a biological impact factor (BIF) (Thomson et al., 2013). This BIF value expresses the overall impact of an exposure or treatment on the entire biological system. Within an experiment, one can express the BIF of each treatment relative to the BIF with the maximum effect. In the context of ENDP assessment, these NPAs and relative BIFs, combined with other endpoints, provide the basis for quantitative

mechanism-by-mechanism comparison of the effects of an ENDP aerosol and CS. Clearly, the same approach enables comparison of the changes induced by switching from cigarette smoking to ENDP use with those induced by smoking cessation.

9.6 SUMMARY AND CONCLUSIONS

The unprecedented advancement of molecular profiling technologies makes it possible to obtain detailed information about the effects of toxicants, pollutants, nutrients, drugs, and physical stressors on a multiomics scale. These data enable assessment of perturbations at the mechanism and system levels, providing a foundation for advances in pharmacology and toxicology/systems toxicology.

While mechanistic toxicology studies have historically taken a reductionist approach for determining

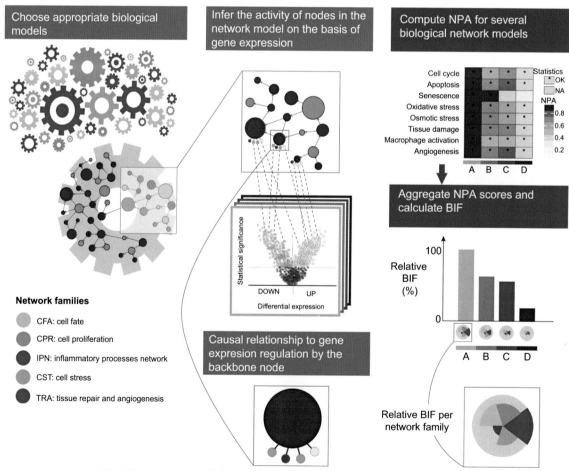

FIG. 9.6 Network perturbation amplitude (NPA) and biological impact factor (BIF).

the precise modes of action of single substances, systems toxicology allows a better understanding of the often multimechanistic effects of complex chemical mixtures. Indeed, assessing the effects of complex mixtures, such as CS and ENDP aerosols, presents numerous challenges, many of which can be addressed through systems toxicology (Iskandar et al., 2019; Szostak et al., 2020; Martin et al., 2016).

As toxicology is moving away from analysis of single targets and toward analysis of adverse outcomes at the pathway level (Leist et al., 2017), the risk assessment community has started to appreciate that the effects of many chemicals converge on similar biological pathways. Therefore, assessment of health effects by examining disrupted pathways will become an increasingly pertinent paradigm. Systems toxicology not only enables identification of AOPs and specific pathways of toxicity but also provides tools for comparing the effects of different exposures on these AOPs (Sturla et al., 2014).

As the AOP framework is being applied across the field of toxicology, pathways of toxicity are emerging that mirror networks from omics-scale systems toxicology experiments (Bell et al., 2016). The AOP framework provides a pertinent bridge between pathways at the molecular and cellular levels and topical toxicities such as skin sensitization. AOPs offer the possibility of regulatory hazard characterization for substances while providing the opportunity to exploit systems toxicology data and endpoints.

International agencies such as the Interagency Coordinating Committee on the Validation of Alternative Methods are promoting the use of new approaches including 21st century systems science for public health protection (ICCVAM, 2018). Health Canada has started to include HTS assays and omics approaches in the toolbox for screening substances of toxicological concern (Carthew et al., 2009). The use of bioactivity—exposure ratios, representing the ratio between doses that demonstrate bioactivity in high-throughput in vitro assays and predicted human exposure levels, is being explored for decision-making. The EU-ToxRisk Initiative 2019 set a mandate for a paradigm shift in toxicological testing toward a comprehensive mechanistic understanding of chemicals on the basis of experimental design spaces, systems toxicology, and human cell—based test systems to deliver testing strategies that enable reliable, animal-free hazard and risk assessment of chemicals (Daneshian et al., 2016).

Outside the field of toxicology, comprehensive systems science—based approaches provide pertinent data at the individual level for precision medicine, at the group level for clinical trials, and, ultimately, at the population level for public health.

REFERENCES

Addona, T.A., Abbatiello, S.E., Schilling, B., Skates, S.J., Mani, D., Bunk, D.M., Spiegelman, C.H., Zimmerman, L.J., Ham, A.-J.L., Keshishian, H., 2009. Multi-site assessment of the precision and reproducibility of multiple reaction monitoring—based measurements of proteins in plasma. Nat. Biotechnol. 27, 633—641.

Aebersold, R., Burlingame, A.L., Bradshaw, R.A., 2013. Western blots versus selected reaction monitoring assays: time to turn the tables? Mol. Cell. Proteom. 12, 2381—2382.

Alexandrov, L.B., Ju, Y.S., Haase, K., van Loo, P., Martincorena, I., Nik-Zainal, S., Totoki, Y., Fujimoto, A., Nakagawa, H., Shibata, T., 2016. Mutational signatures associated with tobacco smoking in human cancer. Science 354, 618—622.

Araki, Y., Mimura, T., 2017. The histone modification code in the pathogenesis of autoimmune diseases. Mediat. Inflamm. 2017.

Baker, M., 2015. Blame it on the antibodies. Nature 521, 274—276.

Barabasi, A.-L., Oltvai, Z.N., 2004. Network biology: understanding the cell's functional organization. Nat. Rev. Genet. 5, 101—113.

Belcastro, V., Cano, S., Marescotti, D., Acali, S., Poussin, C., Gonzalez-Suarez, I., Martin, F., Bonjour, F., Ivanov, N.V., Peitsch, M.C., 2019. GladiaTOX: GLobal assessment of dose-IndicAtor in TOXicology. Bioinformatics 35, 4190—4192.

Bell, S.M., Angrish, M.M., Wood, C.E., Edwards, S.W., 2016. Integrating publicly available data to generate computationally predicted adverse outcome pathways for fatty liver. Toxicol. Sci. 150, 510—520.

Boué, S., Talikka, M., Westra, J.W., Hayes, W., Di Fabio, A., Park, J., Schlage, W.K., Sewer, A., Fields, B., Ansari, S., 2015. Causal biological network database: a comprehensive platform of causal biological network models focused on the pulmonary and vascular systems. Database 2015.

Bruderer, R., Bernhardt, O.M., Gandhi, T., Miladinović, S.M., Cheng, L.-Y., Messner, S., Ehrenberger, T., Zanotelli, V., Butscheid, Y., Escher, C., 2015. Extending the limits of quantitative proteome profiling with data-independent acquisition and application to acetaminophen-treated three-dimensional liver microtissues. Mol. Cell. Proteom. 14, 1400—1410.

Buenrostro, J.D., Wu, B., Chang, H.Y., Greenleaf, W.J., 2015. ATAC-seq: a method for assaying chromatin accessibility genome-wide. Curr. Protoc. Mol. Biol. 109, 21.29.1—21.29.9.

Cai, M., Dai, S., Chen, W., Xia, C., Lu, L., Dai, S., Qi, J., Wang, M., Wang, M., Zhou, L., 2017. Environmental factors, seven GWAS-identified susceptibility loci, and risk of gastric cancer and its precursors in a Chinese population. Cancer Med. 6, 708—720.

Carr, S.A., Abbatiello, S.E., Ackermann, B.L., Borchers, C., Domon, B., Deutsch, E.W., Grant, R.P., Hoofnagle, A.N., Hüttenhain, R., Koomen, J.M., 2014. Targeted peptide measurements in biology and medicine: best practices for mass spectrometry-based assay development using a fit-for-purpose approach. Mol. Cell. Proteom. 13, 907–917.

Carthew, P., Clapp, C., Gutsell, S., 2009. Exposure based waiving: the application of the toxicological threshold of concern (TTC) to inhalation exposure for aerosol ingredients in consumer products. Food Chem. Toxicol. 47, 1287–1295.

Chai, L., Ding, C., Li, J., Yang, Z., Shi, Y., 2019. Multi-omics response of *Pannonibacter phragmitetus* BB to hexavalent chromium. Environ. Pollut. 249, 63–73.

Chauhan, R., Awasthi, S., Indoliya, Y., Chauhan, A.S., Mishra, S., Agrawal, L., Srivastava, S., Dwivedi, S., Singh, P.C., Mallick, S., Chauhan, P.S., Pande, V., Chakrabarty, D., Tripathi, R.D., 2020. Transcriptome and proteome analyses reveal selenium mediated amelioration of arsenic toxicity in rice (*Oryza sativa* L.). J. Hazard Mater. 390, 122122.

Choukrallah, M.-A., Sewer, A., Talikka, M., Sierro, N., Peitsch, M.C., Hoeng, J., Ivanov, N.V., 2018. Epigenomics in tobacco risk assessment: opportunities for integrated new approaches. Curr. Opin. Toxicol. 11, 67–83.

Choukrallah, M.-A., Sierro, N., Martin, F., Baumer, K., Thomas, J., Ouadi, S., Hoeng, J., Peitsch, M.C., Ivanov, N.V., 2019. Tobacco Heating System 2.2 has a limited impact on DNA methylation of candidate enhancers in mouse lung compared with cigarette smoke. Food Chem. Toxicol. 123, 501–510.

Ciaccio, M.F., Wagner, J.P., Chuu, C.P., Lauffenburger, D.A., Jones, R.B., 2010. Systems analysis of EGF receptor signaling dynamics with microwestern arrays. Nat. Methods 7, 148–155.

Clippinger, A.J., Allen, D., Behrsing, H., Berube, K.A., Bolger, M.B., Casey, W., Delorme, M., Gaca, M., Gehen, S.C., Glover, K., Hayden, P., Hinderliter, P., Hotchkiss, J.A., Iskandar, A., Keyser, B., Luettich, K., MA-Hock, L., Maione, A.G., Makena, P., Melbourne, J., Milchak, L., Ng, S.P., Paini, A., Page, K., Patlewicz, G., Prieto, P., Raabe, H., Reinke, E.N., Roper, C., Rose, J., Sharma, M., Spoo, W., Thorne, P.S., Wilson, D.M., Jarabek, A.M., 2018. Pathway-based predictive approaches for non-animal assessment of acute inhalation toxicity. Toxicol. In Vitro 52, 131–145.

Committee on Toxicity Testing and Assessment of Environmental Agents, 2007. Toxicity testing in the twenty-first century: a vision and a strategy. In: Council, N.R. (Ed.). National Academies Press, Washington, DC.

Cui, X., Churchill, G.A., 2003. Statistical tests for differential expression in cDNA microarray experiments. Genome Biol. 4, 210.

Daneshian, M., Kamp, H., Hengstler, J., Leist, M., van de Water, B., 2016. Highlight Report: Launch of a Large Integrated European in vitro Toxicology Project: EU-ToxRisk. Springer.

Dekkers, S., Williams, T.D., Zhang, J., Zhou, J.A., Vandebriel, R., De La Fonteyne, L.J., Gremmer, E., He, S., Guggenheim, E., Lynch, I., 2018. Multi-omics approaches confirm metal ions mediate the main toxicological pathways of metal-bearing nanoparticles in lung epithelial A549 cells. Environ. Sci. J. Integr. Environ. Res.: Nano 5, 1506–1517.

Dellafiora, L., Dall'Asta, C., 2017. Forthcoming challenges in mycotoxins toxicology research for safer food-a need for multi-omics approach. Toxins 9, 18.

Dunbar, S.A., Hoffmeyer, M.R., 2013. Microsphere-based multiplex immunoassays: development and applications using Luminex® xMAP® technology. In: The Immunoassay Handbook: Theory and Applications of Ligand Binding, ELISA and Related Techniques, vol. 157.

Dunn, M.R., Jimenez, R.M., Chaput, J.C., 2017. Analysis of aptamer discovery and technology. Nat. Rev. Chem. 1, 1–16.

Edfors, F., Hober, A., Linderbäck, K., Maddalo, G., Azimi, A., Sivertsson, Å., Tegel, H., Hober, S., Szigyarto, C.A.-K., Fagerberg, L., 2018. Enhanced validation of antibodies for research applications. Nat. Commun. 9, 1–10.

Egelhofer, T.A., Minoda, A., Klugman, S., Lee, K., Kolasinska-Zwierz, P., Alekseyenko, A.A., Cheung, M.-S., Day, D.S., Gadel, S., Gorchakov, A.A., 2011. An assessment of histone-modification antibody quality. Nat. Struct. Mol. Biol. 18, 91–93.

Ekroos, K., 2012. Lipidomics perspective: from molecular lipidomics to validated clinical diagnostics. Lipidom. Technol. Appl. 1–19.

Ekroos, K., Lavrynenko, O., Titz, B., Pater, C., Hoeng, J., Ivanov, N.V., 2020. Lipid-based biomarkers for Cvd, Copd, and aging—a translational perspective. Prog. Lipid Res. 101030.

Eliuk, S., Makarov, A., 2015. Evolution of Orbitrap mass spectrometry instrumentation. Annu. Rev. Anal. Chem. 8, 61–80.

Faner, R., Cruz, T., Casserras, T., Lopez-Giraldo, A., Noell, G., Coca, I., TAL-Singer, R., Miller, B., Rodriguez-Roisin, R., Spira, A., Kalko, S.G., Agusti, A., 2016. Network analysis of lung transcriptomics reveals a distinct B-cell signature in emphysema. Am. J. Respir. Crit. Care Med. 193, 1242–1253.

Filer, D.L., Kothiya, P., Setzer, R.W., Judson, R.S., Martin, M.T., 2017. tcpl: the ToxCast pipeline for high-throughput screening data. Bioinformatics 33, 618–620.

Fluck, J., Madan, S., Ansari, S., Karki, R., Rastegar-Mojarad, M., Catlett, N.L., Hayes, W., Szostak, J., Hoeng, J., Peitsch, M., 2016. Training and evaluation corpora for the extraction of causal relationships encoded in biological expression language (BEL). Database 2016.

Frommer, M., Mcdonald, L.E., Millar, D.S., Collis, C.M., Watt, F., Grigg, G.W., Molloy, P.L., Paul, C.L., 1992. A genomic sequencing protocol that yields a positive display of 5-methylcytosine residues in individual DNA strands. Proc. Natl. Acad. Sci. U S A 89, 1827–1831.

Gage, S.H., Smith, G.D., Ware, J.J., Flint, J., Munafo, M.R., 2016. G = E: what GWAS can tell us about the environment. PLoS Genet. 12.

Gillet, L.C., Navarro, P., Tate, S., Röst, H., Selevsek, N., Reiter, L., Bonner, R., Aebersold, R., 2012. Targeted data extraction of the MS/MS spectra generated by data-independent acquisition: a new concept for consistent and accurate proteome analysis. Mol. Cell. Proteom. 11. O111. 016717.

Gillette, M.A., Carr, S.A., 2013. Quantitative analysis of peptides and proteins in biomedicine by targeted mass spectrometry. Nat. Methods 10, 28–34.

Gonzalez-Suarez, I., Marescotti, D., Martin, F., Scotti, E., Guedj, E., Acali, S., Dulize, R., Baumer, K., Peric, D., Frentzel, S., 2017. In vitro systems toxicology assessment of nonflavored e-cigarette liquids in primary lung epithelial cells. Appl. In Vitro Toxicol. 3, 41–55.

Gormley, P., Winsvold, B.S., Nyholt, D.R., Kallela, M., Chasman, D.I., Palotie, A., 2016. Migraine genetics: from genome-wide association studies to translational insights. Genome Med. 8, 86.

Gross, R.W., Han, X., 2007. Lipidomics in diabetes and the metabolic syndrome. Methods Enzymol. 433, 73–90.

Hartung, T., 2010. Lessons learned from alternative methods and their validation for a new toxicology in the 21st century. J. Toxicol. Environ. Health B Crit. Rev. 13, 277–290.

Hartung, T., Fitzgerald, R.E., Jennings, P., Mirams, G.R., Peitsch, M.C., Rostami-Hodjegan, A., Shah, I., Wilks, M.F., Sturla, S.J., 2017. Systems toxicology: real world applications and opportunities. Chem. Res. Toxicol. 30, 870–882.

Heiskanen, L.A., Suoniemi, M., Ta, H.X., Tarasov, K., Ekroos, K., 2013. Long-term performance and stability of molecular shotgun lipidomic analysis of human plasma samples. Anal. Chem. 85, 8757–8763.

Hennon, G.M.M., Dyhrman, S.T., 2020. Progress and promise of omics for predicting the impacts of climate change on harmful algal blooms. Harmful Algae 91, 101587.

Hoeng, J., Deehan, R., Pratt, D., Martin, F., Sewer, A., Thomson, T.M., Drubin, D.A., Waters, C.A., de Graaf, D., Peitsch, M.C., 2012. A network-based approach to quantifying the impact of biologically active substances. Drug Discov. Today 17, 413–418.

Hoeng, J., Peitsch, M.C., 2015. Computational Systems Toxicology. Springer.

Hoeng, J., Talikka, M., Martin, F., Ansari, S., Drubin, D., Elamin, A., Gebel, S., Ivanov, N.V., Deehan, R., Kogel, U., 2014. Toxicopanomics: applications of genomics, transcriptomics, proteomics, and lipidomics in predictive mechanistic toxicology. In: Hayes' Principles and Methods of Toxicology. CRC Press.

Holmgren, G., Sartipy, P., Andersson, C.X., Lindahl, A., Synnergren, J., 2018. Expression profiling of human pluripotent stem cell-derived cardiomyocytes exposed to doxorubicin-integration and visualization of multi-omics data. Toxicol. Sci. 163, 182–195.

Huang, D.W., Sherman, B.T., Lempicki, R.A., 2009. Systematic and integrative analysis of large gene lists using DAVID bioinformatics resources. Nat. Protoc. 4, 44–57. https://doi.org/10.1038/nprot.2008.211.

ICCVAM, 2018. A Strategic Roadmap for Establishing New Approaches to Evaluate the Safety of Chemicals and Medical Products in the United States. National Toxicology Program. National Institute of Environmental Health.

Iskandar, A.R., Gonzalez-Suarez, I., Majeed, S., Marescotti, D., Sewer, A., Xiang, Y., Leroy, P., Guedj, E., Mathis, C., Schaller, J.-P., 2016. A framework for in vitro systems toxicology assessment of e-liquids. Toxicol. Mech. Methods 26, 392–416.

Iskandar, A.R., Zanetti, F., Marescotti, D., Titz, B., Sewer, A., Kondylis, A., Leroy, P., Belcastro, V., Torres, L.O., Acali, S., 2019. Application of a multi-layer systems toxicology framework for in vitro assessment of the biological effects of Classic Tobacco e-liquid and its corresponding aerosol using an e-cigarette device with MESH™ technology. Arch. Toxicol. 93, 3229–3247.

Joehanes, R., Just, A.C., Marioni, R.E., Pilling, L.C., Reynolds, L.M., Mandaviya, P.R., Guan, W., Xu, T., Elks, C.E., Aslibekyan, S., 2016. Epigenetic signatures of cigarette smoking. Circ. Cardiovasc. Genet. 9, 436–447.

Joshi-Tope, G., Gillespie, M., Vastrik, I., D'Eustachio, P., Schmidt, E., de Bono, B., Jassal, B., Gopinath, G.R., Wu, G.R., Matthews, L., Lewis, S., Birney, E., Stein, L., 2005. Reactome: a knowledgebase of biological pathways. Nucleic Acids Res. 33, D428–D432. https://doi.org/10.1093/nar/gki072.

Jung, H.R., Sylvanne, T., Koistinen, K.M., Tarasov, K., Kauhanen, D., Ekroos, K., 2011. High throughput quantitative molecular lipidomics. Biochim. Biophys. Acta 1811, 925–934.

Kanehisa, M., 2000. KEGG: Kyoto Encyclopedia of Genes and Genomes. Nucleic Acids Res. 28, 27–30. https://doi.org/10.1093/nar/28.1.27.

Kenche, H., Ye, Z.W., Vedagiri, K., Richards, D.M., Gao, X.H., Tew, K.D., Townsend, D.M., Blumental-Perry, A., 2016. Adverse outcomes associated with cigarette smoke radicals related to damage to protein-disulfide isomerase. J. Biol. Chem. 291, 4763–4778.

Khatri, P., Sirota, M., Butte, A.J., 2012. Ten years of pathway analysis: current approaches and outstanding challenges. PLoS Comput. Biol. 8.

Kogel, U., Titz, B., Schlage, W.K., Nury, C., Martin, F., Oviedo, A., Lebrun, S., Elamin, A., Guedj, E., Trivedi, K., 2016. Evaluation of the tobacco heating system 2.2. Part 7: systems toxicological assessment of a mentholated version revealed reduced cellular and molecular exposure effects compared with mentholated and non-mentholated cigarette smoke. Regul. Toxicol. Pharmacol. 81, S123–S138.

Kogelman, L.J., Esserlind, A.-L., Christensen, A.F., Awasthi, S., Ripke, S., Ingason, A., Davidsson, O.B., Erikstrup, C., Hjalgrim, H., Ullum, H., 2019. Migraine polygenic risk score associates with efficacy of migraine-specific drugs. Neurol. Genet. 5, e364.

Kreutz, C., Timmer, J., 2009. Systems biology: experimental design. FEBS J. 276, 923–942.

Krewski, D., Acosta Jr., D., Andersen, M., Anderson, H., Bailar III, J.C., Boekelheide, K., Brent, R., Charnley, G.,

Cheung, V.G., Green Jr., S., 2010. Toxicity testing in the 21st century: a vision and a strategy. J. Toxicol. Environ. Health, Part B 13, 51−138.

Lea, I.A., Gong, H., Paleja, A., Rashid, A., Fostel, J., 2017. CEBS: a comprehensive annotated database of toxicological data. Nucleic Acids Res. 45, D964−D971.

Lee, S.H., Yun, Y., Kim, S.J., Lee, E.-J., Chang, Y., Ryu, S., Shin, H., Kim, H.-L., Kim, H.-N., Lee, J.H., 2018. Association between cigarette smoking status and composition of gut microbiota: population-based cross-sectional study. J. Clin. Med. 7, 282.

Lei, H., Oh, S.P., Okano, M., Juttermann, R., Goss, K.A., Jaenisch, R., Li, E., 1996. De novo DNA cytosine methyltransferase activities in mouse embryonic stem cells. Development 122, 3195−3205.

Leist, M., Ghallab, A., Graepel, R., Marchan, R., Hassan, R., Bennekou, S.H., Limonciel, A., Vinken, M., Schildknecht, S., Waldmann, T., 2017. Adverse outcome pathways: opportunities, limitations and open questions. Arch. Toxicol. 91, 3477−3505.

Leshchiner, I., Alexa, K., Kelsey, P., Adzhubei, I., Austin-Tse, C.A., Cooney, J.D., Anderson, H., King, M.J., Stottmann, R.W., Garnaas, M.K., 2012. Mutation mapping and identification by whole-genome sequencing. Genome Res. 22, 1541−1548.

Lesur, A., Domon, B., 2015. Advances in high-resolution accurate mass spectrometry application to targeted proteomics. Proteomics 15, 880−890.

Li, W., Hu, J., Adebali, O., Adar, S., Yang, Y., Chiou, Y.-Y., Sancar, A., 2017. Human genome-wide repair map of DNA damage caused by the cigarette smoke carcinogen benzo [a] pyrene. Proc. Natl. Acad. Sci. U St A 114, 6752−6757.

Lopes, C.T., Franz, M., Kazi, F., Donaldson, S.L., Morris, Q., Bader, G.D., 2010. Cytoscape Web: an interactive web-based network browser. Bioinformatics 26, 2347−2348.

Lowe, F.J., Luettich, K., Talikka, M., Hoang, V., Haswell, L.E., Hoeng, J., Gaca, M.D., 2017. Development of an adverse outcome pathway for the onset of hypertension by oxidative stress-mediated perturbation of endothelial nitric oxide bioavailability. Appl. In Vitro Toxicol. 3, 131−148.

Ma, B., Stepanov, I., Hecht, S.S., 2019. Recent studies on DNA adducts resulting from human exposure to tobacco smoke. Toxics 7, 16.

Marescotti, D., Mathis, C., Belcastro, V., Leroy, P., Acali, S., Martin, F., Dulize, R., Bornand, D., Peric, D., Guedj, E., 2020. Systems toxicology assessment of a representative e-liquid formulation using human primary bronchial epithelial cells. Toxicol. Rep. 7, 67−80.

Marescotti, D., Suarez, I.G., Acali, S., Johne, S., Laurent, A., Frentzel, S., Hoeng, J., Peitsch, M.C., 2016. High content screening analysis to evaluate the toxicological effects of harmful and potentially harmful constituents (HPHC). JoVE (J. Vis. Exp.) e53987.

Martin, F., Sewer, A., Talikka, M., Xiang, Y., Hoeng, J., Peitsch, M.C., 2014. Quantification of biological network perturbations for mechanistic insight and diagnostics using two-layer causal models. BMC Bioinf. 15, 238.

Martin, F., Talikka, M., Ivanov, N.V., Haziza, C., Hoeng, J., Peitsch, M.C., 2016. Evaluation of the tobacco heating system 2.2. Part 9: application of systems pharmacology to identify exposure response markers in peripheral blood of smokers switching to THS2.2. Regul. Toxicol. Pharmacol. 81, S151−S157.

Mccall, M.N., Bolstad, B.M., Irizarry, R.A., 2010. Frozen robust multiarray analysis (fRMA). Biostatistics 11, 242−253.

Mi, H., Muruganujan, A., Ebert, D., Huang, X., Thomas, P.D., 2019. PANTHER version 14: more genomes, a new PANTHER GO-slim and improvements in enrichment analysis tools. Nucleic Acids Res. 47, D419−D426. https://doi.org/10.1093/nar/gky1038.

Morissette, M.C., Shen, P., Thayaparan, D., Stampfli, M.R., 2015. Disruption of pulmonary lipid homeostasis drives cigarette smoke-induced lung inflammation in mice. Eur. Respir. J. 46, 1451−1460.

Morita, M., Kuba, K., Ichikawa, A., Nakayama, M., Katahira, J., Iwamoto, R., Watanebe, T., Sakabe, S., Daidoji, T., Nakamura, S., Kadowaki, A., Ohto, T., Nakanishi, H., Taguchi, R., Nakaya, T., Murakami, M., Yoneda, Y., Arai, H., Kawaoka, Y., Penninger, J.M., Arita, M., Imai, Y., 2013. The lipid mediator protectin D1 inhibits influenza virus replication and improves severe influenza. Cell 153, 112−125.

National Toxicology Program (NTP), 2004. A National Toxicology Program for the 21st Century: a Roadmap to Achieve the NTP Vision. National Toxicology Program/National Institute of Environmental Health Sciences.

Nishimura, D., 2001. BioCarta. Biotech Software & Internet Rep. 2, 117−120. https://doi.org/10.1089/152791601750294344.

Pfeifer, G.P., Denissenko, M.F., Olivier, M., Tretyakova, N., Hecht, S.S., Hainaut, P., 2002. Tobacco smoke carcinogens, DNA damage and p53 mutations in smoking-associated cancers. Oncogene 21, 7435−7451.

Phillips, B., Veljkovic, E., Boué, S., Schlage, W.K., Vuillaume, G., Martin, F., Titz, B., Leroy, P., Buettner, A., Elamin, A., 2016a. An 8-month systems toxicology inhalation/cessation study in Apoe$^{-/-}$ mice to investigate cardiovascular and respiratory exposure effects of a candidate modified risk tobacco product, THS 2.2, compared with conventional cigarettes. Toxicol. Sci. 149, 411−432.

Phillips, B., Veljkovic, E., Boue, S., Schlage, W.K., Vuillaume, G., Martin, F., Titz, B., Leroy, P., Buettner, A., Elamin, A., Oviedo, A., Cabanski, M., de Leon, H., Guedj, E., Schneider, T., Talikka, M., Ivanov, N.V., Vanscheeuwijck, P., Peitsch, M.C., Hoeng, J., 2016b. An 8-month systems toxicology inhalation/cessation study in Apoe$^{-/-}$ mice to investigate cardiovascular and respiratory exposure effects of a candidate modified risk tobacco product, THS 2.2, compared with conventional cigarettes. Toxicol. Sci. 149, 411−432.

Rahman, I., van Schadewijk, A.A., Crowther, A.J., Hiemstra, P.S., Stolk, J., Macnee, W., de Boer, W.I., 2002. 4-Hydroxy-2-nonenal, a specific lipid peroxidation product, is elevated in lungs of patients with chronic obstructive pulmonary disease. Am. J. Respir. Crit. Care Med. 166, 490−495.

Rajalakshmi, T., Aravindhababu, N., Shanmugam, K., Masthan, K., 2015. DNA adducts-chemical addons. J. Pharm. BioAllied Sci. 7.

Ramaiah, S.K., 2007. A toxicologist guide to the diagnostic interpretation of hepatic biochemical parameters. Food Chem. Toxicol. 45, 1551−1557.

Roberts, J.S., Ostergren, J., 2013. Direct-to-consumer genetic testing and personal genomics services: a review of recent empirical studies. Curr. Genet. Med. Rep. 1, 182−200.

Rovida, C., Alepee, N., Api, A.M., Basketter, D.A., Bois, F.Y., Caloni, F., Corsini, E., Daneshian, M., Eskes, C., Ezendam, J., Fuchs, H., Hayden, P., Hegele-Hartung, C., Hoffmann, S., Hubesch, B., Jacobs, M.N., Jaworska, J., Kleensang, A., Kleinstreuer, N., Lalko, J., Landsiedel, R., Lebreux, F., Luechtefeld, T., Locatelli, M., Mehling, A., Natsch, A., Pitchford, J.W., Prater, D., Prieto, P., Schepky, A., Schuurmann, G., Smirnova, L., Toole, C., van Vliet, E., Weisensee, D., Hartung, T., 2015a. Integrated testing strategies (ITS) for safety assessment. ALTEX 32, 25−40.

Rovida, C., Asakura, S., Daneshian, M., Hofman-Huether, H., Leist, M., Meunier, L., Reif, D., Rossi, A., Schmutz, M., Valentin, J.P., Zurlo, J., Hartung, T., 2015b. Toxicity testing in the 21st century beyond environmental chemicals. ALTEX 32, 171−181.

Santolini, M., Barabási, A.-L., 2018. Predicting perturbation patterns from the topology of biological networks. Proc. Natl. Acad. Sci. U S A 115, E6375−E6383.

Sauer, J.M., Kleensang, A., Peitsch, M.C., Hayes, A.W., 2016. Advancing risk assessment through the application of systems toxicology. Toxicol. Res. 32, 5−8.

Schmidt, D., Wilson, M.D., Spyrou, C., Brown, G.D., Hadfield, J., Odom, D.T., 2009. ChIP-seq: using high-throughput sequencing to discover protein−DNA interactions. Methods 48, 240−248.

Shojaie, A., Michailidis, G., 2009. Analysis of gene sets based on the underlying regulatory network. J. Comput. Biol. 16, 407−426. https://doi.org/10.1089/cmb.2008.0081.

Shreiner, A.B., Kao, J.Y., Young, V.B., 2015. The gut microbiome in health and in disease. Curr. Opin. Gastroenterol. 31, 69.

Simoes, T., Novais, S.C., Natal-da-Luz, T., Devreese, B., de Boer, T., Roelofs, D., Sousa, J.P., van Straalen, N.M., Lemos, M.F.L., 2019. Using time-lapse omics correlations to integrate toxicological pathways of a formulated fungicide in a soil invertebrate. Environ. Pollut. 246, 845−854.

Sturla, S.J., Boobis, A.R., Fitzgerald, R.E., Hoeng, J., Kavlock, R.J., Schirmer, K., Whelan, M., Wilks, M.F., Peitsch, M.C., 2014. Systems toxicology: from basic research to risk assessment. Chem. Res. Toxicol. 27, 314−329.

Subramanian, A., Tamayo, P., Mootha, V.K., Mukherjee, S., Ebert, B.L., Gillette, M.A., Paulovich, A., Pomeroy, S.L., Golub, T.R., Lander, E.S., Mesirov, J.P., 2005. Gene set enrichment analysis: a knowledge-based approach for interpreting genome-wide expression profiles. Proc. Natl. Acad. Sci. U.S.A. 102, 15545−15550. https://doi.org/10.1073/pnas.0506580102.

Sutandy, F., Qian, J., Chen, C.S., Zhu, H., 2013. Overview of protein microarrays. Curr. Protoc. Protein sci. 27 (1), 1−27.1. 16.

Szostak, J., Wong, E.T., Titz, B., Lee, T., Wong, S.K., Low, T., Lee, K.M., Zhang, J., Kumar, A., Schlage, W.K., 2020. A 6-month systems toxicology inhalation study in ApoE$^{-/-}$ mice demonstrates reduced cardiovascular effects of E-vapor aerosols compared with cigarette smoke. Am. J. Physiol. Heart Circ. Physiol. 318, H604−H631.

Talikka, M., Boue, S., Schlage, W.K., 2015. Causal biological network database: a comprehensive platform of causal biological network models focused on the pulmonary and vascular systems. In: Computational Systems Toxicology. Springer.

Thompson, A., Schäfer, J., Kuhn, K., Kienle, S., Schwarz, J., Schmidt, G., Neumann, T., Hamon, C., 2003. Tandem mass tags: a novel quantification strategy for comparative analysis of complex protein mixtures by MS/MS. Anal. Chem. 75, 1895−1904.

Thomson, T.M., Sewer, A., Martin, F., Belcastro, V., Frushour, B.P., Gebel, S., Park, J., Schlage, W.K., Talikka, M., Vasilyev, D.M., 2013. Quantitative assessment of biological impact using transcriptomic data and mechanistic network models. Toxicol. Appl. Pharmacol. 272, 863−878.

Tice, R., Fostel, J., Smith, C., Witt, K., Freedman, J., Portier, C., Dearry, A., Bucher, J., 2007. The National Toxicology Program high throughput screening initiative: current status and future directions. Toxicologist 46, 151.

Titz, B., Boué, S., Phillips, B., Talikka, M., Vihervaara, T., Schneider, T., Nury, C., Elamin, A., Guedj, E., Peck, M.J., 2016a. Effects of cigarette smoke, cessation, and switching to two heat-not-burn tobacco products on lung lipid metabolism in C57BL/6 and Apoe$^{-/-}$ mice—an integrative systems toxicology analysis. Toxicol. Sci. 149, 441−457.

Titz, B., Boue, S., Phillips, B., Talikka, M., Vihervaara, T., Schneider, T., Nury, C., Elamin, A., Guedj, E., Peck, M.J., Schlage, W.K., Cabanski, M., Leroy, P., Vuillaume, G., Martin, F., Ivanov, N.V., Veljkovic, E., Ekroos, K., Laaksonen, R., Vanscheeuwijck, P., Peitsch, M.C., Hoeng, J., 2016b. Effects of cigarette smoke, cessation, and switching to two heat-not-burn tobacco products on lung lipid metabolism in C57BL/6 and Apoe$^{-/-}$ mice-an integrative systems toxicology analysis. Toxicol. Sci. 149, 441−457.

Titz, B., Elamin, A., Martin, F., Schneider, T., Dijon, S., Ivanov, N.V., Hoeng, J., Peitsch, M.C., 2014. Proteomics for systems toxicology. Comput. Struct. Biotechnol. J. 11, 73−90.

Titz, B., Schneider, T., Elamin, A., Martin, F., Dijon, S., Ivanov, N., Hoeng, J., Peitsch, M., 2015. Analysis of proteomic data for toxicological applications. In: Computational Systems Toxicology. Humana Press.

Titz, B., Szostak, J., Sewer, A., Phillips, B., Nury, C., Schneider, T., Dijon, S., Lavrynenko, O., Elamin, A., Guedj, E., 2020. Multi-omics systems toxicology study of mouse lung assessing the effects of aerosols from two heat-not-burn tobacco products and cigarette smoke. Comput. Struct. Biotechnol. J. 18, 1056−1073.

Tyanova, S., Temu, T., Cox, J., 2016. The MaxQuant computational platform for mass spectrometry-based shotgun proteomics. Nat. Protoc. 11, 2301.

U.S.Congress, 2016. Frank R. Lautenberg Chemical Safety for the 21st Century Act. 114th Congress.

Usaj, M.M., Styles, E.B., Verster, A.J., Friesen, H., Boone, C., Andrews, B.J., 2016. High-content screening for quantitative cell biology. Trends Cell Biol. 26, 598–611.

van Meer, G., 2005. Cellular lipidomics. EMBO J. 24, 3159–3165.

van Meer, G., Voelker, D.R., Feigenson, G.W., 2008. Membrane lipids: where they are and how they behave. Nat. Rev. Mol. Cell Biol. 9, 112–124.

Vaughn, C.M., Selby, C.P., Yang, Y., Hsu, D.S., Sancar, A., 2020. Genome-wide single-nucleotide resolution of oxaliplatin–DNA adduct repair in drug-sensitive and-resistant colorectal cancer cell lines. J. Biol. Chem. 013347 jbc. RA120.

Vicari, K., 2013. Targeted proteomics. Nat. Methods 10, 19.

Vulimiri, S.V., Misra, M., Hamm, J.T., Mitchell, M., Berger, A., 2009. Effects of mainstream cigarette smoke on the global metabolome of human lung epithelial cells. Chem. Res. Toxicol. 22, 492–503.

Wang, J., Zibetti, C., Shang, P., Sripathi, S.R., Zhang, P., Cano, M., Hoang, T., Xia, S., Ji, H., Merbs, S.L., 2018. ATAC-Seq analysis reveals a widespread decrease of chromatin accessibility in age-related macular degeneration. Nat. Commun. 9, 1–13.

Wang, P., Ng, Q.X., Zhang, B., Wei, Z., Hassan, M., He, Y., Ong, C.N., 2019. Employing multi-omics to elucidate the hormetic response against oxidative stress exerted by nC60 on *Daphnia pulex*. Environ. Pollut. 251, 22–29.

Weir, J.M., Wong, G., Barlow, C.K., Greeve, M.A., Kowalczyk, A., Almasy, L., Comuzzie, A.G., Mahaney, M.C., Jowett, J.B.M., Shaw, J., Curran, J.E., Blangero, J., Meikle, P.J., 2013. Plasma lipid profiling in a large population-based cohort. JLR (J. Lipid Res.) 54, 2898–2908.

Wenk, M.R., 2006. Lipidomics of host–pathogen interactions. FEBS Lett. 580, 5541–5551.

Wiese, S., Reidegeld, K.A., Meyer, H.E., Warscheid, B., 2007. Protein labeling by iTRAQ: a new tool for quantitative mass spectrometry in proteome research. Proteomics 7, 340–350.

Wilmes, A., Bielow, C., Ranninger, C., Bellwon, P., Aschauer, L., Limonciel, A., Chassaigne, H., Kristl, T., Aiche, S., Huber, C.G., Guillou, C., Hewitt, P., Leonard, M.O., Dekant, W., Bois, F., Jennings, P., 2015. Mechanism of cisplatin proximal tubule toxicity revealed by integrating transcriptomics, proteomics, metabolomics and biokinetics. Toxicol. In Vitro 30, 117–127.

Xia, M., Huang, R., Witt, K.L., Southall, N., Fostel, J., Cho, M.-H., Jadhav, A., Smith, C.S., Inglese, J., Portier, C.J., 2008. Compound cytotoxicity profiling using quantitative high-throughput screening. Environ. Health Perspect. 116, 284–291.

Xu, S., Chen, Y., Ma, Y., Liu, T., Zhao, M., Wang, Z., Zhao, L., 2019. Lipidomic profiling reveals disruption of lipid metabolism in valproic acid-induced hepatotoxicity. Front. Pharmacol. 10, 819.

Zanetti, F., Titz, B., Sewer, A., lo Sasso, G., Scotti, E., Schlage, W.K., Mathis, C., Leroy, P., Majeed, S., Torres, L.O., Keppler, B.R., Elamin, A., Trivedi, K., Guedj, E., Martin, F., Frentzel, S., Ivanov, N.V., Peitsch, M.C., Hoeng, J., 2017. Comparative systems toxicology analysis of cigarette smoke and aerosol from a candidate modified risk tobacco product in organotypic human gingival epithelial cultures: a 3-day repeated exposure study. Food Chem. Toxicol. 101, 15–35.

Zingler, K., Heyse, S., 2008. High content screening—the next challenge: effective data mining and exploration. Drug Discov. World 27–34.

CHAPTER 10

Translational Models for ENDP Assessment

FLORIAN MARTIN • BJOERN TITZ • STEFAN FRENTZEL • WALTER K. SCHLAGE •
NIKOLAI V. IVANOV • JULIA HOENG • MANUEL C. PEITSCH

10.1 INTRODUCTION

The most prevalent smoking-related diseases—cardiovascular disease (CVD), chronic obstructive pulmonary disease (COPD), and lung cancer—generally occur after decades of smoking, and the reduction in risk following smoking cessation and, a fortiori, following switching to electronic nicotine delivery products (ENDPs) (Chapter 2) is slow. This means that clinical health outcome studies based on endpoints that aim to assess the reduction in smoking-related disease risk associated with switching from cigarette smoking to the use of ENDPs are difficult to execute in a premarket setting (Chapter 3). As a consequence, assessment of ENDPs has to rely heavily on nonclinical studies, which require experimental models that are collectively predictive of the risk reduction potential of ENDPs. Therefore, selecting adequate experimental test systems and translational markers is an essential step for ENDP assessment. Most importantly, these systems must be fit for purpose and as relevant as possible to human biology. Nonclinical assessment of ENDPs comprises both in vitro and in vivo studies, each carrying their own challenges that require close attention. Animal models of disease are particularly relevant for assessment of ENDPs, as they allow comparison of the effects of ENDP aerosols with those of cigarette smoke (CS) along the complete causal chain of events linking smoking to disease (CELSD) (Chapter 3) before long-term human studies are/can be performed (Chapter 21).

10.1.1 In Vitro Systems

The most relevant in vitro test systems are those derived from primary human cells that have not been immortalized. While this would be ideal, it is not always possible and, in many cases, immortalized or tumor-derived cell lines are the only available options. A key challenge with in vitro test systems is that they typically lack the natural complexity of a full-body organism and, therefore, reflect neither the structure and cellular composition of organ tissues nor their intercellular communications. It has recently been recognized that extrapolating outcomes from nonanimal approaches to adverse outcomes relevant to chronic tobacco exposure is challenging (Lauterstein et al., 2020). Therefore, in vitro toxicity testing is mainly focused on molecular mechanisms and cellular physiology endpoints. With the development of novel microphysiological and advanced organ-on-a-chip systems, increasingly complex in vitro systems relevant to human biology will become available. This will gradually reduce the need for animal models in toxicity testing (see below) and, hence, ENDP assessment.

10.1.2 In Vivo Systems

While animal models are essential for development of efficacious and safe drugs (Barré-Sinoussi and Montagutelli, 2015) as well as for toxicological assessment of consumer products, they are far from perfect (Bailey et al., 2014; Knight, 2007; Shanks et al., 2009; Wall and Shani, 2008) and have limited negative predictivity (lack of animal event predicting lack of human event) (Clark and Steger-Hartmann, 2018). Conversely, the positive predictivity of many animal models has been confirmed (Clark and Steger-Hartmann, 2018). Importantly, in the field of ENDP assessment, which aims to compare the effects of ENDP aerosols with those of CS and fresh air (Chapter 3), several animal models have consistently shown the adverse effects that CS causes in humans. In these models, CS not only negatively affects the same key mechanisms as those in human smokers but also leads to disease endpoints resembling human smoking–related diseases (see below). It is, however, important to select animal models for ENDP assessment on the basis of several criteria:

1. The animal model must show adverse biological effects in response to CS exposure. These effects must, to a large extent, reverse upon exposure cessation (Chapter 3).
2. The endpoints and biological mechanisms affected by CS exposure must be relevant to the effects observed in humans (Wall and Shani, 2008). This is also clearly stated in the guidance offered by the Organization for Economic Co-operation and Development (OECD, 2014).
3. The animal to human translatability of the model has to be understood, meaning that it is important to understand which aspects of human biology that are affected by CS are replicated in the animal model's biology.

10.1.3 General Aspects of Translatability in Toxicology

10.1.3.1 Conservation of biological processes and translatability

Humans and nonhuman animals are complex adaptive systems shaped by evolutionary processes. Acting on individual components and more complex processes, natural selection results in not only conserved but also divergent functions and traits (Greek and Rice, 2012). Moreover, biological systems are organized and function in a modular and hierarchical fashion. Thus, the question on translatability between species (or, more generally, biological test systems) needs to be phrased specifically, identifying shared functional modules and the right level in the functional hierarchy that allow for informative translation. In some cases, these shared modules are at the lowest level of biological organization—for example, genes, proteins, and other biomolecules. More frequently, these shared functional modules are mechanistic units—for example, pathways and biological networks—of varying complexity. Importantly, basic functional modules, such as cell cycle control, oxidative stress response, cell death, and inflammation, are shared across distantly related species, even if the genes involved in their respective biological networks partially differ, are more distantly related, and/or are not activated in the same manner. The reuse of such basic functional modules along the path of evolution enables comparison of the effect of active substance across species at the function module level. By extension, this also enables mechanism-by-mechanism comparison of the effects of different test items within a species and across species. This is a particularly useful application of systems biology/toxicology in the context of ENDP assessment (Dougherty and Papin, 2020) (Chapter 9).

The basic chemical properties of biomolecules (DNA, proteins, lipids, etc.) are shared across species. For example, Greek and Rice emphasize that the denaturing effect of a strong acid on proteins would not differ much among species (Greek and Rice, 2012). Similarly, exposure of a certain tissue type—for example, the lungs—to reactive oxygen species can be expected to result in similar initial molecular alterations, because of the sufficiently similar basic physicochemical properties of the tissue type shared among species. For example, membrane lipid oxidation and DNA damage induction upon CS exposure have been confirmed in human and rodent lung tissues (Aoshiba et al., 2003; Fahn et al., 1998).

The fundamental cellular mechanisms designed to respond to and detoxify chemical stressors are highly conserved across species. For example, Kirschner and Gerhardt emphasized the conservation of biological processes across phyla and kingdoms, including those involved in cell function and organization, development, and metabolism (Kirschner and Gerhart, 2008). Rather than "inventing" new processes, different species adapt existing processes by tweaking and recombining them in novel ways. For example, cross-species conservation of the core elements of the oxidative stress (Loboda et al., 2016) and DNA damage (Choi and Chung, 2020; Williams and Schumacher, 2017) processes has been emphasized, with specific modulations of the general conserved theme observed in each species (Siauciunaite et al., 2019).

Similar conclusions can be drawn for the conservation of complex systemic processes such as those driven by the immune system (Flajnik and Kasahara, 2010). The ImmGen consortium compared the transcriptional programs of human and mouse immune cells and found general conservation of the global transcriptional profiles (Shay et al., 2013). Especially, for lineage-specific genes, the expression patterns of orthologous genes were conserved. However, not surprisingly, divergent expression patterns of several hundred genes supported specific adaptations for the two species. The same pattern—of a strong core conservation, with specific adaptations—was also identified on the level of immune-related gene sets, which specifically supported a high level of conservation in T-cell and B-cell responses as well as in sepsis-induced immune signatures between humans and mice (Godec et al., 2016).

Recent single-cell analyses have provided further evidence on the conservation of immune processes across species. Zilionis et al. uncovered 25 states of tumor-infiltrating myeloid cells in lung cancer patients and found near-complete congruence of these populations in mice (Zilionis et al., 2019). Crinier et al. identified conserved natural killer cell populations in humans and mice, supporting "the translation of mouse studies to human physiology and disease" (Crinier et al., 2018).

Overall, the immune system is also characterized by a strongly conserved core—for example, between rodents and humans—with species-specific adaptations, such as those exemplified by the human and mouse mononuclear phagocyte networks (Reynolds and Haniffa, 2015).

Aging research offers an opportunity to study the conservation of even more complex biological phenomena. Aging reflects the complex physiological changes of an organism over its lifetime. Many organisms age, and conserved regulators and pathways that affect lifespan have been identified in such diverse organisms as yeast, nematodes, fruit flies, mice, and humans. Strikingly, caloric restriction has been demonstrated to extend the lifespan in organisms ranging from yeast to worms to mice to nonhuman primates (Pifferi et al., 2019). It is highly likely that the overall conservation of this effect is associated with the conservation of the associated signaling pathways (Khan et al., 2019). In particular, the conservation of and effects on lifespan have been studied for the adrenergic system and the 5' adenosine monophosphate-activated protein kinase, insulin/insulin-like growth factor 1, and mammalian target of rapamycin signaling pathways, all signaling pathways with a role in regulating the metabolic state. Interestingly, it has been shown that cigarette smoking causes the phenomenon of "accelerated aging" (Earls et al., 2019; Mamoshina et al., 2019). It has also been shown that smoke exposure accelerates the aging of mouse lungs (Yuan et al., 2015). More recently, using lung gene expression data from several long-term mouse studies, we have confirmed that CS exposure causes a positive age differential, that is, an increase in biological age relative to chronological age (Choukrallah et al., 2020). Importantly, the genes that were dysregulated by aging significantly overlapped with those dysregulated by CS exposure. Moreover, many of these genes are associated with inflammation, which has been shown to be associated with accelerated aging (Sebastiani et al., 2017). Interestingly, cessation of smoke exposure by switching to either fresh air or an ENDP aerosol leads to a gradual reversal of the age differential (Choukrallah et al., 2020).

In conclusion, while each species is adapted to its specific niche, they share core biological processes, which supports the translatability of many findings.

10.1.3.2 Mechanistic models and translatability
The question of conservation has also been addressed more systematically. The International Mouse Phenotyping Consortium aims at generating and phenotyping knockout mouse lines for every protein-coding gene (Muñoz-Fuentes et al., 2018). This resource allows us to ask the basic question: To what extent is the relevance of genes essential for survival of an organism conserved across species? Indeed, Muñoz-Fuentes et al. found that 99.6% of the nonessential genes for embryonic viability in mice were also nonessential in a panel of human cell lines.

While this suggests a general conservation of the relevance of a gene for survival, it represents a rather coarse abstraction of biological functions and, as discussed, the conservation and translatability of a process depends on its position in the modular and hierarchical biological network of the organism. Systems biology attempts to understand biological processes through the complex interactions of the biological components rather than on the basis of individual cellular components, such as single genes. Recently, it has been proposed that the higher level of conceptual understanding obtained through computational systems biology models can also facilitate the translatability of biological processes, and their components, across species (Brubaker and Lauffenburger, 2020). Similarly, computational systems toxicology enables mechanism-by-mechanism comparison of the effects of substance exposure across experimental systems and species (Hoeng et al., 2012). For example, the sbv IMPROVER (Meyer et al., 2012) "Species Translation" challenge demonstrated the potential of machine learning models to translate phosphoproteomic responses to stimuli between rats and humans (Biehl et al., 2015; Poussin et al., 2014b) and shed some light on certain differences between rat and human biology (Bilal et al., 2015; Rhrissorrakrai et al., 2015). Another project, "Found in Translation," established human disease gene prediction models based on mouse transcriptomics data and demonstrated their value in predicting novel disease-associated genes (Normand et al., 2018). Using more mechanistic models, Brubaker et al. bridged mouse and human KRAS signaling by leveraging signaling network models (Brubaker et al., 2019).

Biomarkers are employed to help bridge the effects between animal models and the human situation. By capturing the effects on mechanistic intermediates (or endophenotypes), these biomarkers enable mechanistic translatability. For example, a translational rat–human model for gastrointestinal-related adverse events was established on the basis of citrulline as a marker (Yoneyama et al., 2019). Importantly, these biomarkers not only include molecular measurements but also can, for example, encompass imaging modalities, such as X-ray radiography, magnetic resonance imaging (MRI), and positron emission tomography (PET) (Johansson, 2015). The use of imaging biomarkers has been also proposed specifically for translational toxicology studies (Liachenko, 2020). For example, MRI scans have shown structural brain changes upon heavy metal exposure in animal and clinical studies (Amuno et al., 2020; Beckwith et al., 2018; Feng et al., 2019; Takeuchi et al., 2019), and PET scans have demonstrated increased uptake of ^{18}F-fluorodeoxyglucose upon doxorubicin treatment in the heart of mice and human patients (Bauckneht et al., 2017).

Finally, mechanistic models incorporating biomarker measurements are especially relevant for translation between in vitro systems and the human situation. Relevant, information-rich biomarkers have been found essential for quantitative in vitro to in vivo extrapolation (Hartung, 2018): Biomarkers that are mechanistically linked to the mode of action form the basis for quantitative extrapolation in the context of pathways of toxicity or quantitative adverse outcome pathway models.

10.1.4 Dose Selection and Dose Translation

As outlined in Chapter 3, both in vitro and in vivo test systems must be exposed to ENDP aerosols or CS concentrations that are well-understood, verified, and relevant to human exposure or aimed at determining the highest exposure level at which no, or only very low, adverse effects are observed. This is crucial for proper interpretation of nonclinical data in the context of human toxicity and, therefore, an important criterion when assessing the quality of a study.

ENDP assessment studies are generally aimed at comparing the effects of exposure to an ENDP aerosol with those observed in CS exposure. Such comparative studies require a meaningful reference biomarker that reflects comparable exposure levels between an ENDP aerosol and CS. In clinical studies with ENDPs, exposure doses are usually measured as the number of cigarettes or amount of ENDPs consumed per day, and the reference biomarker of exposure (BoExp) is the quantity of nicotine and its main metabolites found to be present in blood and urine (Haziza et al., 2016; Ludicke et al., 2016) (Chapter 17). For example, single product use pharmacokinetic studies are used to compare the nicotine uptake in smokers with that in smokers who have switched to an ENDP (Chapter 17); in contrast, in more long-term studies, the levels of urinary nicotine and its major metabolites (nicotine equivalents) are used to monitor product exposure (Chapter 17). Similarly, matching nicotine deposition or uptake is commonly used for comparative ENDP assessment studies in vivo or in vitro (Iskandar et al., 2017; Wong et al., 2016; Oviedo et al., 2016; Phillips et al., 2016).

To facilitate translation of comparative toxicity results, the exposure doses used in nonclinical studies should ideally include at least one realistic human-equivalent dose. However, study guidelines require that markedly toxic doses be included. For rodent inhalation toxicity studies, OECD guidance document 116 states: "The highest dose level should be chosen to identify toxic effects including the principal target organs while avoiding severe toxicity, morbidity, or death" (OECD, 2014). For in vitro mutation assays, such as the mouse lymphoma and TK6 genotoxicity assays, OECD TG 490 suggests: "If the maximum concentration is based on cytotoxicity, the highest concentration should aim to achieve between 20% and 10% RTG."[1] This toxicological requirement may lead to unrealistically high concentrations of constituents (relative to those achievable in an exposed organism) if the assay endpoint has low sensitivity and/or the test items have low biological activity. As long as a test item can elicit a measurable response, the concentrations that cause effects equal to those of the reference item can be calculated to quantify their relative toxicity (Gonzalez-Suarez et al., 2016; Kogel et al., 2015). However, this approach is not applicable to assays where no significant response can be achieved with a test item. In any case, relative in vitro toxicity potencies should be interpreted carefully in the context of health risks if the effects have been observed at concentrations far beyond those that can be achieved in an organism. For example, the effects observed in vitro with nicotine concentrations in the millimolar range may not be relevant, given that blood nicotine concentrations in smokers only reach approximately 0.2 μM during a 24-h period (Hukkanen et al., 2005). Therefore, in vitro studies should be conducted as dose–response studies and include at least one human-relevant nicotine concentration.

In animal inhalation studies, the maximum tolerated dose marks the upper limit of exposure. In studies with CS, the concentration of carbon monoxide (CO), rather than that of nicotine, is the limiting factor. In fact, CO inhalation leads to buildup of carboxyhemoglobin (COHb), which may be lethal when its blood concentrations exceed 50%. In contrast, in studies with ENDP aerosols—because of their low CO content—it is possible to achieve aerosol concentrations that can lead to nicotine toxicity. Indeed, nose-only exposure of Sprague Dawley rats to pure nicotine aerosol (6 h/day) was shown to result in a maximum tolerated nicotine concentration of 50–60 μg/L in the

---

[1] RTG: relative total growth.

exposure atmosphere (Phillips et al., 2015a). Under the observed respiratory conditions, a daily delivered dose of 13.6 mg nicotine/kg body weight could be calculated for rats in the 50-μg/L exposure group. The corresponding human-equivalent dose can be calculated on the basis of body surface area by dividing the rat dose by a factor of 6.2 (Center for Drug evaluation and Research (CDER), 2005): 13.6 mg/kg/6.2 = 2.2 mg/kg. This value translates to a daily nicotine dose of 132 mg for a 60-kg adult human, equivalent to smoking approximately 130 cigarettes per day (Phillips et al., 2015a).

For rat inhalation studies with CS (nose-only exposure, 6 h/day), the maximum tolerated concentrations are in the rage of 270—300 μg total particulate matter (TPM)/L, which is equivalent to a nicotine concentration of approximately 23 μg/L (Oviedo et al., 2016; Wong et al., 2016). This is equivalent to smoking approximately 60 cigarettes per day for a 60-kg adult human. Higher smoke concentrations are not well tolerated because of the acute toxicity of CO and other harmful and potentially harmful constituents (HPHCs) present in CS. Similar to the pure nicotine aerosol (Phillips et al., 2015a), a diluted ENDP aerosol could be dosed up to the level of nicotine toxicity (50 μg nicotine/L, corresponding to 370 μg TPM/L) (Oviedo et al., 2016; Phillips et al., 2016), owing to the significantly lower levels of CO and other HPHCs emitted by the ENDP (Chapter 4).

For mouse inhalation studies, the maximum tolerated concentration of CS (whole-body exposure, 3 h/day) is around 600 TPM/L and 30 μg nicotine/L. This is equivalent to smoking 25—30 cigarettes per day for a 60-kg adult human. This dose can be doubled when exposing mice to ENDP aerosols, given their very low CO content. For CS exposure, the 3-h exposure period must be interspersed with intermittent fresh-air breaks to avoid excessive blood COHb levels (Phillips et al., 2015b, 2019). It is important to note that the differences between the nose-only and whole-body exposure setups result in different TPM/nicotine ratios in the diluted aerosols.

In summary, a solid understanding of the exposure dose and how this compares across species is essential to ensure relevant translatability of preclinical findings.

10.1.5 Insights into Translatability from Large-Scale Toxicology Datasets

Large-scale repositories of toxicology data provide the opportunity to systematically evaluate the predictive value of preclinical toxicology for human risk assessment. Several authors have investigated how predictive animal models are for adverse events in humans. Olson et al. reported on the results of a multinational pharmaceutical company survey that aimed at better understanding the concordance between the toxicity of pharmaceuticals observed in humans and experimental animals (Olson et al., 2000). This assessment included data on 150 compounds from 12 pharmaceutical companies. By combining rodent and nonrodent preclinical data, the authors found true positive concordance for human toxicity events in 71% of cases. The highest concordance was identified for cardiovascular, hematological, and gastrointestinal conditions, whereas the lowest concordance was observed for skin conditions. Tamaki et al. evaluated adverse drug reactions for 142 approved drugs and found a concordance of more than 70% with preclinical animal data on hematological disorders, whereas musculoskeletal, respiratory, and neurological adverse drug reactions had a concordance of less than 30% (Tamaki et al., 2013). In the most extensive systematic evaluation of the translatability of animal to human toxicology data, Clark and Steger-Hartmann evaluated the animal—human concordance for over 3000 approved therapeutics by the United States Food and Drug Administration/European Medicines Agency (Clark and Steger-Hartmann, 2018). While the positive predictability of many animal models was confirmed, the negative predictability of animal events for human events was limited.

The European Registration, Evaluation, Authorisation and Restriction of Chemicals legislation requires publication of the toxicology assessment results for each registration dossier by the European Chemical Agency. These data can be mined for toxicological insights (Luechtefeld et al., 2016), and they allowed evaluation of the reproducibility of animal tests conducted in accordance with OECD guidelines: With an 81% balanced accuracy, the same result was observed in a repeat test (Luechtefeld et al., 2018a, 2018b). Interestingly, a read-across-based structure—activity relationship machine learning model could be established, which, by mapping out the chemical similarity space, reached a balanced accuracy of 87% (Hartung, 2019).

Overall, these systematic data evaluations suggest the general translatability of animal data to the human situation. However, the predictions are not perfect because of, for example, the limited negative predictability and differences in concordance depending on the condition. Thus, data from animal studies need to be interpreted with care and always holistically in the context of the totality of evidence, for example, by including computational prediction approaches and in vitro toxicity assessment assays.

10.2 TRANSLATIONAL IN VITRO AND IN VIVO MODELS FOR ENDP ASSESSMENT

As outlined in the introduction, selection of adequate in vitro and in vivo model systems is an important step in the ENDP assessment process. Given the breadth of the deleterious effects of CS, these models must enable comparison of the effects of ENDP aerosols with those of CS across a range of biological mechanisms and organ systems. These systems must be selected to be as representative as possible of human biology, display a response to CS, and be used, as much as possible, in a manner that is representative of human exposure.

In vitro models should preferably employ primary human cells. Clearly, there are assays for which such cells are not available, and, hence, one has to resort to cell lines or even nonhuman model systems. However, with the development of more advanced in vitro technologies—such as pluripotent stem cell–based approaches (Zink et al., 2020), complex multicell type organotypic tissue cultures (Iskandar et al., 2015; Marescotti et al., 2019), organoids (Wörsdörfer et al., 2020), and microphysiological multiorgan-on-a-chip systems (Bovard et al., 2018; Schimek et al., 2020)—increasingly adequate human in vitro model systems will become available and eventually gain regulatory acceptance (Pridgeon et al., 2018) and reduce, or even eliminate, the need for animal models (Shen et al., 2020; Zink et al., 2020).

The use of animal models of disease can be reduced by employing a single model for assessing several disease endpoints. For instance, the $Apoe^{-/-}$ mouse allows us to assess the effects of CS and ENDP aerosols on both atherosclerotic plaque formation (Lietz et al., 2013) and emphysema (Boué et al., 2013). Furthermore, such models not only enable direct comparison between the effects of an ENDP aerosol and CS but also help us benchmark the effects of switching to an ENDP against those of cessation (Boué et al., 2013; Lietz et al., 2013). More recently, such a switching study design was also used with organotypic tissue cultures in vitro (Ito et al., 2020), which shows that in vivo study designs can be successfully reproduced in in vitro systems.

Here, we describe a number of in vitro and in vivo model systems that are useful when assessing ENDPs.

10.2.1 Models for CVD

Smoking is a cause of CVDs (Office of the Surgeon General, 2020). CS causes oxidative stress and vascular inflammation, which, for instance, cause endothelial cell dysfunction and accelerate atherosclerotic plaque formation. This leads to various types of CVDs, such as ischemic heart disease, cerebrovascular disease, peripheral artery disease, and aortic aneurysm (Ambrose and Barua, 2004).

One of the early events in this process is the increase in adhesion of circulating monocytes to the endothelium (Kalra et al., 1994). This event can be measured in vitro by using human primary endothelial cells and a monocytic cell line (Poussin et al., 2014a). This assay also allows us to measure oxidative stress, inflammation, and the cell adhesion markers expressed by monocytic cells exposed to CS extracts. This cell-based assay can also be further developed into a microvessel-on-a-chip assay, in which monocyte adhesion can be measured under flow (Poussin et al., 2020).

However, as there is no current in vitro model that allows assessment of the effects of CS on atherosclerotic plaque development, one has to resort to an animal model of disease. The $Apoe^{-/-}$ mouse is a widely used model for studying atherosclerosis (Lee et al., 2017; Wendler and Wehling, 2010). $Apoe^{-/-}$ mice lack the apolipoprotein E protein, which is required for hepatic lipid uptake. The lack of APOE protein results in elevated plasma cholesterol levels and atherosclerotic plaque formation. Another commonly used mouse model for atherosclerosis is the LDL-receptor knockout mouse, although several other models are available (Lee et al., 2017; Wendler and Wehling, 2010).

Several features of these mouse models resemble the human situation. For instance, $Apoe^{-/-}$ mice demonstrate substantial hypercholesterolemia (Plump and Breslow, 1995), show a shift in plasma lipoprotein profiles toward very-low-density lipoprotein, similar to type II hyperlipidemia in humans (Ghiselli et al., 1981), and spontaneously develop atherosclerotic lesions at various locations in the vasculature. On the other hand, the limitations of this model include its lower LDL levels than those observed in humans (Lo Sasso et al., 2016). In addition, the $Apoe^{-/-}$ model does not capture the process of plaque rupture (Wendler and Wehling, 2010).

While keeping the limitations of these models in mind, the American Heart Association summarized that "although native mice have marked differences in lipoprotein metabolism compared with humans, genetically engineered mice have been invaluable to our understanding of molecular mechanisms and the underlying pathways involved in atherosclerosis" (Daugherty et al., 2017).

10.2.2 Models for COPD

CS exposure directly affects the lungs and is the major risk factor for COPD, which is a global health problem

(López-Campos et al., 2016). COPD is characterized by persistent airflow limitation, which is usually progressive and includes both emphysema and chronic bronchitis (Rabe et al., 2007). The oxidative stress burden and associated inflammatory response induced by CS result in accumulation of structural tissue damage and disease manifestation over time (Titz et al., 2015).

In vitro organotypic epithelial tissue cultures have been established that allow direct exposure of the model system at the apical air–liquid interface (Lacroix et al., 2018). For example, validation of one such in vitro lung exposure system with a test set of 20 compounds has shown a specificity of 83% and sensitivity of 88% with respect to in vivo data (Tsoutsoulopoulos et al., 2019). In the context of ENDP assessment, these models offer the advantage that whole CS or ENDP aerosols can be applied to the apical surface of the tissue culture (Kuehn et al., 2015; Majeed et al., 2014), which is more relevant to human airway exposure than exposing submersed cell cultures to smoke or aerosol fractions and extracts. The translatability of these organotypic systems has been evaluated, and, for instance, organotypic bronchial airway epithelium cultures exposed to CS have been shown to resemble, at the molecular level, the bronchial epithelium of human smokers (Mathis et al., 2013). Furthermore, it has been shown that repeated exposure of organotypic cultures to the CS constituent acrolein (at the air–liquid interface) results in structural and functional changes that recapitulate the pathology of COPD, including the effects on ciliated cells, mucin production, and squamous differentiation (Xiong et al., 2018). Generally, it has been concluded that organotypic systems, resembling the different architectures of the human lungs and possibly integrated in lab-on-a-chip solutions, represent effective models for recreating the complex physiology of the lungs (Evans and Lee, 2020).

Animal models have been established that can effectively recapitulate the key characteristics of COPD, including inflammation, oxidative stress, airway remodeling, emphysema, and impaired lung function (Ghorani et al., 2017; Jones et al., 2017). Guinea pigs, rats, and mice (e.g., A/J and C57Bl/6) have been employed as animal models of disease. In particular, mouse models of CS-induced COPD have been shown to recapitulate characteristics of the human disease (Hautamaki et al., 1997; Phillips et al., 2016), including chronic lung inflammation, emphysema, and thickening of airway epithelium (Ghorani et al., 2017). Indeed, while not all characteristics of emphysema in human COPD are reproduced in animal models, "CS exposure induced emphysema can simulate relatively complex pathological changes and is considered as the most reasonable animal model of COPD at present" (Liang and He, 2019). Especially, multiomics approaches have been demonstrated to broadly cover relevant COPD-associated effects induced by CS exposure, including inflammatory mechanisms and oxidative stress responses (Titz et al., 2020). Moreover, the $Apoe^{-/-}$ mouse is a well-suited model for assessing the effects of CS exposure, because it allows concomitant assessment of the lung and cardiovascular effects (see below) (Lo Sasso et al., 2016).

10.2.3 Models for Lung Cancer

Chronic exposure to CS triggers pathways that lead to accumulation of genetic damages and cause inflammation, which together (Balkwill and Mantovani, 2001) are the two key mechanisms that enable cells to acquire the hallmarks of cancer (Hanahan and Weinberg, 2011) (Chapter 18).

Genetic damage, the first of the two key mechanisms that lead to cancer, can be tested in vitro. Beyond the classical genotoxicity assays (Chapter 13), several other in vitro models can be used to assess cellular responses to the genetic damage induced by CS. For example, an early step in the DNA damage response machinery (Nakamura et al., 2010) can be tested by measuring the abundance of γH2AX in human bronchial epithelial cells (Gonzalez-Suarez et al., 2016; Taylor et al., 2018). Other in vitro models can be employed to measure the more long-term effects of CS on cellular and molecular endpoints linked to carcinogenesis. These include the Bhas 42 cell (mouse fibroblast-derived) transformation assay (Breheny et al., 2017; Taylor et al., 2018) and the long-term exposure assay with human bronchial epithelial BEAS-2B cells, which can be used to demonstrate the functional and molecular changes linked to lung carcinogenesis (van der Toorn et al., 2018).

Inflammation, the second of the two key mechanisms that lead to cancer, can, for instance, be tested by using the human-derived organotypic tissue cultures described above.

Mouse models have been employed for studying the carcinogenicity of chemical compounds and infer the underlying mechanisms of cancer development in humans (Meuwissen and Berns, 2005). In the particular case of carcinogenesis induced by CS (or its constituents), different strains of mice display markedly varied sensitivity to lung tumor development (Gordon and Bosland, 2009). For example, mice of the C57Bl/6, C3H/J, and DBA strains are rather resistant to carcinogen-induced lung tumors, while BALB/c mice are considered intermediate in susceptibility (Vikis et al., 2013). Furthermore, a small number of limited

CS exposure studies have been conducted in B6C3F1 mice (Henry and Kouri, 1986; Hutt et al., 2005); however, given the low-to-intermediate susceptibility of these mice to developing lung tumors in response to CS exposure, such studies require large numbers of animals per group (Hutt et al., 2005). In contrast, the A/J mouse is highly susceptible to lung tumor induction (relative to other mouse strains) and has been widely used in carcinogenicity testing. In this model, *K-ras* oncogene activation is associated with enhanced risk for lung tumor development, illustrated by the presentation of pulmonary adenoma. However, the A/J mouse model, too, has several disadvantages, including that it also develops spontaneous lung tumors and only shows a small increase in the number of lung tumors after exposure to CS. Furthermore, a known pathology of A/J mice is late-onset (4−5 months) progressive muscular dystrophy resulting from a homozygous retro-transposon insertion in the dysferlin (*Dysf*) gene.[2] Myo-fibers in *Dysf^{prmd}* homozygotes undergo degeneration and regeneration, and their nuclei are placed centrally. Proximal muscles are more severely affected than distal muscles (Ho et al., 2004). In addition, because of their high early mortality rate, A/J mice cannot be used in 2-year or longer carcinogenicity bioassays. Nevertheless, study durations of 10−18 months have been shown to be effective for induction of lung tumors upon exposure to CS (Stinn et al., 2013, 2013b).

The list of chemicals that can induce pulmonary tumors in A/J mice is long and ranges from aflatoxin to CS and some of its components, such as polycyclic aromatic hydrocarbons and tobacco-specific nitrosamines (TSNAs) (Hecht et al., 1989; Kim and Lee, 1996; Shimkin and Stoner, 1975; Stoner, 1991). These agents can act as initiators and/or promoters of pulmonary tumorigenesis by accelerating tumor onset and increasing tumor multiplicity (Stinn et al., 2013a). Similar to the spontaneous tumors in mouse lungs, the majority of pulmonary tumors induced by carcinogens are adenomas (Gunning et al., 1991). However, a small proportion (~10%) of tumors have been found to be adenocarcinomas, for example, in A/J mice following treatment with the TSNA 4-methylnitrosamino-1-(3-pyridyl)-1-butanone (NNK) (Lu et al., 2006; Yang et al., 1997), benzo[*a*]pyrene (Estensen et al., 2004), or CS exposure (Stinn et al., 2010, 2013a; Witschi et al., 2004). Furthermore, gene and microRNA expression analysis has demonstrated that lung tumors developing in CS-exposed A/J mice exhibit marked differences to spontaneously arising

tumors and that these differences can be harnessed in the form of a gene expression signature (GES) to potentially predict the extent of CS exposure (Luettich et al., 2014). On the basis of these observations, the A/J mouse can be considered a suitable in vivo model of smoking-related lung cancer that could be employed for assessment of ENDPs relative to cigarettes.

10.2.4 Models for Liver Toxicity

Regarding hepatotoxicity, it has been argued that the standard model systems for drug-induced liver injury do not accurately reflect the molecular markup and functionality of the human liver (Zhou et al., 2019). Hughes found that 38%−51% of hepatotoxic compounds are not identified in preclinical animal tests (Hughes, 2008). More recently, multicell-type organotypic and microphysiological liver systems have started to emerge as promising alternatives for addressing this gap. For example, a recent study evaluated the potential of commercial spheroid cultures of primary human hepatocytes for prediction of hepatotoxicity (Zhou et al., 2019). For a test set of 110 drugs, the authors reported a sensitivity of 59% and specificity of 80%. Another recent study evaluated a liver spheroid model by using chemically defined serum-free conditions and, for a test set of 123 drugs, obtained a sensitivity of 69% and specificity of 100% at an exposure level of 20× the therapeutic concentration detected in patient serum (Vorrink et al., 2018).

Recently, lung−liver-on-a-chip model platforms have been developed (Bovard et al., 2018; Schimek et al., 2020) that will enable assessment of the effects of inhaled substances on both the lungs and liver.

10.3 TRANSLATION IN THE CONTEXT OF THE CELSD

CELSD is the highest level of the adverse outcome pathway of cigarettes smoking (Chapters 3 and 9). The objective of an ENDP assessment program (Chapter 3) is, therefore, to compare the effects of an ENDP aerosol with those of CS and fresh air in as many causally linked events along the CELSD as possible. Moreover, a mechanism-by-mechanism approach enables comparative assessment of the effects of an ENDP aerosol across the many biological mechanisms perturbed by CS. In short, the CELSD provides the breadth of the assessment process, and the mechanism-by-mechanism approach provides the depth of the assessment. To substantiate the risk reduction potential of an ENDP, the results of the assessment studies must, therefore, be coherent with the reduction in toxicant emissions along the CELSD and consistent across studies and mechanisms.

---

[2]The Jackson Laboratory, https://www.jax.org/strain/000646, last accessed Nov. 28, 2019.

All study types in an ENDP assessment program have their limitations, and those of in vitro and in vivo are briefly described in the introduction to this chapter. Moreover, clinical studies are limited by the number and types of samples that can be collected, in addition to other constraints such as time and the number of participants and their adherence to the study group. For this reason, the scientific data collected along the CELSD and across mechanisms will necessarily be a composite image, with contributions from in vitro, in vivo, and clinical studies that support each other in a totality-of-the-evidence approach. Extrapolation of this evidence for human relevance is greatly facilitated by translational biomarkers that can be measured along the CELSD to demonstrate the causal link between connected events, across mechanisms to demonstrate consistency and depth, and across biological systems to demonstrate their relevance. To illustrate this point, we describe a small number of translational markers that act as anchors across the events of the CELSD (Fig. 10.1).

10.3.1 Emissions
The central tenet of tobacco harm reduction is that ENDPs emit significantly lower levels of many toxicants than cigarettes (Chapters 2–4, 6, 7) while delivering nicotine at a level that is satisfying for adult smokers. As toxicological ENDP assessment studies aim to compare the effects of ENDP aerosols with those of CS, it is important to select a minimal set of smoke constituents (i) that distinguish ENDPs from cigarettes on the basis of their emissions and (ii) for which associated BoExps can distinguish biological systems exposed to ENDP aerosols and CS (see next section). A minimal set of HPHCs enabling these distinctions would include the TSNA NNK, CO, and acrylonitrile, all of which are reduced in ENDP emissions. A minimal list should obviously also include nicotine, which is emitted by ENDPs and cigarettes and which serves to compare and calibrate the exposure to ENDP aerosols across all experimental systems. This does not preclude the use of additional HPHCs—for example, acrolein—that are less specific for tobacco products.

10.3.2 Exposure
To demonstrate the causal link between emission and exposure levels in the context of ENDP assessment (the link between the first and second events in the CELSD; see Chapter 3), one should measure BoExps in every study to ascertain that exposure has occurred as intended and to

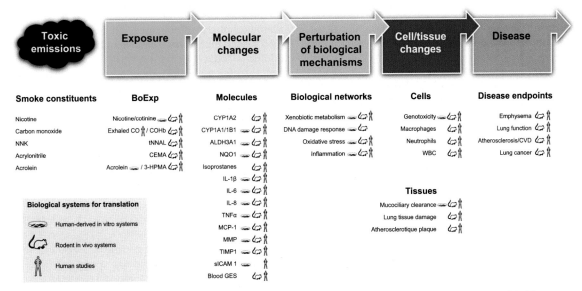

FIG. 10.1 Example of translational markers that serve as anchors for ENDP assessment along the CELSD. *3-HPMA*, 3-hydroxypropylmercapturic acid; *ALDH3A1*, aldehyde dehydrogenase 3A1; *blood GES*, blood-based gene expression signature; *CELSD*, causal chain of events linking smoking to disease; *CEMA*, 2-cyanoethylmercapturic acid; *CO*, carbon monoxide; *COHb*, carboxyhemoglobin; *CVD*, cardiovascular diseases; *CYP1A2*, cytochrome P450 1A2; *CYP1A1/1B1*, cytochrome P450 1A1 and 1B1; *ENDP*, electronic nicotine delivery product; *IL-1β*, interleukin 1β; *IL-6*, interleukin 6; *IL-8*, interleukin 8; *MCP-1*, monocyte chemoattractant protein 1; *MMP*, matrix metalloproteinase; *NNK*, 4-methylnitrosamino-1-(3-pyridyl)-1-butanone; *sICAM-1*, soluble intercellular adhesion molecule 1; *TNFα*, tumor necrosis factor alpha; *tNNAL*, total 4-(methylnitrosamino)-1-(3-pyridyl)-1-butanol; *NQO1*, NAD(P)H dehydrogenase (quinone 1).

enable sound comparisons between exposure groups. The BoExps to the HPHCs in the short list mentioned above are nicotine and its metabolites (e.g., cotinine); total 4-(methylnitrosamino)-1-(3-pyridyl)-1-butanol (tNNAL; metabolite of NNK); exhaled CO or COHb; and 2-cyanoethylmercapturic acid (CEMA; metabolite of acrylonitrile). These BoExps are sufficient to distinguish biological systems exposed to CS from those exposed to an ENDP aerosol, because they allow tracking of nicotine exposure in the context of combustion markers and TSNAs. Many in vitro systems are not suitable for measuring these metabolites, and, in these systems, one can directly measure nicotine and carbonyls to assess exposure (Iskandar et al., 2017). Among the carbonyls, acrolein is of particular value, as it can be measured directly in in vitro systems, and its metabolite 3-hydroxypropylmercapturic acid can be measured in animal (Phillips et al., 2016) and human studies (Chapters 17).

Clearly, clinical exposure reduction studies will include a broader set of BoExps to HPHCs, as these studies are designed to assess the broad effect of reduced emissions and exposure (Chapter 17).

10.3.3 Molecular Changes

To demonstrate the causal link between exposure levels and molecular changes in the context of ENDP assessment (the link between the second and third events in the CELSD; see Chapter 3), one should measure the effect of product exposure on molecular changes in every study where this is sensible in order to (i) ascertain that changes in toxicant exposure levels led to effects at the molecular level and (ii) characterize and quantify these changes in the context of known biological processes. These molecular changes can be measured on a molecule-by-molecule basis, and modern omics platforms (Chapter 9) provide the means to perform these measurements at the genome, proteome, lipidome, and metabolome levels in a very efficient and precise manner. These large-scale datasets can then be analyzed by using computational tools (Chapter 9) to quantify the changes not only in individual molecules but also at the level of functional units or biological mechanisms. Another way to measure molecular changes is to measure their functional changes. For example, one can infer changes at the molecular level from changes at the enzymatic activity level. In the context of ENDP assessment, this is particularly useful for measuring changes in plasma CYP1A2 activity in clinical studies and comparing these changes with gene expression alterations in animal studies (Chapter 18). Changes in enzymatic activities can also be used to (i) confirm that gene and/or protein expression level changes are coherently reflected at the functional level, such as for the matrix metalloproteinases

(MMPs) in the bronchoalveolar lavage fluid (BALF) collected during animal studies (Phillips et al., 2016), and (ii) verify that the changes in MMP expression and activity are consistent across species, even if one study is performed in vivo and the other in vitro (Iskandar et al., 2017; Phillips et al., 2016).

Changes at the molecular level can be representative of biological mechanism perturbations. This means that a change in one particular molecule can be a surrogate for changes that occur within a biological pathway that belongs to a larger biological network. For example, changes in interleukin (IL)-1β levels reflect changes in inflammasome activation, which is a pathway within the broader inflammation network. Only a small number of studies have measured IL-1β levels in the BALF of human smokers and nonsmokers (Kuschner et al., 1996; Song et al., 2020), owing to the invasiveness of the BALF technique; however, this molecule can be readily measured in vitro (Iskandar et al., 2017) and in vivo (Phillips et al., 2016). IL-1β is, therefore, an important translational marker, especially given its key role in inflammation in tumor promotion (Chapter 18). Other markers, such as IL-6, IL-8, and the monocyte chemoattractant protein 1 (Kuschner et al., 1996; Song et al., 2020) can also serve as translational molecular markers for CS-induced lung inflammation (Chapter 18). In the context of vascular inflammation, the soluble intercellular adhesion molecule 1, which plays a key role in neutrophil adhesion to endothelial cells, can be measured in vitro (Poussin et al., 2014a) as well as in human studies (Lüdicke et al., 2015; Peck et al., 2018) (Chapter 17) and, therefore, serves as a translational biomarker in the area of CVD. Furthermore, there are numerous other biomolecules that can serve as translational biomarkers for inflammation, xenobiotic metabolism, and oxidative stress and can be measured in vitro, in vivo, and in human studies: Fig. 10.1 mentions just a few of them.

In the future, it will be necessary to further characterize these biomarkers, identify novel ones, and further develop the area of translational biomarkers to increase the value of nonclinical studies to risk assessment. For example, blood-based GESs—which integrate the expression levels of several genes in a signature that is able to discriminate between exposures—represent a promising new type of biomarker. Indeed, it has been shown that a blood-based GES can discriminate not only smokers from nonsmokers but also smoke-exposed mice from air-exposed mice (Chapter 18). Importantly, such signatures will yield new insights into molecular changes that may eventually shed new light on the mechanisms perturbed by CS.

10.3.4 Biological Mechanism Perturbations

To demonstrate the causal link between molecular changes and perturbation of biological networks in the context of ENDP assessment (the link between the third and fourth events in the CELSD; see Chapter 3), one should analyze large-scale datasets of molecular measurements collected by omics technologies (Chapter 9) through the lens of computable biological networks (Sturla et al., 2014) (Chapter 9). This analysis provides a deep quantitative evaluation of the effects of an ENDP relative to those of CS as well as fresh air across all biological mechanisms affected by CS and also acts as a translational link between in vitro, in vivo, and human studies. Furthermore, these mechanistic perturbations are the causal connectors between molecular changes and the more apical endpoints provided by cell and tissue changes as well as disease manifestations. For example, such an analysis can reveal fine mechanistic details such as the polarization of pulmonary macrophages in different groups of smokers and nonsmokers (Titz et al., 2015).

10.3.5 Cell and Tissue Changes

To demonstrate the causal link between biological network perturbations and cell/tissue changes in the context of ENDP assessment (the link between the fourth and fifth events in the CELSD; see Chapter 3), one should measure a number of cellular and histopathological endpoints, whenever this is feasible. These endpoints provide a solid link between mechanistic perturbations and disease endpoints and allow us to extrapolate from in vitro and animal studies to human health effects. From a translational perspective, lung tissue damage and atherosclerotic plaque formation are two particularly important endpoints, as they are causally linked with disease manifestations. These endpoints, which are the consequence of biological mechanism perturbations driven by the molecular changes induced by CS exposure, can be assessed in both animal models of disease (Phillips et al., 2016) and humans (Chaudhary et al., 2017; Dempsey and Moore, 1992). Similarly, the level of lung inflammation can be assessed by the changes in neutrophil and macrophage counts in the BALF of animal models and human subjects (Kuschner et al., 1996; Song et al., 2020). As the impact of such clinical procedures is unreasonably high in the context of clinical studies, animal models represent a valid alternative for translation, especially because the causal relationship with previous events has been demonstrated.

10.3.6 Disease

As summarized in the introduction to this chapter, clinical health outcome studies based on disease endpoints are difficult to execute with ENDPs in a premarket setting (Chapter 3). Therefore, assessment of ENDPs has to rely on animal models of disease to demonstrate the causal link between cell/tissue changes and disease (the link between the fifth and sixth events in the CELSD; see Chapter 3). These animal models, while far from perfect, have been selected because they develop key aspects of human smoking–related disease. These disease manifestations, such as the loss of lung function, atherosclerotic plaque formation, and lung cancer, resemble the human manifestations of long-term smoking in many relevant ways. In cases where a switching study design was adopted,[3] cessation reduced not only the disease manifestations associated with smoking but also the changes in all previous events of the CELSD across all biological mechanisms that are perturbed by CS exposure. Therefore, this approach is causally consistent and reflects both the principle of toxicology and the epidemiology of smoking and cessation (Chapter 3).

10.4 CONCLUSIONS

ENDP assessment requires a broad range of in vitro and in vivo model systems to enable comparison of the effects of ENDP aerosols with those of CS. By using a combination of adequately selected in vitro and in vivo systems, one can perform the assessment in all events along the CELSD and across the many biological mechanisms affected by CS. These model systems reinforce each other and, thereby, permit the translation of in vivo and in vitro results to the human situation. Importantly, the risk reduction potential of an ENDP is verified if the totality of the evidence of an assessment program is coherent with the reduction in toxicant emissions along the CELSD and consistent across the mechanisms affected by CS.

REFERENCES

Ambrose, J.A., Barua, R.S., 2004. The pathophysiology of cigarette smoking and cardiovascular disease: an update. J. Am. Coll. Cardiol. 43 (10), 1731–1737.

Amuno, S., Rudko, D., Gallino, D., Tuznik, M., Shekh, K., Kodzhahinchev, V., et al., 2020. Altered neurotransmission and neuroimaging biomarkers of chronic arsenic poisoning in wild muskrats (*Ondatra zibethicus*) and red squirrels

---

[3] In a switching study design, animals are first exposed to cigarette smoke and then switched to either fresh air (cessation arm) or an ENDP aerosol (switching arm).

(*Tamiasciurus hudsonicus*) breeding near the City of Yellowknife, Northwest territories (Canada). Sci. Total Environ. 707, 135556.

Aoshiba, K., Koinuma, M., Yokohori, N., Nagai, A., 2003. Immunohistochemical evaluation of oxidative stress in murine lungs after cigarette smoke exposure. Inhal. Toxicol. 15 (10), 1029–1038.

Bailey, J., Thew, M., Balls, M., 2014. An analysis of the use of animal models in predicting human toxicology and drug safety. Altern. Lab. Anim. 42 (3), 181–199.

Balkwill, F., Mantovani, A., 2001. Inflammation and cancer: back to virchow? Lancet 357 (9255), 539–545.

Barré-Sinoussi, F., Montagutelli, X., 2015. Animal models are essential to biological research: issues and perspectives. Future Sci. OA 1 (4), Fso63.

Bauckneht, M., Ferrarazzo, G., Fiz, F., Morbelli, S., Sarocchi, M., Pastorino, P., et al., 2017. Doxorubicin effect on myocardial metabolism as a prerequisite for subsequent development of cardiac toxicity: a translational 18F-FDG PET/CT observation. J. Nucl. Med. 58 (10), 1638–1645.

Beckwith, T.J., Dietrich, K.N., Wright, J.P., Altaye, M., Cecil, K.M., 2018. Reduced regional volumes associated with total psychopathy scores in an adult population with childhood lead exposure. Neurotoxicology 67, 1–26.

Biehl, M., Sadowski, P., Bhanot, G., Bilal, E., Dayarian, A., Meyer, P., et al., 2015. Inter-species prediction of protein phosphorylation in the sbv IMPROVER species translation challenge. Bioinformatics 31 (4), 453–461.

Bilal, E., Sakellaropoulos, T., Melas, I.N., Messinis, D.E., Belcastro, V., Rhrissorrakrai, K., et al., 2015. A crowdsourcing approach for the construction of species-specific cell signaling networks. Bioinformatics 31 (4), 484–491.

Boué, S., De León, H., Schlage, W.K., Peck, M.J., Weiler, H., Berges, A., et al., 2013. Cigarette smoke induces molecular responses in respiratory tissues of ApoE(-/-) mice that are progressively deactivated upon cessation. Toxicology 314 (1), 112–124.

Bovard, D., Sandoz, A., Luettich, K., Frentzel, S., Iskandar, A., Marescotti, D., et al., 2018. A lung/liver-on-a-chip platform for acute and chronic toxicity studies. Lab Chip 18 (24), 3814–3829.

Breheny, D., Oke, O., Pant, K., Gaça, M., 2017. Comparative tumor promotion assessment of e-cigarette and cigarettes using the in vitro Bhas 42 cell transformation assay. Environ. Mol. Mutagen. 58 (4), 190–198.

Brubaker, D.K., Lauffenburger, D.A., 2020. Translating preclinical models to humans. Science 367 (6479), 742–743.

Brubaker, D.K., Paulo, J.A., Sheth, S., Poulin, E.J., Popow, O., Joughin, B.A., et al., 2019. Proteogenomic network analysis of context-specific KRAS signaling in mouse-to-human cross-species translation. Cell Syst. 9 (3), 258–270.e256.

Center for Drug Evaluation and Research (CDER), 2005. Estimating the Maximum Safe Starting Dose in Initial Clinical Trials for Therapeutics in Adult Healthy Volunteers. (Accessed 3 November 2014).

Chaudhary, N., Luettich, K., Peck, M.J., Pierri, E., Felber-Medlin, L., Vuillaume, G., et al., 2017. Physiological and biological characterization of smokers with and without COPD. F1000Research 6.

Choi, J.E., Chung, W.H., 2020. Functional interplay between the oxidative stress response and DNA damage checkpoint signaling for genome maintenance in aerobic organisms. J. Microbiol. 58 (2), 81–91.

Choukrallah, M.A., Hoeng, J., Peitsch, M.C., Martin, F., 2020. Lung transcriptomic clock predicts premature aging in cigarette smoke-exposed mice. BMC Genom. 21 (1), 291.

Clark, M., Steger-Hartmann, T., 2018. A big data approach to the concordance of the toxicity of pharmaceuticals in animals and humans. Regul. Toxicol. Pharmacol. 96, 94–105.

Crinier, A., Milpied, P., Escalière, B., Piperoglou, C., Galluso, J., Balsamo, A., et al., 2018. High-dimensional single-cell analysis identifies organ-specific signatures and conserved NK cell subsets in humans and mice. Immunity 49 (5), 971–986.e975.

Daugherty, A., Tall, A.R., Daemen, M., Falk, E., Fisher, E.A., García-Cardeña, G., et al., 2017. Recommendation on design, execution, and reporting of animal atherosclerosis studies: a scientific statement from the American Heart Association. Arterioscler. Thromb. Vasc. Biol. 37 (9), e131–e157.

Dempsey, R.J., Moore, R.W., 1992. Amount of smoking independently predicts carotid artery atherosclerosis severity. Stroke 23 (5), 693–696.

Dougherty, B.V., Papin, J.A., 2020. Systems biology approaches help to facilitate interpretation of cross-species comparisons. Curr. Opin. Toxicol. 23–24, 74–79.

Earls, J.C., Rappaport, N., Heath, L., Wilmanski, T., Magis, A.T., Schork, N.J., et al., 2019. Multi-omic biological age estimation and its correlation with wellness and disease phenotypes: a longitudinal study of 3,558 individuals. J. Gerontol. A Biol. Sci. Med. Sci. 74 (Suppl. 1), S52–s60.

Estensen, R.D., Jordan, M.M., Wiedmann, T.S., Galbraith, A.R., Steele, V.E., Wattenberg, L.W., 2004. Effect of chemopreventive agents on separate stages of progression of benzo [α]pyrene induced lung tumors in A/J mice. Carcinogenesis 25 (2), 197–201.

Evans, K.V., Lee, J.H., 2020. Alveolar wars: the rise of in vitro models to understand human lung alveolar maintenance, regeneration, and disease. Stem Cells Transl. Med. 9, 867–881. https://doi.org/10.1002/sctm.19-0433. Epub ahead of print 2020/04/10.

Fahn, H.-J., Wang, L.-S., Kao, S.-H., Chang, S.-C., Huang, M.-H., Wei, Y.-H., 1998. Smoking-associated mitochondrial DNA mutations and lipid peroxidation in human lung tissues. Am. J. Respir. Cell Mol. Biol. 19 (6), 901–909.

Feng, C., Liu, S., Zhou, F., Gao, Y., Li, Y., Du, G., et al., 2019. Oxidative stress in the neurodegenerative brain following lifetime exposure to lead in rats: changes in lifespan profiles. Toxicology 411, 101–109.

Flajnik, M.F., Kasahara, M., 2010. Origin and evolution of the adaptive immune system: genetic events and selective pressures. Nat. Rev. Genet. 11 (1), 47–59.

Ghiselli, G., Schaefer, E.J., Gascon, P., Breser, H., 1981. Type III hyperlipoproteinemia associated with apolipoprotein E deficiency. Science 214 (4526), 1239–1241.

Ghorani, V., Boskabady, M.H., Khazdair, M.R., Kianmeher, M., 2017. Experimental animal models for COPD: a methodological review. Tob. Induc. Dis. 15 (1), 25.

Godec, J., Tan, Y., Liberzon, A., Tamayo, P., Bhattacharya, S., Butte, A.J., et al., 2016. Compendium of immune signatures identifies conserved and species-specific biology in response to inflammation. Immunity 44 (1), 194–206.

Gonzalez-Suarez, I., Martin, F., Marescotti, D., Guedj, E., Acali, S., Johne, S., et al., 2016. In vitro systems toxicology assessment of a candidate modified risk tobacco product shows reduced toxicity compared to that of a conventional cigarette. Chem. Res. Toxicol. 29 (1), 3–18.

Gordon, T., Bosland, M., 2009. Strain-dependent differences in susceptibility to lung cancer in inbred mice exposed to mainstream cigarette smoke. Cancer Lett. 275 (2), 213–220.

Greek, R., Rice, M.J., 2012. Animal models and conserved processes. Theor. Biol. Med. Model. 9 (1), 40.

Gunning, W.T., Castonguay, A., Goldblatt, P.J., Stoner, G.D., 1991. Strain A/J mouse lung adenoma growth patterns vary when induced by different carcinogens. Toxicol. Pathol. 19 (2), 168–175.

Hanahan, D., Weinberg, R.A., 2011. Hallmarks of cancer: the next generation. Cell 144 (5), 646–674.

Hartung, T., 2018. Perspectives on in vitro to in vivo extrapolations. Appl. In Vitro Toxicol. 4 (4), 305–316.

Hartung, T., 2019. Predicting toxicity of chemicals: software beats animal testing. EFSA J. 17, e170710.

Hautamaki, R.D., Kobayashi, D.K., Senior, R.M., Shapiro, S.D., 1997. Requirement for macrophage elastase for cigarette smoke-induced emphysema in mice. Science 277 (5334), 2002–2004.

Haziza, C., De La Bourdonnaye, G., Merlet, S., Benzimra, M., Ancerewicz, J., Donelli, A., et al., 2016. Assessment of the reduction in levels of exposure to harmful and potentially harmful constituents in Japanese subjects using a novel tobacco heating system compared with conventional cigarettes and smoking abstinence: a randomized controlled study in confinement. Regul. Toxicol. Pharmacol. 81, 489–499.

Hecht, S.S., Morse, M.A., Amin, S., Stoner, G.D., Jordan, K.G., Choi, C.-I., et al., 1989. Rapid single-dose model for lung tumor induction in A/J mice by 4-(methylnitrosamino)-1-(3-pyridyl)-1-butanone and the effect of diet. Carcinogenesis 10 (10), 1901–1904.

Henry, C.J., Kouri, R.E., 1986. Chronic inhalation studies in mice. II. Effects of long-term exposure to 2R1 cigarette smoke on (C57BL/Cum× C3H/AnfCum) F1 mice. J. Natl. Cancer Inst. 77 (1), 203–212.

Ho, M., Post, C.M., Donahue, L.R., Lidov, H.G., Bronson, R.T., Goolsby, H., et al., 2004. Disruption of muscle membrane and phenotype divergence in two novel mouse models of dysferlin deficiency. Hum. Mol. Genet. 13 (18), 1999–2010.

Hoeng, J., Deehan, R., Pratt, D., Martin, F., Sewer, A., Thomson, T.M., et al., 2012. A network-based approach to quantifying the impact of biologically active substances. Drug Discov. Today 17 (9–10), 413–418.

Hughes, B., 2008. Industry Concern Over EU Hepatotoxicity Guidance. Nature Publishing Group.

Hukkanen, J., Jacob 3rd, P., Benowitz, N.L., 2005. Metabolism and disposition kinetics of nicotine. Pharmacol. Rev. 57 (1), 79–115.

Hutt, J.A., Vuillemenot, B.R., Barr, E.B., Grimes, M.J., Hahn, F.F., Hobbs, C.H., et al., 2005. Life-span inhalation exposure to mainstream cigarette smoke induces lung cancer in B6C3F1 mice through genetic and epigenetic pathways. Carcinogenesis 26 (11), 1999–2009.

Iskandar, A., Titz, B., Sewer, A., Leroy, P., Schneider, T., Zanetti, F., et al., 2017. Systems toxicology meta-analysis of in vitro assessment studies: biological impact of a candidate modified-risk tobacco product aerosol compared with cigarette smoke on human organotypic cultures of the aerodigestive tract. Toxicol. Res. 6 (5), 631–653.

Iskandar, A.R., Xiang, Y., Frentzel, S., Talikka, M., Leroy, P., Kuehn, D., et al., 2015. Impact assessment of cigarette smoke exposure on organotypic bronchial epithelial tissue cultures: a comparison of mono-culture and coculture model containing fibroblasts. Toxicol. Sci. 147 (1), 207–221.

Ito, S., Matsumura, K., Ishimori, K., Ishikawa, S., 2020. In vitro long-term repeated exposure and exposure switching of a novel tobacco vapor product in a human organotypic culture of bronchial epithelial cells. J. Appl. Toxicol. https://doi.org/10.1002/jat.3982.

Johansson, L., 2015. Translational imaging research. In: Principles of Translational Science in Medicine. Elsevier, pp. 189–194.

Jones, B., Donovan, C., Liu, G., Gomez, H.M., Chimankar, V., Harrison, C.L., et al., 2017. Animal models of COPD: what do they tell us? Respirology 22 (1), 21–32.

Kalra, V.K., Ying, Y., Deemer, K., Coates, T.D., Natarajan, R., Nadler, J.L., 1994. Mechanism of cigarette smoke condensate induced adhesion of human monocytes to cultured endothelial cells. J. Cell. Physiol. 160 (1), 154–162.

Khan, A.H., Zou, Z., Xiang, Y., Chen, S., Tian, X.-L., 2019. Conserved signaling pathways genetically associated with longevity across the species. Biochim. Biophys. Acta Mol. Basis Dis. 1865 (7), 1745–1755.

Kim, S.H., Lee, C.S., 1996. Induction of benign and malignant pulmonary tumours in mice with benzo(a)pyrene. Anticancer Res. 16 (1), 465–470.

Kirschner, M., Gerhart, J.C., 2008. The Plausibility of Life: Resolving Darwin's Dilemma. Yale University Press.

Knight, A., 2007. Systematic reviews of animal experiments demonstrate poor human clinical and toxicological utility. Altern. Lab. Anim. 35 (6), 641–659.

Kogel, U., Gonzalez Suarez, I., Xiang, Y., Dossin, E., Guy, P.A., Mathis, C., et al., 2015. Biological impact of cigarette smoke compared to an aerosol produced from a prototypic modified risk tobacco product on normal human bronchial epithelial cells. Toxicol. In Vitro 29, 2102–2115.

Kuehn, D., Majeed, S., Guedj, E., Dulize, R., Baumer, K., Iskandar, A., et al., 2015. Impact assessment of repeated exposure of organotypic 3D bronchial and nasal tissue culture models to whole cigarette smoke. J. Vis. Exp. (96), 52325. https://doi.org/10.3791/52325. Epub ahead of print 2015/03/06.

Kuschner, W., D'alessandro, A., Wong, H., Blanc, P., 1996. Dose-dependent cigarette smoking-related inflammatory responses in healthy adults. Eur. Respir. J. 9 (10), 1989–1994.

Lacroix, G., Koch, W., Ritter, D., Gutleb, A.C., Larsen, S.T., Loret, T., et al., 2018. Air–liquid Interface in vitro models for respiratory toxicology research: consensus workshop and recommendations. Appl. In Vitro Toxicol. 4 (2), 91–106.

Lauterstein, D., Savidge, M., Chen, Y., Weil, R., Yeager, R.P., 2020. Nonanimal toxicology testing approaches for traditional and deemed tobacco products in a complex regulatory environment: limitations, possibilities, and future directions. Toxicol. In Vitro 62, 104684.

Lee, Y.T., Lin, H.Y., Chan, Y.W., Li, K.H., To, O.T., Yan, B.P., et al., 2017. Mouse models of atherosclerosis: a historical perspective and recent advances. Lipids Health Dis. 16 (1), 12.

Liachenko, S., 2020. Translational imaging in toxicology. Curr. Opin. Toxicol. 23–24, 29–38.

Liang, G.B., He, Z.H., 2019. Animal models of emphysema. Chin. Med. J. 132 (20), 2465–2475.

Lietz, M., Berges, A., Lebrun, S., Meurrens, K., Steffen, Y., Stolle, K., et al., 2013. Cigarette-smoke-induced atherogenic lipid profiles in plasma and vascular tissue of apolipoprotein E-deficient mice are attenuated by smoking cessation. Atherosclerosis 229 (1), 86–93.

Lo Sasso, G., Schlage, W.K., Boué, S., Veljkovic, E., Peitsch, M.C., Hoeng, J., 2016. The Apoe–/– mouse model: a suitable model to study cardiovascular and respiratory diseases in the context of cigarette smoke exposure and harm reduction. J. Transl. Med. 14 (1), 146.

Loboda, A., Damulewicz, M., Pyza, E., Jozkowicz, A., Dulak, J., 2016. Role of Nrf2/HO-1 system in development, oxidative stress response and diseases: an evolutionarily conserved mechanism. Cell. Mol. Life Sci. 73 (17), 3221–3247.

López Campos, J.L., Tan, W., Soriano, J.B., 2016. Global burden of COPD. Respirology 21 (1), 14–23.

Lu, G., Liao, J., Yang, G., Reuhl, K.R., Hao, X., Yang, C.S., 2006. Inhibition of adenoma progression to adenocarcinoma in a 4-(methylnitrosamino)-1-(3-pyridyl)-1-butanone–induced lung tumorigenesis model in A/J mice by tea polyphenols and caffeine. Cancer Res. 66 (23), 11494–11501.

Ludicke, F., Haziza, C., Weitkunat, R., Magnette, J., 2016. Evaluation of biomarkers of exposure in smokers switching to a carbon-heated tobacco product: a controlled, randomized, open-label 5-day exposure study. Nicotine Tob. Res. 18 (7), 1606–1613.

Lüdicke, F., Magnette, J., Baker, G., Weitkunat, R., 2015. A Japanese cross-sectional multicentre study of biomarkers associated with cardiovascular disease in smokers and nonsmokers. Biomarkers 20 (6–7), 411–421.

Luechtefeld, T., Maertens, A., Russo, D.P., Rovida, C., Zhu, H., Hartung, T., 2016. Global analysis of publicly available safety data for 9,801 substances registered under REACH from 2008–2014. ALTEX 33 (2), 95.

Luechtefeld, T., Marsh, D., Rowlands, C., Hartung, T., 2018a. Machine learning of toxicological big data enables read-across structure activity relationships (RASAR) outperforming animal test reproducibility. Toxicol. Sci. 165 (1), 198–212.

Luechtefeld, T., Rowlands, C., Hartung, T., 2018b. Big-data and machine learning to revamp computational toxicology and its use in risk assessment. Toxicol. Res. 7 (5), 732–744.

Luettich, K., Xiang, Y., Iskandar, A., Sewer, A., Martin, F., Talikka, M., et al., 2014. Systems toxicology approaches enable mechanistic comparison of spontaneous and cigarette smoke-related lung tumor development in the A/J mouse model. Interdiscipl. Toxicol. 7 (2), 73–84.

Majeed, S., Frentzel, S., Wagner, S., Kuehn, D., Leroy, P., Guy, P.A., et al., 2014. Characterization of the Vitrocell® 24/48 in vitro aerosol exposure system using mainstream cigarette smoke. Chem. Cent. J. 8 (1), 62.

Mamoshina, P., Kochetov, K., Cortese, F., Kovalchuk, A., Aliper, A., Putin, E., et al., 2019. Blood biochemistry analysis to detect smoking status and quantify accelerated aging in smokers. Sci. Rep. 9 (1), 142.

Marescotti, D., Serchi, T., Luettich, K., Xiang, Y., Moschini, E., Talikka, M., et al., 2019. How complex should an in vitro model be? Evaluation of complex 3D alveolar model with transcriptomic data and computational biological network models. ALTEX 36 (3), 388–402.

Mathis, C., Poussin, C., Weisensee, D., Gebel, S., Hengstermann, A., Sewer, A., et al., 2013. Human bronchial epithelial cells exposed in vitro to cigarette smoke at the air-liquid interface resemble bronchial epithelium from human smokers. Am. J. Physiol. Lung Cell Mol. Physiol. 304 (7), L489–L503.

Meuwissen, R., Berns, A., 2005. Mouse models for human lung cancer. Genes Dev. 19 (6), 643–664.

Meyer, P., Hoeng, J., Rice, J.J., Norel, R., Sprengel, J., Stolle, K., et al., 2012. Industrial methodology for process verification in research (IMPROVER): toward systems biology verification. Bioinformatics 28 (9), 1193–1201.

Muñoz-Fuentes, V., Cacheiro, P., Meehan, T.F., Aguilar-Pimentel, J.A., Brown, S.D., Flenniken, A.M., et al., 2018. The International Mouse Phenotyping Consortium (IMPC): a functional catalogue of the mammalian genome that informs conservation. Conserv. Genet. 19 (4), 995–1005.

Nakamura, A.J., Rao, V.A., Pommier, Y., Bonner, W.M., 2010. The complexity of phosphorylated H2AX foci formation and DNA repair assembly at DNA double-strand breaks. Cell Cycle 9 (2), 389–397.

Normand, R., Du, W., Briller, M., Gaujoux, R., Starosvetsky, E., Ziv-Kenet, A., et al., 2018. Found in Translation: a machine learning model for mouse-to-human inference. Nat. Methods 15 (12), 1067–1073.

OECD, 2014. Guidance document 116 on the conduct and design of chronic toxicity and carcinogenicity studies. Supporting Test Guidelines 451, 452 and 453.

Office of the Surgeon General, 2020. Smoking Cessation: A Report of the Surgeon General.

Olson, H., Betton, G., Robinson, D., Thomas, K., Monro, A., Kolaja, G., et al., 2000. Concordance of the toxicity of pharmaceuticals in humans and in animals. Regul. Toxicol. Pharmacol. 32 (1), 56−67.

Oviedo, A., Lebrun, S., Kogel, U., Ho, J., Tan, W.T., Titz, B., et al., 2016. Evaluation of the Tobacco Heating System 2.2. Part 6: 90-day OECD 413 rat inhalation study with systems toxicology endpoints demonstrates reduced exposure effects of a mentholated version compared with mentholated and non-mentholated cigarette smoke. Regul. Toxicol. Pharmacol. 81 (Suppl. 2), S93−S122.

Peck, M.J., Sanders, E.B., Scherer, G., Lüdicke, F., Weitkunat, R., 2018. Review of biomarkers to assess the effects of switching from cigarettes to modified risk tobacco products. Biomarkers 23 (3), 213−244.

Phillips, B., Esposito, M., Verbeeck, J., Boue, S., Iskandar, A., Vuillaume, G., et al., 2015a. Toxicity of aerosols of nicotine and pyruvic acid (separate and combined) in Sprague−Dawley rats in a 28-day OECD 412 inhalation study and assessment of systems toxicology. Inhal. Toxicol. 9 (Early Online), 1−27.

Phillips, B., Szostak, J., Titz, B., Schlage, W.K., Guedj, E., Leroy, P., et al., 2019. A six-month systems toxicology inhalation/cessation study in ApoE(-/-) mice to investigate cardiovascular and respiratory exposure effects of modified risk tobacco products, CHTP 1.2 and THS 2.2, compared with conventional cigarettes. Food Chem. Toxicol. 126, 113−141.

Phillips, B., Veljkovic, E., Boué, S., Schlage, W.K., Vuillaume, G., Martin, F., et al., 2016. An 8-month systems toxicology inhalation/cessation study in Apoe−/− mice to investigate cardiovascular and respiratory exposure effects of a candidate modified risk tobacco product, THS 2.2, compared with conventional cigarettes. Toxicol. Sci. 149 (2), 411−432.

Phillips, B., Veljkovic, E., Boue, S., Schlage, W.K., Vuillaume, G., Martin, F., et al., 2015b. An 8-month systems toxicology inhalation/cessation study in Apoe-/- mice to investigate cardiovascular and respiratory exposure effects of a candidate modified risk tobacco product, THS 2.2, compared with conventional cigarettes. Toxicol. Sci. https://doi.org/10.1093/toxsci/kfv243. Epub ahead of print 2015/11/27.

Pifferi, F., Terrien, J., Perret, M., Epelbaum, J., Blanc, S., Picq, J.-L., et al., 2019. Promoting healthspan and lifespan with caloric restriction in primates. Commun. Biol. 2 (1), 1−3.

Plump, A.S., Breslow, J.L., 1995. Apolipoprotein E and the apolipoprotein E-deficient mouse. Annu. Rev. Nutr. 15 (1), 495−518.

Poussin, C., Gallitz, I., Schlage, W.K., Steffen, Y., Stolle, K., Lebrun, S., et al., 2014a. Mechanism of an indirect effect of aqueous cigarette smoke extract on the adhesion of monocytic cells to endothelial cells in an in vitro assay revealed by transcriptomics analysis. Toxicol. In Vitro 28 (5), 896−908.

Poussin, C., Kramer, B., Lanz, H.L., Van Den Heuvel, A., Laurent, A., Olivier, T., et al., 2020. 3D human microvessel-on-a-chip model for studying monocyte-to-endothelium adhesion under flow - application in systems toxicology. ALTEX 37 (1), 47−63.

Poussin, C., Mathis, C., Alexopoulos, L.G., Messinis, D.E., Dulize, R.H., Belcastro, V., et al., 2014b. The species translation challenge—a systems biology perspective on human and rat bronchial epithelial cells. Sci. Data 1 (1), 1−14.

Pridgeon, C.S., Schlott, C., Wong, M.W., Heringa, M.B., Heckel, T., Leedale, J., et al., 2018. Innovative organotypic in vitro models for safety assessment: aligning with regulatory requirements and understanding models of the heart, skin, and liver as paradigms. Arch. Toxicol. 92 (2), 557−569.

Rabe, K.F., Hurd, S., Anzueto, A., Barnes, P.J., Buist, S.A., Calverley, P., et al., 2007. Global strategy for the diagnosis, management, and prevention of chronic obstructive pulmonary disease: GOLD executive summary. Am. J. Respir. Crit. Care Med. 176 (6), 532−555.

Reynolds, G., Haniffa, M., 2015. Human and mouse mononuclear phagocyte networks: a tale of two species? Front. Immunol. 6, 330.

Rhrissorrakrai, K., Belcastro, V., Bilal, E., Norel, R., Poussin, C., Mathis, C., et al., 2015. Understanding the limits of animal models as predictors of human biology: lessons learned from the sbv IMPROVER species translation challenge. Bioinformatics 31 (4), 471−483.

Schimek, K., Frentzel, S., Luettich, K., Bovard, D., Rütschle, I., Boden, L., et al., 2020. Human multi-organ chip co-culture of bronchial lung culture and liver spheroids for substance exposure studies. Sci. Rep. 10 (1), 7865.

Sebastiani, P., Thyagarajan, B., Sun, F., Schupf, N., Newman, A.B., Montano, M., et al., 2017. Biomarker signatures of aging. Aging Cell 16 (2), 329−338.

Shanks, N., Greek, R., Greek, J., 2009. Are animal models predictive for humans? Philos. Ethics Humanit. Med. 4, 2.

Shay, T., Jojic, V., Zuk, O., Rothamel, K., Puyraimond-Zemmour, D., Feng, T., et al., 2013. Conservation and divergence in the transcriptional programs of the human and mouse immune systems. Proc. Natl. Acad. Sci. U. S. A. 110 (8), 2946−2951.

Shen, J.X., Youhanna, S., Zandi Shafagh, R., Kele, J., Lauschke, V.M., 2020. Organotypic and microphysiological models of liver, gut, and kidney for studies of drug metabolism, pharmacokinetics, and toxicity. Chem. Res. Toxicol. 33 (1), 38−60.

Shimkin, M.B., Stoner, G.D., 1975. Lung tumors in mice: application to carcinogenesis bioassay. Adv. Cancer Res. 21, 1−58.

Siaucicunaite, R., Foulkes, N.S., Calabrò, V., Vallone, D., 2019. Evolution shapes the gene expression response to oxidative stress. Int. J. Mol. Sci. 20 (12), 3040.

Song, M.-A., Freudenheim, J.L., Brasky, T.M., Mathe, E.A., Mcelroy, J.P., Nickerson, Q.A., et al., 2020. Biomarkers of exposure and effect in the lungs of smokers, nonsmokers, and electronic cigarette users. Cancer Epidemiol. Prev. Biomarkers 29 (2), 443−451.

Stinn, W., Arts, J.H., Buettner, A., Duistermaat, E., Janssens, K., Kuper, C.F., et al., 2010. Murine lung tumor response after exposure to cigarette mainstream smoke or its particulate and gas/vapor phase fractions. Toxicology 275 (1), 10−20.

Stinn, W., Berges, A., Meurrens, K., Buettner, A., Gebel, S., Lichtner, R.B., et al., 2013a. Towards the validation of a lung tumorigenesis model with mainstream cigarette smoke inhalation using the A/J mouse. Toxicology 305, 49−64.

Stinn, W., Buettner, A., Weiler, H., Friedrichs, B., Luetjen, S., Van Overveld, F., et al., 2013b. Lung inflammatory effects, tumorigenesis, and emphysema development in a long-term inhalation study with cigarette mainstream smoke in mice. Toxicol. Sci. 131 (2), 596−611.

Stoner, G.D., 1991. Lung tumors in strain A mice as a bioassay for carcinogenicity of environmental chemicals. Exp. Lung Res. 17 (2), 405−423.

Sturla, S.J., Boobis, A.R., Fitzgerald, R.E., Hoeng, J., Kavlock, R.J., Schirmer, K., et al., 2014. Systems toxicology: from basic research to risk assessment. Chem. Res. Toxicol. 27 (3), 314−329.

Takeuchi, H., Taki, Y., Nouchi, R., Yokoyama, R., Kotozaki, Y., Nakagawa, S., et al., 2019. Association of copper levels in the hair with gray matter volume, mean diffusivity, and cognitive functions. Brain Struct. Funct. 224 (3), 1203−1217.

Tamaki, C., Nagayama, T., Hashiba, M., Fujiyoshi, M., Hizue, M., Kodaira, H., et al., 2013. Potentials and limitations of nonclinical safety assessment for predicting clinical adverse drug reactions: correlation analysis of 142 approved drugs in Japan. J. Toxicol. Sci. 38 (4), 581−598.

Taylor, M., Thorne, D., Carr, T., Breheny, D., Walker, P., Proctor, C., et al., 2018. Assessment of novel tobacco heating product THP1. 0. Part 6: a comparative in vitro study using contemporary screening approaches. Regul. Toxicol. Pharmacol. 93, 62−70.

Titz, B., Sewer, A., Schneider, T., Elamin, A., Martin, F., Dijon, S., et al., 2015. Alterations in the sputum proteome and transcriptome in smokers and early-stage COPD subjects. J. Proteomics 128, 306−320.

Titz, B., Szostak, J., Sewer, A., Phillips, B., Nury, C., Schneider, T., et al., 2020. Multi-omics systems toxicology study of mouse lung assessing the effects of aerosols from two heat-not-burn tobacco products and cigarette smoke. Comput. Struct. Biotechnol. J. 18, 1056−1073.

Tsoutsoulopoulos, A, Gohlsch, K, Möhle, N, Breit, A, et al., 2019. Validation of the CULTEX® Radial Flow System for the assessment of the acute inhalation toxicity of airborne particles. Toxicol In Vitro 58, 245−255.

Van Der Toorn, M., Sewer, A., Marescotti, D., Johne, S., Baumer, K., Bornand, D., et al., 2018. The biological effects of long-term exposure of human bronchial epithelial cells to total particulate matter from a candidate modified-risk tobacco product. Toxicol. In Vitro 50, 95−108.

Vikis, H., Rymaszewski, A., Tichelaar, J., 2013. Mouse models of chemically-induced lung carcinogenesis. Front. Biosci. 5, 939.

Vorrink, S.U., Zhou, Y., Ingelman-Sundberg, M., Lauschke, V.M., 2018. Prediction of drug-induced

hepatotoxicity using long-term stable primary hepatic 3D spheroid cultures in chemically defined conditions. Toxicol. Sci. 163 (2), 655−665.

Wall, R.J., Shani, M., 2008. Are animal models as good as we think? Theriogenology 69 (1), 2−9.

Wendler, A., Wehling, M., 2010. The translatability of animal models for clinical development: biomarkers and disease models. Curr. Opin. Pharmacol. 10 (5), 601−606.

Williams, A.B., Schumacher, B., 2017. DNA damage responses and stress resistance: concepts from bacterial SOS to metazoan immunity. Mech. Ageing Dev. 165 (Pt A), 27−32.

Witschi, H., Espiritu, I., Uyeminami, D., Suffia, M., Pinkerton, K.E., 2004. Lung tumor response in strain a mice exposed to tobacco smoke: some dose-effect relationships. Inhal. Toxicol. 16 (1), 27−32.

Wong, E.T., Kogel, U., Veljkovic, E., Martin, F., Xiang, Y., Boue, S., et al., 2016. Evaluation of the tobacco heating system 2.2. Part 4: 90-day OECD 413 rat inhalation study with systems toxicology endpoints demonstrates reduced exposure effects compared with cigarette smoke. Regul. Toxicol. Pharmacol. 81 (Suppl. 2), S59−S81.

Wörsdörfer, P., I, T., Asahina, I., Sumita, Y., Ergün, S., 2020. Do not keep it simple: recent advances in the generation of complex organoids. J. Neural. Transm. https://doi.org/10.1007/s00702-020-02198-8.

Xiong, R., Wu, Q., Muskhelishvili, L., Davis, K., Shemansky, J.M., Bryant, M., et al., 2018. Evaluating mode of action of acrolein toxicity in an in vitro human airway tissue model. Toxicol. Sci. 166 (2), 451−464.

Yang, G.Y., Liu, Z., Seril, D.N., Liao, J., Ding, W., Kim, S., et al., 1997. Black tea constituents, theaflavins, inhibit 4-(methylnitrosamino)-1-(3-pyridyl)-1-butanone (NNK)-induced lung tumorigenesis in A/J mice. Carcinogenesis 18 (12), 2361−2365.

Yoneyama, T., Abdul-Hadi, K., Brown, A., Guan, E., Wagoner, M., Zhu, A.Z., 2019. A citrulline-based translational population system toxicology model for gastrointestinal-related adverse events associated with anticancer treatments. CPT Pharmacometrics Syst. Pharmacol. 8 (12), 951−961.

Yuan, Y.M., Luo, L., Guo, Z., Yang, M., Lin, Y.F., Luo, C., 2015. Smoking, aging, and expression of proteins related to the FOXO3 signaling pathway in lung tissues. Genet. Mol. Res. 14 (3), 8547−8554.

Zhou, Y., Shen, J., Lauschke, V.M., 2019. Comprehensive evaluation of current organotypic and microphysiological liver models for prediction of drug-induced liver injury. Front. Pharmacol. 10, 1093.

Zilionis, R., Engblom, C., Pfirschke, C., Savova, V., Zemmour, D., Saatcioglu, H.D., et al., 2019. Single-cell transcriptomics of human and mouse lung cancers reveals conserved myeloid populations across individuals and species. Immunity 50 (5), 1317−1334.e1310.

Zink, D., Chuah, J.K.C., Ying, J.Y., 2020. Assessing toxicity with human cell-based in vitro methods. Trends Mol. Med. 26 (6), 570−582.

CHAPTER 11

Aerosol Dosimetry and Human-Relevant Exposure

ARKADIUSZ K. KUCZAJ • FRANCESCO LUCCI • ADITYA REDDY KOLLI •
WALTER K. SCHLAGE • PATRICK VANSCHEEUWIJCK • JULIA HOENG

11.1 INTRODUCTION

Estimating human-relevant aerosol exposure and dosimetry is a challenging task. In this chapter, we provide a brief introduction to the aspects that are relevant and currently under research, from long-term toxicity assessments to rapid screening of active pharmaceutical substances, with consideration given to relevant extrapolations between animal and human aerosol exposures. We begin by briefly summarizing the aerosol inhalation process and lung delivery in the context of particle physics and by differentiating exposure from dosimetry. Acute and chronic inhalation exposures, in particular from the perspective of toxicity assessments in rodents, will be discussed and followed by an outline of existing and recently developed approaches to measuring and estimating aerosol exposure. This chapter ends with a short section on the extrapolation of human-relevant doses from rodent data. More comprehensive introductions to all these aspects have been published (Finlay, 2001; Phalen, 2008), which we have extended here in the context of evolving liquid aerosols.

Understanding aerosol dynamics is essential when studying aerosol delivery to the lung. Particular attention will be given here to the processes governing the evolution of liquid aerosols with small (micrometer and submicrometer size) particles of high particle number density, such as evaporation, condensation, and coagulation. Solid-particle (powder) aerosols will not be discussed. In liquid aerosols, the processes related to the thermodynamic state of the aerosol mixture (containing gas and liquid particles) are of key importance, while the particles' shape and physical surface properties are typically irrelevant. The aerosol particles are generally assumed to be spherical, in particular small particles that are not under the influence of significant aerodynamic forces. The particles' surface properties are relevant mainly for their chemical properties (e.g.,

solubility, hydrophilicity) and electrostatic properties (Forsyth et al., 1998; Pc and Hk, 2009; Consta et al., 2018), rather than for physical considerations such as surface roughness, adhesion, or elasticity.

Aerosol evolution, although often driven by distinct chemical or physical forces, leads to alterations in particle size, number density, and phase-partitioning modulations. These alterations modify aerosol deposition during inhalation and, thus, the dosimetry depends strongly on the ability and magnitude of aerosol evolution. In the next section, we discuss various parameters that influence aerosol lung delivery.

11.2 AEROSOL INHALATION AND LUNG DELIVERY

In this section, we discuss aerosol inhalation and lung delivery with respect to the processes underlying alterations in aerosol properties. Tsuda and coworkers have written a comprehensive introduction to particle transport and deposition in the human lungs (Tsuda et al., 2013). During aerosol generation and inhalation, the induced flow leads to changes in the local velocity and dynamic pressure surrounding the particles. The aerosol mixture is either heated or cooled, depending on the aerosol generation mechanisms, reaching a warm and humid-mouth atmosphere temperature of 36.6°C and frequently assumed maximum of 99.5% relative humidity (Longest and Xi, 2008). Apart from temperature-related changes, the immediate availability of water causes condensation, leading to increases in particle size and subsequently increased deposition in the upper respiratory tract by impaction and sedimentation. It is worth noting that aerosols generated by nebulization at room temperature will most likely be heated, while the aerosols generated by thermal nucleation processes, such as that of e-vapor products (EVPs), will be cooled. Although these

Toxicological Evaluation of Electronic Nicotine Delivery Products. https://doi.org/10.1016/B978-0-12-820490-0.00002-X

223

two cases are distinct, the temperature differences are within 10–15°C and the entire process is altered by the mixing of two atmospheres with a large disparity in water content driving the local thermodynamics.

Apart from thermodynamic changes, an important aspect to consider is distinct timescales of processes that depend on the inhalation profile/flow. In immediate inhalation, the aerosol flow will be drawn directly from the upper to the lower respiratory tract. The typical EVP inhalation process consists of consecutive steps in which the consumer takes a puff, which is held in the mouth for a few seconds and then inhaled and exhaled. Frequencies, volumes, flow rates, and measurements of physical aerosol properties have been covered previously (Robinson et al., 2015; Sosnowski and Odziomek, 2018). For aerosols with a high density of particles, the mouth hold provides additional time in which coagulation effects may reduce particle number density but increase particle size. Typical inhalation flow rates will accelerate the local aerosol flow, creating complex airflow patterns caused by the geometrical complexity of the upper respiratory tract. Despite significant velocities, the condensation/evaporation effects are prone to equilibration within milliseconds; consequently, the aerosol entering the human mouth is already altered and equilibrated when passing the trachea. The local velocities, and thus timescales, will differ between the bulk flow and within the boundary layers close to the respiratory tract walls.

Further down, in the lower respiratory tract, the aerosol is decelerated and, therefore, the impaction deposition process is complemented by sedimentation for larger droplets and diffusion for smaller droplets. The local flow velocities depend on the total volumetric flow rate generated by lung expansion and their magnitude is governed by the intrinsic geometry of the lung generations and connecting bifurcations with respect to their diameters, lengths, and angles. Aerosol deposition during lung expansion is not suppressed during lung contraction, leading to total aerosol deposition during the entire inhalation process. Eventually, depending on aerosol size, only a portion of the initial aerosol mass will be deposited, while part will be exhaled (McGrath et al., 2019).

We have discussed already most of the macrophysical transport processes governing aerosol lung delivery that are sufficiently complex to predict aerosol dosimetry. These general bulk transport processes are complemented by intrinsic phase change aerosol dynamics continuously altering the aerosol equilibrium, in particular in the vicinity of the boundary layers close to the respiratory tract walls, terminal ducts, and acini (Feng, 2016; Kleinstreuer

and Zhang, 2010; Grotberg, 2011; Ahookhosh et al., 2020). In these regions, the additional effects that become important are related to significant boundary movements (expansion), the influence of lung surfactant fluid, and moving mucus due to cilia beating in the bronchioles. Complementary to physical processes, aerosol chemistry influences the phase change aerosol dynamics, which is generally understood for aerosols made of a single molecular species. However, for aerosols made of a mixture of chemical species, predicting their phase change/transfer dynamics, and subsequent local aerosol delivery and deposition, becomes a challenge. The governing processes of the multispecies mass transfers from liquid and gas phases are still poorly understood, and various models have been developed (Grasmeijer et al., 2016). The thermodynamic state of the multispecies mixture cannot be generalized, and gas–liquid partitioning of such mixtures depends on their composition (substance affinity driven by material properties that often do not superimpose in a stoichiometric manner between species).

In addition, the dynamics of mass transfer in the vicinity of the liquid particle surface is governed by the species vapor pressures corrected in the multispecies context by their activity coefficients with respect to the liquid mixture. These are dictated by the vapor–liquid equilibrium data that are available only for a limited number of mixtures. Deviations from the ideal stoichiometric solutions given by Raoult's law must often be introduced, and those depend on the concentration of the species. Consequently, the gas–liquid partitioning of species is neither easy to predict nor experimentally measured. In addition, for very small (submicron) liquid particles, the Kelvin effect that modifies the pressure over the curved particle surfaces also induces alterations in the mass transfer and therefore in phase partitioning (Asgari et al., 2019).

Similarly, as particle size distribution describes the number of particles by size class, gas–liquid partitioning defines the amount of the available species to be absorbed from the gas phase. Generally, gas absorption is driven by the diffusion forces governed by Fick's law, relating the gradient of species and its diffusivity to the magnitude of the absorption. Little is known about the concentration of species on the surface of lung tissues, which most likely follows the same law of diffusion within the tissue. Diffusivity for binary species is well understood, but diffusivity in a larger number of species often becomes a nonlinear process, again with limited available data and validated models (Kleinstreuer, 2006).

Theoretical models have been proposed to mechanistically explain the processes of gas absorption and particle deposition in the deep lungs with hypotheses of their sudden reevaporation and condensation (Pankow, 2001; Gowadia and Dunn-Rankin, 2010; Seeman et al., 2004; Seeman and Carchman, 2008). These hypotheses require further verification and potentially experimental validation that is rather impossible in vivo, but certain elements can be tested in vitro, in systems that resemble physiological aspects of lung function when modulating the aerosol. Similarly, tissue species transfer models have been proposed that are based on bulk diffusion forces (Kleinstreuer, 2006), but which also offer a molecular perspective on the transportability of certain species through a complex structure of three-dimensional epithelial tissues.

In summary, lung aerosol delivery is still a fairly unexplored research area that requires synergy between in vitro experimental and computational validation streams, with further advances in biological engineering. This is of particular relevance for the following aspects: particle dynamics of multispecies liquid-evolving aerosols, systems emulating physiological conditions that resemble thermodynamic/physiological lung behavior, the development of standardized epithelial tissues and research in understanding their functioning, and advances in noninvasive in vivo methods for assessing aerosol deposition.

11.3 EXPOSURE AND DOSIMETRY

Aerosol lung delivery involves exposure followed by the subsequent distribution of species along the airways down to the terminating alveolar sacs (acini). Aerosol dosimetry is the measurement of the deposition and species absorption following aerosol exposure, and the related physical and chemical processes. Exposure measurements are often taken to estimate aerosol lung delivery but, in reality, these are just rough approximations of the aerosol dosimetry. Exposure measures the concentration of species having been delivered with a certain flow rate over a defined period of time to an in vitro or in vivo system. Exposure measurements do not recognize the difference between the delivered phases (gas or liquid/solid particles). Thus, they do not take into account the physical processes governing aerosol deposition. In in vivo studies, one generally relies on respiratory minute volumes to estimate aerosol delivery and uptake, but this does not take into account that a fraction of the aerosol is exhaled with each breath. Consequently, only part of the aerosol mixture/species will be delivered to studied systems because deposition forces (e.g., impaction, interception, sedimentation, diffusion) act on the aerosol, limiting delivery to the lung tissue. The delivered dose depends on particle size (aerosol deposition) and species concentration in the gas phase (aerosol gas-phase absorption). The aerosol portion that is not deposited or absorbed will be exhaled (in in vivo systems) or removed (in in vitro systems). For liquid aerosols, a combination of two measurements (liquid/solid aerosol deposition and gas absorption) under physically relevant conditions along the airways uniquely defines the aerosol dosimetry.

Another aspect to consider relates to the significant difference in aerosol delivery between in vitro and in vivo exposures. All commercially available in vitro systems (e.g., Cultex, Hannover, Germany; VITROCELL, Waldkirch, Germany) are based on continuous aerosol delivery in the vicinity of the tissue culture; it is the action of sedimentation and diffusion forces that lead to aerosol deposition. A general limitation of these systems is often related to the fact that their aerosol delivery is not physiologically driven, leading to aerosol dynamics alterations (e.g., size-selective sampling, agglomeration) that can differ from the real-world situation (Steiner et al., 2020). In vivo, the situation is typically more complex and aerosol size-selective sampling also occurs but appears to be a natural consequence of breathing through either the mouth or nose. Furthermore, deposition/absorption mechanisms acting along the respiratory tract can be considered from a filtration perspective as various doses are delivered along that route, directly affecting the transfer rates of species and their bioavailability with respect to several tissues types along the airways (spatial concentration) and, consequently, temporal distribution within the body. Respiratory anatomy and physiology differences between subjects and both population-based and intersubject variability can affect the delivered dose.

Ultimately, simple classification of the administered (generated) and delivered doses may often be insufficient for appropriate calculations and scientific dissemination, including the appropriate understanding and interpretation of the study results. Guidelines issued by the US Environmental Protection Agency (EPA, US EPA, 2014) stratify the term "delivered dose" into the applied, internal, and biologically effective dose. In pharmacology, the administered dose is stratified into the nominal and emitted dose, while the delivered dose is divided into the deposited and systemic dose (Tepper et al., 2016). In summary, the reader should be generally cautious concerning definitions used in the literature in order to avoid generalizations, or even misunderstanding, attributable to the simplifications of dose estimation (see general schema concerning the aerosol delivery process in Fig. 11.1).

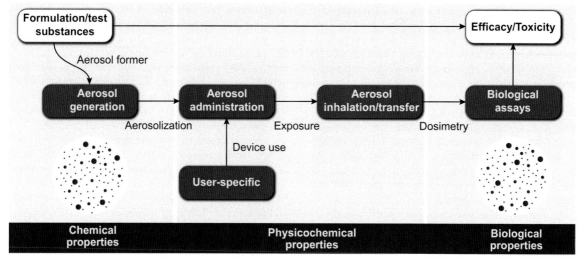

FIG. 11.1 Aerosol delivery route with the importance of the inhalation process and related properties.

11.4 ACUTE AND CHRONIC INHALATION

Safety inhalation studies generally use two distinct (acute and chronic) exposure regimens with their subversions. Following the Organisation for Economic Cooperation and Development (OECD) Test Guidelines (TGs) (OECD, 2018), they span from acute (TG 403), being a single exposure for at least 4 h duration, through subacute (TG 412): 14—28 days (also called a short-term repeated dose), subchronic (TG 413): up to 90 days, and chronic (TG 452): 6—24 months inhalation studies. For a more detailed review see Arts et al. (2008) or refer to particular guidelines that deliver required information to design the inhalation experiments, including, e.g., prerequisites like animal selection criteria, test procedure and conditions, and biological endpoints to be measured or observed.

For pharmacology and toxicity testing, as well as product risk assessment, sophisticated physiologically based pharmacokinetic (PBPK) models are used to calculate absorption, distribution, metabolism, and excretion and to predict the temporal profiles of chemicals, metabolites, or biomarkers in the different compartments of exposed organisms (Kuempel et al., 2015; Phalen and Raabe, 2016). Validation of developed PBPK models requires experimental data that are generated using short inhalation exposures with a fast temporal resolution of the traced substance of interest (i.e., the active substance in the drug discovery process or toxic substance in the toxicity assessment study). The aerosol deposition and dosimetry have the same timescale of action as effective aerosol distribution and exposure-dose measurements, necessitating tight coupling between dosimetry and PBPK modeling. The bridging of aerosol dosimetry and PBPK models has been recently reviewed (Kolli et al., 2019).

Inhalation scenarios require either a single acute dose, multiple doses that are repeated periodically over time (e.g., human-like electronic nicotine delivery product (ENDP) use), or continuous aerosol generation and delivery for chronic exposure. In these studies, the animals are exposed to the aerosol within a specified time and substance concentration interspersed with periods of fresh air delivery that are often imposed by operational or logistical reasons. The previously mentioned OECD TGs (OECD, 2018) provide details on the calculations of required concentrations, exposure time, and methods. In these studies, the concentration of tested substance and duration of exposure are the leading parameters to calculate the dose regimen. Currently, existing guidelines do not refer to more sophisticated methods for predicting aerosol dosimetry. These methods, although probably more accurate, need further development and validation, in particular for evolving liquid aerosols. Luckily, as the processes governing aerosol physics are universal, the aerosol delivery considerations are fundamental. The inclusion of detailed respiratory physiology, linked with lung topology and physicochemical aerosol characteristics during the inhalation process, is required and is subject to ongoing developments in this research field.

11.5 AVAILABLE EXPOSURE AND DOSIMETRY TOOLS

Various approaches can be used to estimate aerosol dosimetry in exposure studies. These are often based on the measured chemical concentration of the substance in the delivered volume of the aerosol flow. The Association of Inhalation Toxicologists recommends that the standard delivered dose calculation be the product of multiplying the substance concentration in the air by the respiratory minute volume and duration of exposure, and divided by the body weight of the exposed subject (Alexander et al., 2008). Such a calculation provides the mass of the substance per kilogram body weight. An additional factor, the inhalable fraction, should be used in the calculations as the proportion of the particles that are inhalable; this factor is often omitted because test aerosols in toxicological studies are normally designed to be inhalable by the subjects. This formula is a global measure of maximum potential dose that can be delivered and must be used cautiously in relation to the various definitions in the literature (US EPA, 1994, 2014). As this definition does not account for the size-selective aerosol sampling, filtration, and deposition that simultaneously occur along the respiratory tract, it will not distinguish between the gas and liquid (particle) delivery phases. Similarly, alterations in the particle size distribution of the delivered aerosol will certainly lead to changes in the deposition pattern and, consequently, in the amount of aerosol exhaled, which is not taken into account here. Aerosol size-selective sampling and exhalation will diminish the actual aerosol dose.

More sophisticated dose calculations that integrate simplified aerosol physics, such as respiratory physiology with the geometry of the airways, can be performed using the so-called whole-lung modeling approach (ICRP, 1994). In this approach, the respiratory minute volume flow is distributed within simplified airway geometry in accordance with the calculated local flows for airway branching, and correlations between aerosol size particles and deposition patterns for selected aerosol physics processes (e.g., sedimentation, impaction, diffusion) are used to estimate regional aerosol deposition. The calculations can be performed in a deterministic average (single-path) manner and then multiplied by the branching number, specified in a multipath more complex geometry-specific manner, and taken as a stochastic process (Hofmann and Sturm, 2004), in particular for the lower respiratory tract down to the terminating alveoli. An overview of various modeling approaches is available in Hofmann (1996, 2011). The best known and publicly available approach is the multiple path particle dosimetry model developed by Applied Research Associates, Inc. (MPPD, 2020; Anjilvel and Asgharian, 1995; Asgharian and Anjilvel, 1998).

The major advantage of such an approach, apart from obtaining detailed information on regional aerosol deposition along the respiratory tract, is the calculation of the aerosol amount that is exhaled. Regional aerosol deposition is particularly important in connection with PBPK models, in which the fast onset of substance transport must be taken into account to obtain the required product profile (see Fig. 11.1 in Kolli et al., 2019 presenting the plot of nicotine concentrations in blood during and after the consumption of cigarettes, oral snuff, chewing tobacco, nicotine gum, nicotine patches, and the Tobacco Heating System 2.2). Whole-lung models, although constructed from physical processes, simplify and accept multiple assumptions on aerosol transport and deposition. There is limited availability of the correlations of aerosol deposition with subject-specific geometries (in particular, for the upper respiratory tract, including mouth and nose), and these are based on the existing limited datasets. Presently, there is no whole-lung model publicly available that accounts for evolving liquid aerosols. For a schematic overview of available methods and approaches concerning dosimetry, see Fig. 11.2.

Modern computational fluid dynamics (CFD) simulations are used to predict upper respiratory tract deposition (Frederix et al., 2018). Various opportunities exist for the computational approach (Rostami, 2009; Kleinstreuer and Zhang, 2010), although the available tools are rather limited in their ability to tackle the complexity of liquid evolving aerosols in the fully thermodynamically coupled multiphase framework. Aero-Solved (AeroSolved, 2020), developed by PMI Research and Development (Fig. 11.3), is a unique CFD tool that can simulate evolving liquid aerosols in a thermodynamically integrated manner. Generally, although delivering detailed aerosol deposition data in circumstances in which the experimental ones are not present or cannot be obtained, CFD methods are limited in application to simulations of the intrinsic geometry of the lower respiratory tract. The natural approach involves the application of CFD simulations to the upper respiratory tract, and their combination in a hybrid model with whole-lung model predictions for the lower respiratory tract (Longest and Holbrook, 2012; Kolanjiyil and Kleinstreuer, 2016, 2017). The required aerosol dosimetry research needs have been articulated in the literature (Phalen and Hoover, 2006; Phalen et al., 2010).

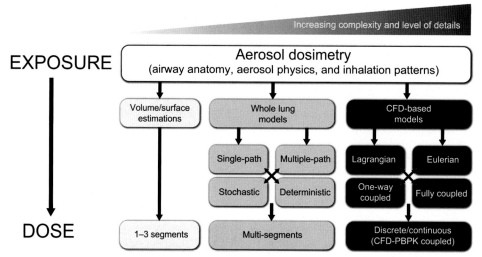

FIG. 11.2 Aerosol dosimetry approaches directly linked with their potential for coupling to PBPK models.

The development of sophisticated and robust dosimetry models, taking into account complex aerosol physics for liquid evolving aerosols, linked with detailed CFD predictions for upper respiratory tract geometries, and validated directly with relevant in vivo studies, in vitro cast deposition experiments and indirectly through PBPK data, is required to advance the understanding and predictions of modern toxicology.

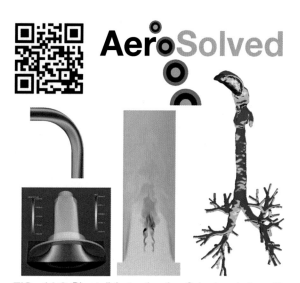

FIG. 11.3 Direct link to the AeroSolved website with snapshots from performed simulations with liquid evolving aerosols (i.e., bent pipe, in vitro aerosol exposure chamber, capillary aerosol generator, and lung cast simulations).

11.6 IN VIVO AEROSOL DELIVERY CONSIDERATIONS FOR LABORATORY ANIMALS

In vivo toxicity testing in laboratory animals requires particular attention be paid to aerosol generation and delivery (Phalen et al., 2008). Small rodents, such as mice and rats, are typically used; these differ from humans in their anatomy of the upper and lower respiratory tract, including airway sizes and their bronchial divisions (Raabe et al., 1976). The same holds true for their respiratory physiology, which is characterized by much larger breathing frequency and smaller respiratory minute volume. Basic respiratory physiology data for rodents have been described elsewhere (Kling, 2011). During inhalation, depending, for example, on the irritation caused by the inhaled substances, both the breathing frequency and respiratory volume can be altered by the animals, to a large extent, which will impact deposited doses. Therefore, it is necessary for the improvement of dose estimations to measure respiratory physiology of exposed animals upon the actual exposure studies for all considered exposure concentrations.

In addition, mice and rats are obligate nose breathers (Wolff and Dorato, 1993), which induces significant filtration of aerosols in the nasal passages. Consequently, the aerosol particle size distribution mass fractions that are inhalable and respirable differ between humans and laboratory rodents (Brown et al., 2013). This is particularly the case for human smoking or the inhalation of ENDP aerosols, which usually occurs through the oral cavity. The inhalable fraction of particles is defined as the mass reaching the nose or mouth, while the respirable fraction is the one that penetrates the unciliated airways, i.e., the bronchioles and beyond (CEN, 1993). In the current OECD guidelines (OECD, 2018), recommendations are given for the mass median aerodynamic diameter to be smaller than 2 μm and a geometric standard deviation within 1−3. For small rodents, aerosols fulfilling these requirements will be inhalable, but perhaps not fully respirable. The size-selective aerosol deposition between the nose, larynx, trachea, and bronchi will affect the distribution of the aerosol. This is of particular importance not only for larger aerosol particles that will be deposited in the nose and upper respiratory tract of small rodents but also for evolving liquid aerosols in which gas−liquid partitioning will dictate the fate of the selected substances by their volatility, with respect to the mixture as a whole and to the characteristics of particle size distribution (see general consideration in Fig. 11.4).

To summarize, in vivo aerosol dosimetry still remains a scientific challenge for accurate regional prediction of the deposition and absorption of aerosols. To remedy this situation, biological response−positive controls with known effects need to be considered to determine whether an exposure study has been appropriate, as planned and expected. Aerosol uptake is confirmed by assessing histopathological changes occurring in the airways and lungs, and by the use of biomarkers of exposure measured in the urine or blood samples (Yeh et al., 1990; Gregg et al., 2013; Peck et al., 2018). In addition, rodent PK studies with known smoke/aerosol constituents can be considered to better understand and verify absorption profiles linked with regional airways and lung aerosol deposition and absorption. Another important aspect requiring detailed validation studies is linked with the use of various in vivo exposure systems with two major distinct types, i.e., whole-body and nose-only systems (Wong, 2007; Phalen et al., 2013; Lucci et al., 2020). Nose-only systems are considered to be better aerosol delivery systems as they avoid uncontrolled aerosol exposure via animal skin and oral consumption due to licking the fur and other present surfaces in the cages. Conversely, they introduce additional stress to the animals constrained in the exposure tubes, which may cause unwanted biological effects (Phalen et al., 2013). Apart from the physical, chemical, and biological considerations concerning aerosol characteristics and its delivery for setting up successful aerosol exposure studies, appropriate logistical and IT-related aspects, like data generation, processing, and governance, including quality control analysis of datasets, must be taken into account when planning the exposure studies. All these steps are necessary and are an integral part of the overall specific animal model validation.

11.7 EXTRAPOLATION OF ANIMAL DOSES TO HUMANS

The predicted dose in in vivo toxicological studies is necessary, but not sufficient, to relate the toxicity induced to human exposure and relevant doses (Nair and Jacob, 2016; Nair et al., 2018). The animal dose must be extrapolated to a human equivalent dose (FDA Center for Drug Evaluation and Research, 2005). Body surface area is recommended as an allometric scaling approach rather than conversion by body mass (Reagan-Shaw et al., 2008). This approach is an empirical scaling based on dose normalization to the body surface area. The conversion is used for estimating human equivalent doses and in interspecies extrapolations for toxicological assessments. Therefore, it is necessary to follow these recommendations to ensure that ENDP assessment studies in animal models of disease are performed with human-relevant doses of ENDP aerosol (Phillips et al., 2016, Phillips et al., 2019; Szostak et al., 2020). These recommendations also permit an understanding of the human relevance of inhalation toxicology studies conducted with an ENDP aerosol (Oviedo et al., 2016; Wong et al., 2016; Phillips et al., 2017) or its components (Ho et al., 2020).

11.8 CONCLUDING REMARKS

Understanding how aerosols are delivered and absorbed through the lung is a highly relevant research topic. Advances in this field will come from the synergy between computational approaches, advances in biological engineering, and in vitro experimental systems. Importantly, computational models will need to be validated using experimental test systems, as well as human (and rodent) pharmacokinetics data.

This field of research is especially important to ENDP assessment as understanding the dynamics of aerosol evolution along the respiratory tract will influence product development processes that are aimed at developing the most satisfying ENDPs with the least possible toxicological effect. Indeed, the efficiency of nicotine delivery, a necessary feature of a satisfying alternative to cigarettes, drives the shape of the nicotine absorption profile. Therefore, it is important to develop ENDPs with aerosol compositions that lead to nicotine pharmacokinetic profiles that resemble as closely as possible that of cigarettes. As outlined in this chapter, aerosol composition is a key driver of aerosol dynamics. Therefore, developing experimentally validated modeling tools that are predictive of nicotine absorption will facilitate the development of ENDPs that meet smoker satisfaction while minimizing the toxicological profile of the aerosol.

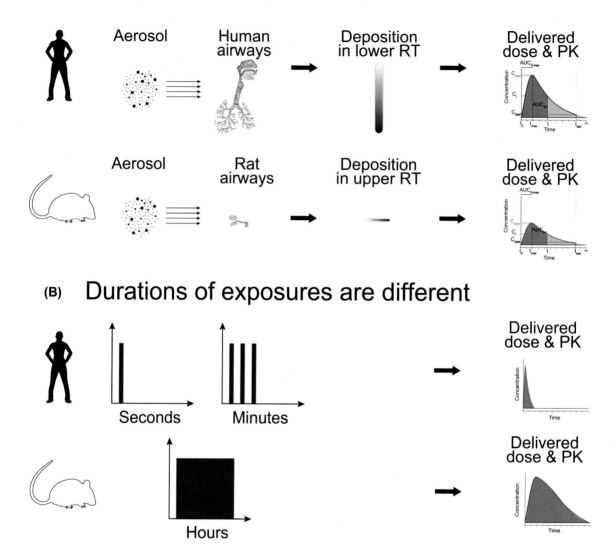

(A)   Aerosol vs. airways diameter ratio

Aerosol — Human airways → Deposition in lower RT → Delivered dose & PK

Aerosol — Rat airways → Deposition in upper RT → Delivered dose & PK

(B)   Durations of exposures are different

Seconds   Minutes → Delivered dose & PK

Hours → Delivered dose & PK

FIG. 11.4 Aerosol dosimetry challenges related to animal to human extrapolations concerning the size of the aerosol particles in comparison to geometrical airway dimensions and flowrates (**A**) and differences in usual exposure regimens (**B**).

Furthermore, locally deposited doses drive the biological responses in the upper respiratory tract and the lung. In the case of cigarette smoking, this is supported by large-scale epidemiology studies (Carter et al., 2015) showing that the smoking-related relative risk of mortality from cancer (RR-MC) increases along the respiratory tract. Indeed, the RR-MC increases from 5.7 in the oral cavity to 13.9 in the larynx and 25.3 in the lung. These differences are mainly driven by the locally

deposited doses of smoke. In this context, understanding the patterns of ENDP aerosol deposition in the respiratory tract could enable a more comprehensive assessment of the long-term relative health risks associated with switching from smoking to ENDP use; this could be achieved before the a posteriori observations that come with epidemiological studies.

Finally, a detailed understanding of the differences in the aerosol evolution and deposition across in vitro models, animal models, and humans is key to the validation of exposure systems, the proper design of nonclinical studies, and the extrapolation of nonclinical study data to human toxicology. There is a need for the harmonization of dosimetry methods to avoid the potential generation of data which are, at best, difficult to compare and, at worst, may result in misleading comparisons and conclusions. As the experimental technologies advance and computational capabilities are continuously growing, more refined methodologies will become available to establish aerosol dosimetry models. These, eventually, should support translation efforts from preclinical to clinical studies, and first-in-human studies. Detailed aerosol dosimetry linked with PBPK modeling will provide quantitative systems pharmacology, a deeper understanding of the acting mechanisms, and, together with the required quality management systems and pertinent certifications, will hopefully support regulatory acceptance efforts, considering the approval of consumer products.

REFERENCES

AeroSolved, 2020. CFD software package. Available at: https://github.com/pmpsa-cfd/aerosolved. (Accessed 16 June 2020).

Ahookhosh, K., et al., 2020. Development of human respiratory airway models: a review. Eur. J. Pharmaceut. Sci. 145, 105233. https://doi.org/10.1016/j.ejps.2020.105233.

Alexander, D.J., et al., 2008. Association of Inhalation Toxicologists (AIT) working party recommendation for standard delivered dose calculation and expression in non-clinical aerosol inhalation toxicology studies with pharmaceuticals. Inhal. Toxicol. 20 (13), 1179–1189. https://doi.org/10.1080/08958370802207318.

Anjilvel, S., Asgharian, B., 1995. A multiple-path model of particle deposition in the rat lung. Toxicol. Sci. 28 (1), 41–50. https://doi.org/10.1093/toxsci/28.1.41.

Arts, J.H.E., et al., 2008. Inhalation toxicity studies: OECD guidelines in relation to REACH and scientific developments. Exp. Toxicol. Pathol. 60 (2–3), 125–133. https://doi.org/10.1016/j.etp.2008.01.011.

Asgari, M., Lucci, F., Kuczaj, A.K., 2019. Multispecies aerosol evolution and deposition in a bent pipe. J. Aerosol Sci. 129, 53–70. https://doi.org/10.1016/j.jaerosci.2018.12.007.

Asgharian, B., Anjilvel, S., 1998. A multiple-path model of fiber deposition in the rat lung. Toxicol. Sci. 44 (1), 80–86. https://doi.org/10.1093/toxsci/44.1.80.

Brown, J.S., et al., 2013. Thoracic and respirable particle definitions for human health risk assessment. Part. Fibre Toxicol. 10 (1), 12. https://doi.org/10.1186/1743-8977-10-12.

Carter, B.D., et al., 2015. Smoking and mortality—beyond established causes. N. Engl. J. Med. 372 (7), 631–640. https://doi.org/10.1056/NEJMsa1407211.

CEN, 1993. EN 481 – Workplace Atmospheres – Size Fraction Definitions for Measurement of Airborne Particles.

Available at: https://standards.globalspec.com/std/969024/EN%20481. (Accessed 17 June 2020).

Consta, S., et al., 2018. Macroion-solvent interactions in charged droplets. J. Phys. Chem. A 122 (24), 5239–5250. https://doi.org/10.1021/acs.jpca.8b01404.

Finlay, W.H., 2001. Introduction. In: The Mechanics of Inhaled Pharmaceutical Aerosols. Elsevier, pp. 1–2. https://doi.org/10.1016/B978-012256971-5/50002-X.

Guidance for Industry: Estimating the Maximum Safe Starting Dose in Initial Clinical Trials for Therapeutics in Adult Healthy Volunteers, 2005. U.S. Department of Health and Human Services Food and Drug Administration Center for Drug Evaluation and Research (CDER), p. 30.

Forsyth, B., Liu, B.Y.H., Romay, F.J., 1998. Particle charge distribution measurement for commonly generated laboratory aerosols. Aerosol. Sci. Technol. 28 (6), 489–501. https://doi.org/10.1080/02786829808965540. Taylor & Francis.

Frederix, E.M.A., et al., 2018. Simulation of size-dependent aerosol deposition in a realistic model of the upper human airways. J. Aerosol Sci. 115, 29–45. https://doi.org/10.1016/j.jaerosci.2017.10.007.

Gowadia, N., Dunn-Rankin, D., 2010. A transport model for nicotine in the tracheobronchial and pulmonary region of the lung. Inhal. Toxicol. 22 (1), 42–48. https://doi.org/10.3109/08958370902862442. Taylor & Francis.

Grasmeijer, N., Frijlink, H.W., Hinrichs, W.L.J., 2016. An adaptable model for growth and/or shrinkage of droplets in the respiratory tract during inhalation of aqueous particles. J. Aerosol Sci. 93, 21–34. https://doi.org/10.1016/j.jaerosci.2015.11.011.

Gregg, E.O., Minet, E., McEwan, M., 2013. Urinary biomarkers of smokers' exposure to tobacco smoke constituents in tobacco products assessment: a fit for purpose approach. Biomarkers 18 (6), 467–486. https://doi.org/10.3109/1354750X.2013.821523.

Grotberg, J.B., 2011. Respiratory fluid mechanics. Phys. Fluids 23 (2), 021301. https://doi.org/10.1063/1.3517737. American Institute of Physics.

Ho, J., et al., 2020. Evaluation of toxicity of aerosols from flavored e-liquids in Sprague-Dawley rats in a 90-day OECD inhalation study, complemented by transcriptomics analysis. Arch. Toxicol. 94 (6), 2179–2206. https://doi.org/10.1007/s00204-020-02759-6.

Hofmann, W., 1996. Modeling techniques for inhaled particle deposition: the state of the art. J. Aerosol Med. 9 (3), 369–388. https://doi.org/10.1089/jam.1996.9.369.

Hofmann, W., 2011. Modelling inhaled particle deposition in the human lung—a review. J. Aerosol Sci. 42 (10), 693–724. https://doi.org/10.1016/j.jaerosci.2011.05.007.

Hofmann, W., Sturm, R., 2004. Stochastic model of particle clearance in human bronchial airways. J. Aerosol Med. 17 (1), 73–89. https://doi.org/10.1089/089426804322994488.

ICRP, 1994. Human Respiratory Tract Model for Radiological Protection, p. 66. Available at: https://journals.sagepub.com/doi/pdf/10.1177/ANIB_24_1-3. (Accessed 16 June 2020).

Kleinstreuer, C., 2006. Biofluid Dynamics: Principles and Selected Applications. CRC Press.

Kleinstreuer, C., Zhang, Z., 2010. Airflow and particle transport in the human respiratory system. Annu. Rev. Fluid Mech. 42 (1), 301−334. https://doi.org/10.1146/annurev-fluid-121108-145453.

Kling, M.A., 2011. A review of respiratory system Anatomy, physiology, and disease in the mouse, rat, hamster, and gerbil. Vet. Clin. Exot. Anim. Pract. 14 (2), 287−337. https://doi.org/10.1016/j.cvex.2011.03.007.

Kolanjiyil, A.V., Kleinstreuer, C., 2016. Computationally efficient analysis of particle transport and deposition in a human whole-lung-airway model. Part I: theory and model validation. Comput. Biol. Med. 79, 193−204. https://doi.org/10.1016/j.compbiomed.2016.10.020.

Kolanjiyil, A.V., Kleinstreuer, C., 2017. Computational analysis of aerosol-dynamics in a human whole-lung airway model. J. Aerosol Sci. 114, 301−316. https://doi.org/10.1016/j.jaerosci.2017.10.001.

Kolli, A.R., et al., 2019. Bridging inhaled aerosol dosimetry to physiologically based pharmacokinetic modeling for toxicological assessment: nicotine delivery systems and beyond. Crit. Rev. Toxicol. 49 (9), 725−741. https://doi.org/10.1080/10408444.2019.1692780.

Kuempel, E.D., et al., 2015. Advances in inhalation dosimetry models and methods for occupational risk assessment and exposure limit derivation. J. Occup. Environ. Hyg. 12 (Suppl. 1), S18−S40. https://doi.org/10.1080/15459624.2015.1060328.

Longest, P.W., Holbrook, L.T., 2012. In silico models of aerosol delivery to the respiratory tract — development and applications. Adv. Drug Deliv. Rev. 64 (4), 296−311. https://doi.org/10.1016/j.addr.2011.05.009.

Longest, P.W., Xi, J., 2008. Condensational growth may contribute to the enhanced deposition of cigarette smoke particles in the upper respiratory tract. Aerosol. Sci. Technol. 42 (8), 579−602. https://doi.org/10.1080/02786820802232964. Taylor & Francis.

Lucci, F., et al., 2020. Experimental and computational investigation of a nose-only exposure chamber. Aerosol. Sci. Technol. 54 (3), 277−290. https://doi.org/10.1080/02786826.2019.1687843. Taylor & Francis.

McGrath, J.A., et al., 2019. Investigation of the quantity of exhaled aerosols released into the environment during nebulisation. Pharmaceutics 11 (2). https://doi.org/10.3390/pharmaceutics11020075.

Feng, Y., 2016. Computational Fluid-Particle Dynamics Modeling for Unconventional Inhaled Aerosols in Human Respiratory Systems | IntechOpen. Available at: https://www.intechopen.com/books/aerosols-science-and-case-studies/computational-fluid-particle-dynamics-modeling-for-unconventional-inhaled-aerosols-in-human-respirat (Accessed 14 July 2020).

Nair, A., Jacob, S., 2016. A simple practice guide for dose conversion between animals and human. J. Basic Clin. Pharm. 7 (2), 27. https://doi.org/10.4103/0976-0105.177703.

Nair, A., Morsy, M.A., Jacob, S., 2018. Dose translation between laboratory animals and human in preclinical and clinical phases of drug development. Drug Dev. Res. 79 (8), 373−382. https://doi.org/10.1002/ddr.21461.

OECD, 2018. Guidance Document on Inhalation Toxicity Studies. Series on Testing and Assessment No.39. OECD. https://www.oecd.org/officialdocuments/publicdisplaydocumentpdf/?cote=env/jm/mono(2009)28/rev1&doclanguage=en. (Accessed 16 June 2020).

Oviedo, A., et al., 2016. Evaluation of the Tobacco Heating System 2.2. Part 6: 90-day OECD 413 rat inhalation study with systems toxicology endpoints demonstrates reduced exposure effects of a mentholated version compared with mentholated and non-mentholated cigarette smoke. Regul. Toxicol. Pharmacol. (RTP) 81 (Suppl. 2), S93−S122. https://doi.org/10.1016/j.yrtph.2016.11.004.

Pankow, J.F., 2001. A consideration of the role of gas/particle partitioning in the deposition of nicotine and other tobacco smoke compounds in the respiratory tract. Chem. Res. Toxicol. 14 (11), 1465−1481. https://doi.org/10.1021/tx0100901. American Chemical Society.

Pc, K., Hk, C., 2009. Electrostatics of pharmaceutical inhalation aerosols. J. Pharm. Pharmacol. 61 (12), 1587−1599. https://doi.org/10.1211/jpp.61.12.0002.

Peck, M.J., et al., 2018. Review of biomarkers to assess the effects of switching from cigarettes to modified risk tobacco products. Biomarkers 23 (3), 213−244. https://doi.org/10.1080/1354750X.2017.1419284. Taylor & Francis.

Phalen, R.F., 2008. Inhalation Studies: Foundations and Techniques, 0 edn. CRC Press. https://doi.org/10.3109/9781420003260.

Phalen, R.F., Hoover, M.D., 2006. Aerosol dosimetry research needs. Inhal. Toxicol. 18 (10), 841−843. https://doi.org/10.1080/08958370600748778.

Phalen, R.F., Raabe, O.G., 2016. The evolution of inhaled particle dose modeling: a review. J. Aerosol Sci. 99, 7−13. https://doi.org/10.1016/j.jaerosci.2015.12.008.

Phalen, R.F., Oldham, M.J., Wolff, R.K., 2008. The relevance of animal models for aerosol studies. Drug Deliv. 21 (1), 113−124. https://doi.org/10.1089/jamp.2007.0673.

Phalen, R.F., Mendez, L.B., Oldham, M.J., 2010. New developments in aerosol dosimetry. Inhal. Toxicol. 22 (Suppl. 2), 6−14. https://doi.org/10.3109/08958378.2010.516031.

Phalen, R.F., Mendez, L.B., Oldham, M.J., 2013. Nose-only exposure systems: design, operation, and performance. Available at: https://escholarship.org/uc/item/7bv1270r. (Accessed 14 July 2020).

Phillips, B., et al., 2016. An 8-month systems toxicology inhalation/cessation study in ApoE$^{-/-}$ mice to investigate cardiovascular and respiratory exposure effects of a candidate modified risk tobacco product, THS 2.2, compared with conventional cigarettes. Toxicol. Sci. 149 (2), 411−432. https://doi.org/10.1093/toxsci/kfv243.

Phillips, B., et al., 2017. Toxicity of the main electronic cigarette components, propylene glycol, glycerin, and nicotine, in Sprague-Dawley rats in a 90-day OECD inhalation study complemented by molecular endpoints. Food Chem. Toxicol. 109 (Pt 1), 315−332. https://doi.org/10.1016/j.fct.2017.09.001.

Phillips, B., et al., 2019. A six-month systems toxicology inhalation/cessation study in ApoE$^{-/-}$ mice to investigate cardiovascular and respiratory exposure effects of modified risk tobacco products, CHTP 1.2 and THS 2.2, compared with conventional cigarettes. Food Chem. Toxicol. 126, 113–141. https://doi.org/10.1016/j.fct.2019.02.008.

Raabe, O.G., et al., 1976. Tracheobronchial Geometry: Human, Dog, Rat, Hamster — A Compilation of Selected Data from the Project Respiratory Tract Deposition Models, UNT Digital Library. Department of Commerce, United States. Available at: https://digital.library.unt.edu/ark:/67531/metadc100754/. (Accessed 16 June 2020).

Reagan-Shaw, S., Nihal, M., Ahmad, N., 2008. Dose translation from animal to human studies revisited. FASEB. J. 22 (3), 659–661. https://doi.org/10.1096/fj.07-9574LSF.

Robinson, R.J., et al., 2015. Electronic cigarette topography in the natural environment. PloS One 10 (6), e0129296. https://doi.org/10.1371/journal.pone.0129296. Public Library of Science.

Rostami, A.A., 2009. Computational modeling of aerosol deposition in respiratory tract: a review. Inhal. Toxicol. 21 (4), 262–290. https://doi.org/10.1080/08958370802448987.

Seeman, J.I., Carchman, R.A., 2008. The possible role of ammonia toxicity on the exposure, deposition, retention, and the bioavailability of nicotine during smoking. Food Chem. Toxicol. 46 (6), 1863–1881. https://doi.org/10.1016/j.fct.2008.02.021.

Seeman, J.I., et al., 2004. On the deposition of volatiles and semivolatiles from cigarette smoke aerosols: relative rates of transfer of nicotine and ammonia from particles to the gas phase. Chem. Res. Toxicol. 17 (8), 1020–1037. https://doi.org/10.1021/tx0300333.

Sosnowski, T.R., Odziomek, M., 2018. Particle size dynamics: toward a better understanding of electronic cigarette aerosol interactions with the respiratory system. Front. Physiol. 9 https://doi.org/10.3389/fphys.2018.00853. Frontiers.

Steiner, S., et al., 2020. Development and testing of a new-generation aerosol exposure system: the independent holistic air-liquid exposure system (InHALES). Toxicol. In Vitro 104909. https://doi.org/10.1016/j.tiv.2020.104909.

Szostak, J., et al., 2020. A 6-month systems toxicology inhalation study in ApoE$^{-/-}$ mice demonstrates reduced cardiovascular effects of E-vapor aerosols compared with cigarette smoke.

Am. J. Physiol. Heart Circ. Physiol. 318 (3), H604–H631. https://doi.org/10.1152/ajpheart.00613.2019.

Tepper, J.S., et al., 2016. Symposium summary: "breathe in, breathe out, its easy: what you need to know about developing inhaled drugs". Int. J. Toxicol. 35 (4), 376–392. https://doi.org/10.1177/1091581815624080.

Tsuda, A., Henry, F.S., Butler, J.P., 2013. Particle transport and deposition: basic physics of particle kinetics. In: Terjung, R. (Ed.), Comprehensive Physiology. John Wiley & Sons, Inc., Hoboken, NJ, USA, pp. 1437–1471. https://doi.org/10.1002/cphy.c100085.

US EPA, 1994. Guidance for Applying Quantitative Data to Develop Data-Derived Extrapolation Factors for Interspecies and Intraspecies Extrapolation. US EPA. Available at: https://www.epa.gov/risk/guidance-applying-quantitative-data-develop-data-derived-extrapolation-factors-interspecies-and. (Accessed 16 June 2020).

US EPA, 2014. Methods for Derivation of Inhalation Reference Concentrations and Application of Inhalation Dosimetry. US EPA. Available at: https://www.epa.gov/risk/methods-derivation-inhalation-reference-concentrations-and-application-inhalation-dosimetry. (Accessed 16 June 2020).

Wolff, R.K., Dorato, M.A., 1993. Toxicologic testing of inhaled pharmaceutical aerosols. Crit. Rev. Toxicol. 23 (4), 343–369. https://doi.org/10.3109/10408449309104076.

Wong, B.A., 2007. Inhalation exposure systems: design, methods and operation. Toxicol. Pathol. 35 (1), 3–14. https://doi.org/10.1080/01926230601060017. SAGE Publications Inc.

Wong, E.T., et al., 2016. Evaluation of the Tobacco Heating System 2.2. Part 4: 90-day OECD 413 rat inhalation study with systems toxicology endpoints demonstrates reduced exposure effects compared with cigarette smoke. Regul. Toxicol. Pharmacol. (RTP) 81 (Suppl. 2), S59–S81. https://doi.org/10.1016/j.yrtph.2016.10.015.

Yeh, H.C., et al., 1990. Comparative evaluation of nose-only versus whole-body inhalation exposures for rats—aerosol characteristics and lung deposition. Inhal. Toxicol. 2 (3), 205–221. https://doi.org/10.3109/08958379009145255. Taylor & Francis.

MPPD (Multiple Path Particle Dosimetry model): A model for human and rat airway particle dosimetry, no date. Available at: http://www.ara.com/products/mppd.htm (Accessed: 16 June 2020).

CHAPTER 12

Systems for Generation of ENDP Aerosols and Their Administration to In Vitro and In Vivo Experimental Models

ANNE MAY • STÉPHANIE BOUÉ • PATRICK VANSCHEEUWIJCK • JULIA HOENG

12.1 INTRODUCTION

The ability to generate, collect, and use aerosols is essential to all electronic nicotine delivery products (ENDPs) assessment activities and to show that the aerosol generated by a specific ENDP (1) emits significantly fewer and lower levels of harmful and potentially harmful constituents (HPHCs) than cigarette smoke (CS), (2) is significantly less toxic than CS in multiple standard in vitro and in vivo toxicology studies, and (3) reduces risk of harm in in vitro and in vivo systems toxicology studies while not presenting new hazards.

ENDP aerosols are qualitatively and quantitatively different from CS, which is generated by tobacco combustion (Chapters 4–7). Furthermore, unlike cigarettes, which constitute a broadly homogeneous product category, ENDPs are more heterogeneous (Chapter 2). This leads to technical and experimental challenges for comparative studies involving ENDP aerosols and/or CS. It should not be assumed that what is known about CS generation, dilution, and delivery to in vitro and in vivo exposure systems will directly apply to ENDP aerosols.

The physical and chemical behaviors of CS and ENDP aerosols are highly variable, both temporally and spatially. For this reason, the design and construction of aerosol generation and exposure systems are likely to alter an aerosol's characteristics (e.g., its particle size distribution [PSD] or the partitioning of its constituents in the solid, liquid, and gas phases) (Chapter 5). This makes the study of these aerosols challenging. For achieving meaningful results when testing aerosols, a key requirement is to understand and control as much as possible the processes that influence aerosol delivery, including aerosol aging, sampling, and deposition in the system.

In this chapter, we focus on the development, validation, and characterization of methods for generating and using aerosols from electrically heated tobacco products (EHTPs) and e-vapor products (EVPs) for in vitro and in vivo assessment. The focus is on mainstream CS and ENDP aerosols that are released during puffing at the mouth end of the product for inhalation. Sidestream CS is the smoke that is released at the lit end of a cigarette; but, ENDPs, by design, do not emit sidestream aerosol.

12.2 PUFFING REGIMENS

While no puffing regimen can be representative of a broad range of human use patterns, standardization is key to providing a basis for enabling meaningful comparisons among different products. To this end, the objective of a standard puffing regimen is to provide a set of conditions under which the product emissions can be compared with those of other products in a meaningful manner.

12.2.1 Puffing Regimens for EHTPs

The World Health Organization Study Group on Tobacco Product Regulation (TobReg) recommended using the Health Canada Intense (HCI) machine smoking regimen, now an ISO intense regimen standard (ISO 20778) (International Organization for Standardization, 2017), for product characterization and hazard assessment (World Health Organization, 2008).

Both the nonintense ISO smoking regimen for cigarettes (ISO 3308) (International Organization for Standardization, 2000a) and the HCI/ISO intense regimen can be used to generate EHTP aerosols, although some requirements cannot be fulfilled for technical reasons. This is the case, for example, in butt length

Toxicological Evaluation of Electronic Nicotine Delivery Products. https://doi.org/10.1016/B978-0-12-820490-0.00017-1

requirement, as tobacco sticks are not consumed by combustion and remain the same size throughout use. Moreover, ventilation blocking can only be applied if the tobacco sticks have ventilation holes; but, tobacco stick filters are generally not perforated.

The HCI/ISO intense regimen has been widely used in EHTP research, mainly because it provides the most relevant comparative basis for evaluating the composition of EHTP aerosols with CS (Belushkin et al., 2018). Moreover, on the basis of puffing topography measurements with two different commercial EHTPs, adult smoker behavior data were shown to be similar to the puff volume and duration of the HCI/ISO intense smoking regimen (Gee et al., 2018; Haziza et al., 2016). However, the debate on the applicability and adaptation of existing smoking standards to EHTPs for regulatory purposes has yet to take place.

12.2.2 Puffing Regimens for EVPs

Human topography studies indicate that EVP usage depends greatly on product design and the individual consumer. Overall, a longer puff duration has been commonly observed among EVP users than cigarette smokers. Among EVP consumers, a wide range of puffing parameters have been reported that might significantly influence e-vapor yields (Farsalinos et al., 2013). It is questionable whether a single puffing regimen is appropriate for all EVP types.

At present, there is no regulatory guidance on EVP puffing regimens for analytical purposes and toxicity testing. As a result, the variety of parameters used in research makes it difficult to evaluate and compare study findings. Standardization is urgently required.

In a 2016 guidance to the industry, the United States (US) Food and Drug Administration recommended using both nonintense and intense regimens for evaluating EVP emissions and testing e-liquids with low and high emission devices; but, the actual parameters were not specified (US Food and Drug Administration, 2016).

ISO Standard 20768:2018 defined the technical requirements, parameters, and standard conditions for routine analytical vaping of EVPs (International Organization for Standardization, 2018).

The standard was developed on the basis of Cooperation Centre for Scientific Research Relative to Tobacco's (CORESTA) recommended method 81 (CORESTA Recommended Method 81; CRM 81) for machine puffing of EVPs (CORESTA, 2015), which aimed at reflecting the puff volume and duration of typical "cig-a-like" EVP users (Vansickel et al., 2018). ISO 20768:2018 and CRM 81 specify a puff volume of 55 mL, a 3-s puff duration, and one puff every 30 s

(55/30/3). A square-shaped profile is recommended, given that a minimum airflow velocity is required for device activation in puff-activated devices. The devices are activated by airflow draw or button.

ISO 20768/CRM 81 may be regarded as reflecting nonintense use. CORESTA has published a technical guide on which criteria can be considered for intense use (CORESTA Guide N° 22 (CORESTA, 2018)). If topography data for the device under study are available, it is recommended to use these as a basis for determining intense usage scenarios. In other cases, the following interdependent parameters should be considered: puff duration, volume, frequency, profile, and number; battery charge; heating element age; voltage and ventilation settings; and device orientation. CORESTA Guide No. 22 stresses that puffing regimens unrepresentative of typical consumer behavior should be avoided, because they might result in generation of by-products that would not occur in real life, as users would experience a self-limiting unpleasant taste.

12.3 AEROSOL GENERATION SYSTEMS
12.3.1 EHTP Aerosol Generation
12.3.1.1 Linear smoking machines
The first machines that allowed smoking of several cigarettes simultaneously or alternately were linear smoking machines (Klus et al., 2016). In a linear smoking machine, individual smoking ports are each coupled to a separate syringe or pump and to an aerosol trapping system such as a Cambridge filter pad (CFP) holder or an impinger (Boué et al., 2020).

These machines allow stick-to-stick or puff-by-puff collection of aerosols for direct analysis or trapping and are, therefore, used for chemical characterization of aerosols (e.g., TNCO [tar, nicotine, and carbon monoxide {CO}] yield determination, or HPHC analyses). A key advantage is that the connection from the smoking port to the trapping system is short, which helps avoid significant changes in aerosol due to surface interference or aging.

Linear smoking machines have been adapted for EHTP aerosol generation. Fig. 12.1 shows a 20-port linear smoking machine type LX20 (Borgwaldt KC GmbH, Hamburg, Germany) adapted for use with the Tobacco Heating System 2.2 (THS), developed by Philip Morris International (PMI). Individual supports made of an aluminum adaptor plate and a Plexiglas adaptor bracket are used to support the tobacco stick holders. An alignment tool, including a stopper, is used to align the support with the smoking port and insert the tobacco stick at the correct distance. The tobacco stick holders are

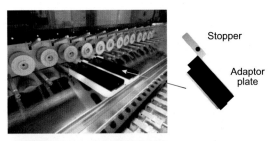

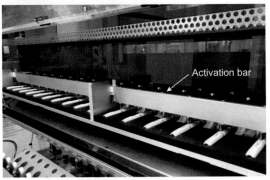

FIG. 12.1 Modified linear smoking machine for THS aerosol generation. *THS*, Tobacco Heating System. (Reproduced from Fig. 4 from Boué, S., Goedertier, D., Hoeng, J., Kuczaj, A., Majeed, S., Mathis, C., et al., 2020. State-of-the-art methods and devices for the generation, exposure, and collection of aerosols from heat-not-burn tobacco products. Toxicol. Res. Appl. 4, 2397847319897869.)

activated either individually or concurrently when an activation bar is used. At the end of a smoking run, the tobacco stick holders are removed manually from the smoking ports, and the tobacco sticks are removed by opening the tobacco stick extractor.

12.3.1.2 Rotary smoking machines

The first prototypes of rotary smoking machines were developed in the mid-1950s as a means to improve the automation of cigarette machine smoking and allow continuous, large-scale aerosol generation (Klus et al., 2016).

Rotary smoking machines are ideally designed for aerosol generation for in vivo exposure studies. They may also be used for large-scale production of aerosol as needed—for example, for analysis of low-yield chemicals (Roemer et al., 2009, 2010).

The rotary smoking machine SM 2000—designed by Philip Morris Research Laboratories (PMRL, Köln, Germany) and manufactured and commercialized by Burghart Messtechnik (Weidel, Germany)—has been widely used in CS research and previously described (Boué et al., 2020; Radtke et al., 2017). The SM 2000 has been adapted for generation of aerosols from THS and the Carbon Heated Tobacco Product (CHTP, PMI, Neuchâtel, Switzerland) (Phillips et al., 2019). Fig. 12.2 shows the SM 2000 THS, a modification of the SM 2000 CS specifically designed by PMI to take into account THS product specificities.

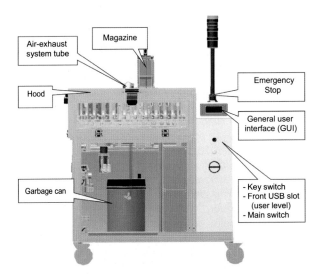

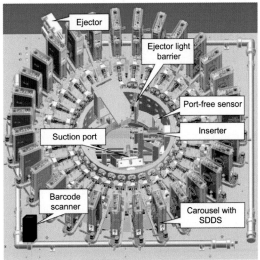

FIG. 12.2 Schematic views of SM 2000 THS. (**A**) Front view. (**B**) Top view. *SDDS*, smoking device docking station; *THS*, Tobacco Heating System. (Modified from Fig. 5 from Boué, S., Goedertier, D., Hoeng, J., Kuczaj, A., Majeed, S., Mathis, C., et al., 2020. State-of-the-art methods and devices for the generation, exposure, and collection of aerosols from heat-not-burn tobacco products. Toxicol. Res. Appl. 4, 2397847319897869.)

Tobacco sticks are inserted into the 30 cigarette ports together with their tobacco stick holders. Each tobacco stick holder is connected to a smoking device docking station (SDDS), which provides energy for recharging the tobacco stick holder battery and acts as an electrical interface between individual tobacco stick holders and the smoking machine controller. Each SDDS consists of a main electronic board with a power supply for recharging and a communication board for interacting with the smoking machine controller (Fig. 12.2).

Insertion and extraction of tobacco sticks into and out of the tobacco stick holders is performed automatically by the smoking machine. An inserter pushes the tobacco stick into the holder. An ejector pulls the head of the tobacco stick holder and grabs and releases the butt. The heating process of the tobacco stick holder is initiated by the smoking machine remotely and controlled by the tobacco stick holder over the preheating and heating periods. Because of the high water content of undiluted THS and CHTP aerosols, condensation may occur when the aerosols come into contact with materials at a lower surface temperature than the aerosol temperature. In order to avoid major condensation effects, the surfaces of the suction port, the programmable dual-syringe pump (PDSP), and all tubes conveying the aerosol up to the dilution system are stabilized at 41°C by using a water warming system (heated water jacket).

For in vitro exposure at the air–liquid interface (ALI), the aerosol is usually generated continuously. Mathis et al. optimized the duration of exposure for organotypic bronchial cell cultures on the basis of their sensitivity to CS exposure, which is likely to have a larger impact on endpoints of interest than THS exposure. The authors exposed normal human bronchial epithelial cells at the ALI to 3R4F CS and found that 28 min of exposure induced the highest concentration of secreted matrix metalloproteinase-1, an indicator of airway cell responsiveness (Mathis et al., 2013).

For in vivo exposure, animals (mice and rats) are exposed to the aerosol for up to 6 h/day for 28 days (subacute toxicity studies (OECD, 2018c)), 90 days (subchronic toxicity studies (OECD, 2018d)), or up to 18 months (chronic inhalation toxicity and tumorigenicity studies (OECD, 2018b)). In studies with CS as a reference, the exposure duration is split into successive 1-h sessions separated by fresh air exposure breaks in order to limit the buildup of carboxyhemoglobin (COHb) concentrations to less than 50% (Phillips et al., 2015).

12.3.2 EVP Aerosol Generation

Different approaches may be used to generate "e-vapors" - defined here as aerosols generated by EVPs. Aerosol may be generated from an EVP e-liquid by using a relevant, standardized puffing regimen, or it may be generated directly from e-liquid solutions by nebulization or using another type of aerosol generator. While it may be argued that aerosol generation from an EVP by using a relevant, standardized puffing regimen is more representative of human consumption, it has several limitations. Given the wide variety of EVP types and devices, any particular device may not be representative of all devices (Williams and Talbot, 2011). Furthermore, poor-quality EVP devices may increase the toxicity of the aerosol, for example, through release of metal ions (Lerner et al., 2015; Mcneill et al., 2018; National Academies of Sciences, 2018; Stephens, 2017; Williams et al., 2013). Moreover, a battery can run out of power, its level of power delivery may vary from one puff to the next, or it may provide a false reading of the applied power. Operating the devices, including charging, refilling, and cleaning, is labor-intensive and a limiting factor when it comes to long-term inhalation studies. According to Werley et al., approximately 27,000 e-cigarettes are required for a 90-day rodent inhalation study (Werley et al., 2016a). Hence, for large-scale production of e-vapors, the use of laboratory nebulizers or aerosol generators simplifies the logistics and eliminates any parameters that could potentially affect reproducibility. However, nebulizers do not allow the study of the effects of substances that may be generated through thermal treatment of the e-liquid; larger-scale aerosol generators may be more suitable for this purpose, as long as the temperature used for aerosolization is representative of that in EVPs.

Thus, the physicochemical characteristics of aerosols generated by these different approaches vary and may result in different toxicity profiles. Therefore, physical and chemical characterization of the aerosol should always be a part of product assessment.

12.3.2.1 E-liquid nebulization (Collison nebulizer)

Nebulization converts a liquid into particles by overcoming the surface tension and mechanicaly "breaking" the liquid into small droplets. Nebulization is widely used in drug delivery devices to administer an active pharmaceutical ingredient inhaled into the lungs. Nebulization does not involve heating, and an aerosol produced by nebulization contains unaltered main e-liquid components.

The Collison nebulizer was first described in the scientific literature by Collison in 1935 (May, 1973). Since then, it has become a recognized technique for nebulizing liquids and suspensions and is commonly used in aerosol generation research.

The Collison nebulizer was shown to be appropriate for delivering nicotine to rodents via inhalation (Shao et al., 2012). Thereafter, it has been used in 28- and 90-day rat inhalation studies on nicotine-containing solutions and shown to be able to continuously generate stable and reproducible aerosols over extended periods (Phillips et al., 2015; Phillips et al., 2017).

In a Collison nebulizer, high-velocity air is used to aspirate a liquid via negative pressure into a siphon and shear it through one or several orifices into small liquid particles, a process known as atomization (Fig. 12.3). Commercial Collison nebulizers (BGI, Butler, NJ, USA; now CH Technologies, USA) possess 1, 3, 6, or 24 orifices to produce the high-speed jet stream. The mass output of the nebulizer is directly proportional to the number of jets present.

The liquid particles (or droplets) produced by this process often have a wide size distribution. To remove larger particles, the jet stream is directed toward the wall of the nebulizer chamber, where large particles with sufficient mass are deposited and drained back to the nebulizer reservoir. Smaller liquid particles leave the reservoir through the aerosol outlet.

A peristaltic pump is used to provide the nebulizer reservoir with a constant supply of e-liquid from an external reservoir in order to maintain the homogeneity of the e-liquid. E-liquid solutions are protected from light in storage at a controlled temperature of 2–8°C. They are equilibrated at room temperature prior to nebulization.

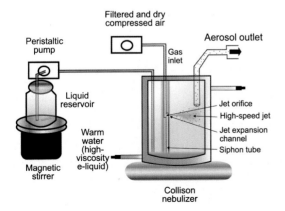

FIG. 12.3 Schematic view of the experimental setup of a Collison nebulizer.

E-liquids typically have high viscosity owing to the presence of propylene glycol (PG) and vegetable glycerin (VG), and their components have different densities. For these reasons, the solution in the external reservoir must be continuously stirred to avoid liquid stratification and maintain a homogeneous feed to the nebulizer.

For high-viscosity solutions, the nebulizer is warmed to 30°C with a water heater in order to decrease viscosity and generate aerosols of required concentrations and particle sizes. The nebulizer should also be warmed when the aerosol is used for cell culture exposure at a temperature matching the exposure chamber temperature (usually 36.6–37°C). This helps minimize changes in the aerosol properties during transportation and delivery.

12.3.2.2 Vaping machines

Given the immense variety in EVPs, vaping machines should allow the use of a variety of designs through custom-designed adaptors. They should also allow the possibility of puff and switch activation of the device and orientation of the product at various degrees. This is necessary for many devices that require an orientation other than horizontal to facilitate efficient wicking of the e-liquid. Vaping machines should also provide external power supply to compensate for potential battery discharge or unreliability (Havel et al., 2017). They should offer the possibility to execute not only standard but also ad-hoc vaping regimens to replicate real-world, human puff profiles.

12.3.2.2.1 Programmable single-syringe pumps. The simplest laboratory vaping machine is a programmable single-syringe pump (PSSP), a linear piston pump with a glass cylinder. The pump is moved by a stepper motor and generates an aerosol by drawing on an EVP device at the inlet valve and delivering the aerosol at the outlet valve. The outlet can be connected to a trapping system or an exposure system.

Fig. 12.4 shows the experimental setup for the continuous generation of e-vapor from two EVP devices using a PSSP (Iskandar et al., 2019).

12.3.2.2.2 Vaping machines. An increasing number of multichannel laboratory vaping machines are becoming commercially available. The EVP vaping machine series CETI (Cerulean, Milton Keynes, UK) is one example of a multichannel linear vaping machine for aerosol trapping and characterization (Fig. 12.5). The machine can be used with puff-activated and switch-activated EVP devices loaded and removed manually. The puff profile (square or sinusoidal), volume,

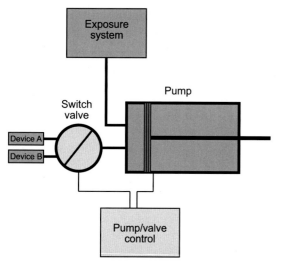

FIG. 12.4 Experimental setup for generation of an aerosol from one type of EVP. Two devices of the same kind are connected to a switch valve, allowing for alternation of aerosol generation from the two devices. *EVP*, e-vapor product.

duration, interval, total number of puffs, and number of conditioning puffs per device can be user defined, including for use in accordance with ISO 20768/CRM 81. The machine also offers the possibility of adjusting the angle at which the device is oriented vertically at 15 degrees intervals between +90 and −90 degrees. Each channel can be combined with a Cambridge filter pad (CFP) holder and/or an impinger for e-vapor fraction collection.

12.3.2.3 Capillary aerosol generator

The capillary aerosol generator (CAG) generates an aerosol from e-liquids by processes that resemble the physical and chemical processes of aerosol generation in an EVP device. The key advantage of the CAG is that it can be used for continuous production of a controlled aerosol similar to e-vapor over several hours (Werley et al., 2016b). Therefore, it is ideal for in vivo inhalation studies.

The CAG was developed by Philip Morris, Inc. and further refined by Virginia Commonwealth University (Gupta et al., 2003; Howell and Sweeney, 1998). The CAG produces a stream of well-controlled aerosol by heating and vaporization of a liquid, followed by nucleation and condensation of the vapor. The physical

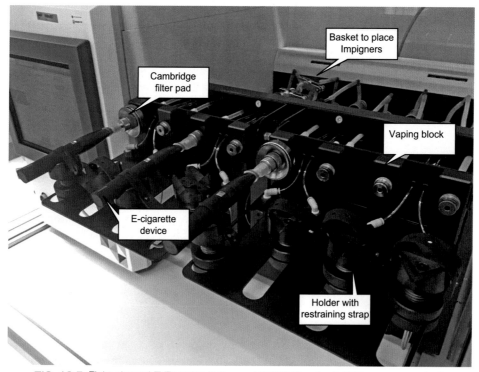

FIG. 12.5 Eight channel EVP vaping instrument CETI8 (Cerulean). *EVP*, e-vapor product.

process of aerosol generation from liquid mixtures in the CAG is complex and follows various stages with varying thermodynamic conditions. The thermodynamic, physical, and chemical properties and conditions of the mixture—such as surface tension, temperature, saturation, equilibrium vapor pressures, and gas-phase concentrations of the constituents—are important to obtain controlled and continuous aerosol delivery at the required particle number density and PSD. Aerosolization by using the CAG helps avoid unintended contamination of the aerosol, for example, by corrosion of the metal heating coil, overheating due to power supply manipulations, or "dry puffing", i.e., overheating due to lack of e-liquid supply for evaporation.

Fig. 12.6 shows the experimental setup and key elements of a CAG.

The CAG described here is a bench-top laboratory device consisting of a stainless steel, heated capillary tube connected to a temperature controller and a liquid reservoir via a peristaltic pump.

E-liquid solutions are prepared and stored as for use with a Collison nebulizer. They are stirred throughout the aerosol generation process to maintain homogeneity. The liquid is supplied via a pump to the capillary tube at a controlled flow rate.

The capillary tube (160 mm; 21 G; stainless steel) is housed in an aluminum block, where it is heated by embedded heating elements. The temperature is set to mimic the temperature of the heating coil during puffing of an EVP, typically 250–275°C (Geiss et al., 2016).

The liquid pumped through the capillary tube is heated, evaporates, and exits the tip of the capillary tube as a supersaturated hot vapor. The vapor is immediately cooled down by mixing with a cooler, filtered air stream around the capillary tube outlet. This leads to homogeneous nucleation of vapors and condensational growth of the generated nuclei, resulting in formation of an aerosol. The flow rate of the filtered air supplied at this point has a strong influence on the PSD (Gupta et al., 2003).

An additional cooling airflow circulates along the capillary tube housing and then along the capillary heating blocks. This airflow prevents vapor from flowing back and coming into contact with the hot surface, thereby avoiding the formation of unwanted degradation products such as carbonyls (Fig. 12.6C).

When used for in vivo inhalation studies, the CAG-generated aerosol is diluted to the target concentration either with conditioned, filtered air at $22 \pm 2°C$ and $60 \pm 5\%$ relative humidity (RH) or with compressed dry air at $22 \pm 2°C$ and 0% RH. The aerosol is delivered via glass tubing to the exposure chamber (Szostak et al., 2020).

The CAG has been shown to produce an aerosol similar to that generated by EVP devices. Werley et al. compared aerosols generated by a prototype EVP and a CAG in terms of chemical composition, chemical by-products, particle size measurements, and port-to-port variability in a nose-only exposure chamber (NOEC) (Werley et al., 2016b). They concluded that the use of the CAG was well justified on the basis of the similarity of its aerosol with that generated by the EVP device and its improved logistics, consistency, and study throughput. When using the CAG to generate an aerosol intended to be representative of the aerosol generated by a specific EVP device, it is important to measure specific chemicals in order to demonstrate similarity and the validity of the approach.

The CAG has been validated prior to application in in vitro and in vivo studies. The impact of various parameters has been assessed, including liquid mixture supply ranging from 0.2 to 1.0 mL/min, capillary temperature ranging from 200°C to 300°C, and air stream of 10–100 L/min. It has been determined that a capillary temperature of 250°C and an air stream of 10 L/min result in a mass median aerodynamic diameter (MMAD) of 1.5 μm and geometric standard deviation (GSD) of 2 (PMI, data not published). For in vivo inhalation studies, a capillary temperature of 250°C and an air stream of 18 L/min, followed by dilution with 260 L/min of filtered air, lead to an MMAD of approximately 1 μm and a GSD of 1.4 when measured in the exposure chamber by using a PIXE cascade impactor.

12.4 COLLECTION OF ENDP AEROSOL FRACTIONS

Collection of aerosol fractions is an indispensable requirement for many applications, spanning routine yield measurements, quantification of constituents, and in vitro toxicity testing.

The collection and fractionation process, while widely used, has several limitations. The methods used for trapping aerosols may exert profound effects on their physical and chemical composition. No single method can efficiently trap all constituents present in the solid, liquid, and gas phases. Analysis of the individual fractions might lead to underestimation of the overall toxicity resulting from the dynamic evolution and interactions among the phases. The stability of the collected materials prior to analysis must be ascertained. The solvents used might react with the constituents of the aerosol fraction or exert biological activity themselves. For in vitro experiments in submerged cell

(A)

Air dilution

CAG

Aerosol
generation

(B)

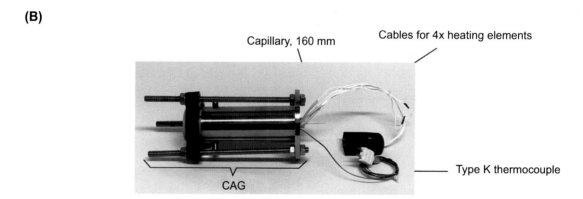

Capillary, 160 mm   Cables for 4x heating elements

CAG

Type K thermocouple

(C)

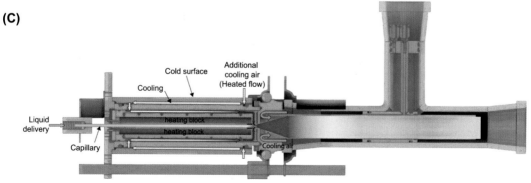

Additional
cooling air
Cold surface   (Heated flow)

Cooling

Liquid
delivery

heating block
heating block

Capillary

Cooling air

FIG. 12.6 CAG. **(A)** Experimental setup. **(B)** CAG capillary and heating elements. **(C)** Cross-sectional
schematic view of the CAG. *CAG*, Capillary aerosol generator.

cultures, the aerosol has to be collected in a biocompatible solvent, which can then be applied to the cells.

Methods for collecting aerosol fractions from THS have been previously described (Boué et al., 2020). Given the qualitative and quantitative differences among CS, EHTP aerosol, and e-vapor, optimization of trapping methods for capturing comparable samples from different products is critical for adequate interpretation and comparison of in vitro exposure assays (Goedertier et al., 2018).

PMI has assessed the impact of various parameters (test item number, sample collection point, trapping solvent volume, trapping temperature, and surface contact material and area) on the efficiency of trapping the aerosol fractions of 3R4F, THS, and EVPs with a view to optimizing them.

Table 12.1 describes the optimal systems and parameters for trapping comparable aerosol fractions from 3R4F, THS, and the EVP P4M3 version 1.0 (P4M3 v 1.0, PMI) for in vitro assays in submersed cell cultures (PMI, data not published).

CS from 3R4F cigarettes was generated on a 20-port Borgwaldt smoking machine (Hamburg, Germany), and test aerosol from THS was generated on a 30-port SM 2000 THS smoking machine (PMI, Neuchâtel, Switzerland) (Boué et al., 2020) in accordance with ISO 20778:2017 (55-mL puff volume, 2-s puff duration, 2-min^{-1} puff frequency, and 100% blocking of filter ventilation holes for 3R4F). Test aerosol from P4M3 was generated on a CETI8 vaping machine in accordance with ISO 20768/CRM 81 (55-mL puff volume, 3-s puff duration, and 2-min^{-1} puff frequency).

12.5 AEROSOL EXPOSURE SYSTEMS FOR IN VITRO STUDIES: EXPOSURE SYSTEMS AT THE ALI

12.5.1 Whole-aerosol Exposure Systems at the ALI

Technical progress has allowed the development of complex, three-dimensional organotypic cell cultures that mimic the physiology of human epithelial tissues. These advanced cellular models can be exposed to aerosols or gases at the ALI. Cells are seeded on porous membranes in culture inserts and supplied with medium from their basal side, while their apical side is in contact with air (Li, 2016; Müller et al., 2012; Paur et al., 2011).

ALI exposure systems are more physiologically relevant than submersed exposure systems for studying tissues exposed to airborne substances, as they better mimic the organization, functionality, and exposure of their human tissue counterparts. In addition, they allow exposure to whole aerosols, bringing the cells into direct contact with the gas–vapor phase (GVP) as well as the particulate phase (Fukano et al., 2004).

However, they present considerable methodological challenges. Aerosol constituents must be transferred from the aerosol to the cell surface to exert an effect on the biological test system. Owing to the complexity of the physical processes governing aerosol transport, dilution, and deposition, the physicochemical characteristics of the aerosol delivered to the biological test system cannot be predicted on the basis of the characteristics of the generated aerosol. Determining the actual delivery efficiency of these exposure systems is, therefore, critical for interpretation and comparison of data from ALI exposure experiments.

TABLE 12.1
Trapping Systems and Parameters for Trapping Aerosol Fractions From 3R4F, THS, and P4M3.

	Test item	# Of test items[a]	# Of puffs	Volume of solvent (mL)	Trapping system
TPM	3R4F	6	61.7	DMSO to a final concentration of 50 mg TPM per mL	CFP 44 mm and elution
	THS	10	120		
	P4M3 v 1.0	1	50		
AE	3R4F	6	61.7	36 mL PBS	Ice cold PBS in impinger
	THS	10	120	40 mL PBS	
	P4M3 v 1.0	1	50	10 mL PBS	
GVP	3R4F	6	61.7	36 mL PBS	CFP 44 mm + ice cold PBS in impinger
	THS	10	120	40 mL PBS	
	P4M3 v 1.0	1	50	10 mL PBS	

AE, aqueous extracts; *CFP*, Cambridge filter pad; *DMSO*, Dimethyl sulfoxide; *GVP*, gas–vapor phase; *PBS*, phosphate-buffered saline; *THS*, Tobacco Heating System; *TPM*, total particulate matter.
a For 3R4F and THS, one test item corresponds to one cigarette or one tobacco stick. For P4M3, one test item corresponds to one e-liquid cap. Reproduced from van der Toorn, M., Koshibu, K., Schlage, W.K., Majeed, S., Pospisil, P., Hoeng, J., et al., 2019. Comparison of Monoamine Oxidase Inhibition by Cigarettes and Modified Risk Tobacco products. (2214–7500 (Electronic)).

A few exposure systems are presently available that enable exposure of cell cultures to CS, EHTP aerosol, and e-vapor at the ALI, including commercial and bespoke systems (Thorne and Adamson, 2013). Each system offers unique advantages and disadvantages. In the next sections, we describe the VITROCELL 24/48 exposure system (VC 24/48; VITROCELL Systems GmbH, Waldkirch, Germany), which has been characterized for use with CS, EHTP aerosols, and e-vapor.

12.5.2 VITROCELL 24/48 Exposure System

The VC 24/48 system has been described previously (Boué et al., 2020) and is schematically represented in Fig. 12.7. Up to 48 wells can be exposed simultaneously in individual exposure chambers grouped into eight rows of six replicate positions.

The test aerosol passes through a dilution/distribution pipe located on top of the base module. The aerosol is diluted with filtered, conditioned fresh air (60 ± 5% RH).

The aerosol is partially sampled by negative pressure—applied by a vacuum pump connected to the cultivation base module—into each individual exposure chamber through trumpet-shaped delivery systems protruding from the dilution/distribution system into the wells. At the end of each dilution row, one exposure chamber allows real-time monitoring of aerosol mass deposition by quartz crystal microbalances (QCMs).

The VC 24/48 exposure system is connected to an aerosol generator. The aerosols are generated as previously described and delivered to the VC 24/48 dilution/distribution system through a fluoroelastomer tube (ISO-Versinic, Saint-Gobain, Courbevoie, France). The distance of the aerosol generator to the cell cultures

is kept as short as possible in order to minimize the influence of aerosol aging processes.

12.5.3 VC 24/48 Exposure System: Characterization

Despite ongoing efforts, limited information and few guidelines are available for characterizing and validating commercial exposure systems (Secondo et al., 2017; Thorne and Adamson, 2013). Flexibility in the design of exposure experiments, unspecified aerosol type—related application, and poorly defined maintenance of the exposure equipment can potentially result in nonreliable and highly variable results. Particular attention must, therefore, be given to understanding how and to what extent the aerosol is modified by the experimental protocol or system before it reaches the exposure site. An appropriate link between the generated and delivered aerosol must be established from the exposure-dose perspective.

Majeed et al. (2014) characterized VC 24/48 for use with CS. They assessed and compared aerosol deposition for different CS concentrations by three different approaches: (1) a WST-1 colorimetric assay, based on a previous observation that WST-1 is reduced upon exposure to CS, presumably because of the high oxidant concentration in CS; (2) determination of eight carbonyls trapped in phosphate-buffered saline (PBS); and (3) QCM-determined particle mass deposition. The authors found that a given concentration of CS reduced WST-1 diluted in Dulbecco's Modified Eagle Medium in all culture inserts to a similar level, as measured by the changes in optical density (OD) at 430 nm. They also observed concentration-dependent changes in OD with different dilution flow rates. Trapped carbonyl concentrations were well correlated with

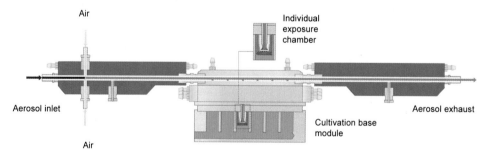

VITROCELL 24/48 – Sectional view

FIG. 12.7 Schematic cross-sectional view of one row of the VC 24/48 exposure system showing the dilution/distribution module, cultivation base module, and individual exposure chambers. (Source: VITROCELL. Modified from Fig. 11 from Boué, S., Goedertier, D., Hoeng, J., Kuczaj, A., Majeed, S., Mathis, C., et al., 2020. State-of-the-art methods and devices for the generation, exposure, and collection of aerosols from heat-not-burn tobacco products. Toxicol. Res. Appl. 4, 2397847319807860.)

the applied CS concentration. The particle mass deposition values measured by QCMs attached to different rows of the dilution/distribution system were also found to be similar at a fixed CS concentration. The authors concluded that the VC 24/48 is well suited for CS exposure of cells growing at the ALI.

However, Steiner et al. demonstrated that the delivery efficiency of individual CS constituents may vary by several orders of magnitude and that, consequently, characterization of the aerosol used in in vitro exposures does not necessarily accurately describe the aerosol fraction that ultimately enters and interacts with the biological test system (Steiner et al., 2018). The authors provided a large set of delivery efficiencies that describe the conversion of an applied dose of CS to a delivered dose during in vitro exposure. These delivery efficiencies provide a simple dose metric tool that allows characterization and comparison of aerosol exposure experiments with respect to the composition of the aerosol presented to the biological test system.

Steiner et al. assessed deposition in cell culture inserts of a fluorescently labeled liquid aerosol generated by a condensation monodisperse aerosol generator (TSI 3475, TSI, Shoreview, MN, USA) (Steiner et al., 2017). The study showed a higher variability in delivery of the liquid aerosol than that when the system was used with CS or EHTP aerosols. Globally, it was found that aerosol delivery to a position of choice in a repetition of choice could reasonably be expected to lie within the range of the average delivery to all positions exposed to the same aerosol concentration $\pm 25\%$. Serial dilution resulted in a clearly discernible dose response; yet, aerosol concentration and aerosol delivery did not generally change by the same factor. The study also showed that QCMs could not report accurate mass deposition of the tested liquid aerosol. The mass of liquid deposits, depending on the thickness of the deposited layer and viscosity of the material, may be underestimated because of viscous energy dissipation into the liquid layer (Voinova et al., 2002; Zhuang et al., 2007).

Frege and colleagues investigated an evolving aerosol inside the VC 24/48 exposure system by online single-photon ionization mass spectrometry to measure in real time the three main constituents of a test aerosol (PG, VG, and nicotine) (Frege et al., 2020). The aerosol was generated from the EVP P4M3 v 1.0 by using a PDSP. The concentrations of PG, VG, and nicotine were measured in the aerosol sampled at the end of each delivery line and at the QCM port in three exposure protocols: (1) no dilution, (2) gradually increasing dilution at each line, and (3) single dilution applied only once at the beginning of the line. The measured concentrations were compared with expected values calculated from the concentrations measured in the aerosol generated by the PDSP and calculated expected changes due to differential phase partitioning, selective sampling, and deposition. The changes in the aerosol as dilution was applied showed not only a reduction in the concentrations of the traced substances but also selective sampling due to evolution of the aerosol and phase partitioning of its constituents. Consequently, the authors recommended that comparative in vitro assessment studies should be conducted with attention to both dilution rates and their actual application in the study design, as these two factors exert direct effects on the delivered doses (Frege et al., 2020).

12.5.4 Aerosol Delivery and Deposition in the VC 24/48 Exposure Chamber

The data presented in the previous section highlight the critical importance of monitoring actual aerosol delivery to and deposition in the individual VC 24/48 exposure chambers. Online and offline approaches may be used to that effect, as described in the following sections.

12.5.4.1 Determination of deposition in the VC 24/48 exposure chamber (PBS experiments)

Actual aerosol deposition in individual exposure chambers can be determined by analyzing deposition in PBS. PBS provides a good model for the thin film of aqueous matrix that commonly covers the surface of cell cultures. Furthermore, because of the stability, low complexity, and lack of metabolic activity and transepithelial transport of PBS, the gross aerosol deposition during PBS exposure experiments can be determined more easily and more accurately than by post-exposure chemical analysis of living cells. Usually, for in situ assessment, each row is loaded with three cell culture and three dummy inserts in randomized positions, for three replicates per aerosol concentration. Immediately after exposure, aliquots of exposed PBS are collected from each steel insert and pooled row-wise into silanized amber glass vials. The samples are stored at $-80°C$ until chemical analysis for quantification of the constituents of interest. PBS deposition can be used to determine the deposition of (for example) carbonyl compounds, nicotine, PG, and VG in VC 24/48 exposure chambers after exposure to CS, EHTP aerosol, or e-vapors.

12.5.4.2 Online aerosol characterization within exposure systems by soft ionization TOFMS (Photonion)

Offline methods like PBS experiments have several limitations. The representativeness and reproducibility of generation and exposure are not guaranteed, as, by definition, they are not performed concurrently with the actual studies. They are time consuming, given the multiple steps required, including trapping, extraction, and measurement. Hence, there is a need for development of methods for sampling and analyzing complex aerosols online during exposure in close proximity to the biological test system.

Photon ionization (PI) time-of-flight mass spectrometry (TOFMS) is an established technology for online, puff-resolved characterization of organic compounds in CS (Adam et al., 2006; Mitschke et al., 2005). The method uses a combination of PI and TOFMS to accelerate and separate ions by mass. Known aerosol constituents can be identified and quantified on the basis of their molecular mass. Many constituents can be detected in real time with single-puff resolution in CS.

Single-PI TOFMS (Photonion GmbH, Schwerin, Germany) can be used with the VC 24/48 system (Boué et al., 2020). Diluted aerosol is sampled from the dilution/distribution system, as shown in Fig. 12.8. A heated (up to 300°C) sampling capillary of 180-μm inner diameter is inserted into the tube, and it samples the aerosol at a rate of 3−5 mL/min. The samples are ionized by vacuum ultraviolet light of 120−160 nm (ionization energy of approximately 10.3 eV) and enter the TOFMS by linear extraction. Mass spectra are reported at a frequency of 1 Hz, and the covered mass range is 10−2000 m/z. Absolute quantification is based on compound-specific cross sections (ionizabilities) relative to toluene, determined by using a 100 ppm reference gas. PI results in only limited fragmentation of analytes; hence, known aerosol constituents can be identified and quantified on the basis of their molecular mass. Yet, the risk of biased quantification in the presence of isobaric molecules should be addressed (e.g., by identifying mass fingerprints for compounds that undergo fragmentation) (Steiner et al., 2017).

12.6 AEROSOL EXPOSURE SYSTEMS FOR ANIMAL INHALATION STUDIES

Despite great progress in the development of complex in vitro surrogate models for in vivo inhalation studies, such as those described earlier in this chapter, these systems cannot yet fully mimic the complex physiological systems of whole living organisms. Animal studies are, therefore, still needed, and rodent inhalation studies are a key element of ENDP assessment.

Animal use in ENDP assessment is restricted to situations where there are no alternatives or where such studies are required by regulation. A well-designed inhalation exposure study can be used to assess the potential toxicity of inhaled products at elevated aerosol exposure concentrations, repeated exposures, and elevated doses over a significant portion of the animals'

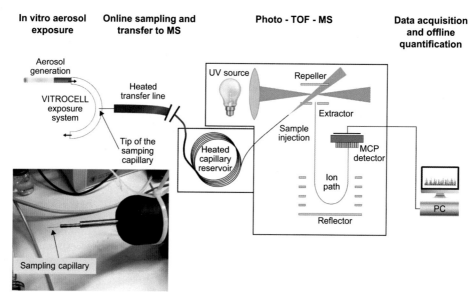

FIG. 12.8 Schematic representation of the Photonion experimental setup. *MCP*, microchannel plate; *MS*, mass spectrometry; *TOF*, time of flight. (Modified from Fig. 13 from Boué, S., Goedertier, D., Hoeng, J., Kuczaj, A., Majeed, S., Mathis, C., et al., 2020. State-of-the-art methods and devices for the generation, exposure, and collection of aerosols from heat-not-burn tobacco products. Toxicol. Res. Appl. 4, 2397847319897869.)

lifetimes and provide a thorough evaluation of the impact on all exposed tissues and organs.

In vivo inhalation studies require exposure systems capable of consistently producing and delivering large volumes of aerosols at concentrations that are stable during prolonged exposure periods and with appropriate physical properties to enable efficient inhalation and uptake.

Today, most inhalation exposure systems are dynamic, single-pass, flow-through exposure systems in which the test atmosphere is continuously delivered to, and removed from, the animal chamber (Dorato, 1990). The aerosol is diluted with conditioned filtered air to obtain the target exposure concentration and volumetric flow rate required by the chamber. In order to avoid particle growth, dilution takes place as soon as possible after aerosol generation (i.e., immediately after the PDSP). To minimize the risk of chemical and physical changes during transportation from the aerosol generator to the exposure chamber, as well as to allow visual inspection of deposition and condensation, the transportation tubing is made of borosilicate glass. The transportation tube length must be kept to a minimum and its route the straightest possible. To avoid experimental artifacts, the transportation routes should be similar for all animal exposure setups used in parallel in a given study.

Various types of chambers have been developed for exposing experimental animals via the inhalation route. These include whole-body exposure chambers (WBECs), head-only exposure chambers, NOECs, and lung-only (intratracheal) and partial-lung exposure systems (Wong, 2007). OECD (Organisation for Economic Co-operation and Development) test guidelines (TGs) expressly mention WBECs and NOECs (OECD, 2018a). Exposure chambers that are used in EHTP research have been extensively described elsewhere, including the 800-L, 24-cage WBEC for mouse inhalation studies, the 64-port NOEC flow-past chamber for rat exposure, and the 60-port NOEC for mice exposure (Boué et al., 2020).

12.6.1 Whole-body Exposure Chambers

WBECs employ chambers in which test animals are free to move in groups or in isolation. Their entire body is immersed in the test atmosphere.

The advantages of WBECs over NOECs include the ability to expose large numbers of animals simultaneously with limited daily animal procedures (no insertion or removal). The animals are unrestrained, which results in minimal stress. On the downside, WBECs require large quantities of test materials and air throughput. Nonhomogeneous distribution of aerosol concentration and particle size is more likely within a large WBEC than in NOECs (Pauluhn and Mohr, 2000). Animals are exposed to the test material via other, confounding routes of exposure, including transdermal uptake following fur deposition and surface contact, oral uptake from grooming, and ocular exposure (Wolff, 2015). When several animals are housed together, they may huddle, leading to varying uptake of the test material, and filtration may occur as rodents breathe through their own or others' fur (Wong, 2007). The test atmosphere may be affected by the differential absorption of aerosol constituents by bedding material and excreta.

12.6.1.1 800-L, 24-cage WBEC for mouse inhalation studies

The 800-L, 24-cage WBEC is a stainless steel and glass inhalation chamber that can house up to 8 mice per cage, for a total of 192 mice (Fig. 12.9).

The aerosol is delivered to the WBEC by three vertical glass pipes running at the back of the chamber. Each vertical glass pipe has eight holes. Each hole is aligned with the top of a cage to deliver the aerosol directly into the cage. Eight sampling ports are available at the back of the WBEC, in the middle row. The aerosol flow rate delivered to the 800-L WBEC after accounting for sampling is ≥ 133 L/min to sustain ≥ 10 air changes per hour (OECD, 2018a). The WBEC is operated under a positive pressure of $20-60$ Pa to help ensure that the entire volume of the WBEC is filled by the test material, thereby improving spatial homogeneity.

Typically, mice are whole-body exposed for $3-4$ h/day, 5 days/week. In order to avoid excessive CO exposure with CS, intermittent exposure may be used, whereby mice are exposed $3-4 \times 1$ h to CS with breaks of $30-60$ min in between, during which the animals are exposed to fresh filtered air.

12.6.2 Nose-only Exposure Chambers

NOECs are designed to expose test animals via the inhalation route while preventing confounding exposure via noninhalation routes. OECD TGs recommend that NOECs be used in inhalation toxicity studies whenever possible (OECD, 2018a). The test animals are held in exposure tubes attached to a central chamber, so that only the nose is exposed to the test atmosphere. The deposition of aerosol particles on the skin and fur of the animals is limited, and aerosol uptake through dermal absorption or ingestion (grooming) is minimized. On the downside, daily animal procedures are highly labor-intensive, de facto limiting the number of animals that can be used in a study. Additionally, the animals may be subjected to higher stress levels in

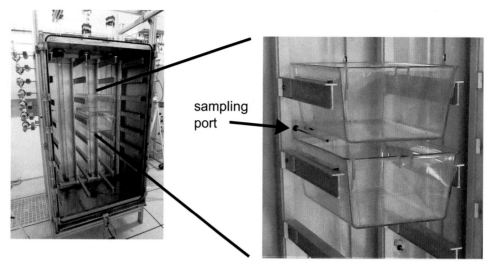

FIG. 12.9 800-L, 24-cage WBEC and sampling ports. *WBEC,* whole-body exposure chamber. (Reproduced from Fig. 18 from Boué, S., Goedertier, D., Hoeng, J., Kuczaj, A., Majeed, S., Mathis, C., et al., 2020. State-of-the-art methods and devices for the generation, exposure, and collection of aerosols from heat-not-burn tobacco products. Toxicol. Res. Appl. 4, 2397847319897869.)

NOECs because of their being restrained and having no access to water throughout the daily exposure period. Stress effects may act as confounding factors for exposure-related study endpoints such as body weight gain and cardiovascular effects (Kogel, in prep).

Fig. 12.10 shows a double-plenum system with an inner and outer plenum built on the so-called "flow-past" model first described by Cannon et al. (1983). The test atmosphere flows vertically downward through an inlet into the inner plenum and is distributed

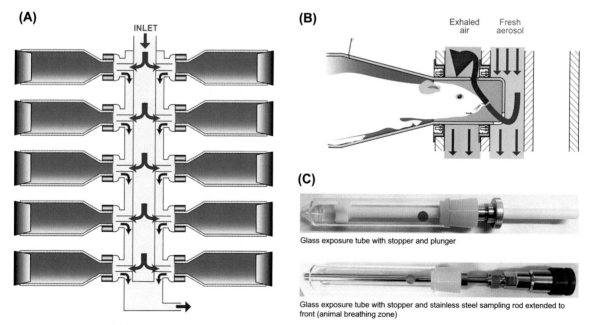

FIG. 12.10 (**A**) Schematic of the principle of a double-plenum FPC. (**B**) Air circulation at the animal breathing zone of the FPC-232. (**C**) Exposure and sampling tubes for the FPC-232 NOEC. *NOEC,* nose-only exposure chamber. (Modified from Fig. 19 from Boué, S., Goedertier, D., Hoeng, J., Kuczaj, A., Majeed, S., Mathis, C., et al., 2020. State-of-the-art methods and devices for the generation, exposure, and collection of aerosols from heat-not-burn tobacco products. Toxicol. Res. Appl. 4, 2397847319897869.)

horizontally through the exposure ports and breathing zone of each animal. Unused aerosol and exhaled air are cleared away with the excess airflow into the outer plenum and then to the chamber exhaust.

NOECs allow sampling of the test atmosphere at the breathing zone of the animals. Closed exposure tubes are fitted with hollow stainless steel sampling rods that extend to the front of the exposure tube to replicate where the animal's nose would be during exposure, so that the samples are representative of what the animal would inhale.

12.6.2.1 The 64-port nose-only flow-past exposure chamber (FPC) for rat inhalation studies

The FPC-232 was designed by PMI (Patent EP2095791A1) and is manufactured by Geraetebau Insul Simsheuser GmbH, Insul, Germany. It is a double-plenum, multilevel, modular chamber made of anodized aluminum for rat inhalation studies.

Typically, the exposure tower is configured with eight levels of eight exposure ports each, for a total of 64 ports. Sampling ports are installed in the exposure ports of the middle row of the tower (row four from the top). Up to five ports are used for sampling and real-time monitoring of parameters such as temperature and chamber pressure.

The volume of the inner chamber is around 4 L and that of the outer chamber is around 12 L. The aerosol flows vertically downward through an inlet into the inner plenum and is distributed horizontally through the exposure ports. Each exposure tube passes through the opening of the exposure port in the outer and inner plenums and extends at least partially into the inner plenum. An airflow of 100 L/min is used to maintain an aerosol flow of 1.2–2 L/min per exposure port. When atmosphere is withdrawn for sampling, the airflow should be adjusted accordingly. The inner plenum is operated under a slight positive pressure of 10–30 Pa, and a pressure differential of 0.5–2 Pa is maintained between the inner and outer plenums to ensure that the aerosol flows from the inner to the outer plenum and not in the reverse direction.

12.6.2.2 The 60-port NOEC for mouse inhalation studies

The 60-port NOEC is a stainless steel, double-plenum, multilevel, modular nose-only exposure system for murine exposure (CH Technologies, Westwood, NJ, USA, Patent 5297502). It consists of individual tiers of 12 exposure ports each. In a typical configuration with 5 tiers and 60 ports, the volume of the inner chamber is around 6 L and that of the outer chamber is around 8 L. The aerosol flows vertically downward through an inlet (16.5-mm diameter in a standard configuration) into the inner plenum and is distributed horizontally through the exposure ports. It exits from the outer plenum through the bottom of the NOEC.

Lucci et al. assessed the aerosol flow characteristics in the chamber using computational flow dynamics and estimated potential particle size–dependent nonuniformities in aerosol sampling at the exposure ports (Lucci et al., 2018). Fig. 12.11 shows the flow through a single tier of a 60-port NOEC (Fig. 12.11A), a visualization of the computed airflow velocity inside the inner plenum (Fig. 12.11B), and computed particle number density in an exposure port (Fig. 12.11C).

The model showed some port variability in airflow velocity, with relatively higher flow through the ports of the lower tiers owing to recirculation of the aerosol after reaching the bottom of the inner plenum. Port variability did not result in significant variability in particle number density. The model also predicted sedimentation of larger particles (>3 μm) inside the exposure ports. However, as the effect was minor and applied to particles beyond the size range recommended for rodent inhalation studies, the authors considered that this sedimentation would not influence the dosimetry of inhaled aerosols (Lucci et al., 2018). Furthermore, the daily rotation of animals across tube positions should prevent artifacts in the data arising from any actual spatial inhomogeneity.

12.6.3 Chamber Equilibration

An exposure chamber approaches and maintains stable equilibrium concentration after an initial buildup of the test material in the chamber (Cheng and Moss, 1995). A positive pressure of 20–60 Pa is applied to achieve a steady state after quasi-saturation of absorbing materials and surfaces. The time to reach 95% equilibrium varies as a function of not only the chamber volume, chamber flow rate, and type of aerosol, but also the presence of bedding, excreta, and fur exposure. Aerosol constituents that exist predominantly in the GVP tend to require shorter durations to reach the equilibrium concentration and display better temporal and spatial homogeneity. Constituents in the liquid or solid phase experience higher depositional losses because of their tendency to impact, coagulate, and deposit. Hence, some components may undergo relatively disproportionate distribution (Achmadi and Pauluhn, 1998; Pauluhn, 2003). Because of their different physicochemical characteristics, different aerosols—such as CS, EHTP aerosols, and e-vapors—are likely to be differently impacted.

The time to reach equilibrium should be kept as short as practically feasible in relation to the total duration of exposure or be adequately taken into account.

Fig. 12.12 shows the concentration–time curves for 3R4F CS CO and nicotine in a WBEC and an NOEC.

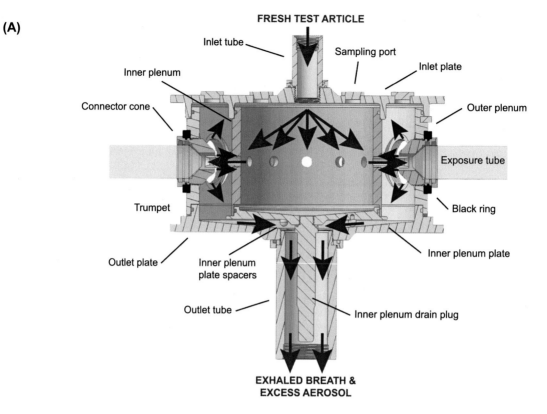

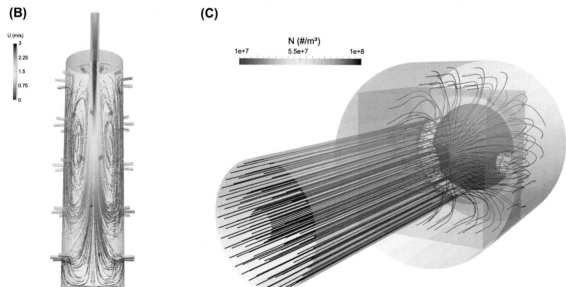

FIG. 12.11 60-port NOEC (**A**) Illustration of flow through the NOEC by using a single tier. (**B**) Computed airflow velocity (U, m/s) in the inner plenum. (**C**) Computed particle number density (N, #/m^3) in the exposure port. *NOEC*, nose-only exposure chamber. (Modified from Fig. 20 from Boué, S., Goedertier, D., Hoeng, J., Kuczaj, A., Majeed, S., Mathis, C., et al., 2020. State-of-the-art methods and devices for the generation, exposure, and collection of aerosols from heat-not-burn tobacco products. Toxicol. Res. Appl. 4, 2397847319897869.)

Because of the smaller chamber volume, smaller internal surface areas, decreased exposure of fur, and absence of bedding and excreta in an NOEC, the time to attain chamber equilibrium is typically shorter and the required volume of test article is lower in NOECs than in large WBECs. Precisely controlled concentrations can be delivered to the breathing zone of each animal, and the concentration in the exposure chamber can be changed rapidly. NOECs also offer less potential for test material chemical instability (e.g., through reaction with excreta or humidity).

12.6.4 Test Atmosphere Sampling and Monitoring

Test atmosphere characterization is critical for understanding and interpreting data from animal inhalation exposure experiments. Achieving the target concentration and target PSD is of primary importance as is their day-to-day reproducibility. OECD TGs provide that an individual measurement in the chamber should not deviate from the mean chamber concentration by more than 10% for gases or by more than 20% for liquid or solid aerosols (OECD, 2018a).

Test atmosphere is sampled at sampling ports close to the animal breathing zone at various frequencies, depending on the parameter and exposure group. Typical sampling and analytical conditions are described in Table 12.2.

12.6.5 Determination of Animal Aerosol Uptake

Even among animals exposed to the same test atmosphere, the volume of material that they inhale and that reaches their respiratory tract can still vary among individuals because of differences in behaviors, respiratory physiology, and anatomical specificities. Hence, aerosol exposure and uptake by the animals should be monitored to demonstrate physiologically relevant exposure and provide a basis for data interpretation and comparison.

Biomarkers of exposure (BoExp) provide quantitative evidence of the presence of HPHCs, or their metabolites, in the body. The US National Academy of Sciences' Institute of Medicine has defined a BoExp as "a constituent or metabolite that is measured in a biological fluid or tissue that has the potential to interact with a biological macromolecule; sometimes considered a measure of internal dose" (Institute of Medicine, 2001). Ideally, a BoExp should be (1) specific to the source of exposure, with other sources being minor or nonexistent, (2) correlated with exposure dose, (3) easily detectable and accurately measurable by using reliable, reproducible, and precise analytical methods, and (4) reflect a specific toxic exposure or be a reliable surrogate of exposure to HPHCs. BoExps may also be of interest for facilitating dosimetric extrapolation from animals to humans.

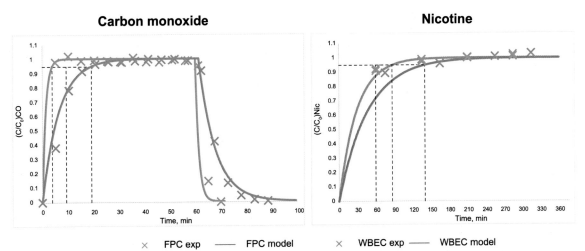

FIG. 12.12 Concentration–time curves for 3R4F CS CO and nicotine in various chambers. *CO*, carbon monoxide; *CS*, cigarette smoke; *FPC*, flow-past chamber. (Modified from Fig. 16 from Boué, S., Goedertier, D., Hoeng, J., Kuczaj, A., Majeed, S., Mathis, C., et al., 2020. State-of-the-art methods and devices for the generation, exposure, and collection of aerosols from heat-not-burn tobacco products. Toxicol. Res. Appl. 4, 2397847319897869.)

TABLE 12.2
Test Atmosphere Sampling Methods.

Parameter	Method	Sampling rate and duration	Sampling rate
Nicotine	EXtrelut cartridges impregnated with 2 mL of 0.5M sulfuric acid and eluted with triethylamine in *n*-butylacetate containing ISTD trimethylamine (Boué et al., 2020) GC	0.4–1.5 L/min 30–60 min	Up to 4 times/day
TPM	44-mm CFP Gravimetry in accordance with ISO 4387:2000 (International Organization for Standardization, 2000b)	0.4–1.5 L/min 30–60 min	Up to 4 times/day
PG, VG (particulate phase and GVP)	44-mm CFP (possibly followed by impinger containing 16 mL of 2-propanol) GC	30–45 min	Up to 4 times/day
Carbonyls[a]	CFP and impinger containing 10 mL of 15 mM 2,4 DNPH in acetonitrile (Boué et al., 2020) LC–MS/MS	0.4–0.7 L/min 15–30 min	Monthly
Flavors	EXtrelut cartridges impregnated with 2 mL of 2-propanol GC–HR–MS	0.7 L/min 30 min	
PSD	APS or PIXE cascade impactor (Boué et al., 2020)	5 L/min (APS) 1 L/min (PIXE) 1.5 min	Weekly or monthly depending on study duration

APS, aerodynamic particle sizer; *CFP*, Cambridge filter pad; *DNPH*, 2,4-dinitrophenylhydrazine; *GC*, gas chromatography; *ISTD*, internal standard; *LC–MS/MS*, liquid chromatography–mass spectrometry/mass spectrometry; *PG*, propylene glycol; *PIXE*, particle-induced X-ray emission; *PSD*, particle size distribution; *VG*, vegetable glycerin.
[a] acetaldehyde, acetone, acrolein, butyraldehyde, crotonaldehyde, formaldehyde, methyl ethyl ketone, and propionaldehyde.

Animal exposure studies typically use BoExps for the particulate and GVP constituents of CS and ENDP aerosols, such as plasma nicotine and cotinine, COHb, and urinary metabolites of representative aerosol constituents. In addition, respiratory measurements, including respiratory frequency, tidal volume, and peak inspiratory flow, may be performed by plethysmography (Boué et al., 2020).

12.7 CONCLUSION

The ability to reproducibly generate, collect, and administer aerosols is critical for characterization and preclinical assessment of ENDPs. The aerosols generated by ENDPs are qualitatively and quantitatively significantly different from CS. This chapter provided detailed information on experimental setups and methods that have been developed to address the technical and experimental challenges of comparing the toxicity of ENDP aerosols with that of CS.

REFERENCES

Achmadi, U.F., Pauluhn, J., 1998. Household insecticides: evaluation and assessment of inhalation toxicity: a workshop summary. Exp. Toxicol. Pathol. 50 (1), 67–72.
Adam, T., Mitschke, S., Streibel, T., Baker, R.R., Zimmermann, R., 2006. Puff-by-puff resolved characterisation of cigarette mainstream smoke by single photon ionisation (SPI) time of flight mass spectrometry (TOFMS):

comparison of the 2R4F research cigarette and pure Burley, Virginia, Oriental and Maryland tobacco cigarettes. Anal. Chim. Acta 572 (2), 219–229.

Belushkin, M., Esposito, M., Jaccard, G., Jeannet, C., Korneliou, A., Tafin Djoko, D., 2018. Role of testing standards in smoke-free product assessments. Regul. Toxicol. Pharmacol. 98, 1–8.

Boué, S., Goedertier, D., Hoeng, J., Kuczaj, A., Majeed, S., Mathis, C., et al., 2020. State-of-the-art methods and devices for the generation, exposure, and collection of aerosols from heat-not-burn tobacco products. Toxicol. Res. Appl. 4, 2397847319897869.

Cannon, W.C., Blanton, E.F., Mcdonald, K.E., 1983. The flow-past chamber: an improved nose-only exposure system for rodents. Am. Ind. Hyg. Assoc. J. 44 (12), 923–928.

Cheng, Y.S., Moss, O.R., 1995. Inhalation exposure systems. In: Henderson, .R.F., McClellan, R.O. (Eds.), Concepts in Inhalation Toxicology, second ed. Taylor & Francis, Washington, DC, pp. 25–66.

CORESTA, 2015. CORESTA Recommended Method No 81. Routine Analytical Machine for e-Cigarette Aerosol Generation and Collection - Definitions and Standard Conditions.

CORESTA, 2018. Guide No. 22. Technical Guide for the Selection of Appropriate Intense Vaping Regimes for e-Vapour Devices.

Dorato, M.A., 1990. Overview of inhalation toxicology. Environ. Health Perspect. 85, 163–170.

Farsalinos, K.E., Romagna, G., Tsiapras, D., Kyrzopoulos, S., Voudris, V., 2013. Evaluation of electronic cigarette use (vaping) topography and estimation of liquid consumption: implications for research protocol standards definition and for public health authorities' regulation. Int. J. Environ. Res. Publ. Health 10 (6), 2500–2514.

Frege, C., Asgari, M., Steiner, S., Ferreira, S., Majeed, S., Lucci, F., et al., 2020. Assessment of single-photon ionization mass spectrometry for online monitoring of in vitro aerosol exposure experiments. Chem. Res. Toxicol. 33 (2), 505–514.

Fukano, Y., Ogura, M., Eguchi, K., Shibagaki, M., Suzuki, M., 2004. Modified procedure of a direct in vitro exposure system for mammalian cells to whole cigarette smoke. Exp. Toxicol. Pathol. 55 (5), 317–323.

Gee, J., Prasad, K., Slayford, S., Gray, A., Nother, K., Cunningham, A., et al., 2018. Assessment of tobacco heating product THP1.0. Part 8: study to determine puffing topography, mouth level exposure and consumption among Japanese users. Regul. Toxicol. Pharmacol. 93, 84–91.

Geiss, O., Bianchi, I., Barrero-Moreno, J., 2016. Correlation of volatile carbonyl yields emitted by e-cigarettes with the temperature of the heating coil and the perceived sensorial quality of the generated vapours. Int. J. Hyg. Environ. Health 219 (3), 268–277.

Goedertier, D.P., Pak, C., Kondylis, A., Vuillaume, G., Hoeng, J., Mathis, C., et al., 2018. Aerosol Trapping, Optimization and Characterization for Comparative in Vitro Assessment of Combustible and Heat-non Burn Tobacco Platforms. Eurotox 2018, Brussels, p. S188.

Gupta, R., Hindle, M., Byron, P.R., Cox, K.A., Mcrae, D.D., 2003. Investigation of a novel condensation aerosol generator: solute and solvent effects. Aerosol Sci. Technol. 37 (8), 672–681.

Havel, C.M., Benowitz, N.L., Jacob 3rd, P., St Helen, G., 2017. An electronic cigarette vaping machine for the characterization of aerosol delivery and composition. Nicotine Tob. Res. 19 (10), 1224–1231.

Haziza, C., De La Bourdonnaye, G., Skiada, D., Ancerewicz, J., Baker, G., Picavet, P., et al., 2016. Evaluation of the Tobacco Heating System 2.2. Part 8: 5-day randomized reduced exposure clinical study in Poland. Regul. Toxicol. Pharmacol. 81, S139–S150.

Howell, T.M., Sweeney, W.R., 1998. Aerosol and a Method and Apparatus for Generating an Aerosol. Philip Morris Incorporated, New York, NY.

Institute of Medicine, 2001. Clearing the Smoke: Assessing the Science Base for Tobacco Harm Reduction. The National Academies Press, Washington, DC.

International Organization for Standardization, 2000a. ISO 3308:2000 Routine Analytical Cigarette-Smoking Machine–Definition and Standard Conditions.

International Organization for Standardization, 2000b. ISO 4387:2000 Cigarettes - Determination of Total and Nicotine-free Dry Particulate Matter Using a Routine Analytical Smoking Machine.

International Organization for Standardization, 2017. ISO 20778:2017 Cigarettes-Routine Analytical Cigarette Smoking Machine-Definitions and Standard Conditions with an Intense Smoking Regime.

International Organization for Standardization, 2018. ISO 20768:2018 Vapour Products – Routine Analytical Vaping Machine – Definitions and Standard Conditions, p. 7.

Iskandar, A.R., Zanetti, F., Kondylis, A., Martin, F., Leroy, P., Majeed, S., et al., 2019. A lower impact of an acute exposure to electronic cigarette aerosols than to cigarette smoke in human organotypic buccal and small airway cultures was demonstrated using systems toxicology assessment. Intern. & Emerg. Med. https://doi.org/10.1007/s11739-019-02055-x.

Klus, H., Boenke-Nimphius, B., Müller, L., 2016. Cigarette mainstream smoke: the evolution of methods and devices for generation, exposure and collection. Beitr. Tabakforsch. Int. 27 (4), 137–274.

Lerner, C.A., Sundar, I.K., Watson, R.M., Elder, A., Jones, R., Done, D., et al., 2015. Environmental health hazards of e-cigarettes and their components: oxidants and copper in e-cigarette aerosols. Environ. Pollut. 198, 100–107.

Li, X., 2016. In vitro toxicity testing of cigarette smoke based on the air-liquid interface exposure: a review. Toxicol. In Vitro 36, 105–113.

Lucci, F., Tan, W.T., Krishnan, S., Hoeng, J., Vanscheeuwijck, P., Jaeger, R., et al., 2018. Characterization of the aerosol flow, sampling, and deposition in a nose only exposure chamber. In: 10th International Aerosol Conference, St. Louis, Missouri, USA.

Majeed, S., Frentzel, S., Wagner, S., Kuehn, D., Leroy, P., Guy, P.A., et al., 2014. Characterization of the Vitrocell(R)

24/48 in vitro aerosol exposure system using mainstream cigarette smoke. Chem. Cent. J. 8 (1), 62.

Mathis, C., Poussin, C., Weisensee, D., Gebel, S., Hengstermann, A., Sewer, A., et al., 2013. Human bronchial epithelial cells exposed in vitro to cigarette smoke at the air-liquid interface resemble bronchial epithelium from human smokers. Am. J. Physiol. Lung Cell Mol. Physiol. 304 (7), L489–L503.

May, K.R., 1973. The collison nebulizer: description, performance and application. J. Aerosol Sci. 4 (3), 235–243.

Mcneill, A., Brose, L.S., Calder, R., Bauld, L., Robson, D., 2018. Evidence Review of e-Cigarettes and Heated Tobacco Products 2018.

Mitschke, S., Adam, T., Streibel, T., Baker, R.R., Zimmermann, R., 2005. Application of time-of-flight mass spectrometry with laser-based photoionization methods for time-resolved on-line analysis of mainstream cigarette smoke. Anal. Chem. 77 (8), 2288–2296.

Müller, L., Comte, P., Czerwinski, J., Kasper, M., Mayer, A.C.R., Schmid, A., et al., 2012. Investigating the potential for different scooter and car exhaust emissions to cause cytotoxic and (pro-)inflammatory responses to a 3D in vitro model of the human epithelial airway. Toxicol. Environ. Chem. 94 (1), 164–180.

National Academies of Sciences, 2018. Public health consequences of e-cigarettes. In: Eaton, D.L., Kwan, L.Y., Stratton, K. (Eds.), Public Health Consequences of e-Cigarettes. National Academies Press (US), Washington (DC).

OECD, 2018a. Guidance Document on Inhalation Toxicity Studies. Series on Testing and Assessment No. 39.

OECD, 2018b. OECD Guidelines for Testing of Chemicals. No. 453: Combined Chronic Toxicity/Carcinogenicity Studies.

OECD, 2018c. OECD Guidelines on the Testing of Chemicals. No. 412. 28-day (Subacute) Inhalation Toxicity Study.

OECD, 2018d. OECD Guidelines on the Testing of Chemicals. No. 413: Subchronic Inhalation Toxicity: 90-day Study.

Pauluhn, J., 2003. Overview of testing methods used in inhalation toxicity: from facts to artifacts. Toxicol. Lett. 140–1, 183–193.

Pauluhn, J., Mohr, U., 2000. Inhalation studies in laboratory animals–current concepts and alternatives. Toxicol. Pathol. 28 (5), 734–753.

Paur, H.-R., Cassee, F.R., Teeguarden, J., Fissan, H., Diabate, S., Aufderheide, M., et al., 2011. In-vitro cell exposure studies for the assessment of nanoparticle toxicity in the lung—a dialog between aerosol science and biology. J. Aerosol Sci. 42 (10), 668–692.

Phillips, B., Esposito, M., Verbeeck, J., Boue, S., Iskandar, A., Vuillaume, G., et al., 2015. Toxicity of aerosols of nicotine and pyruvic acid (separate and combined) in Sprague-Dawley rats in a 28-day OECD 412 inhalation study and assessment of systems toxicology. Inhal. Toxicol. 27 (9), 405–431.

Phillips, B., Szostak, J., Titz, B., Schlage, W.K., Guedj, E., Leroy, P., et al., 2019. A six-month systems toxicology inhalation/cessation study in ApoE$^{-/-}$ mice to investigate cardiovascular and respiratory exposure effects of modified risk tobacco products, CHTP 1.2 and THS 2.2, compared

with conventional cigarettes. Food Chem. Toxicol. 126, 113–141.

Phillips, B., Titz, B., Kogel, U., Sharma, D., Leroy, P., Xiang, Y., et al., 2017. Toxicity of the main electronic cigarette components, propylene glycol, glycerin, and nicotine, in Sprague-Dawley rats in a 90-day OECD inhalation study complemented by molecular endpoints. Food Chem. Toxicol. 109, 315–332.

Radtke, F.S., Ochel, M., Schaffernicht, H.W., 2017. Pump System. European Patent Office.

Roemer, E., Ottmueller, T.H., Urban, H.J., Baillet-Mignard, C., 2010. SKH-1 mouse skin painting: a short-term assay to evaluate the tumorigenic activity of cigarette smoke condensate. Toxicol. Lett. 192 (2), 155–161.

Roemer, E., Ottmueller, T.H., Zenzen, V., Wittke, S., Radtke, F., Blanco, I., et al., 2009. Cytotoxicity, mutagenicity, and tumorigenicity of mainstream smoke from three reference cigarettes machine-smoked to the same yields of total particulate matter per cigarette. Food Chem. Toxicol. 47 (8), 1810–1818.

Secondo, L.E., Liu, N.J., Lewinski, N.A., 2017. Methodological considerations when conducting in vitro, air-liquid interface exposures to engineered nanoparticle aerosols. Crit. Rev. Toxicol. 47 (3), 225–262.

Shao, X.M., Xu, B., Liang, J., Xie, X., Zhu, Y., Feldman, J.L., 2012. Nicotine delivery to rats via lung alveolar region-targeted aerosol technology produces blood pharmacokinetics resembling human smoking. Nicotine Tob. Res. 15 (7), 1248–1258.

Steiner, S., Diana, P., Dossin, E., Guy, P., Vuillaume, G., Kondylis, A., et al., 2018. Delivery efficiencies of constituents of combustion-derived aerosols across the air-liquid interface during in vitro exposures. Toxicol. In Vitro 52, 384–398.

Steiner, S., Majeed, S., Kratzer, G., Vuillaume, G., Hoeng, J., Frentzel, S., 2017. Characterization of the Vitrocell® 24/48 aerosol exposure system for its use in exposures to liquid aerosols. Toxicol. In Vitro 42, 263–272.

Stephens, W.E., 2017. Comparing the cancer potencies of emissions from vapourised nicotine products including e-cigarettes with those of tobacco smoke. Tobac. Contr. https://doi.org/10.1136/tobaccocontrol-2017-053808. Epub ahead of print 2017/08/06.

Szostak, J., Wong, E.T., Titz, B., Lee, T., Wong, S.K., Low, T., et al., 2020. A 6-month systems toxicology inhalation study in ApoE$^{-/-}$ mice demonstrates reduced cardiovascular effects of e-vapor aerosols compared with cigarette smoke. Am. J. Physiol. Heart Circ. Physiol. 318 (3), H604–H631.

Thorne, D., Adamson, J., 2013. A review of in vitro cigarette smoke exposure systems. Exp. Toxicol. Pathol. 65 (7–8), 1183–1193.

US Food and Drug Administration, 2016. Premarket Tobacco Product Applications for Electronic Nicotine Delivery Systems Guidance for Industry, p. 53.

Vansickel, A.R., Edmiston, J.S., Liang, Q., Duhon, C., Connell, C., Bennett, D., et al., 2018. Characterization of puff topography of a prototype electronic cigarette in adult exclusive cigarette smokers and adult exclusive electronic cigarette users. Regul. Toxicol. Pharmacol. 98, 250–256.

Voinova, M.V., Jonson, M., Kasemo, B., 2002. Missing mass effect in biosensor's QCM applications. Biosens. Bioelectron. 17 (10), 835–841.

Werley, M.S., Kirkpatrick, D.J., Oldham, M.J., Jerome, A.M., Langston, T.B., Lilly, P.D., et al., 2016a. Toxicological assessment of a prototype e-cigaret device and three flavor formulations: a 90-day inhalation study in rats. Inhal. Toxicol. 28 (1), 22–38.

Werley, M.S., Miller, J.H., Kane, D.B., Tucker, C.S., Mckinney, W.J., Oldham, M.J., 2016b. Prototype e-cigarette and the capillary aerosol generator (CAG) comparison and qualification for use in subchronic inhalation exposure testing. Aerosol Sci. Technol. 50 (12), 1284–1293.

Williams, M., Talbot, P., 2011. Variability among electronic cigarettes in the pressure drop, airflow rate, and aerosol production. Nicotine Tob. Res. 13 (12), 1276–1283.

Williams, M., Villarreal, A., Bozhilov, K., Lin, S., Talbot, P., 2013. Metal and silicate particles including nanoparticles are present in electronic cigarette cartomizer fluid and aerosol. PLoS One 8 (3), e57987.

Wolff, R.K., 2015. Toxicology studies for inhaled and nasal delivery. Mol. Pharm. 12 (8), 2688–2696.

Wong, B.A., 2007. Inhalation exposure systems: design, methods and operation. Toxicol. Pathol. 35 (1), 3–14.

World Health Organization, 2008. The Scientific Basis of Tobacco Product Regulation. Second report of a WHO study group, p. 289.

Zhuang, H., Lu, P., Lim, S.P., Lee, H.P., 2007. Frequency response of a quartz crystal microbalance loaded by liquid drops. Langmuir 23 (13), 7392–7397.

CHAPTER 13

Toxicological Assessment In Vitro

CARINE POUSSIN • ANITA R. ISKANDAR • CAROLE MATHIS • DANIEL J. SMART •
FILIPPO ZANETTI • MARCO VAN DER TOORN • DAVID BOVARD • REBECCA SAVIOZ •
DAMIAN MCHUGH • WALTER K. SCHLAGE • MANUEL C. PEITSCH •
PATRICK VANSCHEEUWIJCK • JULIA HOENG

13.1 INTRODUCTION

As outlined in Chapter 1, the potential public health benefit of electronic nicotine delivery products (ENDPs), briefly described in Chapter 2, critically depends on their potential to reduce smoking-related disease risk, which needs to be assessed in studies that compare the biological effects of ENDP aerosols with those of cigarette smoke (CS) and fresh air (Chapter 3). Toxicological assessment of an ENDP is the second step in the assessment program outlined in Chapter 3. This step follows analysis of the chemical composition and physical properties of ENDP aerosols, which is aimed at evaluating the degree of reduction in toxicant emissions by ENDPs relative to cigarettes as well as the impact of ENDP use on indoor air quality (Chapters 4–8).

In vitro studies are a major component of this assessment program (Chapter 3) and include a battery of widely accepted regulatory assays as well as more comprehensive and mechanistic systems toxicology–based studies (Chapter 9). Table 13.1 provides an overview of the in vitro studies relevant to ENDP assessment.

In vitro studies are usually designed to investigate certain mechanisms or endpoints in cells and tissues separated from the organism, thereby enabling highly controllable conditions that cannot be achieved in the physiological context of a whole organism. In turn, interpretation of in vitro studies requires extrapolation of their results to the in vivo/in situ context. For example, in vitro mutagenicity data from a very specific and sensitive assay—such as the mouse lymphoma assay (MLA), which involves reverse mutation of an indicator gene—are predictive of a generally elevated mutational risk in an animal rather than of an increase in tumor risk via an acquired oncogene mutation. In the context of product risk assessment, in vitro data

contribute to a body of evidence comprising a multitude of apical and mechanistic endpoints that can be translated between in vitro and in vivo systems, for example, by common molecular mechanisms and functional properties. The significance of the totality of the available scientific evidence for demonstrating the risk reduction potential of ENDPs is discussed in Chapter 18. This chapter focuses on in vitro assessment of ENDPs.

13.2 GENERAL CONSIDERATIONS OF STUDY DESIGN

13.2.1 Product Types and Modes of Exposure

The product type and its intended mode of use will guide the approach for toxicity testing. For ENDPs, which produce inhalable aerosols, the ability to generate, collect, and administer ENDP aerosols is an essential prerequisite to their in vitro assessment (Chapter 12). The Institute of Medicine (Institute of Medicine, 2012) recommends that the comparators for ENDP testing be the leading brands of conventional tobacco products. Among these, today's leading cigarette brands are represented by the reference cigarette 3R4F, which has been recently replaced by the reference cigarette 1R6F (Jaccard et al., 2019). Consequently, as a minimum requirement, the regulatory test battery applicable for CS assessment must be employed to provide evidence that ENDP aerosols have a reduced effect on all endpoints affected by CS. In addition, a variety of mechanistic endpoints relevant to the known health effects of CS should be used to demonstrate the lower toxicity of ENDP aerosols. Because these assays and endpoints are optimized to detect CS-related effects, they are not sufficient to detect any potentially novel effects of ENDP aerosols. Assessment of whether

TABLE 13.1

Overview of the In Vitro Toxicology Studies Performed at PMI for Assessment of ENDPs.

A1. REGULATORY TOXICOLOGY—MONOLAYER (2D) MODELS

Assay type	Purpose	Product/stimulus	Fraction; concentrations/dose	Exposure	Endpoints	Key conclusions [link to intervals page]	References
Regulatory toxicology-based assays (NRU, Ames, and MLA)	Product assessment	THS versus 3R4F	TPM and GVP; various	Direct	- Cell viability: NRU (24 h) - Bacterial mutagenicity (20 min) - Mammalian cell genotoxicity (4 and 24 h)	Cytotoxicity (determined by the NRU assay) and mutagenic potency (mouse lymphoma assay) of THS was reduced by about 90% relative to 3R4F. THS aerosol was not mutagenic in the Ames assay. [https://doi.org/10.26126/intervals.msx63a.1]	Schaller et al. (2016)
Genotoxicity + mode-of-action follow-up assays	Product assessment	Nicotine	n.a; 1.97 −9.86 mM	Direct	In CHO cells: - Micronucleus/ hypodiploid nucleus induction (24 h) - Cell cycle changes (24 h) - Tubulin appearance (24 h) and polymerization (immediate) - DNA damage response markers (e.g., γH2AX) (4 and 24 h)	Nicotine-induced micronuclei formation in CHO cells at >3.95 mM and likely related to tubulin disruption via a lysosomotropic mechanism. Mode-of-action endpoints were not affected, thus casting doubt on the biological relevance of this apparent genotoxicity. Likely irrelevant in the human situation because humans are exposed to much lower levels of nicotine. [n/a in INTERVALS]	Smart et al. (2019b)
Genotoxicity + mode-of-action follow-up assays	Product assessment	Nonflavored e-liquids	n.a.; 1.6%−4% v/v	Direct	In CHO cells: - Micronucleus/ hypodiploid nucleus induction (24 h) - Medium osmolality and pH (immediate) - Cell cycle changes (24 h) - DNA damage response markers (e.g., γH2AX) (4 and 24 h)	Propylene glycol −induced micronuclei formation in CHO cells but likely not biologically relevant, as it had no effect on other mechanistic endpoints. Unlikely to be a genotoxic hazard. [n/a in INTERVALS]	Smart et al. (2019b)

Endpoint	Purpose	Test item	Concentration/dose	Exposure	Assays/readouts	Findings	Reference
NRU assay + follow-up assays	Product assessment	Nonflavored e-liquid + nicotine + other lysosomotropic compounds	n/a; various	Direct	In Balb/c 3T3, A75, A172, A549, and SH-SY5Y cell lines: - Cell viability: NRU, relative cell counts, rezasurin, ATP production, and WST-8 reduction (24 h) - LAMP-1 expression, LysoTracker incorporation (24 h)	Nicotine was confirmed as a lysosomotropic agent and interfered with the readout of the NRU assay. The WST-8 assay is proposed as an alternative assay for assessing the cytotoxic potential of e-liquids. [n/a in INTERVALS]	Cudazzo et al. (2019)

A2. REGULATORY TOXICOLOGY—CELL SUSPENSION

Endpoint	Purpose	Test item	Concentration/dose	Exposure	Assays/readouts	Findings	Reference
Genotoxicity	Assay development	Prototypical genotoxic + nongenotoxic compounds	n/a; various	Direct	In human TK6 cells: - DNA damage response markers (e.g., γH2AX) (4 h) - Micronucleus induction (following a 24-h recovery) - Tk gene mutation (4 weeks posttreatment)	The TK6 cell—based integrated assay represents an in vitro approach that permits comprehensive genotoxicity analysis in a human-relevant test system. [n/a in INTERVALS]	Smart et al. (2020)

B1. SYSTEMS TOXICOLOGY—MONOLAYER (2D) MODELS

Endpoint	Purpose	Test item	Concentration/dose	Exposure	Assays/readouts	Findings	Reference
HCS (13 indicators) and transcriptomics	Mechanistic investigation	Acrolein Formaldehyde Catechol	n/a; nine doses (5–2800 μg/L) n/a; nine doses (2–4500 μg/L) n/a; nine doses (2–300 μg/L)	Direct	In NHBE cells (up to 24h): - HCS assays (cell count; cell membrane permeability; mitochondrial mass; mitochondrial membrane potential; cytochrome C release; apoptosis [caspase 3/7 activity]; cell proliferation [phosphorylation of histone H3, pH3]; cell cycle [DNA content]; cellular stress [phosphorylation of c-Jun]; ROS; oxidative stress [dihydroethidium, DHE]; oxidative stress; GSH content; DNA damage [phosphorylation of H2AX, γH2AX]; nuclear area; DNA structure - Whole-genome transcriptomics findings - RTCA cytotoxicity (cell impedance)	DNA damage/growth arrest, oxidative stress, mitochondrial stress, and apoptosis/necrosis were the most impacted toxicity mechanisms by the highest doses in the HCS assays. At lower doses, changes at the transcriptomics level were detected. The study established that the approach would be suitable for assessing e-liquids and aerosols. [n/a in INTERVALS]	Gonzalez-Suarez et al. (2014)

Continued

TABLE 13.1

Overview of the In Vitro Toxicology Studies Performed at PMI for Assessment of ENDPs.—cont'd

Assay type	Purpose	Product/stimulus	Fraction; concentrations/ dose	Exposure	Endpoints	Key conclusions [link to intervals page]	References
HCS (11 indicators) and transcriptomics	Product assessment; mechanistic investigation	HTP (SMAR or THS) versus 3R4F	AE (smoke-bubbled PBS), TPM and GVP; 3R4F in puffs/L: - AE: 6–200 - TPM: 8–64 - GVP: 6–200 THS 2.2 in puffs/L: - AE: 35–350 - TPM: 75–450 - GVP: 35–350	Direct		Exposure to THS aerosol caused considerably lower biological effects (HCS and transcriptomics) than exposure to 3R4F CS at equal concentrations. Some toxic responses were observed for THS aerosol, but they occurred at concentrations 3 to 18 times higher than those of 3R4F CS. [n/a in INTERVALS]	Kogel et al. (2015), Gonzalez-Suarez et al. (2016)
RTCA, HCS (nine indicators) and transcriptomics	Case study	28 flavoring substances, alone or as a mixture, in base e-liquid	n/a; E-liquids with one flavor or in mixtures: eight concentrations (from 0.0625% to 8%)	Direct		Addition of the flavors enhanced the inherent biological activity of the base solution (on the basis of RTCA and HCS findings), and it increased the network perturbations. Most of the cytotoxic effect was attributed to citronellol. [https://doi.org/10.26126/intervals.lwo6mb.1]	Marescotti et al. (2020b)
RTCA, HCS (six indicators)	Product assessment	MESH base and flavored formulations versus 3R4F	n/a; - E-liquids: 8 doses (22–720 μg nicotine/mL) - 3R4F TPM: Seven doses (4–32 μg nicotine/mL)	Direct		Decreased cell viability was detected following a 24-h incubation with 3R4F TPM at approximately 20-fold lower nicotine concentrations than those of both e-liquids. Incubation of cells with 3R4F TPM or e-liquids resulted in a dose-dependent impact on DNA damage, GSH content, oxidative stress, and stress kinase	Iskandar et al. (2019b)

					phosphorylation (c-Jun). The minimum concentration at which an effect could be observed was >50 times greater with e-liquids than with 3R4F TPM. [https://doi.org/10.26126/intervals.ri2tah.1]	Mathis et al. (2013, 2015)

B2. SYSTEMS TOXICOLOGY—ORGANOTYPIC (3D) MODELS

Microarrays (mRNA and miRNA) and immunoassay (MMP-1)	Assay development	3R4F	Whole smoke; 15% (v/v)	Direct at the ALI	In human bronchial epithelial cultures (7, 14, 21, and 28 min) - mRNA and miRNA changes - MMP-1 release	First, biological perturbations (MMP-1 release and miRNAs associated with inflammation or with cell cycle processes) detected in cultures following exposure to CS were similar to those detected in vivo in smokers' airway epithelium. Second, CS-induced cellular pathways were related to stress responses, inflammation, and proliferation/differentiation. [n/a in INTERVALS]	Mathis et al. (2013, 2015)
LDH release assay; histology; IHC; immunoassay; mRNA microarray; TEER; luminescent CYP activity assay	Assay development	3R4F	Whole smoke; 19.7% and 40.7% (v/v)	Direct at the ALI	In human buccal and gingival epithelial cultures (four cigarettes with a 1-h rest between each cigarette) - Cytotoxicity - Histology/IHC findings, - Secreted inflammatory mediators - mRNA changes - TEER - CYP1A1/1B1 activity	CS exposure increased the secretion of inflammatory mediators, induced CYP activity, and impacted xenobiotic metabolism, which resembled the responses in buccal biopsy samples of smokers. The models are appropriate for assessment of CS-induced adverse effects in the oral cavity. [n/a in INTERVAL]	Schlage W. K. et al. (2014)

Continued

TABLE 13.1
Overview of the In Vitro Toxicology Studies Performed at PMI for Assessment of ENDPs.—cont'd

Assay type	Purpose	Product/stimulus	Fraction; concentrations/ dose	Exposure	Endpoints	Key conclusions [link to intervals page]	References
LDH release assay; histology; IHC; immunoassay; mRNA microarray; CBF; TEER; luminescent CYP activity assay	Assay development	3R4F	Whole smoke; 16 or 16.7% (v/v)	Direct at the ALI	In human bronchial and nasal epithelial cultures (four cigarettes with a 1-h rest between each cigarette) - Cytotoxicity - Histology/IHC findings, - Secreted inflammatory mediators - mRNA changes - CBF - TEER - CYP1A1/1B1 activity	CS exposure increased CYP1A1/ 1B1 activity slightly and altered xenobiotic metabolism, which was similar to the responses observed in the bronchial and nasal epithelial cells of smokers. Nasal and bronchial epithelial tissue cultures are appropriate in vitro models for assessment of CS-induced adverse effects in the respiratory system. [n/ a in INTERVAL]	Talikka et al. (2014), Kuehn et al. (2015)
AK release assay; histology; IHC; immunoassay; mRNA microarray; CBF; TEER; luminescent CYP activity assay	Product assessment	THS versus 3R4F	Whole smoke/ aerosol; THS: three doses in each study (0.14 –0.45 mg nicotine/L aerosol) 3R4F: two doses in each study (0.13 –0.27 mg nicotine/L smoke)	Direct at the ALI	In human bronchial, small airway, and nasal epithelial cultures (28 min, acute) - Cytotoxicity - Histology/IHC findings - Secreted inflammatory mediators - mRNA and miRNA changes - CBF - TEER - Targeted proteomics - CYP1A1/1B1 activity	THS aerosol elicited substantially lower alterations in tissue morphology, lower cytotoxicity, lower secretion of inflammatory mediators, and lower levels of perturbations in the transcriptome and proteome. [Bronchial: https:// www.intervals. science/studies/ #/ths-22-bronchial-organotypic; Nasal: https://www.intervals. science/studies/ #/ths22-organotypic-nasal]	Iskandar et al. (2017c), Iskandar et al. (2017a), Iskandar et al. (2017b)

AK release assay; histology; IHC; immunoassay; mRNA microarray; TEER; luminescent CYP activity assay	Product assessment	THS versus 3R4F	Whole smoke/aerosol; THS: three doses (0.31, 0.46, and 1.09 mg nicotine/L aerosol) 3R4F: two doses (0.32 and 0.51 mg nicotine/L smoke) Whole smoke/aerosol; THS: two doses (54.6, 100.4 μg nicotine/mL PBS) 3R4F: two doses (49.4, 84.6 μg nicotine/mL PBS)	Direct at the ALI	In human buccal epithelial (28 min, acute) and gingival cultures (three times 28 min, repeated) - Cytotoxicity - Histology/IHC - Secretion of inflammatory mediators - mRNA and miRNA changes - Targeted proteomics - Metabolomics - Cytochrome P450s (CYP) 1A1/1B1 activity	Cytotoxicity, pathophysiological alterations, secretion of inflammatory mediators, stress responses, and the impact on transcriptome and metabolome following exposure to THS aerosol exposure were markedly lower than those following exposure to CS. [Buccal: https://www.intervals.science/studies/#/ths-22-buccal-organotypic; Gingival: https://www.intervals.science/studies/#/ths-22-repeated-gingival-organotypic]	Zanetti et al. (2016) Zanetti et al. (2017)
AK release assay; histology; immunoassay; mRNA microarray	Product assessment	MESH base and flavored formulations versus 3R4F	Whole smoke/aerosol; 3D ALI buccal cultures: MESH and Base (28 and 112 min, undiluted) 3R4F (28 min, diluted) 3D ALI small airway cultures: MESH and Base (7 and 28 min, undiluted) 3R4F (28 min, diluted)	Direct at the ALI	In 3D ALI buccal and small airway cultures - Cytotoxicity - Histology - Secretion of inflammatory mediators - CYP1A1/1B1 activity - Targeted proteomics	Relative to 3R4F CS exposure, MESH Classic Tobacco Aerosol exposure did not cause tissue damage and elicited lower changes in the mRNA, miRNA, and protein markers. In the context of tobacco harm reduction strategy. [Buccal: https://www.intervals.science/studies/#/pmi_p4m3_buccal; Small airway: https://www.intervals.science/studies/#/pmi_p4m3_small_airway]	Iskandar et al. (2019b)

Continued

TABLE 13.1
Overview of the In Vitro Toxicology Studies Performed at PMI for Assessment of ENDPs.—cont'd

Assay type	Purpose	Product/stimulus	Fraction; concentrations/ dose	Exposure	Endpoints	Key conclusions [link to intervals page]	References
B3. SYSTEMS TOXICOLOGY—ORGANOTYPIC (3D) COCULTURE MODELS							
AK release assay; histology; immunoassay; mRNA microarray; luminescent CYP activity assay	Assay development	3R4F	Whole smoke/ aerosol; 8% and 15% (v/v)	Direct at the ALI	In human bronchial epithelial monocultures and cocultures with fibroblast (28 min, acute) - Cytotoxicity - Histology findings - mRNA changes - CYP1A1/1B1 activity	In both culture models, similar impact of CS exposure on cytotoxicity, CYP1A1/ 1B1 activity, and tissue histology. A greater number of secreted mediators were significantly altered in the monoculture than in the coculture. The transcriptomic profiles indicated more prominent cellular stress and tissue damage following CS exposure in the monoculture model. The results indicated that the CS-exposed coculture model better reflects the smoking-induced xenobiotic metabolism response. [n/a in INTERVALS]	Iskandar et al. (2015)
B4. SYSTEMS TOXICOLOGY—MECHANISTIC MODELS							
Adhesion assay	Assay development mechanistic investigation	3R4F	AE (smoke-bubbled PBS); 0.015 –0.18 puffs/mL and 0.045 –0.225 puffs/mL	Indirect, direct, and fresh direct	In HUVECs or HCAECs (up to 4 h) - MM6-HUVEC cell adhesion - Adhesion molecules as mRNA and cell surface proteins - mRNA changes - NFκB nuclear translocation In supernatant of MM6 cells (= conditioned medium) TNFα (ELISA)	These studies led to establishment of an adhesion assay and unraveled vascular inflammation- and cytotoxicity-associated mechanisms by which CS AE promotes, directly and indirectly, the adhesion of monocytic cells to human endothelial cells, respectively. [n/ a in INTERVALS]	Poussin et al. (2014, 2015)

Assay	Purpose	Comparison	Extract/dose	Exposure	Endpoints	Findings	Reference
Adhesion assay	Product assessment	THS versus 3R4F	AE (smoke-bubbled PBS) THS: 0.045–2.25 puffs/mL; 3R4F: 0.02–0.225 puffs/mL	Direct, indirect, and fresh direct	In HCAECs (up to 4 h) - MM6-HUVEC cell adhesion - Cell surface adhesion proteins - mRNA changes - High-content screening findings (e.g., NFκB translocation, ICAM-1 quantification, ROS, GSH content, cytotoxicity endpoints) - Cell viability In MM6 cells (= conditioned medium; up to 2 h) - TNFα - Inflammatory mediators (cytokines, chemokines) - mRNA changes	THS AE extract had a lower effect than CS AE on the adhesion of monocytic cells to primary human coronary artery endothelial cells. The assay is relevant to the pathophysiology of atherosclerosis. [n/a in INTERVAL]	Poussin et al. (2016)
Chemotaxis and transmigration assay	Product assessment	THS versus 3R4F	AE (smoke-bubbled medium) 3R4F: 0.01–0.5 puffs/mL; THS: 0.01–3.0 puffs/mL	Direct	In THP-1 and HCAEC cells treated with medium extract migration and TEM of pretreated THP-1 (Boyden Chamber) (up to 4 h) - THP-1 migration - THP-1 with HCAECs (TEM) TEM of pretreated THP-1 (xCelligence; up to 4 h) - THP-1 with HCAECs (TEM) HCAEC adhesion (xCelligence; up to 27 h) - Monitoring HCAECs In MM6 cells (up to 18 h) - TNFα, IL-8 in supernatant - 7AAD (cytotoxicity) TEM of THP-1 and pretreated HCAECs (up to 4 h) - THP-1 with HCAECs - FACS analysis THP-1 (MAC-1 and CD11b) - Migration and TEM	Treatment of THP-1 cells with extracts from CS or THS aerosol –induced concentration-dependent increases in cytotoxicity and inflammation. But, the effects were significantly lower with THS aerosol than with CS. Chemotaxis and TEM were inhibited in extract-treated THP-1 cells. However, extracts from CS were >18 times more potent than those from THS aerosol. [https://www.intervals.science/studies/#/transmigration-assay-ths22]	van der Toorn et al. (2015)

Continued

TABLE 13.1

Overview of the In Vitro Toxicology Studies Performed at PMI for Assessment of ENDPs.—cont'd

Assay type	Purpose	Product/stimulus	Fraction; concentrations/ dose	Exposure	Endpoints	Key conclusions [link to intervals page]	References
Cell transformation assay	Product assessment	THS versus 3R4F	TPM; 3R4F: 7.5 μg/mL THS: 7.5, 37.5, or 150 μg/mL	Direct chronic	In BEAS-2B cells (up to 16 weeks) - High-content screening findings (oxidative stress, GSH content, γH2AX, cell number, cell index, E-cadherin, vimentin) - Luminex protein analysis in supernatant (cytokines, chemokines, MMPs, TIMPs - Gene expression analysis - Epithelial cell invasion - Epithelial–mesenchymal transition (isolated clones were stained for E-cadherin and vimentin)	CS exposure (4 weeks) resulted in crisis and EMT accompanied by decreased barrier function and disrupted cell–cell contacts. By week 8, the cells regained E-cadherin expression, suggesting that EMT was reversible. Increased levels of inflammatory mediators were noted in cells treated with CS but not in cells treated with up to fivefold higher concentrations of THS aerosol. A 20-fold higher concentration of THS aerosol increased oxidative stress and DNA damage and caused reversible EMT. Anchorage-independent growth was seen in cells treated with CS or a high concentration of THS aerosol. CS-exposure–derived clones were invasive, while THS aerosol-exposure–derived clones were not. [https://www.intervals.science/studies/#/long-term-exposure_ths22]	van der Toorn et al. (2018)

B5. SYSTEMS TOXICOLOGY—BIOLOGY-INSPIRED MICROPHYSIOLOGICAL SYSTEMS

Adhesion assay (3D microvessel under flow)	Assay development mechanistic investigation	TNFα	n/a; 50 –10,000 pg/mL	Direct	In HCAECs (up to 8 d): - Junction markers: CD31 and VE-cadherin - HCAEC permeability barrier assay - Adhesion of MM6 cells to the lumen of HCAEC microvessel - ICAM-1 - mRNA changes	A relevant 3D microvessel-on-a-chip model was established for investigating leukocyte–endothelial microvessel adhesion under flow. A case study illustrates how the model can be used for product testing in the context of systems toxicology –based risk assessment. THS aerosol–conditioned medium elicited a reduced effect on monocyte –endothelial adhesion relative to CS-conditioned medium. [https://www.intervals.science/studies/#/microvessel-ths22-mimetas-pmi; and https://www.intervals.science/studies/#/microvessel-ths22-mimetas-pmi]	Poussin et al. (2020)
Adhesion assay (3D microvessel under flow)	Product assessment	THS versus 3R4F	AE (smoke-bubbled PBS); 0.03–2.5 puffs/mL	Indirect	In HCAECs (up to 16 h): - Adhesion of MM6 cells to the lumen of HCAEC microvessels - Adhesion marker: cell surface ICAM-1 protein - Oxidative stress marker: GSH content In supernatant of MM6 cells (= conditioned medium; up to 2 h) - TNFα		

Overview of the in vitro toxicology studies performed at PMI for assessment of ENDPs. *AE*, aqueous extract; *AK*, adenylate kinase; *CBF*, ciliary beating frequency; *CS*, cigarette smoke; *CYP*, cytochrome P450; *GSH*, glutathione; *GVP*, gas–vapor phase; *HCAEC*, human coronary artery endothelial cells; *HCS*, high-content screening; *HUVEC*, human umbilical vein endothelial cells; *ICAM-1*, intercellular adhesion molecule 1; *IHC*, immunohistochemistry; *MM6*, human monocytic cell line Mono Mac 6; *MMP*, matrix metalloproteinases; *NFκB*, nuclear factor kappa-light-chain-enhancer of activated B cells; *NRU*, neural red uptake; *PMI*, Philip Morris International; *ROS*, reactive oxygen species; *RTCA*, real-time cellular analysis; *TEM*, transendothelial migration; *TEER*, transepithelial electrical resistance; *TIMP*, tissue inhibitors of metalloproteinases; *TK*, thymidine kinase; *THP-1*, human monocytic cell line THP-1; *TNF*, tumor necrosis factor; *THS*, Tobacco Heating System 2.2; *TPM*, total particulate matter. In the column "Exposure," the indication DIRECT refers to direct exposure of cells to CS or ENDP aerosol fraction; DIRECT at the ALI refers to direct exposure at the air–liquid interface of cells (generally organotypic cultures) to CS or ENDP aerosol; DIRECT chronic refers to direct chronic exposure of cells to CS or ENDP aerosol fraction (repetitive exposure over time); INDIRECT refers to exposure of cells to conditioned medium and not directly to CS or ENDP aerosol. For the adhesion assay studies, the distinction between FRESH DIRECT and DIRECT is made to differentiate between direct exposure of cells to freshly generated CS or ENDP aerosol fraction or to CS or ENDP aerosol fraction that underwent a specific processing required by the assay protocol before use.

ENDP aerosols cause such novel effects can be achieved by using scientifically robust systems toxicology–based approaches, which are described in greater detail in Chapter 9.

The methods for generating and collecting aerosols are described in detail in Chapter 12. Briefly, CS or ENDP aerosol is generated with aerosol generators or smoking machines, which can be modified to accommodate ENDP specificities. The total particulate matter (TPM) fraction of CS or ENDP aerosol is the most commonly used fraction for in vitro toxicological assessment, as it contains most of the toxicants and nicotine and can be added directly to cell culture media. Likewise, whole CS or ENDP aerosol, or their respective gas–vapor phases (GVPs), can be collected in the form of aqueous extracts (AEs). TPM and AEs are used to expose submersed monolayer cultures or cells in suspension, while whole CS or ENDP aerosol are used to expose organotypic epithelial tissue cultures grown at the air–liquid interface (ALI).

Given the qualitative and quantitative differences between CS and aerosols from ENDPs (Chapter 12), it is important to ensure that the trapping methods for CS and ENDP aerosol will capture comparable samples of the different product types. Therefore, careful analytical characterization and validation of the trapping methods is needed (Chapter 12) (Boué et al., 2020).

13.2.2 Cell Systems and Endpoints

In vitro test systems are chosen on the basis of their relevance to the biological mechanism and target tissues (Chapter 10). For most regulatory assays, specific cell types are determined by design—for example, a set of *Salmonella typhimurium* bacterial strains in the Ames assay or L5178Y mouse lymphoma $Tk^{+/-}$ cells in the MLA. Such assays have been precisely validated for the defined cell type/strain in use, and their relevance to tobacco smoking–related diseases results from the mechanism of toxicity they are able to detect, namely mutagenicity of the major classes of mutagens and carcinogens among the harmful and potentially harmful constituents (HPHCs) of tobacco smoke.

In the context of human respiratory diseases, and to compare the effects of ENDP aerosols with those of CS, one should consider using in vitro systems that represent the human cells/tissues that are directly exposed to CS or ENDP aerosol, such as cells of the aerodigestive tract. These include primary normal human bronchial epithelial (NHBE) and alveolar cells, organotypic tissue cultures of oral, nasal, bronchial, and small airway (bronchiolar) epithelia, as well as cells of the immune system, like lung macrophages and lymphocytes. Cells

cultured as a two-dimensional (2D) monolayer (e.g., NHBEs) are particularly useful for high-content screening (HCS) and real-time cellular analysis (RTCA) endpoints that require optical or impedance measurements (Gonzalez-Suarez et al., 2016). Other applications of 2D lung epithelial cell cultures (e.g., the BEAS-2B cell line) include cell transformation–related assays aimed at measuring changes under long-term repeated exposure conditions (Malinska et al., 2018; van der Toorn et al., 2018). Organotypic epithelial tissue cultures grown at the ALI are three-dimensional (3D) stratified (buccal and gingival) or pseudostratified (nasal, bronchial, and bronchiolar) cultures that resemble the in vivo epithelium. These cultures are suitable for direct exposures to whole CS and ENDP aerosol because they grow at the ALI. These organotypic cultures can be used for morphological, functional, and molecular measurements.

Cigarette smoking causes a continuum of damage patterns along the aerodigestive tract and a field of injury in the lungs and airways (Spira et al., 2007; Sridhar et al., 2008; Steiling et al., 2008). However, in vitro, in spite of broad similarities in damage patterns across organotypic epithelial tissue cultures, studies have reported specific differences in response to CS and ENDP aerosol exposure between buccal and gingival cultures and among nasal, tracheobronchial, and small airway cultures (Iskandar et al., 2017d; Iskandar et al., 2019b; Schlage et al., 2014; Zanetti et al., 2016).

In the context of cardiovascular diseases (CVDs), cells and tissues are indirectly exposed to the inhaled CS or ENDP aerosol constituents or their metabolites. Effector cells, important for smoking-related CVDs, include monocytes and endothelial cells involved in mechanisms leading to atherosclerosis as well as vascular smooth muscle cells involved in abdominal aortic aneurysm. The initial mechanisms of atherosclerosis, such as endothelial cell dysfunction and monocyte-to-endothelial cell adhesion, were investigated in submersed 2D cultures (Poussin et al., 2016), and monocyte invasion through an in vitro endothelium was assessed in 3D transmigration chambers (van der Toorn et al., 2015). In both assays, cells were exposed to aqueous CS and ENDP aerosol extracts, which can be considered as suitable in vitro proxies for an in vivo exposure that allows polar compounds to pass through the alveolar/microvascular barrier into the bloodstream (Poussin et al., 2014). Vascular cell exposure to TPM fractions, however, was not considered in that study because it does not represent the in vivo vascular exposure. More recently, Philip Morris International (PMI) has demonstrated that the monocyte-to-endothelium adhesion assay can be transferred to a microfluidic 96-chip plate format (Poussin et al., 2020). This allows not only investigations with significantly higher throughput than the traditional assay design but also measurement of monocyte adhesion under flow conditions in a configuration that more closely mimics the physiological conditions in blood vessels.

13.2.3 Choice of Exposure and Postexposure Durations

Most in vitro assays assess single/acute exposures that last from approximately 1–24 h; this design is also common for testing CS and ENDP aerosol. Acute exposure allows one to determine primary compound–specific toxic effects that can be interpreted in the context of defined pathophysiological mechanisms leading to smoking-related diseases (e.g., DNA damage and mutation that increase the risk of cancer) or to rank the hazards of various constituents and mixtures. Even shorter exposure periods (e.g., a single 28-min exposure cycle) have been routinely used for direct CS and ENDP aerosol exposure of organotypic cultures at the ALI, with the exception of gingival epithelial cultures, which have also been exposed to a repeated 28-min cycle on 3 consecutive days (Zanetti et al., 2017).

A specific postexposure observation period needs to be considered for each endpoint. For example, ciliary beating frequency measurements can be conducted immediately after the end of an exposure and again at later time points up to 72 h postexposure. Meanwhile, for observing changes in epithelial morphology and the concentrations of inflammatory mediators, longer postexposure time points (e.g., 48 and 72 h) are often preferable (Iskandar et al., 2017d).

A long-term exposure schedule has been successfully applied to cell transformation studies, because stepwise acquisition of neoplastic changes requires ongoing exposure of continuously proliferating cell populations as well as stagnation periods (senescence/crisis). For example, 2D cultures of the immortalized tracheobronchial epithelial cell line BEAS-2B exposed to CS for 12 weeks showed neoplastic changes such as anchorage-independent growth and invasiveness (van der Toorn et al., 2018).

Owing to their longevity, organotypic cultures are, in principle, also suitable for repeated exposure over several weeks or months. For example, a 4-week subchronic exposure study of human organotypic bronchial epithelial cultures exposed to the AE of CS has been reported (Ito et al., 2018). However, in this study, the cultures were exposed to the AE of CS that was added to the basolateral medium, which only represented systemic exposure to the dissolved CS constituents and not direct exposure of the apical surface to whole CS, as it occurs in vivo. A major challenge in performing long-term repeated direct exposure of organotypic cultures to CS/ENDP aerosol at the ALI is maintaining the sterility of the cultures for the long duration of a study. It is, therefore, necessary to develop an exposure setup and associated protocols that are practical for (sub)chronic exposure at the ALI to enable successful chronic in vitro toxicology studies.

13.2.4 Exposure Dose

The concentrations and doses of CS and ENDP aerosol used for exposing in vitro systems should reflect realistic human exposure conditions. This is of particular importance when the studies aim to compare the effects of ENDP aerosols with those of CS and to translate the effects to typical human ENDP use or cigarette smoking. In contrast, mechanistic assays, aimed at determining the toxic potency of a constituent/mixture or uncovering a fundamental mechanism, may need to include doses at higher concentrations than those reasonably observed in humans. Indeed, toxicological testing guidelines typically require that markedly toxic doses/concentrations be included in studies conducted for regulatory submissions. For example, for the neutral red uptake (NRU) assay, the relevant concentration range around the IC50 (i.e., the concentration producing 50% cytotoxicity) should be included. Moreover, for in vitro mutation assays, such as the MLA, OECD (Organisation for Economic Co-operation and Development) Test Guideline (TG) 490 suggests that the highest concentration should aim to achieve between 10% and 20% of the relative total cell growth (80%–90% inhibition) (OECD, 2016b).

In many assessment studies, high concentrations of ENDP are tested to trigger detectable responses. However, this may lead to unrealistically high concentrations of certain constituents compared with those achieved during ENDP use by humans. For example, nicotine concentrations in the millimolar range are used in some in vitro studies, while the blood nicotine concentration in cigarette smokers reaches a plateau of only approximately 30 ng/mL during the day (Benowitz et al., 1983; Hukkanen et al., 2005) and reaches 15–30 ng/mL (venous) and 20–60 ng/mL (arterial) after single use. Hence, the relevance for human health of the biological effects observed at concentrations far beyond realistic exposure in humans is low. Nevertheless, such studies are still suitable for expressing the relative potencies of the tested products. This can be achieved by calculating the ratio of concentrations at which the half-maximum effect is reached, or, for low toxicity test materials, the concentration at which at least a twofold increase in signal above the vehicle is observed (Gonzalez-Suarez et al., 2016, 2017).

For functional in vitro assays using cell types that are systemically exposed to inhaled or ingested substances (e.g., fibroblasts, endothelial cells, muscle cells, and glandular epithelial cells), it is reasonable to test concentrations that correspond to those observed in body fluids for certain compounds (e.g., nicotine). Higher concentrations can also be included (e.g., 3-fold and 10-fold) (Boué et al., 2020) to demonstrate that the test system is responsive to stimuli. A similar rationale can be applied to organotypic 3D ALI epithelial cultures that are exposed to various substances, such as ambient air (respiratory tract epithelium), saliva (oral epithelium), ingested materials (gastrointestinal tract), and urine (kidney and bladder epithelia). The concentration levels can be derived from corresponding in vivo concentrations or from surface doses that represent normal and moderately elevated use levels. The deposited surface dose (g/m^2) and aerosol concentration (ppm, g/m^3) may be relevant, depending on the parameter of reference (TPM, nicotine, or carbonyls). Additionally, the deposited concentration per volume of airway surface liquid (which can be determined in vivo from lung lavage samples) can be used to extrapolate suitable in vitro concentrations. This concept is described in greater detail in an earlier publication (Boue et al., 2020) and in Chapter 12.

In many comparative studies where CS is the reference, nicotine concentrations or doses are used as the basis for matching ENDP aerosol concentrations or doses. With this approach, the doses of CS and ENDP aerosol TPM can remain fundamentally different, because the composition of CS is different from that of ENDP aerosols. The rationale for using nicotine as a unit of comparison is the postulation that ENDP users will titrate their consumption to achieve a similar nicotine intake as they had previously obtained from smoking cigarettes. In fact, clinical studies have demonstrated that cigarette smokers who switched to using the Tobacco Heating System 2.2 (THS), an electrically heated tobacco product (EHTP) (Chapter 2), had a similar nicotine uptake as those who continued to smoke their own brands of cigarettes (Chapter 17).

When CS fractions are used for exposure of submersed cultures, the dosing with TPM can also be matched on the basis of nicotine concentration, because nicotine is almost exclusively present in the particulate phase of CS and ENDP aerosols. However, when matching nicotine concentrations between the AEs of CS and ENDP aerosol, one must consider that the AE of CS retains only a low percentage of hydrophobic particulate matter, which contains most of the CS nicotine. Therefore, the AE of CS contains relatively low levels of nicotine. In contrast, the hydrophilic TPM of ENDP aerosols dissolves very well in an aqueous medium and, therefore, contains most of the nicotine. Consequently, the proportion of nicotine to other aerosol constituents is different in the AE of ENDP aerosol than in the AE of CS; this would lead to underdosing of the AE of ENDP aerosol when matched to the nicotine content of the AE of CS. Therefore, dose matching on the basis of puffs per volume of AE (or number of items extracted per volume) could be a preferable measure, as long as the puff volumes, numbers of puffs per item, and nicotine delivery per puff/item are similar. The primary guidance can come from the doses a consumer typically would inhale (e.g., number of puffs or total volume of puffs per day).

13.3 REGULATORY TOXICOLOGY

13.3.1 Battery of Assays

The battery of in vitro regulatory toxicology assays used by PMI for assessment of ENDPs is similar to that historically and currently used for evaluation of conventional cigarettes. It includes the

1. Bacterial reverse mutation test (or Ames assay) for assessing mutagenicity;
2. MLA for assessing mammalian cell mutagenicity;
3. In vitro micronucleus (MNvit) assay for assessing mammalian cell genotoxicity; and
4. NRU assay for assessing cytotoxicity.

These assays were selected on the basis of scientific literature and recommendations from different authorities (IARC, 1986, 1999; The United States Department of Health and Human Services, 1993; The US Centers for Disease Control and Prevention, 2012; The US Food and Drug Administration, 2000). Widely accepted United States (US) and international guidelines that define the testing requirements for regulatory product approvals also influenced the selection process (International Conference on Harmonisation, 1995, 1997, 2010; OECD, 1981). Each assay should follow these important criteria:

1. The assay must be responsive to at least some of the CS fractions (TPM, GVP, and AE).
2. The assay must deliver quantitative results.
3. The assay must be sufficiently sensitive to distinguish between different products.
4. The assay must be validated to ensure the robustness of the results.

5. The biological principles of the assay must be relevant to CS/ENDP aerosol assessment.

Because no single assay can detect all classes of genotoxic compounds and all types of genotoxic effects, our test battery includes several genotoxicity assays. The Ames assay, which measures mutagenicity in prokaryotic cells, is an important element of the battery, as it can identify compounds with carcinogenic potential (Benigni, 2012; Kirkland et al., 2011; Pfuhler et al., 2010; Tennant et al., 1987). However, it may not be appropriate for classes of compounds that interfere specifically with the mammalian replication system. Moreover, mammalian cells differ from prokaryotic cells in their substance uptake, metabolism, chromosome structure, and DNA repair processes. For these reasons, mammalian cell genotoxicity tests are usually used to complement the bacterial mutation assay in a first tier of in vitro genotoxicity testing for regulatory purposes (Cimino, 2006; Dybing et al., 1997).

13.3.1.1 Ames assay
Mutagenicity is strongly related to carcinogenicity (Klaunig and Kamendulis, 2008; Preston and Hoffmann, 2008). Indeed, although mutations may also occur at later stages in carcinogenesis, they represent a necessary first step for the action of many carcinogens, in particular, if occurring in proto-oncogenes and/or tumor suppressor genes. The Ames assay is widely used to determine the mutagenic potential of chemicals and drugs and is frequently a part of regulatory submissions for registration or acceptance of new chemicals, including drugs and biocides. In the tobacco industry, the Ames assay has been used to demonstrate that CS is mutagenic and to differentiate between the mutagenic potential of smoke from different tobaccos. In this context, the Ames assays were shown to be reproducible (CORESTA, 2007; Oldham et al., 2012; Rickert et al., 2007; Roemer et al., 2002), discriminatory (CORESTA, 2007; Oldham et al., 2012), and predictive of rodent carcinogenicity (Benigni, 2012; Kirkland et al., 2011; Pfuhler et al., 2010; Tennant et al., 1987). Moreover, the Ames assay readily detects mutations and frame-shifts, which have been identified at various chromosomal sites in lung cancer tissues of smokers (The US Centers for Disease Control and Prevention, 2010).

The Ames assay is performed in accordance with OECD TG 471 (OECD, 1997) and OECD Good Laboratory Practices (GLP) quality standards. For evaluation of the mutagenic activity of ENDP aerosols, the Ames assay is performed with TPM or native e-liquid in five strains of *Salmonella typhimurium* (TA98, TA100, TA102, TA1535, and TA1537) that have been genetically engineered to be incapable of synthesizing the essential amino acid histidine. The test detects mutations induced by the test substance that revert the mutations present in the test strains and restore the ability to synthesize the amino acid. The revertant bacteria are detected by their ability to grow in the absence of the amino acid required by the parent strain. Furthermore, the Ames assay is performed also with an exogenous metabolic activation system (S9 mix) to detect promutagens.

13.3.1.2 Mouse lymphoma assay
The MLA is a frequently used mammalian genotoxicity assay for testing industrial chemicals, pharmaceutical drugs, and consumer products (The US Food and Drug Administration, 2000). The MLA can detect most of the mutational events known to be associated with the etiology of cancer and other human diseases. These events include point mutations and several different types of chromosomal damage, recombinations, and deletions (Applegate et al., 1990; Chen et al., 2002; Clive et al., 1979; Honma et al., 2001; Liechty et al., 1998; Zeiger, 2010).

The MLA has also been the method of choice for assessing the genotoxic potential of tobacco products because of its ability to differentiate between different cigarette types, for example, for assessment of manufacturing processes, tobacco varieties, and novel tobacco products (Combes et al., 2012; Schramke et al., 2006; Thorne et al., 2019a; Werley et al., 2008). In addition, over the past years, an increasing number of academic and governmental researchers have also recommended the use of the MLA for assessing the in vitro genotoxicity of tobacco smoke (Albert, 1983; Clive et al., 1979; Guo et al., 2011; Mitchell et al., 1981).

The MLA is performed in accordance with OECD TG 490 (OECD, 2016b) and OECD GLP quality standards. The assay detects mutagenic and clastogenic events at the thymidine kinase (TK) locus of L5178Y mouse lymphoma $Tk^{+/-}$ cells. Mutant $Tk^{-/-}$ cells—deficient in TK enzyme activity because of a mutation from $Tk^{+/-}$ to $Tk^{-/-}$ induced by a test chemical—are resistant to the cytostatic effects of the pyrimidine analog trifluorothymidine (TFT). When these cells are grown in a selective medium containing TFT, wild-type $Tk^{+/-}$ cells die, but the mutant $Tk^{-/-}$ cells, which cannot incorporate TFT into their DNA, survive to form colonies that may be large (indicative of gene mutation) or small (indicative of gross chromosomal damage) in nature.

13.3.1.3 In vitro micronucleus assay
The MNvit assay is the second in vitro mammalian genotoxicity assay included in the assay battery. This assay

detects micronuclei distinct from the main nucleus of cells. Micronuclei may originate because of acentric chromosome fragments (i.e., chromosomes lacking a centromere) or whole chromosomes that are unable to migrate to the poles (spindle poisoning) during cell division. Therefore, the MNvit assay can detect both aneugens and clastogens in cells that have undergone cell division during or after exposure to a test chemical (OECD, 2016a). The Life Sciences Research Office has also mentioned that a micronucleus frequency assay is a useful component of an in vitro assay battery for ENDP assessment because it provides a simple and efficient method for characterizing product-induced chromosomal damage (The Life Sciences Research Office, 2007). This assay has also been applied successfully by others to assess the reduced genotoxicity of ENDPs (Thorne et al., 2019b).

The MNvit assay is performed in accordance with OECD TG 487 (OECD, 2016a) and OECD GLP quality standards by using Chinese hamster ovary (CHO) cells. The CHO-WBL cell line is considered acceptable for use, as it has been used for 32 years for genotoxicity testing at Merck Research Laboratories (Lorge et al., 2016). Moreover, throughout this time, the karyotype has remained stable and the levels of polyploidy low, and there has been no change in growth rate, modal number, or background levels of chromosome aberrations or micronuclei.

13.3.1.4 Neutral red uptake assay
Cytotoxicity is a major manifestation of tobacco smoke exposure and can be assumed to be involved in many, if not all, smoking-related diseases. Cytotoxicity may lead to morphological changes and inflammation, may contribute to tumorigenesis, and has been associated with tissue destruction in smoking-induced pulmonary emphysema and endothelial dysfunction (Dey et al., 2010; Milara and Cortijo, 2012; Siasos et al., 2014; Tesfamariam and DeFelice, 2007). Owing to their pivotal importance, assays that measure cytotoxicity have been included in most assay batteries for evaluation of tobacco products. Moreover, academic and governmental researchers have considered a cytotoxicity assay as a key element of an in vitro assay battery for assessing tobacco products (Andreoli et al., 2003; Putnam et al., 2002; Thorne et al., 2014; Yauk et al., 2012).

The NRU cytotoxicity assay has long been used to assess the cytotoxic potency of tobacco smoke and smokeless tobacco products because of its accuracy, reproducibility (CORESTA, 2007; Oldham et al., 2012), and discriminatory power (Richter et al., 2010; Roemer et al., 2004, 2008, 2014; Zenzen et al., 2012).

This has largely contributed to its wide acceptance, and, today, the results of the NRU assay are considered a statutory requirement for tobacco products (Health Canada, 2004). Therefore, the NRU cytotoxicity assay is a valuable component of a weight-of-evidence evaluation of the risk reduction potential of ENDPs.

The NRU assay is performed in accordance with INVITTOX protocol 3a (Health Canada, 2004; INVITTOX, 1990) and OECD GLP quality standards. The assay is based on the uptake of the supravital dye neutral red by mouse embryo BALB/c 3T3 cells, where it accumulates in the lysosomes/endosomes of living cells but not in dead/dying cells. The amount of neutral red taken up by cells is proportional to the cell number.

13.3.2 Application of the Test Battery to Toxicological Assessment of ENDPs
The assays described above have been applied for characterizing different EHTPs (Schaller et al., 2016; Thorne et al., 2018) and e-vapor products (EVPs) (Thorne et al., 2019a,b); their results are summarized below.

13.3.2.1 Ames assay
TPM fractions of 3R4F smoke and THS aerosol (Chapter 12) were tested in the Ames assay with *S. typhimurium* strains TA98, TA100, TA102, TA1535, and TA1537 both in the presence and absence of S9. After overnight growth, the bacteria were incubated for 20 min in the presence of various concentrations of TPM from THS (0.1–10 mg/plate) or 3R4F (0.2–1.0 mg/plate) with or without an S9 enzymatic metabolizing fraction. Revertant colonies were counted after 2 days of growth on minimal glucose agar base plates at 37°C (Schaller et al., 2016).

Three of the five *S. typhimurium* tester strains—TA98, TA100, and TA1537—showed mutagenic response in the presence of the S9 fraction in the Ames test with TPM from the 3R4F reference cigarette. In contrast, despite treatment with 5–10 mg/plate of TPM from THS, none of the tester strains showed mutagenicity under the conditions of this assay (Schaller et al., 2016).

13.3.2.2 Mouse lymphoma assay
The MLA was used to assess the mutagenicity of both TPM and GVP derived from THS aerosol and 3R4F reference CS (Schaller et al., 2016). L5178Y cells were exposed to 14 concentrations of TPM and GVP from THS (range, 45–1200 µg/mL for TPM and 40–1980 µg TPM equivalent/mL for GVP) or 3R4F (range, 2.5–54 µg/mL for TPM and 3–168 µg TPM equivalent/mL for GVP). The cells were exposed at 37°C for 4 and 24 h in the presence or absence of S9

metabolic activation (±S9). Relative total growth and mutation frequency, calculated in accordance with a published method (Clements, 2000), were used to determine the in vitro mutagenicity of the CS and THS aerosol fractions under each treatment condition and to compare their lowest observable genotoxic effect levels (LOGEL) (Guo et al., 2016).

On a per-mg TPM basis, the LOGEL values of THS aerosol were between 15.4- and 29.6-fold higher than those of 3R4F CS for TPM and between 8.3- and 23.6-fold higher for the GVP. Similarly, on a per-mg nicotine basis, the LOGEL values of THS-derived TPM were between 9.1- and 21.9-fold higher than those of 3R4F-derived TPM (Schaller et al., 2016).

13.3.2.3 In vitro micronucleus assay

CHO cells were exposed to several concentrations of TPM and GVP from THS (range, 1000–3200 μg TPM/mL for TPM and 1000–5000 μg TPM equivalent/mL for GVP) or 3R4F CS (range, 40–300 μg TPM/mL for TPM and 100–550 μg TPM equivalent/mL for GVP) for 4 and 24 h with or without S9 (Smart and McHugh, 2018). Nuclei and micronuclei were harvested and analyzed by using a flow cytometry method (Bryce et al., 2007). Cytotoxicity (relative population doubling) and genotoxicity (micronucleus frequency [%MN]) data were used to determine the relative in vitro genotoxicity of the CS and THS aerosol fractions and to compare their LOGELs. In this study, the LOGEL was defined as the lowest concentration that (1) induced a statistically significant increase in %MN relative to the concurrent solvent-treated controls; (2) was part of a statistically significant, positive trend in %MN induction; and (3) was above the +95% control limit of the laboratory's historical solvent-treated control %MN distribution.

Because some of the experiments failed to produce significant genotoxicity, it was not possible to derive the LOGELs for all test items under all treatment conditions. On those occasions where LOGELs could be derived, the LOGEL was at least 7.7-fold higher for THS-derived GVP than for its counterpart fraction from 3R4F and at least 15.1-fold higher for THS TPM than 3R4F TPM (Smart and McHugh, 2018).

13.3.2.4 Neutral red uptake assay

BALB/c 3T3 cells were incubated for 23 ± 1 h with several concentrations of TPM or GVP from THS (range, 2–95 items/L for TPM and 5–95 items/L for GVP) or 3R4F (range, 0.2–5.5 items/L for TPM and 0.5–6 items/L for GVP). NRU was determined by spectrophotometry of cell lysates. The concentrations that reduced the number of viable cells by 50% (EC_{50}) were determined, and $1/EC_{50}$ values (expressed on per-item and per-mg nicotine basis) were used to compare the relative cytotoxicity of the THS aerosol and 3R4F CS fractions (Schaller et al., 2016).

The results showed that the cytotoxic potencies of TPM and GVP from THS aerosol were significantly lower than those of the corresponding 3R4F smoke fractions. This reduction reached 91%–95% when expressed on a per-item basis and 85%–92% when expressed on a per-mg nicotine basis (Schaller et al., 2016). Importantly, these results were coherent with the relative levels of toxicants emitted by THS and 3R4F (Chapter 4).

13.3.2.5 Studies performed by others

British American Tobacco (BAT) assessed the TPM from its commercially available tobacco heating product 1.0 (THP1.0) in comparison with those from the 3R4F cigarette and PMI's THS by the Ames, NRU, and mouse lymphoma assays (Thorne et al., 2018). The NRU assay was performed in accordance with the Interagency Coordinating Committee on the Validation of Alternative Methods (ICCVAM) guidelines (ICCVAM, 2006). Balb/c 3T3 cells were exposed for 24 h to eight TPM concentrations. In the Ames assay, five tester strains of *S. typhimurium*—TA98, TA100, TA1535, TA1537, and TA102—were exposed to eight TPM concentrations in the presence and absence of S9 in accordance with OECD TG 471 (OECD, 1997). In the MLA, eight TPM concentrations from the three products were assessed under three test conditions—for 3 h with and without S9 and for 24 h without S9—in accordance with OECD TG 490 (OECD, 2016b). Both EHTPs showed very similar results; they were noncytotoxic up to the highest tested TPM concentration (240 μg/mL) in the NRU assay, nonmutagenic in the Ames assay at up to 2400 μg/plate, and nonmutagenic in the MLA at up to 240 μg/mL. Conversely, TPM from 3R4F produced dose-dependent responses in all three assays. As a complement, whole aerosols from the three test products were also assessed by the Ames assay (tester strains TA98, TA100, TA1535, TA97, and TA102 with S9) in accordance with OECD TG 471, by using a scaled-down, and previously described, methodology (Kilford et al., 2014; Thorne et al., 2015; Thorne et al., 2014). Whole aerosols from THP1.0 and THS were nonmutagenic in all tester strains exposed to diluting airflows of 12, 8, 4, and 1 L/min for 3 h, whereas whole smoke from 3R4F was deemed positive for mutagenicity in tester strains TA98 and TA100 at the same diluting airflows for only 24 min (Thorne et al., 2018).

Furthermore, BAT also showed that neither the basic e-liquid nor its aerosol induced marked genotoxicity in the MLA (Thorne et al., 2019a) or MNvit assay (Thorne et al., 2019b).

13.3.2.6 Conclusions

Overall, preclinical assessment of ENDPs by using a battery of in vitro regulatory toxicology assays demonstrated that the toxicological activity of aerosols generated from such products is significantly lower than that of CS (Table 13.2).

13.3.3 Mode-of-Action Investigations—Follow-up on Assay Battery Results

While the battery of in vitro assays is important for characterizing ENDPs from a regulatory toxicology perspective, it can also generate unexpected findings that require further investigation. It is widely recognized that genotoxicity assays conducted in mammalian cell cultures are highly sensitive and, consequently, prone to false-positive results (Cimino, 2006; Eastmond et al., 2009). Mode-of-action (MoA) investigations are recommended for providing a mechanistic context for such data and shedding light on their biological relevance (Kirkland et al., 2007). We have so far conducted three follow-up MoA experiments, which were essential to further understanding the initial findings.

Example 1: To address the dearth of modern-day genotoxicity data on nicotine, we conducted an MNvit study in a recommended cell line (CHO-WBL with known provenance) using a state-of-the-art flow cytometry—based assay in compliance with the current revision of OECD TG 487 and under GLP study conditions (Smart et al., 2019b). Nicotine induced an apparent genotoxic response at concentrations >3.95 mM; furthermore, mechanistic signals in the assay—for example, induction

of hypodiploid nuclei—indicated a possible aneugenic MoA. Follow-up experiments revealed a number of effects, including cellular vacuolization and accompanying distortions in α-tubulin—related microtubules at micronucleus-inducing concentrations (Smart et al., 2019b). We deduced that the vacuoles likely originated from acidic compartments, such as lysosomes, while genotoxicity was suppressed by alkalizing chemicals, such as ammonium chloride. However, the negligible changes in the phosphorylated histones H2AX and H3 cast doubt on the biological relevance of this apparent genotoxicity. On the basis of these results as well as those obtained with the major nicotine metabolites and by taking into account the effective concentration range (i.e., >3.95 mM), we were able to conclude that the observed effects were likely to be of minimal physiological relevance for nicotine consumers.

Example 2: With the goal of understanding the effects of nonflavored e-liquids (NFELs) in the MNvit assay, we conducted a similar study to the one described earlier but using six NFEL variants (Smart et al., 2019). We sought to establish a baseline of effects that could serve as a reference point for future assessment of flavored e-liquids and, ultimately, e-liquid aerosols. Propylene glycol (PG)-predominant e-liquids showed significant genotoxic responses, while e-liquids with higher proportions of vegetable glycerin (VG) were nongenotoxic. However, all six NFELs induced extreme cell culture conditions (i.e., increases in pH and osmolality), indicating that the micronucleus effects were not related to these phenomena. Analysis of mechanistic endpoints, such as cell cycle changes and changes in phosphorylated histones H2AX and H3, revealed no biologically relevant effects. Importantly, nicotine was found not to interfere with DNA damage response signaling in cells exposed to genotoxins, thus ruling out any masking effects of nicotine. On this basis, we concluded that the apparent

TABLE 13.2
Summary of Findings Generated From Assessment of EHTPs by Regulatory-Based Toxicology Assays.

		Cytotoxicity	Bacterial mutagenicity	Mammalian cell mutagenicity	Mammalian cell genotoxicity
EHTPs versus cigarette	TPM	>90% lower[a, b]	Not mutagenic[a, b]	Lower by at least a factor 15[a, b]	Lower by at least a factor 15[c]
	GVP	>90% lower[a]	Not mutagenic[a]	Lower by at least a factor 8[a]	Lower by at least a factor 7[c]
	Whole aerosol	n/a	Not mutagenic[b]	n/a	n/a

Summary of findings generated from assessment of EHTPs by regulatory-based toxicology assays. *EHTP*, electronic nicotine delivery product; *GVP*, gas—vapor phase; *n/a*, not applicable; *TPM*, total particulate matter.
[a] (Schaller et al., 2016).
[b] (Thorne et al., 2018).
[c] (Smart and McHugh, 2018).

DNA damage induced by the PG-predominant e-liquids is potentially misleading and of negligible biological relevance. In view of this extensive NFEL characterization, future e-liquid–related assessments that reveal additional adverse changes in these endpoints might indicate the presence of a possible genotoxic hazard and would prompt further investigation for exploring their biological relevance.

Example 3: In the context of EVP assessment, we implemented an NRU assay–based screening program to evaluate the cytotoxic potency of e-liquids, the matrices that are ultimately aerosolized by EVP devices (Cudazzo et al., 2019). E-liquids induced a biphasic response in the BALB/c 3T3 cell–based assay; NRU initially increased in a concentration-dependent manner before decreasing upon treatment with higher concentrations of e-liquids, until it was abolished (Fig. 13.1A). In light of this unusual response profile, follow-up experiments were performed to characterize the mechanism underlying the biphasic signal. Nicotine alone was found to induce the same biphasic effects in the NRU assay while inducing a monotonic decrease in relative cell counts (Fig. 13.1B). Imaging—targeting the LAMP-1 protein—and flow cytometry data generated with the LysoTracker reagent revealed that the increases in NRU likely resulted from nicotine-induced vacuolization via a lysosomotropic mechanism.

Given the potential distorting effects of this biphasic NRU profile on the interpolation of accurate potency metrics (such as EC_{50}), we explored other endpoints of cytotoxicity—such as resazurin, adenosine triphosphate production, and water-soluble tetrazolium salt (WST)-8 reduction—and, importantly, found that they were not compromised by nicotine's lysosomotropic effects. On the basis of this evidence, we were able to recommend the adoption of the WST-8 assay for assessing the cytotoxic potency of nicotine-containing e-liquids.

13.3.4 Integrated In Vitro Mammalian Genotoxicity Assessment of the Future

It is commonly accepted that no single genotoxicity assay among those currently available is sufficient to detect all types of DNA damage that can be inflicted upon a genome, and, therefore, a battery of genotoxicity assays is required. Importantly, for registration of different types of chemicals, such as pharmaceuticals and cosmetic ingredients, regulatory bodies around the world mandate combinations of data from these assays (Scientific Committee on Consumer Safety, 2018; The International Council for Harmonisation, 2011; US Food and Drug Administration Center for Devices and Radiological Health, 2016). However, where two in vitro mammalian assays covering gene mutation and chromosome damage endpoints are required (e.g., for plant protection products) (Commission Regulation 283/2013, 3AD), data complementarity might be suboptimal, given the possibility that different mammalian cell models and diverse experimental conditions, such as distinct test chemical concentration

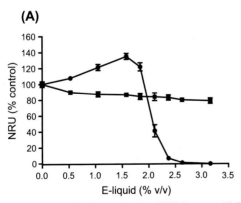
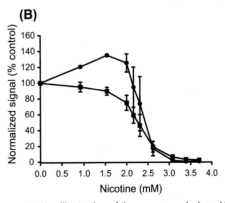

FIG. 13.1 **Biphasic Effects in the NRU Assay.** (A) Representative illustration of the responses induced by nicotine-containing (●) and nicotine-free (■) e-liquids after 24 h in the BALB/c 3T3 cell-based NRU assay (mean ± SEM, n = 6). (B) Nicotine-induced concentration-dependent changes in NRU (●) and RCC (■) in the same cells following 24-h treatment (mean ± SEM, n = 3). *NRU,* neutral red uptake; *RCC,* relative cell count; *SEM,* standard error of mean. (Adapted from Fig. 1 of Cudazzo, G., Smart, D.J., Mchugh, D., Vanscheeuwijck, P., 2019. Lysosomotropic-related limitations of the BALB/c 3T3 cell-based neutral red uptake assay and an alternative testing approach for assessing e-liquid cytotoxicity. Toxicol. In Vitro 61, 104647, published under CC-BY license.)

ranges, may be employed. Furthermore, there is also evidence to suggest that rodent cell–based assays are potentially less specific than counterpart assays in human cells (Whitwell et al., 2015). Thus, considering this information, there is an obvious utility in adopting an approach where both endpoints are evaluated in one human cell–based assay. To this end, we have developed an integrated assay in human TK6 cells that not only addresses gene mutation and chromosome damage endpoints but also provides data on genotoxic MoA through biomarkers of the cellular DNA damage response (Smart et al., 2020). In a proficiency-type study using a subset of prototypical genotoxic and nongenotoxic substances, the assay was found to accurately detect both clastogenic and aneugenic DNA damage while also correctly reporting a lack of effects induced by the nongenotoxic agents. Although there are no granular regulations in the context of genetic toxicology data for ENDPs in 2020, a prominent role can be foreseen for this integrated assay for characterizing the genotoxic potential of these products in a comprehensive manner as well as for regulatory purposes.

13.4 IN VITRO SYSTEMS TOXICOLOGY

Steadily accumulating evidence indicates that using systems data alongside conventional histopathology and clinical chemistry data enables better and more informed decision-making than data obtained by traditional safety assessment methods. The US National Research Council, commissioned by the US Environmental Protection Agency, has developed a vision for toxicity testing in the 21st century, called Tox 21-c. It postulates that there will be a shift from traditional toxicity testing toward efforts focused on exploring and improving our understanding of the signaling pathways that are perturbed by biologically active substances or their metabolites, potentially leading to adverse health effects in humans (Hartung, 2010; Krewski et al., 2010).

Systems toxicology is an approach intended to help gain a more comprehensive understanding of the biological effects of active substances and leverage this understanding in product assessment (Chapter 9). It is a highly interdisciplinary approach that uses advanced analytical and computational tools to integrate classical toxicology and quantitative analysis of large networks of molecular and functional changes occurring across multiple levels of biological organization. Systems toxicology depends on extensive datasets produced by using omics technologies, such as transcriptomics, metabolomics, and proteomics (Hoeng et al., 2014a). The approach enables integration of quantitative

systems-wide molecular changes in the context of chemical exposure measurements and a causal chain of events linking exposures with toxicity and disease (Sturla et al., 2014).

The objective of systems toxicology is to generate a comprehensive overview of the effects of an exposure and, thereby, help gain a deep understanding of the biological networks that are perturbed by the exposure (Hoeng et al., 2012; Sturla et al., 2014). In contrast to a battery of assays selected according to the properties of a reference product (usually CS), an untargeted systems biology/toxicology approach offers the opportunity to detect potentially novel effects that are not caused by the reference product. Furthermore, in the context of ENDP assessment, systems biology/toxicology approaches can reveal biological changes occurring along the causal chain of events linking smoking to disease. This knowledge is then applied to a mechanism-by-mechanism comparison of the effects of an ENDP aerosol with those of CS.

In the context of ENDP assessment, numerous nonclinical studies have been conducted by using in vitro laboratory models ranging from simple 2D cell cultures to 3D culture models and microphysiologically inspired models. An overview of the different models, along with their respective advantages and limitations, is presented in Fig. 13.2. A list of these studies and their key conclusions are presented in Table 13.1. Generally, most assay models currently lack a standardized protocol. One opportunity to standardize the protocols is for suppliers to develop kits for development/preparation and use of the models. Furthermore, if primary cells are used, the number of cultures/models that can be generated from the same donor is limited. Donor-specific responses may be observed in certain endpoints.

13.4.1 Application of Systems Toxicology by Using 2D Monolayer Culture Systems

13.4.1.1 System establishment

Within the ENDP assessment framework, we use submersed cell monolayer (simple 2D) cultures, typically composed of epithelial cells or fibroblasts, primarily as an early screening tool. In such systems, a large number of experimental conditions, including multiple concentrations and time points, can easily be tested simultaneously, and multiparametric indicators of cellular toxicity can be assessed by RTCA and HCS. This approach is also suitable for investigating the MoA of various test materials, from individual CS constituents to aerosols generated from ENDPs, because the HCS data can be complemented with whole-transcriptome analysis. The transcriptome analysis will

Models		Advantages	Limitations	Recommendations
Celluar models	**Primary respiratory, cardiovascular, and other 2D cell cultures** 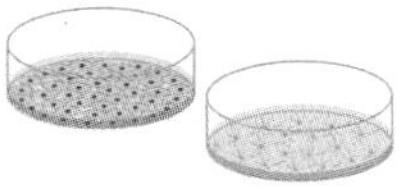	- Use primary cells of different donors - Simple - High throughput	- Cross-talk among cell types cannot be studied - Generally suitable for short-term experiments - Need to generate aerosol fractions (unsuitable for whole-aerosol exposure experiments)	- Protocols should be standardized across laboratories
	Organotypic 3D cell cultures 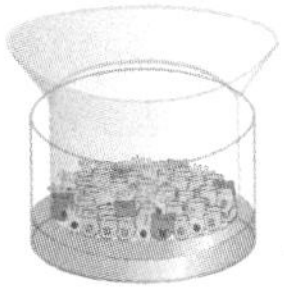	- Use primary cells of different donors - Better recapitulate the morphology and physiology of the in vivo situation than 2D cell cultures - Medium throughput - For airway epithelial cultures, the air–liquid interface setup allows for direct aerosol exposure - Cross-talk among cell types can be studied - Some cultures can be maintained for several months (potentially suitable for chronic exposure studies)	- Often lack immune cells - Long-term culturing is not possible for all models - Lack of protocol standardization across laboratories	- Protocols should be standardized across laboratories
Mechanistic models	**2D adhesion assay** 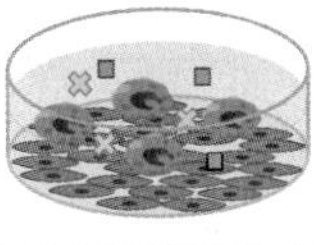	- Uses primary cells of different donors - Simple - High throughput - Cross-talk among cell types can be studied	- 2D model - Suitable only for short-term experiments - Need to generate aerosol fractions (unsuitable for whole-aerosol exposure experiments)	- Protocols should be standardizecd across laboratories - The number of monocytes adherent to endothelial cells and the number of endothelial cells in the same wells should be reported to support data interpretation
	Transmigration assay 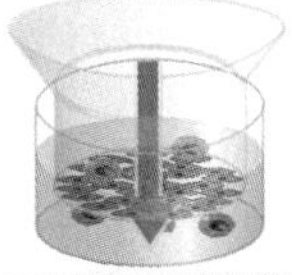	- Uses primary cells of different donors - Cross-talk among cell types can be studied - Real-time measurement - Label-free detection	- Low throughput - Unsuitable for non-adherent monocytes	- Protocols should be standardized across laboratories - Chemotaxis and transendothelial migration assays (using Boyden chamber) should be run in parallel
Microphysiology-based models	**Microvessel-on-a-chip adhesion assay** 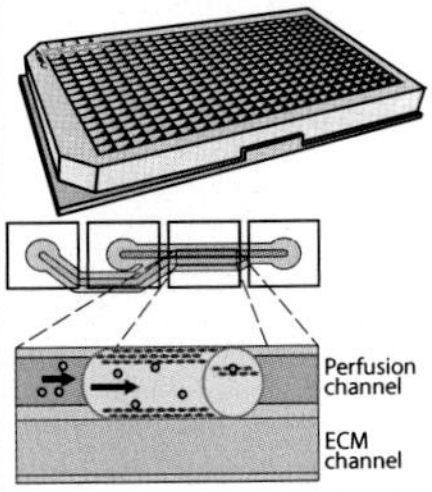	- Uses primary cells of different donors - Easy to use - High throughput - Cross-talk among cell types can be studied - Recapitulates the physiology of the in vivo situation by adding flow to the system - Can be maintained up to 8 days (potentially suitable for repeated exposure studies) - Accomodates other assays (e.g., leukocyte adhesion and transmigration, angiogenesis)	- Cannot simulate different shear stress levels/patterns	- Protocols should be standardized across laboratories - The integrity of the microvessels should be monitored by measuring the cell count or their permeability
	Lung–liver-on-a-chip system 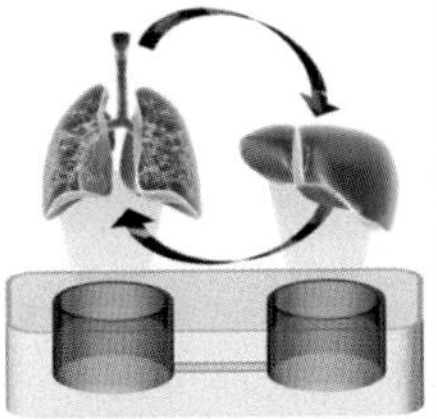	- Uses primary cells of different donors - Useful to assess the toxicity of compounds on both lung and liver models - Useful to assess the cross talk between tissue models (e.g., the toxicity of compounds metabolized by the liver on the lungs can be studied) - Can be maintained up to 28 days - Includes various models of organ systems (modular system) - The air–liquid interface of the lung model allows for direct aerosol exposure - Incorporates flow in the system (multiple flow options)	- Low throughput - Because of the large volume of culture media circulating in the system, the concentrations of mediators/metabolites might not be measurable	- Protocols should be standardized across laboratories - Should be used in later stages of preclinical studies

Increasing complexity

Perfusion channel
ECM channel

FIG. 13.2 **Overview of Laboratory Models With Their Respective Advantages and Limitations.** *N/A,* not applicable.

identify toxicity pathways and evaluate the risk associated with the test product by using systems toxicology approaches.

Primary NHBE cells are the preferred cell type for simple 2D airway test systems. In the lungs, they constitute a cell layer that is directly exposed to the inhaled

HPHCs present in CS and play a key role in the development of smoking-related diseases. Exposure to CS has been shown to cause a complex array of responses in lung epithelial cells. These responses include changes in gene expression mapped to molecular pathways related to xenobiotic metabolism and detoxification, oxidative stress response, inflammation, DNA damage response, apoptosis, and cell cycle regulation (Jorgensen et al., 2004; Mathis et al., 2013; Nyunoya et al., 2014; Pickett et al., 2010; Sen et al., 2007; Yauk et al., 2012). The use of human primary cells offers an important advantage because it minimizes the risk that genetic modifications (which are always present in immortalized cell lines) may act as confounding factors when identifying perturbations in specific molecular pathways by whole-genome transcriptomics analyses.

We previously established an HCS method using a simple 2D culture of primary NHBE cells, in which we evaluated three well-known HPHCs of tobacco smoke, namely acrolein, formaldehyde, and catechol (Gonzalez-Suarez et al., 2014). We evaluated a wide range of concentrations, each applied for 4, 8, and 24 h. The HCS assays, covering 13 different indicators of toxicity, and the whole-genome transcriptomics analysis revealed that DNA damage/growth arrest, oxidative stress, mitochondrial stress, and apoptosis/necrosis were the most impacted mechanisms of toxicity. These data demonstrate that such a model provides robust insights into the molecular mechanisms of toxicity and enables MoA investigations. Similar approaches have been followed for testing a broader selection of test materials, including e-liquids and aerosols, in the context of ENDP assessment.

13.4.1.2 EHTP assessment

The biological impacts of three different aerosol fractions of THS were compared with those of the same fractions of 3R4F CS in a simple 2D airway test system that employed primary NHBE cells (Gonzalez-Suarez et al., 2016). The CS and THS aerosol fractions tested were (1) AEs of whole smoke/aerosol, (2) TPM, and (3) GVP (for details of sample generation, see Chapter 12). These fractions were mixed with the culture medium. Eleven different toxicity endpoints as well as biological network perturbations based on systems-wide transcriptomics data were quantified in cells exposed to various concentrations of these fractions for 4 and 24 h. Exposure of cells to the 3R4F CS fractions resulted in a dose-dependent response in most toxicity endpoints. Significant levels of perturbations were observed in multiple biological pathways, particularly in those related to cellular stress. In contrast, the THS aerosol

fractions had considerably smaller biological effects (HCS and transcriptomics assays) on NHBE cells than the 3R4F CS fractions at comparable concentrations. Responses were detected against the aerosol fractions in some endpoints, but only at concentrations between 3 and 15 times higher than those of the 3R4F fractions (Gonzalez-Suarez et al., 2016).

13.4.1.3 EVP assessment

We have proposed a multilayer systems toxicology—based framework for in vitro assessment of e-liquids to complement the battery of classical assays for mutagenicity and genotoxicity testing (Iskandar et al., 2016). Briefly, the first layer of the framework is aimed at screening e-liquids for potential cytotoxicity by, for example, impedance-based RTCA in a simple 2D airway test system using NHBE cells. This is followed, in the second layer, by toxicity-related mechanistic investigation of selected e-liquids by HCS assays with the same test system as that in the first layer. Finally, the third layer of the framework focuses on toxicity-related mechanistic investigation of the corresponding aerosols by using 3D airway culture systems grown at the ALI (further elaborated in Section 13.4.2). As highlighted in Chapter 16, a fast, high-throughput in vitro screening test system is particularly useful for evaluating the flavoring substances used in e-liquids, as over 8000 flavor mixtures are currently available on the market, with new ones appearing every month (Bals et al., 2019; Tierney et al., 2016).

In a case study aimed at developing a flavor toolbox, we followed the framework to assess 28 flavoring substances commonly used in e-liquid formulations (Chapter 16; Marescotti et al., 2020b). The effects of these 28 different flavors, added individually or as a mixture, were compared with those of a flavorless base e-liquid. The flavor content of the e-liquid with the mixture reached 5.7%, which exceeds the reported total proportion of flavors usually present in e-liquids (1%—4%). The base e-liquid had a minor effect on cell viability, mainly because of a dose-dependent increase in osmolality induced by PG and VG. Addition of the flavor mixture significantly increased the cytotoxicity of the e-liquid without increasing its osmolality. Each individual flavor was also assessed, and the results revealed that citronellol was the main contributor to the cytotoxicity of the mixture and that interaction effects were at play. The base e-liquid had a limited impact on phenotypic changes (HCS endpoints) and network perturbations (gene expression analyses) in NHBE cells. When NHBE cells were exposed for 24 h to the 28-flavor mixture, the levels of indicators of (for example) cellular stress, apoptosis, necrosis, proliferation, and inflammation were significantly higher than those when the cells were exposed to the base e-liquid. This study highlights the benefits of testing both individual flavoring substances and mixtures within a framework covering a broad range of endpoints beyond cytotoxicity. Further considerations and conclusions regarding the flavor toolbox approach are discussed in Chapter 16.

This multilayer systems toxicology framework for in vitro assessment of e-liquids was also applied to evaluate the biological impact of the *MESH* Classic Tobacco e-liquid in comparison with the flavorless base e-liquid and TPM from the 3R4F reference cigarette (Iskandar et al., 2019b). The first assessment layer showed decreased NHBE cell viability following a 24-h incubation with 3R4F TPM at approximately 20-fold lower nicotine concentrations than those of both e-liquids. The second assessment layer revealed that the base e-liquid and *MESH* e-liquid had similar, minor effects. However, incubation of cells with 3R4F TPM resulted in a dose-dependent impact on DNA damage, glutathione (GSH) content, oxidative stress, and phosphorylation of the stress kinase c-Jun. The minimum concentration at which an effect could be observed was >50 times greater for both e-liquids than for 3R4F TPM.

Overall, the simple airway 2D model used within the ENDP assessment framework is a robust and useful approach for screening numerous e-liquids and finished products for potential reduced toxicity relative to cigarettes, as it covers a wide range of toxicological endpoints and allows rapid testing of multiple concentrations and time points. However, 2D models have limitations, as they do not reflect the in vivo situation. Indeed, they neither reflect the structure nor cell composition and differentiation of the epithelium. Furthermore, they do not permit an in vivo-like exposure to whole CS/ENDP aerosols, as CS/ENDP aerosol fractions must be dissolved in the culture medium. These limitations can be addressed, at least in part, with more sophisticated in vitro models, which are presented and discussed in the following sections.

13.4.1.4 Studies performed by others
In a study published by BAT, TPM from another EHTP, THP1.0, was tested in 2D NHBE cell cultures, and its effects compared with those of TPM from THS and 3R4F (Taylor et al., 2018). The same HCS endpoints were evaluated as those in an earlier publication (Gonzalez-Suarez et al., 2016). The results showed that 3R4F TPM elicited a moderate response, mainly in endpoints related to oxidative stress, whereas neither THP1.0 nor THS TPM induced signals in any of the HCS endpoints at similar concentrations (Taylor et al., 2018).

Furthermore, Munakata and colleagues (Munakata et al., 2018) used BEAS-2B cells to assess the effects of exposure to the AE fractions of (1) 3R4F CS, (2) a commercially available EHTP, (3) an EVP, and (4) a novel tobacco vapor product (NTV from Japan Tobacco Inc. [Tokyo, Japan]). Using a battery of assays, including a cell viability assay, GSH quantification, an NRF2 reporter gene assay, and cytokine (interleukin [IL]-8 and granulocyte—macrophage colony-stimulating factor [GM-CSF]) measurements, they found that all endpoints were perturbed by exposure to each AE, but the effective dose ranges of CS and the ENDP aerosols were different. Indeed, in the cell viability assay, the EC_{50} determined after a 24-h exposure to 3R4F AE (0.045 puffs/mL) was 10 times lower than the EC_{50} of the EHTP (0.518 puffs/mL) (EC_{50} values were not determined for the other AEs). The lowest AE concentrations that caused a statistically significant decrease in the GSH/GSSG (glutathione disulfide) ratio relative to untreated controls were 0.0225, 0.12, 4.5, and 9 puffs/mL for 3R4F, EHTP, NTV, and EVP, respectively. NRF2 reporter activity was increased in a dose-dependent manner under all exposures. The lowest concentration that caused a significant increase in NRF2 reporter activity was observed with 3R4F AE (0.015 puffs/mL), while much higher concentrations were needed with the EHTP and the EVP (0.12 and 2.25 puffs/mL, respectively). For the NTV, none of the tested doses (0.9—18.0 puffs/mL) induced a significant increase in NRF2 activation relative to the control. The concentrations of secreted inflammatory cytokines (IL-8 and GM-CSF) were increased after a 6-h exposure to each test product AE. The highest level of IL-8 was detected following exposure to 0.03 puffs/mL of 3R4F AE, 0.36 puffs/mL of the EHTP AE, and 18 puffs/mL of the NTV and EVP AEs. The authors concluded that the assays used in this study were suitable for detecting differences among products.

13.4.2 Application of Systems Toxicology by Using 3D Culture Systems Grown at the ALI

13.4.2.1 Models for aerosol assessment
Epithelial cultures grown at the ALI provide the unique advantage that cells normally exposed to air can be exposed to inhaled aerosols. Furthermore, an experimental setup designed for whole CS and ENDP aerosol exposure to the ALI can better simulate a dosimetry that is relevant to human exposure. This enables better extrapolation of test results to the in vivo situation than can be achieved with 2D cellular systems (Polk et al., 2016).

Primary basal airway cells obtained from human donors can be expanded and further cultured on specially designed tissue culture inserts to expose the apical side of the cells to air. Under these conditions, the basal pluripotent cells will differentiate into ciliated epithelial cells, goblet cells (in case of nasal and bronchial epithelium), and club cells (in case of small airway epithelium) forming, after a few weeks, a pseudostratified epithelium resembling the human lung epithelium. Models that incorporate multiple cell types (e.g., submucosal fibroblasts and immune cells) are also available (Iskandar et al., 2015; Marescotti et al., 2019). These morphological properties support the relevance of such culture models as a potential gold standard for assessment of inhaled aerosols.

Similarly, reconstituted organotypic tissues of the oral cavity, such as 3D cultures of the oral mucosa grown at the ALI (e.g., from suppliers such as MatTek and SkinEthic) express characteristics of differentiated epithelial tissue like those observed in vivo (Klausner et al., 2007; Schlage et al., 2014). The relevance of using oral epithelial tissue cultures for cigarette and ENDP toxicity testing is obvious, as the oral mucosa is exposed to the fresh CS/ENDP aerosol leaving the cigarette/ENDP mouthpiece.

In the context of ENDP assessment, it has been shown that exposure to CS creates a field of injury in epithelial cells lining the respiratory tract (Sridhar et al., 2008). Therefore, human organotypic tissue cultures that are grown at the ALI and represent the various epithelia of the respiratory tract are relevant for assessing the effects of ENDP aerosol exposure (Fig. 13.3).

13.4.2.2 Cigarette smoke exposure investigation studies for model establishment

The utility of human organotypic ALI airway epithelial culture models for assessing the toxicological impact of inhaled aerosols has been demonstrated (Upadhyay and Palmberg, 2018). We have also conducted various studies in which the effects of exposure to whole CS were investigated in vitro and compared to the known effects of CS exposure on smokers' airways in vivo. The following sections summarize the relevant work in this field.

First, following acute exposure (7, 14, 21, and 28 min) of human 3D bronchial epithelial tissue cultures to CS (15% dilution with air), a dose-dependent increase in matrix metalloproteinase-1 (MMP-1) release was measured in the basal culture medium. This was in agreement with the known effect of cigarette smoking on MMP-1 gene expression in tissues from smokers (Mathis et al., 2013). In this study, using a gene set enrichment analysis (GSEA) approach, Mathis and colleagues further observed a significant enrichment of human smokers' bronchial epithelium gene signatures derived from different clinical datasets in CS-exposed organotypic bronchial epithelium cultures. The genes affected by CS exposure in 3D ALI bronchial cultures were negatively correlated with those affected by smoking cessation. Comparison of in vitro miRNA profiles with available miRNA data from healthy smokers also highlighted various highly

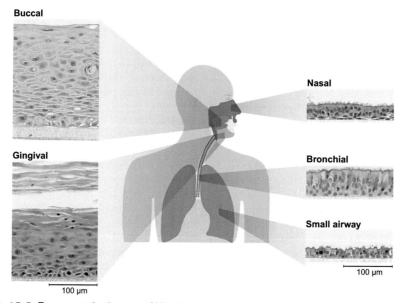

Buccal

Nasal

Gingival

Bronchial

Small airway

100 μm

100 μm

FIG. 13.3 Representative images of histological culture sections covering the respiratory tract.

translatable miRNAs associated with inflammation or cell cycle processes that are known to be perturbed by CS in lung tissue.

In a follow-up study which used additional computational approaches (i.e., GSEA and reverse causal reasoning analysis), the biological impact of CS exposure on organotypic bronchial epithelium cultures was further dissected at the gene expression level (at both mRNA and miRNA levels) (Mathis et al., 2015). This study provided the first supporting evidence that the effects observed in organotypic tissue cultures directly exposed to CS in vitro can be translated to the known effects of CS in smokers (e.g., cell stress, inflammatory responses, and cell proliferation changes).

Second, a study was conducted to compare the effects of CS exposure on an organotypic bronchial epithelial culture (the monoculture) with those on a coculture of the same organotypic culture maintained together with fibroblasts (the coculture) (Iskandar et al., 2015). The results demonstrated that CS exposure had similar effects on cytotoxicity, cytochrome P450 (CYP) 1A1/1B1 activity, and tissue histology in both models. However, a greater number of secreted mediators were identified in the basolateral medium of the monoculture than in that of the coculture. Furthermore, analyses indicated that cellular stress responses and tissue damage following CS exposure were more prominent in the monoculture than in the coculture. Finally, our results indicated that the in vivo CS-induced xenobiotic metabolism response of bronchial epithelial cells was better reflected by the CS-exposed coculture than the monoculture.

The effects of repeated exposures (each corresponding to smoking one cigarette, separated by a 1-h interval) have been investigated by using human organotypic bronchial, nasal, buccal, and gingival epithelium cultures (Schlage et al., 2014; Talikka et al., 2014) (Fig. 13.4A). The proportions of the different cell types (e.g., p63-positive basal cells) constituting the tissue cultures as well as the levels of secreted inflammatory mediators were altered in a similar manner in both bronchial and nasal cultures (Talikka et al., 2014). The results indicated that repeated CS smoke exposure induced an inflammatory response, despite causing only mild effects on culture morphology and cellular staining characteristics (Talikka et al., 2014). CS exposure also induced an inflammatory response in buccal and gingival cultures, while barely affecting tissue integrity (Schlage et al., 2014). Furthermore, CS exposure led to an increase in CYP1A1 and 1B1 levels in all culture types (nasal,

bronchial, buccal, and gingival) relative to their corresponding air-exposed controls (Kuehn et al., 2015; Schlage et al., 2014; Talikka et al., 2014). CYP1A1 and CYP1B1, which belong to phase I xenobiotic metabolizing enzymes, are known to be responsible for the degradation as well as metabolic activation of tobacco smoke constituents (Guengerich, 2000; Port et al., 2004; Rendic and Guengerich, 2012). Ciliary beating frequency, another functional endpoint specific to ciliated epithelia, was also found to be useful when investigating the impact of CS exposure, especially because the measurements could be conducted longitudinally (Kuehn et al., 2015). Transcriptomics data analysis of both nasal and bronchial cultures by using network-based approaches (described in greater detail in Chapter 9) showed that CS exposure perturbs both similar and diverse biological processes. Furthermore, comparison of differentially expressed genes in human smokers' bronchial and nasal epithelial cells with these in vitro datasets highlighted similarities in the response to CS exposure (Talikka et al., 2014). Interestingly, using a similar approach, a gene set analysis revealed that the pathways induced by CS exposure in the in vitro buccal cultures resembled those in the in vivo samples obtained from buccal tissue biopsies of smokers (Schlage et al., 2014). These results further support the relevance of using human organotypic airways tissue cultures to assess CS-induced adverse effects in the respiratory system, pointing to common patterns that are independent of the donors who were used to generate the organotypic models.

A recent study reported on efforts to establish a robust and longer-term repeated exposure pattern by using organotypic tissue cultures. Ito et al. performed a 40-day repeated exposure study using human organotypic bronchial epithelial cultures (Ito et al., 2020); however, the authors only tested TPM fractions. The cultures were first exposed to CS TPM daily for 20 days and subsequently subjected to either air exposure (cessation) or ENDP aerosol TPM exposure (switching) for another 20 days. The authors found that the cultures could recover from the damage induced by CS TPM exposure even when they were switched to an ENDP aerosol TPM. They also noticed that repeated exposure to TPM from an ENDP aerosol induced negligible toxic effects in the tissue cultures, while CS TPM exposure led to cumulative adverse effects. This is the first example of an in vitro study conducted with organotypic airway epithelial cultures that included not only long-term CS and ENDP aerosol fractions exposures but also an ENDP switching arm as well as a smoking cessation arm.

(A)

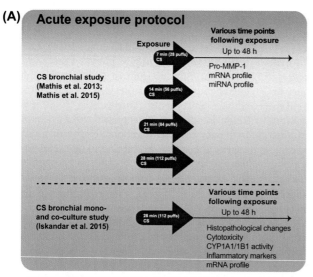

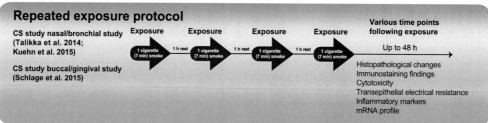

(B)

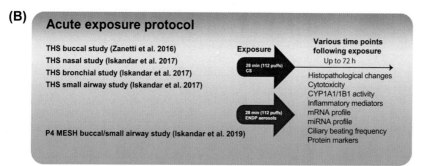

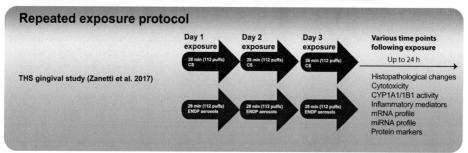

FIG. 13.4 **Exposure Protocols in Various Organotypic Studies.**   Protocols used in different published studies where (**A**) the effects of whole mainstream CS exposure were used to demonstrate the utility of human organotypic cultures as a key cellular model for assessing the toxicological impact of inhaled aerosol exposure, and (**B**) the effects of ENDP aerosols were investigated by using human organotypic culture models. Representative, nonexhaustive endpoints are indicated. *CS*, cigarette smoke; *THS*, Tobacco Heating System 2.2.

13.4.2.3 EHTP assessment

The relative effects of THS aerosol and CS exposure were evaluated in several studies using human organotypic cultures of buccal, gingival, nasal, bronchial, and small airway epithelia. The systems toxicology approach included cellular assays (i.e., cytotoxicity and cytochrome P450 activity assays), measurement of secreted inflammatory markers, histopathological analysis, and comprehensive molecular investigations of the buccal epithelial transcriptome (mRNA and miRNA) by using computational network biology.

Human organotypic oral (buccal) epithelium cultures were exposed for 28 min to 3R4F CS or THS aerosol at two nicotine-matched concentrations and one higher THS concentration and monitored for up to 72 h postexposure (Zanetti et al., 2016). CS exposure led to typical concentration-related adaptive and proinflammatory effects, while THS aerosol exposure led to responses that were predominantly not significant (Figs. 13.5 and 13.6A).

An organotypic gingival epithelium culture was also used to compare the impact of repeated exposure to THS aerosol (daily for 3 days) with that of repeated exposure to CS (Zanetti et al., 2017). CS exposure resulted in visible tissue damage; but, no such findings were detected in cultures exposed repeatedly to THS aerosol (Fig. 13.5). On the basis of the profiles of secreted inflammatory markers and metabolomics and transcriptomics findings (Fig. 13.6B), the study demonstrated that THS aerosol exposure had a broadly and significantly lower impact than CS exposure.

Furthermore, in another study, human organotypic nasal epithelium cultures exposed to CS or THS aerosol were analyzed for cytotoxicity, cytochrome P450 activity, secreted proinflammatory factors, histological characteristics, and ciliary beating frequency, and these findings were complemented by a computational network biology analysis of global mRNA and miRNA changes (Iskandar et al., 2017b). At comparable nicotine concentrations, THS aerosol—exposed cultures had significantly lower functional (cilia beating frequency) and toxic responses than 3R4F CS-exposed cultures, and the pattern of biological impact in the network models was diminished for THS aerosol exposure (Figs. 13.5 and 13.6C).

Similar investigations were performed by using human organotypic bronchial (Iskandar et al., 2017c) and small airway (Iskandar et al., 2017a) epithelium cultures. These studies demonstrated concentration-dependent CS toxicity and biological network perturbations (cell death, inflammatory processes, cell proliferation, and cell stress), which were significantly lower in THS aerosol—exposed cultures at comparable nicotine concentrations (see Figs. 13.5 and 13.6D,E).

A systems toxicology metaanalysis (Iskandar et al., 2017d) was conducted in the context of in vitro assessment of THS aerosol by using three human organotypic epithelial cultures of the aerodigestive tract (buccal, bronchial, and nasal epithelia). All cultures showed lower toxicity following exposure to THS aerosol than after CS exposure. Because of their morphological differences, buccal cultures (stratified epithelium) showed a smaller exposure impact than bronchial and nasal cultures (pseudostratified epithelium). However, the results of causal network enrichment approach supported a similar mechanistic impact of CS across the three cultures, including the impact on xenobiotic, oxidative stress, and inflammatory responses. At comparable nicotine concentrations, THS aerosol exposure elicited reduced and more transient effects on these processes. The metaanalysis demonstrated the overall reduced impact of THS aerosol exposure relative to CS exposure.

Furthermore, another group (Haswell et al., 2018) conducted an in vitro toxicogenomics-based assessment of two commercially available EHTPs (THS and THP1.0) and the 3R4F reference cigarette by using human organotypic bronchial epithelial cultures. The study found decreases in ciliary beating frequency and transepithelial electrical resistance in cultures exposed to CS but not in those exposed to THS or THP1.0 aerosols. Using RNA-sequencing (i.e., 3R4F vs. air; THS vs. air; THP1.0 vs. air) and qPCR analyses, the authors found that exposure to CS elicited the strongest differential gene expression response. This study demonstrated the reduced impact of exposure to aerosols of EHTPs on lung epithelial cultures relative to the impact of exposure to CS.

13.4.2.4 EVP assessment

A recent study investigated the toxicity profiles of both the e-liquid and the corresponding aerosol of the EVP MESH Classic Tobacco flavor by following the three-layer systems toxicology assessment framework described earlier (Iskandar et al., 2016, 2019b). The third layer of the framework focuses on systems toxicology studies using organotypic culture systems grown at the ALI. The study demonstrated that, unlike CS exposure, the MESH Classic Tobacco aerosol did not cause cytotoxicity or tissue damage in buccal or small airway epithelium cultures (Iskandar et al., 2019b) (Fig. 13.7).

According to the global gene expression profiles, exposure to MESH Classic Tobacco aerosol impacted processes related to inflammatory response. However,

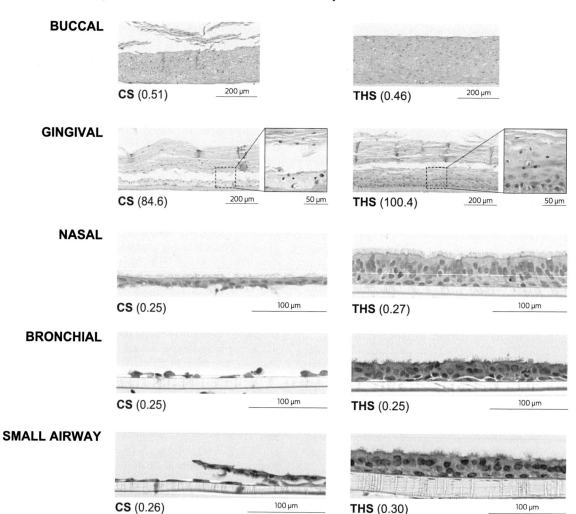

FIG. 13.5 **Postexposure Culture Histological Findings.** Representative images of hematoxylin—eosin- and Alcian blue—stained sections of buccal, nasal, bronchial, and small airway cultures observed at the 72-h time point following exposure and gingival cultures observed at the 24-h time point following exposure. *CS*, cigarette smoke; *THS*, Tobacco Heating System 2.2 aerosol. The number in parentheses reflects the nicotine concentrations (mg/L) in the aerosol or deposited in the exposure chamber. (Adapted from Fig. 3 of Zanetti, F., Sewer, A., Mathis, C., Iskandar, A.R., Kostadinova, R., Schlage, W.K., et al., 2016. Systems toxicology assessment of the biological impact of a candidate modified risk tobacco product on human organotypic oral epithelial cultures. Chem. Res. Toxicol. 29(8), 1252—1269 published under an ACS AuthorChoice License; and from Fig. 2 of Zanetti, F., Titz, B., Sewer, A., Lo Sasso, G., Scotti, E., Schlage, W.K., et al., 2017. Comparative systems toxicology analysis of cigarette smoke and aerosol from a candidate modified risk tobacco product in organotypic human gingival epithelial cultures: a 3-day repeated exposure study. Food Chem. Toxicol. 101, 15—35, Fig. 3 of Iskandar, A.R., Mathis, C., Martin, F., Leroy, P., Sewer, A., Majeed, S., et al., 2017b. 3-D nasal cultures: systems toxicological assessment of a candidate modified-risk tobacco product. ALTEX 34(1), 23—48, Fig. 2 of Iskandar, A.R., Mathis, C., Schlage, W.K., Frentzel, S., Leroy, P., Xiang, Y., et al., 2017c. A systems toxicology approach for comparative assessment: biological impact of an aerosol from a candidate modified-risk tobacco product and cigarette smoke on human organotypic bronchial epithelial cultures. Toxicol. In Vitro 39, 29—51 and Fig. 3 of Iskandar, A.R., Martinez, Y., Martin, F., Schlage, W.K., Leroy, P., Sewer, A., et al., 2017a. Comparative effects of a candidate modified-risk tobacco product Aerosol and cigarette smoke on human organotypic small airway cultures: a systems toxicology approach. Toxicol. Res. (Camb). 6(6), 930—946, published under CC-BY license.)

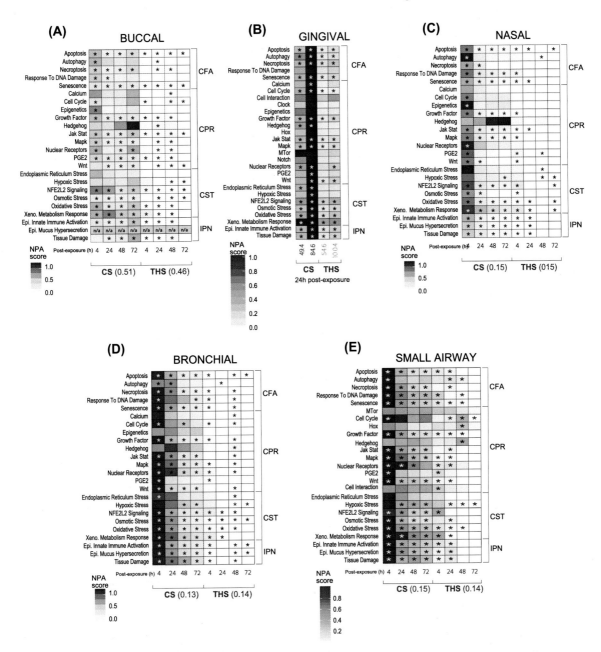

FIG. 13.6 Heatmaps of Network Perturbation Amplitude (NPA) Scores. Impact of CS or THS aerosol exposure on biological network perturbations in (**A**) buccal, (**B**) gingival, (**C**) nasal, (**D**) bronchial, and (**E**) small airway organotypic tissues. *, Statistically significant perturbations. The numbers in parentheses (for buccal, nasal, bronchial and small airway) or colored in red and grey (gingival) indicate nicotine concentrations (in mg/L) in smoke/aerosol or deposited in the exposure chamber. *CFA*, cell fate; *CPR*, cell proliferation; *CS*, cigarette smoke; *CST*, cellular stress; *Epi.*, epithelial; *IPN*, inflammatory process network; *THS*, Tobacco Heating System 2.2; *Xeno.*, xenobiotic. (Adapted from Fig. 7 of Zanetti, F., Sewer, A., Mathis, C., Iskandar, A.R., Kostadinova, R., Schlage, W.K., et al., 2016. Systems toxicology assessment of the biological impact of a candidate modified risk tobacco product on human organotypic oral epithelial cultures. Chem. Res. Toxicol. 29(8), 1252–1269 published under an ACS AuthorChoice License; and from Fig. 3 of Zanetti, F., Titz, B., Sewer,

the impact decreased with postexposure duration, suggesting that the cultures eventually recovered (Fig. 13.8). In addition, the impacts were also much lower than those elicited by CS exposure. The study also demonstrated tissue-specific response. For example, decreased chemokine (C-X-C motif) ligand 1 (CXCL1) and increased IL-1β secretion were detected following CS exposure in buccal epithelial cultures but not in small airway epithelial cultures. In addition, increased secretion of VEGFA (vascular endothelial growth factor A), IL-8, and TIMP-1 (tissue inhibitor of metalloproteinase 1) was observed following CS exposure in small airway epithelial cultures but not in buccal cultures. The secretion of tissue-specific soluble factors was expected; an earlier study reported that this specific response is important for conditioning the local environment against stimuli or pathogens (Hu and Pasare, 2013).

Another study was conducted to understand the potential reduced impact of EVP use in human oral and lung epithelia (Iskandar et al., 2019a) relative to cigarette smoking. In this study, the impact of acute exposure to undiluted EVP aerosols was compared with that of acute exposure to diluted CS at a matching puff number (112 puffs) on human organotypic buccal epithelium and small airway epithelium cultures. The EVP aerosols were generated from prototype e-liquids Test Mix (PG, VG, nicotine, and flavors), Base (PG, VG, and nicotine), and Carrier (PG and VG only) by using EVP devices. Importantly, to avoid overt tissue damage following exposure to 112 puffs, diluted 3R4F CS was applied to the cultures.

The study found significantly lower toxicity (tissue damage and ciliary beating frequency changes) following exposure to undiluted EVP aerosols (Test Mix, Base, and Carrier) than after exposure to diluted 3R4F CS at a matching puff number. In buccal cultures, exposure to Test Mix and Base aerosols did not cause tissue damage, despite resulting in deposited nicotine concentrations nearly double that of 3R4F CS. In small airway cultures, exposure to Test Mix and Base aerosols did not affect tissue integrity or ciliary beating frequency, even at deposited nicotine concentrations 10–20 times that of 3R4F CS.

Furthermore, the study found that exposure to the EVP aerosols caused molecular and cellular changes. Test Mix, Base, and Carrier aerosol exposure elicited changes in gene expression and affected the profiles of secreted inflammatory mediators. However, most alterations were much smaller than those detected following exposure to diluted CS. The data did not reveal meaningful and biologically relevant differences in the overall impacts of the Test Mix, Base, and Carrier aerosols.

The number of puffs and puff duration used in this study (112 puffs, 5-s puffs) were similar to the median puff number and duration (132 puffs/day, 4-s puffs) measured in a group of 135 French EVP users (Dautzenberg and Bricard, 2015). A 5-s puff duration was also used in a previous study (Werley et al., 2016). Therefore, a study conducted with human organotypic cultures exposed to realistic doses of whole CS/ENDP aerosol is more relevant to human exposure than studies that only test e-liquids or EVP fractions (Alqarni et al., 2018; Anderson et al., 2016; Barber et al., 2016; Manna et al., 2018; Putzhammer et al., 2016; Schaal et al., 2018; Schweitzer et al., 2015; Teasdale et al., 2016).

13.4.3 Mechanistic Models for Cardiovascular Effects

Smoking is a major risk factor for the development of cardiovascular disorders (Messner and Bernhard, 2014; The United States Department of Health and Human Services, 2010). However, vascular cells and tissues are not directly exposed to inhaled CS or ENDP aerosol, and, thus, exposure of submersed cultures to AEs of CS or ENDP aerosols can be considered a suitable surrogate of in vivo exposure. Indeed, it has been argued that predominantly GVP constituents, such as carbonyls

A., Lo Sasso, G., Scotti, E., Schlage, W.K., et al., 2017. Comparative systems toxicology analysis of cigarette smoke and aerosol from a candidate modified risk tobacco product in organotypic human gingival epithelial cultures: a 3-day repeated exposure study. Food Chem. Toxicol. 101, 15–35, Fig. 8 of Iskandar, A.R., Mathis, C., Martin, F., Leroy, P., Sewer, A., Majeed, S., et al., 2017b. 3-D nasal cultures: systems toxicological assessment of a candidate modified-risk tobacco product. ALTEX 34(1), 23–48, Fig. 8 of Iskandar, A.R., Mathis, C., Schlage, W.K., Frentzel, S., Leroy, P., Xiang, Y., et al., 2017c. A systems toxicology approach for comparative assessment: biological impact of an aerosol from a candidate modified-risk tobacco product and cigarette smoke on human organotypic bronchial epithelial cultures. Toxicol. In Vitro. 39, 29–51. and Fig. 7 of Iskandar, A.R., Martinez, Y., Martin, F., Schlage, W.K., Leroy, P., Sewer, A., et al., 2017a. Comparative effects of a candidate modified-risk tobacco product Aerosol and cigarette smoke on human organotypic small airway cultures: a systems toxicology approach. Toxicol. Res. (Camb). 6(6), 930–946, published under CC-BY license.)

A Hematoxylin–eosin-stained sections (Buccal epithelial cultures)

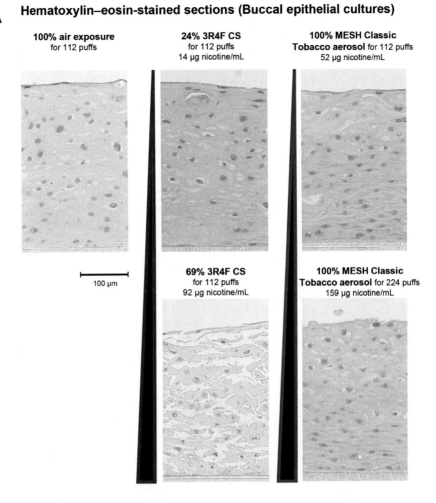

100% air exposure
for 112 puffs

24% 3R4F CS
for 112 puffs
14 µg nicotine/mL

100% MESH Classic
Tobacco aerosol for 112 puffs
52 µg nicotine/mL

100 µm

69% 3R4F CS
for 112 puffs
92 µg nicotine/mL

100% MESH Classic
Tobacco aerosol for 224 puffs
159 µg nicotine/mL

B Hematoxylin–eosin- and Alcian Blue-stained sections (Small airway epithelial cultures)

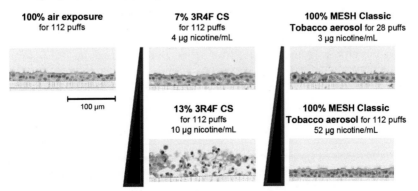

100% air exposure
for 112 puffs

7% 3R4F CS
for 112 puffs
4 µg nicotine/mL

100% MESH Classic
Tobacco aerosol for 28 puffs
3 µg nicotine/mL

100 µm

13% 3R4F CS
for 112 puffs
10 µg nicotine/mL

100% MESH Classic
Tobacco aerosol for 112 puffs
52 µg nicotine/mL

FIG. 13.7 **Histological Findings in Human Buccal and Small Airway Epithelial Cultures Following Acute Exposure to 3R4F CS, MESH Classic Tobacco Aerosol, Base Aerosol or Air.** (A) Representative images of hematoxylin–eosin-stained buccal culture sections and (B) hematoxylin–eosin- and Alcian blue–stained

and peroxynitrite-like oxidants that are trapped in AEs, can increase the permeability of and pass through the alveolar epithelial—endothelial barrier. From there, they enter the systemic circulation via the pulmonary circulation and increase systemic oxidative damage, leading to the development of cigarette smoking—related diseases such as atherosclerosis (Horinouchi et al., 2016; Yamaguchi et al., 2007; Zhang et al., 2010). Over time, smokers accumulate oxidants in blood and develop low-grade inflammation through the increase of circulating molecules such as cytokines and eicosanoids (Libby et al., 2002). In vivo, chronic exposure of the endothelium to low concentrations of inflammatory molecules concomitant with the oxidants present in circulating blood plasma can alter its functions (e.g., vasotone regulation, endothelial permeability, and coagulation) (Favero et al., 2014; Libby, 2002; Yanbaeva et al., 2007). Dysfunctional endothelial cells express surface adhesion molecules that favor the adhesion and subsequent transendothelial migration (TEM) of monocytic cells, eventually leading to the formation of foam cells. This sequence of events (Fig. 13.9) is thought to initiate and accelerate the formation of atherosclerotic plaque, which, over time, continues to grow and can ultimately result in destabilization and disruption, leading to cardiovascular adverse events (Favero et al., 2014; Libby et al., 2002; Messner and Bernhard, 2014; Yanbaeva et al., 2007).

The impact of ENDPs on key processes involved in the initiation of atherosclerosis has been investigated in recently established in vitro models of monocyte-to-endothelial cell adhesion and transmigration and in comparative assessment studies.

13.4.3.1 Adhesion assay

13.4.3.1.1 Model establishment. A systems toxicology approach combined with a functional in vitro adhesion assay was used to investigate the impact of CS in the form of AE on monocyte—endothelial cell adhesion and understand the underlying molecular mechanisms driving this process (Poussin et al., 2014, 2015). The exposure design mimicked to some extent the in vivo situation where both interacting cell types—circulating monocytic cells and endothelial cells

covering the arterial walls—are exposed to polar CS constituents that pass the lung barrier into the blood plasma (Yamaguchi et al., 2007; Zhang et al., 2010). The adhesion assay involved enumerating fluorescently labeled monocytic cells attached to a monolayer of nuclear dye-stained endothelial cells after AE exposure. The study design included both indirect and direct exposure of human umbilical vein endothelial cells or disease-relevant primary coronary arterial endothelial cells to 3R4F CS AE. The designated indirect treatment involved treating endothelial cells with conditioned media (CM) prepared by treating the human monocytic cell line Mono Mac 6 (MM6) with different concentrations of freshly generated 3R4F CS AE. This first mode of exposure was used to understand the combined effects of inflammatory molecules secreted by CS AE-treated monocytic cells and CS oxidants (i.e., stable smoke-derived chemicals) on endothelial cells. This mode of exposure was designed to mimic, in a simple and controlled system, some of the characteristics of smokers' blood and the impact of exposure on endothelial cells. Direct exposure of ECs to different concentrations of 3R4F unconditioned media (UM; generated by using the same protocol as that used to prepare CM, except by excluding MM6 cells) or freshly prepared 3R4F AE was designated direct treatment and fresh direct treatment, respectively. These modes of exposure were intended for investigating the direct effects of stable and unstable smoke-derived chemicals on endothelial cells and for deconvoluting the effects observed with indirect and direct exposures.

Functional (i.e., adhesion assay) and molecular (i.e., transcriptomic) investigations revealed that the 3R4F AE promoted the adhesion of MM6 cells to endothelial cells through distinct direct and indirect concentration-dependent mechanisms. Indirect treatment promoted an inflammatory response in endothelial cells at low concentrations of 3R4F CM. The CM was shown to contain inflammatory mediators, such as TNFα released by TACE (tumor necrosis factor alpha converting enzyme)-dependent shedding, and new transcripts from MM6 cells exposed to freshly prepared 3R4F AE. These inflammatory mediators,

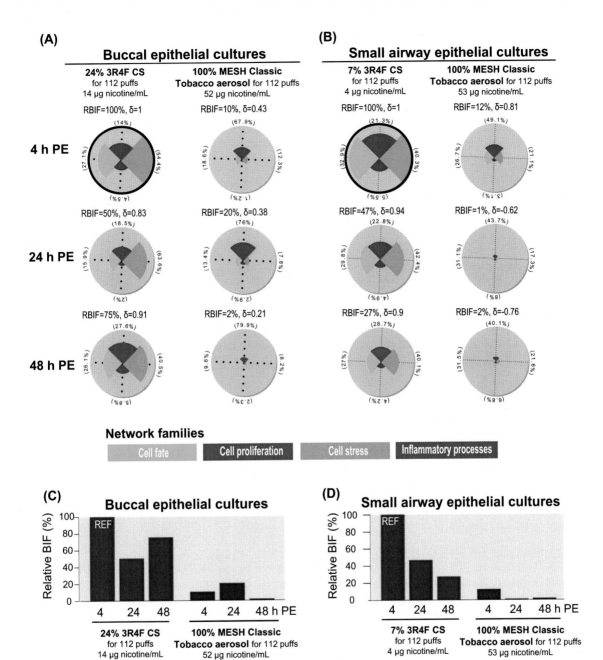

FIG. 13.8 **Causal Network Enrichment Analysis of Transcriptome Profiles.** From the global gene expression changes between test item—exposed and air-exposed control samples, we used a collection of toxicological causal biological network models to deduce the biological impact of an exposure on a given network by using an NPA algorithm. The overall impact, termed BIF, can be deduced, as the BIF takes into account the overall perturbations of all analyzed networks. The perturbations in network families in **(A)** buccal and **(B)** small airway cultures 4, 24, and 48 h following exposure to 3R4F CS or MESH Classic Tobacco aerosol for 112 puffs are shown as pie charts. For a given culture type, the contrast with the highest perturbation is marked with a thick black line (taken as 100% BIF, or the reference REF). The overall BIF for the corresponding PE time points are shown in **(C)** and **(D)** for buccal and small airway cultures, respectively. *BIF,* biological impact factor; *CS,* cigarette smoke; *PE,* postexposure; *RBIF,* relative BIF. (Adapted from Fig. 5 of Iskandar, A.R., Zanetti, F., Marescotti, D., Titz, B., Sewer, A., Kondylis, A., et al., 2019b. Application of a multi-layer systems toxicology framework for in vitro assessment of the biological effects of classic tobacco e-liquid and its corresponding aerosol using an e-cigarette device with MESH technology. Arch. Toxicol. 93(11), 3229—3247, published under CC-BY license.)

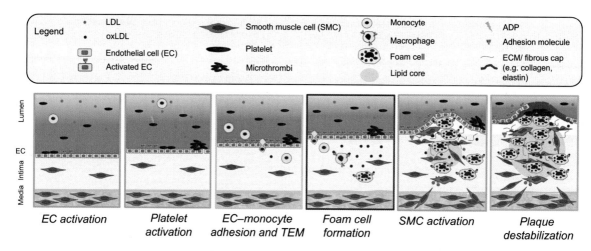

FIG. 13.9 **Key Biological Processes at Play During Atherogenesis.** *EC*, endothelial cell; *ECM*, extracellular matrix; *LDL*, low-density lipoprotein; *SMC*, smooth muscle cell; *TEM*, transendothelial migration.

through a paracrine effect, activated NFκB (nuclear factor kappa-light-chain-enhancer of activated B cells) translocation and increased the expression of adhesion molecules at the transcript and protein levels in endothelial cells, leading to the binding of MM6 cells at the surface of endothelial cells. Stable smoke-derived chemicals present in CM and UM triggered an oxidative stress response in endothelial cells following indirect and direct treatment; however, they were not responsible for the observed adhesion of MM6 cells to endothelial cells at low concentrations of 3R4F CM. Fresh direct treatment of endothelial cells triggered toxicity at high concentrations of 3R4F AE, which led to cell death through necrosis and apoptosis (Poussin et al., 2018). Oxidative stress—induced apoptotic endothelial cells have been previously shown to express at their surface "eat-me" molecules (Szczepanski et al., 2012), recognized by macrophages that engulf apoptotic cells (Kristof et al., 2013). This mechanism may explain the observed increase in MM6—endothelial cell adhesion at high concentrations of 3R4F AE upon fresh direct treatment. The stable and unstable smoke-derived chemicals present in the fresh fraction were responsible for the measured effect. All findings of these mechanistic studies have been discussed in greater detail in previous publications (Poussin et al., 2014, 2015).

13.4.3.1.2 Assessment of THS in the adhesion assay.
A systems toxicology approach combined with a functional in vitro adhesion assay was used to assess the effects of THS aerosol and 3R4F CS on the adhesion of monocytic cells to human coronary artery endothelial cells (HCAEC). HCAECs were treated for 4 h with CM from MM6 cells that had been incubated with low and high concentrations of AEs of THS aerosol and 3R4F CS for 2 h (indirect treatment), UM (direct treatment), or fresh AEs of THS aerosol and 3R4F CS (fresh direct treatment) (Poussin et al., 2016). Functional and molecular investigations revealed that the 3R4F CS AE promoted the adhesion of MM6 cells to HCAECs through distinct direct and indirect concentration-dependent mechanisms. Using the same approach, we found that compared with 3R4F AE, THS aerosol AE had significantly smaller effects on the adhesion of MM6 cells to HCAECs and caused less pronounced molecular changes in endothelial cells and monocytic cells. A THS aerosol AE concentration 10 times higher than the 3R4F AE concentration in fresh direct exposure mode or 20 times higher than the 3R4F AE concentration in indirect exposure mode was required to produce effects similar to those induced by 3R4F AE (Fig. 13.10; Schlage et al., 2020). Our systems toxicology study, using the adhesion of monocytic cells to HCAECs as a surrogate for pathophysiologically relevant events in atherogenesis, showed that an AE of THS aerosol had weaker effects than an AE of 3R4F CS.

The observations were supported by the less pronounced molecular changes triggered by the THS AE relative to 3R4F AE in the ECs and MCs. Effects similar to those measured with 3R4F AE were observed with THS AE only when the concentrations were shifted to 10-fold (direct treatment) and 20-fold (indirect treatment) higher levels.

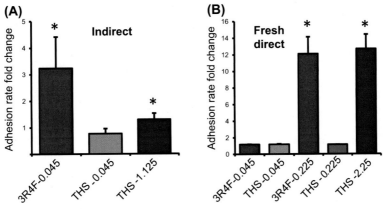

FIG. 13.10 **Cardiovascular Effects In Vitro.** (A) Adhesion of monocytic cells to coronary arterial endothelial cells treated with the CM from monocytes treated with AEs of 3R4F CS or THS aerosol (indirect exposure). (B) Adhesion of monocytic cells to coronary arterial endothelial cells treated with freshly prepared AEs of 3R4F CS and THS aerosol (fresh direct exposure). Data are expressed as the mean ± SEM of at least three independent experiments (*P value < .05). *CM*, conditioned medium; *SEM*, standard error of the mean; *THS*, Tobacco Heating System 2.2; *TNF*, tumor necrosis factor. (Adapted from Fig. 10 of Schlage, W., Titz, B., Iskandar, A., Poussin, C., Van Der Toorn, M., Wong, E.T., et al., 2020. Comparing the preclinical risk profile of inhalable candidate and potential candidate modified risk tobacco products: a bridging use case. Toxicol. Rep. 7, 1187-1206, published under CC-BY license.)

13.4.3.2 Assessment of THS in a chemotaxis and TEM assay

In vitro methods for studying monocyte intra- and extravasation, where monocytic cells cross the endothelial barrier, allow investigation of migratory behavior, which is currently impossible to accomplish in organisms (Muller and Luscinskas, 2008). A functional, real-time in vitro TEM assay was used to investigate the direct effects of exposure to AEs of THS aerosol or 3R4F CS on monocytic cell migration, which allowed us to assess cellular behavior on a minute-to-minute basis. The assay was conducted by using cell invasion/migration (CIM) plates and a real-time cell analyzer dual-plate (RTCA-DP) xCELLigence instrument (Bucher Biotec, Basel, Switzerland).

HCAECs were plated on CIM plates and grown to full confluence, after which a monocytic cell line (THP-1) was seeded on top the HCAEC monolayer. Serum-free medium with or without CXCL12, a chemokine involved in diverse cellular functions including chemotaxis, was added to the bottom chamber of the CIM in independent experiments. The effects of exposure to THS aerosol and 3R4F CS AEs on the migratory behavior of THP-1 cells was monitored in real time by the xCELLigence instrument for up to 4 h (van der Toorn et al., 2015). The results show that the inhibitory effects of THS aerosol AE on TEM were ~18 times less than the inhibitory effects of the 3R4F smoke AE (Fig. 13.11; Schlage et al., 2020).

Next, we tested the integrity of the HCAEC monolayer against exposure to THS aerosol and 3R4F CS AEs using

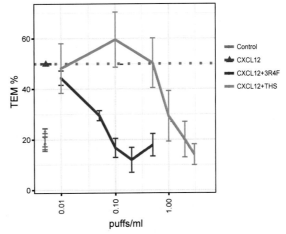

FIG. 13.11 **Effects of AEs of 3R4F CS and THS Aerosol on Real-Time Impedance-Based Transendothelial Migration.** Real-time impedance-based TEM of THP-1 cells migrating across a layer of human coronary artery endothelial cells when exposed to increasing concentrations of AEs of 3R4F CS or THS aerosol in cell invasion/migration chambers. The CXCL12 concentration that induced 50% migration was used in these assays. Data are expressed as the mean ± SEM of at least three independent experiments (*P value < .05). *CXCL12*, C-X-C motif chemokine 12; *SEM*, standard error of the mean; *TEM*, transendothelial migration; *THS*, Tobacco Heating System 2.2. (Adapted from Fig. 10 of Schlage, W., Titz, B., Iskandar, A., Poussin, C., Van Der Toorn, M., Wong, E.T., et al., 2020. Comparing the preclinical risk profile of inhalable candidate and potential candidate modified risk tobacco products: a bridging use case. Toxicol. Rep. 7, 1187-1206, published under CC-BY license.)

the RTCA xCELLigence instrument and E-plates. An E-plate is a cell culture plate covered with a gold microelectrode network, which generates an impedance signal upon cell adhesion. Changes in cell index (impedance) were recorded and measured in real time during cell growth. HCAECs seeded in E-plates were grown to full confluence, stimulated with various concentrations of freshly prepared AEs, and monitored for 4 h. The results showed that treatment of a confluent monolayer of HCAECs with AEs of 3R4F CS and THS aerosol caused a decrease in electrical impedance in a concentration-dependent manner, suggesting disruption of intercellular junctions in the HCAEC monolayer. The AE of 3R4F CS was more potent than that of THS aerosol in reducing the impedance. The concentrations of THS aerosol AE required to affect HCAEC adhesion were at least an order of magnitude higher than those of 3R4F CS AE required to induce the same effect.

Finally, cytotoxic and inflammatory responses to the AEs of 3R4F CS and THS aerosol were tested. THP-1 cells were stimulated for 18 h with various concentrations of freshly prepared AEs, and the effects of exposure were assessed by flow cytometry and ELISA. The results showed that the AEs induced concentration-dependent cytotoxic and inflammatory effects. The effects of 3R4F CS AE were more than one order of magnitude stronger than those of the THS aerosol AE on all examined endpoints. The data indicated that the aerosol of THS posed a lower risk of CVD than 3R4F smoke (van der Toorn et al., 2015).

13.4.4 Assessment of THS in a Cell Transformation Assay

Many cellular and molecular processes of carcinogenesis can be modeled adequately in cell culture systems. An in vitro model was established which mimicked the chronic exposure of smokers' airways to CS. This model involved continuous exposure of the human bronchial epithelial cell line BEAS-2B (LGC Standards GmbH, Wesel, Germany) to TPM from 3R4F CS or THS aerosol for 12 weeks (van der Toorn et al., 2018). TPM was used as the test item to investigate the effects of the mixture of cancer-causing chemicals present in CS and to compare these effects with those of the TPM from THS aerosol. To gain a better mechanistic understanding of the stepwise transformation of immortalized but phenotypically benign airway epithelial cells to full malignancy, several endpoints including proliferation, DNA damage, oxidative stress, epithelial—mesenchymal transition (EMT), and wound repair were assessed.

Furthermore, a systems toxicology approach was used to gain deeper mechanistic insights. The in vitro cell transformation assay (CTA)—which closely mimics the in vivo conversion of normal cells into a transformed phenotype that is characteristic of tumorigenic cells—was performed at the end of the exposure period. Transformed cells show reduced requirements for extracellular growth–promoting factors, and their proliferation is anchorage-independent (growth in soft agar), while normal cells require extracellular growth factors and cell—substratum contact. Cells that formed colonies in the CTA were collected for assessment of cell invasion, a process commonly observed in cancer metastasis.

In this study (van der Toorn et al., 2018), the cells showed increased oxidative stress and DNA damage within the first 2 weeks of 3R4F TPM treatment; but these effects subsided thereafter, indicating adaptation. 3R4F TPM treatment for 4 weeks resulted in crisis and EMT (loss of cell—cell contact and E-cadherin expression and de novo vimentin expression). By week 8, the cells had regained E-cadherin expression, suggesting that the EMT was reversible. Increased MMP levels and wound repair were noted in 3R4F TPM-treated cells at week 12. However, these changes were not observed following prolonged treatment of BEAS-2B cells with the same or a 5-fold higher concentration of THS TPM, although a 20-fold higher concentration of THS TPM also led to increased oxidative burden and DNA damage and caused reversible EMT. In addition, cellular transformation was observed in 3R4F TPM-treated BEAS-2B cells and in cells treated with a 20-fold higher concentration of THS TPM. 3R4F TPM-derived clones were invasive, while THS TPM-derived (all concentrations) clones were not. Systems toxicological analysis indicated an overall smaller biological impact of THS compared with 3R4F TPM, confirming a differential effect of the TPM fractions of the EHTP and reference cigarette. These experiments show that repeated exposure of bronchial epithelial cells to CS TPM induces progressive alterations in gene expression as well as phenotypic changes related to tumorigenesis.

13.4.5 Microphysiological Systems

The 3R principles (replacement, reduction, and refinement) encourage the scientific community to develop more physiologically relevant models that recapitulate the cell composition, geometry, and physiological complexity of tissues/organs (Burden et al., 2015). The emergence of a wide range of engineered microfluidic systems and techniques enabling cell culture under flow and in three dimensions has advanced the innovation of in vitro perfusable models (Marx et al., 2016, 2020).

Following these principles, we developed an endothelial microvessel-on-a-chip model by using a microfluidic platform technology with the 96-chip OrganoPlate (Mimetas BV, Leiden, NL). The assay allows measurement of the adhesion of monocytic cells to the lumen of perfused microvessels and provides insights into molecular changes through high-content imaging and gene expression analyses. We performed a comparative assessment of THS aerosol and 3R4F CS (administered as CM) on the adhesion of MM6 cells to HCAEC microvessels, which mimics a key event in atherogenesis (Poussin et al., 2020). To investigate oxidative status in the microenvironment, GSH content was also measured after the exposure. Our results showed that THS aerosol-CM had a reduced effect on monocyte—endothelium adhesion relative to 3R4F smoke-CM. Given the biological robustness of the model and its ease of implementation, the microvessel-on-a-chip model provides perspectives for vascular disease research and drug discovery.

In the context of inhalation toxicology, the lung tissue can partially metabolize certain compounds, thus generating new metabolites that will reach the blood circulation together with unmetabolized compounds. These will finally reach the liver, where the major metabolic transformation of xenobiotic compounds occurs. To study such phenomena, different groups have developed various multi-organ-on-a-chip (MOC) models, combining several organs on a single system (chip) (Lee and Sung, 2017; Marx et al., 2016; Materne et al., 2015). These platforms generally connect one (or more) organ(s) with, in most cases, a liver organ or "compartment," which acts as the primary organ for compound metabolization (Choe et al., 2017; Maschmeyer et al., 2015; Oleaga et al., 2016).

To better evaluate the potential toxicity of inhaled aerosols, we have recently developed a system connecting a human organotypic bronchial epithelium model with liver spheroid cultures to produce a lung/liver-on-a-chip platform (Bovard et al., 2018). This technology consists of a plate that allows joint cultivation of representative in vitro models of various human organs. Through a pump incorporated in the model, the culture medium can circulate among the different tissue models/compartments, allowing cross-talk (Fig. 13.12).

Using this platform, we have demonstrated that the functionality, morphology, and viability of human organotypic bronchial epithelium cultures and 3D liver spheroids can be maintained over 28 days (Bovard et al., 2018). The capacity of the liver spheroids to metabolize the compounds present in the medium and modulate their toxicity was proven by using aflatoxin B1. The toxicity of aflatoxin B1 in the organotypic bronchial cultures decreased when the liver spheroids were present in the same chip circuit, proving that liver-mediated detoxification was protecting/decreasing because of aflatoxin B1—mediated cytotoxicity. This lung/liver-on-a-chip platform offers new opportunities to study the toxicity of inhaled aerosols or demonstrate the safety and efficacy of new drug candidates targeting the human lungs.

The interconnected microphysiological platform will be used to support the safety testing of aerosols from ENDS and will potentially provide a framework for efficacy and safety assessments of pharmaceuticals and neutraceuticals. These advancements will substantiate nonanimal approaches in accordance with the 3R principles, in line with many international efforts (3R, ICH, ECVAM) to reduce animal experimentation in the future.

13.5 INDEPENDENT PEER REVIEW AND TRANSPARENCY OF IN VITRO TOXICOLOGICAL ASSESSMENT STUDIES

The evidence supporting the risk reduction potential of ENDPs should be reviewed by independent experts who are experienced in the methodologies that were used. Importantly, and especially in the area of ENDP assessment, these experts should have no vested interest in the outcome of the review. Such a review would increase confidence in the conclusions derived from the available evidence.

We invited a two-tier, independent scientific peer review of the methods, data, and results from the toxicological and exposure assessment studies on the EHTP THS, which included chemical analyses of aerosol composition and in vitro and in vivo toxicological studies as well as clinical studies. The overall principles, scope, and procedure of the peer-review process are outlined in Chapter 3, and the complete peer-review methodology and results have been published (Boue et al., 2019).

The in vitro toxicological studies on THS included in the peer-review package were the

1. Ames, NRU, and mouse lymphoma assays (Schaller et al., 2016; Section 13.3.2),
2. TEM assay (van der Toorn et al., 2015; Section 13.4.3.2),
3. monocyte—endothelial cell adhesion assay (Poussin et al., 2016; Section 13.5.3.1.2),
4. assessment of THS aerosol in organotypic tissue cultures of the oral, nasal and bronchial epithelium

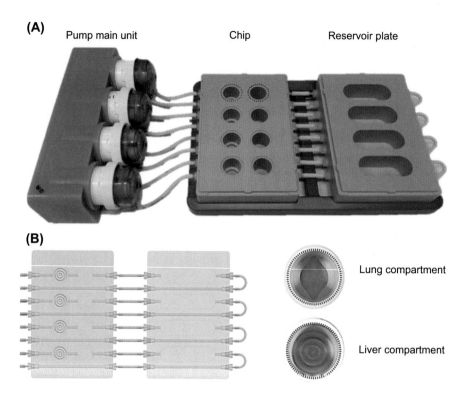

FIG. 13.12 **The Lung/Liver-on-a-Chip Platform.** (**A**) A photograph of the chip system, comprising the pump main unit with four pump heads, the PEEK chip, and the reservoir plate. (**B**) A schematic view of the chip, comprising four circuits; each circuit includes two compartments, one each for housing the lung and liver tissues. The cross-section schemas of the plates show the path of the tubes and channels and the relative depth of each well. (**C**) A close-up view of the two compartments, showing the groove pattern on the bottom of the wells. *PEEK*, polyetheretherketone. (Adapted from Fig. 1 of Bovard, D., Sandoz, A., Luettich, K., Frentzel, S., Iskandar, A., Marescotti, D., et al., 2018. A lung/liver-on-a-chip platform for acute and chronic toxicity studies. Lab Chip. 18(24), 3814–3829, published under CC-BY license.)

(Iskandar et al., 2017b; Zanetti et al., 2017; Section 13.4.1.2).

Briefly, for the first-tier review, five panels of 5 to 12 independent, anonymous scientific experts were provided the data package on an online platform and asked to answer a questionnaire of 30 items addressing the study design, methods used, results obtained, and interpretation of the results. This was followed by a second tier of review by two panels of nine experts each, who were asked to reach overarching conclusions on the data package as a whole and on the peer-review process itself. Answers had to be given on a Likert scale, with the options ranging from "not confident at all" or "not convincing" to "very confident" or "very convincing." The whole process was double-blinded (PMI, as the sponsor, and the experts were anonymized to each other).

Tier 1 reviewers rated the choice of models and study designs positively, which was judged to be convincing or moderately convincing by tier 2 reviewers. All tier 2 reviewers were confident that state-of-the-art methods had been used. Regarding the added value of the systems toxicology approaches, the answers ranged from "not at all confident" to "very confident" (one reviewer each), with the majority being "confident" or "moderately confident." Furthermore, the reviewers had the opportunity to add free-text comments, which led to a number of recommendations, with extending the study durations, using multiple doses, using alternative exposure modes, and conducting comparative studies by using additional human cell lines being among the most frequently mentioned. These recommendations were mainly driven by scientific interests and have been partly addressed by further research conducted at PMI.

Furthermore, our assessment studies aim to provide robust evidence that THS is less harmful than cigarettes. Overall, the results of the peer review were supportive of the study design, results, and interpretation of the results. While 65% percent of the reviewers were "convinced" or "very convinced" by the evidence that switching to THS had comparable effects to smoking cessation, 53% of them judged the evidence that THS was likely to have the potential for reduced risk relative to conventional cigarettes to be "convincing" or "very convincing."

13.6 ADVANTAGES AND CHALLENGES OF TOXICOLOGICAL ASSESSMENT IN VITRO

13.6.1 Advantages

The advantage in testing ENDPs by using in vitro regulatory toxicology assays is the availability of guidance documents, which help ensure that such methods are well designed, robust, validated, and reliable for human safety assessment. In a tiered approach, results from such regulatory toxicology assays determine whether further testing, including in vivo and clinical studies are required.

Unlike assays implemented for regulatory use, systems toxicology–based assays mostly rely on in vitro models that aim to mimic the human physiology. Therefore, these assays are also useful for studying the underlying mechanisms of toxicity. For example, our group has developed various mechanistic disease assays and used systems toxicology–based approaches to understand CS/ENDP aerosols-induced perturbations. With such investigations, it is possible to identify novel ENDP-related effects that might not be detectable by using the classic cell-based assays traditionally used for CS assessment.

The use of human cells and 3D reconstructed tissues/vessels is not only in line with the 3R principles but also facilitates extrapolation of mechanistic findings from the in vitro to the human situation. The European Union Reference Laboratory for alternatives to animal testing (EURL ECVAM) indeed refers to mechanistically driven toxicology as an optimal way to inform chemical hazard assessment by using data from alternative methods (Zuang and Dura, 2019). In combination with computational modeling, systems toxicology–based assays can further facilitate extrapolation from in vitro to in vivo disease mechanisms, species-to-species translation, and identification of relevant biomarkers for clinical studies (Hoeng et al., 2014a,b; Sauer et al., 2016).

13.6.2 Challenges
13.6.2.1 Regulatory acceptance and validation
Models and test systems for toxicity testing have been continuously evolving. Regulatory agencies have gradually started accepting data generated by using novel in vitro assays. The 3R principles have become a part of the regulations in Europe (Commission Regulation, 2015/282, 2015; Directive, 2010/63/EU, 2010; Regulation, 1907/2006, 2006); however, the full transition from animal to nonanimal alternative procedures depends on method validation, which lies at the interface of method development and regulatory acceptance (Burden et al., 2015; NACD, 2016). The EURL ECVAM in the EU and ICCVAM in the US have developed clear roadmaps for effective validation of alternative methods (Vinken, 2020), and it is foreseeable that toxicological evaluation of ENDPs may not require any in vivo testing in the future.

One major challenge for regulatory acceptance of alternative methods and mechanistic assays is the lack of reporting guidelines. However, efforts are ongoing to harmonize the evaluation and reporting of such data (Krebs et al., 2019).

13.6.2.2 Long-term versus short-term exposure
Among the current challenges for long-term cell culture exposure is the fact that many 2D cell cultures have limited long-term stability (i.e., they need to be kept in a proliferative, nonconfluent state), primary cells have limited passage numbers, and many ALI exposure systems are not sterile, which increases the risk of contamination of tissue cultures. Hence, in vitro assays are typically limited to assessing the effects of a single or repeated exposure within 24 h. Although such experimental procedures can reveal acute toxicity effects, they are not optimal for assessing the pathophysiological changes that occur slowly, such as those potentially associated with long-term exposure to ENDP aerosols (exposure to ENDP aerosols in humans is usually chronic).

Furthermore, despite the difficulty in maintaining the sterility of organotypic cultures, our group successfully performed a 3-day repeated ALI exposure study using organotypic oral epithelium cultures (Zanetti et al., 2017). Alternatively, aerosol fractions could be applied onto the apical surface of such cultures. Finally, even though exposure at the ALI better mimics the actual exposure in human smokers, long-term basolateral treatment of ALI cultures has been demonstrated. For example, Ito and collaborators successfully applied CS AE to the basolateral medium of organotypic bronchial cultures over a 4-week period (Ito et al., 2018).

13.6.2.3 The tradeoff between model complexity and high throughput

Although simplicity is generally considered to be a shortcoming of in vitro models, the simpler the model the better the control. Therefore, the use of a simple model can improve the reproducibility of the results. For example, in vitro assays, such as the NRU assay and RTCA, are simple and well defined and can, therefore, be conducted in a large-scale/high-throughput mode. Furthermore, upscaling is easier to implement when the endpoints can be automated (i.e., do not require extensive human intervention), such as microscopic cell counting.

A higher level of complexity is inherent to assays in which two or more cell types are used (e.g., for studying monocyte—endothelial cell adhesion, assessing monocyte chemotaxis, and investigating invasion). Similarly, RNA and protein detection by microscopy image analysis (e.g., in HCS assays) generally has low throughput.

Direct aerosol exposure to organotypic cultures grown at the ALI requires a sophisticated apparatus. Exposure doses are more difficult to control in these systems than in submerged 2D cell cultures, where the test substance/mixture is simply added to the culture medium. Additionally, the cellular composition of organotypic cultures is heterogeneous—generally comprising several cell types—and may vary between culture inserts. Moreover, many endpoints in organotypic cultures cannot be measured simultaneously in multiple inserts, which necessitates labor-intensive studies (e.g., cultures must be handled one-by-one during RNA isolation and histological processing). Recently, some HCS endpoints previously established for 2D monolayer cultures have been successfully adapted for organotypic bronchial epithelium cultures. Such improvement will gradually increase the versatility of these models (Marescotti et al., 2020a).

Lab-on-a-chip and MOC technologies are designed to address some of the shortcomings of classical in vitro systems and eventually lead to replacement of animal studies. These technologies allow, for example, assessment of cell—cell interactions (cell adhesion assay under flow conditions), differentiation processes (endothelial tube formation), and complex endpoints (immunohistochemistry findings and RNA and protein expression) and can be developed for medium to high throughput. They, however, have their own challenges, including identification of tissue culture media that are compatible with all cells in the system, standardization, and automation (Bovard et al., 2018; Poussin et al., 2020).

13.6.2.4 Single versus multiple cell donors

Response to exposure at a population level cannot be easily replicated in vitro, because cells from a single donor do not represent an entire population. Different primary cells can be obtained from numerous donors; however, it is currently not feasible to obtain a sufficient number of donors who can reflect the diversity of the population. Therefore, studying the impact of the sex, age, smoking status, and disease status of the donors on the response of the cultures to stimuli is not straightforward. These limitations also apply to any cell line that has been derived from the cells of a single donor and has been cloned often and, thereby, represents the progeny of a single cell from a single donor. A recent study reported that differences in individual donors' genetic background and experimental variability contribute to the variation in induced pluripotent stem cell models. They can impact the differentiation potency, cellular heterogeneity, morphology, and transcript and protein abundance (Volpato and Webber, 2020).

Nonetheless, efforts have been initiated to address multidonor diversity. Various publications have discussed approaches for obtaining various human tissue/cell sources and the methods of isolation that are currently available for researchers (Ashok et al., 2020; Geurts et al., 2020; Hayden, 2020; Schutgens and Clevers, 2020). In addition, a small number of commercially available models have been developed by including several donors; examples include DonorPlex hepatocytes (Lonza Walkersville, Inc., Walkersville, MD, USA), 3D InSight Human Liver Microtissues (InSphero AG, Schlieren, Switzerland), and the MucilAir nasal epithelium models (Epithelix Sarl, Geneva, Switzerland) that are generated from a pool of primary nasal epithelial cells from multiple donors. Therefore, it can be expected that more sophisticated cellular models will become available that might reflect the diversity of the responses attributed to population diversity.

13.6.2.5 Reproducibility

The use of primary cells from a single donor is particularly preferable for development of organotypic cultures; but, it is often debated as being a major limitation, because the results may not be generalizable to other donors. This challenge has also been highlighted for cloned cell lines. Moreover, the prospect of using cultures from several donors—although possible in assays using primary cultures—has limited possibility, or is even impossible, if a specific cloned cell line is needed in a particular assay. Nonetheless, the results from in vitro experiments are specific and correct for the particular cell type and conditions used. Therefore, they are useful for deducing certain mechanisms. Finally, systems toxicology approaches may offer an opportunity to predict the response in the population from in vitro data on the basis of common patterns of response (Mathis et al., 2013; Schlage et al., 2014).

Moreover, considering the complexity of organotypic cultures, most studies using such cultures have been conducted with a limited number of replicates. This increases intra-assay variability, which might eventually compromise assay reproducibility. The reproducibility of the key findings obtained in three human organotypic cultures of the aerodigestive tract (buccal, bronchial, and nasal epithelia) exposed to CS or EHTP aerosols over approximately 2 years has been investigated in a metaanalysis (Iskandar et al., 2017d). This metaanalysis showed that the mechanistic impact of CS and THS aerosols across the three cultures was similar.

Cytotoxicity results (mainly IC_{50} values) obtained in various cell lines have shown good reproducibility not only in testing cosmetics ingredients (Barker-Treasure et al., 2015) but also in assays that used CHO cells to assess the toxicity of CS or an aerosol of carbon heated tobacco products (Fields et al., 2017). In-house investigations on the reproducibility of these assays have demonstrated variation coefficients in the range of 10%–20% for the MLA (Schramke et al., 2006), less than 10% for the Ames assay (strain TA98) (Roemer et al., 1998), less than 10% for the NRU assay with CS TPM, and 20% for the NRU assay with CS GVP (Tewes et al., 2003).

These examples demonstrate that quantitatively reproducible results (from simple, standardized in vitro assays) and qualitatively reproducible results (from complex tissue culture systems with functional and systems toxicological endpoints) should ideally complement each other.

13.7 CONCLUSIONS

The desire to move away from animal testing has been the impetus for developing advanced in vitro models, although findings from in vitro studies may not be interpreted in, or extrapolated to, the in vivo context in a straightforward manner. Thus, relevant biological test systems are needed to facilitate accurate identification of biomarkers of exposure, response, and disease. Advanced test methods that rely on systems biology/ toxicology endpoints paired with quantitative network modeling enable identification of the biological networks perturbed by CS and ENDP aerosol exposure.

These emerging methodologies and transparency protocols presented here will lead to significant improvements in the 21st century risk assessment of complex mixtures and ENDPs.

In this chapter, we have summarized the results from in vitro regulatory toxicology assays and systems toxicology–based approaches. The results collectively demonstrate that ENDP aerosols have a considerably reduced biological impact relative to an equivalent CS exposure. It was possible to induce toxic effects with ENDP aerosols, but only when they were tested at significantly higher exposure concentrations than CS. These conclusions, in particular for THS, were judged to be robust by independent scientific experts through an advanced, tiered peer-review process.

REFERENCES
Albert, R.E., 1983. Comparative carcinogenic potencies of particulates from diesel engine exhausts, coke oven emissions, roofing tar aerosols and cigarette smoke. Environ. Health Perspect. 47, 339–341.

Alqarni, A., Brand, O., Pasini, A., Alshehri, M., Pang, L., 2018. Effect of e-cigarette vapour extraction on vasoactive gene expression in human pulmonary artery smooth muscle and endothelial cells. Eur. Respir. J. 52 (Suppl. 62), PA3110. https://doi.org/10.1183/13993003.congress-2018.PA3110.

Anderson, C., Majeste, A., Hanus, J., Wang, S., 2016. E-cigarette aerosol exposure induces reactive oxygen species, DNA damage, and cell death in vascular endothelial cells. Toxicol. Sci. 154 (2), 332–340.

Andreoli, C., Gigante, D., Nunziata, A., 2003. A review of in vitro methods to assess the biological activity of tobacco smoke with the aim of reducing the toxicity of smoke. Toxicol. In Vitro 17 (5–6), 587–594.

Applegate, M., Moore, M., Broder, C., Burrell, A., Juhn, G., Kasweck, K., et al., 1990. Molecular dissection of mutations at the heterozygous thymidine kinase locus in mouse lymphoma cells. Proc. Natl. Acad. Sci. U. S. A. 87 (1), 51–55.

Ashok, A., Choudhury, D., Fang, Y., Hunziker, W., 2020. Towards manufacturing of human organoids. Biotechnol. Adv. 39, 107460.

Bals, R., Boyd, J., Esposito, S., Foronjy, R., Hiemstra, P.S., Jimenez-Ruiz, C.A., et al., 2019. Electronic cigarettes: a task force report from the European Respiratory Society. Eur. Respir. J. 53 (2), 1801151.

Barber, K.E., Yin, W., Rubenstein, D.A., 2016. Electronic cigarette extracts alter endothelial cell inflammatory responses. FASEB J. 30 (Suppl. 1), 722–7288.

Barker-Treasure, C., Coll, K., Belot, N., Longmore, C., Bygrave, K., Avey, S., et al., 2015. Non-animal replacements for acute toxicity testing. Altern. Lab. Anim. 43 (3), 199–203.

Benigni, R., 2012. Alternatives to the carcinogenicity bioassay for toxicity prediction: are we there yet? Expet Opin. Drug Metabol. Toxicol. 8 (4), 407–417.

Benowitz, N.L., Kuyt, F., Jacob 3rd, P., Jones, R.T., Osman, A.L., 1983. Cotinine disposition and effects. Clin. Pharmacol. Ther. 34 (5), 604–611.

Boué, S., Goedertier, D., Hoeng, J., Kuczaj, A., Majeed, S., Mathis, C., et al., 2020. State-of-the-art methods and devices for the generation, exposure, and collection of aerosols from heat-not-burn tobacco products. Toxicol. Res. & Appl. 4, 2397847319897869.

Boue, S., Schlage, W.K., Page, D., Hoeng, J., Peitsch, M.C., 2019. Toxicological assessment of tobacco heating system 2.2: findings from an independent peer review. Regul. Toxicol. Pharmacol. 104, 115–127.

Bovard, D., Sandoz, A., Luettich, K., Frentzel, S., Iskandar, A., Marescotti, D., et al., 2018. A lung/liver-on-a-chip platform for acute and chronic toxicity studies. Lab Chip 18 (24), 3814–3829.

Bryce, S.M., Bemis, J.C., Avlasevich, S.L., Dertinger, S.D., 2007. In vitro micronucleus assay scored by flow cytometry provides a comprehensive evaluation of cytogenetic damage and cytotoxicity. Mutat. Res. 630 (1–2), 78–91.

Burden, N., Chapman, K., Sewell, F., Robinson, V., 2015. Pioneering better science through the 3Rs: an introduction to the national centre for the replacement, refinement, and reduction of animals in research (NC3Rs). J. Am. Assoc. Lab. Anim. Sci. 54 (2), 198–208.

Chen, T., Harrington-Brock, K., Moore, M.M., 2002. Mutant frequencies and loss of heterozygosity induced by N-ethyl-N-nitrosourea in the thymidine kinase gene of L5178Y/Tk$^{+/-}$ −3.7.2C mouse lymphoma cells. Mutagenesis 17 (2), 105–109.

Choe, A., Ha, S.K., Choi, I., Choi, N., Sung, J.H., 2017. Microfluidic gut-liver chip for reproducing the first pass metabolism. Biomed. Microdevices 19 (1), 4.

Cimino, M.C., 2006. Comparative overview of current international strategies and guidelines for genetic toxicology testing for regulatory purposes. Environ. Mol. Mutagen. 47 (5), 362–390.

Clements, J., 2000. The mouse lymphoma assay. Mutat. Res. 455 (1–2), 97–110.

Clive, D., Johnson, K., Spector, J., Batson, A., Brown, M., 1979. Validation and characterization of the L5178Y/TK$^{+/-}$ mouse lymphoma mutagen assay system. Mutat. Res. Fund Mol. Mech. Mutagen 59 (1), 61–108.

Combes, R., Scott, K., Dillon, D., Meredith, C., Mcadam, K., Proctor, C., 2012. The effect of a novel tobacco process on the in vitro cytotoxicity and genotoxicity of cigarette smoke particulate matter. Toxicol. In Vitro 26 (6), 1022–1029.

Commission Regulation 283/2013, 3.4.2013. Commission regulation (EU) No. 283/2013 of 1 March 2013 setting out the data requirements for active substances, in accordance with regulation (EC) No 1107/2009 of the European parliament and of the council concerning the placing of plant protection products on the market L93. OJEU 1–84.

Commission Regulation 2015/282, 21.02.2015. Commission regulation (EU) 2015/282 of 20 February 2015 amending annexes VIII, IX and X to regulation (EC) No 1907/2006. L50 Off. J. Eur. Union 1–6.

Cooperation Centre for Scientific Research Relative to Tobacco, 2007. In Vitro Toxicology Task Force. Report on interlaboratory study of the in vitro toxicity of particulate matter of four cigarettes. Available at: https://www.coresta.org/sites/default/files/technical_documents/main/IVT_TF_Report_Particulate_Matter_Tox.pdf (Accessed 19 May 2020).

Cudazzo, G., Smart, D.J., Mchugh, D., Vanscheeuwijck, P., 2019. Lysosomotropic-related limitations of the BALB/c 3T3 cell-based neutral red uptake assay and an alternative testing approach for assessing e-liquid cytotoxicity. Toxicol. Vitro 61, 104647.

Dautzenberg, B., Bricard, D., 2015. Real-time characterization of e-cigarettes use: the 1 million puffs study. J. Addiction Res. Ther. 6, 4172.

Dey, N., Das, A., Ghosh, A., Chatterjee, I.B., 2010. Activated charcoal filter effectively reduces p-benzosemiquinone from the mainstream cigarette smoke and prevents emphysema. J. Biosci. 35 (2), 217–230.

Directive 2010/63/Eu, 20.10.2010. Directive 2010/63/eu of the European Parliament and of the council of 22 September 2010 on the protection of animals used for scientific purposes. L276 Off. J. Eur. Union 33–79.

Dybing, E., Sanner, T., Roelfzema, H., Kroese, D., Tennant, R.W., 1997. T25: a simplified carcinogenic potency index: description of the system and study of correlations between carcinogenic potency and species/site specificity and mutagenicity. Pharmacol. Toxicol. 80 (6), 272–279.

Eastmond, D.A., Hartwig, A., Anderson, D., Anwar, W.A., Cimino, M.C., Dobrev, I., et al., 2009. Mutagenicity testing for chemical risk assessment: update of the WHO/IPCS Harmonized Scheme. Mutagenesis 24 (4), 341–349.

Favero, G., Paganelli, C., Buffoli, B., Rodella, L.F., Rezzani, R., 2014. Endothelium and its alterations in cardiovascular diseases: life style intervention. BioMed Res. Int. 2014, 801896.

Fields, W., Fowler, K., Hargreaves, V., Reeve, L., Bombick, B., 2017. Development, qualification, validation and application of the neutral red uptake assay in Chinese Hamster Ovary (CHO) cells using a VITROCELL® VC10® smoke exposure system. Toxicol. In Vitro 40, 144–152.

Geurts, M.H., De Poel, E., Amatngalim, G.D., Oka, R., Meijers, F.M., Kruisselbrink, E., et al., 2020. CRISPR-based adenine editors correct nonsense mutations in a cystic fibrosis organoid biobank. Cell Stem Cell 26, 503–510.e7.

González-Suárez, I., Marescotti, D., Martin, F., Scotti, E., Guedj, E., Acali, S., et al., 2017. In vitro systems toxicology assessment of nonflavored e-cigarette liquids in primary lung epithelial cells. Appl. In Vitro Toxicol. 3, 41–55.

Gonzalez-Suarez, I., Martin, F., Marescotti, D., Guedj, E., Acali, S., Johne, S., et al., 2016. In vitro systems toxicology assessment of a candidate modified risk tobacco product shows reduced toxicity compared to that of a conventional cigarette. Chem. Res. Toxicol. 29 (1), 3–18.

Gonzalez-Suarez, I., Sewer, A., Walker, P., Mathis, C., Ellis, S., Woodhouse, H., et al., 2014. Systems biology approach for evaluating the biological impact of environmental toxicants in vitro. Chem. Res. Toxicol. 27 (3), 367–376.

Guengerich, F.P., 2000. Metabolism of chemical carcinogens. Carcinogenesis 21 (3), 345–351.

Guo, X., Heflich, R.H., Dial, S.L., Richter, P.A., Moore, M.M., Mei, N., 2016. Quantitative analysis of the relative mutagenicity of five chemical constituents of tobacco smoke in the mouse lymphoma assay. Mutagenesis 31 (3), 287–296.

Guo, X., Verkler, T.L., Chen, Y., Richter, P.A., Polzin, G.M., Moore, M.M., et al., 2011. Mutagenicity of 11 cigarette smoke condensates in two versions of the mouse lymphoma assay. Mutagenesis 26 (2), 273–281.

Hartung, T., 2010. Lessons learned from alternative methods and their validation for a new toxicology in the 21st century. J. Toxicol. Environ. Health B Crit. Rev. 13 (2–4), 277–290.

Haswell, L.E., Corke, S., Verrastro, I., Baxter, A., Banerjee, A., Adamson, J., et al., 2018. In vitro RNA-seq-based toxicogenomics assessment shows reduced biological effect of tobacco heating products when compared to cigarette smoke. Sci. Rep. 8 (1), 1145.

Hayden, P.J., 2020. Cell sources and methods for producing organotypic in vitro human tissue models. In: Organ-on-a-Chip. Elsevier, pp. 13–45.

Health Canada, January 30, 2004. Health Canada (HC) Official Method T-502. Neutral Red Uptake Assay for Mainstream Tobacco Smoke. Department of Health dated.

Hoeng, J., Deehan, R., Pratt, D., Martin, F., Sewer, A., Thomson, T.M., et al., 2012. A network-based approach to quantifying the impact of biologically active substances. Drug Discov. Today 17 (9–10), 413–418.

Hoeng, J., Talikka, M., Martin, F., Ansari, S., Drubin, D., Elamin, A., et al., 2014a. Toxicopanomics: Applications of Genomics, Transcriptomics, Proteomics, and Lipidomics in Predictive Mechanistic Toxicology, pp. 295–332.

Hoeng, J., Talikka, M., Martin, F., Sewer, A., Yang, X., Iskandar, A., et al., 2014b. Case study: the role of mechanistic network models in systems toxicology. Drug Discov. Today 19 (2), 183–192.

Honma, M., Momose, M., Sakamoto, H., Sofuni, T., Hayashi, M., 2001. Spindle poisons induce allelic loss in mouse lymphoma cells through mitotic non-disjunction. Mutat. Res. Genet. Toxicol. Environ. Mutagen. 493 (1–2), 101–114.

Horinouchi, T., Higashi, T., Mazaki, Y., Miwa, S., 2016. Carbonyl compounds in the gas phase of cigarette mainstream smoke and their pharmacological properties. Biol. Pharm. Bull. 39 (6), 909–914.

Hu, W., Pasare, C., 2013. Location, location, location: tissue-specific regulation of immune responses. J. Leukoc. Biol. 94 (3), 409–421.

Hukkanen, J., Jacob 3rd, P., Benowitz, N.L., 2005. Metabolism and disposition kinetics of nicotine. Pharmacol. Rev. 57 (1), 79–115.

International Agency for Research on Cancer, 1986. Monographs on the Evaluation of Carcinogenic Risks to Humans: Tobacco Smoking. volume 38. IARC Monographs. IARC, Lyon, France.

International Agency for Research on Cancer, 1999. Monographs on the Evaluation of Carcinogenic Risks to Humans: Re-evaluation of Some Organic Chemicals, Hydrazine and Hydrogen Peroxide. Volume 71 (Part 1). IARC Monographs (Lyon, France).

Interagency Coordinating Committee on the Validation of Alternative Methods, 2006. Test Method Protocol for the BALB/c 3T3 NRU Cytotoxicity Test Method. Appendix C1. NIH Publication No. 07e4519.

Institute of Medicine, 2012. Scientific Standards for Studies on Modified Risk Tobacco Products. The National Academies Press, Washington, DC.

International Conference on Harmonisation, 1995. Guidance on specific aspects of regulatory genotoxicity tests for pharmaceuticals: S2A. In: International Conference on Harmonisation of Technical Requirements for Registration of Pharmaceuticals for Human Use.

International Conference on Harmonisation, 1997. Genotoxicity: a standard battery for genotoxicity testing of pharmaceuticals: S2B. In: International Conference on Harmonisation of Technical Requirements for Registration of Pharmaceuticals for Human Use.

International Conference on Harmonisation, 2010. Guidance for Industry: M3(R2) Nonclinical Safety Studies for the Conduct of Human Clinical Trials and Marketing Authorization for Pharmaceuticals. U.S. Department of Health and Human Services, FDA.

INVITTOX, 1990. INVITTOX ERGATT/FRAME. The FRAME Modified Neutral Red Uptake Cytotoxicity Test. Nottingham: INVITTOX Protocol No. 3a, 1990, INVITTOX: THE ERGATT/FRAME Data Bank of In Vitro Techniques in Toxicology.

Iskandar, A.R., Gonzalez-Suarez, I., Majeed, S., Marescotti, D., Sewer, A., Xiang, Y., et al., 2016. A framework for in vitro systems toxicology assessment of e-liquids. Toxicol. Mech. Methods 26 (6), 389–413.

Iskandar, A.R., Martinez, Y., Martin, F., Schlage, W.K., Leroy, P., Sewer, A., et al., 2017a. Comparative effects of a candidate modified-risk tobacco product aerosol and cigarette smoke on human organotypic small airway cultures: a systems toxicology approach. Toxicol. Res. (Camb.) 6 (6), 930–946.

Iskandar, A.R., Mathis, C., Martin, F., Leroy, P., Sewer, A., Majeed, S., et al., 2017b. 3-D nasal cultures: systems toxicological assessment of a candidate modified-risk tobacco product. ALTEX 34 (1), 23–48.

Iskandar, A.R., Mathis, C., Schlage, W.K., Frentzel, S., Leroy, P., Xiang, Y., et al., 2017c. A systems toxicology approach for comparative assessment: biological impact of an aerosol from a candidate modified-risk tobacco product and cigarette smoke on human organotypic bronchial epithelial cultures. Toxicol. In Vitro 39, 29–51.

Iskandar, A.R., Titz, B., Sewer, A., Leroy, P., Schneider, T., Zanetti, F., et al., 2017d. Systems toxicology meta-analysis of in vitro assessment studies: biological impact of a candidate modified-risk tobacco product aerosol compared with cigarette smoke on human organotypic cultures of the aerodigestive tract. Toxicol. Res. (Camb). 6 (5), 631–653.

Iskandar, A.R., Xiang, Y., Frentzel, S., Talikka, M., Leroy, P., Kuehn, D., et al., 2015. Impact assessment of cigarette smoke exposure on organotypic bronchial epithelial tissue cultures: a comparison of mono-culture and coculture model containing fibroblasts. Toxicol. Sci. 147 (1), 207–221.

Iskandar, A.R., Zanetti, F., Kondylis, A., Martin, F., Leroy, P., Majeed, S., et al., 2019a. A lower impact of an acute exposure to electronic cigarette aerosols than to cigarette smoke in human organotypic buccal and small airway cultures was demonstrated using systems toxicology assessment. Intern. Emerg. Med. 14 (6), 863–883.

Iskandar, A.R., Zanetti, F., Marescotti, D., Titz, B., Sewer, A., Kondylis, A., et al., 2019b. Application of a multi-layer systems toxicology framework for in vitro assessment of the biological effects of classic tobacco e-liquid and its corresponding aerosol using an e-cigarette device with MESH technology. Arch. Toxicol. 93 (11), 3229–3247.

Ito, S., Ishimori, K., Ishikawa, S., 2018. Effects of repeated cigarette smoke extract exposure over one month on human bronchial epithelial organotypic culture. Toxicol. Rep. 5, 864–870.

Ito, S., Matsumura, K., Ishimori, K., Ishikawa, S., 2020. In vitro long-term repeated exposure and exposure switching of a novel tobacco vapor product in a human organotypic culture of bronchial epithelial cells. J. Appl. Toxicol. https://doi.org/10.1002/jat.3982. Epub ahead of print 2020/04/23.

Jaccard, G., Djoko, D.T., Korneliou, A., Stabbert, R., Belushkin, M., Esposito, M., 2019. Mainstream smoke constituents and in vitro toxicity comparative analysis of 3R4F and 1R6F reference cigarettes. Toxicol. Rep. 6, 222–231.

Jorgensen, E.D., Dozmorov, I., Frank, M.B., Centola, M., Albino, A.P., 2004. Global gene expression analysis of human bronchial epithelial cells treated with tobacco condensates. Cell Cycle 3 (9), 1154–1168.

Kilford, J., Thorne, D., Payne, R., Dalrymple, A., Clements, J., Meredith, C., et al., 2014. A method for assessment of the genotoxicity of mainstream cigarette-smoke by use of the bacterial reverse-mutation assay and an aerosol-based exposure system. Mutat. Res. Genet. Toxicol. Environ. Mutagen 769, 20–28.

Kirkland, D., Reeve, L., Gatehouse, D., Vanparys, P., 2011. A core in vitro genotoxicity battery comprising the Ames test plus the in vitro micronucleus test is sufficient to detect rodent carcinogens and in vivo genotoxins. Mutat. Res. 721 (1), 27–73.

Kirkland, D.J., Aardema, M., Banduhn, N., Carmichael, P., Fautz, R., Meunier, J.R., et al., 2007. In vitro approaches to develop weight of evidence (WoE) and mode of action (MoA) discussions with positive in vitro genotoxicity results. Mutagenesis 22 (3), 161–175.

Klaunig, J.E., Kamendulis, L.M., 2008. Chemical carcinogenesis. In: Klaassen, C.D. (Ed.), Casarett & Doull's Toxicology, 7 ed. McGraw-Hill Companies, New York, NY, pp. 329–379.

Klausner, M., Ayehunie, S., Breyfogle, B.A., Wertz, P.W., Bacca, L., Kubilus, J., 2007. Organotypic human oral tissue models for toxicological studies. Toxicol. In Vitro 21 (5), 938–949.

Kogel, U., Gonzalez Suarez, I., Xiang, Y., Dossin, E., Guy, P.A., Mathis, C., et al., 2015. Biological impact of cigarette smoke compared to an aerosol produced from a prototypic

modified risk tobacco product on normal human bronchial epithelial cells. Toxicol. In Vitro 29 (8), 2102–2115.

Krebs, A., Waldmann, T., Wilks, M.F., Van Vugt-Lussenburg, B.M., Van Der Burg, B., Terron, A., et al., 2019. Template for the description of cell-based toxicological test methods to allow evaluation and regulatory use of the data. ALTEX Altern. Anim. Exp. 36 (4), 682–699.

Krewski, D., Acosta Jr., D., Andersen, M., Anderson, H., Bailar 3rd, J.C., Boekelheide, K., et al., 2010. Toxicity testing in the 21st century: a vision and a strategy. J. Toxicol. Environ. Health B Crit. Rev. 13 (2–4), 51–138.

Kristof, E., Zahuczky, G., Katona, K., Doro, Z., Nagy, E., Fesus, L., 2013. Novel role of ICAM3 and LFA-1 in the clearance of apoptotic neutrophils by human macrophages. Apoptosis 18 (10), 1235–1251.

Kuehn, D., Majeed, S., Guedj, E., Dulize, R., Baumer, K., Iskandar, A., et al., 2015. Impact assessment of repeated exposure of organotypic 3D bronchial and nasal tissue culture models to whole cigarette smoke. J. Vis. Exp. 96 https://doi.org/10.3791/52325.

Lee, S.H., Sung, J.H., 2017. Microtechnology-based multi-organ models. Bioengineering 4 (2).

Libby, P., 2002. Inflammation in atherosclerosis. Nature 420 (6917), 868–874.

Libby, P., Ridker, P.M., Maseri, A., 2002. Inflammation and atherosclerosis. Circulation 105 (9), 1135–1143.

Liechty, M.C., Scalzi, J.M., Sims, K.R., Crosby Jr., H., Spencer, D.L., Davis, L.M., et al., 1998. Analysis of large and small colony L5178Y tk$^{-/-}$ mouse lymphoma mutants by loss of heterozygosity (LOH) and by whole chromosome 11 painting: detection of recombination. Mutagenesis.

Lorge, E., Moore, M.M., Clements, J., O'donovan, M., Fellows, M.D., Honma, M., et al., 2016. Standardized cell sources and recommendations for good cell culture practices in genotoxicity testing. Mutat. Res. 809, 1–15.

Malinska, D., Szymanski, J., Patalas-Krawczyk, P., Michalska, B., Wojtala, A., Prill, M., et al., 2018. Assessment of mitochondrial function following short- and long-term exposure of human bronchial epithelial cells to total particulate matter from a candidate modified-risk tobacco product and reference cigarettes. Food Chem. Toxicol. 115, 1–12.

Manna, S., Waring, A., Papanicolaou, A., Hall, N.E., Bozinovski, S., Dunne, E.M., et al., 2018. The transcriptomic response of Streptococcus pneumoniae following exposure to cigarette smoke extract. Sci. Rep. 8 (1), 15716.

Marescotti, D., Bovard, D., Morelli, M., Sandoz, A., Luettich, K., Frentzel, S., et al., 2020a. In vitro high-content imaging-based phenotypic analysis of bronchial 3D organotypic air-liquid interface cultures. SLAS Technol. https://doi.org/10.1177/2472630319895473.

Marescotti, D., Mathis, C., Belcastro, V., Leroy, P., Acali, S., Martin, F., et al., 2020b. Systems toxicology assessment of a representative e-liquid formulation using human primary bronchial epithelial cells. Toxicol. Rep. 7, 67–80.

Marescotti, D., Serchi, T., Luettich, K., Xiang, Y., Moschini, E., Talikka, M., et al., 2019. How complex should an in vitro model be? Evaluation of complex 3D alveolar model with transcriptomic data and computational biological network models. ALTEX 36 (3), 388–402.

Marx, U., Akabane, T., Andersson, T.B., Baker, E., Beilmann, M., Beken, S., et al., 2020. Biology-inspired microphysiological systems to advance patient benefit and animal welfare in drug development. ALTEX. https://doi.org/10.14573/altex.2001241. Epub ahead of print 2020/03/01.

Marx, U., Andersson, T.B., Bahinski, A., Beilmann, M., Beken, S., Cassee, F.R., et al., 2016. Biology-inspired microphysiological system approaches to solve the prediction dilemma of substance testing. ALTEX 33 (3), 272–321.

Maschmeyer, I., Lorenz, A.K., Schimek, K., Hasenberg, T., Ramme, A.P., Hubner, J., et al., 2015. A four-organ-chip for interconnected long-term co-culture of human intestine, liver, skin and kidney equivalents. Lab Chip 15 (12), 2688–2699.

Materne, E.M., Maschmeyer, I., Lorenz, A.K., Horland, R., Schimek, K.M., Busek, M., et al., 2015. The multi-organ chip–a microfluidic platform for long-term multi-tissue coculture. J. Vis. Exp. 98, e52526. https://doi.org/10.3791/52526. Epub ahead of print 2015/05/21.

Mathis, C., Gebel, S., Poussin, C., Belcastro, V., Sewer, A., Weisensee, D., et al., 2015. A systems biology approach reveals the dose- and time-dependent effect of primary human airway epithelium tissue culture after exposure to cigarette smoke in vitro. Bioinf. Biol. Insights 9, 19–35.

Mathis, C., Poussin, C., Weisensee, D., Gebel, S., Hengstermann, A., Sewer, A., et al., 2013. Human bronchial epithelial cells exposed in vitro to cigarette smoke at the air-liquid interface resemble bronchial epithelium from human smokers. Am. J. Physiol. Lung Cell Mol. Physiol. 304 (7), L489–L503.

Messner, B., Bernhard, D., 2014. Smoking and cardiovascular disease: mechanisms of endothelial dysfunction and early atherogenesis. Arterioscler. Thromb. Vasc. Biol. 34 (3), 509–515.

Milara, J., Cortijo, J., 2012. Tobacco, inflammation, and respiratory tract cancer. Curr. Pharmaceut. Des. 18 (26), 3901–3938.

Mitchell, A., Evans, E., Jotz, M., Riccio, E., Mortelmans, K., Simmon, V., 1981. Mutagenic and carcinogenic potency of extracts of diesel and related environmental emissions: in vitro mutagenesis and DNA damage. Environ. Int. 5, 393–401.

Muller, W.A., Luscinskas, F.W., 2008. Assays of transendothelial migration in vitro. Methods Enzymol. 443, 155–176.

Munakata, S., Ishimori, K., Kitamura, N., Ishikawa, S., Takanami, Y., Ito, S., 2018. Oxidative stress responses in human bronchial epithelial cells exposed to cigarette smoke and vapor from tobacco- and nicotine-containing products. Regul. Toxicol. Pharmacol. 99, 122–128.

NCAD, 2016. The Netherlands National Committee for the Protection of Animals Used for Scientific Purposes (NCad). NCad Opinion Transition to Non-Animal Research. Available at: https://www.ncadierproevenbeleid.nl/documenten/rapport/2016/12/15/ncad-opinion-transition-to-non-animal-research (Accessed 08 May 2020).

Nyunoya, T., Mebratu, Y., Contreras, A., Delgado, M., Chand, H.S., Tesfaigzi, Y., 2014. Molecular processes that drive cigarette smoke-induced epithelial cell fate of the lung. Am. J. Respir. Cell Mol. Biol. 50 (3), 471–482.

OECD, 1981. Organisation for Economic Co-operation and Development. Guidelines for the Testing of Chemicals. OECD, Paris, France.

OECD, 1997. Organisation for Economic Co-operation and Development. Test No. 471: Bacterial Reverse Mutation Test. https://doi.org/10.1787/9789264071247-en.

OECD, 2016a. Organisation for Economic Co-operation and Development. Test No. 487: In Vitro Mammalian Cell Micronucleus Test. https://doi.org/10.1787/9789264264861-en.

OECD, 2016b. Organisation for Economic Co-operation and Development. Test No. 490: In Vitro Mammalian Cell Gene Mutation Tests Using the Thymidine Kinase Gene. https://doi.org/10.1787/9789264264908-en.

Oldham, M.J., Haussmann, H.J., Gomm, W., Rimmer, L.T., Morton, M.J., Mckinney Jr., W.J., 2012. Discriminatory power of standard toxicity assays used to evaluate ingreints added to cigarettes. Regul. Toxicol. Pharmacol. 62 (1), 49–61.

Oleaga, C., Bernabini, C., Smith, A.S., Srinivasan, B., Jackson, M., Mclamb, W., et al., 2016. Multi-organ toxicity demonstration in a functional human in vitro system composed of four organs. Sci. Rep. 6, 20030.

Pfuhler, S., Kirst, A., Aardema, M., Banduhn, N., Goebel, C., Araki, D., et al., 2010. A tiered approach to the use of alternatives to animal testing for the safety assessment of cosmetics: genotoxicity. A COLIPA analysis. Regul. Toxicol. Pharmacol. 57 (2–3), 315–324.

Pickett, G., Seagrave, J., Boggs, S., Polzin, G., Richter, P., Tesfaigzi, Y., 2010. Effects of 10 cigarette smoke condensates on primary human airway epithelial cells by comparative gene and cytokine expression studies. Toxicol. Sci. 114 (1), 79–89.

Polk, W.W., Sharma, M., Sayes, C.M., Hotchkiss, J.A., Clippinger, A.J., 2016. Aerosol generation and characterization of multi-walled carbon nanotubes exposed to cells cultured at the air-liquid interface. Part. Fibre Toxicol. 13, 20.

Port, J.L., Yamaguchi, K., Du, B., De Lorenzo, M., Chang, M., Heerdt, P.M., et al., 2004. Tobacco smoke induces CYP1B1 in the aerodigestive tract. Carcinogenesis 25 (11), 2275–2281.

Poussin, C., Gallitz, I., Schlage, W.K., Steffen, Y., Stolle, K., Lebrun, S., et al., 2014. Mechanism of an indirect effect of aqueous cigarette smoke extract on the adhesion of monocytic cells to endothelial cells in an in vitro assay revealed by transcriptomics analysis. Toxicol. In Vitro 28 (5), 896–908.

Poussin, C., Kramer, B., Lanz, H.L., Van Den Heuvel, A., Laurent, A., Olivier, T., et al., 2020. 3D human microvessel-on-a-chip model for studying monocyte-to-endothelium adhesion under flow - application in systems toxicology. ALTEX 37 (1), 47–63.

Poussin, C., Laurent, A., Kondylis, A., Marescotti, D., Van Der Toorn, M., Guedj, E., et al., 2018. In vitro systems toxicology-based assessment of the potential modified risk tobacco product CHTP 1.2 for vascular inflammation- and cytotoxicity-associated mechanisms promoting adhesion of monocytic cells to human coronary arterial endothelial cells. Food Chem. Toxicol. 120, 390–406.

Poussin, C., Laurent, A., Peitsch, M.C., Hoeng, J., De Leon, H., 2015. Systems biology reveals cigarette smoke-induced concentration-dependent direct and indirect mechanisms that promote monocyte-endothelial cell adhesion. Toxicol. Sci. 147 (2), 370–385.

Poussin, C., Laurent, A., Peitsch, M.C., Hoeng, J., De Leon, H., 2016. Systems toxicology-based assessment of the candidate modified risk tobacco product THS2.2 for the adhesion of monocytic cells to human coronary arterial endothelial cells. Toxicology 339, 73–86.

Preston, R.J., Hoffmann, G.R., 2008. Genetic toxicology. In: Klaassen, C.D. (Ed.), Casarett & Doull's Toxicology, pp. 329–379, 7 ed. McGraw-Hill Companies, New York, NY. pp. 381–413.

Putnam, K.P., Bombick, D.W., Doolittle, D.J., 2002. Evaluation of eight in vitro assays for assessing the cytotoxicity of cigarette smoke condensate. Toxicol. In Vitro 16 (5), 599–607.

Putzhammer, R., Doppler, C., Jakschitz, T., Heinz, K., Förste, J., Danzl, K., et al., 2016. Vapours of US and EU market leader electronic cigarette brands and liquids are cytotoxic for human vascular endothelial cells. PLoS One 11 (6) e0157337-e0157337.

Regulation 1907/2006, 30.12.2006. Regulation (EC) no 1907/2006 of the European Parliament and of the council of 18 December 2006 concerning the Registration, Evaluation, Authorisation and Restriction of Chemicals (REACH). L396 Off. J. Eur. Union 1–849

Rendic, S., Guengerich, F.P., 2012. Contributions of human enzymes in carcinogen metabolism. Chem. Res. Toxicol. 25 (7), 1316–1383.

Richter, P.A., Li, A.P., Polzin, G., Roy, S.K., 2010. Cytotoxicity of eight cigarette smoke condensates in three test systems: comparisons between assays and condensates. Regul. Toxicol. Pharmacol. 58 (3), 428–436.

Rickert, W.S., Trivedi, A.H., Momin, R.A., Wright, W.G., Lauterbach, J.H., 2007. Effect of smoking conditions and methods of collection on the mutagenicity and cytotoxicity of cigarette mainstream smoke. Toxicol. Sci. 96 (2), 285–293.

Roemer, E., Dempsey, R., Hirter, J., Deger Evans, A., Weber, S., Ode, A., et al., 2014. Toxicological assessment of kretek cigarettes part 6: the impact of ingredients added to kretek cigarettes on smoke chemistry and in vitro toxicity. Regul. Toxicol. Pharmacol. 70 (Suppl. 1), S66–S80.

Roemer, E., Meisgen, T.J., Tewes, F.J., Solana, R.P., 1998. Discrimination of cigarette mainstream smoke condensates with the Salmonella reverse mutation assay. Toxicol. Sci. 42 (1), 295.

Roemer, E., Stabbert, R., Rustemeier, K., Veltel, D.J., Meisgen, T.J., Reininghaus, W., et al., 2004. Chemical composition, cytotoxicity and mutagenicity of smoke from US commercial and reference cigarettes smoked under two sets of machine smoking conditions. Toxicology 195 (1), 31–52.

Roemer, E., Stabbert, R., Veltel, D., Muller, B.P., Meisgen, T.J., Schramke, H., et al., 2008. Reduced toxicological activity of cigarette smoke by the addition of ammonium magnesium phosphate to the paper of an electrically heated cigarette: smoke chemistry and in vitro cytotoxicity and genotoxicity. Toxicol. In Vitro 22 (3), 671–681.

Roemer, E., Tewes, F.J., Meisgen, T.J., Veltel, D.J., Carmines, E.L., 2002. Evaluation of the potential effects of ingredients added to cigarettes. Part 3: in vitro genotoxicity and cytotoxicity. Food Chem. Toxicol. 40 (1), 105–111.

Sauer, J.M., Kleensang, A., Peitsch, M.C., Hayes, A.W., 2016. Advancing risk assessment through the application of systems toxicology. Toxicol. Res. 32 (1), 5–8.

Schaal, C., Bora-Singhal, N., Kumar, D., Chellappan, S., 2018. Regulation of Sox2 and stemness by nicotine and electronic-cigarettes in non-small cell lung cancer. Mol. Cancer 17, 149.

Schaller, J.P., Keller, D., Poget, L., Pratte, P., Kaelin, E., Mchugh, D., et al., 2016. Evaluation of the Tobacco Heating System 2.2. Part 2: chemical composition, genotoxicity, cytotoxicity, and physical properties of the aerosol. Regul. Toxicol. Pharmacol. 81 (Suppl. 2), S27–S47.

Schlage, W.K., Iskandar, A.R., Kostadinova, R., Xiang, Y., Sewer, A., Majeed, S., et al., 2014. In vitro systems toxicology approach to investigate the effects of repeated cigarette smoke exposure on human buccal and gingival organotypic epithelial tissue cultures. Toxicol. Mech. Methods 24 (7), 470–487.

Schlage, W., Titz, B., Iskandar, A., Poussin, C., Van Der Toorn, M., Wong, E.T., et al., 2020. Comparing the preclinical risk profile of inhalable candidate and potential candidate modified risk tobacco products: a bridging use case. Toxicol. Rep. 7, 1187–1206.

Schramke, H., Meisgen, T.J., Tewes, F.J., Gomm, W., Roemer, E., 2006. The mouse lymphoma thymidine kinase assay for the assessment and comparison of the mutagenic activity of cigarette mainstream smoke particulate phase. Toxicology 227 (3), 193–210.

Schutgens, F., Clevers, H., 2020. Human organoids: tools for understanding biology and treating diseases. Annu. Rev. Pathol. 15, 211–234.

Schweitzer, K.S., Chen, S.X., Law, S., Van Demark, M., Poirier, C., Justice, M.J., et al., 2015. Endothelial disruptive proinflammatory effects of nicotine and e-cigarette vapor exposures. Am. J. Physiol. Lung Cell Mol. Physiol. 309 (2), L175–L187.

Scientific Committee on Consumer Safety, 2018. SCCS/1602/18: the SCCP notes of guidance for the testing of cosmetic ingredients and their safety evaluation (10th revision). In: Adopted by the SCCP During Its Plenary Meeting on 24–25 October.

Sen, B., Mahadevan, B., Demarini, D.M., 2007. Transcriptional responses to complex mixtures: a review. Mutat. Res. 636 (1–3), 144–177.

Siasos, G., Tsigkou, V., Kokkou, E., Oikonomou, E., Vavuranakis, M., Vlachopoulos, C., et al., 2014. Smoking and atherosclerosis: mechanisms of disease and new therapeutic approaches. Curr. Med. Chem. 21 (34), 3936–3948.

Smart, D.J., Helbling, F.R., Mchugh, D., Vanscheeuwijck, P., 2019. Baseline effects of non-flavored e-liquids in the in vitro micronucleus assay. Toxicol. Res. & Appl. 3.

Smart, D.J., Helbling, F.R., Verardo, M., Huber, A., Mchugh, D., Vanscheeuwijck, P., 2020. Development of an integrated assay in human TK6 cells to permit comprehensive genotoxicity analysis in vitro. Mutat. Res. 849, 503129.

Smart, D.J., Helbling, F.R., Verardo, M., Mchugh, D., Vanscheeuwijck, P., 2019b. Mode-of-action analysis of the effects induced by nicotine in the in vitro micronucleus assay. Environ. Mol. Mutagen. 60 (9), 778−791.

Smart, D.J., McHugh, D., 2018. Determination of the Genotoxicity of the Mainstream Aerosol Fractions Generated from the Test Item, Tobacco Heating System Tobacco Sticks, and the Mainstream Smoke Fractions Generated from the Reference Item, 3R4F, in the In Vitro Micronucleus Assay. (PMI Internal Report. Unpublished work).

Spira, A., Beane, J.E., Shah, V., Steiling, K., Liu, G., Schembri, F., et al., 2007. Airway epithelial gene expression in the diagnostic evaluation of smokers with suspect lung cancer. Nat. Med. 13 (3), 361−366.

Sridhar, S., Schembri, F., Zeskind, J., Shah, V., Gustafson, A.M., Steiling, K., et al., 2008. Smoking-induced gene expression changes in the bronchial airway are reflected in nasal and buccal epithelium. BMC Genom. 9, 259.

Steiling, K., Ryan, J., Brody, J.S., Spira, A., 2008. The field of tissue injury in the lung and airway. Cancer Prev. Res. (Phila). 1 (6), 396−403.

Sturla, S.J., Boobis, A.R., Fitzgerald, R.E., Hoeng, J., Kavlock, R.J., Schirmer, K., et al., 2014. Systems toxicology: from basic research to risk assessment. Chem. Res. Toxicol. 27 (3), 314−329.

Szczepanski, M., Kamianowska, M., Kamianowski, G., 2012. Effects of fluorides on apoptosis and activation of human umbilical vein endothelial cells. Oral Dis. 18 (3), 280−284.

Talikka, M., Kostadinova, R., Xiang, Y., Mathis, C., Sewer, A., Majeed, S., et al., 2014. The response of human nasal and bronchial organotypic tissue cultures to repeated whole cigarette smoke exposure. Int. J. Toxicol. 33 (6), 506−517.

Taylor, M., Thorne, D., Carr, T., Breheny, D., Walker, P., Proctor, C., et al., 2018. Assessment of novel tobacco heating product THP1.0. Part 6: a comparative in vitro study using contemporary screening approaches. Regul. Toxicol. Pharmacol. 93, 62−70.

Teasdale, J.E., Newby, A.C., Timpson, N.J., Munafò, M.R., White, S.J., 2016. Cigarette smoke but not electronic cigarette aerosol activates a stress response in human coronary artery endothelial cells in culture. Drug Alcohol Depend. 163, 256−260.

Tennant, R.W., Margolin, B.H., Shelby, M.D., Zeiger, E., Haseman, J.K., Spalding, J., et al., 1987. Prediction of chemical carcinogenicity in rodents from in vitro genetic toxicity assays. Science 236 (4804), 933−941.

Tesfamariam, B., Defelice, A.F., 2007. Endothelial injury in the initiation and progression of vascular disorders. Vasc. Pharmacol. 46 (4), 229−237.

Tewes, F.J., Meisgen, T.J., Veltel, D.J., Roemer, E., Patskan, G., 2003. Toxicological evaluation of an electrically heated cigarette. Part 3: genotoxicity and cytotoxicity of mainstream smoke. J. Appl. Toxicol. 23 (5), 341−348.

The International Council for Harmonisation, 2011. ICH technical requirements for registration of pharmaceuticals for human use. In: Guidance on Genotoxicity Testing and Data Interpretation for Pharmaceuticals Intended for Human Use. S2(R1).

The Life Sciences Research Office, 2007. The Life Sciences Research Office (LSRO) Report on Biological Effects Assessment in the Evaluation of Potential Reduced-Risk Tobacco Products. Life Sciences Research Office, Bethesda, Maryland, 9650 Rockville Pike.

The United States Department of Health and Human Services, 1993. U.S. Consumer Product Safety Commission. Toxicity Testing Plan. Volume 5. Available at: https://www.cpsc.gov/s3fs-public/testing1.pdf (Accessed 19 May 2020).

The United States Department of Health and Human Services, 2010. The Surgeon General's Vision for a Healthy and Fit Nation. Office of the Surgeon General.

The U.S. Centers for Disease Control and Prevention, 2010. How Tobacco Smoke Causes Disease: The Biology and Behavioral Basis for Smoking-Attributable Disease: A Report of the Surgeon General.

The U.S. Centers for Disease Control and Prevention, 2012. NIOSH Carcinogen List. Revised May 2, 2012. Available at: http://www.cdc.gov/niosh/topics/cancer/npotocca.html (Accessed 19 May 2020).

The U.S. Food and Drug Administration, 2000. Guidance for industry and other stakeholders toxicological principles for the safety assessment of food ingredients. Redbook. Available at: https://www.fda.gov/media/79074/download (Accessed 19 May 2020).

Thorne, D., Breheny, D., Proctor, C., Gaca, M., 2018. Assessment of novel tobacco heating product THP1.0. Part 7: comparative in vitro toxicological evaluation. Regul. Toxicol. Pharmacol. 93, 71−83.

Thorne, D., Kilford, J., Hollings, M., Dalrymple, A., Ballantyne, M., Meredith, C., et al., 2015. The mutagenic assessment of mainstream cigarette smoke using the Ames assay: a multi-strain approach. Mutat. Res. Genet. Toxicol. Environ. Mutagen. 70, 9−17.

Thorne, D., Kilford, J., Payne, R., Haswell, L., Dalrymple, A., Meredith, C., et al., 2014. Development of a BALB/c 3T3 neutral red uptake cytotoxicity test using a mainstream cigarette smoke exposure system. BMC Res. Notes 7, 367.

Thorne, D., Leverette, R., Breheny, D., Lloyd, M., Mcenaney, S., Whitwell, J., et al., 2019a. Genotoxicity evaluation of tobacco and nicotine delivery products: Part One. Mouse lymphoma assay. Food Chem. Toxicol. 132, 110584.

Thorne, D., Leverette, R., Breheny, D., Lloyd, M., Mcenaney, S., Whitwell, J., et al., 2019b. Genotoxicity evaluation of tobacco and nicotine delivery products: Part Two. In vitro micronucleus assay. Food Chem. Toxicol. 132, 110546.

Tierney, P.A., Karpinski, C.D., Brown, J.E., Luo, W., Pankow, J.F., 2016. Flavour chemicals in electronic cigarette fluids. Tobac. Contr. 25 (e1), e10−15.

Upadhyay, S., Palmberg, L., 2018. Air-liquid interface: relevant in vitro models for investigating air pollutant-induced pulmonary toxicity. Toxicol. Sci. 164 (1), 21−30.

U.S. Food and Drug Administration Center for Devices and Radiological Health, 2016. Use of International Standard ISO 10993-1. Biological Evaluation of Medical Devices - Part 1: Evaluation and Testing within a Risk Management Process.

van der Toorn, M., Frentzel, S., De Leon, H., Goedertier, D., Peitsch, M.C., Hoeng, J., 2015. Aerosol from a candidate modified risk tobacco product has reduced effects on chemotaxis and transendothelial migration compared to combustion of conventional cigarettes. Food Chem. Toxicol. 86, 81–87.

van der Toorn, M., Sewer, A., Marescotti, D., Johne, S., Baumer, K., Bornand, D., et al., 2018. The biological effects of long-term exposure of human bronchial epithelial cells to total particulate matter from a candidate modified-risk tobacco product. Toxicol. In Vitro 50, 95–108.

Vinken, M., 2020. 3Rs toxicity testing and disease modeling projects in the European horizon 2020 research and innovation program. EXCLI J. 19, 775–784.

Volpato, V., Webber, C., 2020. Addressing variability in iPSC-derived models of human disease: guidelines to promote reproducibility. Dis. Model. Mech. 13 (1).

Werley, M.S., Freelin, S.A., Wrenn, S.E., Gerstenberg, B., Roemer, E., Schramke, H., et al., 2008. Smoke chemistry, in vitro and in vivo toxicology evaluations of the electrically heated cigarette smoking system series K. Regul. Toxicol. Pharmacol. 52 (2), 122–139.

Werley, M.S., Kirkpatrick, D.J., Oldham, M.J., Jerome, A.M., Langston, T.B., Lilly, P.D., et al., 2016. Toxicological assessment of a prototype e-cigaret device and three flavor formulations: a 90-day inhalation study in rats. Inhal. Toxicol. 28 (1), 22–38.

Whitwell, J., Smith, R., Jenner, K., Lyon, H., Wood, D., Clements, J., et al., 2015. Relationships between p53 status, apoptosis and induction of micronuclei in different human and mouse cell lines in vitro: implications for improving existing assays. Mutat. Res. Genet. Toxicol. Environ. Mutagen 789–90, 7–27.

Yamaguchi, Y., Nasu, F., Harada, A., Kunitomo, M., 2007. Oxidants in the gas phase of cigarette smoke pass through the lung alveolar wall and raise systemic oxidative stress. J. Pharmacol. Sci. 103 (3), 275–282.

Yanbaeva, D.G., Dentener, M.A., Creutzberg, E.C., Wesseling, G., Wouters, E.F., 2007. Systemic effects of smoking. Chest 131 (5), 1557–1566.

Yauk, C.L., Williams, A., Buick, J.K., Chen, G., Maertens, R.M., Halappanavar, S., et al., 2012. Genetic toxicology and toxicogenomic analysis of three cigarette smoke condensates in vitro reveals few differences among full-flavor, blonde, and light products. Environ. Mol. Mutagen. 53 (4), 281–296.

Zanetti, F., Sewer, A., Mathis, C., Iskandar, A.R., Kostadinova, R., Schlage, W.K., et al., 2016. Systems toxicology assessment of the biological impact of a candidate modified risk tobacco product on human organotypic oral epithelial cultures. Chem. Res. Toxicol. 29 (8), 1252–1269.

Zanetti, F., Titz, B., Sewer, A., Lo Sasso, G., Scotti, E., Schlage, W.K., et al., 2017. Comparative systems toxicology analysis of cigarette smoke and aerosol from a candidate modified risk tobacco product in organotypic human gingival epithelial cultures: a 3-day repeated exposure study. Food Chem. Toxicol. 101, 15–35.

Zeiger, E., 2010. Historical perspective on the development of the genetic toxicity test battery in the United States. Environ. Mol. Mutagen. 51 (8–9), 781–791.

Zenzen, V., Diekmann, J., Gerstenberg, B., Weber, S., Wittke, S., Schorp, M.K., 2012. Reduced exposure evaluation of an Electrically Heated Cigarette Smoking System. Part 2: smoke chemistry and in vitro toxicological evaluation using smoking regimens reflecting human puffing behavior. Regul. Toxicol. Pharmacol. 64 (2 Suppl. 1), S11–S34.

Zhang, J., Juedes, N., Narayan, V.M., Yue, B., Rockwood, A.L., Palma, N.L., et al., 2010. A cellular model to mimic exhaled cigarette smokeinduced lung microvascular endothelial cell injury and death. Int. J. Clin. Exp. Med. 3 (3), 223–232.

Zuang, V., Dura, A., 2019. EURL ECVAM Status Report on the Development, Validation and Regulatory Acceptance of Alternative Methods and Approaches. Publications Office of the European Union, Luxembourg. https://doi.org/10.2760/25602.

CHAPTER 14

Toxicological Assessment of ENDPs In Vivo

ULRIKE KOGEL • BLAINE W. PHILLIPS • EE TSIN WONG • STÉPHANIE BOUÉ • PATRICK VANSCHEEUWIJCK • MANUEL C. PEITSCH

14.1 INHALATION TOXICOLOGY STUDIES FOR ENDPS

Toxicological assessment of electronic nicotine delivery products (ENDPs) may include preclinical inhalation toxicology studies performed in rodents. The Organisation for Economic Co-operation and Development (OECD) provides guidance on how to design 28- and 90-day inhalation studies for toxicological assessment. Such studies mostly focus on respiratory tract organs, as they are the most sensitive and likely to be affected by exposure to inhaled toxicants. These studies provide the first level of in vivo data for comparing the effects of ENDP aerosols with those of cigarette smoke (CS), and, where applicable, their different modes of action.

14.1.1 Aerosol Generation for ENDP Testing

A prerequisite for conducting inhalation toxicology studies is the ability to generate stable and well-monitored test atmospheres for animal exposure. These test atmospheres must be consistent throughout the study and across studies to ensure repeatability and comparability of study results. Therefore, it is preferred to employ automated means of aerosol generation (Chapter 12). The nature of the test article, be it liquids or sticks that require heating/combustion, will dictate the means of generating aerosols for inhalation studies. While standard, commercially available rotary smoking machines have been used for CS exposure studies for many years, electrically heated tobacco products (EHTPs) require customized rotary aerosol generation machines, which are not widely available (Chapter 12). Moreover, liquid-based test items, such as e-liquids for e-vapor products (EVPs), require very different means of aerosol generation.

First, nebulizers can be used to generate a fine, inhalable aerosol by using compressed air. The liquid formulation is drawn up by a peristaltic pump and delivered to the reservoir of a commercially available nebulizer (e.g., collison jet) (Chapter 12). Under the pressure generated by compressed dry air, the droplets are expanded through small orifices of the nebulizer, resulting in the production of a fine aerosol. This allows assessment of e-liquid formulations separately from their respective devices as well as assessment of other liquid-based compound formulations. Second, aerosols can be generated from liquids by using capillary aerosol generators (CAGs). CAGs generate aerosols by passing liquids through a capillary tube heated to a user-defined temperature. This temperature can be set to mimic the temperature of an EVP heating coil, typically 250−275°C (Chapter 12). CAGs permit continuous and effective production of aerosols from liquids and are, therefore, suitable for assessment of aerosols generated by heating of e-liquid solutions in subacute (28-day), subchronic (90-day), or more extended study designs (Werley et al., 2016b).

While nebulizers generate aerosols at ambient temperature, which is appropriate for many liquid-based test items, CAGs generate heated aerosols that are more representative of EVP aerosols. Indeed, for evaluating the toxicity of an e-liquid-based aerosol generated by a heating device such as a coil in EVPs, it is important to use such a device or a CAG, because thermal treatment of the e-liquid might (slightly) alter its chemical composition. Molecules newly generated by such thermal treatment include carbonyls (Chapter 4), which are toxicologically relevant.

Ideally, the test item (tobacco sticks for CS or EHTPs or liquid constituents for EVPs) as well as the aerosol will have been chemically well characterized and validated before any inhalation exposure is started. During such performance verification experiments, it should be

Toxicological Evaluation of Electronic Nicotine Delivery Products. https://doi.org/10.1016/B978-0-12-820490-0.00014-6

demonstrated that the expected aerosols are effectively and stably generated and have been delivered to the breathing zone of the exposure chambers.

14.1.2 Subacute and Subchronic OECD Inhalation Studies (28- and 90-Day Studies)

Traditional inhalation toxicological assessment approaches preferably follow internationally recognized testing guidelines, such as the "OECD Guidelines for the Testing of Chemicals." These guidelines are important for protocol standardization and incorporate aspects of animal welfare and regulatory needs and requirements. In particular, Test Guidelines (TG) 412

and 413 have been designed for fully characterizing test article toxicity by the inhalation route for a subacute or subchronic duration (i.e., 28 or 90 days, respectively) and for providing robust data for quantitative inhalation risk assessment (OECD, 2018a,b). The guidelines advise on the study design and endpoints that should be included, and are regularly reviewed and updated.

According to the OECD guidelines for subacute or subchronic inhalation toxicology testing, the recommended study design includes both male and female rodents, preferably rats (a minimum of 5 male and 5 female rodents for a 28-day inhalation study and 10 male and 10 female rodents for a 90-day inhalation study) (Fig. 14.1). The preferred mode of exposure is

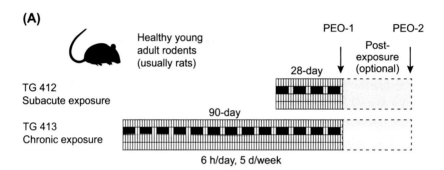

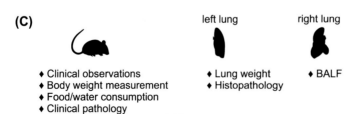

FIG. 14.1 Key principles of the OECD TG 412 and TG 413 guidelines. **(A)** Exposure schedule. **(B)** Groups included in the study for one test substance. **(C)** Endpoints to be included. *BALF*, bronchoalveolar lavage fluid; *PEO*, postexposure observations; *TG*, test guideline.

nose-only exposure (which includes head-only, nose-only, or snout-only) in dynamic inhalation chambers, which have adequate airflow. Importantly, the aerosol should be delivered in a carefully controlled manner and monitored continuously (Chapter 12). Monitoring includes measurement of key parameters, such as temperature and humidity, and the concentrations of key aerosol constituents. These measurements should be recorded regularly during each exposure. Particulate aerosols must have mass median aerodynamic diameters ≤ 2 μm, with geometric standard deviations (σg) ranging from 1 to 3. The rodents are exposed to the test atmospheres for 6 h per day for 5 days per week at three or more concentrations.

The target concentrations of the test aerosols should be confirmed following a dose range—finding study to ensure that the animals can tolerate the highest concentration without experiencing unnecessary stress. Ideally, the highest concentration used should elicit toxic effects. Concurrent negative (air) control animals should be handled identically to the test group animals, except that they are exposed to filtered air rather than to the test aerosol. It is important to consider all potential constituents in the aerosol when designing a study, including any chemical that might be used as an excipient or a vehicle. When a vehicle other than water is used to assist in generating the test atmosphere, a vehicle control group should be used and can replace the air control group (OECD, 2018a,b). Animals should be clinically monitored before, during, and after each exposure period as well as during the postexposure period(s), and the findings should be individually recorded. This includes individual body weight measurements and food consumption. It is particularly important to evaluate the respiratory physiology of the animals (head-out plethysmography for rats), as this parameter is directly linked to the delivered dose (Alexander et al., 2008). An aerosol which is an irritant will negatively impact the breathing frequency (lower frequency) and, usually, the respiratory minute volume of a conscious animal in the exposure chamber. This might result in lower aerosol uptake than expected following exposure to increased aerosol concentrations. This must be considered when interpreting the results of the study.

Importantly, correct exposure of the animals to the test items should be confirmed by measuring appropriately selected biomarkers of exposure (BoExp) to key aerosol constituents. In ENDP assessment studies, it is advisable to measure plasma and/or urinary concentrations of nicotine and its major metabolites. Furthermore, in studies designed for comparing the toxicity of an ENDP aerosol with that of CS, one should also measure BoExps to typical CS toxicants (Chapter 17), such as carboxyhemoglobin (COHb, BoExp to carbon monoxide), 2-cyanoethylmercapturic acid (CEMA, BoExp to acrylonitrile), total 4-(methylnitrosamino)-1-(3-pyridyl)-1-butanol (tNNAL, BoExp to 4-methylnitrosamino-1-(3-pyridyl)-1-butanone), 3-hydroxypropylmercapturic acid (3-HPMA, BoExp to acrolein), and S-phenylmercapturic acid (S-PMA, BoExp to benzene). These measurements provide a solid basis for distinguishing animals exposed to CS from those exposed to ENDP aerosols (Chapters 4 and 17).

Beyond exposure, the test guidelines provide clear directions on the technical requirements and endpoints to be considered during and after terminal necropsy. Additional parameters that will best characterize the test chemical's toxicity may be added on the basis of the dose range—finding study results. At the scheduled necropsy time point, the animals are sacrificed within 24 h after the end of the last exposure day. Pulmonary findings, including pulmonary inflammation and histopathological findings in the lungs and other respiratory tract organs, are of particular importance for inhalation studies. As bronchoalveolar lavage (BALF) and lung histological analyses are mandatory endpoints, the lungs are typically partitioned for multiple endpoint modalities: The left lung is used for histopathological analysis, while the right lung is used for BALF analysis. In addition to the effects on respiratory tract organs, systemic toxicological effects are also evaluated, including clinical (hematological and clinical chemistry analysis and optional urinalysis) and gross pathological parameters and organ weights as well as histopathological parameters, with particular attention to the respiratory tract, other relevant target organs, and gross lesions.

14.1.3 Acute and Chronic OECD Inhalation Studies

In addition to the TGs for subacute and subchronic inhalation studies, three other TGs are available for acute inhalation toxicity studies, namely TG 403—acute inhalation toxicity (i.e., a traditional LC50 protocol and a concentration x time [C x t] protocol) (OECD, 2009a); TG 433—acute inhalation toxicity (fixed concentration procedure) (OECD, 2018c); and TG 436—acute inhalation toxicity (acute toxic class method) (OECD, 2009b). These TGs are, however, not applied in the current ENDP assessment.

There are no chronic or carcinogenicity TGs specifically for the inhalation route. The following three TGs may be used for any route of administration, including inhalation: TG 451—carcinogenicity studies (OECD, 2018d), TG 452—chronic toxicity studies (OECD, 2018e), and TG 453—combined chronic toxicity/carcinogenicity studies (OECD, 2018f). TGs 412 and 413 should be specifically consulted in the design of longer-term inhalation studies.

Although rats are typically used in studies that follow TG 453, it is also possible to use the A/J mouse, which is a model for CS-induced lung cancer. The A/J mouse also develops emphysema upon CS exposure, allowing simultaneous evaluation of two lung diseases, which makes this mouse model very valuable for ENDP assessment (Chapter 15).

14.1.4 OECD Inhalation Studies in the 21st Century (OECD-Plus)

The OECD studies described above are classical toxicological risk assessment studies using apical endpoints. In the vision of 21st century toxicology, studies are foreseen to move away from solely evaluating apical endpoints and turn toward identifying toxicity pathways and adverse outcome pathways (National Research Council, 2007). Experience demonstrates that toxicological markers are only detectable after substantial damage has already occurred and, therefore, are considered to lack sensitivity (Ellinger-Ziegelbauer et al., 2011). Combining omics technologies with classical toxicology has been shown to be a useful tool for mechanistic investigation and identification of putative biomarkers (Cutler et al., 1999; Ellinger-Ziegelbauer et al., 2011).

OECD studies can also be supplemented with additional investigations using systems toxicology approaches in order to gain a mechanistic understanding of the changes that occur upon exposing rodents to aerosols (Ho et al., 2020; Kogel et al., 2014, 2016; Oviedo et al., 2016; Phillips et al., 2015, 2017; Sewer et al., 2016; Titz et al., 2018; Wong et al., 2016). In the context of ENDP assessment, this additional experimental arm, referred to as OECD-plus, allows us to determine the total biological effect of aerosols or inhaled substances on key events along the causal chain of events linking smoking to disease (CELSD) (Chapter 3) and across the numerous biological mechanisms affected by CS (Fig. 14.2). Chapter 9 describes in detail how systems toxicology data can be analyzed to reveal key biological networks and pathways that are perturbed by various stimuli.

14.1.5 In Vivo Genotoxicity Testing

Genetic toxicology tests are often used as a part of test batteries consisting of in vitro and in vivo tests, each focusing on different aspects of genotoxic events (Eastmond et al., 2009; Kirkland et al., 2019). The mutagenicity and genotoxicity of CS and ENDP aerosol are typically assessed by microbial mutagenesis assays (the Ames test) or mammalian cell–based assays, such as the in vitro micronucleus and mouse lymphoma assays (Schaller et al., 2016; Taylor et al., 2018) (Chapter 13). In vivo genotoxicity tests are often conducted to follow-up on positive in vitro findings

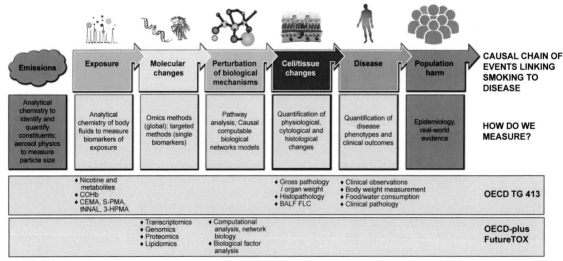

FIG. 14.2 OECD-plus concept *and the CELSD*: Addition of systems toxicology endpoints to OECD studies. *3-HPMA,*
3-hydroxypropylmercapturic acid; *CELSD*, causal chain of events linking smoking to disease; *CEMA*,
2-cyanoethylmercapturic acid; *COHb*, carboxyhomoglobin; *FLC*, free lung cells; *S-PMA*, S-phenylmercapturic acid; *tNNAL*, total 4-(methylnitrosamino)-1-(3-pyridyl)-1-butanol.

(Eastmond et al., 2009; Kirkland et al., 2019). There are four commonly used guidelines for in vivo mutagenesis tests: TG 474—mammalian erythrocyte micronucleus test (OECD, 2016a), TG 475—mammalian bone marrow chromosomal aberration test (OECD, 2016b), TG 489—in vivo mammalian alkaline comet assay (OECD, 2016c), and TG 488—transgenic rodent gene mutation assays (OECD, 2013).

The in vivo micronucleus test is used for detection of genotoxicity due to chromosomal DNA damage or impairment of the mitotic apparatus in erythroblasts. As with other in vivo genotoxicity assays, factors of in vivo metabolism, pharmacokinetics, and DNA repair will contribute to the assay outcomes.

The other in vivo genotoxicity assays are less commonly used for CS exposure studies. However, one alternative mutagenesis assay, the *Pig-a* gene mutation assay, offers greater ease of rapid detection of in vivo gene mutation and at a lower cost than the transgenic rodent gene mutation assay. Another advantage is that this assay can be performed with peripheral blood samples. It can thus be integrated in, for example, a 90-day inhalation study and does not require additional animals (except for a positive control). This assay relies on detection of cells that carry inactivating mutations of the X-linked gene *Pig-a* leading to the loss of expression of glycosylphosphatidylinositol anchors on the cell surface, which can then be detected by antibody labeling (typically CD59 for rats or CD24 for mice) (Bryce et al., 2008; Phonethepswath et al., 2008). "Although the *Pig-a* gene mutation assay does not have an OECD Test guideline, it is a promising new in vivo mutation test that is sensitive and less costly than the transgenic rodent gene mutation assay, and it can be integrated into repeat-dose standard toxicology tests" (US EPA OPP, 2012). The *Pig-a* assay is applicable to many animal models. The low blood volume requirement also enables longitudinal data collection and integration into long-term studies.

14.2 RESULTS OF OECD AND OECD-PLUS EVP ASSESSMENT STUDIES

Several studies have been conducted in accordance with OECD guidelines and proven to be suitable for assessing heated tobacco products (HTPs), EVPs, and single components or mixtures used in ENDPs.

While EVPs have been tested in very few OECD inhalation studies (Werley et al., 2016a), the toxicity of the main compounds of EVPs, such as nicotine (Phillips et al., 2015; Werley et al., 2014), propylene glycol (PG) (Suber et al., 1989; Werley et al., 2011), and glycerin (Renne et al., 1992), have been individually assessed in separate in vivo OECD inhalation studies. Furthermore, mixtures of the main EVP aerosol, with or without a flavor mixture, have also recently been studied in such studies (Ho et al., 2020; Phillips et al., 2017).

Exposure of Sprague Dawley rats for 90 days (6 h/day, 5 days/week) to test atmosphere concentrations of 0.0, 0.16, 1.0, or 2.2 mg/L PG led to a significant increase in the number of goblet cells or an increase in mucin content in existing goblet cells in the nasal passages, nasal hemorrhage, and ocular discharge in a high proportion of animals. This was attributed to the potential dehydration of the nares and eyes (Suber et al., 1989). Additionally, the body weight as well as food consumption in female rats exposed to 2.2 mg/L PG was significantly lower than those in the control animals. The lower concentrations of PG (0.16 and 1.0 mg/L air) had no effect on any parameter (Suber et al., 1989).

In a 28-day study Sprague Dawley rats were exposed to up to 30 mg/L PG aerosol for up to 120 min/day. The target exposure concentrations and durations were selected to attain the following dose depositions in the lungs: 7.2, 21.6, 72.0, and 216.0 mg/kg/day. The only biologically relevant findings included clinical signs of ocular and nasal irritation (described as minor bleeding around the eyes and nose (Werley et al., 2011)) and minimal laryngeal squamous metaplasia. However, the former is likely attributed to stress-related Harderian gland secretion, as observed in previously conducted studies using nose-only exposure aerosol delivery (Phillips et al., 2017), and the latter is a lesion commonly observed in many inhalation studies and probably related to the unique sensitivity at a specific site of the larynx and its capacity for efficient aerosol deposition and/or impaction. Under the conditions of these studies, the no-observed-effect level (NOEL) for the rats was determined to be 20 mg/kg/day in the 28-day study (Werley et al., 2011).

Renne et al. studied aerosolized glycerol in a 2-week exposure study with test atmosphere concentrations of 1.00 ± 0.08, 1.93 ± 0.123, or 3.91 ± 0.458 mg/L glycerol. The results of this study showed that rats exposed for 6 h/day for 10 days exhibited minimal to mild squamous metaplasia of the epithelium lining at the base of the epiglottis at all three glycerol concentrations (Renne et al., 1992). Furthermore, exposure to glycerol aerosol for 13 consecutive weeks (mean aerosol concentrations: 0, 0.033 ± 0.0046, 0.167 ± 0.023, or 0.662 ± 0.085 mg glycerol/L of air) resulted in minimal to mild squamous metaplasia of the epithelium lining at the base of the epiglottis only in rats exposed to the highest concentration of glycerol (Renne et al., 1992). As described above for PG, this finding is associated with the unique sensitivity of this anatomical region to aerosol deposition and impaction.

The toxicity of nebulized nicotine (and nicotine/pyruvic acid mixtures) was characterized in a 28-day inhalation study (6 h/day, 5 days/week) by Phillips et al. In this study, seven groups of animals were exposed to filtered air, saline, nicotine (50 μg/L), sodium pyruvate (33.9 μg/L), or three concentrations of an equimolar nicotine/pyruvate mixture (18, 25, and 50 μg nicotine/L) (Phillips et al., 2015). Only rats exposed to nicotine-containing aerosols exhibited decreased body weight gain and a concentration-dependent increase in liver weight relative to fresh air–exposed animals. The only histopathological finding in nonrespiratory tract organs was increased liver vacuolation, which occurred in a nicotine (at 50 μg/L nicotine) dose-dependent manner.

Respiratory tract findings following nicotine exposure (but also some phosphate-buffered saline aerosol effects) were observed only in the larynx and were limited to adaptive changes. Following hematological and clinical chemistry–based blood profiling, it was noted that neutrophil counts were increased, and lymphocyte counts were decreased; the activities of alkaline phosphatase and alanine aminotransferase were increased, and the levels of cholesterol and glucose had decreased (Phillips et al., 2015). Additional transcriptomics and lipidomics analyses (OECD-plus analysis) showed very weak gene expression changes in the lungs and liver, lower plasma lipid (including cholesteryl ester and free cholesterol) levels, and lower phospholipid and sphingolipid levels in the liver (Phillips et al., 2015). Thus, a few effects were seen at the molecular level in the nicotine/pyruvic acid (high) group, but they were not reflected in the endpoints of toxicity.

Waldum et al. examined the effect of long-term (2 years, 20 h/day, 5 days/week) inhalation of nicotine on rats. The authors used a nicotine concentration that amounted to twice the plasma nicotine concentration recorded in heavy smokers. These rats showed no increase in mortality, atherosclerosis, or frequency of tumors relative to the controls; but, throughout the study, the bodyweight of the nicotine-exposed rats was lower than that of the control animals (Waldum et al., 1996).

In another study in Sprague Dawley rats, only very limited biological effects were detected when the inhalation toxicity of a nebulized mixture of PG and vegetable glycerin (VG) was compared with that of a nebulized vehicle (saline) (Phillips et al., 2017). Importantly, no toxicologically relevant effects of PG/VG aerosols (up to 1.520 mg PG/L + 1.890 mg VG/L) were observed (Phillips et al., 2017). Addition of nicotine to the PG/VG aerosols resulted in effects that were in line with the nicotine effects observed in previous studies conducted with nicotine-containing aerosols. These effects included upregulation of xenobiotic enzymes (Cyp1a1) in the lungs and metabolic effects such as reduced serum lipid concentrations and changes in hepatic metabolic enzyme expression (Oviedo et al., 2016; Phillips et al., 2015; Wong et al., 2016). No adverse effects were observed with PG/VG/nicotine mixtures at concentrations up to 438/544/6.6 mg/kg/day (Phillips et al., 2017) (Fig. 14.3).

This study demonstrated how complementary systems toxicology analyses can reveal, even in the absence of phenotypic adverse effects, subtoxic and adaptive responses to pharmacologically active compounds such as nicotine.

In a first step toward characterizing the combined toxicity of flavoring substances, a 90-day inhalation study was performed by using three concentrations of a specifically designed flavor substance mixture (a flavor tool box, as defined in Chapter 16) dissolved in a base solution composed of PG, VG, and nicotine. The test atmosphere concentration of the base solution was constant across the groups (nicotine at 23 μg/L, PG at 1520 μg/L, and VG at 1890 μg/L). Furthermore, nonflavored and nicotine-free test atmospheres were included as references (Ho et al., 2020). The aerosols were generated with nebulizers at ambient temperature. The flavor substance mixture was produced by grouping 178 flavors into 26 distinct chemical groups on the basis of structural similarity and potential metabolic and biological effects (Chapter 16). Flavoring substances predicted to show the highest toxicological effect from each group were selected as flavor group representatives. The biological effects induced by exposure to the flavor substance mixture were limited and mainly nicotine-related and included changes in hematological and blood chemistry parameters as well as organ weight. In this subchronic inhalation study, inhalation of a nebulized (nonthermally treated) flavoring substance mixture did not cause significant additive biological changes beyond the known effects of nicotine.

To date, the 90-day study by Werley et al. is the only OECD study that used a (prototype) EVP. The authors studied exposure to low-, medium-, and high-dose levels of aerosols with flavors (18.1% glycerol, 62.3% PG, 2.0% nicotine, and 17.6% proprietary flavor mixture) or without flavors (22.5% glycerol, 75.5%

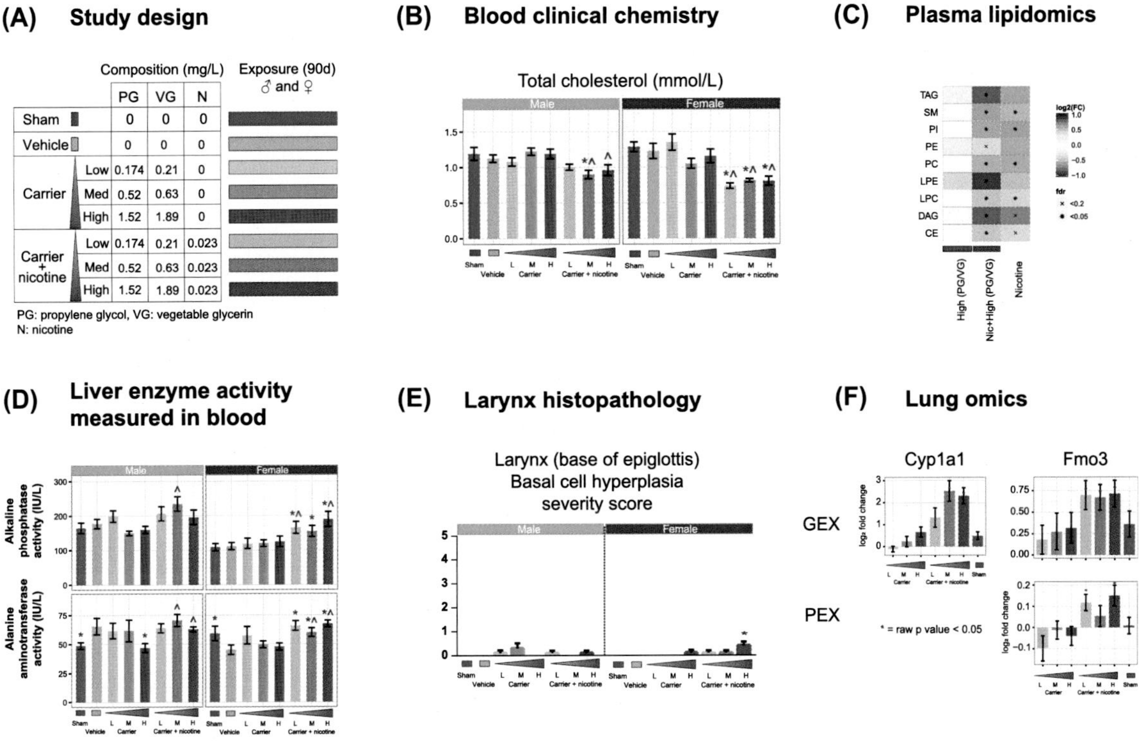

(A) Study design

(B) Blood clinical chemistry

(C) Plasma lipidomics

(D) Liver enzyme activity measured in blood

(E) Larynx histopathology

(F) Lung omics

FIG. 14.3 Results of a PG/VG/nicotine OECD-plus experiment. (A) Study design showing exposure groups and target concentrations in the test atmospheres of the 90-day OECD TG413 inhalation toxicity study. (B) From the blood clinical chemistry, the total cholesterol concentrations are shown (mean ± SEM). Statistically significant differences from the vehicle group are represented by *asterisks* (*); statistically significant differences between groups with and without nicotine (at the same PG/VG concentration) are represented by *carets* (ˆ) (P-value < .05). (C) Plasma lipid changes measured by lipidomics. Log2 fold-change of lipid classes compared with vehicle group or for nicotine effect is color-coded, and statistically significant changes are marked. (D) Liver enzyme activities of alkaline phosphatase and alanine aminotransferase measured in blood (mean ± SEM). Statistically significant differences from the vehicle group are represented by *asterisks* (*); statistically significant differences between groups with and without nicotine (at the same PG/VG concentration) are represented by *carets* (ˆ) (P-value < .05). (E) Histopathology of the larynx (mean scores ± SEM). Statistically significant differences from the vehicle group are represented by *asterisks* (*); no statistically significant differences between groups with and without nicotine (at the same PG/VG concentration) were found (P-value < .05). (F) Gene expression (GEX) and protein expression (PEX) profiles for Cyp1a1 and Fmo3. Differences compared with the vehicle group with a raw P-value < .05 are marked (*). Note that the average nicotine effect for these changes is significant (FDR-adjusted P-value < .05) and that Cyp1a1 was only detected by GEX. *CE*, cholesteryl esters; *CYP1A1*, Cytochrome P450, family 1, subfamily A, polypeptide 1; *DAG*, diacylglycerol; *Fmo3*, Flavin containing monooxygenase 3; *LPC*, lyso-phosphatidylcholine; *LPE*, lyso-phosphatidylethanolamine; *PC*, phosphatidylcholine; *PE*, phosphatidylethanolamine; *PI*, phosphatidylinositol; *SM*, sphingomyelin; *TAG*, triacylglycerol. (Adapted from Phillips, B., Titz, B., Kogel, U., Sharma, D., Leroy, P., Xiang, Y., Vuillaume, G., Lebrun, S., Sciuscio, D., Ho, J., et al. 2017. Toxicity of the main electronic cigarette components, propylene glycol, glycerin, and nicotine, in Sprague-Dawley rats in a 90-day OECD inhalation study complemented by molecular endpoints. Food Chem. Toxicol. 109, 315–332.)

PG, and 2.0% nicotine). The control aerosol contained 23% glycerol and 77% PG (Werley et al., 2016a). The study also included a commercially available EVP and applied daily targeted aerosol total particulate matter (TPM) doses of 3.2, 9.6, and 32.0 mg/kg/day. The treatment-related effects following 90 days of exposure included changes in body weight, food consumption, and respiratory rate. Dose-related decreases in thymus, spleen, and lung weights were observed. BALF analysis revealed increased lactate dehydrogenase, total protein, alveolar macrophage, and neutrophil levels. Histopathological evaluations revealed sporadic increases in epithelial hyperplasia and vacuolization at nasal sections 1–4. The authors specified that smoking-related respiratory tract effects are generally more adverse (in terms of increased incidence and severity) than those observed in their study, although they did not perform a side-by-side comparison with CS. The NOEL based on body weight decrease was found to be the mid-dose level for each formulation, equivalent to a daily TPM exposure dose of approximately 9.6 mg/kg/day (Werley et al., 2016a).

14.3 RESULTS OF OECD AND OECD-PLUS HTP ASSESSMENT STUDIES

In contrast to EVPs, HTPs contain tobacco, and, therefore, their aerosol is more complex than that of EVPs (Chapter 4).

The toxicological profiles of several HTPs have been compared with those of reference cigarettes in OECD inhalation studies. The first rat subchronic inhalation study (1 h/day, 5 days/week, 13 weeks in total) with an HTP was conducted 20 years ago with a carbon-heated tobacco product (CHTP) (Ayres et al., 2001). The authors compared the biological activity of mainstream aerosol from a cigarette that primarily heats tobacco ("Eclipse") at test atmosphere concentrations of 0, 0.16, 0.32, or 0.64 mg/L wet TPM (WTPM) with that of mainstream smoke from the 1R4F reference cigarette at matched concentrations. Plethysmography results indicated that respiratory rates were decreased at all concentrations of 1R4F smoke, but only at the highest concentration of Eclipse aerosol. In addition to a slight body weight decrease, the only treatment-related effect seen in organ weights was an increase in heart weight among female rats in the Eclipse high-concentration exposure group; this was attributed to the higher CO concentrations in the Eclipse aerosol exposure atmosphere. The higher CO levels resulted from the lower dilution of Eclipse aerosol required to maintain WTPM concentrations equal to those of 1R4F smoke and not from a higher CO yield by Eclipse aerosol. Nasal epithelial hyperplasia and ventral laryngeal squamous metaplasia were noted after exposure, but the degree of change was less in Eclipse aerosol-exposed rats. Lung macrophage numbers were increased to a similar extent in the Eclipse aerosol- and 1R4F smoke-exposed groups. Brown/gold-pigmented macrophages were detected in the lungs of rats exposed to

1R4F smoke but not in those exposed to Eclipse aerosol. In summary, these findings indicated that the overall biological activity of Eclipse aerosol was lower than that of 1R4F smoke at comparable exposure concentrations (Ayres et al., 2001).

In 2003, the effects of an electrically heated cigarette (EHC) with controlled combustion were compared with those of the same reference cigarette (1R4F). The exposure lasted 90 days for 6 h/day, 7 days/week, and basically conformed with OECD TG 413 (version of 1981) (Terpstra et al., 2003). Two exposure doses were chosen for the EHC, because the anticipated results were within the dynamic range of the 1R4F dose–response curve (four concentrations) for most endpoints. The TPM concentrations were 40 and 90 μg/L for the EHC and 40–170 μg/L for 1R4F. Exposure-related histopathological findings in the respiratory tract included epithelial cell hyperplasia, squamous metaplasia, atrophy, and accumulation of pigmented alveolar macrophages. These changes were mostly concentration-dependent, more pronounced in the upper than lower respiratory tract, and completely or partially reversed after 6 weeks of recovery. Qualitatively, the biological effects seen with the EHC and 1R4F were comparable and similar to those observed in other mainstream smoke inhalation studies. Quantitatively, the biological activity of the EHC mainstream aerosol was, on average, 65% lower than that of the 1R4F mainstream smoke on an equal cigarette basis and equivalent on an equal TPM basis (Terpstra et al., 2003).

The first generation of EHCs that was assessed by Terpstra et al. had high formaldehyde yields; therefore, a second generation of EHCs was developed with a cigarette paper containing ammonium magnesium phosphate, in part, to address this increase in formaldehyde levels (Moennikes et al., 2008). Many of the typical smoke exposure–related changes were found to be less pronounced after 90 days of exposure to aerosol from a second-generation EHC relative to aerosol from a first-generation EHC or 1R4F smoke, when compared on a particulate matter or nicotine basis (Moennikes et al., 2008).

A 90-day nose-only inhalation study in rats showed a reduction in pulmonary inflammation and other biological activity, including histopathological endpoints, when the Electrically Heated Cigarette Smoking System Series K was compared with the 2R4F reference cigarette (Werley et al., 2014).

The first OECD study with integrated molecular toxicology endpoints (OECD-plus) was a 28-day rat inhalation study performed with a CHTP prototype. This study not only compared the effects of the CHTP aerosol with those of smoke from the 3R4F reference cigarette but also investigated the molecular perturbations that accompany the histopathological changes caused by the test items (Kogel et al., 2014). Concentration-dependent gene expression changes were observed following 3R4F smoke exposure, while much smaller changes were observed in CHTP aerosol-exposed animals. A computational modeling approach based on tissue-specific causal biological network models (Chapter 9) identified cell stress, inflammation, proliferation, and senescence as the molecular mechanisms most perturbed by 3R4F smoke exposure. These perturbations were correlated with the histopathological observations. Only weak perturbations were observed with CHTP aerosol exposure. This study demonstrated that correlative evaluation of classical histopathological endpoints together with gene expression–based computational network model analyses might facilitate a systems toxicology–based risk assessment (Kogel et al., 2014).

Another study by Fujimoto et al. analyzed the biological effects of another CHTP and compared them with those of the 3R4F cigarette. After a 13-week exposure (200, 600, or 1000 μg/L WTPM for 1 h/day, 7 days/week), the histopathological changes in the respiratory tract were significantly lower in the CHTP groups, and the lesions were completely or partially reversed after a 13-week recovery period (Fujimoto et al., 2015).

More recently, a 90-day nose-only inhalation study compared the toxicity of an EHTP, the Tobacco Heating System 2.2 (THS), with that of the 3R4F reference cigarette by combining classical and systems toxicology approaches (Wong et al., 2016). The THS aerosol-exposed groups showed significantly less pronounced lung inflammation, histopathological findings in respiratory tract organs, and reduction in respiratory minute volume relative to the 3R4F smoke-exposed groups. Transcriptomics data from nasal epithelium and lung parenchyma showed concentration-dependent differential gene expression following 3R4F smoke exposure. These changes were less pronounced in the THS aerosol-exposed groups. Molecular network analysis showed that inflammatory processes were the most affected by 3R4F smoke exposure, while the effects of THS aerosol exposure were much lower. Most other evaluated toxicological endpoints showed no exposure-related effects in THS aerosol-exposed animals (Wong et al., 2016).

In another study, the toxicity of a mentholated version of the THS (THS-M) was characterized in a 90-day OECD inhalation study. Differential gene and protein expression analyses of nasal epithelium and lung tissue were also performed to record exposure effects at the molecular level. Systemic toxicity and alterations in the respiratory tract were significantly lower in THS-M aerosol-exposed rats than in rats exposed to smoke from a mentholated reference cigarette and the 3R4F cigarette. Pulmonary inflammation and the magnitude of changes in gene and protein expression observed after THS-M aerosol exposure were also dramatically lower than those following exposure to smoke from the reference cigarettes (Oviedo et al., 2016). Extended analysis of the systems toxicology data complemented and reconfirmed the results from the classical toxicological endpoints (Kogel et al., 2016) (Fig. 14.4).

14.4 RESULTS OF GENOTOXICITY TESTS IN VIVO

Sensitivity to CS-induced micronucleated cell formation is species- and strain-specific, as an increase in micronucleus-positive cells is not detected in Sprague Dawley rats but has been observed in some mouse strains (Lee et al., 1990; Van Miert et al., 2008). CS exposure induces an increase in micronucleated polychromatic erythrocytes or normochromatic red blood cells in various mouse strains (e.g., BDF1, Swiss albino, B6C3F$_1$, and ICR) (Balansky et al., 1987; Coggins et al., 2008; Nakamura et al., 2015). One mouse inhalation study that compared the impact of aerosol from HTP with that of CS did not show any difference in the occurrence of micronucleated cells (Coggins et al., 2008). However, these results should be interpreted with caution: Often, erythropoiesis is stimulated by CS exposure, and stress erythropoiesis, caused by both handling and exposure, is sufficient to cause a modest increase in micronucleated cells in the absence of a chemical genotoxicant (Tweats et al., 2007).

Other in vivo genotoxicity assays are less commonly used for CS-exposure studies and have shown variable degrees of success (Coggins et al., 2008; Dalrymple et al., 2016; Lee et al., 1990).

A positive relationship was found between mutant *Pig-a* frequency and smoking expressed as cigarette pack-years (Cao et al., 2016). As demonstrated in a 90-day inhalation study in Sprague Dawley rats, for 4-(methylnitrosamino)-1-(3-pyridyl)-1-butanone (NNK)—a known carcinogen present in CS—the applied dose of 7.8 mg/kg was the maximum tolerated dose, but it was unable to induce *Pig-a* positive red blood cells or reticulocytes. The negative in vivo result is likely due to insufficient bone marrow exposure (Mittelstaedt et al., 2019). Hence, the choice of target tissue,

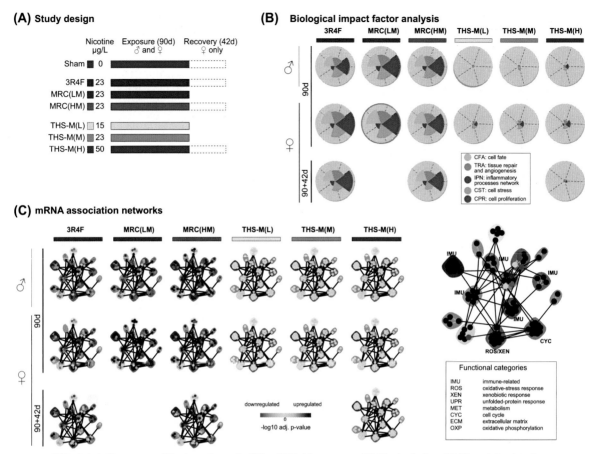

FIG. 14.4 Response of the lung tissue to CS or THS-M exposure. (**A**) Study design. (**B**) Star plots showing relative network-level biological impact factors (RBIFs) for each exposure group relative to the sham groups. The total area of each star plot represents the RBIF of each comparison relative to the comparison with the MRC(LM), females, 90-days group. (**C**) Functional association clustering of transcriptomics data of the lung tissue. Functional clusters affected by the exposure conditions were identified and compared across the clusters. Lower panel shows the identified clusters and their associated functional categories (see key). Each *node* represents a gene, and *lines* represent functional associations. The identified gene clusters are grouped and circled. The top panel shows the differential expression response for each gene in the association network. The node color represents the −log10 adjusted *P* value (see color key). *H*, high; *HM*, high menthol; *L*, low; *LM*, low menthol; *M*, medium; *MRC*, menthol reference cigarette. (Adapted from Figs. 1 and 4 from Kogel et al. (2016).)

level of exposure of the target tissue, and metabolic activity of the organ should be considered when planning genotoxicity studies. The assessment of micronucleus and *Pig-a* in solid tissues offers alternatives to the blood- and bone marrow–type assays (Avlasevich et al., 2018; Dertinger et al., 2019; Khanal et al., 2018). It remains to be proven whether the *Pig-a* assay is suitable for assessment of ENDPs (Dalrymple et al., 2016; Mittelstaedt et al., 2019; Van Miert et al., 2008).

14.5 CONCLUSIONS

Several rat inhalation studies that followed OECD guidelines have assessed the effects of HTPs, the ingredients of e-liquids, as well as EVPs.

In comparison with CS, the aerosol of the latest generation EHTP caused very low or no pulmonary inflammation, as evaluated by (i) free lung cell counts in BALF, (ii) multiplexed cytokine analysis, and (iii) histopathology analyses. Systemic findings included liver vacuolation, changes in liver enzyme levels, some hematological and clinical chemistry findings, and changes in organ weights. These changes were interpreted as mainly stress-related and mostly nicotine-dependent and found to be reversible following a recovery phase.

In general, only minimal or sporadic findings were observed following inhalation exposure to e-liquid aerosols. These findings were shown to be reversible during the recovery phase of the respective studies and appeared to be mainly nicotine-related.

Inclusion of OECD-plus groups in inhalation studies enables mechanism-by-mechanism comparison of the effects of ENDP aerosol exposure with those of CS exposure. The results of the OECD-plus studies conducted with the latest generation EHTP showed that the EHTP aerosols had significantly lower effects on the biological mechanisms affected by CS. In the context of the CELSD, these results were coherent with the relative toxicant exposure levels of the tested groups and predictive of the cell and tissue changes (toxicological endpoints).

The available data show that, overall, HTP and EVP aerosols are less toxic than CS in subacute and subchronic inhalation studies.

REFERENCES

Alexander, D.J., Collins, C.J., Coombs, D.W., Gilkison, I.S., Hardy, C.J., Healey, G., Karantabias, G., Johnson, N., Karlsson, A., Kilgour, J.D., 2008. Association of Inhalation Toxicologists (AIT) working party recommendation for standard delivered dose calculation and expression in non-clinical aerosol inhalation toxicology studies with pharmaceuticals. Inhal. Toxicol. 20, 1179–1189.

Avlasevich, S.L., Khanal, S., Singh, P., Torous, D.K., Bemis, J.C., Dertinger, S.D., 2018. Flow cytometric method for scoring rat liver micronuclei with simultaneous assessments of hepatocyte proliferation. Environ. Mol. Mutagen. 59, 176–187.

Ayres, P.H., Hayes, J.R., Higuchi, M.A., Mosberg, A.T., Sagartz, J.W., 2001. Subchronic inhalation by rats of mainstream smoke from a cigarette that primarily heats tobacco compared to a cigarette that burns tobacco. Inhal. Toxicol. 13, 149–186.

Balansky, R.M., Blagoeva, P.M., Mircheva, Z.I., 1987. Investigation of the mutagenic activity of tobacco smoke. Mutat. Res. 188, 13–19.

Bryce, S.M., Bemis, J.C., Dertinger, S.D., 2008. In vivo mutation assay based on the endogenous Pig-a locus. Environ. Mol. Mutagen. 49, 256–264.

Cao, Y., Yang, L., Feng, N., Shi, O., Xi, J., You, X., Yin, C., Yang, H., Horibata, K., Honma, M., et al., 2016. A population study using the human erythrocyte Pig-a assay. Environ. Mol. Mutagen. 57, 605–614.

Coggins, C.R.E., Doolittle, D.J., Lee, C.K., Ayres, P.H., Mosberg, A.T., Bolin, D.C., Burger, G.T., Hayes, A.W., 2008. Histopathology, urine mutacenicity, and bone marrow cytocenetics of mice exposed nose-only to smoke from cigarettes that burn or heat tobacco. Inhal. Toxicol. 2, 407–431.

Cutler, P., Bell, D.J., Birrell, H.C., Connelly, J.C., Connor, S.C., Holmes, E., Mitchell, B.C., Monte, S.Y., Neville, B.A., Pickford, R., et al., 1999. An integrated proteomic approach to studying glomerular nephrotoxicity. Electrophoresis 20, 3647–3658.

Dalrymple, A., Ordonez, P., Thorne, D., Walker, D., Camacho, O.M., Buttner, A., Dillon, D., Meredith, C., 2016. Cigarette smoke induced genotoxicity and respiratory tract pathology: evidence to support reduced exposure time and animal numbers in tobacco product testing. Inhal. Toxicol. 28, 324–338.

Dertinger, S.D., Avlasevich, S.L., Torous, D.K., Singh, P., Khanal, S., Kirby, C., Drake, A., MacGregor, J.T., Bemis, J.C., 2019. 3Rs friendly study designs facilitate rat liver and blood micronucleus assays and Pig-a gene mutation assessments: proof-of-concept with 13 reference chemicals. Environ. Mol. Mutagen. 60, 704–739.

Eastmond, D.A., Hartwig, A., Anderson, D., Anwar, W.A., Cimino, M.C., Dobrev, I., Douglas, G.R., Nohmi, T., Phillips, D.H., Vickers, C., 2009. Mutagenicity testing for chemical risk assessment: update of the WHO/IPCS Harmonized Scheme. Mutagenesis 24, 341–349.

Ellinger-Ziegelbauer, H., Adler, M., Amberg, A., Brandenburg, A., Callanan, J.J., Connor, S., Fountoulakis, M., Gmuender, H., Gruhler, A., Hewitt, P., et al., 2011. The enhanced value of combining conventional and "omics" analyses in early assessment of drug-induced hepatobiliary injury. Toxicol. Appl. Pharmacol. 252, 97–111.

Fujimoto, H., Tsuji, H., Okubo, C., Fukuda, I., Nishino, T., Lee, K.M., Renne, R., Yoshimura, H., 2015. Biological responses in rats exposed to mainstream smoke from a heated cigarette compared to a conventional reference cigarette. Inhal. Toxicol. 27, 224–236.

Ho, J., Sciuscio, D., Kogel, U., Titz, B., Leroy, P., Vuillaume, G., Talikka, M., Martin, E., Pospisil, P., Lebrun, S., et al., 2020. Evaluation of toxicity of aerosols from flavored e-liquids in Sprague-Dawley rats in a 90-day OECD inhalation study, complemented by transcriptomics analysis. Arch. Toxicol. 94, 2179–2206.

Khanal, S., Singh, P., Avlasevich, S.L., Torous, D.K., Bemis, J.C., Dertinger, S.D., 2018. Integration of liver and blood micronucleus and Pig-a gene mutation endpoints into rat 28-day repeat-treatment studies: proof-of-principle with diethylnitrosamine. Mutat. Res. 828, 30–35.

Kirkland, D., Uno, Y., Luijten, M., Beevers, C., van Benthem, J., Burlinson, B., Dertinger, S., Douglas, G.R., Hamada, S., Horibata, K., et al., 2019. In vivo genotoxicity testing strategies: report from the 7th International Workshop on Genotoxicity Testing (IWGT). Mutat. Res. 847, 403035.

Kogel, U., Schlage, W.K., Martin, F., Xiang, Y., Ansari, S., Leroy, P., Vanscheeuwijck, P., Gebel, S., Buettner, A., Wyss, C., et al., 2014. A 28-day rat inhalation study with an integrated molecular toxicology endpoint demonstrates reduced exposure effects for a prototypic modified risk tobacco product compared with conventional cigarettes. Food Chem. Toxicol. 68, 204–217.

Kogel, U., Titz, B., Schlage, W.K., Nury, C., Martin, F., Oviedo, A., Lebrun, S., Elamin, A., Guedj, E., Trivedi, K., et al., 2016. Evaluation of the Tobacco Heating System 2.2. Part 7: systems toxicological assessment of a mentholated version revealed reduced cellular and molecular exposure effects compared with mentholated and non-mentholated cigarette smoke. Regul. Toxicol. Pharmacol. 81 (Suppl. 2), S123–S138.

Lee, C.K., Brown, B.G., Reed, E.A., Lowe, G.D., McKarns, S.C., Fulp, C.W., Coggins, C.R., Ayres, P.H., Doolittle, D.J., 1990. Analysis of cytogenetic effects in bone-marrow cells of rats subchronically exposed to smoke from cigarettes which burn or only heat tobacco. Mutat. Res. 240, 251–257.

Mittelstaedt, R.A., Dobrovolsky, V.N., Revollo, J.R., Pearce, M.G., Wang, Y., Dad, A., McKinzie, P.B., Rosenfeldt, H., Yucesoy, B., Yeager, R., et al., 2019. Evaluation of 4-(methylnitrosamino)-1-(3-pyridyl)-1-butanone (NNK) mutagenicity using in vitro and in vivo Pig-a assays. Mutat. Res. Genet. Toxicol. Environ. Mutagen 837, 65–72.

Moennikes, O., Vanscheeuwijck, P., Friedrichs, B., Anskeit, E., Patskan, G., 2008. Reduced toxicological activity of cigarette smoke by the addition of ammonia magnesium phosphate to the paper of an electrically heated cigarette: subchronic inhalation toxicology. Inhal. Toxicol. 20, 647–663.

Nakamura, T., Ishida, Y., Ainai, K., Nakamura, S., Shirata, S., Murayama, K., Kurimoto, S., Saigo, K., Murashige, R., Tsuda, S., et al., 2015. Genotoxicity-suppressing effect of aqueous extract of Connarus ruber cortex on cigarette smoke-induced micronuclei in mouse peripheral erythrocytes. Gene Environ. Off. J. Jpn. Environ. Mutagen Soc. 37, 17.

National Research Council, 2007. Toxicity Testing in the 21st Century: A Vision and a Strategy. National Academies Press.

OECD, 2009a. Test No. 403: Acute Inhalation Toxicity.

OECD, 2009b. Test No. 436: Acute Inhalation Toxicity – Acute Toxic Class Method.

OECD, 2013. OECD Test No. 488: The Transgenic Somatic and Germ Cell Gene Mutation Assays.

OECD, 2016a. OECD Test No. 474: Mammalian Erythrocyte Micronucleus Test.

OECD, 2016b. OECD Test No. 475: The Mammalian Bone Marrow Chromosomal Aberration Test.

OECD, 2016c. OECD Test No. 489: The In Vivo Mammalian Alkaline Comet Assay.

OECD, 2018a. Test No. 412: Subacute Inhalation Toxicity: 28-Day Study.

OECD, 2018b. Test No. 413: Subchronic Inhalation Toxicity: 90-Day Study.

OECD, 2018c. Test No. 433: Acute Inhalation Toxicity: Fixed Concentration Procedure.

OECD, 2018d. Test No. 451: Carcinogenicity Studies.

OECD, 2018e. Test No. 452: Chronic Toxicity Studies.

OECD, 2018f. Test No. 453: Combined Chronic Toxicity/Carcinogenicity Studies.

Oviedo, A., Lebrun, S., Kogel, U., Ho, J., Tan, W.T., Titz, B., Leroy, P., Vuillaume, G., Bera, M., Martin, F., et al., 2016. Evaluation of the Tobacco Heating System 2.2. Part 6: 90-day OECD 413 rat inhalation study with systems toxicology endpoints demonstrates reduced exposure effects of a mentholated version compared with mentholated and non-mentholated cigarette smoke. Regul. Toxicol. Pharmacol. 81 (Suppl. 2), S93–S122.

Phillips, B., Esposito, M., Verbeeck, J., Boué, S., Iskandar, A., Vuillaume, G., Leroy, P., Krishnan, S., Kogel, U., Utan, A., et al., 2015. Toxicity of aerosols of nicotine and pyruvic acid (separate and combined) in Sprague-Dawley rats in a 28-day OECD 412 inhalation study and assessment of systems toxicology. Inhal. Toxicol. 27, 405–431.

Phillips, B., Titz, B., Kogel, U., Sharma, D., Leroy, P., Xiang, Y., Vuillaume, G., Lebrun, S., Sciuscio, D., Ho, J., et al., 2017. Toxicity of the main electronic cigarette components, propylene glycol, glycerin, and nicotine, in Sprague-Dawley rats in a 90-day OECD inhalation study complemented by molecular endpoints. Food Chem. Toxicol. 109, 315–332.

Phonethepswath, S., Bryce, S.M., Bemis, J.C., Dertinger, S.D., 2008. Erythrocyte-based Pig-a gene mutation assay: demonstration of cross-species potential. Mutat. Res. 657, 122–126.

Renne, R., Wehner, A., Greenspan, B., Deford, H., Ragan, H., Westerberg, R., Buschbom, R., Burger, G., Hayes, A., Suber, R., et al., 1992. 2-week and 13-week inhalation studies of aerosolized glycerol in rats. Inhal. Toxicol. 4, 95–111.

Schaller, J.P., Keller, D., Poget, L., Pratte, P., Kaelin, E., McHugh, D., Cudazzo, G., Smart, D., Tricker, A.R., Gautier, L., et al., 2016. Evaluation of the Tobacco Heating System 2.2. Part 2: chemical composition, genotoxicity, cytotoxicity, and physical properties of the aerosol. Regul. Toxicol. Pharmacol. 81 (Suppl. 2), S27–S47.

Sewer, A., Kogel, U., Talikka, M., Wong, E.T., Martin, F., Xiang, Y., Guedj, E., Ivanov, N.V., Hoeng, J., Peitsch, M.C., 2016. Evaluation of the Tobacco Heating System 2.2 (THS2.2). Part 5: microRNA expression from a 90-day rat inhalation study indicates that exposure to THS2.2 aerosol causes reduced effects on lung tissue compared with cigarette smoke. Regul. Toxicol. Pharmacol. 81 (Suppl. 2), S82–S92.

Suber, R., Deskin, R., Nikiforov, I., Fouillet, X., Coggins, C., 1989. Subchronic nose-only inhalation study of propylene glycol in Sprague-Dawley rats. Food Chem. Toxicol. 27, 573–583.

Taylor, M., Thorne, D., Carr, T., Breheny, D., Walker, P., Proctor, C., Gaca, M., 2018. Assessment of novel tobacco heating product THP1.0. Part 6: a comparative in vitro study using contemporary screening approaches. Regul. Toxicol. Pharmacol. 93, 62–70.

Terpstra, P.M., Teredesai, A., Vanscheeuwijck, P.M., Verbeeck, J., Schepers, G., Radtke, F., Kuhl, P., Gomm, W., Anskeit, E., Patskan, G., 2003. Toxicological evaluation of an electrically heated cigarette. Part 4: subchronic inhalation toxicology. J. Appl. Toxicol. 23, 349—362.

Titz, B., Kogel, U., Martin, F., Schlage, W.K., Xiang, Y., Nury, C., Dijon, S., Baumer, K., Peric, D., Bornand, D., et al., 2018. A 90-day OECD TG 413 rat inhalation study with systems toxicology endpoints demonstrates reduced exposure effects of the aerosol from the carbon heated tobacco product version 1.2 (CHTP1.2) compared with cigarette smoke. II. Systems toxicology assessment. Food Chem. Toxicol. 115, 284—301.

Tweats, D.J., Blakey, D., Heflich, R.H., Jacobs, A., Jacobsen, S.D., Morita, T., Nohmi, T., O'Donovan, M.R., Sasaki, Y.F., Sofuni, T., et al., 2007. Report of the IWGT working group on strategies and interpretation of regulatory in vivo tests I. Increases in micronucleated bone marrow cells in rodents that do not indicate genotoxic hazards. Mutat. Res. 627, 78—91.

US EPA OPP, 2012. US Environmental Protection Agency, Office of Pesticide Programs: Advances in Genetic Toxicology and Integration of In Vivo Testing into Standard Repeat Dose Studies. Guidance statement. https://www.epa.gov/pesticide-science-and-assessing-pesticide-risks/advances-genetic-toxicology-and-integration-vivo.

Van Miert, E., Vanscheeuwijck, P., Meurrens, K., Gomm, W., Terpstra, P.M., 2008. Evaluation of the micronucleus assay in bone marrow and peripheral blood of rats for the determination of cigarette mainstream-smoke activity. Mutat. Res. 652, 131—138.

Waldum, H.L., Nilsen, O.G., Nilsen, T., Rørvik, H., Syversen, V., Sanvik, A.K., Haugen, O.A., Torp, S.H., Brenna, E., 1996. Long-term effects of inhaled nicotine. Life Sci. 58, 1339—1346.

Werley, M.S., Jerome, A.M., Oldham, M.J., 2014. Toxicological evaluation of aerosols of a tobacco extract formulation and nicotine formulation in acute and short-term inhalation studies. Inhal. Toxicol. 26, 207—221.

Werley, M.S., Kirkpatrick, D.J., Oldham, M.J., Jerome, A.M., Langston, T.B., Lilly, P.D., Smith, D.C., McKinney Jr., W.J., 2016a. Toxicological assessment of a prototype e-cigaret device and three flavor formulations: a 90-day inhalation study in rats. Inhal. Toxicol. 28, 22—38.

Werley, M.S., McDonald, P., Lilly, P., Kirkpatrick, D., Wallery, J., Byron, P., Venitz, J., 2011. Non-clinical safety and pharmacokinetic evaluations of propylene glycol aerosol in Sprague-Dawley rats and Beagle dogs. Toxicology 287, 76—90.

Werley, M.S., Miller, J.H., Kane, D.B., Tucker, C.S., McKinney, W.J., Oldham, M.J., 2016b. Prototype e-cigarette and the capillary aerosol generator (CAG) comparison and qualification for use in subchronic inhalation exposure testing. Aerosol. Sci. Technol. 50, 1284—1293.

Wong, E.T., Kogel, U., Veljkovic, E., Martin, F., Xiang, Y., Boue, S., Vuillaume, G., Leroy, P., Guedj, E., Rodrigo, G., et al., 2016. Evaluation of the Tobacco Heating System 2.2. Part 4: 90-day OECD 413 rat inhalation study with systems toxicology endpoints demonstrates reduced exposure effects compared with cigarette smoke. Regul. Toxicol. Pharmacol. 81 (Suppl. 2), S59—S81.

CHAPTER 15

Assessment of ENDPs in Animal Models of Disease

BLAINE W. PHILLIPS • EE TSIN WONG • JUSTYNA SZOSTAK • STÉPHANIE BOUÉ •
ULRIKE KOGEL • KARSTA LUETTICH • WALTER K. SCHLAGE •
PATRICK VANSCHEEUWIJCK • JULIA HOENG • MANUEL C. PEITSCH

15.1 INTRODUCTION

Electronic nicotine delivery products (ENDPs), such as e-vapor products (EVPs) and electrically heated tobacco products (EHTPs), emit significantly lower levels of harmful or potentially harmful constituents (HPHCs) (Chapter 4) and other substances of toxicological concern (Chapters 6 and 7) than cigarettes. According to the ENDP assessment framework (Chapter 3), which is based on the epidemiology of smoking and cessation as well as the fundamental principle of toxicology, this reduction in toxicant emission should lead to a reduction in toxicant exposure and, hence, a reduction in adverse health effects. However, smoking-related diseases generally occur after decades of smoking, and the reduction in excess risk following smoking cessation and, a fortiori, following switching to ENDPs is slow (Chapter 3). Therefore, epidemiological and clinical health outcome studies, based on definitive disease endpoints, that aim to assess the reduction in disease risk associated with switching from cigarette smoking to the use of ENDPs are difficult to execute and will require time (Chapter 3). Therefore, animal models are critical to the comparative evaluation of ENDPs against both continued smoking and cessation within a relatively short timeframe.

A toxicological approach following standardized experimental guidelines is an important first step in comparative evaluation of ENDPs and cigarettes (Chapters 13 and 14). These toxicological studies can be enhanced with systems toxicology—based approaches (Chapter 9) to compare the effects of these products on the mechanisms involved in disease initiation or progression (Chapters 13 and 14). Cigarette smoke (CS) has been linked to development of diseases or pathologies in multiple systems, including many outside of the classically considered diseases of the respiratory system (Office of the Surgeon General, 2014). While animal models are available for many smoking-related diseases, this chapter will focus on chronic obstructive pulmonary disease (COPD), cardiovascular disease (CVD), and lung cancer. The studies summarized hereafter have been conducted within the ENDP assessment program outlined in Chapter 3 and were aimed at collecting data relevant to most events along the causal chain of events linking smoking to disease (CELSD) (Chapter 3) and across most biological mechanisms that are affected by CS.

There are important technical challenges associated with assessment of ENDPs in animal models. As ENDPs are consumed by inhalation, it is important that inhalation is the route of ENDP aerosol administration in any animal model study designed for assessing their in vivo toxicology and effects on smoking-related disease progression. Therefore, it is necessary to generate aerosols that are equivalent to those to which human consumers would be exposed (Chapter 11). The generation of aerosols by using automated smoking machines (for cigarettes, such as the 3R4F reference cigarette), modified machines for EHTPs, or capillary aerosol generators, which produce aerosols similar to those from EVPs, is described in Chapter 12. The aerosols are diluted and then conveyed to exposure chambers, where conscious animals will be either placed in open cage—based whole-body exposure chambers or restrained in individual exposure tubes in a nose-only exposure chamber. Importantly, although both exposure systems are considered to cause stress, the greater restraint associated with nose-only exposure will induce higher stress than whole-body exposure, thus necessitating adequate habituation to the treatment itself as well as adequate sham exposure controls. In addition, certain models might be impacted by exposure-related stress, and it is, therefore, essential to pretest the models and their suitability for inhalation studies.

Toxicological Evaluation of Electronic Nicotine Delivery Products. https://doi.org/10.1016/B978-0-12-820490-0.00024-9

15.2 ANIMAL MODELS OF COPD

COPD is considered to be a major contributor to global mortality and disease burden (Mathers and Loncar, 2006). COPD is a common preventable disease that is characterized by persistent respiratory symptoms and airflow limitation due to airway and/or alveolar abnormalities usually caused by significant exposure to noxious particles or gases (GOLD, 2020). Chronic inflammation is considered to be an important causative mechanism of the structural changes and airway narrowing as well as a contributor to lung parenchymal damage, ultimately resulting in the combined loss of alveolar attachment and changes to the elastic recoil of the lungs (GOLD, 2020). Cigarette smoking is an important causative factor in the development and continued progression of this largely preventable disorder (Rennard and Vestbo, 2006). Importantly, smoking duration and intensity appear to be important predictors of COPD development and progression, with cessation positively influencing the course of the disease and culminating in a lower death rate and symptom severity (Bai et al., 2017) (Chapter 18). Therefore, demonstrating the risk mitigation effects of switching from cigarette smoking to using alternative nicotine delivery devices such as EVPs and EHTPs is of high interest. However, because of the timescale of COPD development and dearth of validated, early predictive biomarkers, many researchers resort to using in vivo models of disease to understand these effects within a reasonable timeframe compared to what can be achieved by long-term clinical studies or epidemiology.

Studies with animal models of COPD, mainly focusing on signs of emphysema, have been conducted by using numerous animal species (mice, rats, pigs, guinea pigs, dogs, and livestock), reviewed in Fricker et al. (2014), Liang and He (2019). Animal model selection will be based on a balance between aspects that are most relevant to the human disease—for example, inflammatory processes and cytokine production, proteolytic imbalance, emphysema, lung function—and ethical as well as logistical concerns—for example, the ability to conduct studies to scale (where small rodent models would have a clear advantage). Therefore, the focus of this discussion will be on mouse models, which are the most commonly used animal models for studying emphysema and COPD.

An important consideration is the strain of mouse to use as a model for smoke-induced COPD studies. Being inbred, it is natural that there might be subtle differences and sensitivities to the induction of COPD or emphysema in different mouse strains. Indeed, high variability in emphysematous changes were noted in a smoke-induced COPD model that used different strains, where AKR/j mice were highly susceptible to the smoke challenge, while, at the other end of the scale, NZWLac/J mice showed relatively poor susceptibility in terms of COPD indications. Other evaluated strains were shown to have intermediate susceptibility (including C57Bl/6 and A/J mice) (Guerassimov et al., 2004). In our laboratory, we have observed consistent development of emphysematous changes following smoke exposure in multiple laboratory mouse strains, including C57Bl/6, $Apoe^{-/-}$, and A/J. The finding that multiple mouse strains are capable of developing smoke-induced emphysema allows the possibility of combining emphysema with other disease modalities in order to optimize the time and resources required for executing a mouse study in COPD. Accordingly, and in line with the 3R principle or animal welfare, we conduct COPD studies in $Apoe^{-/-}$ mice, enabling analysis of additional cardiovascular endpoints (Phillips et al., 2016) (Section 15.3), and in A/J mice to enable analysis of lung cancer endpoints (Stinn et al., 2013a) (Section 15.4).

There are several commonly used mouse models of emphysema categorized in terms of acute (chemically induced), chronically induced, and genetic models of COPD and emphysema, which will be discussed in turn.

15.2.1 Chemically Induced COPD

Early in vivo models of emphysema involved administration of elastase into the lungs by an intranasal or intratracheal route of administration (Snider et al., 1986). Initially conducted mainly with hamsters (Lucey et al., 1998), such studies now more commonly use mice as a test system. The elastase model is used to simulate emphysematous lung tissue destruction, thereby supporting the mechanistic evaluation of this aspect of emphysema. Chemically induced models are also used to study factors that might exacerbate the impact of the elastase administration, such as air pollution (Moreira et al., 2020) or other environmental factors, including CS. In addition, because of the relatively short timeframe needed for chemically induced COPD models (several weeks), they are commonly used to test the efficacy of potentially therapeutic compounds or aerosols.

Following intratracheal delivery of elastase to the lungs, the resulting response develops in separate phases. Initially, there is an inflammatory response, where free lung cell (FLC) numbers in a bronchoalveolar lavage sample are highly elevated 24 h postelastase challenge, although they return to normal or control conditions within 1 week postchallenge (Kawakami et al., 2008). This initial period of inflammation is followed by tissue destruction, for which microcomputed tomography (μCT) measurements of areas of low tissue density are supported by lung morphometric assessment of (for example) mean chord length, bronchiolar attachment, and destructive index to show the progression of tissue destruction for approximately 3 weeks. With similarity to human emphysema, elastase treatment results in nonhomogeneous distribution of affected areas of the lungs.

While this is an interesting model to use for short-term induction of certain aspects of emphysema, there are currently no examples of research using this model to evaluate the impact of exposure to ENDP aerosols. A limited number of articles have studied combinatorial induction with elastase and CS, with the expected outcome that CS exacerbated the histopathological endpoint of emphysema (mean chord length) and caused increased expression of proteolytic enzymes (Rodrigues et al., 2017). Despite this, CS exposure–based induction of COPD in conscious, breathing mice has been the preferred model system for studying the mechanistic aspects of CS exposure.

15.2.2 Genetic Models of COPD

There has been interest in genetic models (mutant as well as transgenic) of COPD for many years, when mice with spontaneous predisposition to the development of COPD-like symptoms first emerged (Perez-Rial et al., 2015; Shapiro, 2007). In more recent times, the most common means of genetic manipulation for inducing symptomatic features of COPD are typically by overexpression of cytokines or proteolytic enzymes in mice (Liang and He, 2019). In many cases, targeted expression strategies have been used, whereby inflammatory cytokines are overexpressed in the lungs, often by using the surfactant protein C promoter (SPC). This approach has been employed for overexpression of TGFβ (transforming growth factor β; SPC–TGFβ construct) (Hardie et al., 1997; Korfhagen et al., 1994) as well as PDGF (platelet-derived growth factor; SPC–PDGF-B) (Hoyle et al., 1999) in the lungs. In both cases, this targeted overexpression of the specific cytokine was associated with hallmark characteristics of COPD, including lung inflammation, increased expression of matrix metalloproteinases (MMPs), and adverse impact on lung function. However, these effects were progressive, in some cases taking 6 months to reach full penetrance in a population of animals. Various mutants have been investigated as susceptible mouse models of COPD features, such as the pallid mouse (C57Bl/6J, pa+/+), which has a severe α1 antitrypsin (αl-AT) deficiency (De Santi et al., 1995;

Martorana et al., 1993), while the C57Bl/6 wildtype strain (particularly female mice) has a mild α1-AT deficiency (Bartalesi et al., 2005). Mechanisms of adaptive immune response can be addressed in the AKR mouse featuring an MHC haplotype with enhanced T-cell response (Guerassimov et al., 2004).

However, these models are more often combined with other more traditional models of COPD, such as the elastase or CS-exposure models, to study the contribution of the impacted gene or pathway in mechanistic studies. Such models are thus less frequently used for studies on toxicological or pharmacological interventions against COPD.

15.2.3 CS-exposure Models of COPD and Emphysema

Cigarette smoking is an important contributing factor to COPD in general and emphysema in particular. It is, therefore, physiologically justifiable that using chronic or subchronic CS exposure to induce emphysematous changes would have the most clinical relevance for testing the mechanisms of COPD development as well as to test potential therapeutic compounds. CS-exposure models of COPD have been used since the 1990s, when guinea pigs were first exposed to CS, with the resultant pathophysiological changes resembling aspects of emphysema (Wright and Churg, 1990, 2002); these studies were then extended to mouse models that responded to CS (Churg and Wright, 2007; March et al., 1999). Of note, rats were less prone to CS-induced emphysema, and Wistar rats appeared to be more sensitive than Fischer F-344 rats (Cendon et al., 1997; Escolar et al., 1995; Ke et al., 2020; March et al., 1999; Xiao et al., 2011). This led to multiple laboratories employing CS (or other noxious aerosol) administration for inducing COPD-like or emphysematous changes to respiratory tract organs, particularly in mice (Schleef et al., 2006; Vlahos and Bozinovski, 2014). Advances in exposure regimens, animal species, and timelines have also improved the outcomes, as factors such as aerosol or smoke concentration, exposure duration per day, and overall length of the study have been progressively optimized (Boue et al., 2013; Phillips et al., 2015; Wong, 2007).

The experimental endpoints in animal models of COPD focus on human-relevant disease indicators, with emphasis on lung inflammation and histopathological findings. Histopathological analysis is particularly important, as it is a way to observe and quantify physical manifestations in the lungs that are linked to lung function changes, which are important for translation to the human disease.

With regard to airway obstruction by small airway remodeling and mucus overproduction—another hallmark of human COPD (Burgel et al., 2011)—guinea pig models have been used preferentially over rat and mouse models (Fricker et al., 2014; Hoang et al., 2016; Ke et al., 2020; Stebbins et al., 2010; Vlahos and Bozinovski, 2015; Wright and Churg, 2010; Xiao et al., 2011).

15.2.3.1 Aerosol administration

When reviewing publications using animal models of COPD, it is always important to consider the technical details of smoke or aerosol generation, method of delivery to the animals, and amount of aerosol sampling conducted in each study. We study CS generated from the 3R4F reference cigarette (University of Kentucky, 2003) as our inductive agent for modeling chronic emphysema development in various mouse models. Aerosol generation is ideally performed by using automated machines in order to ensure stable aerosols that are reproducible from study to study (described in detail in Chapter 12). It is also important that an appropriate exposure chamber is selected for the animals, to ensure reproducible aerosol delivery at all chamber positions, balanced by a reduction in procedural stress (Ansari et al., 2016; Wong, 2007). The use of whole-body exposure chambers may be preferred for two reasons: First, to minimize restraint-related stress, which might impact model performance when using nose-only restraint, and, second, nose-only exposure results in logistic limitations to the study size owing to the technical aspects of loading and observing the animals during the daily exposures (Phillips et al., 2019, 2015). There is, however, precedence for using nose-only exposure in a CS model of emphysema and EVP assessment (Lee et al., 2018). The exposure parameters are also important considerations when using a CS-induced COPD model. The objective is to achieve the target daily dose of CS within the constraints of tolerability to the CS or any of its constituents. We typically use a 4 h/day exposure regimen, with target total particulate matter (TPM) concentrations of up to 750 µg/L in C57Bl/6 mice, corresponding to nicotine concentrations of approximately 35−40 µg/L. Other strains such as $Apoe^{-/-}$ have lower tolerance to CS exposure and are, therefore, exposed for a shorter duration (3 h/day) and to a lower target CS concentration (600 µg/L TPM, with corresponding nicotine concentrations of approximately 30−35 µg/L). The daily exposure protocol consists of four (three) 1-h exposure sessions separated by 30- and 60-min fresh air breaks in order to avoid buildup of excessive carboxyhemoglobin

(COHb) concentrations (Phillips et al., 2015). With such an experimental design, we have observed progressive development of the characteristic clinical manifestations of COPD (mainly markers of emphysema) (Phillips et al., 2015), as assessed by lung inflammation, lung function changes, and histopathological changes.

15.2.3.2 Lung inflammation

Chronic lung inflammation is a major feature of COPD development, where recruitment of both innate and adaptive immune cells is associated with the release of inflammatory cytokines and degradative proteolytic enzymes, contributing to the overall lung tissue destruction associated with the disease (Hoenderdos and Condliffe, 2013). In rodent models, lung inflammation can be evaluated by several different methods. Bronchoalveolar lavage fluid (BALF) may be evaluated for FLC number and composition by determining the differential cell counts, usually by flow cytometry. The remaining cell-free BALF can then be used to assess the concentrations of key inflammatory cytokines or matrix-degrading proteases. Finally, these cell/molecular results are then verified through histopathological assessment of inflammatory cell numbers and composition in the lungs.

For collecting BALF, the test animals are anesthetized and intubated. The lungs are then lavaged (flushed) for up to five cycles with 1 mL of a buffer that will support FLC viability (for example, phosphate-buffered saline [PBS] with bovine serum albumin, fetal calf serum, or just PBS for cell-free BALF analysis) (Boue et al., 2013; Van Hoecke et al., 2017). The resulting BALF can then be processed by centrifugation to recover the FLCs (pellet) for differential inflammatory cell count, and the cell-free BALF (supernatant) is used to quantify inflammatory cytokines or proteolytic enzymes.

FLCs in a healthy mouse will be mainly composed of resident alveolar macrophages and only a small number of other cell types, such as neutrophils and lymphocytes. CS exposure results in increased numbers of all types of inflammatory cells in the lung interstitium and bronchioloalveolar luminal space—the so-called FLC (macrophages, neutrophils, and lymphocytes)—although with a net relative increase in neutrophils and lymphocytes. This increase in the number of inflammatory cells is accompanied by a corresponding increase in the release of inflammatory cytokines and proteolytic enzymes. Therefore, analysis of FLCs and cell-free BALF collectively can indicate the severity of the inflammatory response and provide a mechanistic understanding for disease progression linked to aerosol exposure or other stimuli. For example, the presence or upregulation of MMPs or other proteolytic enzymes may explain the destructive process or emphysema development (Elkington and Friedland, 2006).

As routinely observed in murine models of COPD, CS exposure results in an increase in the number of inflammatory cells in BALF after just 1 month, with the total FLC counts increasing from a baseline level of approximately $3-4 \times 10^5$ cells to as high as 25×10^5 cells after CS exposure, representing an approximately sevenfold increase (Phillips et al., 2016, 2015). The pulmonary inflammatory response is primarily driven by an influx of neutrophils, though there are also exposure-dependent increases in lymphocytes and macrophages. This is associated with an increase in the concentrations of many inflammatory cytokines and mediators. We have observed increased levels of various inflammatory analytes and mediators, with consistently elevated levels of myeloperoxidase, macrophage inflammatory proteins (MIP)-1, -2, and -3, monocyte chemoattractant proteins (MCP)-1, -2, and -5, interleukins, granulocyte—macrophage colony stimulating factor (GM-CSF), and interferon gamma (IFNγ). Finally, MMP-2 and MMP-9, key members of the MMP family of proteolytic enzymes, along with tissue inhibitor of metalloproteinases 1 (TIMP-1), a major inhibitor, are also consistently elevated in CS-exposed mice of various strains, including C57Bl/6 (Phillips et al., 2015), $Apoe^{-/-}$ (Phillips et al., 2019, 2016), and A/J mice (Stinn et al., 2013b). These changes are indicative of disruption of the protease—inhibitor balance, tipping toward tissue destruction.

15.2.3.3 Lung tissue changes
Histopathological evaluation of the lung tissue is the key endpoint for evaluating emphysematous changes in animal models. Important for accurate histopathological assessment of the lungs is the careful preparation of this fragile tissue. During lung preparation, physical isolation of the lungs results in their collapse, as the pleural cavity is breached during dissection. Quantitative evaluation of the characteristic features of lung damage due to emphysema requires inflation of the lungs to constant pressure during histological preparation (Fawell and Lewis, 1971; Hsia et al., 2010; Muhlfeld and Ochs, 2013; Ochs and Muhlfeld, 2013). This process is complicated by any treatment-related physiological effect on the elastance or compliance of the lung tissue, which can result in overinflation (emphysema) or underinflation (fibrosis) of the lungs at fixed pressure. Additional technical effects which may impact the evaluation of lung tissue is the shrinkage due to the processing with organic solvents for paraffin block embedding (Schneider and Ochs, 2014).

Histopathological evaluation of the lungs can be conducted by several methods. Pathological evaluation by a certified pathologist provides an overall assessment of the degree of emphysematous changes in the tissue, including semiquantitative, subjective scoring of tissue destruction and inflammatory findings with an ordinal scale (e.g., from 0 [no finding] to 5 [severe alteration]). This evaluation is performed in a blinded fashion (without knowledge of the exposure status of the specimen); however, an initial calibration can be done with sections from the sham control group and a high exposure group, to adjust the scores to the full range of effects (Fig. 15.1). In addition, these findings may be supported by morphometric analysis of the lungs, traditionally including such measurements as mean chord intercept length (MCL), destructive index, and bronchiolar attachment. In particular, MCL has been commonly used as a finding and is typically measured by drawing an overlay of parallel lines over a representative section of the lungs (Knudsen et al., 2010). The intercept points (where the lines cross an area of parenchyma) are then marked, and the average distance between parenchymal areas are quantified, thereby indirectly measuring the average length of the spaces between the parenchyma.

MCL is a volume-dependent morphometric parameter, in that the results are affected by any factor that impacts lung volume, be it treatment-related or a technical aspect of histological preparation (as described above). To circumvent these technical issues, additional methods have been developed to supplement the classical methods of lung morphometry. For example, the dissector method has been used to directly measure the destruction of parenchymal regions. This includes quantification of parenchymal, airspace, and alveolar volumes and alveolar number. Collectively, these measurements constitute a volume-independent means for comparing normal and potentially diseased tissue (Muhlfeld et al., 2015; Ochs, 2014).

15.2.3.4 Lung function
Functional measurements are essential for confirming that the molecular, cellular, and histopathological changes described in the previous subsections are associated with changes in lung function, which is the primary endpoint used for evaluating COPD in humans. In humans, spirometry parameters—such as the reduction in forced expiratory volume during 1 s (FEV$_1$)—are used to assess lung function, and changes in these parameters are associated with COPD. However, such a test, involving forced expiration, is not possible in rodent systems. Nevertheless, changes to key lung parameters can be analyzed by studying pressure—volume

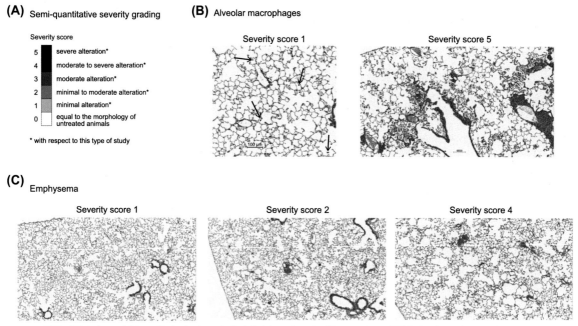

(A) Semi-quantitative severity grading

Severity score

5	severe alteration*
4	moderate to severe alteration*
3	moderate alteration*
2	minimal to moderate alteration*
1	minimal alteration*
0	equal to the morphology of untreated animals

* with respect to this type of study

(B) Alveolar macrophages

Severity score 1   Severity score 5

(C) Emphysema

Severity score 1   Severity score 2   Severity score 4

FIG. 15.1 Lung histopathological analysis following chronic CS exposure. **(A)** Typical 5-point scoring scale used for pathological severity scoring. **(B)** Representative scoring images for normal (score 0) and severe (score 5) increase in alveolar macrophages. **(C)** Representative images depicting severity scores for lung emphysema (scores 1, 2, and 4, respectively).

(P—V) relationships in the lungs of sedated rodents by using controlled ventilation (flow and volumes) and sensors for determining the intrapulmonary pressure during these maneuvers. Tissue destruction is associated with general loss of resistance and increased elastance. The simplest maneuvers (snapshot perturbations) that reflect the elastance and resistance of the lungs are controlled inflation/deflation cycles at fixed flow rates. More sophisticated measurements of lung function will evaluate parameters of the deep lungs and lower bronchioles by using adjusted flow rates (primewave-8 modeling) to provide information about the peripheral loss of elastance in the airways and lung tissue. The overall functioning and tonicity of the lungs may be summarized by measuring a net P—V relationship— that is, by evaluating, in a maneuver, the relationship between the volume of air and a progressively increasing pressure up to that corresponding to a 30-cm water column. As the pressure increases, emphysematous lungs with reduced elastance will have increased volume capacity relative to healthy lungs. This results in a leftward and upward shift in the overall PV loop, which is highly characteristic of emphysematous tissue (Vanoirbeek et al., 2010).

In our studies, the pulmonary inflammation caused by 3R4F smoke exposure was accompanied by emphysematous changes, as reflected by lung function parameters such as changes in elastance and resistance and the characteristic upward—leftward shifts in the PV loops. These changes were fairly mild after 1 month and become progressively more pronounced until stabilizing after approximately 5 months of exposure. These findings are consistent with the finding in the elastase chemically induced emphysema model, where similar changes to lung function parameters were noted (Vanoirbeek et al., 2010).

15.2.3.5 Systems toxicology

The effects of inhaled substances on the respiratory tract can be further evaluated at the mechanistic level by a deep analysis of systems toxicology data (Chapter 9). Chronic CS exposure is consistently associated with changes in both protein and mRNA levels in tissues throughout the respiratory tract (nasal epithelia and lung tissue) (Ansari et al., 2016; Elamin et al., 2016; Phillips et al., 2019). Transcriptional changes can be mapped onto carefully curated transcriptional networks (Hoeng et al., 2012) (Chapter 9); this process has consistently revealed that the majority of transcriptional effects of CS exposure lie within the inflammatory networks (>50%). Also represented, though to a lesser extent, were networks defining cell fate, tissue repair and angiogenesis, and cell stress (Phillips et al., 2016, 2015). This highly sensitive molecular methodology is highly confirmatory of the apical changes observed in the lungs following CS exposure, all consistent with the development and progression of emphysematous lesions.

15.2.4 Postexposure Recovery (Cessation) in the CS-induced Model of COPD

An important application of rodent CS exposure models is the study of the effects of smoking cessation and, thereby, modeling of the biological processes that might occur when human smokers quit smoking. Such studies would include not only a long-term CS exposure group but also a cessation group, where, after a certain time, CS exposure is replaced with fresh air exposure.

We have included cessation groups in multiple studies (Phillips et al., 2019, 2016, 2015) to demonstrate the biological consequence of cessation compared with that of continued CS exposure. There are certain endpoints which show rapid recovery upon cessation, with the CS-induced effects returning to or approaching baseline (sham control) levels within the first or second month of cessation. This notably includes rapid recovery of most lung inflammation endpoints, with the exception of the histologically observed pigmented alveolar nests, which persist for up to 13 months following cessation (Stinn et al., 2013a). The total FLC counts typically return to control levels within 3 months of cessation, with neutrophils being cleared more rapidly than lymphocytes (Phillips et al., 2016). These findings are further confirmed by the reestablishment of basal levels of inflammatory cytokines and matrix modulatory enzymes in the cell-free BALF. However, other endpoints show slower or even no recovery (persistence) following cessation of CS exposure. For instance, the emphysema score, assessed during histopathological evaluation, neither worsens nor recovers to the control (untreated group) levels after the point of cessation (Phillips et al., 2019, 2016, 2015). Therefore, the CS-induced emphysematous changes in the lungs appear to be largely irreversible. Yet, emphysematous changes did no longer worsen when the animals were switched from CS to fresh air. This persistence of emphysematous changes induced by CS exposure was also observed in functional tests, where the changes in lung elastance and resistance only partially recovered and did not reach sham control levels even 6 months after switching from CS exposure to fresh air (Phillips et al., 2016). Previous studies in A/J mice also showed a lower number of inflammatory cells in BALF

upon 8 weeks of cessation after CS exposure for 20 weeks. However, the airway enlargement, lung function effects, and pigmented macrophages in the lung tissue sections persisted even after the 8-week cessation period (Braber et al., 2010). Overall, these findings are consistent with clinical findings suggesting the persistence of irreversible changes in alveolar enlargement and emphysema following periods of smoking abstinence (Jeffery, 2001; Saetta et al., 2001).

Importantly, animal studies that include a cessation group provide an important benchmark—cessation is the gold standard for ENDP assessment studies (Chapter 3)—for ENDP switching studies, where, instead of switching to fresh air, the animals are switched to the aerosol of an ENDP. Thereby, the effects of switching from CS to ENDP aerosol exposure can be compared with continued CS exposure and benchmarked against cessation, as outlined in Chapter 3 (Fig. 3.1 in Section 3.2.1).

15.2.5 Effects of ENDP Aerosols on Emphysema

Currently, the majority of studies evaluating the effects of ENDP aerosols on lung emphysema development are using the CS-induced model of disease development in mice. We have used this model to examine the pulmonary effects of chronic exposure (ranging from 6 to 8 months) to two subcategories of heated tobacco products (HTPs): an EHTP, the Tobacco Heating System 2.2 (THS) (Phillips et al., 2016) and a carbon heated tobacco product (CHTP) (Phillips et al., 2019, 2015). The pulmonary effects of EVP aerosol exposure were also studied in this model (Lee et al., 2018; Madison et al., 2019; Olfert et al., 2018).

The effects of ENDP aerosol exposure are generally compared with those of CS exposure (from a reference cigarette such as 3R4F) and fresh air controls (Fig. 15.2A). When executing studies with multiple types of products (cigarettes and ENDPs), it is important to normalize the exposures in order to effectively compare the disease endpoints. For experiments conducted in our laboratory, exposures are normalized on the basis of nicotine content (with target nicotine concentrations ranging from 29 to 34 µg/L in recent studies). The results are then evaluated on the basis of several important comparisons: First, the effects of ENDP aerosol exposure are compared with those of CS and sham (fresh air) exposure. This means that the results may be interpreted in terms of risk reduction potential relative to CS exposure or the potential to cause risk relative to the control (comparison with sham control). Second, additional groups may be included to examine the effects of switching from CS to an ENDP aerosol or fresh air, as described above (Section 15.2.4).

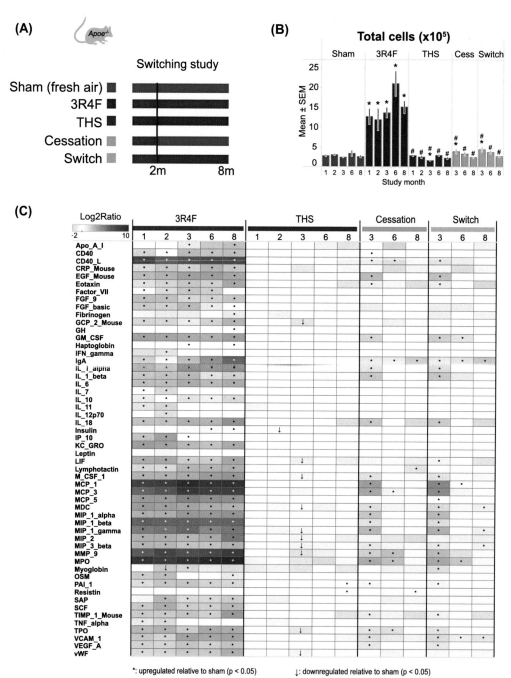

FIG. 15.2 Inflammation assessment in *Apoe*⁻/⁻ mice in a switching study with THS. A. Study design for a typical chronic exposure study, including cessation and switching arms. B. Total free lung cells in BALF collected at months 1, 2, 3, 4, 6, and 8 post-exposure. Statistics depicted as *$P < 0.05$ compared with the sham groups and #$P < 0.05$ compared with the 3R4F group. C. Multianalyte profiling showing relative protein levels of inflammatory cytokines in each of the treatment groups. The color intensity corresponds to the fold difference in protein levels relative to the sham (fresh air)-exposed group at each time point. (Adapted from Phillips, B., Veljkovic, E., Boue, S., Schlage, W.K., Vuillaume, G., Martin, F., et al., 2016. An 8-month systems toxicology inhalation/cessation study in Apoe⁻/⁻ mice to investigate cardiovascular and respiratory exposure effects of a candidate modified risk tobacco product, THS 2.2, compared with conventional cigarettes. Toxicol. Sci. 151 (2), 462–464.)

15.2.5.1 Lung inflammation

Lung inflammation, a key driver of emphysema, is an important early indicator of the potential for exposure-related disease causation. In contrast to CS exposure, exposure to nicotine-matched HTP aerosols led to consistently low levels of lung inflammation across our studies (Phillips et al., 2019, 2016) (Fig. 15.2B and C). Irrespective of which HTP was evaluated, exposure to their aerosols did not affect the number or composition of BALF FLCs relative to sham control. Similar results have been reported in studies in which mice were exposed to EVP aerosols (Lee et al., 2018; Madison et al., 2019). These studies showed that continuous exposure to EVP aerosols had minimal impact on lung inflammation, although exposure-related effects were described for macrophages and attributed to exposure-induced changes in lipid metabolism in one study with EVP aerosol (Madison et al., 2019; Olfert et al., 2018).

15.2.5.2 Lung tissue changes and function

In our studies, the absence of inflammatory response to HTP aerosol exposure was accompanied by minimal lung tissue (histopathological) or lung function changes. The histopathological and morphological findings in HTP aerosol–exposed animals were closely aligned with the scores and measurements noted in sham-exposed animals (Fig. 15.3A). The PV loops following chronic exposure to HTPs were similar to those of fresh air–exposed animals; in contrast, CS exposure caused a characteristic upward–leftward shift in the PV loop associated with emphysema (Fig. 15.3B). Similarly, Olfert and coauthors (Olfert et al., 2018) showed that EVP aerosol exposure did not lead to lung tissue (histopathological) changes or negative effects on respiratory physiology.

There are a limited number of published results in which some degree of emphysematous changes have been observed following exposure to EVP aerosols. In one study (Reinikovaite et al., 2018), Sprague Dawley rats exposed to aerosols of an e-cigarette (in two daily exposure blocks over a 5-week study duration) showed a degree of tissue destruction (airspace enlargement and loss of peripheral vasculature). A reference group that received subcutaneously administered nicotine also exhibited airway destruction, though to a lesser extent than the aerosol-exposed animals (all relative to fresh air controls) (Reinikovaite et al., 2018), indicating a potentially systemic effect of nicotine rather than an acute inflammatory process triggered in the lungs. These results are difficult to interpret, as the actual aerosol concentrations of nicotine and other constituents in the exposure chambers were not provided. Garcia-Arcos and colleagues exposed A/J mice for 1 h per day to EVP carrier aerosol

(composed of propylene glycol [PG] and vegetable glycerin [VG]) with or without nicotine (Garcia-Arcos et al., 2016). In this study, animals exposed to the nicotine-containing aerosol, but not those exposed to the carrier aerosol, exhibited a higher mean linear intercept than the animals in the fresh air group. Changes in lung inflammation (restricted to the nicotine-containing aerosol group) were noted at the 14-day time point but were not different from those in sham or carrier aerosol groups at the 4-month time point. Finally, in another study, a sex difference was noted in C57Bl/6 mice whole-body exposed to an e-liquid aerosol for 2 h/day for 3 days. While there was a minimal effect on FLC counts in general, only female mice showed a higher neutrophil count (Wang et al., 2019). These results are not in agreement with those obtained in our and other laboratories. Indeed, we observed neither lung inflammation nor histopathological changes in Sprague Dawley rats exposed to e-liquid aerosols (OECD TG413 study) with or without nicotine (Phillips et al., 2017). We also did not observe lung inflammation or lung tissue changes in A/J mice exposed to e-liquid aerosols (Wong et al., in preparation) or in C57Bl/6 or $Apoe^{-/-}$ mice exposed to HTP aerosols (Phillips et al., 2019, 2016, 2015), even after up to 8 months of exposure. The inflammation might, therefore, reflect an acute inflammatory response which is detectable in short-term exposure (3 days) but not present in extended exposure periods of up to 8 months.

The variability of lung inflammation results reported in the literature might, in part, be due to technical differences in aerosol generation and delivery. Indeed, exposure duration and aerosol concentrations in the inhalation chambers will have profound effects on endpoint severity and must be carefully considered when comparing results across studies. ENDPs might be particularly sensitive to the technical aspects of aerosol delivery, as differences in aerosol generation methodology may lead to certain contaminants such as metals (from metal heater coils) and aldehydes (from thermal degradation of e-liquids) being delivered to the animals. Furthermore, it is challenging to deliver reproducible and stable aerosols by using commercial e-cigarette devices, and there are more adequate methodologies for this purpose (Chapter 12).

15.2.6 Conclusions for COPD

The mouse model of emphysema has limitations, particularly as it may only reflect the early stages of human COPD resembling the low GOLD grades (Churg and Wright, 2007) and does not take into account the multiple exacerbations (mostly by bacterial and viral infections) that usually drive the worsening of human COPD (Brown and Braman, 2020; Higham et al.,

(A)

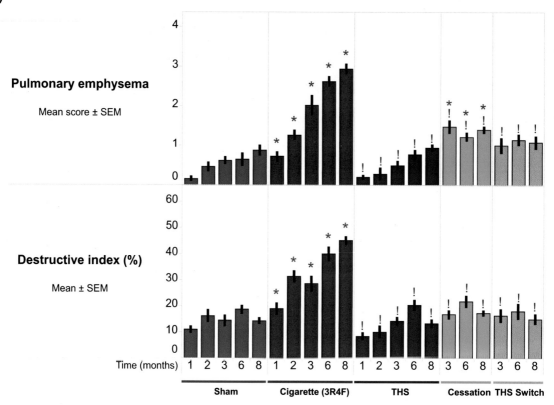

Pulmonary emphysema

Mean score ± SEM

Destructive index (%)

Mean ± SEM

Time (months)   1 2 3 6 8   1 2 3 6 8   1 2 3 6 8   3 6 8   3 6 8

Sham   Cigarette (3R4F)   THS   Cessation   THS Switch

(B)

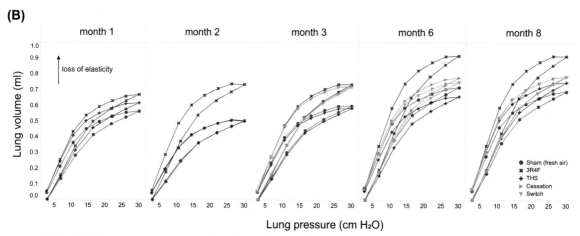

FIG. 15.3 Emphysema assessment in an *Apoe*$^{-/-}$ switching study with THS. (A) Histopathological scores for lung emphysema and destructive index following blinded assessment by a board-certified pathologist. (B) Pressure–volume relationships were assessed by using flexiVent respirator equipment (Scireq, Montreal, Canada). Inflation and deflation cycles were graphed for each treatment group. *, $p < 0.05$ compared with the sham groups, !, $p < 0.05$ significant versus 3R4F groups. *SEM*, standard error of the mean; *THS*, tobacco heating system 2.2. (Adapted from Phillips, B., Veljkovic, E., Boue, S., Schlage, W.K., Vuillaume, G., Martin, F., et al., 2016. An 8-month systems toxicology inhalation/cessation study in Apoe$^{-/-}$ mice to investigate cardiovascular and respiratory exposure effects of a candidate modified risk tobacco product, THS 2.2, compared with conventional cigarettes. Toxicol. Sci. 151 (2), 462–464.)

2019). Nevertheless, animal models of COPD and emphysema remain an important means to study the mechanisms of emphysema development and progression and to assess the effects of ENDP aerosol exposure in comparison with those of CS exposure.

We have shown that chronic CS exposure (3R4F exposure, 5 days per week for up to 8 months) leads to reproducible effects across different mouse strains and similar endpoint severities in C57Bl/6, $Apoe^{-/-}$, and A/J mice. CS exposure resulted in lung inflammation, reflected by elevated cell counts, increased inflammatory mediator levels in BALF, and upregulation of inflammatory transcription networks (detected through systems toxicology analyses). This chronic CS-induced lung inflammation led to emphysematous changes in the lungs, identified through histopathological assessment and further supported by stereological analysis of several parameters of lung morphometry. These histopathological changes were reflected by lung function changes, highlighted by a characteristic upward—leftward shift in the PV loops. In contrast, exposure to HTP aerosols did not cause notable abnormalities in the lungs relative to sham exposure. Importantly, switching from CS to an EHTP aerosol exposure resulted in recovery of lung inflammation, stabilization of the histopathological findings, and arrest of the decline in lung function from the time of switching. These results were similar to those induced by discontinuation of CS exposure. Furthermore, exposure to EVP aerosols did not lead to lung inflammation, lung tissue changes, or lung function changes in several mouse studies. These results, which are coherent along the CELSD (Chapter 3), indicate that ENDP aerosols are less likely to cause emphysema and COPD than CS.

15.3 ANIMAL MODELS OF CVD

15.3.1 Introduction

Smoking is an important modifiable risk factor for the development of CVDs such as coronary artery disease, stable angina, acute coronary syndromes, sudden death syndrome, stroke, peripheral vascular disease, congestive heart failure, erectile dysfunction, and aortic aneurysms via initiation and progression of atherosclerosis (Daiber et al., 2017). The toxicants in CS cause chronic oxidative stress, vascular inflammation, and endothelial dysfunction, the critical drivers of CVD (Carnevale et al., 2016; Tayyarah and Long, 2014). Atherosclerosis remains asymptomatic until the atherosclerotic plaque becomes large enough to obstruct the lumen and cause ischemic pain. This may further escalate to the atherosclerotic plaque rupturing, causing myocardial infarction, stroke, or peripheral artery disease (Blankstein et al., 2019; Daiber et al., 2017; De Leon et al., 2014; Geovanini and Libby, 2018). Accumulation and internalization of cholesterol-rich, apolipoprotein B-containing lipoproteins in the intima represent the earliest step of atherosclerosis. In the intima, the oxidation process leads to lipoprotein modifications and activation of proinflammatory signaling. The activated endothelium expresses increasing levels of adhesive molecules such as vascular cell adhesion protein 1 (VCAM-1) and intercellular adhesion molecule 1 (ICAM-1), which recruit circulating immune cells such as monocytes and T-cells. Within the intima, monocytes differentiate into macrophages and ingest modified lipoproteins, becoming cholesterol-laden foam cells (Libby et al., 2011). At this stage, the release of inflammatory molecules increases and potentiates the inflammation mediated by immune cells in the arterial wall. The inflammatory signals degrade the extracellular matrix, thus increasing plaque vulnerability and increasing the eventual risk of rupture, leading to platelet aggregation, blood coagulation, and thrombus formation (Libby et al., 2011).

15.3.2 Cardiovascular Risk Assessment in the Regulatory Framework

Atherosclerosis plaque formation, an important indicator of CVD, occurs through a complex mechanism that requires endothelial cells, inflammatory cells, as well as smooth muscle cells. Currently, there are no available in vitro models that can recapitulate the complex interactions involved in atherosclerosis, such as complex mixed cultures of endothelial cells, smooth muscle cells, and inflammatory cells. Therefore, it is challenging to assess the relative effects of ENDP aerosols and CS exposure on atherosclerosis. Nevertheless, several in vitro systems that represent the key mechanisms involved in atherosclerosis can be used to overcome some of these limitations. For instance, in vitro models based on endothelial cell monolayer cultures as well as more complex models including a novel human microvessel-on-a-chip model can be used to study endothelial dysfunction, cell adhesion, and oxidative stress (Navab et al., 1988; Poussin et al., 2015, 2018; Robert et al., 2013) (Chapter 13). However, animal models of CVD constitute the best means for assessing atherosclerosis plaque development in a fully functional and complex system.

Inhalation toxicology studies conducted in accordance with widely accepted testing guidelines, such as those described in Chapter 14, enable comparison of the effects of ENDP aerosols with those of CS on both respiratory tract and systemic tissues and organs, including the heart. These studies, however, do not address disease development. In the context of CVD, and more particularly atherosclerosis, in vivo animal models subjected to chronic CS or ENDP aerosol exposure are essential to demonstrate the causal molecular and biological links between exposure and disease outcomes. The $Apoe^{-/-}$ mouse model of atherosclerosis is particularly suited for evaluation of ENDPs. This model has been established and widely applied for investigating atherosclerosis development and treatment. In the context of ENDP assessment, this animal model allows comparison of the effects of CS and ENDP aerosol exposure on atherosclerosis development, cardiovascular function, and oxidative stress (Lo Sasso et al., 2016). As described earlier (Section 15.2), it is also suitable for comparing the effects of inhaled CS and ENDP aerosols on lung inflammation, emphysematous changes to the lung tissue, and lung function in the same study.

15.3.3 Animal Models of Atherosclerosis

Atherosclerosis in humans is a complex disease, and numerous risk factors, including hypertension, diabetes, and aging, could contribute positively to atherosclerosis progression through endothelial dysfunction and immunometabolic dysregulation. For studying the molecular mechanisms that drive disease progression, mouse models that mimic the human pathophysiology have been engineered (Fig. 15.4). Indeed, wild-type mice do not develop atherosclerosis and, therefore, require genetic modification and/or supplementation with high-fat diet to recapitulate key aspects of the human disease (Emini Veseli et al., 2017).

15.3.3.1 Animal models of dyslipidemia for study of atherosclerosis

High levels of circulating plasma low-density lipoprotein cholesterol (LDL-C), very-low-density lipoprotein cholesterol (VLDL-C), and triglycerides and low levels of high-density lipoprotein cholesterol (HDL-C) are required for atherosclerosis development. To mimic human hypercholesterolemia in mouse models, dietary or genetic adaptations are necessary because of several aspects of mouse physiology that make them refractory to spontaneous atherosclerosis. In mice, cholesterol circulation is predominantly based on HDLs. In addition, mice lack the gene encoding the cholesteryl ester transfer protein (CETP), which is associated with low VLDL-C and LDL-C levels. Consequently, most wild-type mouse strains are resistant to dyslipidemia and, thereby, afforded protection from atherosclerosis. Dietary manipulations have, therefore, been developed to generate mouse models that present a proatherogenic lipid profile similar to that in humans.

In comparison to the BALB/c and C3H3 strains, C57Bl/6 mice present a reduced level of HDL-C, which makes them a suitable background model for dyslipidemia. The C57BL/6 strain was used by Paigen and collaborators to evaluate the effect of the lipid components of the diet on atherosclerosis and plasma lipids (Paigen et al., 1985). They showed that 0.5% and 1% of cholesterol and 0.1% and 0.5% of cholic acid administered separately did not cause atherosclerotic lesions. However, a mixed diet containing 1% cholesterol and 0.5% cholic acid increased the development of small fatty streak lesions in the proximal aorta, which was correlated with the percentage of saturated fatty acid content in the fat source (diet) and inversely correlated with the quantity of monounsaturated fatty acids (Getz and Reardon, 2006; Nishina et al., 1990, 1993; Paigen et al., 1985).

In addition to dietary modification, genetic engineering strategies have been employed to enhance dyslipidemia. The most commonly used models were generated through deletion of the genes encoding apolipoprotein E ($Apoe^{-/-}$) or the low-density lipoprotein receptor ($Ldlr^{-/-}$) (Schreyer et al., 1998).

APOE is part of the structure of the chylomicron remnants VLDL and HDL, and it binds to the LDLR, VLDL receptor (VLDLR), and LDLR-related protein in the liver to facilitate the clearance of plasma chylomicrons and VLDL remnants. Genetic deletion of APOE in mice, therefore, results in a decrease in lipoprotein clearance, causing accumulation of cholesterol in plasma (Getz and Reardon, 2016; Lee et al., 2018; Lo Sasso et al., 2016). $Apoe^{-/-}$ knockout mice have higher total plasma cholesterol levels than wild-type mice, with the concentrations in $Apoe^{-/-}$ mice ranging from 400 to 600 mg/dL, in contrast to a range of 75–110 mg/dL in wild-type mice (fed a standard chow diet) (Fig. 15.4). The elevated plasma cholesterol level has the consequence of hypercholesterolemia under normal diet, resulting in the development of spontaneous atherosclerotic lesions (Nakashima et al., 1994) as well as hypercholesterolemia and hypertriglyceridemia (Huszar et al., 2000; Knouff et al., 2004; Plump et al., 1992; Powell-Braxton et al., 1998; Schreyer et al., 1998; Van Ree et al., 1994). Providing $Apoe^{-/-}$ mice with a high-cholesterol diet further increases their plasma cholesterol levels above 1000 mg/dL, thus driving an extensive and accelerated atherosclerosis development process. $Apoe^{-/-}$ mice have a different lipoprotein profile from humans, because the majority of plasma cholesterol is carried by VLDL and chylomicron particles, whereas, in humans, cholesterol is mainly transported by LDL. Another limitation of this mouse model is that its stable characteristics of

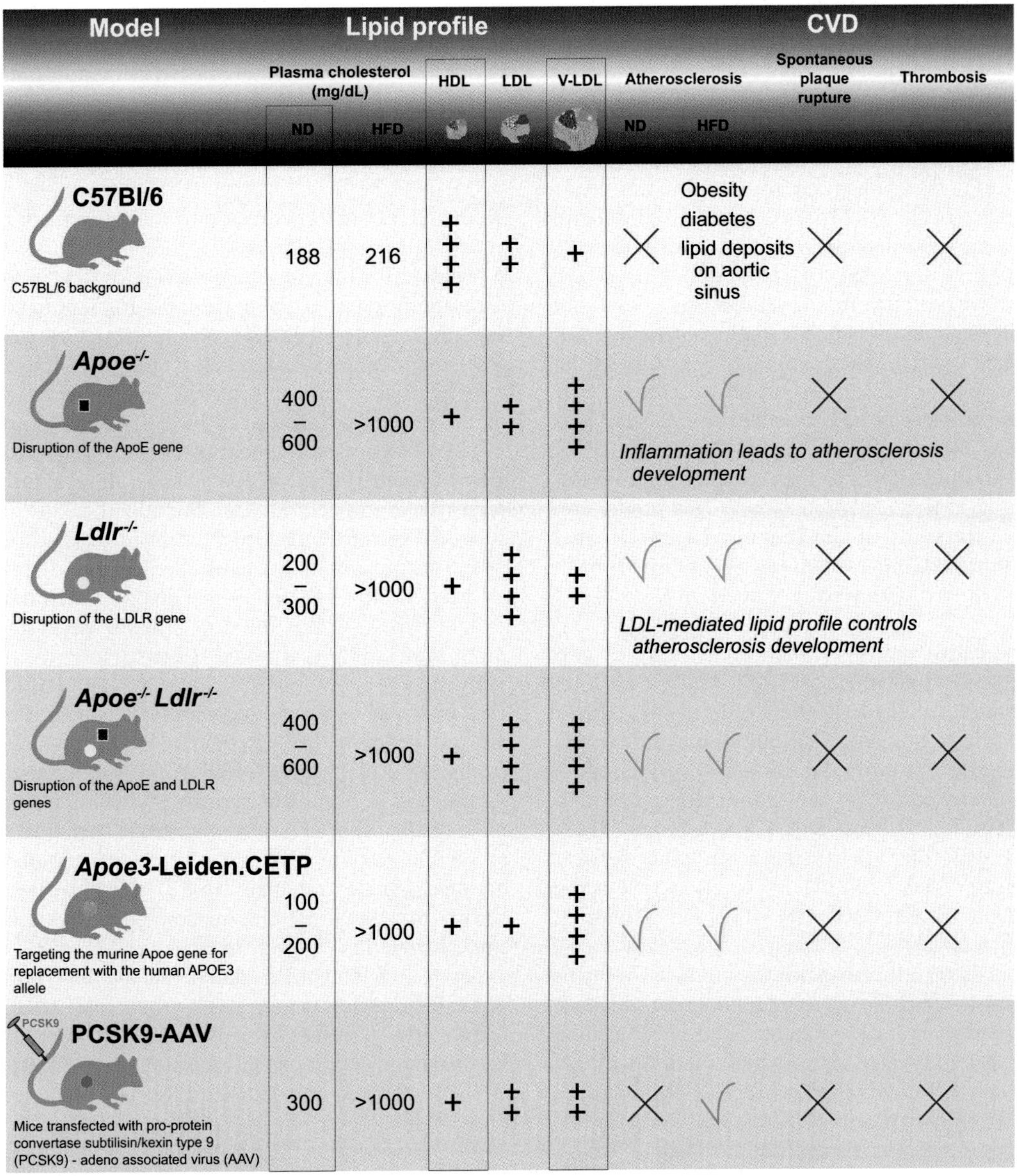

Model	Plasma cholesterol (mg/dL)		HDL	LDL	V-LDL	Atherosclerosis		Spontaneous plaque rupture	Thrombosis
	ND	HFD				ND	HFD		
C57Bl/6 — C57BL/6 background	188	216	++++	++	+	Obesity diabetes lipid deposits on aortic sinus		✗	✗
Apoe⁻ᐟ⁻ — Disruption of the ApoE gene	400–600	>1000	+	++	++++	✓	✓	✗	✗
						Inflammation leads to atherosclerosis development			
Ldlr⁻ᐟ⁻ — Disruption of the LDLR gene	200–300	>1000	+	+++	++	✓	✓	✗	✗
						LDL-mediated lipid profile controls atherosclerosis development			
Apoe⁻ᐟ⁻ Ldlr⁻ᐟ⁻ — Disruption of the ApoE and LDLR genes	400–600	>1000	+	+++	+++	✓	✓	✗	✗
Apoe3-Leiden.CETP — Targeting the murine Apoe gene for replacement with the human APOE3 allele	100–200	>1000	+	+	+++	✓	✓	✗	✗
PCSK9-AAV — Mice transfected with pro-protein convertase subtilisin/kexin type 9 (PCSK9) - adeno associated virus (AAV)	300	>1000	+	++	++	✗	✓	✗	✗

FIG. 15.4 Lipid profile in mouse models of atherosclerosis. *HFD*, high-fat diet; *ND*, normal diet.

atherosclerotic lesions differ from those in humans. In *Apoe*⁻ᐟ⁻ mice, there is no apparent thrombosis or vascular occlusion upon plaque rupture or erosion, as these lesions are repaired by overgrowth with another intimal layer, as observed in histological sections of older plaques (Smith and Breslow, 1997). The same

limitation also applies to the other murine atherosclerosis models (Fig. 15.4).

The *Ldlr* knockout mouse (*Ldl*⁻ᐟ⁻) is another commonly used model for studying atherosclerosis. LDLR, a membrane receptor located on the surface of many cell types, mediates endocytosis of circulating

LDL. Similar to APOE deletion, genetic deletion of LDLR increases the cholesterol levels to 200–300 mg/dL on chow diet and to about 1000 mg/dL on an atherogenic diet (Fig. 15.4). The elevated lipid levels in plasma lead to the development of atherosclerotic lesions in the proximal aorta at early stages and along the distal aorta at more advanced stages (Ishibashi et al., 1994; Tangirala et al., 1995). As in humans, cholesterol in $Ldlr^{-/-}$ mice is transported by LDL particles (Defesche, 2004). In humans, over 600 mutations of the $Ldlr$ gene have been reported, several of them that cause familial hypercholesterolemia, a frequent genetic disorder associated with high levels of LDL-C and atherosclerosis development (Goldstein and Brown, 2001).

Another suitable model for atherosclerosis study is the $Apoe^{-/-}$*3-Leiden.CETP mouse line (Fig. 15.4), which has been designed to carry a mutation from human familial dysbetalipoproteinemia. This model presents overexpression of the human cholesteryl ester transfer protein (CETP), which causes a drastic shift in the distribution of cholesterol from HDL-C to VLDL-C/LDL-C.

An alternative strategy, developed recently by two different groups, makes use of $PCSK9$-AAV mouse lines (Bjorklund et al., 2014; Roche-Molina et al., 2015). These mice have no genetic modifications and express APOE and LDLR at normal levels. However, introduction of a mouse or human gain-of-function proprotein convertase subtilisin/kexin type 9PCSK9 mutant leads to an increase in total plasma cholesterol (over 1000 mg/dL), VLDL-C, and LDL-C levels as well as the development of atherosclerosis when fed a high-fat diet (Fig. 15.4).

High-fat diets and sucrose-rich diets induce obesity in C57Bl/6 mice, which favors the development of type-2 diabetes (Parekh et al., 1998; Surwit et al., 1988); these mice are, therefore, often used in combination with genetic models of atherosclerosis. $Ldlr^{-/-}$ and $Apoe^{-/-}$ mice are largely used to study atherosclerosis and cardiometabolic diseases. In comparison to $Apoe^{-/-}$ mice, $Ldlr^{-/-}$ mice are more susceptible to developing diabetes when fed high-fat diets (Schreyer et al., 2002). With high-fat diets, $Ldlr^{-/-}$ mice display an increase in body weight caused by accumulation of subcutaneous adipose tissue and have high glucose levels, which causes insulin resistance (Collins et al., 2001; Parekh et al., 1998; Phillips et al., 2003). Similar to other strains, $Apoe^{-/-}$*3-Leiden.CETP mice fed a high-fat high-cholesterol diet for 6 months mimic the changes in lipid profiles observed in humans suffering from the metabolic syndrome and may, therefore, be the preferred model for studying age-related changes in lipid metabolism and reverse cholesterol transport (Kuhnast et al., 2015; Paalvast et al., 2017). Altogether, these data demonstrate that a high-fat diet aggravates the lipid profile and causes metabolic changes associated with insulin resistance and aggravation of atherosclerosis.

15.3.3.2 Sex differences and development of atherosclerosis

A review of the literature does not demonstrate a consistent significant effect of sex on atherosclerotic plaque size in mouse atherosclerosis studies. Comparative assessment of sex impact on plaque progression revealed that female mice have a similar lesion area as male mice (Lloyd-Jones et al., 2009; Zhou et al., 2017). Chen and colleagues observed extensive progression of lesions in the aortic sinus in $Apoe^{-/-}$ mice in response to concentrated ambient particulate matter ($PM_{2.5}$) exposure but no difference in plaque size between female and male mice (Chen et al., 2013). Interestingly, Smith et al. and others demonstrated that the female $Apoe^{-/-}$ mice develop atherosclerotic lesions more aggressively than males (Kunitomo et al., 2009; Smith and Breslow, 1997; Zhang et al., 2002). Caliguiri et al. observed larger and more advanced atherosclerotic lesions in young female than in male $Apoe^{-/-}$ mice (Caligiuri et al., 1999); however, no significant difference in lesion size or maturity was discerned in older mice (Caligiuri et al., 1999). Scientific literature tends to highlight some differences in plaque composition between female and male $Apoe^{-/-}$ mice. It has been shown that neutral lipid, macrophage, and vascular smooth muscle cell levels were reduced by 47%, 41%, and 44% in female mice relative to male mice, and plaque calcification was increased in male mice relative to female $Apoe^{-/-}$ mice (Laniado-Laborin, 2009). A high-fat diet significantly increased plaque size (Rangasamy et al., 2009); however, no sex difference was observed on plaque progression in $Apoe^{-/-}$ mice (Yang et al., 2006). Although some recent publications encourage scientists to use biological sex as an experimental variable to account for the potential effect of sex hormones (Bracke et al., 2006; Hutt et al., 2005; Koul et al., 2003; Shein and Jeschke, 2019; Witschi et al., 1997a), this is not always feasible because of logistical constraints during study execution or in the context of animal use reduction (the 3Rs principle). It is common, therefore, to study only one sex in order to reduce the number of animals while performing an in-depth investigation of the cardiorespiratory system at molecular, structural, and functional levels.

15.3.4 Endothelial Dysfunction, Inflammation, and Atherosclerotic Plaque Formation

Hypercholesterolemia favors an oxidation process and causes an increase in superoxide and hydrogen peroxide production by increasing NAD(P)H (nicotinamide adenine dinucleotide phosphate) oxidase levels (Warnholtz et al., 1999). The increase in superoxide levels interferes with nitric oxide (NO) signaling, resulting in reduced endothelial NO synthase (eNOS) coupling and NO bioavailability, leading to generation of additional oxidation products and reactive oxygen species (ROS). ROS induce oxidation of lipids, proteins, and DNA, which cause cell damage, necrosis, and cell apoptosis. As summarized by Meyrelles and coworkers (Meyrelles et al., 2011), aged $Apoe^{-/-}$ mice (50- to 70-week-old) that exhibit both hypercholesterolemia and established atherosclerosis have been reported to show endothelial dysfunction, evidenced by a significantly blunted aorta relaxation response to acetylcholine. CS exposure has been shown to cause endothelial dysfunction, one of the primary effects leading to atherosclerosis development. Circulating cigarette toxicants such as free radicals and reactive glycation products can react with endothelial cells and cause vascular impairment (Cerami et al., 1997). Celermajer and others were able to show that continuous smoking impairs flow-mediated dilation (FMD), a marker of endothelial function (Celermajer et al., 1992; Zeiher et al., 1995). In addition, cigarette smoking induces an inflammatory state, as indicated by increases in white blood cell, adhesion molecule, and cytokine levels, ROS production, and lipid peroxidation (Cerami et al., 1997; Heitzer et al., 1996; Lavi et al., 2007). These mechanisms contribute to impaired eNOS dimerization, leading to the decrease in endothelium-dependent vasodilation observed in active smokers (even in young, healthy adults) and passive smokers (Warnholtz et al., 1999).

Endothelial dysfunction leads to activation of proinflammatory chemokines and cytokines such as VCAM-1 and ICAM-1, favoring recruitment and engulfment of inflammatory cells by the endothelial layer (Manning-Tobin et al., 2009; Nakashima et al., 1994; Park et al., 2009; Sheedy et al., 2013; Tian et al., 2005). These proinflammatory cells home in on atherosclerotic lesions, where they propagate the innate and adaptive immune response by expressing high levels of proinflammatory mediators, cytokines, and chemokines (Blankstein et al., 2019; Geovanini and Libby, 2018; Libby et al., 2011). Numerous inflammatory cells, such as macrophages and lymphocytes, are key

effectors in the modulation of inflammatory response and plaque progression. A variety of studies have proven that cigarette smoking induces oxidative stress, vascular inflammation, platelet coagulation, and vascular dysfunction, impairs serum lipid profile in smokers, and has detrimental effects on the cardiovascular system (Golbidi et al., 2020; Grassi et al., 2010; Han et al., 2012; Kunitomo et al., 2009; Lietz et al., 2013; Siasos et al., 2014; Von Holt et al., 2009). In the context of CS exposure, we have observed that CS exposure causes an increase in cell adhesion and inflammation (Poussin et al., 2015, 2018, 2016) (Chapter 13) and leads to dysregulation of genes involved in the oxidative processes that favor atherosclerosis progression (Szostak et al., 2017, 2020a,b).

15.3.5 Cardiovascular Assessment of EHTP Aerosols

THS was the first ENDP assessed in the $Apoe^{-/-}$ mouse model (Phillips et al., 2016). The study had the dual objective of assessing both the respiratory and cardiovascular effects of THS aerosol in comparison with those of CS and fresh air control. This study also compared the effects of switching from CS to THS aerosol exposure with those of cessation of CS exposure. This study confirmed that CS exposure led to acceleration in atherosclerotic plaque growth in this model, whereas an 8-month exposure to THS aerosol did not (Phillips et al., 2016). These results were confirmed in a 6-month follow-up study in the same mouse model (Phillips et al., 2019). Furthermore, switching from CS to THS aerosol exposure slowed the progression of atherosclerotic plaque formation similarly to cessation of CS exposure. A comparative transcriptomics analysis of the effects of CS and THS aerosol on the heart showed that CS exposure led to time-dependent transcriptomics changes in the heart tissue in these mice. The differentially expressed genes indicated that CS exposure causes downregulation of genes involved in cytoskeleton organization and the contractile function of the heart. However, these effects were not observed in mice exposed to THS aerosol (Szostak et al., 2017).

15.3.6 Cardiovascular Assessment of EVP Aerosols

In order to assess the impact of chronic EVP aerosol exposure on CVD, we conducted a 6-month inhalation study in $Apoe^{-/-}$ mice. The objective was to compare atherosclerotic plaque progression, systodiastolic function, arterial stiffness as a marker of endothelial dysfunction, and gene expression signatures in response to 3R4F CS and EVP aerosol exposure (Szostak et al.,

2020b) relative to fresh air or carrier aerosol (composed of PG and VG) exposure (control groups). This work was part of a comprehensive inhalation study that also included assessment of systemic and respiratory effects.

Female mice were allocated to five exposure groups: fresh air (sham), 3R4F CS ("3R4F"), PG/VG ("carrier"), PG/VG/nicotine ("base"), and PG/VG/nicotine/flavoring ("test"). The aerosol for the base group contained PG, VG, and 4% nicotine, while that for the test group contained PG, VG, 4% nicotine, and flavor mix. The animals were exposed to 3R4F CS or aerosolized (with a capillary aerosol generator, as described in Chapter 12) e-liquids for 3 h/day, 5 days per week, in whole-body exposure chambers for up to 6 months. The base and test group exposures were configured to deliver a nicotine concentration of 35 μg/L (equivalent to the nicotine level in 560 μg/L TPM from 3R4F CS). The mice were terminally dissected at months 3 and 6 to evaluate atherosclerotic plaque progression, systo-diastolic function, and vascular stiffness (Fig. 15.5).

Daily characterization of nicotine and TPM concentrations in the test atmosphere demonstrated that CS and aerosol delivery to the exposure chambers were reproducible. To verify the aerosolization and stable

delivery of flavoring substances during the 6-month exposure, the test atmosphere was analyzed for the presence of guaiacol, which was part of the test mixture. The concentrations of selected toxicants, including CO, formaldehyde, acrolein, and acetaldehyde, were significantly reduced in EVP aerosols relative to 3R4F CS (Szostak et al., 2020b).

15.3.6.1 Oxidative stress following EVP aerosol exposure

During the past decade, research has revealed the widespread involvement of oxidative stress in a number of disease processes, including CVD, atherosclerosis, diabetes, arthritis, neurodegenerative disorders, and pulmonary, renal, and hepatic diseases (Granger and Kvietys, 2015; Negre-Salvayre et al., 2010; Valko et al., 2007). Thus, oxidative stress markers are important tools for assessing the biological redox status, which may be indicative of disease state. Lipid oxidation end-product analysis is a widely used marker of oxidative stress. Malondialdehyde (MDA) and 4-hydroxy-2-nonenal (HNE) represent the most investigated end products of lipid oxidation (Sousa et al., 2017). HNE can be detected by high-performance liquid chromatography (HPLC) directly or as a derivatized product with

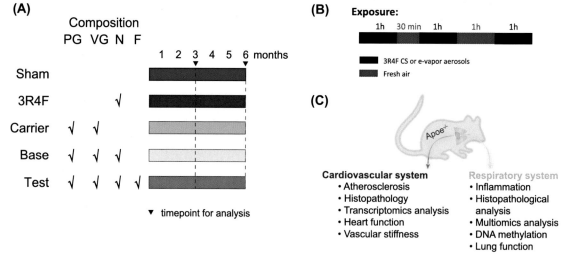

FIG. 15.5 Study design, groups, and exposure. **(A)** Timeline of the study showing the different groups. 3R4F is the standard reference cigarette; carrier, base, and test represent ENDP aerosols from the test formulation. "Carrier" represents the PG/VG group; "base," the PG/VG/N group; and "test," the PG/VG/N/F group. **(B)** Whole-body exposure protocol. The *black boxes square* represent exposure time. The *blue boxes* represent exposure breaks. **(C)** Key cardiovascular and respiratory endpoints assessed in the study. *F*, flavors; *N*, nicotine; *PG*, propylene glycol; *VG*, vegetable glycerin. (Adapted from Szostak, J., Wong, E.T., Titz, B., Lee, T., Wong, S.K., Low, T., et al., 2020b. A 6-month systems toxicology inhalation study in ApoE(-/-) mice demonstrates reduced cardiovascular effects of E-vapor aerosols compared with cigarette smoke. Am. J. Physiol. Heart Circ. Physiol. 318 (3), H604–H631.)

2,4-dinitrophenylhydrazine or 1,3-cyclohexanedione by gas chromatography coupled with mass spectroscopy (GC−MS).

Our study results showed that the levels of MDA and prostaglandin F2 alpha (PGF2α; both products of lipid peroxidation and radical-mediated oxidation of arachidonic acid) as well as 2,3-di-PGF2α (a β-oxidation product of PGF2α) were significantly higher in the urine of 3R4F CS-exposed mice than in sham-exposed mice ($P < .05$) (Szostak et al., 2020b). The presence of higher levels of these oxidation products is in line with the levels of HPHCs in CS and indicative of a CS-dependent increase in oxidative stress levels. In contrast to CS exposure, exposure to EVP aerosols did not cause significant changes in oxidative stress parameters (Fig. 15.6) (Szostak et al., 2017, 2020a).

15.3.6.2 Cardiovascular functions following EVP aerosol exposure

With improvements in spatial and temporal resolution, echocardiography became an indispensable tool for measuring cardiovascular dysfunction in animal models. Arterial stiffness, estimated by pulse wave velocity (PWV), is an independent predictor of cardiovascular morbidity and mortality. The pulse wave is transmitted through the arterial system, and its speed is inversely related to the distensibility of the arterial wall itself (Laurent et al., 2006). Assessment of PWV is considered the "gold standard" measurement of aortic stiffness, as it is a simple, noninvasive, and reproducible method supported by clinical evidence demonstrating the predictive value of aortic stiffness for cardiovascular events (Di Lascio et al., 2014, 2017).

Previous data have shown that CS exposure reduces the distensibility of both medium-sized muscular arteries as well as large elastic arteries, thereby causing systemic arterial stiffening (Karakaya et al., 2006; Mahmud and Feely, 2003). Acute cigarette smoking increases arterial stiffness in large arteries in healthy young smokers, and these changes are more prominent in chronic smokers. In addition, resting blood flow and endothelium-dependent FMD of brachial and epicardial arteries are significantly impaired in smokers (Carnevale et al., 2016). Impairment of FMD and increased intima−media thickness are related to the duration and number of cigarettes smoked. Thus, smoking is associated with dose- and/or time-related impairment of FMD and increased intima−media thickness in large human arteries. Recent investigations demonstrated that exposure to ENDP aerosol caused some impairment of vascular relaxation, leading to an increase in PWV. This was observed in acute human trials in which

aortic stiffness was determined up to 1 h after use of cigarettes or e-cigarettes relative to a control group (Franzen et al., 2018; Ikonomidis et al., 2018; Vlachopoulos et al., 2016). Higher PWV was also observed following CS or e-vapor exposure relative to fresh air in C57Bl/6 mice in a chronic inhalation study (5 days/week for 6 months) (Olfert et al., 2018).

In our study, echocardiography was used to assess the exposure impact on cardiovascular tissue function. In murine vascular tissue, we analyzed the impact of CS or EVP on PWV and PPV (pulse propagation velocity) as markers of endothelial dysfunction (Szostak et al., 2020b). CS exposure resulted in higher ($P < .05$) PPV in the abdominal aorta and PWV compared with control exposure. Interestingly exposure to EVP aerosols containing nicotine (base and test) also caused a significant increase ($P < .05$) in PPV and PWV. Nevertheless, in comparison with 3R4F CS-exposed mice, mice exposed to the base and test aerosols had a significantly lower PWV (reduction of 7.5% and 8.1%, respectively; $P < .05$). In contrast, exposure to carrier aerosol had no impact on PWV or PPV (Fig. 15.7).

Echocardiography was combined with Doppler measurements to determine heart systodiastolic function as well as the morphological impact of EVP aerosols on the heart. To evaluate the global systolic function of the left ventricle (LV), we measured the LV ejection fraction (EF) and LV fractional shortening (FS). Transmitral inflow Doppler measurements obtained in an apical four-chamber view or LV long-axis view were used to evaluate the LV diastolic function (Du et al., 2008; Peter et al., 2007; Schaefer et al., 2003; Schmidt et al., 2002). The Doppler indexes included the ratio of peak velocity of early to late filling of mitral inflow (E/A), deceleration time (DT) of early filling of mitral inflow, isovolumetric relaxation time (IVRT), and isovolumetric contraction time (IVCT). Pulse-wave Doppler- or tissue Doppler-derived myocardial performance index (MPI) is a useful index for assessing cardiac systolic and diastolic function in mice. It can be calculated by using the ratio of isovolumetric contraction and relaxation time to ejection time (IVRT + IVCT)/ET. Increased MPI indicates diastolic dysfunction. Because this index is based on the ratio of several parameters, all evaluated within the same cardiac cycle, MPI is independent of heart rate and LV shape (Broberg et al., 2003; Schaefer et al., 2005). Numerous studies have shown that the evaluation of systodiastolic dysfunction with echocardiography is useful for detecting and monitoring the development of cardiac pathologies (Peter et al., 2007).

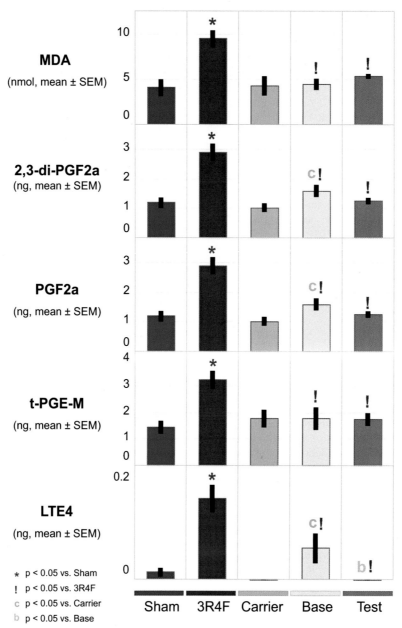

FIG. 15.6 Effect of EVP aerosols and 3R4F CS exposure on urinary biomarkers of oxidative stress and inflammation at 4 months of exposure. Absolute values of MDA, 2,3-di-PGF2α, 8-iso-PGF2α, t-PGE-M, and LTE4 (n = 7−8). *$P < .05$ significant versus sham group; !$P < .05$ significant versus 3R4F group; cp < .05 significant versus carrier group; bp < .05 significant versus base group. (n = 8). *LTE4*, leukotriene E4; *MDA*, malondialdehyde; *PGF2α*, prostaglandin F2 alpha; *SEM*, standard deviation of the mean; *t-PGE-M*, tetranor-prostaglandin D metabolite. (Adapted from Szostak, J., Wong, E.T., Titz, B., Lee, T., Wong, S.K., Low, T., et al., 2020b. A 6-month systems toxicology inhalation study in ApoE$^{(-/-)}$ mice demonstrates reduced cardiovascular effects of E-vapor aerosols compared with cigarette smoke. Am. J. Physiol. Heart Circ. Physiol. 318 (3), H604−H631.)

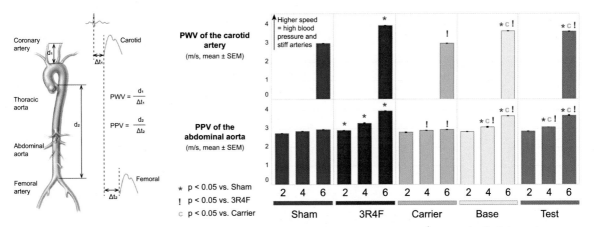

FIG. 15.7 Effect of EVP aerosols and 3R4F CS on PWV and PPV in *Apoe*^{−/−} mice. (Left) Schematic representation of PWV and PPV acquisition area. (Right) Abdominal aorta PPV at 2, 4, and 6 months of exposure (n = 8–12). (c) Carotid artery PWV at 6 months (n = 10–12). *$P < .05$ significant vs. sham group; !$P < .05$ significant vs. 3R4F group; c$p < .05$ significant vs. carrier group; b$p < .05$ significant vs. base group. *CS*, 3R4F cigarette smoke; *PPV*, pulse propagation velocity; *PWV*, pulse wave velocity. (Adapted from Szostak, J., Wong, E.T., Titz, B., Lee, T., Wong, S.K., Low, T., et al., 2020b. A 6-month systems toxicology inhalation study in ApoE^(−/−) mice demonstrates reduced cardiovascular effects of E-vapor aerosols compared with cigarette smoke. Am. J. Physiol. Heart Circ. Physiol. 318 (3), H604–H631.)

Our investigations on the heart function in *Apoe*^{−/−} mice demonstrated that, relative to sham exposure, CS exposure caused significant ($P < .05$) impairment of EF (−15.5%), FS (−20.1%), and cardiac output (−18.7 mL/min) after 6 months of exposure ($P < .05$; Fig. 15.8). In mice exposed to EVP aerosols at similar levels of nicotine to that in CS exposure, no significant changes relative to sham were observed in EF, FS, or cardiac output.

We also assessed, both by conventional ultrasonic and tissue Doppler imaging, the impact of EVP aerosols and 3R4F CS on isovolumic relaxation time, reliable indices of diastolic function, and isovolumic contraction time, an additional parameter of systolic performance. After 6 months of exposure, the isovolumic contraction and relaxation times in CS-exposed mice were significantly higher, by 25.9% and 37.2%, respectively, than those in sham-exposed mice (Fig. 15.8). In comparison with sham exposure, EVP aerosol exposure caused no change in isovolumic contraction time. However, mice exposed to the base and test aerosols showed an increase in isovolumic relaxation time (34.3% and 23%, respectively; $P < .05$) relative to sham-exposed mice after 6 months of exposure (Fig. 15.8).

To assess the global impact of EVP aerosols and 3R4F CS exposure on heart function, we derived the MPI from four-chamber Doppler and tissue Doppler imaging data. Four-chamber Doppler ultrasound analysis demonstrated

that, relative to sham exposure, 3R4F CS exposure caused a significant increase in MPI after 2 (by 18.8%; $P < .05$), 4 (by 20.3%; $P < .05$), and 6 (by 50.5%; $P < .05$) months of exposure. Similarly, tissue Doppler analysis confirmed a significant increase in MPI at 6 months of exposure in the 3R4F CS group, relative to the sham group. To a lesser extent, it was observed that exposure to the EVP aerosols had a slight impact on the MPI. Tissue Doppler analysis revealed a small but significant ($P < .05$) increase in MPI in the base and test groups relative to the carrier and sham groups at 6 months.

15.3.6.3 Atherosclerosis progression following EVP aerosol exposure

Different methods are used to assess the extent of atherosclerotic plaque burden. One standard method involves serial sectioning of the heart and aortic root (Paigen et al., 1987) and subsequent histopathological analysis to score and measure atherosclerotic lesions. Another method employs Sudan IV staining to determine the extent of atherosclerosis affecting the intimal surface in the aorta, which is commonly known as the "en face" technique (Collins et al., 2001; Tangirala et al., 1995). Other ex vivo techniques that have been used to detect and quantify plaque volume include high-resolution MRI (magnetic resonance imaging) (McAteer et al., 2004) and μCT (Lloyd et al., 2011).

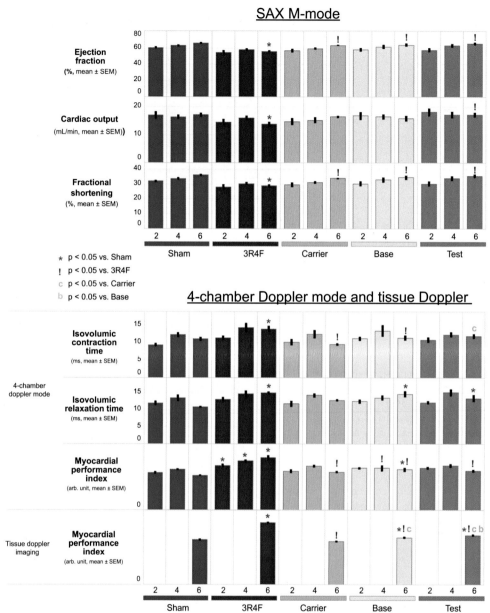

FIG. 15.8 Echocardiographic evaluation of left ventricular systodiastolic function in response to EVP aerosols and 3R4F CS exposure. (Top panel) SAX M-mode: Percentage ejection fraction, cardiac output, and percentage of fractional shortening at 3 and 6 months after exposure to EVP carrier, base, or test aerosol or 3R4F CS ($n = 10–12$). (Lower panel) Four-chamber Doppler mode: Isovolumic contraction time, isovolumic relaxation time, and myocardial performance index at 3 and 6 months after exposure to EVP carrier, base, or test aerosol or 3R4F CS ($n = 10–12$). Tissue Doppler imaging: Myocardial performance index as an index of global systodiastolic dysfunction. $*P < .05$ significant versus sham group; $!P < .05$ significant versus 3R4F group; $cp < .05$ significant versus carrier group; $bp < .05$ significant versus base group. *M-mode*, one dimensional echocardiography; *SAX*, short-axis; SEM, standard deviation of the mean. (Adapted from Szostak, J., Wong, E.T., Titz, B., Lee, T., Wong, S.K., Low, T., et al., 2020b. A 6-month systems toxicology inhalation study in ApoE$^{(-/-)}$ mice demonstrates reduced cardiovascular effects of E-vapor aerosols compared with cigarette smoke. Am. J. Physiol. Heart Circ. Physiol. 318 (3), H604–H631.)

CS exposure significantly and consistently increased atherosclerotic plaque progression across several studies in $Apoe^{-/-}$ mice. This was the case for both mainstream CS (Boue et al., 2012; Lietz et al., 2013; Phillips et al., 2016; Szostak et al., 2020a; Von Holt et al., 2009) and sidestream CS (Dong et al., 2010; Gairola et al., 2001, 2010; Han et al., 2012). However, as summarized earlier, exposure to HTP and EVP aerosols led to plaque sizes that were comparable to those in sham-exposed animals (Boue et al., 2012; Phillips et al., 2016; Szostak et al., 2020a).

In our chronic EVP exposure study, analysis of the aortic arch by using the en face method revealed that mice exposed to 3R4F CS showed a significant ($P < .05$) increase in aortic arch area covered by atherosclerotic plaque relative to sham-exposed mice (2.1-fold increase after 3 months and 1.4-fold increase after 6 months; $P < .05$) (Szostak et al., 2020b). No significant difference in plaque surface area was observed between mice exposed to EVP aerosols and sham-exposed mice (Fig. 15.9A and B). In comparison with 3R4F CS-exposed mice, mice exposed to the carrier, base, and test aerosols had smaller plaque areas.

Additionally, a quantitative μCT investigation was performed on the thoracic aorta of a separate cohort of mice (n = 16) (Fig. 15.9C and D). Consistent with the planimetry findings, the atherosclerotic plaque surface and volume were greater in 3R4F CS-exposed mice than in sham-exposed mice after 6 months of exposure (Fig. 15.9D). No significant difference in plaque surface area or volume were observed among mice exposed to EVP aerosols (Fig. 15.9D). Mice exposed to EVP aerosols presented lower plaque surface area than 3R4F CS-exposed mice (Fig. 15.9D). Similarly, a lower plaque volume was observed in mice exposed to EVP aerosols than in 3R4F CS-exposed mice ($P < .05$) at 3 and 6 months of exposure (Fig. 15.9D).

(A)   Representative lesions at 6 months

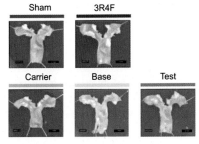

(B)   Planimetry

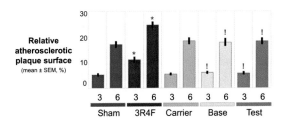

(C)   Representative CT images of atherosclerotic lesions in thoracic aorta

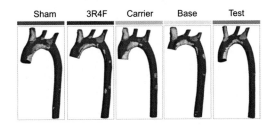

(D)   μCT quantification

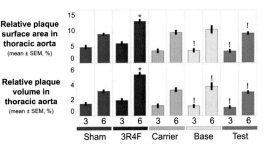

FIG. 15.9 Effect of EVP aerosols and 3R4F CS exposure on atherosclerotic plaque area and volume in $Apoe^{-/-}$ mice. **(A)** Representative images of atherosclerotic lesions in the aortic arch, with measurements acquired by planimetry at 6 months. **(B)** Relative atherosclerotic plaque surface area in the aortic arch, evaluated by planimetry (n = 19−20). **(C)** Representative images of atherosclerotic lesions in the thoracic aorta acquired by CT. **(D)** Relative atherosclerotic plaque volume and relative atherosclerotic plaque surface evaluated by μCT (n = 15−16). $*P < .05$ significant versus sham group; $!P < .05$ significant versus 3R4F group. (Adapted from Szostak, J., Wong, E.T., Titz, B., Lee, T., Wong, S.K., Low, T., et al., 2020b. A 6-month systems toxicology inhalation study in ApoE$^{(-/-)}$ mice demonstrates reduced cardiovascular effects of E-vapor aerosols compared with cigarette smoke. Am. J. Physiol. Heart Circ. Physiol. 318 (3), H604−H631.)

Our results from the $Apoe^{-/-}$ model are comparable with the findings in chronic smokers in clinical studies, which have demonstrated that smoking is associated with increased atherosclerosis progression in carotid, femoral, and brachial arteries (Esen et al., 2004; Poredos et al., 1999; van den Berkmortel et al., 2000). Therefore, it can be assumed that the lower plaque progression following exposure to ENDP (EHTP and EVP) aerosols in the $Apoe^{-/-}$ mouse model indicates that ENDPs are likely to have a lower proatherosclerotic potential than cigarettes.

15.3.6.4 Systems toxicology assessment of ENDP aerosol exposure

To capture cardiovascular toxicity and disease-relevant mechanisms in the $Apoe^{-/-}$ inhalation model, we complemented the in vivo atherosclerosis progression and cardiac function endpoints with in-depth systems toxicology analyses (Chapter 9) and compared these endpoints among sham-, CS-, and ENDP aerosol-exposed mice. Heart tissue and the thoracic aorta were collected for investigating the effects of ENDP aerosol exposure on gene expression and biological network perturbations in three studies, which assessed the aerosols from two HTPs (Szostak et al., 2017, 2020a,b) and one EVP (Szostak et al., 2020b).

15.3.6.4.1 Analysis of gene sets. In the myocardial tissue, 3R4F CS exposure substantially dysregulated the genes involved in collagen formation and extracellular matrix organization, integrin signaling, inflammatory signaling, xenobiotic metabolism, and mitochondrial responses. In particular, mechanisms related to extracellular matrix organization, extracellular matrix receptor interaction, collagen formation, and related integrin components (such as the integrin 1 pathway) were significantly downregulated after 3 and 6 months of exposure. Mechanisms such as xenobiotic metabolism, glutathione conjugation, and ABC family protein-mediated transport were significantly upregulated in the 3R4F group at 3 and 6 months (Szostak et al., 2017, 2020a, 2020b).

In the thoracic aorta, significant gene dysregulation was observed in response to 6 months of 3R4F CS exposure, particularly in three gene sets related to circadian pathways (specifically, BMAL1:CLOCK, NPAS2 activates circadian gene expression, circadian rhythm-mammal, and circadian pathway) (Fig. 15.10).

15.3.6.4.2 Pathway analysis. We further analyzed the gene expression data to identify primary biological functions, pathways, and upstream regulators affected by exposure to CS and ENDP aerosols in the heart ventricle. CS exposure significantly affected processes related to cell assembly, organization, and function of the heart ventricle (Szostak et al., 2020b) (Fig. 15.11). Biological functions such as cytoplasm organization, cytoskeleton organization, neuron development, microtubule dynamics, formation of cellular protrusions, and cell-to-cell contact were significantly altered in response to CS exposure for 3 and 6 months (Z scores <-2). In parallel, mechanisms related to cell movements (lymphocyte movement, cell invasion, spread, and migration) were predicted to be negatively regulated, whereas organismal death and weight loss were predicted to be positively regulated in response to CS exposure at 3 and 6 months (Szostak et al., 2020b). None of these biological functions or processes were identified in the animals exposed to EVP aerosols. Overall, the transcriptomic analysis indicated that 3R4F CS exposure altered the cardiac transcriptome, but exposure to ENDP aerosols did not (Fig. 15.11).

15.3.7 Conclusions for CVD

Although a variety of mouse models are used for evaluating atherosclerosis (e.g., $Apoe^{-/-}$, $Ldlr^{-/-}$, and double knockouts), it should be recognized that all these models have limitations and may not represent the exact characteristics of the human disease. Indeed the atherosclerotic lesions are developed in different vessel types and locations and have different severity (Hajek et al., 2014) owing to some mechanistic differences between humans and mice. However, historical data as well as our investigations have demonstrated that the $Apoe^{-/-}$ mouse model is a relevant model for assessing the impact of CS exposure on atherosclerotic disease progression. Our studies demonstrated that, compared with CS exposure, ENDP aerosol exposure leads to significantly lower levels of oxidative stress, a lower impact on gene dysregulation, lower atherosclerotic plaque progression, and a lower impact on heart function. These results, which are coherent along the CELSD (Chapter 3), indicate that ENDPs are likely to have lower cardiovascular effects than cigarettes.

15.4 ANIMAL MODELS FOR LUNG CANCER

Smoking is the primary risk factor for developing lung cancer. Lung cancer initiation and progression can be enhanced by genome instability and mutations that are caused by exposure to the various carcinogens

(A)

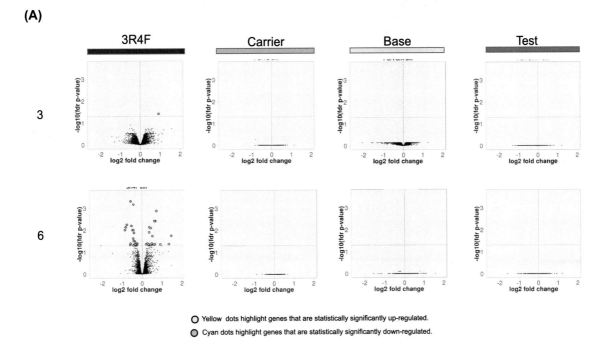

○ Yellow dots highlight genes that are statistically significantly up-regulated.

○ Cyan dots highlight genes that are statistically significantly down-regulated.

(B)

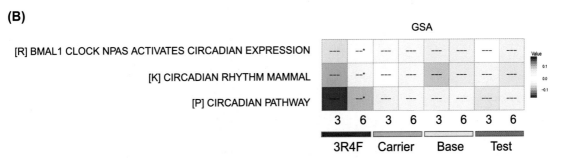

FIG. 15.10 Molecular dysregulation in the thoracic aorta, assessed through a systems toxicology approach. **(A)** Volcano plot representing the changes in gene expression groups in the thoracic aorta after exposure to EVP aerosols (carrier, base, or test) or 3R4F CS (at 3 and 6 months) (n = 6–10; total, n = 139). Yellow indicates significantly upregulated genes, and cyan indicates significantly downregulated genes (FDR P < .05). **(B)** GSA analysis. The average fold change of the gene sets is represented by the color scale. Significant enrichment (FDR-adjusted P value < .05) for three different methods is indicated: Camera/Q1(*–), Roast/Q2 (-*-), and ORA (–*). *FDR*, false discovery rate; *GSA*, gene set analysis. (Adapted from Szostak, J., Wong, E.T., Titz, B., Lee, T., Wong, S.K., Low, T., et al., 2020b. A 6-month systems toxicology inhalation study in ApoE$^{(-/-)}$ mice demonstrates reduced cardiovascular effects of E-vapor aerosols compared with cigarette smoke. Am. J. Physiol. Heart Circ. Physiol. 318 (3), H604–H631.)

(such as tobacco-specific nitrosamines [TSNA]), free radicals, and solid carbon-based nanoparticles present in CS. The HPHCs contained in CS also cause chronic inflammation, the key process that promotes COPD and lung cancer development (Balkwill and Mantovani, 2001; Hecht, 2012; Hoeng et al., 2019; Office of the Surgeon General, 2014). There is a strong link between COPD and increased risk of lung cancer development in smokers (Brenner et al., 2012; de-Torres et al., 2015; Durham and Adcock, 2015). The chronic inflammatory state in COPD further fuels lung cancer development and progression (Adcock et al., 2011; Houghton,

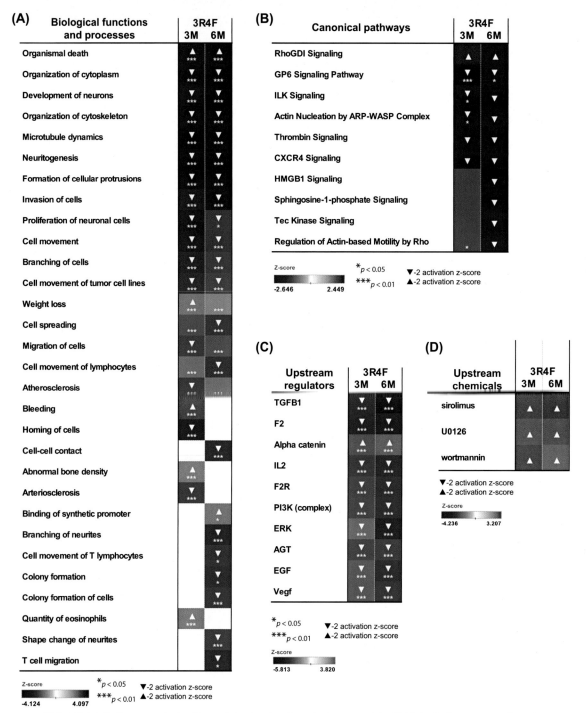

FIG. 15.11 Pathways analysis of transcriptomics data from the heart ventricle. (A) Biological processes affected by CS and EVP aerosol exposure (B), canonical pathways (C), top 10 upstream regulators (D), and top three chemical upstream regulators significantly impacted in the 3R4F, carrier, base, and test groups (n = 9–10). *P < .05; ***P < .01. Blue indicates "predicated as downregulated," and orange indicates "predicated as upregulated." The intensity of coloring varies with Z score value. Z scores >2 are indicated by ▲; Z scores < −2 are indicated by ▼. ((Adapted from Szostak, J., Wong, E.T., Titz, B., Lee, T., Wong, S.K., Low, T., et al., 2020b. A 6-month systems toxicology inhalation study in ApoE(−/−) mice demonstrates reduced cardiovascular effects of E-vapor aerosols compared with cigarette smoke. Am. J. Physiol. Heart Circ. Physiol. 318 (3), H604–H631.)

2018). Assessment of lung inflammation by using animal models of ENDP aerosol inhalation (Madison et al., 2019; Olfert et al., 2018; Phillips et al., 2017; Werley et al., 2016) will provide evidence for the potential of ENDPs to reduce the risk of lung cancer development compared to cigarettes.

15.4.1 Preclinical Approach to Assess the Lung Cancer Risk ENDPs

Assessing the potential of an ENDP to reduce the risk of lung cancer is challenging because of the long latency of disease manifestation, heterogeneous nature of the disease, and presence of several histological types of lung cancers. Nevertheless, both in vitro and in vivo studies can be used for assessing the key biological mechanisms associated with COPD and lung carcinogenesis by leveraging systems toxicology approaches (Hoeng et al., 2019; Smith et al., 2016). Therefore, the holistic approach taken for assessing ENDPs for their potential to reduce the risk of lung cancer encompasses assessment of genetic damage, lung inflammation, and lung cancer development (Hoeng et al., 2019) (Chapter 18). In combination with aerosol chemistry analyses (Chapter 4, 6–7) and analysis of biomarkers of exposure to toxicants (Chapters 14 and 17), ENDP assessments will include the link from reduction in emission of carcinogenic toxicants to reduction in exposure to carcinogenic toxicants and to biological outcomes (COPD and lung carcinogenesis). In vivo animal models are valuable for demonstrating the biological and molecular links from aerosol exposure to disease outcomes (Chapter 3). Genetic toxicology tests are frequently performed with cell-based assays (Chapter 13), and the advantages and limitations of in vivo genetic toxicity tests are discussed in Chapter 14. The use of mouse models for studying the impact of CS and aerosol from ENDPs on lung tumor development and on mechanisms linking chronic lung inflammation, emphysema, and lung cancer will be discussed here. Alongside nonclinical studies, clinical ENDP assessment will evaluate the impact of switching from cigarette smoking to ENDP use on the potentially reduced toxicant exposure as well as potentially positive changes in the various biomarkers of potential harm (BoPH) (Chapter 17). Using an approach based on the inhalation unit risks of the most important carcinogenic toxicants in CS, Stephens compared the cancer potencies of various ENDP emissions and their lifetime cancer risks on the basis of daily product consumption estimates (Stephens, 2017). As the emission of HPHCs is markedly reduced in ENDP aerosols relative to CS (Chapter 4), smokers who switch completely from cigarette smoking to ENDP use will be exposed to markedly lower levels of

these toxicants/carcinogens (Chapter 17). Therefore, switching completely from cigarette smoking to ENDP use is likely to reduce the risk of lung cancer for smokers.

15.4.2 Animal Models of Lung Cancer

There are two major types of lung cancer, small cell lung cancer (SCLC) and non-small cell lung cancer (NSCLC). The latter can be further classified on the basis of histological characteristics into adenocarcinoma (AC), squamous cell carcinoma (SCC), and large cell carcinoma. CS exposure is associated with all types of lung cancer. Despite histological differences between murine and human lung tumors, mouse models have been useful for studying the carcinogenicity of chemicals and the biology underlying lung tumor development in humans (Akbay and Kim, 2018; Nikitin et al., 2004; Witschi, 2005). Various chemical-induced lung tumor models may be suitable for comparative testing of tumorigenesis following inhalation of CS and ENDP aerosols and will be described here in relation to human smoker lung cancers. Genetic models of lung tumors are valuable for elucidating distinct molecular events and processes in tumor initiation and progression. The genetically modified models may be suitable for evaluating lung tumor progression in the context of CS exposure and exposure to aerosols from ENDPs. Details of genetically modified models of lung tumors are reviewed elsewhere (Gazdar et al., 2016; Kellar et al., 2015; Kwon and Berns, 2013) and will be discussed here mainly in their potential relevance for ENDP testing.

15.4.3 Mouse Models of SCLC

SCLC is a fast progressing and mostly lethal lung tumor characterized by rapid growth and early metastasis. It accounts for approximately 15% of all lung cancers in the United States (National Cancer Institute). The occurrence of SCLC is high among heavy smokers (Alexandrov et al., 2016; Khuder, 2001; Khuder and Mutgi, 2001). These tumor cells express markers of neuroendocrine differentiation and are thought to arise from the neuroendocrine cells located at the junctions of the bronchi (Semenova et al., 2015). Murine models of SCLC have been focused on genetic models for understanding the key molecular players in tumorigenesis rather than assessing complete tumor formation. No known complete chemical- or CS- induced SCLC model has been reported thus far.

There are two histological subgroups of human SCLC. Most frequent is the classic SCLC, which is characterized by small cells with high nuclear to cytoplasmic ratios and fine granular chromatin (Gazdar et al., 1985). In contrast, the variant SCLCs have larger cells with prominent cytoplasm and nucleoli (Gazdar et al., 1985). By using mouse and human gene expression data, biologically distinct subtypes of classic and variant SCLCs can be defined (Rudin et al., 2019). The high occurrence of C>A transversion in SCLCs is consistent with CS exposure. Inactivating mutations in *TP53* and *RB1* are highly prevalent in the tumors (Peifer et al., 2012; Pleasance et al., 2010; Rudin et al., 2012). Most genetically modified models of SCLC are based on the conditional loss of Trp53 and Rb1 expression (Table 15.1) and related reviews (Akbay and Kim, 2018; Semenova et al., 2015). Additional genetic events that drive the development of certain SCLC subtypes are known (George et al., 2015) (see also Table 15.1 and reviews (Rudin et al., 2019; Semenova et al., 2015)). Genetically engineered mouse models are pivotal for identification of the key genetic drivers of SCLC development. SCLC arises from different cell types (neuroendocrine and basal cells) that influence its evolution (Table 15.1). By using distinct promoters to target genetic mutations in mouse models, defined populations of lung cells have been identified as the origin of distinct lung cancer types.

Because of the complex genetics of tumorigenesis, expression pattern changes during development/tumorigenesis, and distinct cellular origin of SCLC

development, single transgenic mouse models overexpressing human papillomavirus-16 E6/E7 (Carraresi et al., 2001), simian virus large T antigen (Magdaleno et al., 1997; Wikenheiser et al., 1992), c-myc with EGF (Ehrhardt et al., 2001), and Raf-1 (Kerkhoff et al., 2000) using constitutively expressed or cell type-targeted promoters had resulted in lung adenocarcinoma instead of SCLC in mice. To our knowledge, the conditional and targeted mouse models of SCLC (Table 15.1) using Cre recombinase expression have not been tested for the role of CS in tumor progression.

15.4.4 Mouse Models of Adenocarcinoma

AC is the most frequent lung cancer type ($\sim$45%) (National Cancer Institute) and occurs in both smokers and nonsmokers (Sun et al., 2007). Most ACs arise from type 2 pneumocytes in the alveoli of the lung tissue (Travis et al., 2013; Xu et al., 2012). Smoking-associated ACs exhibit high mutation rates, specifically more of C>A transversions than C>T transitions (Cancer Genome Atlas Research, 2014; Govindan et al., 2012). Mutations in certain oncogenes and tumor suppressor genes (e.g., *KRAS*, *BRAF*, *FAK2/3*, *TP53*, and *STK11*) are significantly correlated with smoking-associated AC (Cancer Genome Atlas Research, 2014; Govindan et al.,

TABLE 15.1
Key Genetic Drivers in Distinct Subtypes of Small Cell Lung Cancers (Mouse Models).

GEMM	Promoter driving Cre expression	Neuroendocrine gene expression	Potential targeted cell population	References
Trp53 lox/lox, Rb1 lox/lox	CMV	ASCL1-high	Multiple cell types. Tumors of mainly SCLC	Meuwissen et al. (2003)
Trp53 lox/lox, Rb1 lox/lox, Rbl2 lox/lox	CMV	ASCL1-high	Multiple cell types. Predominantly SCLC at late time points	Schaffer et al. (2010)
Trp53 lox/lox, Rb1 lox/lox, PTEN lox/lox	CGRP	ASCL1-high	Neuroendocrine cells; mainly LCNEC mixed with SCLC and adenocarcinoma	McFadden et al. (2014), Song et al. (2012)
Trp53 lox/lox, Rb1 lox/lox, Rbl2 lox/lox, PTEN lox/lox	Keratin K5	ASCL1-high	Basal cells	Lazaro et al. (2019)
Trp53 lox/lox, Rb1 lox/lox, MycT58A	CGRP	NeuroD1-high	Neuroendocrine cells	Mollaoglu et al. (2017)
Trp53 lox/lox, Rb1 lox/lox, Rbl2 lox/lox, NICD	CMV, CGRP	ASCL1-low/ NeuroD1-low	Multiple cell types	Lim et al. (2017)

ASCL1/ASH1, achaete-scute homologue 1; *CGRP*, calcitonin gene-related peptide; *CMV*, cytomegalovirus; *GEMM*, genetically engineered mouse model; *LCNEC*, large cell neuroendocrine carcinoma; *NeuroD1*, neurogenic differentiation factor 1; *NICD*, Notch intracellular domain; *SCLC*, squamous cell lung cancer.

2012). Both chemically induced and genetic models of mouse AC have been the most studied among the major histological subtypes of this cancer. Spontaneous lung tumors in susceptible mice are similar in morphology, histopathology, and molecular characteristics to human ACs (Meuwissen and Berns, 2005). Tumors arising in the peripheral lung parenchyma are the most common primary proliferative lesions in aging mice. The majority of murine lung lesions are classified as hyperplasias and adenomas, which is in contrast to the prevalence of ACs in humans (Nikitin et al., 2004). In addition, histological heterogeneity in a single tumor is rather uncommon in experimental animals, unlike the frequently observed combination of different histological types in human lung carcinomas (Franklin et al., 2004). The relevance of mouse models for AC to testing CS and ENDP aerosols will be discussed.

15.4.4.1 Chemically induced lung AC

The majority of chemical- and CS-induced lung tumors in mice are adenomas with low frequency progressing into AC within a year. The mutations seen in chemically induced adenocarcinoma parallel those seen in smoking-related AC. The carcinogens benzo[*a*]pyrene and urethane induce C>A transversions and T>A transversions, respectively, in *Kras* (Kirsten rat sarcoma viral oncogene homolog), leading to G12 and Q61 mutations, respectively (Westcott et al., 2015; You et al., 1989). The TSNA 4-(methylnitrosamino)-1-(3-pyridyl)-1-butanone (NNK) and methylnitrosourea induce C>T transitions in *Kras*, leading to G12 mutations (Kawano et al., 1996; Ronai et al., 1993; You et al., 1992).

The frequency and latency of spontaneous and chemically induced lung AC vary depending on the inbred strain used (Manenti and Dragani, 2005; Shimkin and Stoner, 1975)—the A and A/J strains are the most sensitive; the Swiss, BALB/c, and FVB strains have intermediate susceptibility, while the DBA, C57BL, and C57L strains are the most resistant. The A/J mouse is highly susceptible to spontaneous and induced lung adenoma and AC development due to spontaneous *Kras* activation (You et al., 1989). Increased lung tumor development in A/J mice was shown in response to known tobacco-derived carcinogens (Hecht et al., 1994; Singh et al., 1998; Wang et al., 1992; You et al., 1989) and CS exposure (Coggins, 1998; Stinn et al., 2010, 2005; Witschi et al., 2002, 2004).

Early studies on reproducing the tumor-promoting activity of CS in mice have failed (Coggins, 2010; Witschi, 2005). In NNK-treated mice, exposure to CS did not increase lung tumor development (Finch et al., 1996; Witschi et al., 1997b). This could possibly be because of CS-induced toxicity and stress (observed weight loss in response to CS exposure) as well as CS-mediated inhibition of the metabolic activation of NNK (Brown et al., 1999). Inclusion of a recovery phase (4 months) following a 5-month environmental tobacco smoke surrogate (ETSS) or CS exposure was necessary to observe CS-mediated enhancement of lung tumor development (Curtin et al., 2004; Gordon and Bosland, 2009; Stinn et al., 2005, 2010; Witschi, 2005). The biological relevance of such an exposure regimen for assessment of smoking-induced tumorigenesis remains to be established. To better mirror the lung tumor development in chronic smokers, a lifetime CS-exposure regimen without a recovery phase were applied successfully in female F344 rats, female B6C3F1, A/J, and Swiss mice (Balansky et al., 2007; Hutt et al., 2005; Mauderly et al., 2004; Stinn et al., 2013a,b). In A/J mice, lung tumor multiplicity and incidence were concentration-dependent and reproducibly enhanced following CS exposure for 18 months, which demonstrated the validity and reproducibility of the cancer model (Stinn et al., 2013a,b). This lifetime exposure schedule fulfills the requirements of the OECD guideline TG 453—Combined Chronic Toxicity\Carcinogenicity Studies (OECD, 2018, https://www.oecd-ilibrary.org/content/publication/9789264071223-en).

CS- and chemically induced lung tumor development did not show consistent sex-related differences in tumor multiplicity (Maronpot et al., 1986; Shimkin and Stoner, 1975). CS-exposed A/J mice developed pronounced lung inflammation, emphysematous changes, and altered lung function. The A/J mouse is, therefore, a suitable model for studying the pathogenesis and underlying molecular changes in smoking-induced COPD and lung cancer (Cabanski et al., 2015; Stinn et al., 2013b). Furthermore, systems toxicology—based analyses demonstrated that lung tumors developing in CS-exposed A/J mice exhibit marked differences from spontaneously arising tumors and that these differences can be harnessed to potentially predict differences in exposure on the basis of unique molecular signatures (e.g., metabolic and DNA damage response) in the tumor cells (Luettich et al., 2014). On the basis of these observations, we consider the A/J mouse to be a suitable in vivo model of smoking-related lung cancer for assessment of ENDPs relative to combustible tobacco products. The results from studies with the A/J AC model for investigating lung cancer development in response to aerosol from THS will be further described (Section 15.4.6).

15.4.4.2 Genetic models of lung AC

The *KRAS* mutations in lung AC are strongly associated with smoking and are the key oncogenic drivers in lung cancer progression (Cancer Genome Atlas Research, 2014; Govindan et al., 2012). Genetically engineered mouse models of lung AC are, therefore, frequently based on mutant *Kras*, either singly or in combination with loss of specific tumor suppressor genes (reviewed in Akbay and Kim, 2018; Kwon and Berns, 2013). Furthermore, CS exposure has been applied to genetically modified *Kras* models for investigating the molecular mechanisms of tumor progression. In the transgenic rasH2 (c-Ha-*ras* gene) mouse model, CS exposure (a 20-week exposure followed by a 16-week recovery period) enhanced the development of lung tumors relative to air exposure (control) (Curtin et al., 2004). The activating glycine-to-aspartic acid mutation at codon 12 of *Kras* in the *Kras*$^{LA2+/-}$ mouse model, when combined with intermittent CS exposure (3 months of CS exposure over a span of 5 months, followed by a 4-month recovery period), resulted in increased lung adenoma multiplicity and size (Takahashi et al., 2010). In this mutant *Kras* model, lung inflammation triggered by CS exposure promotes tumor cell proliferation and lung tumor progression (Takahashi et al., 2010).

15.4.5 Mouse Models of SCCs

SCCs account for approximately 23% of human lung cancers (National Cancer Institute) and are strongly associated with smoking history (Alexandrov et al., 2016; Khuder, 2001; Khuder and Mutgi, 2001). Lung SCCs originate from the keratin 5-positive basal cells of the pseudostratified bronchial epithelial cells in the lungs, and SCC cells display markers of squamous cell differentiation (e.g., keratin deposition, p63, keratin 5/6, and SOX2 expression) (Ferone et al., 2016). Lung SCCs are of two subtypes—central and peripheral—according to the primary site of tumor development. CS-associated SCCs are mainly of the central type, especially in patients who smoke cigarettes with high tar content (Brooks et al., 2005). Mutations and copy number changes are common in various oncogenes and tumor suppressors (e.g., *TP53, CDKN2A, PTEN, RB1, PIK3CA, NOTCH1, SOX2, PDGFRA, KIT, EGFR, MYC,* and *PTEN*) (Cancer Genome Atlas Research, 2014) and are reviewed elsewhere (Akbay and Kim, 2018). The tumors frequently show alterations in the PI3K, RAS, receptor tyrosine kinase, and NOTCH pathways. Unlike lung AC, murine models of SCC have been the least studied owing to technical challenges and complex genetics of the disease.

15.4.5.1 Chemically induced lung SCC

Intratracheal administration of methylcholanthrene (Henry et al., 1981), methyl carbamate (Nettesheim and Hammons, 1971), or benzo[a]pyrene with charcoal powder (Yoshimoto et al., 1977, 1980) for 16–40 weeks led to development of mostly SCCs, mixed with adenomas. Technical challenges and the reproducibility of these SCC models have largely limited their common use. Repeated cutaneous (skin painting) application of N-nitroso-bis-chloroethylurea (Rehm et al., 1991) or N-nitroso-tris-chloroethylurea (NTCU) led to hyperplasia of bronchiole epithelia, squamous metaplasia—squamous dysplasia, SCC in situ, adenosquamous carcinoma, and invasive carcinoma in susceptible mouse strains (NIH Swiss, A/J, and SWR/J mice) within 23–43 weeks. The role of inflammation in enhancing invasive lung SCC development was demonstrated in an A/J mouse model by using simultaneous intranasal lipopolysaccharide and NTCU administration (Song et al., 2015). CS-exposed A/J mice developed adenomas and AC (Coggins, 2010), while CS-exposed newborn Swiss mice developed a mix of SCC, AC, and adenosquamous carcinoma following the treatment (Balansky et al., 2007). In contrast, Swiss mice exposed to mainstream CS starting from the usual age (10–13 weeks) with a 5-month exposure and 4-month recovery schedule developed exclusively bronchioloalveolar adenoma (89%) and bronchioloalveolar AC (11%) (Stinn et al., 2010). It would be interesting to investigate if sequential or concurrent inhalation of CS and NTCU cause enhanced SCC relative to NTCU or CS inhalation alone.

15.4.5.2 Genetic models of lung SCC

In genetically modified mouse models, conditional biallelic knockout of both *Lkb1* and *Pten* tumor suppressor genes by administration of adenovirus-Cre via intranasal instillation led to SCC development within 40–50 weeks (Xu et al., 2014a). In the ubiquitously expressing IKKα kinase-dead mouse model (IKKαK44A), spontaneous SCC developed in the skin and lungs at 4–10 months of age (Xiao et al., 2013), and early euthanasia because of severe skin phenotypes resulted in only 20% of the mutant mice having developed lung tumors. In this model, all mice developed lung SCCs within 4–6 months of age when the skin phenotypes were rescued by concurrent expression of wild-type IKKα by using the skin-specific loricrin promoter. Other genetically modified mouse models of SCC are based on targeted (tissue-specific promoter with localized delivery of adenovirus/lentivirus-Cre) overexpression of *Sox2* with or without loss of tumor suppressors (*LKB1*, *PTEN*, and *CDKN2ab*) (Ferone et al., 2016; Mukhopadhyay et al., 2014). Because of the complex genetic crosses and requirements of targeted Cre recombinase expression, such genetically modified mouse models of SCC are less preferred for studying lung tumorigenesis due to CS exposure. The Sox2 and Notch signaling pathways play important roles in lung cancer development, promoting squamous hyperplasia instead of adenocarcinoma in KRAS carcinogenesis (Xu et al., 2014b) and may be exploited for investigating the role of CS and CS carcinogen exposure in SCC development.

15.4.6 Carcinogenicity of ENDPs

The effects of exposure to EVP aerosols (composed of PG, VG, nicotine, and flavor mixtures) or their individual key components have been tested in in vivo models of lung cancer. Early chronic exposure studies with PG and glycerin were based on noninhalational routes of administration. The absence of carcinogenicity noted in long-term cutaneous or oral studies on PG and glycerin in mice and rats (Gaunt et al., 1972; Morris et al., 1974; Stenbäck and Shubik, 1974; Wilson et al., 1978) was consistent with the minimal toxicity of PG and glycerin administered via the inhalational route (Renne et al., 2009; Renne et al., 1992; Robertson et al., 1947; Suber et al., 1989). In a 2-year study in rats, inhaled nicotine did not show enhanced carcinogenicity (Waldum et al., 1996). Even though ENDPs are considered safer and contain significantly reduced levels of toxicants/carcinogens relative to CS (National Academies of Sciences, 2018; Polosa and Caponnetto, 2016), uncertainties from impurities, thermal degradation products, as well as the consequences of uncharacterized inhalation of flavoring ingredients (Farsalinos et al., 2015; Kosmider et al., 2014; Laino et al., 2011; Mravec et al., 2020; National Academies of Sciences, 2018) necessitate further testing of their lung cancer risk. In a 54-week inhalation study, male FVB/N mice exposed to e-vapor containing nicotine showed a higher incidence of lung AC than mice exposed to the PG- and VG-containing vehicle control (Tang et al., 2019). The concentrations of TSNAs and other HPHCs in the e-vapor were not measured, and the sham-exposed group lacked statistical power because of its small group size at termination. As a CS-exposed group was not included in the study setup, comparison of lung cancer risk of the e-vapor exposure relative to CS exposure was not possible in this study. At this time (June 2020), a state-of-the-art lung carcinogenesis study for EVP aerosols is still pending.

With regard to EHTP aerosol carcinogenicity, we have conducted a lifetime (18-month) inhalation study in A/J mice to compare lung tumor incidence and multiplicity, extent of lung inflammation, emphysematous changes, and gene expression, miRNA, and protein signatures in response to exposure to CS from 3R4F reference cigarettes and aerosol from the THS (Titz et al., 2020; Wong et al., 2020; Xiang et al., 2020). In alignment with the OECD Test Guideline 453 for combined chronic toxicity/carcinogenicity studies (OECD, 2018), female A/J mice were whole-body exposed for 6 h per day continuously, 5 days per week, for up to 18 months to filtered air (sham), CS at 13.4 µg/L nicotine, or one of three concentrations of aerosol from the THS (THS Low (L), THS Medium (M), and THS High (H), corresponding to 6.7, 13.4, and 26.8 µg/L nicotine, respectively). Male A/J mice were exposed to air or THS (H) aerosol. The decision to omit the CS group in male mice was made on the basis of earlier findings that (i) female mice and rats are more sensitive to CS toxicity (Vanscheeuwijck et al., 2002; Wong et al., 2016); (ii) lung tumor multiplicities are equal in male and female CS-exposed A/J mice (Stinn et al., 2013a); and (iii) the levels of HPHCs in THS aerosol are significantly reduced relative to CS (Mallock et al., 2018; Schaller et al., 2016a,b). Interim dissections of female mice at months 1, 5, and 10 were conducted to evaluate lung inflammation, emphysema, and lung function. Histopathological evaluation and systems toxicology–based analyses were conducted at interim dissections and at the end of lifetime exposure to characterize lung tumor development and systems toxicology changes.

Daily characterization of nicotine and TPM concentrations in the test atmospheres demonstrated that CS and aerosol delivery to the exposure chambers were consistent and reproducible. Consistent with the lower concentrations of HPHCs in THS aerosol, the concentrations of selected toxicants, including carbon monoxide (CO), formaldehyde, acrolein, and acetaldehyde, were significantly reduced in THS aerosol relative to 3R4F CS (Wong et al., 2020).

The uptake of nicotine and reduced uptake of selected toxicants/carcinogens present in THS aerosol were demonstrated by quantification of biomarkers of exposure in the blood or urine samples of the exposed A/J mice (Fig. 15.12). Consistent with the nicotine concentrations in THS aerosol, plasma nicotine, plasma cotinine, and urine total nicotine metabolites showed a concentration-dependent increase across the three female THS groups. Exposure- and sex-dependent

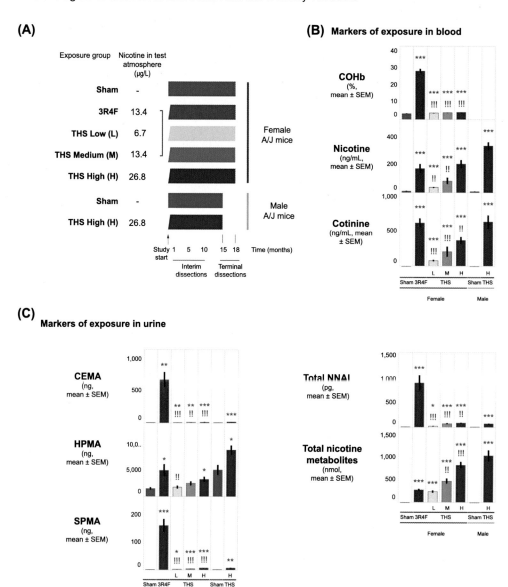

FIG. 15.12 Study design and biomarkers of exposure. **(A)** Study design. **(B)** COHb concentration in blood, cotinine, and nicotine concentrations in plasma, and **(C)** absolute levels of CEMA, HPMA, SPMA, total NNAL, and total nicotine metabolites in 24-h urine samples. Blood was collected within 15 min after the end of daily exposure (selected data collected at months 12 to 15 are shown). The 24-h urine samples consisted of urine collected during the 6-h exposure and during approximately 18 h postexposure (selected data at month 14 are shown). *, **, and *** represent statistically significant differences between the treatment and sham groups at $P \leq .05$, $P \leq .01$, and $P \leq .001$, respectively. !, !!, and !!! represent statistically significant differences between the THS and 3R4F groups at $P \leq .05$, $P \leq .01$, and $P \leq .001$, respectively. *CEMA*, 2-cyanoethylmercapturic acid; *H*, high; *HPMA*, 3-hydroxypropylmercuric acid; *L*, low; *M*, medium; *NNAL*, 4-(methylnitrosamino)-1-(3-pyridyl)-1-butanol; *SPMA*, S-phenylmercapturic acid; *THS*, Tobacco Heating System. (Adapted from Wong, E.T., Luettich, K., Krishnan, S., Wong, S.K., Lim, W.T., Yeo, D., et al., 2020. Reduced chronic toxicity and carcinogenicity in A/J mice in response to life-time exposure to aerosol from a heated tobacco product compared with cigarette smoke. Toxicol. Sci. https://doi.org/10.1093/toxsci/kfaa131. Epub ahead of print.)

differences in plasma nicotine and cotinine concentrations were also noted. Consistent with the CO concentrations in the test atmospheres, the average levels of COHb in the THS aerosol—exposed animals were lower than those in the 3R4F CS—exposed mice. Also consistent with the exposure item and chemical composition of the aerosol (Schaller et al., 2016a), the urinary levels of 2-cyanoethylmercapturic acid (CEMA), total 4-(methyl-nitrosamino)-1-(3-pyridyl)-1-butanol (NNAL), 3-hydroxypropylmercuric acid (HPMA), and S-phenylmercapturic acid (SPMA) in mice exposed to THS aerosol were much lower than those in 3R4F CS exposed mice.

Evaluation of lung inflammation was performed by enumeration of FLCs, analysis of MMP activity, quantification of soluble analytes in BALF, and histopathological evaluation (Fig. 15.13). 3R4F CS—exposed female mice showed extensive lung inflammation, as evidenced by their higher total FLC counts, inflammatory mediator concentrations, and MMP activity in BALF and increased macrophage, neutrophilic granulocyte, and lymphocyte infiltrates in the lungs relative to those in sham mice. In contrast, the THS aerosol—exposed groups showed no or minimal changes in these parameters. The reduced lung inflammation in THS aerosol—exposed A/J mice is consistent with the data from other THS studies in $Apoe^{-/-}$ mice (Phillips et al., 2019, 2016) and Sprague Dawley rats (Oviedo et al., 2016; Wong et al., 2016).

Emphysematous changes and altered lung functions were observed in CS-exposed mice but not in THS aerosol—exposed female A/J mice (Wong et al., 2020) (Fig. 15.14). The absence of emphysematous changes following long-term exposure to THS aerosol is consistent with the findings of our past THS inhalation studies in female $Apoe^{-/-}$ mice (Phillips et al., 2019, 2016).

Pulmonary proliferative lesions were classified in accordance with the International Classification of Rodent Tumors (Dungworth et al., 2001) and International Harmonization of Nomenclature and Diagnostic Criteria (Renne et al., 2009). At terminal dissection, all experimental groups had a group size of at least 50 animals to ensure sufficient statistical power, and tumor data were survival-adjusted to account for early deaths in accordance with the OECD guidance document 116 (OECD, 2012). Preneoplastic and neoplastic lesions of the lungs in A/J mice exclusively included nodular hyperplasia of the alveolar epithelium, bronchioloalveolar adenoma, and bronchioloalveolar AC. Exposure of A/J mice to THS aerosol did not increase the incidence or multiplicity of lung bronchioloalveolar adenomas or carcinomas relative to sham exposure (Fig. 15.15). The incidence and multiplicity of lung tumors were higher in the 3R4F group than in the sham and THS aerosol groups.

In summary, lung inflammation, emphysema, and lung tumor incidence and multiplicity were not increased following long-term exposure of A/J mice to THS aerosol, even when the mice were exposed to double the nicotine concentration used in the CS-exposed group and at a human equivalent dose of ca. 1—2 packs of cigarettes a day. This is in stark contrast to the effect of CS exposure. The findings are consistent with the significantly reduced levels of known carcinogens and noxious irritant chemicals in THS aerosol and, hence, the lower uptake of these carcinogens and proinflammatory compounds by the THS aerosol—exposed A/J mice in this study. The significantly reduced genotoxicity (Schaller et al., 2016a), lung inflammation, and emphysematous changes upon chronic exposure to THS aerosol compared to CS exposure collectively point to the absence of a tumor-promoting environment and potential favorable lung cancer risk reduction of this ENDP relative to CS. The data further support previous findings demonstrating that the A/J mouse is a suitable animal model for studying CS exposure—related pulmonary tumorigenesis and chronic toxicity, with the added value of assessing the impact of ENDP aerosol exposure on tumor development.

15.4.7 Systems Toxicology Assessment of EHTP Aerosol Exposure

To capture toxicity- and disease-relevant mechanisms in the A/J inhalation study, we complemented the in vivo lung inflammation and emphysema endpoints with in-depth systems toxicology analyses and compared these endpoints among the sham, 3R4F CS- and THS aerosol—exposed mice. Respiratory nasal epithelia (RNE), the larynx, and lung tissues were collected for investigating the effects of THS aerosol exposure on gene, miRNA, and protein expression in these tissues (Titz et al., 2020).

3R4F CS exposure resulted in a clear differential expression response, with more differentially expressed genes/miRNAs/proteins in the RNE, larynx, and lung tissues relative to the sham group (FDR < 0.05). In contrast, the differential expression response due to THS aerosol exposure was much more limited (Fig. 15.16). Next, the gene expression changes were compared in the context of curated, biologically relevant causal network models (Boue et al., 2015) to derive the network perturbation amplitude (NPA) for each causal network, and the NPA values were aggregated to derive overall relative biological impact factors (RBIF) (Hoeng et al., 2014) (Chapter 9). The results of

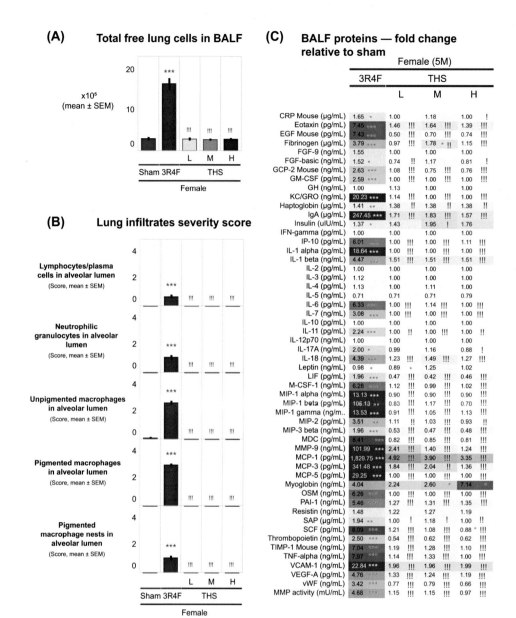

FIG. 15.13 Evaluation of lung inflammation in female mice at month 5. **(A)** Total free lung cell counts in BALF. **(B)** Severity scores of macrophage, neutrophilic granulocyte, and lymphocyte lung infiltrates. **(C)** Changes in inflammatory mediator concentrations and MMP activity in BALF. The concentrations of BALF inflammatory mediators are shown as fold change relative to the sham group. The extent of histopathological findings was scored in accordance with a defined severity scale from 0 to 5, with 0 indicating findings within normal limits; score 1, minimal changes; score 2, minimal to moderate changes; score 3, moderate changes; score 4, moderate to severe changes; and score 5, severe changes. *, **, and *** represent statistically significant differences between the treatment and sham groups at P ≤ .05, P ≤ .01, and P ≤ .001, respectively. !, !!, and !!! represent statistically significant differences between the THS and 3R4F groups at P ≤ .05, P ≤ .01, and P ≤ .001, respectively. *BALF*, bronchoalveolar lavage fluid; *H*, high; *L*, low; *M*, medium; *MMP*, matrix metalloproteinase; *SEM*, standard error of the mean; *THS*, Tobacco Heating System. (Adapted from Wong, E.T., Luettich, K., Krishnan, S., Wong, S.K., Lim, W.T., Yeo, D., et al., 2020. Reduced chronic toxicity and carcinogenicity in A/J mice in response to life-time exposure to aerosol from a heated tobacco product compared with cigarette smoke. Toxicol. Sci. https://doi.org/10.1093/toxsci/kfaa131. Epub ahead of print.)

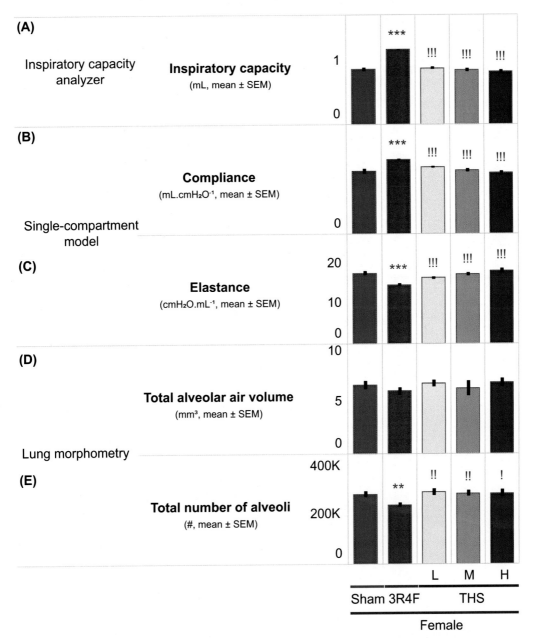

(A) Inspiratory capacity analyzer — **Inspiratory capacity** (mL, mean ± SEM)

(B) Single-compartment model — **Compliance** (mL.cmH₂O⁻¹, mean ± SEM)

(C) **Elastance** (cmH₂O.mL⁻¹, mean ± SEM)

(D) Lung morphometry — **Total alveolar air volume** (mm³, mean ± SEM)

(E) **Total number of alveoli** (#, mean ± SEM)

L   M   H

Sham   3R4F   THS

Female

FIG. 15.14 Evaluation of lung function and emphysema in female mice at month 5. **(A)** Inspiratory capacity, **(B)** compliance, **(C)** elastance, **(D)** total air (alveolar and ductal) volume, and **(E)** total number of alveoli in the sham, 3R4F, and THS groups. *, **, and *** represent statistically significant differences between the treatment and sham groups at $P \leq .05$, $P \leq .01$, and $P \leq .001$, respectively. !, !!, and !!! represent statistically significant differences between the THS and 3R4F groups at $P \leq .05$, $P \leq .01$, and $P \leq .001$, respectively. *H*, high; *L*, low; *M*, medium; *SEM*, standard error of the mean; *THS*, Tobacco Heating System. (Adapted from Wong, E.T., Luettich, K., Krishnan, S., Wong, S.K., Lim, W.T., Yeo, D., et al., 2020. Reduced chronic toxicity and carcinogenicity in A/J mice in response to life-time exposure to aerosol from a heated tobacco product compared with cigarette smoke. Toxicol. Sci. https://doi.org/10.1093/toxsci/kfaa131. Epub ahead of print. Epub ahead of print.)

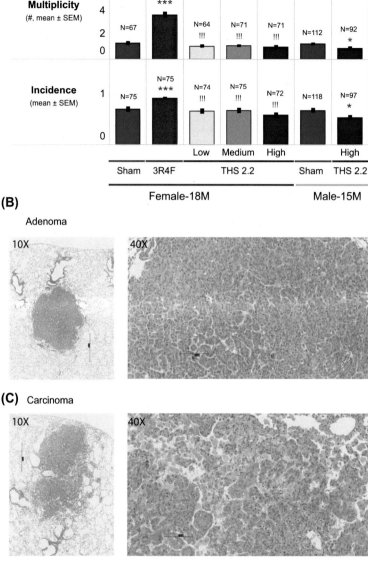

FIG. 15.15 Neoplastic lesions in the lungs. **(A)** Survival-adjusted multiplicity and incidence of bronchioloalveolar adenoma and bronchioloalveolar carcinoma combined are shown for female (month 18; 18M) and male (month 15; 15M) animals. A power of 3 in the poly-k analysis (k = 3) was used for survival-adjustment of tumor incidence. A power of 2 (X = 2) as well as thresholds (T) of study days 400 for female mice and 240 for male mice were used for survival-adjustment of tumor multiplicity. **(B)** Representative images of adenoma. **(C)** Representative images of carcinoma. *, **, and *** represent statistically significant differences between the treatment and sham groups at $P \leq .05$, $P \leq .01$, and $P \leq .001$, respectively. !, !!, and !!! represent statistically significant differences between the THS and 3R4F groups at $P \leq .05$, $P \leq .01$, and $P \leq .001$, respectively. H, high; L, low; M, medium; SEM, standard error of the mean; THS, Tobacco Heating System; ♂, male; ♀, female. (Adapted from Wong, E.T., Luettich, K., Krishnan, S., Wong, S.K., Lim, W.T., Yeo, D., et al., 2020. Reduced chronic toxicity and carcinogenicity in A/J mice in response to life-time exposure to aerosol from a heated tobacco product compared with cigarette smoke. Toxicol. Sci. https://doi.org/10.1093/toxsci/kfaa131. Epub ahead of print.)

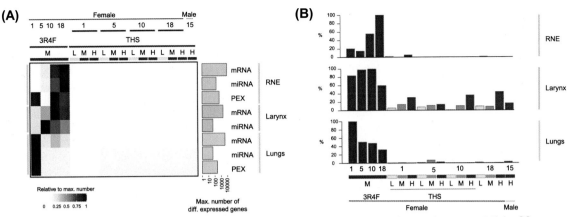

FIG. 15.16 THS aerosol exposure induces fewer molecular changes in the respiratory tract than CS exposure. **(A)** Number of differentially expressed molecules in the respiratory tract. The heatmap shows the number of differentially expressed molecules per exposure group (columns) and data type (rows) relative to the maximum number of significantly affected molecules for the data type (bar chart). Note that miRNA and protein (PEX) expression in the lungs were only measured after 1 month. **(B)** Relative biological impact factors in the three tissues calculated from transcriptomic data and causal biological network models. Relative biological impact factors are represented for each group versus sham. RNE, respiratory nasal epithelia; Exposure months 1, 5, 10, 15, and 18 are indicated. *H*, high; *L*, low; *M*, medium; *THS*, Tobacco Heating System. (Adapted from Titz, B., Sewer, A., Luettich, K., Wong, E.T., Guedj, E., Nury, C., et al., 2020. Respiratory effects of exposure to aerosol from the candidate modified-risk tobacco product THS 2.2 in an 18-month systems toxicology study with A/J mice. Toxicol. Sci. https://doi.org/10.1093/toxsci/kfaa132. Epub ahead of print.)

the calculated RBIFs confirmed the observed differential expression profiles: 3R4F CS exposure strongly perturbed the evaluated biological mechanisms (higher RBIF), whereas the effects of THS aerosol exposure were much milder (Fig. 15.16). Multiomics factor analysis (MOFA) of protein and gene expression has been further discussed previously (Titz et al., 2020). 3R4F CS exposure induced a clear immune response in the RNE, larynx, and lung tissues. In the RNE, antimicrobial peptides were strongly expressed following exposure to 3R4F CS but not to THS aerosol. In the larynx, downregulation of T cell- and B cell–related gene sets were observed following 3R4F CS exposure. In the lungs, activation of neutrophil and macrophage signaling networks was observed following 3R4F CS exposure. Perturbation of oxidative stress and xenobiotic metabolism response networks in the RNE, larynx, and lung tissues was much less or absent following THS aerosol exposure, relative to 3R4F CS exposure. Distinct miRNA response profiles were observed following 3R4F CS exposure in the three respiratory tissues, while miRNA responses to THS aerosol exposure were limited to only the laryngeal tissues. Overall, the integrative analysis of molecular changes confirmed the substantially lower impact of THS aerosol than 3R4F CS on toxicologically and disease-relevant molecular

processes such as immune responses, oxidative stress responses, and xenobiotic metabolism (Titz et al., 2020).

15.4.8 Molecular Signatures of Lung Tumors in CS- and EHTP Aerosol–Exposed A/J Mice

Lung tissues were also collected, processed, and subjected to microarray analysis to gain insights into the molecular makeup of spontaneously arising and exposure-related lung tumors (Xiang et al., 2020). We have previously identified a 50-gene expression signature that distinguished spontaneous and CS-induced lung tumors in A/J mice (Luettich et al., 2014). Furthermore, we derived a 1-class classifier comprising the 13 highest ranked genes from the prior A/J mouse CS-exposure study: *Scgb3a1*, *Iglv1*, *Ighv1-14*, *Bex1*, *Ighg3*, *Chia1*, *Ighm*, *Ighg2b*, *Iglc1*, *Saa3*, *Acoxl*, *Itih4*, and *Ighg1*[1]. As the THS aerosol contains significantly lower levels of HPHCs than CS, it is hypothesized that lung tumors from THS aerosol–exposed mice would show

---

[1]Section 10.3.4 (Lung Tumor Gene Signature) of SR 15020 AJ LC Transcriptomics_Release in Full.pdf. In: August 30, 2018 Amendment: Submission of Finalized In Vivo Study. Available at https://digitalmedia.hhs.gov/tobacco/static/mrtpa/PMP/August%2030%2C%202018.zip

differential effects in their molecular makeup relative to tumors arising in CS-exposed mice. The 13-gene signature classifier—when applied along with Mahalanobis distance calculations to the data from this study—was able to distinguish lung tumors in CS-exposed animals from spontaneous lung tumors; lung tumors in THS aerosol—exposed female mice were significantly different from those in CS-exposed mice but not from the tumors in sham mice (Xiang et al., 2020).

This gene signature was also applied to human lung AC gene expression data (Cancer Genome Atlas Research, 2014) and was able to discriminate cancers in never-smokers from those in ever-smokers (Xiang et al., 2020). Former smokers exhibited a median distance closer to the current smokers than to the never-smokers. In conclusion, the gene signature derived from the mouse lung tumor data is translatable for distinguishing lung AC in current smokers and never-smokers.

15.4.9 Conclusions for Lung Cancer
While only few animal models are suitable for assessing the effects of CS and ENDP aerosols on lung cancer, the A/J mouse model has proven its value for this purpose. The study conducted in this mouse model with the EHTP THS has shown that THS aerosol causes significantly less lung inflammation, emphysematous changes, and lung function alterations than CS. Furthermore, in contrast to CS exposure, exposure to THS aerosol does not cause an increase in tumor incidence or multiplicity in this model. Importantly, these results are coherent with the reduced exposure of THS aerosol—exposed mice to HPHCs and other toxicants relative to CS-exposed mice. Furthermore, the differential effects of CS and THS aerosol on lung inflammation, emphysematous changes, and lung function are consistent across animal models and studies. These results, which are coherent along the CELSD (Chapter 3), indicate that THS aerosol is less likely to cause lung cancer than CS.

15.5 OVERALL CONCLUSIONS
In vivo models of disease have been shown to be suitable for assessment of ENDPs and for demonstrating their potential to reduce the risk of key smoking-related diseases relative to cigarettes. While it is important to be aware of the limitations of each disease model, one should also value their contribution in deciphering the molecular mechanisms induced by CS, as this knowledge is highly relevant for mechanism-based comparison of the effects of CS and

ENDP aerosols. It is also important to stress that CS-induced diseases take a considerable time to develop in humans and that animal models of disease are indispensable for assessing ENDPs in a decent time frame.

The studies summarized in this chapter have collectively shown that exposure to the aerosol of an ENDP caused less harm than exposure to CS in all events along the CELSD. Importantly, these reductions in biological effects were consistent across studies and coherent with the reduced emission of toxicants by the tested ENDP relative to cigarettes. In short, these studies have demonstrated that the reduced exposure to CS toxicants leads to reduced molecular changes, which leads to reduced biological network perturbations, which, in turn, lead to reduced cell/tissue changes and, finally, reduced disease manifestations. These studies also demonstrated that integration of large multiomics datasets with apical endpoints provides a uniquely powerful approach for evaluating the relative risk of ENDPs and cigarettes along the CELSD and across the many biological mechanisms affected by CS. Furthermore, studies in certain animal models of disease can be conducted according to a "switching design," in which the effects of switching to an ENDP can be compared with those of continued smoking and benchmarked against those of smoking cessation, which is the "gold standard" for ENDP assessment (Chapter 3).

REFERENCES
Adcock, I.M., Caramori, G., Barnes, P.J., 2011. Chronic obstructive pulmonary disease and lung cancer: new molecular insights. Respiration 81 (4), 265–284.
Akbay, E.A., Kim, J., 2018. Autochthonous murine models for the study of smoker and never-smoker associated lung cancers. Transl. Lung Cancer Res. 7 (4), 464–486.
Alexandrov, L.B., Ju, Y.S., Haase, K., Van Loo, P., Martincorena, I., Nik-Zainal, S., et al., 2016. Mutational signatures associated with tobacco smoking in human cancer. Science 354 (6312), 618–622.
Ansari, S., Baumer, K., Boue, S., Dijon, S., Dulize, R., Ekroos, K., et al., 2016. Comprehensive systems biology analysis of a 7-month cigarette smoke inhalation study in C57BL/6 mice. Sci. Data 3, 150077.
Bai, J.W., Chen, X.X., Liu, S., Yu, L., Xu, J.F., 2017. Smoking cessation affects the natural history of COPD. Int. J. Chronic Obstr. Pulm. Dis. 12, 3323–3328.
Balansky, R., Ganchev, G., Iltcheva, M., Steele, V.E., D'agostini, F., De Flora, S., 2007. Potent carcinogenicity of cigarette smoke in mice exposed early in life. Carcinogenesis 28 (10), 2236–2243.
Balkwill, F., Mantovani, A., 2001. Inflammation and cancer: back to Virchow? Lancet 357 (9255), 539–545.

Bartalesi, B., Cavarra, E., Fineschi, S., Lucattelli, M., Lunghi, B., Martorana, P.A., et al., 2005. Different lung responses to cigarette smoke in two strains of mice sensitive to oxidants. Eur. Respir. J. 25 (1), 15–22.

Bjorklund, M.M., Hollensen, A.K., Hagensen, M.K., Dagnaes-Hansen, F., Christoffersen, C., Mikkelsen, J.G., et al., 2014. Induction of atherosclerosis in mice and hamsters without germline genetic engineering. Circ. Res. 114 (11), 1684–1689.

Blankstein, R., Libby, P., Bhatt, D.L., 2019. Arterial inflammation: the heat before the storm. J. Am. Coll. Cardiol. 73 (12), 1383–1385.

Boue, S., De Leon, H., Schlage, W.K., Peck, M.J., Weiler, H., Berges, A., et al., 2013. Cigarette smoke induces molecular responses in respiratory tissues of ApoE$^{(-/-)}$ mice that are progressively deactivated upon cessation. Toxicology 314 (1), 112–124.

Boue, S., Talikka, M., Westra, J.W., Hayes, W., Di Fabio, A., Park, J., et al., 2015. Causal biological network database: a comprehensive platform of causal biological network models focused on the pulmonary and vascular systems. Database (Oxford) 2015, bav030.

Boue, S., Tarasov, K., Janis, M., Lebrun, S., Hurme, R., Schlage, W., et al., 2012. Modulation of atherogenic lipidome by cigarette smoke in apolipoprotein E-deficient mice. Atherosclerosis 225 (2), 328–334.

Braber, S., Henricks, P.A., Nijkamp, F.P., Kraneveld, A.D., Folkerts, G., 2010. Inflammatory changes in the airways of mice caused by cigarette smoke exposure are only partially reversed after smoking cessation. Respir. Res. 11, 99.

Bracke, K.R., D'hulst A, I., Maes, T., Moerloose, K.B., Demedts, I.K., Lebecque, S., et al., 2006. Cigarette smoke-induced pulmonary inflammation and emphysema are attenuated in CCR6-deficient mice. J. Immunol. 177 (7), 4350–4359.

Brenner, D.R., Boffetta, P., Duell, E.J., Bickeböller, H., Rosenberger, A., Mccormack, V., et al., 2012. Previous lung diseases and lung cancer risk: a pooled analysis from the International Lung Cancer Consortium. Am. J. Epidemiol. kws151.

Broberg, C.S., Pantely, G.A., Barber, B.J., Mack, G.K., Lee, K., Thigpen, T., et al., 2003. Validation of the myocardial performance index by echocardiography in mice: a noninvasive measure of left ventricular function. J. Am. Soc. Echocardiogr. 16 (8), 814–823.

Brooks, D.R., Austin, J.H., Heelan, R.T., Ginsberg, M.S., Shin, V., Olson, S.H., et al., 2005. Influence of type of cigarette on peripheral versus central lung cancer. Cancer Epidemiol. Biomark. Prev. 14 (3), 576–581.

Brown, B.G., Chang, C.J., Ayres, P.H., Lee, C.K., Doolittle, D.J., 1999. The effect of cotinine or cigarette smoke co-administration on the formation of O6-methylguanine adducts in the lung and liver of A/J mice treated with 4-(methylnitrosamino)-1-(3-pyridyl)-1-butanone (NNK). Toxicol. Sci. 47 (1), 33–39.

Brown, S.A.W., Braman, S., 2020. Recent advances in the management of acute exacerbations of chronic obstructive pulmonary disease. Med. Clinics 104 (4), 615–630.

Burgel, P.R., Bourdin, A., Chanez, P., Chabot, F., Chaouat, A., Chinet, T., et al., 2011. Update on the roles of distal airways in COPD. Eur. Respir. Rev. 20 (119), 7–22.

Cabanski, M., Fields, B., Boue, S., Boukharov, N., Deleon, H., Dror, N., et al., 2015. Transcriptional profiling and targeted proteomics reveals common molecular changes associated with cigarette smoke-induced lung emphysema development in five susceptible mouse strains. Inflamm. Res. 64 (7), 471–486.

Caligiuri, G., Nicoletti, A., Zhou, X., Tornberg, I., Hansson, G.K., 1999. Effects of sex and age on atherosclerosis and autoimmunity in apoE-deficient mice. Atherosclerosis 145 (2), 301–308.

Cancer Genome Atlas Research, N., 2014. Comprehensive molecular profiling of lung adenocarcinoma. Nature 511 (7511), 543–550.

Carnevale, R., Sciarretta, S., Violi, F., Nocella, C., Loffredo, L., Perri, L., et al., 2016. Acute impact of tobacco vs electronic cigarette smoking on oxidative stress and vascular function. Chest 150 (3), 606–612.

Carraresi, L., Tripodi, S.A., Mulder, L.C., Bertini, S., Nuti, S., Schuerfeld, K., et al., 2001. Thymic hyperplasia and lung carcinomas in a line of mice transgenic for keratin 5-driven HPV16 E6/E7 oncogenes. Oncogene 20 (56), 8148–8153.

Celermajer, D.S., Sorensen, K.E., Gooch, V.M., Spiegelhalter, D.J., Miller, O.I., Sullivan, I.D., et al., 1992. Non-invasive detection of endothelial dysfunction in children and adults at risk of atherosclerosis. Lancet 340 (8828), 1111–1115.

Cendon, S.P., Battlehner, C., Lorenzi Filho, G., Dohlnikoff, M., Pereira, P.M., Conceicao, G.M., et al., 1997. Pulmonary emphysema induced by passive smoking: an experimental study in rats. Braz. J. Med. Biol. Res. 30 (10), 1241–1247.

Cerami, C., Founds, H., Nicholl, I., Mitsuhashi, T., Giordano, D., Vanpatten, S., et al., 1997. Tobacco smoke is a source of toxic reactive glycation products. Proc. Natl. Acad. Sci. U.S.A. 94 (25), 13915–13920.

Chen, T., Jia, G., Wei, Y., Li, J., 2013. Beijing ambient particle exposure accelerates atherosclerosis in ApoE knockout mice. Toxicol. Lett. 223 (2), 146–153.

Churg, A., Wright, J.L., 2007. Animal models of cigarette smoke-induced chronic obstructive lung disease. Contrib. Microbiol. 14, 113–125.

Coggins, C.R., 1998. A review of chronic inhalation studies with mainstream cigarett smoke in rats and mice. Toxicol. Pathol. 26 (3), 307–314.

Coggins, C.R., 2010. A further review of inhalation studies with cigarette smoke and lung cancer in experimental animals, including transgenic mice. Inhal. Toxicol. 22 (12), 974–983.

Collins, A.R., Meehan, W.P., Kintscher, U., Jackson, S., Wakino, S., Noh, G., et al., 2001. Troglitazone inhibits formation of early atherosclerotic lesions in diabetic and nondiabetic low density lipoprotein receptor-deficient mice. Arterioscler. Thromb. Vasc. Biol. 21 (3), 365–371.

Curtin, G.M., Higuchi, M.A., Ayres, P.H., Swauger, J.E., Mosberg, A.T., 2004. Lung tumorigenicity in A/J and rasH2 transgenic mice following mainstream tobacco smoke inhalation. Toxicol. Sci. 81 (1), 26–34.

Daiber, A., Steven, S., Weber, A., Shuvaev, V.V., Muzykantov, V.R., Laher, I., et al., 2017. Targeting vascular (endothelial) dysfunction. Br. J. Pharmacol. 174 (12), 1591–1619.

De-Torres, J.P., Wilson, D.O., Sanchez-Salcedo, P., Weissfeld, J.L., Berto, J., Campo, A., et al., 2015. Lung cancer in patients with chronic obstructive pulmonary disease. Development and validation of the COPD Lung Cancer Screening Score. Am. J. Respir. Crit. Care Med. 191 (3), 285–291.

De Leon, H., Boue, S., Schlage, W.K., Boukharov, N., Westra, J.W., Gebel, S., et al., 2014. A vascular biology network model focused on inflammatory processes to investigate atherogenesis and plaque instability. J. Transl. Med. 12, 185.

De Santi, M., Martorana, P.A., Cavarra, E., Lungarella, G., 1995. Pallid mice with genetic emphysema. Neutrophil elastase burden and elastin loss occur without alteration in the bronchoalveolar lavage cell population. Lab. Invest. 73 (1), 40–47.

Defesche, J.C., 2004. Low-density lipoprotein receptor–its structure, function, and mutations. Semin. Vasc. Med. 4 (1), 5–11.

Di Lascio, N., Kusmic, C., Stea, F., Faita, F., 2017. Ultrasound-based pulse wave velocity evaluation in mice. J. Vis. Exp. 120 https://doi.org/10.3791/54362.

Di Lascio, N., Stea, F., Kusmic, C., Sicari, R., Faita, F., 2014. Non-invasive assessment of pulse wave velocity in mice by means of ultrasound images. Atherosclerosis 237 (1), 31–37.

Dong, A., Caicedo, J., Han, S.G., Mueller, P., Saha, S., Smyth, S.S., et al., 2010. Enhanced platelet reactivity and thrombosis in Apoe$^{-/-}$ mice exposed to cigarette smoke is attenuated by P2Y12 antagonism. Thromb. Res. 126 (4), e312–317.

Du, J., Liu, J., Feng, H.Z., Hossain, M.M., Gobara, N., Zhang, C., et al., 2008. Impaired relaxation is the main manifestation in transgenic mice expressing a restrictive cardiomyopathy mutation, R193H, in cardiac TnI. Am. J. Physiol. Heart Circ. Physiol. 294 (6), H2604–H2613.

Dungworth, D.L., Rittinghausen, S., Schwartz, L., Harkema, J.R., Hayashi, Y., Kittel, B., Lewis, D., Miller, R.A., Mohr, U., Rehm, S., Slayter, M.V., 2001. Respiratory system and mesothelium. In: Mohr, U. (Ed.), International Classification of Rodent Tumors. The Mouse. Springer, Berlin, Heidelberg, pp. 87–139.

Durham, A.L., Adcock, I.M., 2015. The relationship between COPD and lung cancer. Lung Cancer 90 (2), 121–127.

Ehrhardt, A., Bartels, T., Geick, A., Klocke, R., Paul, D., Halter, R., 2001. Development of pulmonary bronchiolo-alveolar adenocarcinomas in transgenic mice overexpressing murine c-myc and epidermal growth factor in alveolar type II pneumocytes. Br. J. Cancer 84 (6), 813–818.

Elamin, A., Titz, B., Dijon, S., Merg, C., Geertz, M., Schneider, T., et al., 2016. Quantitative proteomics analysis using 2D-PAGE to investigate the effects of cigarette smoke and aerosol of a prototypic modified risk tobacco product on the lung proteome in C57BL/6 mice. J. Proteomics 145, 237–245.

Elkington, P.T., Friedland, J.S., 2006. Matrix metalloproteinases in destructive pulmonary pathology. Thorax 61 (3), 259–266.

Emini Veseli, B., Perrotta, P., De Meyer, G.R.A., Roth, L., Van Der Donckt, C., Martinet, W., et al., 2017. Animal models of atherosclerosis. Eur. J. Pharmacol. 816, 3–13.

Escolar, J.D., Martínez, M.N., Rodríguez, F.J., Gonzalo, C., Escolar, M.A., Roche, P.A., 1995. Emphysema as a result of involuntary exposure to tobacco smoke: morphometrical study of the rat. Exp. Lung Res. 21 (2), 255–273.

Esen, A.M., Barutcu, I., Acar, M., Degirmenci, B., Kaya, D., Turkmen, M., et al., 2004. Effect of smoking on endothelial function and wall thickness of brachial artery. Circ. J. 68 (12), 1123–1126.

Farsalinos, K.E., Gillman, I.G., Melvin, M.S., Paolantonio, A.R., Gardow, W.J., Humphries, K.E., et al., 2015. Nicotine levels and presence of selected tobacco-derived toxins in tobacco flavoured electronic cigarette refill liquids. Int. J. Environ. Res. Publ. Health 12 (4), 3439–3452.

Fawell, J.K., Lewis, D.J., 1971. A simple apparatus for the inflation fixation of lungs at constant pressure. Lab. Anim. 5 (2), 267–270.

Ferone, G., Song, J.Y., Sutherland, K.D., Bhaskaran, R., Monkhorst, K., Lambooij, J.P., et al., 2016. SOX2 is the determining oncogenic switch in promoting lung squamous cell carcinoma from different cells of origin. Cancer Cell 30 (4), 519–532.

Finch, G.L., Nikula, K.J., Belinsky, S.A., Barr, E.B., Stoner, G.D., Lechner, J.F., 1996. Failure of cigarette smoke to induce or promote lung cancer in the A/J mouse. Cancer Lett. 99 (2), 161–167.

Franklin, W.A., Wistuba, I.I., Geisinger, K., Lam, S., Hirsch, F.R., Muller, K.M., et al., 2004. Pathology and Genetics of Tumours of the Lung, Pleura, Thymus and Heart. IARC.

Franzen, K.F., Willig, J., Cayo Talavera, S., Meusel, M., Sayk, F., Reppel, M., et al., 2018. E-cigarettes and cigarettes worsen peripheral and central hemodynamics as well as arterial stiffness: a randomized, double-blinded pilot study. Vasc. Med. 23 (5), 419–425.

Fricker, M., Deane, A., Hansbro, P.M., 2014. Animal models of chronic obstructive pulmonary disease. Expet Opin. Drug Discov. 9 (6), 629–645.

Gairola, C.G., Drawdy, M.L., Block, A.E., Daugherty, A., 2001. Sidestream cigarette smoke accelerates atherogenesis in apolipoprotein E$^{-/-}$ mice. Atherosclerosis 156 (1), 49–55.

Gairola, C.G., Howatt, D.A., Daugherty, A., 2010. Dietary coenzyme Q10 does not protect against cigarette smoke-augmented atherosclerosis in apoE-deficient mice. Free Radic. Biol. Med. 48 (11), 1535–1539.

Garcia-Arcos, I., Geraghty, P., Baumlin, N., Campos, M., Dabo, A.J., Jundi, B., et al., 2016. Chronic electronic cigarette exposure in mice induces features of COPD in a nicotine-dependent manner. Thorax. https://doi.org/10.1136/thoraxjnl-2015-208039.

Gaunt, I.F., Carpanini, F.M., Grasso, P., Lansdown, A.B., 1972. Long-term toxicity of propylene glycol in rats. Food Cosmet. Toxicol. 10 (2), 151–162.

Gazdar, A.F., Carney, D.N., Nau, M.M., Minna, J.D., 1985. Characterization of variant subclasses of cell lines derived from small cell lung cancer having distinctive biochemical, morphological, and growth properties. Cancer Res. 45 (6), 2924–2930.

Gazdar, A.F., Hirsch, F.R., Minna, J.D., 2016. From mice to men and back: an assessment of preclinical model systems for the study of lung cancers. J. Thorac. Oncol. 11 (3), 287–299.

George, J., Lim, J.S., Jang, S.J., Cun, Y., Ozretic, L., Kong, G., et al., 2015. Comprehensive genomic profiles of small cell lung cancer. Nature 524 (7563), 47–53.

Geovanini, G.R., Libby, P., 2018. Atherosclerosis and inflammation: overview and updates. Clin. Sci. (Lond.) 132 (12), 1243–1252.

Getz, G.S., Reardon, C.A., 2006. Diet and murine atherosclerosis. Arterioscler. Thromb. Vasc. Biol. 26 (2), 242–249.

Getz, G.S., Reardon, C.A., 2016. ApoE knockout and knockin mice: the history of their contribution to the understanding of atherogenesis. J. Lipid Res. 57 (5), 758–766.

Golbidi, S., Edvinsson, L., Laher, I., 2020. Smoking and endothelial dysfunction. Curr. Vasc. Pharmacol. 18 (1), 1–11.

GOLD, 2020. Global Strategy for the Diagnosis, Management, and Prevention of Chronic Obstructive Pulmonary Disease (Updated 2020). Report. https://goldcopd.org/wp-content/uploads/2019/12/GOLD-2020-FINAL-ver1.2-03Dec19_WMV.pdf.

Goldstein, J.L., Brown, M.S., 2001. Molecular medicine. The cholesterol quartet. Science 292 (5520), 1310–1312.

Gordon, T., Bosland, M., 2009. Strain-dependent differences in susceptibility to lung cancer in inbred mice exposed to mainstream cigarette smoke. Cancer Lett. 275 (2), 213–220.

Govindan, R., Ding, L., Griffith, M., Subramanian, J., Dees, N.D., Kanchi, K.L., et al., 2012. Genomic landscape of non-small cell lung cancer in smokers and never-smokers. Cell 150 (6), 1121–1134.

Granger, D.N., Kvietys, P.R., 2015. Reperfusion injury and reactive oxygen species: the evolution of a concept. Redox Biol. 6, 524–551.

Grassi, D., Desideri, G., Ferri, L., Aggio, A., Tiberti, S., Ferri, C., 2010. Oxidative stress and endothelial dysfunction: say NO to cigarette smoking! Curr. Pharmaceut. Des. 16 (23), 2539–2550.

Guerassimov, A., Hoshino, Y., Takubo, Y., Turcotte, A., Yamamoto, M., Ghezzo, H., et al., 2004. The development of emphysema in cigarette smoke-exposed mice is strain dependent. Am. J. Respir. Crit. Care Med. 170 (9), 974–980.

Hajek, P., Etter, J.F., Benowitz, N., Eissenberg, T., Mcrobbie, H., 2014. Electronic cigarettes: review of use, content, safety, effects on smokers and potential for harm and benefit. Addiction 109 (11), 1801–1810.

Han, S.G., Howatt, D.A., Daugherty, A., Gairola, C.G., 2012. Atherogenic and pulmonary responses of ApoE- and LDL receptor-deficient mice to sidestream cigarette smoke. Toxicology 299 (2–3), 133–138.

Hardie, W.D., Bruno, M.D., Huelsman, K.M., Iwamoto, H.S., Carrigan, P.E., Leikauf, G.D., et al., 1997. Postnatal lung function and morphology in transgenic mice expressing transforming growth factor-alpha. Am. J. Pathol. 151 (4), 1075–1083.

Hecht, S.S., 2012. Lung carcinogenesis by tobacco smoke. Int. J. Cancer 131 (12), 2724–2732.

Hecht, S.S., Isaacs, S., Trushin, N., 1994. Lung tumor induction in A/J mice by the tobacco smoke carcinogens 4-(methylnitrosamino)-1-(3-pyridyl)-1-butanone and benzo[a]pyrene: a potentially useful model for evaluation of chemopreventive agents. Carcinogenesis 15 (12), 2721–2725.

Heitzer, T., Just, H., Munzel, T., 1996. Antioxidant vitamin C improves endothelial dysfunction in chronic smokers. Circulation 94 (1), 6–9.

Henry, C.J., Billups, L.H., Avery, M.D., Rude, T.H., Dansie, D.R., Lopez, A., et al., 1981. Lung cancer model system using 3-methylcholanthrene in inbred strains of mice. Cancer Res. 41 (12 Pt 1), 5027–5032.

Higham, A., Quinn, A.M., Cancado, J.E.D., Singh, D., 2019. The pathology of small airways disease in COPD: historical aspects and future directions. Respir. Res. 20 (1), 49.

Hoang, L.L., Nguyen, Y.P., Aspee, R., Bolton, S.J., Shen, Y.H., Wang, L., et al., 2016. Temporal and spatial expression of transforming growth factor-beta after airway remodeling to tobacco smoke in rats. Am. J. Respir. Cell Mol. Biol. 54 (6), 872–881.

Hoenderdos, K., Condliffe, A., 2013. The neutrophil in chronic obstructive pulmonary disease. Am. J. Respir. Cell Mol. Biol. 48 (5), 531–539.

Hoeng, J., Deehan, R., Pratt, D., Martin, F., Sewer, A., Thomson, T.M., et al., 2012. A network-based approach to quantifying the impact of biologically active substances. Drug Discov. Today 17 (9–10), 413–418.

Hoeng, J., Maeder, S., Vanscheeuwijck, P., Peitsch, M.C., 2019. Assessing the lung cancer risk reduction potential of candidate modified risk tobacco products. Intern. Emerg. Med. https://doi.org/10.1007/s11739-019-02045-z.

Hoeng, J., Talikka, M., Martin, F., Sewer, A., Yang, X., Iskandar, A., et al., 2014. Case study: the role of mechanistic network models in systems toxicology. Drug Discov. Today 19 (2), 183–192.

Houghton, A.M., 2018. Common mechanisms linking chronic obstructive pulmonary disease and lung cancer. Ann. Am. Thorac. Soc. 15 (Suppl. 4), S273–S277.

Hoyle, G.W., Li, J., Finkelstein, J.B., Eisenberg, T., Liu, J.Y., Lasky, J.A., et al., 1999. Emphysematous lesions, inflammation, and fibrosis in the lungs of transgenic mice overexpressing platelet-derived growth factor. Am. J. Pathol. 154 (6), 1763–1775.

Hsia, C.C., Hyde, D.M., Ochs, M., Weibel, E.R., 2010. An offi-cial research policy statement of the American Thoracic So-ciety/European Respiratory Society: standards for quantitative assessment of lung structure. Am. J. Respir. Crit. Care Med. 181 (4), 394–418.

Huszar, D., Varban, M.L., Rinninger, F., Feeley, R., Arai, T., Fairchild-Huntress, V., et al., 2000. Increased LDL choles-terol and atherosclerosis in LDL receptor-deficient mice with attenuated expression of scavenger receptor B1. Arte-rioscler. Thromb. Vasc. Biol. 20 (4), 1068–1073.

Hutt, J.A., Vuillemenot, B.R., Barr, E.B., Grimes, M.J., Hahn, F.F., Hobbs, C.H., et al., 2005. Life-span inhalation exposure to mainstream cigarette smoke induces lung can-cer in B6C3F1 mice through genetic and epigenetic pathways. Carcinogenesis 26 (11), 1999–2009.

Ikonomidis, I., Vlastos, D., Kourea, K., Kostelli, G., Varoudi, M., Pavlidis, G., et al., 2018. Electronic cigarette smoking in-creases arterial stiffness and oxidative stress to a lesser extent than a single conventional cigarette: an acute and chronic study. Circulation 137 (3), 303–306.

Ishibashi, S., Goldstein, J.L., Brown, M.S., Herz, J., Burns, D.K., 1994. Massive xanthomatosis and atherosclerosis in cholesterol-fed low density lipoprotein receptor-negative mice. J. Clin. Invest. 93 (5), 1885–1893.

Jeffery, P.K., 2001. Remodeling in asthma and chronic obstruc-tive lung disease. Am. J. Respir. Crit. Care Med. 164 (10 Pt 2), S28–S38.

Karakaya, O., Barutcu, I., Esen, A.M., Kaya, D., Turkmen, M., Melek, M., et al., 2006. Acute smoking-induced alterations in Doppler echocardiographic measurements in chronic smokers. Tex. Heart Inst. J. 33 (2), 134–138.

Kawakami, M., Matsuo, Y., Yoshiura, K., Nagase, T., Yamashita, N., 2008. Sequential and quantitative analysis of a murine model of elastase-induced emphysema. Biol. Pharm. Bull. 31 (7), 1434–1438.

Kawano, R., Takeshima, Y., Inai, K., 1996. Effects of K-ras gene mutations in the development of lung lesions induced by 4-(N-methyl-n-nitrosamino)-1-(3-pyridyl)-1-butanone in A/J mice. Jpn. J. Cancer Res. 87 (1), 44–50.

Ke, Q., Yang, L., Cui, Q., Diao, W., Zhang, Y., Xu, M., et al., 2020. Ciprofibrate attenuates airway remodeling in cigarette smoke-exposed rats. Respir. Physiol. Neurobiol. 271, 103290.

Kellar, A., Egan, C., Morris, D., 2015. Preclinical murine models for lung cancer: clinical trial applications. BioMed Res. Int. 2015, 621324.

Kerkhoff, E., Fedorov, L.M., Siefken, R., Walter, A.O., Papadopoulos, T., Rapp, U.R., 2000. Lung-targeted expres-sion of the c-Raf-1 kinase in transgenic mice exposes a novel oncogenic character of the wild-type protein. Cell Growth Differ. 11 (4), 185–190.

Khuder, S.A., 2001. Effect of cigarette smoking on major histo-logical types of lung cancer: a meta-analysis. Lung Cancer 31 (2–3), 139–148.

Khuder, S.A., Mutgi, A.B., 2001. Effect of smoking cessation on major histologic types of lung cancer. Chest 120 (5), 1577–1583.

Knouff, C., Briand, O., Lestavel, S., Clavey, V., Altenburg, M., Maeda, N., 2004. Defective VLDL metabolism and severe

atherosclerosis in mice expressing human apolipoprotein E isoforms but lacking the LDL receptor. Biochim. Biophys. Acta 1684 (1–3), 8–17.

Knudsen, L., Weibel, E.R., Gundersen, H.J., Weinstein, F.V., Ochs, M., 2010. Assessment of air space size characteristics by intercept (chord) measurement: an accurate and efficient stereological approach. J. Appl. Physiol. (1985) 108 (2), 412–421.

Korfhagen, T.R., Swantz, R.J., Wert, S.E., Mccarty, J.M., Kerlakian, C.B., Glasser, S.W., et al., 1994. Respiratory epithelial cell expression of human transforming growth factor-alpha induces lung fibrosis in transgenic mice. J. Clin. Invest. 93 (4), 1691–1699.

Kosmider, L., Sobczak, A., Fik, M., Knysak, J., Zaciera, M., Kurek, J., et al., 2014. Carbonyl compounds in electronic cigarette vapors: effects of nicotine solvent and battery output voltage. Nicotine Tob. Res. 16 (10), 1319–1326.

Koul, A., Singh, A., Sandhir, R., 2003. Effect of alpha-tocopherol on the cardiac antioxidant defense system and atherogenic lipids in cigarette smoke-inhaling mice. Inhal. Toxicol. 15 (5), 513–522.

Kuhnast, S., Van Der Tuin, S.J., Van Der Hoorn, J.W., Van Klinken, J.B., Simic, B., Pieterman, E., et al., 2015. Anacetra-pib reduces progression of atherosclerosis, mainly by reducing non-HDL-cholesterol, improves lesion stability and adds to the beneficial effects of atorvastatin. Eur. Heart J. 36 (1), 39–48.

Kunitomo, M., Yamaguchi, Y., Kagota, S., Yoshikawa, N., Nakamura, K., Shinozuka, K., 2009. Biochemical evidence of atherosclerosis progression mediated by increased oxida-tive stress in apolipoprotein E-deficient spontaneously hyperlipidemic mice exposed to chronic cigarette smoke. J. Pharmacol. Sci. 110 (3), 354–361.

Kwon, M.C., Berns, A., 2013. Mouse models for lung cancer. Mol. Oncol. 7 (2), 165–177.

Laino, T., Tuma, C., Curioni, A., Jochnowitz, E., Stolz, S., 2011. A revisited picture of the mechanism of glycerol dehydration. J. Phys. Chem. 115 (15), 3592–3595.

Laniado-Laborin, R., 2009. Smoking and chronic obstruc-tive pulmonary disease (COPD). Parallel epidemics of the 21 century. Int. J. Environ. Res. Publ. Health 6 (1), 209–224.

Laurent, S., Cockcroft, J., Van Bortel, L., Boutouyrie, P., Giannattasio, C., Hayoz, D., et al., 2006. Expert consensus document on arterial stiffness: methodological issues and clinical applications. Eur. Heart J. 27 (21), 2588–2605.

Lavi, S., Prasad, A., Yang, E.H., Mathew, V., Simari, R.D., Rihal, C.S., et al., 2007. Smoking is associated with epicar-dial coronary endothelial dysfunction and elevated white blood cell count in patients with chest pain and early coro-nary artery disease. Circulation 115 (20), 2621–2627.

Lazaro, S., Perez-Crespo, M., Lorz, C., Bernardini, A., Oteo, M., Enguita, A.B., et al., 2019. Differential development of large-cell neuroendocrine or small-cell lung carcinoma upon inactivation of 4 tumor suppressor genes. Proc. Natl. Acad. Sci. U.S.A. 116 (44), 22300–22306.

Lee, K.M., Hoeng, J., Harbo, S., Kogel, U., Gardner, W., Oldham, M., et al., 2018. Biological changes in C57BL/6 mice following 3 weeks of inhalation exposure to cigarette smoke or e-vapor aerosols. Inhal. Toxicol. 30 (13–14), 553–567.

Liang, G.B., He, Z.H., 2019. Animal models of emphysema. Chin. Med. J. (Engl.) 132 (20), 2465–2475.

Libby, P., Ridker, P.M., Hansson, G.K., 2011. Progress and challenges in translating the biology of atherosclerosis. Nature 473 (7347), 317–325.

Lietz, M., Berges, A., Lebrun, S., Meurrens, K., Steffen, Y., Stolle, K., et al., 2013. Cigarette-smoke-induced atherogenic lipid profiles in plasma and vascular tissue of apolipoprotein E-deficient mice are attenuated by smoking cessation. Atherosclerosis 229 (1), 86–93.

Lim, J.S., Ibaseta, A., Fischer, M.M., Cancilla, B., O'young, G., Cristea, S., et al., 2017. Intratumoural heterogeneity generated by Notch signalling promotes small-cell lung cancer. Nature 545 (7654), 360–364.

Lloyd-Jones, D., Adams, R., Carnethon, M., De Simone, G., Ferguson, T.B., Flegal, K., et al., 2009. Heart disease and stroke statistics–2009 update: a report from the American Heart Association Statistics Committee and stroke statistics subcommittee. Circulation 119 (3), 480–486.

Lloyd, D.J., Helmering, J., Kaufman, S.A., Turk, J., Silva, M., Vasquez, S., et al., 2011. A volumetric method for quantifying atherosclerosis in mice by using microCT: comparison to en face. PLoS One 6 (4), e18800.

Lo Sasso, G., Schlage, W.K., Boue, S., Veljkovic, E., Peitsch, M.C., Hoeng, J., 2016. The Apoe$^{(-/-)}$ mouse model: a suitable model to study cardiovascular and respiratory diseases in the context of cigarette smoke exposure and harm reduction. J. Transl. Med. 14 (1), 146.

Lucey, E.C., Goldstein, R.H., Stone, P.J., Snider, G.L., 1998. Remodeling of alveolar walls after elastase treatment of hamsters. Results of elastin and collagen mRNA in situ hybridization. Am. J. Respir. Crit. Care Med. 158 (2), 555–564.

Luettich, K., Xiang, Y., Iskandar, A., Sewer, A., Martin, F., Talikka, M., et al., 2014. Systems toxicology approaches enable mechanistic comparison of spontaneous and cigarette smoke-related lung tumor development in the A/J mouse model. Interdiscipl. Toxicol. 7 (2), 73–84.

Madison, M.C., Landers, C.T., Gu, B.H., Chang, C.Y., Tung, H.Y., You, R., et al., 2019. Electronic cigarettes disrupt lung lipid homeostasis and innate immunity independent of nicotine. J. Clin. Invest. 129 (10), 4290–4304.

Magdaleno, S.M., Wang, G., Mireles, V.L., Ray, M.K., Finegold, M.J., Demayo, F.J., 1997. Cyclin-dependent kinase inhibitor expression in pulmonary Clara cells transformed with SV40 large T antigen in transgenic mice. Cell Growth Differ. 8 (2), 145–155.

Mahmud, A., Feely, J., 2003. Effect of smoking on arterial stiffness and pulse pressure amplification. Hypertension 41 (1), 183–187.

Mallock, N., Boss, L., Burk, R., Danziger, M., Welsch, T., Hahn, H., et al., 2018. Levels of selected analytes in the emissions of "heat not burn" tobacco products that are relevant to assess human health risks. Arch. Toxicol. 92 (6), 2145–2149.

Manenti, G., Dragani, T.A., 2005. Pas1 haplotype-dependent genetic predisposition to lung tumorigenesis in rodents: a meta-analysis. Carcinogenesis 26 (5), 875–882.

Manning-Tobin, J.J., Moore, K.J., Seimon, T.A., Bell, S.A., Sharuk, M., Alvarez-Leite, J.I., et al., 2009. Loss of SR-A and CD36 activity reduces atherosclerotic lesion complexity without abrogating foam cell formation in hyperlipidemic mice. Arterioscler. Thromb. Vasc. Biol. 29 (1), 19–26.

March, T.H., Barr, E.B., Finch, G.L., Hahn, F.F., Hobbs, C.H., Menache, M.G., et al., 1999. Cigarette smoke exposure produces more evidence of emphysema in B6C3F1 mice than in F344 rats. Toxicol. Sci. 51 (2), 289–299.

Maronpot, R.R., Shimkin, M.B., Witschi, H.P., Smith, L.H., Cline, J.M., 1986. Strain A mouse pulmonary tumor test results for chemicals previously tested in the National Cancer Institute carcinogenicity tests. J. Natl. Cancer Inst. 76 (6), 1101–1112.

Martorana, P.A., Brand, T., Gardi, C., Van Even, P., De Santi, M.M., Calzoni, P., et al., 1993. The pallid mouse. A model of genetic alpha 1-antitrypsin deficiency. Lab. Invest. 68 (2), 233–241.

Mathers, C.D., Loncar, D., 2006. Projections of global mortality and burden of disease from 2002 to 2030. PLoS Med. 3 (11), e442.

Mauderly, J.L., Gigliotti, A.P., Barr, E.B., Bechtold, W.E., Belinsky, S.A., Hahn, F.F., et al., 2004. Chronic inhalation exposure to mainstream cigarette smoke increases lung and nasal tumor incidence in rats. Toxicol. Sci. 81 (2), 280–292.

Mcateer, M.A., Schneider, J.E., Clarke, K., Neubauer, S., Channon, K.M., Choudhury, R.P., 2004. Quantification and 3D reconstruction of atherosclerotic plaque components in apolipoprotein E knockout mice using ex vivo high-resolution MRI. Arterioscler. Thromb. Vasc. Biol. 24 (12), 2384–2390.

Mcfadden, D.G., Papagiannakopoulos, T., Taylor-Weiner, A., Stewart, C., Carter, S.L., Cibulskis, K., et al., 2014. Genetic and clonal dissection of murine small cell lung carcinoma progression by genome sequencing. Cell 156 (6), 1298–1311.

Meuwissen, R., Berns, A., 2005. Mouse models for human lung cancer. Genes Dev. 19 (6), 643–664.

Meuwissen, R., Linn, S.C., Linnoila, R.I., Zevenhoven, J., Mooi, W.J., Berns, A., 2003. Induction of small cell lung cancer by somatic inactivation of both Trp53 and Rb1 in a conditional mouse model. Cancer Cell 4 (3), 181–189.

Meyrelles, S.S., Peotta, V.A., Pereira, T.M., Vasquez, E.C., 2011. Endothelial dysfunction in the apolipoprotein E-deficient mouse: insights into the influence of diet, gender and aging. Lipids Health Dis. 10, 211.

Mollaoglu, G., Guthrie, M.R., Bohm, S., Bragelmann, J., Can, I., Ballieu, P.M., et al., 2017. MYC drives progression of small cell lung cancer to a variant neuroendocrine subtype with vulnerability to Aurora kinase inhibition. Cancer Cell 31 (2), 270–285.

Moreira, A.R., Pereira De Castro, T.B., Kohler, J.B., Ito, J.T., De Franca Silva, L.E., Lourenco, J.D., et al., 2020. Chronic exposure to diesel particles worsened emphysema and increased M2-like phenotype macrophages in a PPE-induced model. PLoS One 15 (1), e0228393.

Morris, H.J., Nelson, A.A., Calvery, H.O., 1974. Observations on the chronic toxicities of propylene glycol, ethylene glycol, diethylene glycol, ethylene glycol, mono-ethyl-ether, and diethylene glycol monoethyl-ether. J. Pharmacol. Exp. Therapeut. 74 (3), 266−273.

Mravec, B., Tibensky, M., Horvathova, L., Babal, P., 2020. E-cigarettes and cancer risk. Cancer Prev. Res. (Phila.) 13 (2), 137−144.

Muhlfeld, C., Hegermann, J., Wrede, C., Ochs, M., 2015. A review of recent developments and applications of morphometry/stereology in lung research. Am. J. Physiol. Lung Cell Mol. Physiol. 309 (6), L526−L536.

Muhlfeld, C., Ochs, M., 2013. Quantitative microscopy of the lung: a problem-based approach. Part 2: stereological parameters and study designs in various diseases of the respiratory tract. Am. J. Physiol. Lung Cell Mol. Physiol. 305 (3), L205−L221.

Mukhopadhyay, A., Berrett, K.C., Kc, U., Clair, P.M., Pop, S.M., Carr, S.R., et al., 2014. Sox2 cooperates with Lkb1 loss in a mouse model of squamous cell lung cancer. Cell Rep. 8 (1), 40−49.

Nakashima, Y., Plump, A.S., Raines, E.W., Breslow, J.L., Ross, R., 1994. ApoE-deficient mice develop lesions of all phases of atherosclerosis throughout the arterial tree. Arterioscler. Thromb. 14 (1), 133−140.

National Academies of Sciences, 2018. Public Health Consequences of E-Cigarettes.

National Cancer Institute, Surveillance, epidemiology, and end results program. Cancer Stat facts: lung and bronchus.https://seer.cancer.gov/statfacts/html/lungb.html. Available at: https://seer.cancer.gov/statfacts/html/lungb.html.

Navab, M., Hough, G.P., Stevenson, L.W., Drinkwater, D.C., Laks, H., Fogelman, A.M., 1988. Monocyte migration into the subendothelial space of a coculture of adult human aortic endothelial and smooth muscle cells. J. Clin. Invest. 82 (6), 1853−1863.

Negre-Salvayre, A., Auge, N., Ayala, V., Basaga, H., Boada, J., Brenke, R., et al., 2010. Pathological aspects of lipid peroxidation. Free Radic. Res. 44 (10), 1125−1171.

Nettesheim, P., Hammons, A.S., 1971. Induction of squamous cell carcinoma in the respiratory tract of mice. J. Natl. Cancer Inst. 47 (3), 697−701.

Nikitin, A.Y., Alcaraz, A., Anver, M.R., Bronson, R.T., Cardiff, R.D., Dixon, D., et al., 2004. Classification of proliferative pulmonary lesions of the mouse: recommendations of the mouse models of human cancers consortium. Cancer Res. 64 (7), 2307−2316.

Nishina, P.M., Lowe, S., Verstuyft, J., Naggert, J.K., Kuypers, F.A., Paigen, B., 1993. Effects of dietary fats from animal and plant sources on diet-induced fatty streak lesions in C57BL/6J mice. J. Lipid Res. 34 (8), 1413−1422.

Nishina, P.M., Verstuyft, J., Paigen, B., 1990. Synthetic low and high fat diets for the study of atherosclerosis in the mouse. J. Lipid Res. 31 (5), 859−869.

Ochs, M., 2014. Estimating structural alterations in animal models of lung emphysema. Is there a gold standard? Ann. Anat. 196 (1), 26−33.

Ochs, M., Muhlfeld, C., 2013. Quantitative microscopy of the lung: a problem-based approach. Part 1: basic principles of lung stereology. Am. J. Physiol. Lung Cell Mol. Physiol. 305 (1), L15−L22.

OECD, 2012. Guidance document 116 on the conduct and design of chronic toxicity and carcinogenicity studies. Support. Test Guidel. 451, 452−453.

OECD, 2018. OECD test guideline 453: Combined Chronic Toxicity/Carcinogenicity Studies.

Office of the Surgeon General, 2014. The Health Consequences of Smoking—50 Years of Progress: A Report of the Surgeon General. Centers for Disease Control and Prevention, Atlanta, US.

Olfert, I.M., Devallance, E., Hoskinson, H., Branyan, K.W., Clayton, S., Pitzer, C.R., et al., 2018. Chronic exposure to electronic cigarettes results in impaired cardiovascular function in mice. J. Appl. Physiol. (1985) 124 (3), 573−582.

Oviedo, A., Lebrun, S., Kogel, U., Ho, J., Tan, W.T., Titz, B., et al., 2016. Evaluation of the Tobacco Heating System 2.2. Part 6: 90-day OECD 413 rat inhalation study with systems toxicology endpoints demonstrates reduced exposure effects of a mentholated version compared with mentholated and non-mentholated cigarette smoke. Regul. Toxicol. Pharmacol. 81 (Suppl. 2), S93−S122.

Paalvast, Y., Gerding, A., Wang, Y., Bloks, V.W., Van Dijk, T.H., Havinga, R., et al., 2017. Male apoE*3-Leiden.CETP mice on high-fat high-cholesterol diet exhibit a biphasic dyslipidemic response, mimicking the changes in plasma lipids observed through life in men. Phys. Rep. 5 (19).

Paigen, B., Morrow, A., Brandon, C., Mitchell, D., Holmes, P., 1985. Variation in susceptibility to atherosclerosis among inbred strains of mice. Atherosclerosis 57 (1), 65−73.

Paigen, B., Morrow, A., Holmes, P.A., Mitchell, D., Williams, R.A., 1987. Quantitative assessment of atherosclerotic lesions in mice. Atherosclerosis 68 (3), 231−240.

Parekh, P.I., Petro, A.E., Tiller, J.M., Feinglos, M.N., Surwit, R.S., 1998. Reversal of diet-induced obesity and diabetes in C57BL/6J mice. Metabolism 47 (9), 1089−1096.

Park, Y.M., Febbraio, M., Silverstein, R.L., 2009. CD36 modulates migration of mouse and human macrophages in response to oxidized LDL and may contribute to macrophage trapping in the arterial intima. J. Clin. Invest. 119 (1), 136−145.

Peifer, M., Fernandez-Cuesta, L., Sos, M.L., George, J., Seidel, D., Kasper, L.H., et al., 2012. Integrative genome analyses identify key somatic driver mutations of small-cell lung cancer. Nat. Genet. 44 (10), 1104−1110.

Perez-Rial, S., Giron-Martinez, A., Peces-Barba, G., 2015. Animal models of chronic obstructive pulmonary disease. Arch. Bronconeumol. 51 (3), 121−127.

Peter, P.S., Brady, J.E., Yan, L., Chen, W., Engelhardt, S., Wang, Y., et al., 2007. Inhibition of p38 alpha MAPK rescues cardiomyopathy induced by overexpressed beta 2-

adrenergic receptor, but not beta 1-adrenergic receptor. J. Clin. Invest. 117 (5), 1335–1343.

Phillips, B., Szostak, J., Titz, B., Schlage, W.K., Guedj, E., Leroy, P., et al., 2019. A six-month systems toxicology inhalation/cessation study in ApoE$^{(-/-)}$ mice to investigate cardiovascular and respiratory exposure effects of modified risk tobacco products, CHTP 1.2 and THS 2.2, compared with conventional cigarettes. Food Chem. Toxicol. 126, 113–141.

Phillips, B., Titz, B., Kogel, U., Sharma, D., Leroy, P., Xiang, Y., et al., 2017. Toxicity of the main electronic cigarette components, propylene glycol, glycerin, and nicotine, in Sprague-Dawley rats in a 90-day OECD inhalation study complemented by molecular endpoints. Food Chem. Toxicol. 109 (Pt 1), 315–332.

Phillips, B., Veljkovic, E., Boue, S., Schlage, W.K., Vuillaume, G., Martin, F., et al., 2016. An 8-month systems toxicology inhalation/cessation study in Apoe$^{-/-}$ mice to investigate cardiovascular and respiratory exposure effects of a candidate modified risk tobacco product, THS 2.2, compared with conventional cigarettes. Toxicol. Sci. 151 (2), 462–464.

Phillips, B., Veljkovic, E., Peck, M.J., Buettner, A., Elamin, A., Guedj, E., et al., 2015. A 7-month cigarette smoke inhalation study in C57BL/6 mice demonstrates reduced lung inflammation and emphysema following smoking cessation or aerosol exposure from a prototypic modified risk tobacco product. Food Chem. Toxicol. 80, 328–345.

Phillips, J.W., Barringhaus, K.G., Sanders, J.M., Yang, Z., Chen, M., Hesselbacher, S., et al., 2003. Rosiglitazone reduces the accelerated neointima formation after arterial injury in a mouse injury model of type 2 diabetes. Circulation 108 (16), 1994–1999.

Pleasance, E.D., Stephens, P.J., O'meara, S., Mcbride, D.J., Meynert, A., Jones, D., et al., 2010. A small-cell lung cancer genome with complex signatures of tobacco exposure. Nature 463 (7278), 184–190.

Plump, A.S., Smith, J.D., Hayek, T., Aalto-Setala, K., Walsh, A., Verstuyft, J.G., et al., 1992. Severe hypercholesterolemia and atherosclerosis in apolipoprotein E-deficient mice created by homologous recombination in ES cells. Cell 71 (2), 343–353.

Polosa, R., Caponnetto, P., 2016. The health effects of electronic cigarettes. N. Engl. J. Med. 375 (26), 2608.

Poredos, P., Orehek, M., Tratnik, E., 1999. Smoking is associated with dose-related increase of intima-media thickness and endothelial dysfunction. Angiology 50 (3), 201–208.

Poussin, C., Laurent, A., Kondylis, A., Marescotti, D., Van Der Toorn, M., Guedj, E., et al., 2018. In vitro systems toxicology-based assessment of the potential modified risk tobacco product CHTP 1.2 for vascular inflammation- and cytotoxicity-associated mechanisms promoting adhesion of monocytic cells to human coronary arterial endothelial cells. Food Chem. Toxicol. 120, 390–406.

Poussin, C., Laurent, A., Peitsch, M.C., Hoeng, J., De Leon, H., 2015. Systems biology reveals cigarette smoke-induced concentration-dependent direct and indirect mechanisms that promote monocyte-endothelial cell adhesion. Toxicol. Sci. 147 (2), 370–385.

Poussin, C., Laurent, A., Peitsch, M.C., Hoeng, J., De Leon, H., 2016. Systems toxicology-based assessment of the candidate modified risk tobacco product THS2.2 for the adhesion of monocytic cells to human coronary arterial endothelial cells. Toxicology 339, 73–86.

Powell-Braxton, L., Veniant, M., Latvala, R.D., Hirano, K.I., Won, W.B., Ross, J., et al., 1998. A mouse model of human familial hypercholesterolemia: markedly elevated low density lipoprotein cholesterol levels and severe atherosclerosis on a low-fat chow diet. Nat. Med. 4 (8), 934–938.

Rangasamy, T., Misra, V., Zhen, L., Tankersley, C.G., Tuder, R.M., Biswal, S., 2009. Cigarette smoke-induced emphysema in A/J mice is associated with pulmonary oxidative stress, apoptosis of lung cells, and global alterations in gene expression. Am. J. Physiol. Lung Cell Mol. Physiol. 296 (6), L888–L900.

Rehm, S., Lijinsky, W., Singh, G., Katyal, S.L., 1991. Mouse bronchiolar cell carcinogenesis. Histologic characterization and expression of Clara cell antigen in lesions induced by N-nitrosobis-(2-chloroethyl) ureas. Am. J. Pathol. 139 (2), 413–422.

Reinikovaite, V., Rodriguez, I.E., Karoor, V., Rau, A., Trinh, B.B., Deleyiannis, F.W., et al., 2018. The effects of electronic cigarette vapour on the lung: direct comparison to tobacco smoke. Eur. Respir. J. 51 (4).

Rennard, S.I., Vestbo, J., 2006. COPD: the dangerous underestimate of 15%. Lancet 367 (9518), 1216–1219.

Renne, R., Brix, A., Harkema, J., Herbert, R., Kittel, B., Lewis, D., et al., 2009. Proliferative and nonproliferative lesions of the rat and mouse respiratory tract. Toxicol. Pathol. 37 (7 Suppl. l), 5S–73S.

Renne, R., Wehner, A., Greenspan, B., Deford, H., Ragan, H., Westerberg, R., et al., 1992. 2-Week and 13-week inhalation studies of aerosolized glycerol in rats. Inhal. Toxicol. 4 (2), 95–111.

Robert, J., Weber, B., Frese, L., Emmert, M.Y., Schmidt, D., Von Eckardstein, A., et al., 2013. A three-dimensional engineered artery model for in vitro atherosclerosis research. PLoS One 8 (11), e79821.

Robertson, O.H., Loosh, C.G., Puck, T.T., Wise, H., Lemon, H.M., Lester, W., 1947. Tests for the chronic toxicity of propylene glycol and trlethylene glycol on monkeys and rats by vapor inhalation and oral administration. J. Pharmacol. Exp. Therapeut. 91, 51–76.

Roche-Molina, M., Sanz-Rosa, D., Cruz, F.M., Garcia-Prieto, J., Lopez, S., Abia, R., et al., 2015. Induction of sustained hypercholesterolemia by single adeno-associated virus-mediated gene transfer of mutant hPCSK9. Arterioscler. Thromb. Vasc. Biol. 35 (1), 50–59.

Rodrigues, R., Olivo, C.R., Lourenco, J.D., Riane, A., Cervilha, D.a.B., Ito, J.T., et al., 2017. A murine model of elastase- and cigarette smoke-induced emphysema. J. Bras. Pneumol. 43 (2), 95–100.

Ronai, Z.A., Gradia, S., Peterson, L.A., Hecht, S.S., 1993. G to A transitions and G to T transversions in codon 12 of the Ki-ras oncogene isolated from mouse lung tumors induced by 4-(methylnitrosamino)-1-(3-pyridyl)-1-butanone (NNK) and related DNA methylating and pyridyloxobutylating agents. Carcinogenesis 14 (11), 2419–2422.

Rudin, C.M., Durinck, S., Stawiski, E.W., Poirier, J.T., Modrusan, Z., Shames, D.S., et al., 2012. Comprehensive genomic analysis identifies SOX2 as a frequently amplified gene in small-cell lung cancer. Nat. Genet. 44 (10), 1111–1116.

Rudin, C.M., Poirier, J.T., Byers, L.A., Dive, C., Dowlati, A., George, J., et al., 2019. Molecular subtypes of small cell lung cancer: a synthesis of human and mouse model data. Nat. Rev. Cancer 19 (5), 289–297.

Saetta, M., Turato, G., Maestrelli, P., Mapp, C.E., Fabbri, L.M., 2001. Cellular and structural bases of chronic obstructive pulmonary disease. Am. J. Respir. Crit. Care Med. 163 (6), 1304–1309.

Schaefer, A., Klein, G., Brand, B., Lippolt, P., Drexler, H., Meyer, G.P., 2003. Evaluation of left ventricular diastolic function by pulsed Doppler tissue imaging in mice. J. Am. Soc. Echocardiogr. 16 (11), 1144–1149.

Schaefer, A., Meyer, G.P., Hilfiker-Kleiner, D., Brand, B., Drexler, H., Klein, G., 2005. Evaluation of Tissue Doppler Tei index for global left ventricular function in mice after myocardial infarction: comparison with Pulsed Doppler Tei index. Eur. J. Echocardiogr. 6 (5), 367–375.

Schaffer, B.E., Park, K.S., Yiu, G., Conklin, J.F., Lin, C., Burkhart, D.L., et al., 2010. Loss of p130 accelerates tumor development in a mouse model for human small-cell lung carcinoma. Cancer Res. 70 (10), 3877–3883.

Schaller, J.P., Keller, D., Poget, L., Pratte, P., Kaelin, E., Mchugh, D., et al., 2016a. Evaluation of the Tobacco Heating System 2.2. Part 2: chemical composition, genotoxicity, cytotoxicity, and physical properties of the aerosol. Regul. Toxicol. Pharmacol. 81 (Suppl. 2), S27–S47.

Schaller, J.P., Pijnenburg, J.P., Ajithkumar, A., Tricker, A.R., 2016b. Evaluation of the Tobacco Heating System 2.2. Part 3: influence of the tobacco blend on the formation of harmful and potentially harmful constituents of the Tobacco Heating System 2.2 aerosol. Regul. Toxicol. Pharmacol. 81 (Suppl. 2), S48–S58.

Schleef, R., Vanscheeuwijck, P., Schlage, W., Borzelleca, J., Coggins, C., Haussmann, H., 2006. Animal Models for Three Major Cigarette-Smoke-Induced Diseases. Inhal Toxicol. CRC Press, Boca Raton, FL, pp. 851–873.

Schmidt, A.G., Gerst, M., Zhai, J., Carr, A.N., Pater, L., Kranias, E.G., et al., 2002. Evaluation of left ventricular diastolic function from spectral and color M-mode Doppler in genetically altered mice. J. Am. Soc. Echocardiogr. 15 (10 Pt 1), 1065–1073.

Schneider, J.P., Ochs, M., 2014. Alterations of mouse lung tissue dimensions during processing for morphometry: a comparison of methods. Am. J. Physiol. Lung Cell Mol. Physiol. 306 (4), L341–L350.

Schreyer, S.A., Vick, C., Lystig, T.C., Mystkowski, P., Leboeuf, R.C., 2002. LDL receptor but not apolipoprotein E deficiency increases diet-induced obesity and diabetes in mice. Am. J. Physiol. Endocrinol. Metabol. 282 (1), E207–E214.

Schreyer, S.A., Wilson, D.L., Leboeuf, R.C., 1998. C57BL/6 mice fed high fat diets as models for diabetes-accelerated atherosclerosis. Atherosclerosis 136 (1), 17–24.

Semenova, E.A., Nagel, R., Berns, A., 2015. Origins, genetic landscape, and emerging therapies of small cell lung cancer. Genes Dev. 29 (14), 1447–1462.

Shapiro, S.D., 2007. Transgenic and gene-targeted mice as models for chronic obstructive pulmonary disease. Eur. Respir. J. 29 (2), 375–378.

Sheedy, F.J., Grebe, A., Rayner, K.J., Kalantari, P., Ramkhelawon, B., Carpenter, S.B., et al., 2013. CD36 coordinates NLRP3 inflammasome activation by facilitating intracellular nucleation of soluble ligands into particulate ligands in sterile inflammation. Nat. Immunol. 14 (8), 812–820.

Shein, M., Jeschke, G., 2019. Comparison of free radical levels in the aerosol from conventional cigarettes, electronic cigarettes, and heat-not-burn tobacco products. Chem. Res. Toxicol. https://doi.org/10.1021/acs.chemrestox.9b00085.

Shimkin, M.B., Stoner, G.D., 1975. Lung tumors in mice: application to carcinogenesis bioassay. Adv. Cancer Res. 21, 1–58.

Siasos, G., Tsigkou, V., Kokkou, E., Oikonomou, E., Vavuranakis, M., Vlachopoulos, C., et al., 2014. Smoking and atherosclerosis: mechanisms of disease and new therapeutic approaches. Curr. Med. Chem. 21 (34), 3936–3948.

Singh, S.V., Benson, P.J., Hu, X., Pal, A., Xia, H., Srivastava, S.K., et al., 1998. Gender-related differences in susceptibility of A/J mouse to benzo[a]pyrene-induced pulmonary and forestomach tumorigenesis. Cancer Lett. 128 (2), 197–204.

Smith, J.D., Breslow, J.L., 1997. The emergence of mouse models of atherosclerosis and their relevance to clinical research. J. Intern. Med. 242 (2), 99–109.

Smith, M.R., Clark, B., Ludicke, F., Schaller, J.P., Vanscheeuwijck, P., Hoeng, J., et al., 2016. Evaluation of the tobacco heating system 2.2. Part 1: description of the system and the scientific assessment program. Regul. Toxicol. Pharmacol. 81 (Suppl. 2), S17–S26.

Snider, G.L., Lucey, E.C., Stone, P.J., 1986. Animal models of emphysema. Am. Rev. Respir. Dis. 133 (1), 149–169.

Song, H., Yao, E., Lin, C., Gacayan, R., Chen, M.H., Chuang, P.T., 2012. Functional characterization of pulmonary neuroendocrine cells in lung development, injury, and tumorigenesis. Proc. Natl. Acad. Sci. U.S.A. 109 (43), 17531–17536.

Song, J.M., Qian, X., Teferi, F., Pan, J., Wang, Y., Kassie, F., 2015. Dietary diindolylmethane suppresses inflammation-driven lung squamous cell carcinoma in mice. Cancer Prev. Res. (Phila.) 8 (1), 77–85.

Sousa, B.C., Pitt, A.R., Spickett, C.M., 2017. Chemistry and analysis of HNE and other prominent carbonyl-containing lipid oxidation compounds. Free Radic. Biol. Med. 111, 294–308.

Stebbins, K.J., Broadhead, A.R., Baccei, C.S., Scott, J.M., Truong, Y.P., Coate, H., et al., 2010. Pharmacological blockade of the DP2 receptor inhibits cigarette smoke-induced inflammation, mucus cell metaplasia, and epithelial hyperplasia in the mouse lung. J. Pharmacol. Exp. Therapeut. 332 (3), 764–775.

Stenbäck, F., Shubik, P., 1974. Lack of toxicity and carcinogenicity of some commonly used cutaneous agents. Toxicol. Appl. Pharmacol. 30 (1), 7–13.

Stephens, W.E., 2017. Comparing the cancer potencies of emissions from vapourised nicotine products including e-cigarettes with those of tobacco smoke. Tobac. Contr. https://doi.org/10.1136/tobaccocontrol-2017-053808.

Stinn, W., Arts, J.H., Buettner, A., Duistermaat, E., Janssens, K., Kuper, C.F., et al., 2010. Murine lung tumor response after exposure to cigarette mainstream smoke or its particulate and gas/vapor phase fractions. Toxicology 275 (1–3), 10–20.

Stinn, W., Berges, A., Meurrens, K., Buettner, A., Gebel, S., Lichtner, R.B., et al., 2013a. Towards the validation of a lung tumorigenesis model with mainstream cigarette smoke inhalation using the A/J mouse. Toxicology 305, 49–64.

Stinn, W., Buettner, A., Weiler, H., Friedrichs, B., Luetjen, S., Van Overveld, F., et al., 2013b. Lung inflammatory effects, tumorigenesis, and emphysema development in a long-term inhalation study with cigarette mainstream smoke in mice. Toxicol. Sci. 131 (2), 596–611.

Stinn, W., Teredesai, A., Kuhl, P., Knorr-Wittmann, C., Kindt, R., Coggins, C., et al., 2005. Mechanisms involved in A/J mouse lung tumorigenesis induced by inhalation of an environmental tobacco smoke surrogate. Inhal. Toxicol. 17 (6), 263–276.

Suber, R.L., Deskin, R., Nikiforov, I., Fouillet, X., Coggins, C.R., 1989. Subchronic nose-only inhalation study of propylene glycol in Sprague-Dawley rats. Food Chem. Toxicol. 27 (9), 573–583.

Sun, S., Schiller, J.H., Gazdar, A.F., 2007. Lung cancer in never smokers–a different disease. Nat. Rev. Cancer 7 (10), 778–790.

Surwit, R.S., Kuhn, C.M., Cochrane, C., Mccubbin, J.A., Feinglos, M.N., 1988. Diet-induced type II diabetes in C57BL/6J mice. Diabetes 37 (9), 1163–1167.

Szostak, J., Boue, S., Talikka, M., Guedj, E., Martin, F., Phillips, B., et al., 2017. Aerosol from Tobacco Heating System 2.2 has reduced impact on mouse heart gene expression compared with cigarette smoke. Food Chem. Toxicol. 101, 157–167.

Szostak, J., Titz, B., Schlage, W.K., Guedj, E., Sewer, A., Phillips, B., et al., 2020a. Structural, functional, and molecular impact on the cardiovascular system in ApoE$^{(-/-)}$ mice exposed to aerosol from candidate modified risk tobacco products, Carbon Heated Tobacco Product 1.2 and Tobacco Heating System 2.2, compared with cigarette smoke. Chem. Biol. Interact. 315, 108887.

Szostak, J., Wong, E.T., Titz, B., Lee, T., Wong, S.K., Low, T., et al., 2020b. A 6-month systems toxicology inhalation study in ApoE$^{(-/-)}$ mice demonstrates reduced cardiovascular effects of E-vapor aerosols compared with cigarette smoke. Am. J. Physiol. Heart Circ. Physiol. 318 (3), H604–H631.

Takahashi, H., Ogata, H., Nishigaki, R., Broide, D.H., Karin, M., 2010. Tobacco smoke promotes lung tumorigenesis by triggering IKKbeta- and JNK1-dependent inflammation. Cancer Cell 17 (1), 89–97.

Tang, M.S., Wu, X.R., Lee, H.W., Xia, Y., Deng, F.M., Moreira, A.L., et al., 2019. Electronic-cigarette smoke induces lung adenocarcinoma and bladder urothelial hyperplasia in mice. Proc. Natl. Acad. Sci. U.S.A. 116 (43), 21727–21731.

Tangirala, R.K., Rubin, E.M., Palinski, W., 1995. Quantitation of atherosclerosis in murine models: correlation between lesions in the aortic origin and in the entire aorta, and differences in the extent of lesions between sexes in LDL receptor-deficient and apolipoprotein E-deficient mice. J. Lipid Res. 36 (11), 2320–2328.

Tayyarah, R., Long, G.A., 2014. Comparison of select analytes in aerosol from e-cigarettes with smoke from conventional cigarettes and with ambient air. Regul. Toxicol. Pharmacol. 70 (3), 704–710.

Tian, J., Pei, H., James, J.C., Li, Y., Matsumoto, A.H., Helm, G.A., et al., 2005. Circulating adhesion molecules in apoE-deficient mouse strains with different atherosclerosis susceptibility. Biochem. Biophys. Res. Commun. 329 (3), 1102–1107.

Titz, B., Sewer, A., Luettich, K., Wong, E.T., Guedj, E., Nury, C., et al., 2020. Respiratory effects of exposure to aerosol from the candidate modified-risk tobacco product THS 2.2 in an 18-month systems toxicology study with A/J mice. Toxicol. Sci. https://doi.org/10.1093/toxsci/kfaa132. Epub ahead of print.

Travis, W.D., Brambilla, E., Riely, G.J., 2013. New pathologic classification of lung cancer: relevance for clinical practice and clinical trials. J. Clin. Oncol. 31 (8), 992–1001.

University of Kentucky, 2003. University of Kentucky Tobacco Research and Development Center: The Reference Cigarette.

Valko, M., Leibfritz, D., Moncol, J., Cronin, M.T., Mazur, M., Telser, J., 2007. Free radicals and antioxidants in normal physiological functions and human disease. Int. J. Biochem. Cell Biol. 39 (1), 44–84.

Van Den Berkmortel, F.W., Smilde, T.J., Wollersheim, H., Van Langen, H., De Boo, T., Thien, T., 2000. Intima-media thickness of peripheral arteries in asymptomatic cigarette smokers. Atherosclerosis 150 (2), 397–401.

Van Hoecke, L., Job, E.R., Saelens, X., Roose, K., 2017. Bronchoalveolar lavage of murine lungs to analyze inflammatory cell infiltration. J. Vis. Exp. 123 https://doi.org/10.3791/55398.

Van Ree, J.H., Van Den Broek, W.J., Dahlmans, V.E., Groot, P.H., Vidgeon-Hart, M., Frants, R.R., et al., 1994. Diet-induced hypercholesterolemia and atherosclerosis in heterozygous apolipoprotein E-deficient mice. Atherosclerosis 111 (1), 25–37.

Vanoirbeek, J.A., Rinaldi, M., De Vooght, V., Haenen, S., Bobic, S., Gayan-Ramirez, G., et al., 2010. Noninvasive and invasive pulmonary function in mouse models of obstructive and restrictive respiratory diseases. Am. J. Respir. Cell Mol. Biol. 42 (1), 96−104.

Vanscheeuwijck, P.M., Teredesai, A., Terpstra, P.M., Verbeeck, J., Kuhl, P., Gerstenberg, B., et al., 2002. Evaluation of the potential effects of ingredients added to cigarettes. Part 4: subchronic inhalation toxicity. Food Chem. Toxicol. 40 (1), 113−131.

Vlachopoulos, C., Ioakeimidis, N., Abdelrasoul, M., Terentes-Printzios, D., Georgakopoulos, C., Pietri, P., et al., 2016. Electronic cigarette smoking increases aortic stiffness and blood pressure in young smokers. J. Am. Coll. Cardiol. 67 (23), 2802−2803.

Vlahos, R., Bozinovski, S., 2014. Recent advances in pre-clinical mouse models of COPD. Clin. Sci. (Lond.) 126 (4), 253−265.

Vlahos, R., Bozinovski, S., 2015. Preclinical murine models of chronic obstructive pulmonary disease. Eur. J. Pharmacol. 759, 265−271.

Von Holt, K., Lebrun, S., Stinn, W., Conroy, L., Wallerath, T., Schleef, R., 2009. Progression of atherosclerosis in the Apo $E^{-/-}$ model: 12-month exposure to cigarette mainstream smoke combined with high-cholesterol/fat diet. Atherosclerosis 205 (1), 135−143.

Waldum, H.L., Nilsen, O.G., Nilsen, T., Rorvik, H., Syversen, V., Sanvik, A.K., et al., 1996. Long-term effects of inhaled nicotine. Life Sci. 58 (16), 1339−1346.

Wang, Q., Khan, N.A., Muthumalage, T., Lawyer, G.R., Mcdonough, S.R., Chuang, T.D., et al., 2019. Dysregulated repair and inflammatory responses by e-cigarette-derived inhaled nicotine and humectant propylene glycol in a sex-dependent manner in mouse lung. FASEB Bioadv. 1 (10), 609−623.

Wang, Z.Y., Hong, J.Y., Huang, M.T., Reuhl, K.R., Conney, A.H., Yang, C.S., 1992. Inhibition of N-nitrosodiethylamine- and 4-(methylnitrosamino)-1-(3-pyridyl)-1-butanone-induced tumorigenesis in A/J mice by green tea and black tea. Cancer Res. 52 (7), 1943−1947.

Warnholtz, A., Nickenig, G., Schulz, E., Macharzina, R., Brasen, J.H., Skatchkov, M., et al., 1999. Increased NADH-oxidase-mediated superoxide production in the early stages of atherosclerosis: evidence for involvement of the renin-angiotensin system. Circulation 99 (15), 2027−2033.

Werley, M.S., Kirkpatrick, D.J., Oldham, M.J., Jerome, A.M., Langston, T.B., Lilly, P.D., et al., 2016. Toxicological assessment of a prototype e-cigaret device and three flavor formulations: a 90-day inhalation study in rats. Inhal. Toxicol. 28 (1), 22−38.

Westcott, P.M., Halliwill, K.D., To, M.D., Rashid, M., Rust, A.G., Keane, T.M., et al., 2015. The mutational landscapes of genetic and chemical models of Kras-driven lung cancer. Nature 517 (7535), 489−492.

Wikenheiser, K.A., Clark, J.C., Linnoila, R.I., Stahlman, M.T., Whitsett, J.A., 1992. Simian virus 40 large T antigen directed by transcriptional elements of the human surfactant protein C gene produces pulmonary adenocarcinomas in transgenic mice. Cancer Res. 52 (19), 5342−5352.

Wilson, J., Clapp, M.J., Conning, D.M., 1978. Effect of glycerol on local and systemic carcinogenicity of topically applied tobacco condensate. Br. J. Cancer 38 (2), 250−257.

Witschi, H., 2005. The complexities of an apparently simple lung tumor model: the A/J mouse. Exp. Toxicol. Pathol. 57 (Suppl. 1), 171−181.

Witschi, H., Espiritu, I., Dance, S.T., Miller, M.S., 2002. A mouse lung tumor model of tobacco smoke carcinogenesis. Toxicol. Sci. 68 (2), 322−330.

Witschi, H., Espiritu, I., Maronpot, R.R., Pinkerton, K.E., Jones, A.D., 1997a. The carcinogenic potential of the gas phase of environmental tobacco smoke. Carcinogenesis 18 (11), 2035−2042.

Witschi, H., Espiritu, I., Peake, J.L., Wu, K., Maronpot, R.R., Pinkerton, K.E., 1997b. The carcinogenicity of environmental tobacco smoke. Carcinogenesis 18 (3), 575−586.

Witschi, H., Espiritu, I., Uyeminami, D., Suffia, M., Pinkerton, K.E., 2004. Lung tumor response in strain a mice exposed to tobacco smoke: some dose-effect relationships. Inhal. Toxicol. 16 (1), 27−32.

Wong, B.A., 2007. Inhalation exposure systems: design, methods and operation. Toxicol. Pathol. 35 (1), 3−14.

Wong, E.T., Kogel, U., Veljkovic, E., Martin, F., Xiang, Y., Boue, S., et al., 2016. Evaluation of the Tobacco Heating System 2.2. Part 4: 90-day OECD 413 rat inhalation study with systems toxicology endpoints demonstrates reduced exposure effects compared with cigarette smoke. Regul. Toxicol. Pharmacol. 81 (Suppl. 2), S59−S81.

Wong, E.T., Luettich, K., Krishnan, S., Wong, S.K., Lim, W.T., Yeo, D., et al., 2020. Reduced chronic toxicity and carcinogenicity in A/J mice in response to life-time exposure to aerosol from a heated tobacco product compared with cigarette smoke. Toxicol. Sci. https://doi.org/10.1093/toxsci/kfaa131. Epub ahead of print.

Wright, J.L., Churg, A., 1990. Cigarette smoke causes physiologic and morphologic changes of emphysema in the Guinea pig. Am. Rev. Respir. Dis. 142 (6 Pt 1), 1422−1428.

Wright, J.L., Churg, A., 2002. Animal models of cigarette smoke-induced COPD. Chest 122, 301s−306s.

Wright, J.L., Churg, A., 2010. Animal models of cigarette smoke-induced chronic obstructive pulmonary disease. Expert Rev. Respir. Med. 4 (6), 723−734.

Xiang, Y., Luettich, K., Martin, F., Battey, J.N.D., Trivedi, D.K., Neau, L., et al., 2020. Discriminating Spontaneous from Cigarette Smoke and THS 2.2 Aerosol Exposure-Related Proliferative Lung Lesions in A/J Mice Using Gene Expression and Mutation Spectrum Data. Submitted.

Xiao, J., Wang, K., Feng, Y.L., Chen, X.R., Xu, D., Zhang, M.K., 2011. Role of extracellular signal-regulated kinase 1/2 in cigarette smoke-induced mucus hypersecretion in a rat model. Chin. Med. J. (Engl.) 124 (20), 3327−3333.

Xiao, Z., Jiang, Q., Willette-Brown, J., Xi, S., Zhu, F., Burkett, S., et al., 2013. The pivotal role of IKKalpha in the development of spontaneous lung squamous cell carcinomas. Cancer Cell 23 (4), 527−540.

Xu, C., Fillmore, C.M., Koyama, S., Wu, H., Zhao, Y., Chen, Z., et al., 2014a. Loss of Lkb1 and Pten leads to lung squamous cell carcinoma with elevated PD-L1 expression. Cancer Cell 25 (5), 590−604.

Xu, X., Huang, L., Futtner, C., Schwab, B., Rampersad, R.R., Lu, Y., et al., 2014b. The cell of origin and subtype of K-

Ras-induced lung tumors are modified by Notch and Sox2. Genes Dev. 28 (17), 1929–1939.

Xu, X., Rock, J.R., Lu, Y., Futtner, C., Schwab, B., Guinney, J., et al., 2012. Evidence for type II cells as cells of origin of K-Ras-induced distal lung adenocarcinoma. Proc. Natl. Acad. Sci. U.S.A. 109 (13), 4910–4915.

Yang, S.R., Chida, A.S., Bauter, M.R., Shafiq, N., Seweryniak, K., Maggirwar, S.B., et al., 2006. Cigarette smoke induces proinflammatory cytokine release by activation of NF-kappaB and posttranslational modifications of histone deacetylase in macrophages. Am. J. Physiol. Lung Cell Mol. Physiol. 291 (1), L46–L57.

Yoshimoto, T., Hirao, F., Sakatani, M., Nishikawa, H., Ogura, T., 1977. Induction of squamous cell carcinoma in the lung of C57BL/6 mice by intratracheal instillation of benzo[a]pyrene with charcoal powder. Gan 68 (3), 343–352.

Yoshimoto, T., Inoue, T., Iizuka, H., Nishikawa, H., Sakatani, M., Ogura, T., et al., 1980. Differential induction of squamous cell carcinomas and adenocarcinomas in mouse lung by intratracheal instillation of benzo(a)pyrene and charcoal powder. Cancer Res. 40 (11), 4301–4307.

You, M., Candrian, U., Maronpot, R.R., Stoner, G.D., Anderson, M.W., 1989. Activation of the Ki-ras protooncogene in spontaneously occurring and chemically induced lung tumors of the strain A mouse. Proc. Natl. Acad. Sci. U.S.A. 86 (9), 3070–3074.

You, M., Wang, Y., Lineen, A.M., Gunning, W.T., Stoner, G.D., Anderson, M.W., 1992. Mutagenesis of the K-ras protooncogene in mouse lung tumors induced by N-ethyl-N-nitrosourea or N-nitrosodiethylamine. Carcinogenesis 13 (9), 1583–1586.

Zeiher, A.M., Schachinger, V., Minners, J., 1995. Long-term cigarette smoking impairs endothelium-dependent coronary arterial vasodilator function. Circulation 92 (5), 1094–1100.

Zhang, J., Liu, Y., Shi, J., Larson, D.F., Watson, R.R., 2002. Side-stream cigarette smoke induces dose-response in systemic inflammatory cytokine production and oxidative stress. Exp. Biol. Med. 227 (9), 823–829.

Zhou, B., Wang, X., Li, F., Wang, Y., Yang, L., Zhen, X., et al., 2017. Mitochondrial activity and oxidative stress functions are influenced by the activation of AhR-induced CYP1A1 overexpression in cardiomyocytes. Mol. Med. Rep. 16 (1), 174–180.

CHAPTER 16

Toxicological Assessment of Flavors Used in E-vapor Products

DIEGO MARESCOTTI • CAROLE MATHIS • ANNE MAY • DAVIDE SCIUSCIO • MANUEL C. PEITSCH • JULIA HOENG

16.1 INTRODUCTION

E-vapor products (EVPs) are designed to be potentially less harmful than cigarettes (Chapter 2). The majority of the EVPs contain nicotine. These EVPs deliver nicotine while significantly reducing or eliminating the toxicants present in cigarette smoke (CS). To enable successful and complete switching from cigarettes to EVPs and thus reduce the health risks of smoking, an EVP must provide a satisfying experience and be sensorially acceptable to current smokers (Farsalinos et al., 2018; Polosa et al., 2013). This experience can be augmented by using flavoring substances that appeal to current adult smokers. Therefore, flavoring substances represent an important group of ingredients in EVPs.

Compared with CS, the nicotine-containing aerosols of EVPs (Chapter 2) are fundamentally different, being simpler in their composition, with propylene glycol (PG) and/or vegetable glycerin (VG), water, and nicotine (Chapter 2) as their main constituents. These constituents, alone and in combination, have been demonstrated to have a low toxicity profile at consumer-relevant doses (Chapters 13–15). Therefore, EVPs emit significantly lower levels of harmful and potentially harmful constituents (Chapter 4) and other toxicants (Chapters 6 and 7) than cigarettes. While a significant reduction in toxicant emissions leads to a reduction in toxicity (Chapters 3, 13–15), it is important to ensure that EVPs do not present novel health risks for consumers.

The flavors that are added to the e-liquids in EVPs may influence the toxicological profiles of EVP aerosols and, hence, may present health risks. Therefore, it is important to assess these substances and their combinations from a toxicological perspective.

More than 7,700 flavors were already commercially available in early 2014 (Zhu et al., 2014). However, only a small number of studies have focused on the inhalation toxicology of flavors, flavored e-liquids, and their corresponding aerosols. Therefore, there is a pressing need to develop adequate scientific methods for assessing the safety of flavors for use in EVPs.

Flavors are volatile organic compounds, usually with well-characterized chemical structures carrying a single functional group, and of low molecular weight (<300 g/mol). Approximately 2,500 chemically defined flavors are in use in Europe or the United States (US) (Munro et al., 1999). These substances can be either synthetic or extracted from natural sources.

While most of the flavors used in today's EVPs are on the US Food and Drug Administration's (FDA) generally recognized as safe (GRAS) list, this does not necessarily mean that they are safe for inhalation and, hence, for use in EVPs (FEMA, 2018). Indeed, the GRAS certification generally applies only to ingestion, and most chemicals on this list have not been tested for safety by inhalation. Therefore, the US Flavor and Extract Manufacturers Association (FEMA) recommends that manufacturers of EVPs should test the safety of flavors used in EVPs (FEMA, 2018). Indeed, the biological activity of a substance can be markedly different when inhaled rather than ingested, especially following long-term exposure. One example for this difference is 2,3-butanedione (diacetyl), a flavor that is safe for ingestion but highly toxic when inhaled. This substance has an intensely buttery flavor, and manufacturers use it to flavor a number of food products, including margarine and popcorn. Chronic workplace exposure to high levels of diacetyl have led to respiratory diseases in popcorn factory workers, including subclinical decline in lung function, airway obstruction, and, eventually, life-threatening bronchiolitis obliterans (a.k.a. "popcorn lung"), an irreversible respiratory disease

Toxicological Evaluation of Electronic Nicotine Delivery Products. https://doi.org/10.1016/B978-0-12-820490-0.00019-5

(Klager et al., 2017; Kreiss et al., 2002; Rose, 2017; Wallace, 2017). The National Institute for Occupational Safety and Health and the American Conference of Governmental Industrial Hygienists have since implemented occupational exposure limits for diacetyl. Likewise, inhalation of other flavors used by the food industry, including acetoin, 2,3-pentanedione, 2,3-heptanedione, 2,3-hexanedione, and 3,4-hexanedione, is also known to cause respiratory hazards (Hubbs et al., 2019; Morgan et al., 2016, 2019).

These examples highlight the need for assessing the flavors used in EVPs. However, given the large number of available flavors and the even larger number of possible flavor mixtures, this is a daunting task which calls for a pragmatic yet precise flavor assessment strategy. Here, we will introduce a flavor assessment strategy and use cases to provide a scientific basis for future research in this field.

16.2 E-LIQUID AND EVP AEROSOL ASSESSMENT STUDIES

E-liquid constituents and flavors are typically selected on the basis of previous knowledge. For example, ingredients known to have toxic properties or likely to exert toxicity are excluded. Most manufacturers rely on the GRAS status of flavors to justify the safety of the ingredients. However, strategies have been proposed for selecting ingredients on the basis of additional scientific evidence. In 2015, Costigan and Meredith suggested that the ingredients should have certain purity criteria, should not be carcinogenic, mutagenic, or reprotoxic (CMR), and should not act as respiratory sensitizers (Costigan and Meredith, 2015). Furthermore, in 2017, Costigan and Lopez-Belmonte suggested that selection of flavors could also be based on their potential as respiratory allergens (Costigan and Lopez-Belmonte, 2017). In 2019, Stevenson and colleagues proposed a selection of flavors by using a Genomic Allergen Rapid Detection approach, which classifies flavors on the basis of their sensitizing potential (Stevenson et al., 2019). In addition, our group has proposed a multilayer systems toxicology framework for in vitro assessment of e-liquids that is meant to complement the battery of classical assays for mutagenicity and genotoxicity testing (Iskandar et al., 2016).

Despite the absence of standardized methods for toxicological assessment of the flavors used in EVPs, several publications have reported significant efforts for characterizing flavored e-liquids and their corresponding aerosols (Table 16.1).

Among these publications, the FDA-commissioned study (Hung et al., 2020) is noteworthy because it uses alternative testing methods as prioritization tools for studying the genotoxic mode of action of 150 flavors. To our knowledge, this is the first high-content and high-throughput genotoxicity screening study on EVP flavors. In this study, clastogen-sensitive (γH2AX

TABLE 16.1
Nonexhaustive List of Studies Investigating the Toxicity of Flavored E-liquids and Their Corresponding Aerosols.

Study Type	Publication References
In vitro assessment of flavorings and flavored e-liquids (cytotoxicity, oxidative responses, high-content screening, etc.)	Muthumalage et al. (2017) Sherwood and Boitano (2016) Iskandar et al. (2019b) Sassano et al. (2018) Behar et al. (2016) Bahl et al. (2012) Farsalinos K. E. et al. (2013) Farsalinos K. E. et al. (2013) Lerner et al. (2015) Gerloff et al. (2017) Marescotti et al. (2020) Cudazzo et al. (2019) Hung et al., 2020
In vitro assessment of flavored aerosol fractions	Ji et al. (2016)
Exposure of organotypic tissue cultures at the air–liquid interface	Lerner et al. (2015) Leigh et al. (2016) Bengalli et al. (2017) Iskandar et al. (2019b) Iskandar et al. (2019a) Muthumalage et al. (2019)
In vitro assessment of serum from flavored e-cigarette users	Lee et al. (2019)
In vivo inhalation studies	Werley et al. (2016) Lerner et al. (2015) Reumann et al. (2020) Reumann et al. (2020) Szostak et al. (2020) Lee et al. (2018)

and p53) and aneugen-sensitive (p-H3 and polyploidy) biomarkers of DNA damage in human TK6 cells were aggregated by using a supervised machine learning prediction model to prioritize chemicals on the basis of their genotoxic potential. With this in vitro approach, 25 flavors were identified as positive for genotoxicity (15 clastogenic, 8 aneugenic, and 2 with a mixed mode of action [clastogenic and aneugenic]). In addition, in silico quantitative structure–activity relationship (QSAR) models were used to predict the genotoxic and carcinogenic potential of the flavors. The QSAR models predicted 31% of the 150 compounds to be mutagenic, clastogenic, or carcinogenic in rodents and 49% to be negative for all three endpoints; the remaining compounds had no prediction.

In the context of EVPs, research on flavors is particularly difficult because of the abundance and diversity of the flavors and the plethora of possible combinations that can be used. Therefore, the classical approach of evaluating the toxicity of single flavors and then testing every possible combination of flavoring substances is impracticable, and only a very limited number of e-liquids available on the market have been tested to date. Furthermore, flavor assessment faces a number of methodological challenges. First, the methods used to identify the threshold of toxicity are not standardized. Second, the toxicity of a single compound may not reflect the toxicity of the same compound when it is a part of a mixture, as chemical interactions among substances may generate new and unknown compounds. Third, the long-term effects of flavors are difficult to assess, and, hence, most studies only report the acute effects of flavors. Finally, extrapolating the results of in vitro toxicity studies to humans is not straightforward.

16.3 TOXICITY ASSESSMENT OF E-LIQUIDS AND EVP AEROSOLS

EVPs emit significantly lower levels and fewer numbers of the toxicants found in CS (Chapters 4, 6–7). Therefore, the aerosols generated by EVPs are significantly less toxic than CS in both acute and longer-term toxicology studies (Chapters 13–15). However, the long-term health risks of EVPs have not yet been assessed (Tobacco Advisory Group of the Royal College of Physicians, 2016). The National Academies of Sciences, Engineering, and Medicine conducted a comprehensive review of emerging evidence on EVPs and health and suggested that "e-cigarettes are not without physiological activity in humans" and that further investigations

are needed (National Academies of Sciences E., and Medicine, 2018; National Academies of Sciences E. et al., 2018). Because epidemiological evidence on the health effects of long-term EVP use will take decades to become available, there is a need for short- and mid-term assessment of the potential health impacts associated with EVP use. In the absence of standards for manufacturing and toxicity testing of EVPs, Philip Morris International has developed an integrated in vitro systems toxicology assessment framework for e-liquids and their associated aerosols (Fig. 16.1) (Iskandar et al., 2016).

The core of this framework, intended to complement the battery of assays for standard toxicity testing (Chapter 13), consists of three experimental layers.

In the first layer, a broad range of e-liquid formulations that have passed the standard toxicity testing battery are subjected to high-throughput cytotoxicity screening in primary human cell monolayer (2D) culture systems, such as aortic endothelial cells and bronchial epithelial cells.

In the second layer, e-liquids that have passed the first layer of assessment are tested for their effects on toxicity-related mechanisms by using an array of pathophysiologically relevant high-content screening (HCS) endpoints in the same human primary 2D culture systems.

In the third layer, whole EVP aerosols generated from e-liquids that have passed the first two layers of testing are assessed in organotypic tissue cultures that are derived from human primary airway epithelial cells and grown at the air–liquid interface (ALI). These cultures are exposed directly to whole EVP aerosol at the ALI by using a dedicated exposure system (Chapter 12). This step is necessary to account for the potential changes in aerosol composition caused by the EVP heating engine, such as a coil, and to mimic the direct effect of inhaled EVP aerosols on airway epithelia. In parallel, extensive physicochemical characterization of the aerosol and determination of regional deposition in the human respiratory tract are conducted to enable in vitro-to-in vivo dose extrapolation.

In the second and third layers, omics analyses complement the targeted functional and physiological endpoints in a systems toxicology–based approach (Chapter 13). This deepens the mechanistic understanding of exposure effects and—because of its untargeted nature—enables detection of potential novel effects that are not observed in targeted assays of CS toxicity (CS is the default benchmark for assessing EVP aerosol effects).

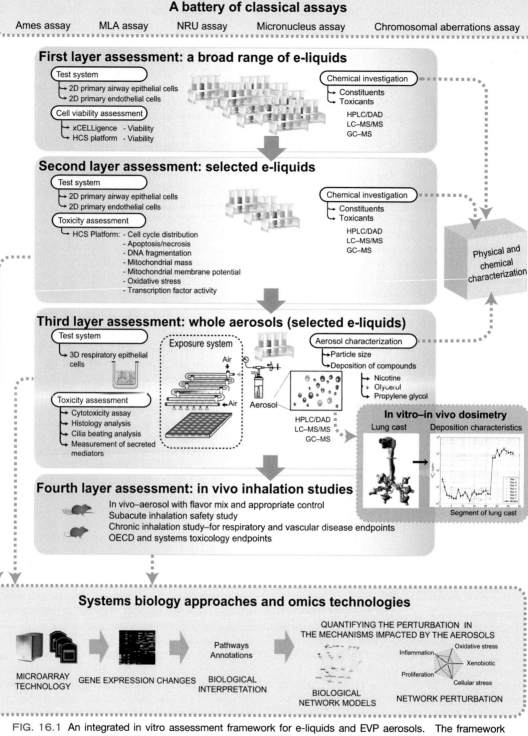

FIG. 16.1 An integrated in vitro assessment framework for e-liquids and EVP aerosols. The framework complements and extends the battery of classical assays for toxicity testing of tobacco products with mechanistic, functional, and molecular assays in a three-layered systems toxicology approach. The framework can be extended to address specific scientific questions, such as evaluating the effects of heating power or puff topography for specific EVPs or specifically assessing the effects of flavor compounds. Dosimetry can be leveraged for estimating human equivalent exposure doses. (Modified from Iskandar, A.R., Gonzalez-Suarez, I., Majeed, S., Marescotti, D., Sewer, A., Xiang, Y., et al. 2016. A framework for in vitro systems toxicology assessment of e-liquids. Toxicol. Mech. Method. 26(6), 389—413.)

In all three layers, chemical analysis of the exposure media will be necessary to verify e-liquid and/or aerosol deposition (Chapter 12).

While this framework is limited to in vitro studies, it provides an effective way for selecting candidate e-liquid formulations on the basis of both toxicological and mechanistic endpoints. Selected formulations may be further assessed in in vivo inhalation studies, if necessary (Chapter 14). It is obvious that effective selection of suitable e-liquid formulations by using in vitro approaches helps avoid unnecessary in vivo testing (the 3R principles (Balls et al., 2012)).

Moreover, in the third layer of the framework, the aerosol is generated by a standardized device, thereby ruling out any influence from specific EVP devices. This limits the variability of aerosol compositions to the variability inherent to the e-liquid formulations. In case the influence of the e-liquid–device combination is the primary objective of the assessment, the design of the exposure in the third layer can be easily adapted (Chapter 12).

16.3.1 Use Case 1: Application of the in Vitro Assessment Framework

As illustrated in Fig. 16.1, the first layer of this workflow involved real-time cellular analysis (RTCA) in 2D cultures of normal human bronchial epithelial (NHBE) cells to determine the cytotoxicity of a flavored e-liquid relative to its base e-liquid without flavors and the carrier e-liquid without flavors or nicotine (Iskandar et al., 2019b). The cytotoxicity of the flavored e-liquid was similar to that of the base EVP liquid, but its EC_{50} was reached at a 20-fold higher nicotine concentration than with 3R4F CS TPM, demonstrating that the flavors in the e-liquid did not increase the cytotoxicity of the base e-liquid and that both formulations were markedly less cytotoxic than CS TPM.

In the second layer, the same culture model was used to explore changes in specific markers by using HCS assays to identify potential toxicity-related mechanisms induced by the flavored and base e-liquids in comparison with those induced by 3R4F CS TPM. NHBE cells were incubated for 4 and 24 h with the flavored e-liquid, base e-liquid, or 3R4F CS TPM at different concentrations. Fig. 16.2 shows the ratios of minimal effective concentrations. It shows that a 4-h incubation with 3R4F CS TPM had dose-dependent impact on DNA damage, glutathione content, oxidative stress, and stress kinase (c-Jun) phosphorylation, with the impact being more pronounced when the cells were incubated for 24 h. Changes in these markers were

also detected after incubation with the flavored or base e-liquid, but only at much higher nicotine concentrations and without an obvious flavor effect. The similarity between the flavored and unflavored e-liquids can also be seen in the aggregated response of these parameters: To reach the effects of a 24-h incubation with 3R4F CS TPM, we needed to incubate the NHBE cells with the flavored e-liquid at an approximately 51-fold higher concentration than that of 3R4F CS TPM, while a ~52-fold higher concentration of base e-liquid was needed for the same effects.

The third layer of the framework focuses on investigation of the toxicity-related mechanism of EVP aerosols, not e-liquids, compared with those of whole CS by using human organotypic buccal and small airway epithelial cultures grown at the ALI. To fairly compare the effects of exposure, the doses of flavored and base aerosols applied to the cultures are those that resulted in nicotine depositions (in the exposure chamber) at least similar to or higher than 3R4F CS. In these organotypic cultures, no cytotoxicity was observed with either undiluted EVP aerosol, while, with diluted 3R4F CS, the cytotoxicity reached 30% at the same puff number. No pronounced histological alterations were seen in buccal or small airway cultures 48 h after exposure to the undiluted flavored or unflavored aerosols (nicotine concentrations, up to 159 [buccal] and 54 [small airway] µg/mL). In contrast, marked effects were seen in buccal and small airway cultures after diluted CS exposure at nicotine concentrations of 92 and 10 µg/mL, respectively (Iskandar et al., 2019b).

The omics investigations involved a genome-wide transcriptomics analysis that leveraged causal biological networks to identify molecular mechanisms of toxicity (Chapter 9) and a targeted protein analysis of secreted inflammatory mediators and selected markers in epithelial cells. The exposure doses were 112 puffs of undiluted EVP aerosol and 112 puffs of CS, which was diluted to 24% (buccal) or 7% (small airway) to avoid overt cell damage in CS-exposed cultures. Gene expression profiles were projected into causal biological network models representing molecular mechanisms across a wide range of biological processes relevant to human respiratory physiology, including cell fate, cell stress, cell proliferation, and inflammation (Boué et al., 2015; Hoeng et al., 2012). Biological impact factor (BIF) values were calculated to aggregate the perturbations in the biological networks investigated; BIF values can be decomposed into their mechanistic components, expressed as network perturbation amplitudes (Martin et al., 2014). For comparative purposes, the

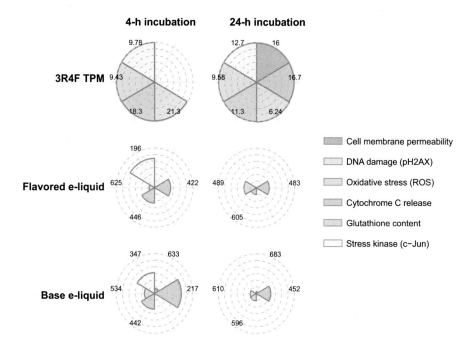

FIG. 16.2 High-content screening: Ratios of minimal effective concentrations relative to the concentrations of 3R4F CS TPM that elicited a response. *3R4F TPM*, total particulate matter of 3R4F reference CS; *pH2AX*, phosphorylated histone H2AX; *ROS*, reactive oxygen species. (From Iskandar, A.R., Zanetti, F., Marescotti, D., Titz, B., Sewer, A., Kondylis, A., et al., 2019. Application of a multi-layer systems toxicology framework for in vitro assessment of the biological effects of Classic Tobacco e-liquid and its corresponding aerosol using an e-cigarette device with MESH technology. Arch. Toxicol. 93 (11), 3229–3247.)

highest BIF value can be set as 100%, and the BIF values of other exposure conditions are expressed as relative BIFs (RBIF).

In buccal epithelial cells, the RBIFs for both undiluted EVP aerosols were lower than those for diluted 3R4F CS at all three time points, with an attenuation at 48 h, while the RBIF for CS declined by 50% from 4 to 24 h postexposure and rose to 75% again at 48 h. According to the global gene expression profiles, among the four network families tested, the Inflammatory Process Network (IPN) family was the one most impacted by exposure to the undiluted flavored aerosol. Nonetheless, at the 48-h postexposure time point, the perturbations in the IPN family following exposure to undiluted flavored or base aerosols were less than those following diluted 3R4F CS exposure in both buccal and small airway cultures (Iskandar et al., 2019b). These results suggested that exposure to the flavored and base aerosols triggered an early inflammatory response, although the cultures could finally recover. Interestingly, in

buccal cultures, exposure to the base aerosol resulted in slightly higher overall perturbations (up to ~40% RBIF) than exposure to the flavored aerosol (up to ~20% RBIF). These slightly higher RBIF scores of the base aerosol compared with those of the flavored aerosol in buccal cells were, however, not supported by other endpoints in this study, including the secreted inflammatory mediator levels.

In conclusion, this study has showcased how the multilayer systems toxicology framework can be applied to assess the potential toxicity of an e-liquid formulation and its aerosol. In the first layer of the assessment, we determined that the cytotoxicity levels of the flavored and base e-liquids were similar and much lower than that of the 3R4F CS TPM fraction. Additionally, in the second layer of the assessment, treatment with the flavored e-liquid elicited no distinct molecular changes compared with base e-liquid treatment, as determined by HCS assays, while 3R4F CS TPM elicited substantial effects at much lower nicotine concentrations. Finally, in the third layer of the assessment, we found that the impact of aerosol exposure was not substantially influenced by the presence of flavors, and it was markedly lower than that of 3R4F CS exposure. This study demonstrated that the in vitro assessment framework (Fig. 16.1) could be useful in assessing the potential impact of flavored e-liquids relative to unflavored base e-liquids and in acquiring—beyond typical in vitro endpoints—mechanistic information that can be helpful when extrapolating in vitro findings to potential clinical outcomes.

16.4 DEVELOPING A FLAVOR ASSESSMENT STRATEGY FOR EVPS

Considering the range of different flavors used in e-liquids and the resulting flavor mixtures, it is practically impossible, or scientifically and ethically undesirable (considering the thousands of experimental animals required for in vivo studies), to test all possible flavor combinations for inhalation toxicity. To add to the complexity of investigating the potential human health effects of EVPs in preclinical settings, there is currently no harmonization of research methodologies, which makes interpretation and comparison of findings from different studies difficult and may explain the sometimes controversial results. There is an urgent need to harmonize EVP aerosol research strategy and testing protocols, including e-liquid preparation guidelines, aerosol generation and physicochemical characterization methods, and preclinical and clinical toxicity studies (Breland et al., 2017; McNeill et al., 2018; Noel et al., 2018; Orr, 2014).

Here, we propose a pragmatic "flavor toolbox" approach for selecting flavors, evaluating their toxicity when inhaled, and determining their acceptable use levels (AULs) (Fig. 16.3).

16.4.1 Generating a List of Candidate Flavors

The first step of the "flavor toolbox" approach is to generate a list of candidate flavors on the basis of desirable sensorial properties, analysis of the flavors used in existing EVPs, and historical use in cigarettes. This list should explicitly exclude all oils and crude plant extracts because their composition may greatly vary across geographies, seasons, and suppliers. Moreover, as a practical way of minimizing risks from potential contaminants, the list should include only high-purity, food grade flavors. In general, the use of food grade flavors ensures that the flavors are not CMR. However, there are exceptions because classification criteria may

differ among regions and because some flavors have been grandfathered on the basis of historic use. Therefore, known respiratory sensitizers and ingredients classified as group 1, 2A, or 2B carcinogens in the International Agency for Research on Cancer (IARC) classification or classified as CMR by the FDA should be excluded.

For each flavor in the list, available toxicology data (in vitro and in vivo) should be collected from well-established databases, such as the European Chemicals Agency (ECHA)[1] and Toxplanet.[2] Furthermore, additional in vitro data may be generated to characterize the mode of action of each flavor. Finally, toxicological properties predicted by using computational toxicology software could be used to fill information gaps.

16.4.2 Grouping Flavors

The second step of the "flavor toolbox" approach is to group substances into flavor groups on the basis of their structural, toxicological, and metabolic properties. For example, read-across is a valuable technique for predicting the toxicological properties of chemicals on the basis of known toxicity of structurally similar chemicals. An outstanding example of this approach has been elaborated by the European Food and Safety Authority (EFSA) to determine flavors that are acceptable for use in foods. In particular, the EFSA, in its Flavorings Group Evaluation approach, has defined groups of flavors with similar structural and metabolic properties. In this approach, defined in Commission Regulation No. 1565/2000 (European Commission, 2000), read-across principles were applied for evaluation of data-poor substances every time toxicological data were available for a data-rich substance considered similar enough.

Other examples of flavor grouping/clustering can be found in the literature. Recently, Date and coworkers developed a robust, tiered system for chemical classification of fragrances on the basis of (i) organic functional group, (ii) structural similarity and reactivity features of the hydrocarbon skeletons, (iii) predicted or experimentally verified phase I and phase II metabolism, and (iv) expert pruning to consider these variables in the context of specific toxicity endpoints (Date et al., 2020). Date and coworkers described the application of this clustering scheme to the Research Institute for Fragrance Materials inventory and demonstrated how this approach improves read-across analog searches for safety assessment of fragrances.

---

[1]https://echa.europa.eu/fr/information-on-chemicals.
[2]https://www.toxplanet.com/default.aspx.

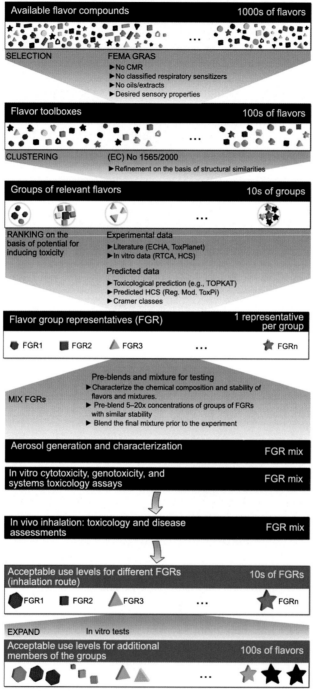

FIG. 16.3 The "flavor toolbox" approach. *CMR*, substances that are carcinogenic, mutagenic, or toxic to reproduction; *ECHA*, European Chemicals Agency; *FEMA GRAS*, generally recognized as safe by the flavor and extract manufacturers association of the United States; *FGR*, flavor group gepresentative; *HCS*, high-content screening; *Reg. Mod. ToxPi*, regression model toxicological priority index; *RTCA*, real-time cellular analysis.

By using such approaches, the list of candidate flavors that may be used in EVPs should be clustered into flavor groups by taking into account their structural, metabolic, and physicochemical properties.

16.4.3 Selecting Flavor Group Representatives

The third step of the "flavor toolbox" approach is to identify the substance that can represent each flavor group. This can be achieved by ranking each substance within a flavor group on the basis of the available experimental and predicted toxicological data. Then, an objective scoring system and a computational procedure should be used to select the representative flavor—the flavor with the worst predicted toxicological profile—for each flavor group.

These flavor group representatives (FGRs) should be then combined to create a mixture representing the "flavor toolbox." This representative flavor mixture (RFM) should then be tested in vitro and, if necessary, in vivo. These preclinical investigations will lead to a better understanding of the hazards and chronic toxicity of the RFM and provide the basis to define AULs for the different FGRs.

16.4.4 In Vitro Assessment of Flavor Mixtures

The fourth step of the "flavor toolbox" approach is to assess the toxicity of the RFM in vitro. In these studies, the RFM is dissolved in a base e-liquid (composed of PG, VG, and nicotine), which also serves as a reference.

This process starts by applying the battery of standard in vitro assays used for ENDP assessment (Chapter 13). This battery includes the Ames and mouse lymphoma assays for mutagenicity testing, in vitro micronucleus assay (MNvit) for assessing mammalian cell genotoxicity, and neutral red uptake (NRU) assay for cytotoxicity.

The next phase of the in vitro assessment leverages the integrated in vitro assessment framework for e-liquids and EVP aerosols (Section 16.3, Fig. 16.1) (Iskandar et al., 2016) and is designed to allow screening of many flavored e-liquids for potential toxicity in primary NHBE cells prior to whole aerosol assessment in human organotypic tissue cultures. This approach has the potential to greatly improve our knowledge of the toxicity of inhaled flavors, as shown in a recent study conducted with an RFM containing 26 FGRs, which represented 180 individual substances (Marescotti et al., 2020) (Chapter 13). As outlined in use case 1, this approach can also be applied for evaluating commercial e-liquids in comparison with their corresponding base e-liquids (Iskandar et al., 2019a, 2019b) (Chapter 13).

To take full advantage of this approach, studies should use multiple donors of primary NHBE cells. Furthermore, commercially available EVPs contain PG and VG in different proportions with various nicotine concentrations, and one should eventually assess whether the toxicity profiles of certain flavors could be affected by such differences.

Finally, the effects of aerosols generated from flavored e-liquids with EVP devices can only be assessed by using organotypic tissue cultures and whole-aerosol exposure systems, as explained in Chapter 13 and in our previous publications (Hayes et al., 2019; Iskandar et al., 2016, 2019a).

16.4.5 In Vivo Assessment of Flavor Mixtures

In its 2018 report, the US National Academies of Sciences (National Academies of Sciences E. et al., 2018) pointed out the lack of long-term data from repeated inhalation exposures and recommended conducting "long-term animal studies, using inhalation exposure to e-cigarette aerosol, to better understand risks from inhaling complex mixtures containing reactive carbonyl compounds, flavoring substances, and additives." In line with this recommendation, inhalation studies involving classic subchronic/chronic rat inhalation toxicity investigations (Chapter 14, Section 16.4.7.7) should be complemented with studies in mouse models of the corresponding disease to assess the impact of EVP aerosols on smoking-related diseases (Chapter 15) (Reumann et al., 2020; Szostak et al., 2020).

16.4.6 Establishing AULs for Flavors in EVPs

AULs for flavors are established on the basis of the results of the in vitro and, if necessary, in vivo testing described above. Basically, if a given flavor causes toxicological perturbations less than/equal to those of the FGR of its flavor group, the AUL identified in previous in vivo studies could be applied to it as well. In contrast, if a flavor of a specific group causes more toxicological perturbations than its corresponding FGR, additional in vitro and, eventually, dedicated in vivo studies should be performed to define its AUL.

In the "flavor toolbox" approach, a flavored e-liquid composed of an RFM dissolved in a base e-liquid (composed of water, PG, VG, and nicotine) is tested by using a panel of in vitro tests and compared head-to-head with the base e-liquid tested in chronic in vivo studies at its "no observed adverse effect level"/benchmark dose level 10 (NOAEL/BMDL10) concentration. Results from different toxicological endpoints should be used to compare the effects of the flavored e-liquid with those of the base e-liquid. If the result of this comparison shows that the flavored e-liquid has toxicity lower than/equal to that of the base e-liquid at its NOAEL/BMDL10 concentration, the flavored e-liquid could be released for use in EVPs. In contrast, if the flavored e-liquid has higher toxicity than the base e-liquid at its NOAEL/BMDL10 concentration, the flavored e-liquid formulation should be discarded.

16.4.7 Use Case 2: Applying the Flavor Toolbox Approach

In this use case, an exemplary flavor toolbox of approximately 200 commonly used EVP flavors, represented by 38 FGRs (the most biologically active flavors of each group), was assembled in accordance with the proposed workflow (Section 16.4, Fig. 16.3). These 38 FGRs were combined to create a proxy of the full "toolbox" flavor mixture. This RFM was tested in preclinical (in vitro and in vivo) toxicity studies. The results of these studies will be used to gain a better understanding of the toxicity of flavor compounds in e-liquids and EVP aerosols and, finally, to set their respective AULs.

16.4.7.1 Flavor selection, characterization, and grouping

For this work, 245 candidate flavors were initially screened for quality, purity, and FEMA GRAS status. This was followed by a comprehensive review of the available toxicity data. Flavors classified as group 1, 2A, or 2B carcinogens in the IARC classification and any flavoring classified as CMR by the EU were excluded.

The remaining flavors were assigned to groups on the basis of their chemical structure, initially by using the 34 chemical groups defined in Commission Regulation (EC) No. 1565/2000 (European Commission, 2000). Further subdivision of the groups on the basis of their structural similarities and the resulting metabolic and biological behavior led to 38 final groups being defined.

16.4.7.2 Toxicological read-across and FGRs

By applying the read-across principles, the ECHA[1] and Toxplanet[2] databases were screened for available toxicity data, with a preference for ECHA data when a flavor was included in both databases. For many flavors,

information was missing and/or route-specific data were absent, which precluded intragroup comparisons and identification of the most biologically active FGR within each group. The data gaps were filled with computational toxicological predictions and new in vitro data generated by following the integrated in vitro assessment framework described in Section 16.3 (Fig. 16.1) (Iskandar et al., 2016).

Finally, Cramer classes were assigned to each flavoring substance to define the threshold of toxicological concern for inhalation toxicity, whereby chemicals assigned to Cramer class I are predicted to be less toxic than those assigned to Cramer class III, both at the local (respiratory) and systemic levels (Carthew et al., 2009; Costigan and Meredith, 2015). For selecting the FGR—that is, the flavor with the highest calculated toxicological potential in the group—all predicted and experimental toxicity attributes were coded numerically and aggregated to derive a final scoring index.

16.4.7.3 Stability of flavor mixtures

E-liquids used for experimental purposes must be stable at least for the duration of the study. One approach for maximizing stability and simplifying the preparation of e-liquids for long-term inhalation studies is to use stable concentrated flavor mixture preblends, which are then mixed to prepare final e-liquid formulations with the desired flavors. These preblends can be designed on the basis of criteria such as chemical structure, solubility, and chemical reactivity of the flavors (i.e., unreactive, electrophilic, nucleophilic, basic, and acidic) (Fig. 16.4) to maximize their stability; the stability of these preblends should, however, be confirmed by appropriate testing.

16.4.7.4 In vitro assessment of the combined FGRs

Prior to in vivo testing, the representative flavors were tested for in vitro cytotoxicity and genotoxicity. The flavors were mixed in a carrier (PG/VG) to prepare the test mixtures (up to 18% flavor load), with and without nicotine. The test mixtures were subjected to a standard battery of in vitro cytotoxicity (NRU) and genotoxicity (Ames and MNvit) assays. The test mixtures (with and without nicotine) were negative in the Ames mutagenicity assay but cytotoxic in the NRU assay. To further identify the flavor ingredient(s) potentially responsible for the cytotoxic response in the NRU assay, we tested the six preblends separately. The results suggested that preblends containing certain flavor ingredients—for example, ethyl maltol and furaneol—were more cytotoxic, which is consistent with previously published

Grouping into stable pre-blends

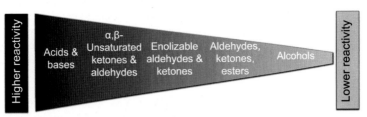

FIG. 16.4 Criteria for generating concentrated preblend formulations.

findings on these ingredients being cytotoxic/irritant in vitro (Hua et al., 2019). In addition to the NRU assay, RTCAs were performed to confirm the cytotoxicity of the mixtures and assess single flavors to identify the main contributing individual flavors.

In the MNvit genotoxicity assay, the test mixture with nicotine was negative, but the test mixture without nicotine showed equivocal results. In addition to the MNvit assay, a γH2AX DNA repair assay was performed to assess the DNA-damaging properties of the mixtures and selected individual flavor ingredients. While the mixture had a significant effect on γH2AX levels, the individual flavors produced variable responses. In a complementary approach to these genotoxicity tests, the individual flavors and flavor mixtures were assessed for their genotoxic and nongenotoxic properties by the in vitro ToxTracker assay (Hendriks et al., 2016). ToxTracker employs a panel of mammalian stem cell lines possessing different fluorescent reporters responsive to induction of DNA damage, oxidative stress, and protein damage. The differential induction of these fluorescent reporters and the cytotoxicity of test compounds are determined by flow cytometry. Control compounds are included in each test to determine the technical performance and reproducibility of the Tox-Tracker assay. Selected flavors were analyzed in the absence and presence of the S9 rat liver extract–based metabolizing system. Seven flavor compounds and both flavor mixtures (with and without nicotine) caused DNA damage (positive ToxTracker results).

16.4.7.5 Transfer of flavors from e-liquids to aerosols

Because the in vitro testing described above was performed with e-liquids, it was necessary to assess the e-liquid-to-aerosol transfer rates of the flavors prior to in vivo inhalation toxicity testing.

Clearly, the flavor and nicotine concentrations in the mixtures described above are defined by their respective amounts added to the carrier e-liquid composed of water, PG, and VG. However, aerosol generation might influence their relative concentrations in the corresponding aerosols because of their respective physicochemical properties, such as vapor pressure (Chapter 12). In an aerosol generated by a nebulizer, an e-liquid with its dissolved ingredients is disrupted into small droplets with the same composition as the bulk volume, and only a partial redistribution of volatile substances into the gas phase of the aerosol will occur. Upon exposure to both the particulate and gas phases of this aerosol, a biological system (animal or in vitro culture system) will receive the same proportions of inhaled substances as if exposed to the liquid. However, EVPs and experimental devices, such as the capillary aerosol generator (CAG) (Chapter 12), vaporize the e-liquid, and this vapor subsequently condenses into an aerosol composed of liquid droplets and a gas phase. This process requires heating of the e-liquid to temperatures high enough to reach the boiling points of the carrier e-liquid constituents (PG and VG). This process may not lead to quantitative transfer of all e-liquid constituents to the aerosol, and, hence, the transfer efficiency of flavors must be determined prior to in vivo inhalation testing.

To this end, we generated aerosols from e-liquids containing the 38 FGRs by using a CAG with the capillary temperature set at 250°C, which is the typical temperature of e-cigarette coils (Geiss et al., 2016). The aerosol was trapped and analyzed, as described in Chapter 12.

After verifying that the physicochemical properties and aerosol concentrations of the base e-liquid constituents (PG, VG, and nicotine) were not changed by the addition of flavors, the transfer efficiency of the flavors from the e-liquid to the diluted aerosol was quantified in an exposure chamber. 12 compounds were transferred efficiently from the CAG to the inhalation chamber, with transfer rates above 85%. Minor losses were observed for seven compounds during the transfer, with transfer rates between 70% and 85%. High losses were determined for 13 flavors, with transfer rates ranging from 50% to 70%. No transfer values were obtained for four compounds—namely, isobutyraldehyde, *p*-menth-8-thiol-3-one, 1-penten-3-one, and acetal—because they were not trapped efficiently by the Extrelut NT 3 cartridges (Chapter 12).

These transfer efficiencies were taken into account when calculating the flavor exposure levels in in vivo inhalation studies.

16.4.7.6 Inhalation toxicity of the RFM in a 5-week A/J mouse tolerability study

The e-liquid containing the 38 FGRs was subjected to in vivo inhalation testing in a dose-range-finding study in A/J mice, with an emphasis on subacute toxicity and respiratory tract irritation and inflammation. The results from this study were intended to help select appropriate exposure concentrations of the flavor mixtures for a subsequent 18-month chronic inhalation study in A/J mice.

A/J mice were whole-body exposed (6 h/day, 5 days/week) to fresh air (sham), aerosol from the base e-liquid (PG and VG with 2% nicotine), aerosols from the flavor mixture (base e-liquid with up to 18% of flavors), or smoke from the 3R4F reference cigarette for 5 weeks. The aerosols were well tolerated by the mice, with no signs of severe acute toxicity. Exposure to the flavored aerosols, even at the highest flavor concentration (18% of the e-liquid), did not cause lung inflammation, as evidenced by the absence of immune cell infiltration in bronchoalveolar lavage fluid and histopathological analysis. In contrast, exposure to smoke from the 3R4F cigarette resulted in lung inflammation and moderate to severe adaptive changes in nasal and laryngeal epithelia.

In summary, neither the mixture of 38 FGRs nor the base e-liquid (PG, VG, and nicotine) elicited significant subacute toxicity or respiratory tract irritation/inflammation, and both were considered suitable for use in a subsequent chronic inhalation study in A/J mice.

16.4.7.7 90-day rat inhalation study

A subchronic rat inhalation study was conducted in accordance with OECD test guideline 413 to characterize the toxicity of an EVP aerosol containing a flavor mix of 26 FGRs, representing 178 flavors allocated to 26 groups, dissolved in a PG/VG/nicotine base e-liquid. Nonflavored e-liquids, with and without nicotine, were used as references to identify potential additive or synergistic effects between nicotine and the flavors

(Ho et al., 2020). In this study, the aerosols were generated with nebulizers, thus avoiding thermal transformation of the e-liquid constituents (Chapter 12). Groups of 18 male and 18 female rats were exposed for 91 days (6 h/day, 5 days/week, nose-only) to three different concentrations of the flavored aerosols, the two reference aerosols, or phosphate-buffered saline (control). For selected groups of rats (eight male and eight female per group), a 42-day postexposure recovery period was included to investigate the reversibility, persistence, and delayed occurrence of exposure effects. Within each group of rats exposed for 91 days, 10 rats were allocated to the endpoints listed in the OECD test guideline, and the remaining 8 rats were allocated to systems toxicology investigations (the OECD-plus approach described in Chapter 14). The exposure concentrations of nicotine, PG, and VG in the base aerosol were 23, 1520, and 1890 µg/L, respectively, and the flavor mix was added at low, medium, and high concentration levels. The low flavor mix concentration levels were selected on the basis of potential use levels of each FGR in EVPs defined by odor thresholds and sensorial properties. The high flavor mix concentration levels were set by the maximum solubility of each FGR, and the medium flavor mix concentration was chosen as an intermediate point (for most FGRs, this was two-thirds of the high level).

The respiratory tract (nose, larynx, and lungs) and systemic toxic effects resulting from inhalation of the flavored e-liquid aerosols were minimal. No remarkable clinical (in-life) effects were observed in rats exposed to the flavored e-liquid aerosol. The biological effects of exposure to the FGR mixture were limited and mainly nicotine-mediated, including changes in hematological and blood chemistry parameters, body weight, and organ weight. Moreover, there were no significant additive biological effects caused by exposure to the nebulized FGR mixture above the nicotine effects, which resembled those observed in previous inhalation studies with nicotine-containing aerosols (Phillips et al., 2015, 2016, 2017). Likewise, transcriptomics analysis of the nasal epithelium revealed minimal flavor-related effects (only three differentially expressed genes [DEGs]) and a weak nicotine effect (23 DEGs in female rats only). Furthermore, no flavor-related effects and only minimal nicotine-related effects (2 DEGs in female and 7 DEGs in male rats) were observed in the lungs, and no flavor-related effect was observed in the liver. However, consistent with the findings of the previous nicotine aerosol inhalation studies mentioned above, the liver showed 764 DEGs in female rats and 426 DEGs in male rats. Gene set enrichment analysis indicated mainly upregulation in gene sets related to cholesterol biosynthesis and xenobiotic metabolism and downregulation in gene sets related to antigen processing and presentation.

In conclusion, the FGR mixture did not increase the inhalation toxicity of an EVP aerosol containing nicotine, PG, and VG, even at exaggerated concentrations. Although the presence of nicotine was associated with several adaptive changes, no major adverse effects were caused by the FGRs in the aerosol, and there were no apparent additive or synergistic toxic effects among the FGRs in this mixture, which represented a total of 178 flavors allocated to 26 groups.

As noted above, in this study, the aerosols were generated with a nebulizer, which helps avoid thermal effects during aerosolization. In a planned follow-up study with the same exposure design, aerosols will be generated with a CAG to mimic the thermal effects of EVPs. These results, in combination with those obtained with a nebulizer, will allow us to estimate the contribution of heating to the toxicity (if any) of flavored EVP aerosols.

16.4.7.8 Chronic inhalation toxicity and carcinogenicity study in A/J mice

The "toolbox" of 38 flavors was recently subjected to in vivo inhalation testing in a dose-range-finding study in A/J mice, with an emphasis on subacute toxicity and respiratory tract irritation and inflammation. It is important to address the long-term toxicity and carcinogenic risk of the aerosolized toolbox flavors in a complementary chronic inhalation toxicity and carcinogenicity study, according to OECD TG 453 (OECD, 2018). This study involved exposure of A/J mice to aerosol from the base e-liquid (PG and VG with 2% nicotine), aerosols from the flavor mixture (base e-liquid with up to 18% of flavors), or smoke from the 3R4F reference cigarette for 18 months. At the time of writing, this study was still ongoing and we will publish its results in due course.

16.5 CHALLENGES AND PRINCIPLES OF EVP TESTING

16.5.1 Interactions Between Flavors and the Base E-liquid

E-liquids can be chemically unstable, with reactions occurring between flavors and the base e-liquid. According to Erythropel et al. these reactions occur immediately after mixing at room temperature, and the resulting compounds may have toxicological properties that differ from those of the flavor or vehicle

(Erythropel et al., 2019). Synergistic and/or antagonistic interactions may occur, and some interactions may mask or dampen the effect of a flavor. One example illustrating this point comes from a situation where individual flavors and their mixtures were assessed in vitro in NHBE cells (Marescotti et al., 2020). Twenty-six flavors, when tested individually, showed low cytotoxicity in exposed cells (measured by RTCA). However, when tested as a mixture, the flavors showed a much higher toxicity, suggesting that they may have additive and/or synergistic effects that might result from their interactions. Hence, testing of individual flavors should be complemented with approaches for obtaining information on their potential contribution in more complex mixtures. Furthermore, Erythropel et al. (Erythropel et al., 2019) suggested that, to comprehensively assess the risk of e-liquids, it is important to consider the complete life cycle of the e-liquid constituents, from mixing through storage, heating, and oxidation in EVP devices, and their stability in biological environments (e.g., mouth, airways, and lungs).

16.5.2 Testing e-Liquids versus Testing E-vapors

Given the number of commercially available flavored e-liquids, several authors have suggested testing e-liquids as a first screen (i.e., before testing the aerosol) to identify flavoring substances and/or chemical constituents that have a higher toxicological potential and, therefore, should be subjected to additional studies (Iskandar et al., 2016; Sassano et al., 2018). E-liquid testing would constitute a less expensive, faster, and less labor-intensive approach than EVP aerosol testing, at least as a justifiable first-pass screening.

Yet, any complete risk assessment of an EVP should ultimately include evaluation of the heated and aerosolized e-liquid by using its corresponding EVP device or an aerosolization system that can mimic the operational conditions of the EVP under investigation. This is particularly important for flavors because they are volatile compounds. As pointed out by Romagna et al. it is unlikely that flavors in e-liquids will still be present in the aerosol in the same amounts and proportions (Farsalinos et al., 2013). This was confirmed in our transfer efficiency study summarized above.

Second, e-liquid testing will not provide information on the products generated by thermal degradation of their constituents. Chemical reactions during heating and aerosolization of the flavors and constituents of the base e-liquid may result in the formation of new compounds. For example, Khlystov and Samburova have suggested that the formation of aldehydes during e-cigarette use is related to the concentration of flavors (Khlystov and Samburova, 2016). However, this finding was not observed in other studies (Farsalinos et al., 2017). Sucrose, a sweetener and flavor enhancer found in e-liquids, has also been suggested as a potential ingredient that may thermally degrade to produce carbonyl compounds (Kubica et al., 2014). For instance, saccharides degrade and produce furans and aldehydes when heated (Soussy et al., 2016). Moreover, a study on 28 e-liquids identified more than 140 volatile flavoring substances at concentrations varying from 1% to 5% (10–50 mg/mL) and detected the formation of aldehydes (Hutzler et al., 2014). However, the aerosols of closed-system EVPs contain much lower levels of carbonyls than CS (Belushkin et al., 2020).

16.5.3 Dose Calculations and Human-Relevant Exposures

The present in vitro experiments have provided useful information about the hazards associated with flavors, including mechanistic details of the biological effects they elicit. However, because of the nature of these tests, the flavor concentrations used in vitro are often one or more orders of magnitude higher than those achievable in vivo and in EVP consumers (Chapter 12). In the in vivo studies, animals were exposed to flavor mixtures containing up to 38 different flavors; however, commercial e-liquids do not typically contain more than 20 flavors. Furthermore, the flavors in the mixtures reached up to 18% of the e-liquid mass, while, in commercial e-liquids, they commonly account for a much lower mass fraction (typically 5%). Therefore, and because the 38 FGRs are the most biologically active flavors in their respective groups, we consider this a hypothetical worst-case scenario. However, each flavor in the mixture was tested at concentrations relevant to human exposure, taking into account the maximum flavor use levels in commercial EVPs. In particular, to derive the concentrations of the flavors in the formulation suitable for a mouse inhalation study, we assumed a human e-liquid consumption of 4 mL/day. On this basis, we calculated the equivalent animal dose and derived the concentration of each individual flavor ingredient in the test atmosphere (Alexander et al., 2008) by considering body surface extrapolation in accordance with the Center for Drug Evaluation and Research recommendations (CDER, 2005). Finally, we calculated the concentration of each flavor in the stock formulation used for aerosolization by using an average transfer rate (60%, on the basis of the above transfer studies) and the CAG output and aerosol dilution factors necessary for achieving the desired nicotine concentrations in the test atmospheres.

16.6 CONCLUSIONS

Flavors are an important group of ingredients of e-liquids and EVP aerosols. While many, if not most, flavor ingredients used in inhalable EVPs are GRAS for oral consumption, they may frequently have insufficient safety data concerning inhalation exposure. However, scientific studies focusing on the toxicological effects of flavoring substances via inhalation are still scarce, and most of the methods and approaches used for assessing their inhalation risks provide only limited evidence relevant to specific flavors and AULs. Therefore, there is a pressing need to identify proper scientific methods for assessing the safety of flavors used in EVPs and to establish appropriate safety standards for their development.

Here, we have presented a pragmatic approach for evaluating the inhalation toxicology of flavors and determining their AULs. While this work is only beginning, the several use cases we have presented to exemplify how this challenge could be addressed may provide a basis for future discussion and research into the safety of inhaled flavors.

REFERENCES

Alexander, D.J., Collins, C.J., Coombs, D.W., Gilkison, I.S., Hardy, C.J., Healey, G., et al., 2008. Association of Inhalation Toxicologists (AIT) working party recommendation for standard delivered dose calculation and expression in non-clinical aerosol inhalation toxicology studies with pharmaceuticals. Inhal. Toxicol. 20 (13), 1179–1189.

Bahl, V., Lin, S., Xu, N., Davis, B., Wang, Y.H., Talbot, P., 2012. Comparison of electronic cigarette refill fluid cytotoxicity using embryonic and adult models. Reprod. Toxicol. 34 (4), 529–537.

Balls, M., Combes, R.D., Bhogal, N., 2012. The use of integrated and intelligent testing strategies in the prediction of toxic hazard and in risk assessment. In: Balls, M., Combes, R.D., Bhogal, N. (Eds.), New Technologies for Toxicity Testing. Springer US, New York, NY, pp. 221–253.

Behar, R.Z., Luo, W., Lin, S.C., Wang, Y., Valle, J., Pankow, J.F., et al., 2016. Distribution, quantification and toxicity of cinnamaldehyde in electronic cigarette refill fluids and aerosols. Tobac. Contr. 25 (Suppl. 2), ii94–ii102.

Belushkin, M., Tafin Djoko, D., Esposito, M., Korneliou, A., Jeannet, C., Lazzerini, M., et al., 2020. Selected harmful and potentially harmful constituents levels in commercial e-cigarettes. Chem. Res. Toxicol. 33 (2), 657–668.

Bengalli, R., Ferri, E., Labra, M., Mantecca, P., 2017. Lung toxicity of condensed aerosol from E-CIG liquids: influence of the flavor and the in vitro model used. Int. J. Environ. Res. Publ. Health 14 (10).

Boué, S., Talikka, M., Westra, J.W., Hayes, W., Di Fabio, A., Park, J., et al., 2015. Causal Biological Network Database:

A Comprehensive Platform of Causal Biological Network Models Focused on the Pulmonary and Vascular Systems. Database.

Breland, A., Soule, E., Lopez, A., Ramôa, C., El-Hellani, A., Eissenberg, T., 2017. Electronic cigarettes: what are they and what do they do? Ann. N. Y. Acad. Sci. 1394 (1), 5.

Carthew, P., Clapp, C., Gutsell, S., 2009. Exposure based waiving: the application of the toxicological threshold of concern (TTC) to inhalation exposure for aerosol ingredients in consumer products. Food Chem. Toxicol. 47 (6), 1287—1295.

Cder, 2005. Guidance for Industry Estimating the Maximum Safe Starting Dose in Initial Clinical Trials for Therapeutics in Adult Healthy Volunteers from. https://www.fda.gov/media/72309/download. (Accessed 22 July 2020).

Costigan, S., Lopez-Belmonte, J., 2017. An approach to allergy risk assessments for e-liquid ingredients. Regul. Toxicol. Pharmacol. 87, 1—8.

Costigan, S., Meredith, C., 2015. An approach to ingredient screening and toxicological risk assessment of flavours in e-liquids. Regul. Toxicol. Pharmacol. 72 (2), 361—369.

Cudazzo, G., Smart, D.J., Mchugh, D., Vanscheeuwijck, P., 2019. Lysosomotropic-related limitations of the BALB/c 3T3 cell-based neutral red uptake assay and an alternative testing approach for assessing e-liquid cytotoxicity. Toxicol. In Vitro 61, 104647.

Date, M.S., O'brien, D., Botelho, D.J., Schultz, T.W., Liebler, D.C., Penning, T.M., et al., 2020. Clustering a chemical inventory for safety assessment of fragrance ingredients: identifying read-across analogs to address data gaps. Chem. Res. Toxicol. https://doi.org/10.1021/acs.chemrestox.9b00518.

Erythropel, H.C., Jabba, S.V., Dewinter, T.M., Mendizabal, M., Anastas, P.T., Jordt, S.E., et al., 2019. formation of flavorant-propylene glycol adducts with novel toxicological properties in chemically unstable E-cigarette liquids. Nicotine Tob. Res. 21 (9), 1248—1258.

European Commission, 2000. Commission Regulation (EC) No 1565/2000 from. https://eur-lex.europa.eu/legal-content/EN/TXT/PDF/?uri=CELEX:32000R1565&from=EN. (Accessed 22 July 2020).

Farsalinos, K., et al., 2018. Patterns of Flavored E-Cigarette Use Among Adults Vapers in the United States: An Internet Survey. Submitted to: Docket No. FDA-2017-N-6565 for "Regulation of Flavors in Tobacco Products".

Farsalinos, K., Gillman, G., Kistler, K., Yannovits, N., 2017. Comment on "flavoring compounds dominate toxic aldehyde production during E cigarette vaping". Environ. Sci. Technol. 51 (4), 2491—2492.

Farsalinos, K.E., Romagna, G., Allifranchini, E., Ripamonti, E., Bocchietto, E., Todeschi, S., et al., 2013. Comparison of the cytotoxic potential of cigarette smoke and electronic cigarette vapour extract on cultured myocardial cells. Int. J. Environ. Res. Publ. Health 10 (10), 5146—5162.

Fema, 2018. Safety Assessment and Regulatory Authority to Use Flavors — Focus on Electronic Nicotine Delivery Systems and Flavored Tobacco Products from. https://www.femaflavor.org/sites/default/files/2018-05/FEMAGRAS%20Ecig%2004302018.pdf. (Accessed 14 July 2020).

Geiss, O., Bianchi, I., Barrero-Moreno, J., 2016. Correlation of volatile carbonyl yields emitted by e-cigarettes with the temperature of the heating coil and the perceived sensorial quality of the generated vapours. Int. J. Hyg Environ. Health 219 (3), 268—277.

Gerloff, J., Sundar, I.K., Freter, R., Sekera, E.R., Friedman, A.E., Robinson, R., et al., 2017. Inflammatory response and barrier dysfunction by different e-cigarette flavoring chemicals identified by gas chromatography-mass spectrometry in e-liquids and e-vapors on human lung epithelial cells and fibroblasts. Appl. In Vitro Toxicol. 3 (1), 28—40.

Hayes, A.W., Li, R., Hoeng, J., Iskandar, A.R., Peitsch, M.C., Dourson, M.L., 2019. New approaches to risk assessment of chemical mixtures. Toxicol. Res. Appl. 3, 1—10.

Hendriks, G., Derr, R.S., Misovic, B., Morolli, B., Calléja, F.M., Vrieling, H., 2016. The extended ToxTracker assay discriminates between induction of DNA damage, oxidative stress, and protein misfolding. Toxicol. Sci. 150 (1), 190—203.

Ho, J., Sciuscio, D., Kogel, U., Titz, B., Leroy, P., Vuillaume, G., et al., 2020. Evaluation of toxicity of aerosols from flavored e-liquids in Sprague-Dawley rats in a 90-day OECD inhalation study. Complement. Trans. Analysis 94 (6), 2179—2206.

Hoeng, J., Deehan, R., Pratt, D., Martin, F., Sewer, A., Thomson, T.M., et al., 2012. A network-based approach to quantifying the impact of biologically active substances. Drug Discov. Today 17 (9), 413—418.

Hua, M., Omaiye, E.E., Luo, W., Mcwhirter, K.J., Pankow, J.F., Talbot, P., 2019. Identification of cytotoxic flavor chemicals in top-selling electronic cigarette refill fluids. Sci. Rep. 9 (1), 2782.

Hubbs, A.F., Kreiss, K., Cummings, K.J., Fluharty, K.L., O'connell, R., Cole, A., et al., 2019. Flavorings-related lung disease: a brief review and new mechanistic data. Toxicol. Pathol. 47 (8), 1012—1026.

Hung, P.H., Savidge, M., De, M., Kang, J., Healy, S.M., Valerio Jr., L.G., 2020. In vitro and in silico genetic toxicity screening of flavor compounds and other ingredients in tobacco products with emphasis on ENDS. J. Appl. Toxicol. 40 (11), 1566—1587.

Hutzler, C., Paschke, M., Kruschinski, S., Henkler, F., Hahn, J., Luch, A., 2014. Chemical hazards present in liquids and vapors of electronic cigarettes. Arch. Toxicol. 88 (7), 1295—1308.

Iskandar, A.R., Gonzalez-Suarez, I., Majeed, S., Marescotti, D., Sewer, A., Xiang, Y., et al., 2016. A framework for in vitro systems toxicology assessment of e-liquids. Toxicol. Mech. Method. 26 (6), 389—413.

Iskandar, A.R., Zanetti, F., Marescotti, D., Titz, B., Sewer, A., Kondylis, A., et al., 2019a. Application of a multi-layer systems toxicology framework for in vitro assessment of the biological effects of Classic Tobacco e-liquid and its corresponding aerosol using an e-cigarette device with MESH technology. Arch. Toxicol. 93 (11), 3229—3247.

Iskandar, A.R., Zanetti, F., Kondylis, A., Martin, F., Leroy, P., Majeed, S., et al., 2019b. A lower impact of an acute exposure to electronic cigarette aerosols than to cigarette smoke in human organotypic buccal and small airway cultures was demonstrated using systems toxicology assessment. Intern. Emerg. Med 14 (6), 863–883.

Ji, E.H., Sun, B., Zhao, T., Shu, S., Chang, C.H., Messadi, D., et al., 2016. Characterization of electronic cigarette aerosol and its induction of oxidative stress response in oral keratinocytes. PloS One 11 (5), e0154447.

Khlystov, A., Samburova, V., 2016. Flavoring compounds dominate toxic aldehyde production during E-cigarette vaping. Environ. Sci. Technol. 50 (23), 13080–13085.

Klager, S., Vallarino, J., Macnaughton, P., Christiani, D.C., Lu, Q., Allen, J.G., 2017. Flavoring chemicals and aldehydes in E-cigarette emissions. Environ. Sci. Technol. 51 (18), 10806–10813.

Kreiss, K., Gomaa, A., Kullman, G., Fedan, K., Simoes, E.J., Enright, P.L., 2002. Clinical bronchiolitis obliterans in workers at a microwave-popcorn plant. N. Engl. J. Med. 347 (5), 330–338.

Kubica, P., Wasik, A., Kot-Wasik, A., Namiesnik, J., 2014. An evaluation of sucrose as a possible contaminant in e-liquids for electronic cigarettes by hydrophilic interaction liquid chromatography-tandem mass spectrometry. Anal. Bioanal. Chem. 406 (13), 3013–3018.

Lee, K.M., Hoeng, J., Harbo, S., Kogel, U., Gardner, W., Oldham, M., et al., 2018. Biological changes in C57BL/6 mice following 3 weeks of inhalation exposure to cigarette smoke or e-vapor aerosols. Inhal. Toxicol. 30 (13–14), 553–567.

Lee, W.H., Ong, S.G., Zhou, Y., Tian, L., Bae, H.R., Baker, N., et al., 2019. Modeling cardiovascular risks of E-cigarettes with human-induced pluripotent stem cell-derived endothelial cells. J. Am. Coll. Cardiol. 73 (21), 2722–2737.

Leigh, N.J., Lawton, R.I., Hershberger, P.A., Goniewicz, M.L., 2016. Flavourings significantly affect inhalation toxicity of aerosol generated from electronic nicotine delivery systems (ENDS). Tobac. Contr. 25 (Suppl. 2), ii81–ii87.

Lerner, C.A., Sundar, I.K., Yao, H., Gerloff, J., Ossip, D.J., Mcintosh, S., et al., 2015. Vapors produced by electronic cigarettes and e-juices with flavorings induce toxicity, oxidative stress, and inflammatory response in lung epithelial cells and in mouse lung. PloS One 10 (2), e0116732.

Marescotti, D., Mathis, C., Belcastro, V., Leroy, P., Acali, S., Martin, F., et al., 2020. Systems toxicology assessment of a representative e-liquid formulation using human primary bronchial epithelial cells. Toxicol. Rep. 7, 67–80.

Martin, F., Sewer, A., Talikka, M., Xiang, Y., Hoeng, J., Peitsch, M.C., 2014. Quantification of biological network perturbations for mechanistic insight and diagnostics using two-layer causal models. BMC Bioinf. 15 (1), 238.

Mcneill, A., Brose, L.S., Calder, R., Bauld, L., Robson, D., 2018. Evidence review of e-cigarettes and heated tobacco products 2018. In: A Report Commissioned by Public Health England. Public Health England, London, p. 6.

Morgan, D.L., Flake, G.P., Gwinn, W.M., Johnson, C.L., 2019. NTP Research Report on Respiratory Tract Toxicity of the Flavoring Agent 2,3-Hexanedione in Mice Exposed by Inhalation. NTP Research Reports. National Toxicology Program, Research Triangle Park (NC). Research Report 10.

Morgan, D.L., Jokinen, M.P., Johnson, C.L., Price, H.C., Gwinn, W.M., Bousquet, R.W., et al., 2016. Chemical reactivity and respiratory toxicity of the α-diketone flavoring agents: 2,3-butanedione, 2,3-pentanedione, and 2,3-hexanedione. Toxicol. Pathol. 44 (5), 763–783.

Munro, I.C., Kennepohl, E., Kroes, R., 1999. A procedure for the safety evaluation of flavouring substances. Joint FAO/WHO Expert Committee on Food Additives. Food Chem. Toxicol. 37 (2–3), 207–232.

Muthumalage, T., Lamb, T., Friedman, M.R., Rahman, I., 2019. E-cigarette flavored pods induce inflammation, epithelial barrier dysfunction, and DNA damage in lung epithelial cells and monocytes. Sci. Rep. 9 (1), 19035.

Muthumalage, T., Prinz, M., Ansah, K.O., Gerloff, J., Sundar, I.K., Rahman, I., 2017. Inflammatory and oxidative responses induced by exposure to commonly used e-cigarette flavoring chemicals and flavored e-liquids without nicotine. Front. Physiol. 8, 1130.

National Academies of Sciences, E., and Medicine, 2018. Public Health Consequences of E-Cigarettes. The National Academies Press, Washington DC.

National Academies of Sciences, E., Medicine, Health, Medicine, D., Board on Population, H., Public Health, P., et al., 2018. In: Eaton, D.L., Kwan, L.Y., Stratton, K. (Eds.), Public Health Consequences of E-Cigarettes. National Academies Press (US), Washington (DC). Copyright 2018 by the National Academy of Sciences. All rights reserved.

Noel, A., Verret, C.M., Hasan, F., Lomnicki, S., Morse, J., Robichaud, A., et al., 2018. Generation of electronic cigarette aerosol by a third-generation machine-vaping device: application to toxicological studies. J. Vis. Exp. (138) https://doi.org/10.3791/58095.

Oecd, 2018. Test No. 453: Combined Chronic Toxicity/Carcinogenicity Studies.

Orr, M.S., 2014. Electronic cigarettes in the USA: a summary of available toxicology data and suggestions for the future. Tobac. Contr. 23 (Suppl. 2), ii18–22.

Phillips, B., Esposito, M., Verbeeck, J., Boué, S., Iskandar, A., Vuillaume, G., et al., 2015. Toxicity of aerosols of nicotine and pyruvic acid (separate and combined) in Sprague-Dawley rats in a 28-day OECD 412 inhalation study and assessment of systems toxicology. Inhal. Toxicol. 27 (9), 405–431.

Phillips, B., Titz, B., Kogel, U., Sharma, D., Leroy, P., Xiang, Y., et al., 2017. Toxicity of the main electronic cigarette components, propylene glycol, glycerin, and nicotine, in Sprague-Dawley rats in a 90-day OECD inhalation study complemented by molecular endpoints. Food Chem. Toxicol. 109 (Pt 1), 315–332.

Phillips, B., Veljkovic, E., Boué, S., Schlage, W.K., Vuillaume, G., Martin, F., et al., 2016. An 8-month systems toxicology inhalation/cessation study in apoe-/- mice to investigate cardiovascular and respiratory exposure effects of a candidate modified risk tobacco product, THS 2.2, compared with conventional cigarettes. Toxicol. Sci. 149 (2), 411–432.

Polosa, R., Rodu, B., Caponnetto, P., Maglia, M., Raciti, C., 2013. A fresh look at tobacco harm reduction: the case for the electronic cigarette. Harm Reduct. J. 10 (1), 19.

Reumann, M.K., Schaefer, J., Titz, B., Aspera-Werz, R.H., Wong, E.T., Szostak, J., et al., 2020. E-vapor aerosols do not compromise bone integrity relative to cigarette smoke after 6-month inhalation in an ApoE(-/-) mouse model. Arch. Toxicol. https://doi.org/10.1007/s00204-020-02769-4.

Rose, C.S., 2017. Early detection, clinical diagnosis, and management of lung disease from exposure to diacetyl. Toxicology 388, 9–14.

Sassano, M.F., Davis, E.S., Keating, J.E., Zorn, B.T., Kochar, T.K., Wolfgang, M.C., et al., 2018. Evaluation of e-liquid toxicity using an open-source high-throughput screening assay. PLoS Biol. 16 (3), e2003904.

Sherwood, C.L., Boitano, S., 2016. Airway epithelial cell exposure to distinct e-cigarette liquid flavorings reveals toxicity thresholds and activation of CFTR by the chocolate flavoring 2,5-dimethypyrazine. Respir. Res. 17 (1), 57.

Soussy, S., El-Hellani, A., Baalbaki, R., Salman, R., Shihadeh, A., Saliba, N.A., 2016. Detection of 5-hydroxymethylfurfural and furfural in the aerosol of electronic cigarettes. Tobac. Contr. 25 (Suppl. 2), ii88–ii93.

Stevenson, M., Czekala, L., Simms, L., Tschierske, N., Larne, O., Walele, T., 2019. The use of Genomic Allergen Rapid Detection (GARD) assays to predict the respiratory and skin sensitising potential of e-liquids. Regul. Toxicol. Pharmacol. 103, 158–165.

Szostak, J., Wong, E.T., Titz, B., Lee, T., Wong, S.K., Low, T., et al., 2020. A 6-month systems toxicology inhalation study in ApoE(-/-) mice demonstrates reduced cardiovascular effects of E-vapor aerosols compared with cigarette smoke. Am. J. Physiol. Heart Circ. Physiol. 318 (3), H604–H631.

Tobacco Advisory Group of the Royal College of Physicians, 2016. Nicotine Without Smoke—Tobacco Harm Reduction. (Accessed 25 April 2018).

Wallace, K.B., 2017. Future perspective of butter flavorings-related occupational lung disease. Toxicology 388, 7–8.

Werley, M.S., Kirkpatrick, D.J., Oldham, M.J., Jerome, A.M., Langston, T.B., Lilly, P.D., et al., 2016. Toxicological assessment of a prototype e-cigaret device and three flavor formulations: a 90-day inhalation study in rats. Inhal. Toxicol. 28 (1), 22–38.

Zhu, S.H., Sun, J.Y., Bonnevie, E., Cummins, S.E., Gamst, A., Yin, L., et al., 2014. Four hundred and sixty brands of e-cigarettes and counting: implications for product regulation. Tobac. Contr. 23 (Suppl. 3) iii3-9.

CHAPTER 17

Clinical Assessment of ENDPs

SANDRINE POULY • CHRISTELLE HAZIZA • MICHAEL J. PECK •
MANUEL C. PEITSCH

17.1 A CLINICAL STRATEGY FOR ENDP ASSESSMENT

As outlined in Chapter 1, the potential public health benefit of using electronic nicotine delivery products (ENDPs), briefly described in Chapter 2, depends both on their potential to reduce smoking-related disease risk and their acceptability as alternatives to cigarettes by adult smokers. The clinical assessment strategy is, therefore, focused on assessing the disease risk reduction potential of ENDPs and leveraging the clinical studies to gather early insights into the acceptability of ENDPs as alternatives to cigarettes for current adult smokers. Importantly, this assessment strategy must take into account both the ENDP assessment framework and the causal chain of events linking smoking to disease (CELSD) (Chapter 3) to mitigate some of the key challenges faced by the clinical assessment of ENDPs:

1. The most prevalent smoking-related diseases—that is, cardiovascular disease (CVD), chronic obstructive pulmonary disease (COPD), and lung cancer (Carter et al., 2015)—generally occur after decades of smoking, whereas the reduction in excess risk following smoking cessation and, a fortiori, following switching to ENDPs is progressive and slow. This means that long-term clinical health outcome and epidemiological studies for quantifying the disease risk reduction associated with switching from cigarette smoking to ENDP use are impracticable in a premarket setting (Chang et al., 2019; Hoeng et al., 2019). Indeed, as smoking-related diseases often take decades to manifest, epidemiological studies will, unfortunately, take decades. Therefore, an approach that leverages short- to mid-term clinical evidence across various studies is needed to estimate the long-term risk reduction potential of ENDPs. Consequently, clinical studies conducted in a premarket setting can only measure endpoints of the earlier events of the CELSD, mainly from exposure to cell/tissue changes and a limited number of physiological changes.

2. Smoking affects several organ systems and multiple biological mechanisms, so that no single endpoint can inform, on its own, about the relative risk of ENDPs in comparison with that of cigarettes. Therefore, a number of biomarkers that address the multifaceted biological impact of cigarette smoke should be considered in combination in the risk assessment of ENDPs. However, there are a limited number of clinically validated biomarkers that can be used to assess the biological effects of smoking cessation and, therefore, switching to ENDPs in healthy smokers.

3. Clinical ENDP assessment studies for assessing short- to mid-term effects are typically conducted with healthy adult volunteer smokers who have smoked at least 10 cigarettes per day for at least 10 years. Hence, the study population will generally cover a range of smoking histories as well as a broad age range. As a consequence, the effects of smoking on biomarkers of potential harm (BoPHs) are quite variable, both at baseline and post-cessation/switching. In addition, with the enrollment of a smoking population in good health, the effects of switching and cessation on BoPHs that are generally indicative of diseases are expected to be small. It is, therefore, important to compare the effects of switching with those of cessation to contextualize the magnitudes of the effects of switching with those of cessation, which is the maximum achievable effect in smokers.

4. Self-reported product use by study participants is intrinsically inaccurate during ambulatory clinical studies with ENDPs. It is, therefore, key to verify self-reported product use with measurements of biomarkers of exposure (BoExps) that are sensitive and specific enough to detect when a few cigarettes have been smoked. Evaluation of cigarette smoking on top of ENDP use is critical to understanding the true effect of switching in comparison with ongoing smoking and/or cessation.

17.2 A CLINICAL ASSESSMENT PROGRAM FOR ENDPS

The overall objective of the clinical assessment program is to measure the relevance of changes induced by switching from cigarette smoking to ENDP use at multiple steps of the CELSD and compare the effects of switching with those of continued smoking and benchmark them against the effects of cessation as outlined in Chapter 3. These considerations led to a clinical assessment program that is based on the following study types: pharmacokinetics/pharmacodynamics (PK/PD), reduced exposure, and exposure-response studies.

17.2.1 Pharmacokinetics/ Pharmacodynamics Studies

For ENDPs to contribute effectively to harm reduction at the population level, they must not only reduce risk but also be sufficiently acceptable to cigarette smokers and, thereby, enable them to switch (Chapter 1). Therefore, ENDPs are developed to minimize the emission of toxicants while maximizing the acceptability of the product to a smoker. Both the nicotine delivery profile and rewarding subjective effects of tobacco products are critical components of product satisfaction and, hence, actual use. This means that ENDPs should both deliver nicotine and elicit subjective effects in a manner similar to cigarettes. The purpose of PK/PD studies is to compare, after a 1-day washout period, the nicotine absorption profile and related short-term subjective effects of an ENDP in comparison with those of the smokers' own brand of cigarettes after single use. Consequently, these studies should be designed not only to assess the nicotine absorption profile but also to gain first insights into how the ENDP is perceived.

17.2.1.1 Background on nicotine absorption and distribution: nicotine PK

The amount and speed of nicotine uptake are dependent on the route of administration and rate of absorption across biological membranes. When nicotine is delivered via inhalation, droplet size is considered a key parameter that influences uptake and distribution. Inhaled nicotine is rapidly absorbed when it reaches the lungs, after which nicotine concentrations rapidly increase in the blood to reach a maximum plasma concentration (Benowitz et al., 2009).

Nicotine reaches the brain approximately 5–7 s after the first puff, with maximum accumulation in the brain occurring in about 4–5 min, without puff-associated peaks and troughs of nicotine concentration (Rose et al., 2010). The rapid rise in plasma and brain nicotine levels permits the smoker to titrate the level of nicotine

during smoking. On average, about 1 mg (with a range of 0.3–2 mg) of nicotine present in cigarette smoke is absorbed systemically during the smoking of one cigarette, leading to an observed maximum concentration of nicotine (C_{max}) ranging from 15 to 30 (venous) and 20 to 60 (arterial) ng/mL following use of a single cigarette (Hukkanen et al., 2005). After absorption, nicotine is distributed extensively to body tissues (e.g., the liver, kidney, spleen, and lungs (Benowitz et al., 2009)) and heavily metabolized, with cotinine being a major metabolite (Benowitz et al., 2009).

Overall, nicotine metabolism is a complex phenomenon which can be influenced by multiple factors, such as sex, age, genetics, hormonal drugs, and race. Besides nicotine metabolism itself, the amount of nicotine uptake can vary among smokers even if they smoke the same type of cigarettes. The amount of nicotine inhaled with a cigarette also depends on how the cigarette is smoked (e.g., depth of inhalation, puff volume, and rate and intensity of puffing). In the context of ENDP assessment, it is critical to understand the PK parameters of nicotine uptake, as the speed and amount of nicotine absorption are key factors in the acceptance of the new products as long-term replacement for cigarettes and achievement of full switching.

17.2.1.1.1 Intrinsic and extrinsic factors and impact on clinical pharmacology.
Nicotine is a high-affinity substrate for cytochrome P450 2A6 (CYP2A6), a hepatic enzyme responsible for converting nicotine into cotinine and further metabolizing cotinine into 3′-hydroxycotinine. Nicotine clearance is primarily driven by the liver blood flow, while the rate of cotinine clearance is mainly driven by the activity of metabolizing enzymes in the liver. Both CYP2A6 activity and liver blood flow are influenced by several factors, such as age, sex, race, (concomitant) medications, and smoking.

17.2.1.1.1.1 Age. Clearance of nicotine is dependent on age, with the total clearance of nicotine shown to be lower by 23% and renal clearance lower by 49% in the elderly (aged 65 years and above) in comparison with young adults (Molander et al., 2001). It is hypothesized that this lower nicotine metabolism in the elderly is due to reduced liver blood flow, as no age-related decrease in CYP2A6 protein levels or nicotine metabolism in liver microsomes has been reported (Messina et al., 1997).

17.2.1.1.1.2 Sex. Sex effects on nicotine and cotinine metabolism are well established in the literature (Benowitz et al., 2009). Clearance of infused deuterium-labeled nicotine and cotinine has been shown to be

13% and 24% higher, respectively, in women not using oral contraceptives than in men (Benowitz et al., 2006). Similar results have been observed in smokers (Johnstone et al., 2006; Kandel et al., 2007).

In addition, oral contraceptive use in women induces an increase in nicotine and cotinine clearance by 28% and 30%, respectively. These results suggest that CYP2A6 activity is induced by sex hormones, which is in line with the estrogen-induced CYP2A6 activity in in vitro studies (Higashi et al., 2007).

17.2.1.1.1.3 Race.
Race and ethnicity are reported to be critical factors that influence nicotine and cotinine metabolism, in particular among African American and Caucasian populations (Benowitz et al., 1999; Pérez-Stable et al., 1998). The total clearance of cotinine is significantly lower in African Americans (0.57 mL/min/kg) than in Caucasians (0.76 mL/min/kg). Slower metabolism of cotinine has also been described in African Americans than in Caucasians, as evidenced by the slower rate of nicotine and cotinine glucuronidation and presence of higher cotinine levels in the former (Caraballo et al., 1998; English et al., 1994; Wagenknecht et al., 1990).

Japanese and Chinese Americans are reported to have a significantly lower total clearance of nicotine and cotinine (slower metabolism) as well as a lower nicotine intake than Latinos and Caucasians (Benowitz et al., 2002; Domino et al., 2003); no difference in glucuronidation was detected in this study. However, it is worth mentioning that another study indicated no relevant differences in nicotine PK parameters among Asians, Blacks, and Caucasians or a statistically significant association between CYP2A6 activity and nicotine PK parameters, as the intersubject variability in this study was greater than the interrace variability (Dempsey et al., 2013).

Racial differences have been shown to be highly correlated with polymorphic CYP2A6 allele variations and the related impairment of nicotine and cotinine metabolism.

17.2.1.1.1.4 Diet, meals, and exercise.
As clearance of nicotine is dependent on liver blood flow, factors that are known to influence this parameter (e.g., diet, drug intake, and exercise) should be considered as parameters that can affect nicotine metabolism.

Gries et al. showed that consumption of meals during a steady-state infusion of nicotine resulted in a consistent decline in plasma nicotine concentration, with the maximal effect seen 30–60 min after the end of a meal. This is suggested to be due to an increase in liver blood flow of approximately 30% and a resulting increase in nicotine clearance of about 40% after a meal (Gries et al., 1996; Lee et al., 1989). Grapefruit juice is also well known to inhibit CYP2A6 activity, while watercress could impact the glucuronidation process of both nicotine and cotinine (Hukkanen et al., 2006; Runkel et al., 1997), leading to lower nicotine metabolism.

Compared with rest, exercise can lead to increased nicotine absorption (for example) from transdermal nicotine patches, possibly because of exercise-induced increase in peripheral blood flow at the site of the transdermal patch. For example, Lenz and Gillespie (2011) reported an increase in plasma nicotine levels during physical exercise. Furthermore, exercise decreases liver blood flow. After 40 min of exercise, with at least 20 min at 75% of the maximal heart rate, portal vein flow was reported to be decreased by 74% in healthy subjects (Ersoz and Ersoz, 2003). Decreased liver blood flow due to exercise is, therefore, expected to limit the clearance of nicotine.

17.2.1.1.1.5 Medication.
Several drugs have been shown to have an inducing or inhibiting effect on CYP2A6 activity in human primary hepatocyte cultures. Inducers include drugs such as antibiotics (e.g., rifampicin), steroids (e.g., dexamethasone), and barbiturates (e.g., phenobarbital), with a wide interindividual variability reported in the literature (Benowitz et al., 2002; Dempsey et al., 2013; Domino et al., 2003; English et al., 1994; Gries et al., 1996; Hukkanen et al., 2006; Lee et al., 1989; Runkel et al., 1997; Wagenknecht et al., 1990). Inhibitors of CYP2A6-mediated nicotine metabolism include, among others, antidepressants (e.g., tranylcypromine), systemic psoralens (e.g., 8-methoxypsoralen), tryptamine, and coumarin (Le Gal, 2003; MacDougall et al., 2003; Nakajima et al., 1996a, 1996b; Zhang et al., 2001).

17.2.1.1.1.6 Inhibiting effects of smoking on nicotine metabolism.
Some of the constituents present in cigarette smoke appear to interact with key components involved in nicotine metabolism and, thus, modulate the process. First, nicotine clearance is significantly slower in cigarette smokers than nonsmokers (Benowitz and Jacob, 1993). Second, a contrario, a short period (4−7 days) of smoking abstinence has the opposite effect of cigarette smoking and results in an increase of 14% −36% in nicotine clearance (Benowitz and Jacob, 2000).

The potential causes hypothesized in the literature are either inhibition of CYP2A6 activity or downregulation of CYP2A6 gene expression. A study by Denton et al. (2004) has found that β-nicotyrine, a minor tobacco alkaloid, inhibited CYP2A6 in in vitro testing.

Another in vivo study showed that administration of nicotine to monkeys for 21 days caused a decrease in CYP2A6 activity by downregulation of *CYP2A6* mRNA and protein in the liver (Schoedel et al., 2003).

Some constituents present in cigarette smoke (nicotine, cotinine, 4-methylnitrosamino-1-(3-pyridyl)-1-butanone (NNK), and 1,3-butadiene) are well-established substrates for CYP2A6 (Raunio et al., 2001). As an example, up to 80% of nicotine inhaled in the body is metabolized via CYP2A6 into cotinine, and several procarcinogens, such as NNK, can be metabolically activated by CYP2A6. Beyond these findings, smoke constituents that have a true effect on nicotine metabolism have not been fully identified nor have their mechanisms of action.

17.2.1.2 Nicotine metabolism
17.2.1.2.1 Metabolic pathways and quantification.
Nicotine is extensively metabolized to a number of metabolites by the liver. Six primary metabolites of nicotine have been identified in humans. Quantitatively, the most important metabolite of nicotine in most mammalian species is cotinine.

Quantitative aspects of the pattern of nicotine metabolism have been fairly well elucidated in humans. About 90% of a systemic dose of nicotine can be accounted for as nicotine and metabolites in urine (Benowitz et al., 1994). On the basis of studies involving simultaneous infusion of labeled nicotine and cotinine, it has been determined that 70%—80% of nicotine is converted to cotinine (Benowitz et al., 1994), and about 4%—7% of nicotine is excreted as nicotine-*N*-oxide and 3%—5% as nicotine glucuronide (Benowitz et al., 1994; Byrd et al., 1992). Cotinine is excreted unchanged in urine to a small degree (10% —15% of the nicotine and metabolites in urine), with the remainder converted to metabolites, primarily *trans*-3′-hydroxycotinine (33%—40%), cotinine glucuronide (12%—17%), and *trans*-3′-hydroxycotinine glucuronide (7%—9%) (Hukkanen et al., 2005).

Approximately 85% of the total nicotine uptake and excretion in smokers can be accounted for by the molar sum of nicotine, cotinine, and *trans*-3′-hydroxycotinine concentrations as well as the concentrations of their respective glucuronide conjugates, expressed as nicotine equivalents (NEQs) in 24-h urine (Benowitz and Jacob, 1994). NEQs are a well-established, robust, and valid biomarker of nicotine exposure to cigarette smoke (Tricker, 2006), representing the major metabolic pathways of nicotine. To obtain a comprehensive understanding of the switching process from cigarettes to an ENDP in smokers, urinary NEQ levels provide valuable

insights into the effects of potential adaptation processes in product use patterns over time as well as metabolic activity when assessed in combination with product consumption per day, human puffing topography (HPT), and CYP2A6 activity.

17.2.1.2.2 Genetic variations and impact on nicotine metabolism.
Genetic variations in CYP2A6-related genes result in absent, reduced, increased, or normal CYP2A6 enzymatic activity (Hukkanen et al., 2005; Malaiyandi et al., 2006).

More than 20 established alleles (polymorphisms) of *CYP2A6* have been identified, and, owing to these genetic variations, CYP2A6 enzymatic activity and the associated decrease/increase in nicotine metabolism vary both among individuals of the same ethnicity/race and across ethnicities/races. The frequency of these variations is substantially higher in Japanese and Chinese populations than in Caucasians or populations of any other race/ethnicity (Hukkanen et al., 2005; Malaiyandi et al., 2006). A *CYP2A6* allele variation (*CYP2A6*17*) leading to decreased enzymatic activity which appears to be specific to the African American population has been reported (Hukkanen et al., 2005).

The *trans*-3′-hydroxycotinine/cotinine molar ratio (*trans*-3′-hydroxycotinine/cotinine) in plasma has been evaluated as a noninvasive measure of CYP2A6 activity (Dempsey et al., 2004) and can be used to phenotype nicotine metabolism and CYP2A6 enzyme activity (Johnstone et al., 2006; Kandel et al., 2007; Lerman et al., 2006; Patterson et al., 2008).

17.2.1.2.3 Effect of menthol on nicotine metabolism and smoking behavior.
The Tobacco Products Scientific Advisory Committee (TPSAC) stated in their report on menthol and public health (Tobacco Products Scientific Advisory Committee (TPSAC), 2011) that the evidence is sufficient to conclude that it is at least as likely as not that menthol inhibits the metabolism of nicotine in smokers. However, TPSAC further concluded that it is unlikely that such a metabolic difference would have much, if any, effect on smoking behavior.

This conclusion is supported by a study from Strasser et al. (2013), which suggested that menthol has minimal impact on smoking behaviors, exposure to smoke constituents, and subjective ratings of menthol versus nonmenthol cigarettes. The mean urinary concentrations of nicotine and cotinine were comparable for the own brand, menthol, and nonmenthol periods between the experimental and control groups. Comparison of nicotine and cotinine levels between the experimental and control group in this study revealed no significant condition or interaction effects. Caucasians had significantly higher cotinine levels than non-Caucasian participants but showed no differences in nicotine levels. There were no significant interaction effects with race. Total puff volume, the sum of all puffs taken during smoking and mouth-level exposure, tended to increase by 11% when the experimental group switched from menthol to nonmenthol cigarettes; however, there was no corresponding increase in cigarette consumption or exposure to smoke constituents. Subjective ratings related to taste and smell decreased during the nonmenthol period relative to the menthol period.

17.2.1.3 Background on the subjective effects of nicotine: nicotine pharmacodynamics

Evaluation of the PD effects associated with an ENDP, including the effects of nicotine as well as the taste, ritual, and sensorial experience during and after use, is important for understanding the potential of such a product as an acceptable substitute for cigarettes. Subjective effect measures—in particular, assessment of the reinforcing and aversive effects of smoking, such as relief from urge to smoke, craving, and withdrawal symptoms, as well as assessment of (for example) psychological reward through validated questionnaires—are well established and widely used as outcomes in the context of assessment of PD effects.

17.2.1.3.1 Reinforcing and aversive effects of product use.
Reinforcement refers to the observation that behaviors increase or decrease according to whether a person associates a particular behavior (e.g., smoking) with a positive or negative experience. In the context of cigarette smoking or ENDP use, an example of positive reinforcement would be the strengthening of a certain behavior because of its rewarding effects, such as pleasurable sensory cues, euphoria, etc. In contrast, an example of negative reinforcement could be illustrated by the withdrawal symptoms and urge to smoke that a smoker may experience during smoking abstinence. Such a negative stimulus perceived by a smoker may trigger relapse to cigarette smoking in order to alleviate this aversive state.

It is recognized that nicotine intake and its related psychostimulant and pharmacological effects are the main drivers for its behavioral reinforcement effects. However, recently, additional factors such as psychological and sensorimotor factors during product use experience, have also been suggested as playing a

role in smoking behavior (including persistent smoking) (Bozinoff and Le Foll, 2018; Rupprecht et al., 2015). Unfortunately, these factors have been investigated to a very limited extent and are poorly understood.

The reinforcing and aversive effects of smoking are critical factors in the context of switching from cigarette smoking to ENDP use and will partly determine the adoption and predict future use of a nicotine-containing product other than cigarette.

17.2.1.3.2 Urge to smoke.
The urge to smoke is a subjective motivational state which is, among other aversive effects, held responsible for maintenance of abstinence from cigarette use or relapse. In the context of ENDP assessment, evaluation of urge to smoke has been recommended as a key outcome measure for demonstrating that an ENDP can reduce the risk and harm of smoking at the population level (Breland et al., 2002; Cobb et al., 2010; Hanson et al., 2009; IOM (Institute of Medicine), 2012; Rosenberg, 2009). If an ENDP cannot suppress aversive withdrawal symptoms like urge to smoke, smokers who try an ENDP may relapse to cigarette use or change their product use pattern in a way that reduces or eliminates the potential beneficial effect of ENDP use (e.g., dual use).

Recent clinical studies have indicated that urge to smoke is strongly associated with factors other than nicotine alone and that, therefore, the reduction in urge to smoke observed for an ENDP must be considered linked to multiple factors, such as behavioral, sensory, and contextual factors, and go beyond conventional pharmacological factors (Hanson et al., 2009). In other words, there is evidence that urge to smoke does not emerge from the addictive characteristics of nicotine alone. Therefore, the results determined for urge to smoke cannot be limited to the effects of nicotine and should be interpreted not in isolation but in the context of a set of measures for assessing the effect of nicotine as well as the impact of, for example, taste, ritual, and sensory experience.

The most widely used self-reported questionnaire for measuring urge to smoke is the Questionnaire of Smoking Urges (QSU) in its brief version (QSU-brief) (Cox et al., 2001), which is derived from the initial QSU 32-item questionnaire (Tiffany and Drobes, 1991) and provides a multidimensional measure for assessing the urge to smoke with two-factor scores and a total score derived from 10 questionnaire items. The 10 items have to be rated on a 7-point scale, ranging from 1 (strongly disagree) to 7 (strongly agree), and are calculated as Factor 1 or Factor 2:

- Factor 1: A positive reinforcement factor reflecting intention and desire to smoke and anticipation of pleasure from smoking.
- Factor 2: A negative reinforcement factor reflecting the anticipation of relief from negative affect and nicotine withdrawal and an urgent and overwhelming desire to smoke.

The total score is the average of Factor 1 and Factor 2. Higher scores in this questionnaire indicate a greater urge to smoke.

17.2.1.3.3 Product evaluation.

The modified Cigarette Evaluation Questionnaire (mCEQ) is the most widely used validated tool for assessing the reinforcing and aversive effects of smoking (Cappelleri et al., 2007; Hanson et al., 2009). The 12-item mCEQ measures (1) smoking satisfaction (satisfying, tastes good, and smoking is enjoyable), (2) psychological rewards (calms down, more awake, less irritable, helps concentration, and reduces hunger), (3) aversion (dizziness and nausea), (4) enjoyment of respiratory tract sensations (single-item assessment), and (5) craving reduction (single-item assessment). Each item is rated on a 7-point scale, with 1 = not at all and 7 = extremely.

The mCEQ has been commonly applied in clinical studies to evaluate if pharmacological treatments may decrease the reinforcing effects of smoking (Cappelleri et al., 2007). In the context of ENDP assessment, the mCEQ has been used to evaluate how close an ENDP may come to the profile of the reinforcing and aversive effects observed with cigarettes and may, therefore, allow an estimate on adoption and future use of the new product.

17.2.1.3.4 Craving and withdrawal symptoms.

In order to assess whether an ENDP may be a satisfactory substitute for cigarettes, one needs to evaluate the effect of the ENDP on the relief from withdrawal symptoms upon switching.

The Minnesota Nicotine Withdrawal Scale (MNWS) is one of the instruments indicated in the European Medicines Agency (EMA) guidelines on the development of medicinal products for treatment of smoking (EMA (European Medicines Agency), 2008). It is one of the most widely used and validated measures of withdrawal symptoms from cigarette smoking (Hughes and Hatsukami, 1986) and has been shown to be of equal reliability as other nicotine withdrawal scales, such as the Mood and Physical Symptoms Scale, Shiffman Scale, Wisconsin Smoking Withdrawal Scale, and Cigarette Withdrawal Scale (West et al., 2006). Many

of the constituent items have demonstrated sensitivity to deprivation and nicotine replacement therapy (NRT) (Hanson et al., 2009; Shiffman et al., 2004).

A revised version (MNWS-R) proposed by the authors of the original scale (Hughes and Hatsukami, 2012) includes 15 items (symptoms) for assessing nicotine-related symptom withdrawal and are scored from 0 (none) to 4 (severe).

17.2.2 Reduced Exposure Studies

The central tenet of tobacco harm reduction (THR) is that ENDPs emit significantly reduced levels of toxicants, also known as harmful and potentially harmful constituents (HPHC), than cigarettes (Chapters 2 and 4). This reduction in toxicant emissions should lead to a reduction in toxicant exposure when smokers switch to ENDP use. The degree of this exposure reduction should be coherent with the degree of reduction in emissions (measured by aerosol chemistry analyses) by the tested ENDP. This is the first causal link in the CELSD (Chapter 3).

The purpose of reduced exposure studies is to assess this causal link. Importantly, the reduction in exposure resulting from switching to ENDP use should be as close as possible to that resulting from smoking cessation, as this will define the performance of the product as a less harmful alternative to cigarettes.

BoExps to HPHCs are the primary endpoints of reduced exposure studies. A BoExp is a chemical, its metabolite(s), or the product of a reaction between the chemical and some target molecule that is measured in a compartment of an organism. To enable comparison of the effects of switching on toxicant exposure with those of ongoing smoking and cessation, reduced exposure studies should ideally be conducted with adult healthy smokers who are allocated (randomized or not) to three groups: (1) continued smoking, (2) switching to the ENDP, and (3) smoking abstinence.

Reduced exposure studies can be conducted both in confinement and ambulatory settings. The advantage of confinement studies—although they are generally of short duration (e.g., 1 week of exposure)—is that product use can be tightly supervised and controlled. Such settings offer the advantage of accurate monitoring of adherence to the allocated product use/regimen. Thereby, these studies provide the data necessary for evaluating the maximum exposure reduction an ENDP can achieve in comparison with continued smoking by using smoking cessation as a benchmark. Besides product use and the inherent characteristics of the subjects themselves, environmental factors such as diet, among others, can influence the levels of BoExps. Therefore, this type of a study is ideally complemented with longer-term (e.g., 3 months of exposure) ambulatory studies. Such studies are aimed at confirming that the reduced exposure observed in confinement is sustained for a longer period in a real-world setting. Furthermore, such studies allow gathering of valuable insights into product use patterns, acceptance/satisfaction, and, importantly, safety data related to ENDP use.

17.2.2.1 Selecting BoExps for heated tobacco products

Cigarette smoke is a complex mixture of more than 6000 identified compounds (Rodgman and Perfetti, 2013). Regulatory authorities have established lists of HPHCs recommended to be measured and reported for tobacco products (FDA-18; United States [US] Food and Drug Administration) (FDA (Food and Drug Administration), 2012) or recommended for mandated lowering in cigarette smoke (WHO-9; World Health Organization) (WHO Study Group et al., 2008) (Table 17.1). These lists serve as the main references for selecting HPHCs to be assessed in clinical studies.

BoExps to HPHCs are used to quantify the degree of exposure to smoke toxicants. They provide direct quantitative evidence of the presence of HPHCs or their metabolites in the body. The BoExps to be used in reduced exposure studies need to be fit for purpose and follow these criteria:

1. The BoExps must be representative of a broad range of HPHC classes contained in cigarette smoke, such as carbonyls, mono- and poly-cyclic aromatic hydrocarbons (PAH), aromatic amines, and tobacco-specific nitrosamines, as outlined in Table 17.2.
2. The BoExps must represent HPHCs of known toxic effects, including carcinogens, cardiovascular toxicants, respiratory toxicants, reproductive and developmental toxicants, and addictive constituents.
3. Each BoExp must reflect a specific toxic exposure or be a reliable surrogate of exposure to a class of HPHCs. For example, total 1-hydroxypyrene (1-OHP), the BoExp for pyrene, is broadly representative for exposure to PAHs, as there is a strong positive association between the levels of pyrene and total PAHs generated during cigarette combustion in the same way that there is a strong positive association between the levels of benzo[a] pyrene (B[a]P) and total PAHs (Vu et al., 2015).
4. The BoExps must cover a broad range of HPHC formation temperatures. For example, when assessing a heated tobacco product (HTP), one should measure BoExps to HPHCs that are typically generated during tobacco combustion, such as acrylonitrile.

5. The BoExps should represent HPHCs that are specific to smoking, with other sources being minor or nonexistent. Typical examples are BoExps to tobacco-specific nitrosamines, which are naturally present in tobacco and passively transferred into cigarette smoke.

TABLE 17.1
Lists of HPHCs in cigarette smoke.

Abbreviated name of the list	Description of the list	References
FDA-93	Established list of 93 HPHCs in tobacco products	(U.S. Department of Health and Human Services and FDA (Food and Drug Administration), 2012)
FDA-18	Abbreviated list of 18 HPHCs to be reported to the FDA	(FDA (Food and Drug Administration), 2012)
PMI-58	List of 58 HPHCs measured by PMI	(Roemer et al., 2004, 2012)[a]
HC	List of 44 constituents in the mainstream smoke of tobacco products to be reported to Health Canada[b]	(Health Canada, 2013; Health Canada, Modified, 2011)
WHO-39	Nonexhaustive list of 39 priority toxic constituents and emissions of tobacco products	(WHO Study Group et al., 2015)[b]
WHO-18	Initial list of 18 priority toxicants	WHO Study Group et al. (2008)
WHO-9	Mandated lowering list of 9 toxicants	WHO Study Group et al. (2008)

FDA, United States Food and Drug Administration; *HC*, Health Canada; *HPHC*, harmful and potentially harmful constituents of tobacco smoke; *PMI*, Philip Morris International; *WHO*, World Health Organization.
[a] Partially listed.
[b] Based on the Hoffmann analytes list (Hoffmann and Wynder, 1986; Rodgman and Perfetti, 2013).

6. The BoExps should be reliably measurable by using validated, reproducible, and precise analytical methods.
7. A BoExp to an HPHC must have a half-life that is suitable for the duration of the study and measurement time points.

On the basis of these criteria, Philip Morris International (PMI) selected several HPHCs for clinical assessment of its electrically heated tobacco product (EHTP), the Tobacco Heating System 2.2 (THS) (Chapter 2). Table 17.2 provides information on their allocation to chemical classes, presence in the gas–vapor phase (GVP) and total particulate matter (TPM) fraction, and risk categorization by the FDA. Because there is no regulatory framework listing which HPHCs should be measured in reduced exposure studies, the selection of HPHCs in studies on HTPs may vary among different academic groups or companies. However, most of these HPHCs have been assessed in all published studies on such products (Section 17.5).

PMI's reduced exposure studies measured 16 BoExps to HPHCs as well as nicotine and its metabolites (Table 17.3). These included BoExps for 14 of the 18 HPHCs currently mandated for reporting to the FDA (Table 17.1) (FDA (Food and Drug Administration), 2012). The four HPHCs that were excluded are acetaldehyde, ammonia, formaldehyde, and isoprene, because they cannot be measured reliably and reproducibly in body fluids (selection criterion 6).

17.2.2.2 Selecting biomarkers of exposure for e-cigarettes

Although e-vapor products (EVPs) deliver nicotine, they do not contain tobacco (Chapter 2). Therefore, the list

TABLE 17.2
List of HPHCs covered in PMI's clinical reduced exposure studies.

PMI's list of HPHCs covered in clinical studies	BOEXP COVERAGE OF FDA TOXICITY CLASSES					
	None	CA[a]	CT[a]	RT[a]	RDT[a]	AD[a]
Gas: Carbon monoxide (GVP)	–	–	–	–	●	–
Aliphatic dienes: 1,3-butadiene (GVP)	–	●	●	–	●	–
Carbonyls: Acrolein (GVP)	–	–	●	●	–	–
Crotonaldehyde (GVP)	–	●	–	–	–	–
Acid derivatives: Acrylonitrile (GVP)	–	●	–	●	–	–
Epoxides: Ethylene oxide (GVP)	–	●	–	●	●	–
Monocyclic aromatic hydrocarbons: Benzene (GVP)	–	●	●	●	●	–
Toluene (GVP/PP)	–	–	–	●	●	–
Aromatic amines: 1-NA (PP)	–	●	–	–	–	–
2-NA (PP)	–	●	–	–	–	–
4-ABP (PP)	–	●	–	–	–	–
o-Toluidine (PP)	–	●	–	–	–	–
N-nitrosamines: NNK (PP)	–	●	–	–	–	–
NNN (PP)	–	●	–	–	–	–
Polycyclic aromatic hydrocarbons: B[a]P (PP)	–	●	–	–	–	–
Pyrene (PP)[b]	●	–	–	–	–	–
Alkaloids: Nicotine (TPM)	–	–	–	–	●	●

1-NA, 1-aminonaphthalene; 2-NA, 2-aminonaphthalene; 4-ABP, 4-aminobiphenyl; B[a]P, benzo[a]pyrene; FDA, Food and Drug Administration; GVP, gas–vapor phase; HPHC, harmful and potentially harmful constituents; NNK, 4-(methylnitrosamino)-1-(3-pyridyl)-1-butanone; NNN, N-nitrosonornicotine; PMI, Philip Morris International; PP, particulate phase; TPM, total particulate matter.
[a] CA, carcinogen; CT, cardiotoxicant; RT, respiratory toxicant; RDT, reproductive and developmental toxicant; AD, addictive.
[b] Pyrene is not listed as an HPHC by the US FDA but is nevertheless listed here, because its metabolite 1-OHP serves as a surrogate for PAHs in general, complementing B[a]P.
PMI (Based on the FDA-93 list referenced in Table 17.1).

TABLE 17.3
List of HPHCs selected by PMI, with their corresponding BoExps.

HPHC	WHO-9	FDA-18	PMI's selection of BoExps for clinical studies
Acrolein	●	●	3-hydroxypropylmercapturic acid (3-HPMA)
Acrylonitrile		●	2-cyanoethylmercapturic acid (CEMA)
4-Aminobiphenyl		●	4-aminobiphenyl (4-ABP)
Benzene	●	●	S-phenylmercapturic acid (S-PMA)
Benzo[a]pyrene	●	●	total 3-hydroxybenzo[a]pyrene (3-OH-B[a]P)
1,3-Butadiene	●	●	monohydroxybutenylmercapturic acid (MHBMA)
Carbon monoxide (CO)	●	●	blood carboxyhemoglobin (COHb)[a] and exhaled CO[a] (COex)[a]
Crotonaldehyde		●	3-hydroxy-1-methylpropylmercapturic acid (3-HMPMA)
Ethylene oxide			2-hydroxyethylmercapturic acid (HEMA)
1-Aminonaphthalene		●	1-aminonaphthalene (1-NA)
2-Aminonaphthalene		●	2-aminonaphthalene (2-NA)
Nicotine		●	nicotine equivalents (NEQs) Plasma nicotine and continine[a]
NNK	●	●	total 4-(methylnitrosamino)-1-(3-pyridyl)-1-butanol (total NNAL)
NNN	●	●	total N-nitrosonornicotine (total NNN)
o-Toluidine			o-toluidine
Pyrene[b]			total 1-hydroxypyrene (1-OHP)
Toluene		●	S-benzylmercapturic acid (S-BMA)

FDA, Food and Drug Administration; HPHC, harmful and potentially harmful constituents of tobacco smoke; PMI, Philip Morris International; WHO; World Health Organization.
[a] These BoExps are the only ones not measured in urine.
[b] Pyrene is not listed as an HPHC by FDA but is nevertheless listed here, because its metabolite 1-OHP serves as a surrogate for PAHs in general. PMI (Based on the WHO-9 and FDA-18 lists referenced in Table 17.1).

of HPHCs relevant for EVP assessment should be coherent with the characteristics of these products. A recently released document by the FDA has listed at least 33 chemical compounds that need to be measured in the aerosol of EVPs (FDA (Food and Drug Administration), 2019). This list, together with the lists of HPHCs provided in Table 17.1, can serve as the basis for selection of HPHCs and associated BoExps to be measured in reduced exposure studies on e-cigarettes. Selection of BoExps to e-cigarettes should follow the same principles as those used for assessment of HTPs

(Section 17.2.2.1). As the chemical composition of an EVP aerosol is typically simpler than that of an HTP aerosol (Chapter 4), the possibility to select fit-for-purpose BoExps to EVPs is more limited. Nevertheless, the list of BoExps should ideally represent the most important HPHCs emitted by EVPs, such as carbonyls, metals, and certain flavor ingredients (Belushkin et al., 2019; Gaur and Agnihotri, 2019).

Among the HPHCs listed in this recently released guidance (FDA (Food and Drug Administration), 2019), six have BoExps that are measurable and can be readily assessed: acrolein, acrylonitrile, benzene, crotonaldehyde, NNK, and *N*-nitrosonornicotine (NNN), with their respective BoExps being 3-hydroxypropylmercapturic acid (3-HPMA), 2-cyanoethylmercapturic acid (CEMA), S-phenylmercapturic acid (S-PMA), 3-hydroxy-1-methylpropyl-mercapturic acid (3-HMPMA), total4-(methylnitrosamino)-1-(3-pyridyl)-1-butanol (total NNAL), and total NNN. Other toxicants, such as metals, should be included on the basis of the composition of the e-liquid, cartridge, and heating device and by considering at least the following criteria: (1) specificity of the toxicant to the e-cigarette, (2) detectable amounts in the aerosol of the e-cigarette, and (3) half-lives of the associated BoExps.

17.2.3 Exposure Response Studies

An ENDP that emits significantly reduced levels of toxicants relative to cigarettes and consequently leads to an expected and coherent degree of exposure reduction in smokers who switch to it should induce positive changes in BoPHs (Chang et al., 2019) similar to those observed upon quitting. These positive changes in BoPHs can be assessed along the CELSD and are both prerequisites and indicators of the risk reduction potential of an ENDP (Chapter 3). Given the first challenge outlined above and in Chapter 3, exposure response studies are the most practicable studies for assessing the biological effects of switching to an ENDP that can be conducted in a premarket setting. The purpose of these studies is to assess whether the reduction in toxicant exposure caused by switching to an ENDP leads to positive changes in BoPHs and, hence, indicate that a reduction in toxicant exposure leads to a risk and harm reduction. These BoPHs must be selected to reflect the effects of cigarette smoke on different organ systems and biological mechanisms. These biomarkers must also be responsive to smoking cessation within the duration of the study, and measurable by validated methods. Therefore, the duration of these studies must be aligned with the time it takes for the measured BoPHs to undergo positive changes upon smoking cessation, which is typically longer than the duration of reduced exposure studies (6 months or longer). For interpretation of the results, adaptation to the product during the switching process needs to be taken into consideration. In these switching studies, not all study participants can be expected to fully adhere to the product over time. Therefore, it is important to get a realistic picture of the average number of cigarettes smoked together with the number of ENDPs used by an individual on a daily basis to understand how much cigarette smoking can modify the BoPH response. It is then crucial to implement a self-reporting tool to capture a

subject's cumulative product use during the entire study to further classify the subjects according to categories of product use patterns (e.g., complete switcher, dual user, cigarette smoker, or other use) at the time of analysis.

Moreover, it is necessary to also measure at least some BoExps to ensure that the causal link between exposure reduction and positive changes in BoPHs can be established within exposure response studies. Furthermore, given the limited reliability of self-reported product use patterns, measurement of BoExps specific for cigarette smoking is necessary to ensure biochemical verification of both switching and cessation (Chapter 3).

17.2.3.1 Selecting disease mechanisms

The first step in selecting BoPHs is to identify the key mechanisms underlying the major smoking-related diseases. The 2010 US Surgeon General's Report titled "How Tobacco Smoke Causes Diseases" identifies inflammation and oxidative stress, among others, as key mechanisms underlying all major smoking-related diseases (U.S. Department of Health and Human Services, 2010). There is ample evidence showing that both mechanisms are intricately linked to each other and to disease development in smokers.

Cigarette smoking is causally linked to the development of CVDs, contributing to endothelial injury and dysfunction, a proatherogenic lipid profile, chronic inflammation, and an abnormally increased tendency toward coagulation. Evidence gathered from in vitro and in vivo studies as well as population-based observational studies has led to the recognition that vascular inflammatory processes are central to all stages of atherogenesis, from local endothelial dysfunction to plaque development and rupture (Libby et al., 2002; Ross, 1999). In addition, multiple lines of evidence suggest that reactive oxygen species (ROS) are key contributors to molecular signaling pathways underlying the development of atherosclerosis (Harrison et al., 2003; Madamanchi et al., 2005) and play a central role in modifying most of the known main risk factors for CVDs, including hypertension, hypercholesterolemia, obesity, and diabetes (Asmat et al., 2016; Ceriello and Motz, 2004; Keaney et al., 2003; Rodriguez-Porcel et al., 2001).

COPD is a respiratory disease characterized by progressive airflow limitation and associated with an abnormal inflammatory response of the lungs to noxious particles and gases (Global Initiative for Chronic Obstructive Lung Disease (GOLD), 2020). Development of COPD in smokers has been linked to a number of sustained cellular stress responses, including endoplasmic reticulum, hypoxic, and auto-phagic stress (Chen et al., 2008; Hengstermann and Müller, 2008; Hwang et al., 2010). Most of these responses are the result of oxidative insults that arise from direct exposure to cigarette smoke and cause tissue injury through oxidative stress. Concomitantly, cigarette smoke—related oxidative stress also attracts and activates immune and inflammatory cells and induces the release of proinflammatory mediators which, in turn, produce a number of (endogenous) oxidative stressors capable of perpetuating an inflammatory response.

Cigarette smoking is the major cause of lung cancer in most human populations (Doll and Peto, 1981; Harris et al., 2004; R. et al., 2004; Wakai et al., 2006; Zhang Hong and Cai, 2003). Most of the inflammatory processes identified in smokers with COPD can also be observed in smokers with lung cancer, which suggests a shared etiology; it has also been shown that COPD is a risk factor for development of lung cancer in smokers (Viegi et al., 2001; Watson et al., 1993). In addition to inflammatory processes promoting a micro-environment that favors tumor formation, direct damage to DNA, proteins, and lipids by ROS and reactive nitrogen species is a key initiating factor for events that ultimately lead to lung cancer (Fearon et al., 2011; Halliwell, 2007). Furthermore, ROS can also act as second messengers and mediate processes such as proliferation, cell survival, angiogenesis, and cell transformation (Federico et al., 2007; Storz, 2005), thus contributing to tumor promotion and progression.

In summary, chronic exposure to HPHCs affects multiple organ systems, disease pathways, and mechanisms such as inflammation, oxidative stress, platelet activation, and lipid metabolism, which occur simultaneously and cannot be expressed by a single endpoint. Hence, no single biomarker or clinical risk endpoint can be considered as a surrogate measure for the adverse health effects associated with smoking-related diseases and, *a fortiori*, for the relative risk of ENDPs in comparison with cigarettes. Therefore, a number of biomarkers that address the multifaceted biological impact of cigarette smoke must be considered in combination for risk assessment of ENDPs. In addition, there is a limited number of clinically validated biomarkers that can be used to assess the biological effects of smoking cessation in healthy smokers. Despite the recent growing interest in identifying BoPHs that are fit for purpose in the context of ENDP risk assessment, there is, to date, no consensus within the scientific community and/or regulatory bodies (Chang et al., 2019; Scherer, 2018). Consequently, exposure response studies should assess a panel of BoPHs and endpoints to provide collective

evidence about the risk and harm reduction profile of ENDPs (Chang et al., 2019).

17.2.3.2 Selecting BoPHs

There is increasing interest in using multiple biomarkers in a predisease state to better identify people at risk, in particular for CVDs (Wang et al., 2006), and for assessing major smoking-related diseases such as CVDs, COPD, and lung cancer (Cagle et al., 2013; Doyle et al., 2012; Nozaki et al., 2009). Considering all these elements, PMI decided to use a framework of coherent, reliable, and mutually supportive BoPHs that are indicative of various mechanistic pathways underlying smoking-related diseases and are altered by smoking, to substantiate the relative reduction in risk of harm of THS compared with continued smoking. PMI initiated a thorough and comprehensive review of the available literature on smoking cessation from published clinical and epidemiological research to identify (1) the main pathways involved in the main diseases attributable to smoking and (2) the BoPHs indicative of these pathways. The following criteria, based on Hill's approach, were to be met to distinguish association "by chance" versus causation (Hill, 1965):

- Epidemiological evidence suggesting a robust relationship between each BoPH and at least one known smoking-related disease. The BoPH can be either directly involved in the pathophysiological mechanisms of the disease or indirectly involved as an indicator of the pathological pathway,
- Consistency of epidemiological and clinical evidence linking cigarette smoking to the BoPH, and
- Consistency of epidemiological and clinical evidence linking smoking cessation to the BoPH and evidence indicating that the BoPH is reversible within 6—12 months following smoking cessation.

The justification for the selection of pathways, their related BoPHs, and the link to smoking-attributable disease has previously been published (Peck et al., 2018). This process resulted in the identification of 25 BoPHs (Table 17.4).

Of these 25 BoPHs, not all had the same robust evidence of a relationship with all of Hill's criteria. To further refine the selection, the BoPHs were also required to fulfill the following criteria:

- Reflect a common pathway across multiple smoking-related disease pathways (e.g., oxidative stress and inflammation) or for which association with one specific smoking-related disease was strong (e.g., lung function for COPD),
- Be measurable but with limited invasiveness: robust and available validated analytical methods fit for

TABLE 17.4
Identification of BoPHs linked to morbidity and mortality attributable to smoking, Following systematic smoking cessation literature review.

Biomarker	Change caused by smoking	Relationship to smoking	Relationship to cessation	DISEASE RELATED TO THE BIOMARKER		Time to normalize
				Resp	CVD	
Forced expiratory volume (FEV₁)	↓	+++	++	+++	−	Months
Iso-prostaglandin (8-iso-PGF$_{2\alpha}$)	↑	+	+/−	+/−	++	Weeks
Thromboxane B2 (11-DTXB2)	↑	++	+	−	++	Days–weeks
C-reactive protein (CRP)	↑	++	+/−	−	+++	Years
White blood cell count (WBC)	↑	++	++	++	+++	Weeks–months
Soluble intracellular adhesion molecule (s-ICAM-1)	↑	++	+	++	+ +	Weeks
Fibrinogen (FBG)	↓↑	+/−	+/−	++	+ +	−
Tumor necrosis factor (TNFα)	↓↑	+	+/−	++	++	−
Myeloperoxidase (MPO)	↓↑	+/−	+/−	+++	+++	−
Exhaled nitric oxide (FeNO)	↓	+	+	++	−	−
Sputum neutrophils	↑	+	+/−	++	−	No change
Phospholipase A2 (Lp-PLA2)	↑	+/−	−	−	++	Months
Albumin (ALB)	↑	+	+	−	+	Months–years
Low-density lipoprotein cholesterol (LDL-C)	↓↑	++	+/−	−	+++	−
High-density lipoprotein cholesterol (HDL-C)	↓	+++	+++	+/−	+ + +	Months
Apolipoprotein AI (ApoAI)	↓	+	+	−	+ +	Weeks–months
Oxysterols (OxS)	↑?	−	−	−	++	−
Homocysteine (HCY)	↑	−	−	−	+/−	Months
P-selectin (P-Sel)	↑	+	+/−	−	+	Weeks–months
Thiocyanate (SCN)	↑	++	+	+	++	Weeks
Von Willebrand factor (vWF)	↑	+	+	−	+	Weeks
Glycated hemoglobin (HbAlc)	↑	++	++	−	++	Weeks–months
Carboxyhemoglobin (COHb)	↑	+++	+++	+	+++	Days
Wheeze, cough, and sputum (W/C/S)	↑	+++	++	+++	−	Months–years

TABLE 17.4
Identification of BoPHs linked to morbidity and mortality attributable to smoking, Following systematic smoking cessation literature review.—cont'd

| Biomarker | Change caused by smoking | Relationship to smoking | Relationship to cessation | DISEASE RELATED TO THE BIOMARKER | | Time to normalize |
				Resp	CVD	
4-(methylnitrosamino)-1-(3-pyridyl)-l-butanol (NNAL)	↓	+++	+++	(Cancer)	−	Weeks—months

CVD, cardiovascular disease; Resp, respiratory diseases; arrows indicate increase or decrease in biomarker levels caused by smoking; time to normalize is an indication of how long following smoking cessation the biomarker returns to normal levels (for some biomarkers this is not clear from the literature).
Peck MJ, Sanders EB, Scherer G, Ludicke F, Weitkunat R. Review of biomarkers to assess the effects of switching from cigarettes to modified risk tobacco products. Biomarkers. 2018:1–32.

purpose in the context of use, that do not require invasive sample collection, and

- Have indications on the magnitude of effect and variability between cigarette smokers and quitters.

By further applying these criteria, eight coherent, plausible, and mutually supportive BoPHs were selected that were representative of multiple mechanisms and consistently reported to change upon smoking and quitting (Table 17.5). They have since then been part of the BoPH risk assessment framework in clinical studies conducted by PMI.

These eight BoPHs, when tested together, are likely to reflect the effect of exposure to multiple HPHCs and be predictive of long-term clinical outcomes attributable to smoking as follows:

- Lipid metabolism (high-density lipoprotein cholesterol [HDL-C]),
- Endothelial dysfunction (soluble intercellular adhesion molecule-1 [sICAM-1]),
- Inflammation (white blood cell [WBC] count),
- Oxidative stress (8-epi-prostaglandin-F2α [8-epi-PGF2α]),
- Platelet activation (11-dehydrothromboxane B2 [11-DTX-B2]) and oxygen transport (carboxyhemoglobin [COHb]),
- Lung function (forced expiratory volume in 1 s [FEV₁]), and
- Exposure to carcinogens (total NNAL).

Table 17.5 further provides the matrix in which they were measured and their timeframe of reversibility.

The BoPHs selected by PMI have also been reported by external researchers. Of the eight BoPHs tested as coprimary endpoints in the exposure response study, six were also reported in another comprehensive review that evaluated BoPHs for their suitability in clinical studies on nicotine-containing products (Scherer, 2018).

TABLE 17.5
Coprimary biomarkers of potential harm.

BoPH	Mechanism	Matrix/function	Timeframe of reversibility upon smoking cessation
CARDIOVASCULAR DISEASE			
HDL-C	Lipid metabolism	Serum	Within 3 months
sICAM-1	Endothelial dysfunction	Serum	Within 4 weeks
COHb	Oxygen transport	Blood	Within 1–7 days
11-DTX-B2	Platelet activation	Urine	Within 2–4 weeks
RESPIRATORY DISEASE			
FEV₁	Lung function	Lung function	Within 6–12 months
SMOKING-RELATED DISEASE			
WBC (total count)	Inflammation	Blood	Within 6–12 months
8-epi-PGF2α	Oxidative stress	Urine	Within 1–2 weeks
GENOTOXICITY			
Total NNAL	Carcinogen exposure	Urine	Within 3 months

11-DTX-B2, 11-dehydrothromboxane B2; 8-epi-PGF2α, 8-epi-prostaglandin F2α; COHb, carboxyhemoglobin; FEV₁, forced expiratory volume in 1 s; HDL-C, high-density lipoprotein cholesterol; NNAL, 4-(methylnitrosamino)-1-(3-pyridyl)-1-butanol; sICAM-1, soluble intercellular adhesion molecule 1; WBC, white blood cells.

The authors followed a similar systematic approach, taking into consideration various parameters: (1) association with a disease, (2) difference between smokers and nonsmokers, (3) dose—response relationship, (4) reversibility, and (5) kinetics following smoking cessation. Each BoPH was ranked for the five parameters on a 3-level scale (0, 0.5, and 1). The following were rated the highest among all the other identified BoPHs: FEV_1, HDL-C, 11-DBX2, and WBC = 4; s-ICAM-1 and 8-epi-PGF2α = 3.5.

British American Tobacco (BAT) has considered a comparable selection approach for their study, which is also aimed at evaluating the effects of switching from cigarette smoking to using a tobacco heating product on health effect indicators in healthy subjects (Newland et al., 2019). In their primary objective, however, they are considering three endpoints: total NNAL, 8-Epi-PGF2α type III, and augmentation index. They plan to compare changes from baseline between study arms by specific contrasts in mixed models while performing study-wise multiple comparison adjustments to account for a multiplicity of time points and comparisons within time points (Camacho et al., 2020).

Such a combination of endpoints for assessing the potential risk reduction when switching to a novel product seems to be further endorsed by the FDA, as suggested by a summary published in 2019 of a public workshop sponsored by the FDA in 2016, which reports promising BoPHs to be evaluated in assessing the reduced risk of candidate modified risk tobacco products (MRTPs) for CVD, COPD, and lung cancer (Chang et al., 2019). This publication evaluates the following as adequate and promising BoPHs in accordance with Hill's criteria: s-ICAM-1, 8-epi-PGF2α, and HDL for CVD; FEV_1 for COPD; and total NNAL for its association with subsequent cancer risk. These were all part of the endpoints assessed in the primary objective of PMI's exposure response study. Fibrinogen, high-sensitivity C-reactive protein, platelet-derived biomarkers, and hemoglobin A1c, also mentioned in this publication, were measured as secondary endpoints in PMI's exposure response study to provide supporting evidence to the BoPH risk assessment framework. In addition, this publication concludes that "for the major tobacco-related diseases (CVD, pulmonary disease, and cancer), a set of biomarkers, rather than a single biomarker, could better represent the multiple mechanisms by which tobacco causes these diseases. One possible approach is to improve disease risk prediction by combining multiple markers into a composite variable" (Chang et al., 2019).

In conclusion, it appears that selecting a rigorous BoPH risk assessment framework is in line with regulatory recommendations, and combination of several endpoints is the best possible approach to date to provide, as early as possible, an overall metric of clinical significance in the absence of epidemiological evidence.

17.2.3.3 Product compliance or smoking abstinence

Subject compliance is a crucial aspect in studies assessing reduced exposure or reduced risk when switching to an ENDP product, as the effects of dual use (i.e., use of the ENDP product plus a certain number of cigarettes) on the magnitude of effects for the different endpoints is unknown. Subject adherence to the assigned product is, thus, extremely important for assessment of changes in BoExps and BoPHs during such studies.

Self-report of tobacco use has its limitations, particularly in an ambulatory setting. Self-reports from studies with a high demand for abstinence have been shown to be biased (Blank et al., 2016; IARC (International Agency for Research on Cancer), 2008; Scheuermann et al., 2017). Misclassification of self-reported cigarette use by adult smokers who have been advised to quit has been observed in clinical studies. This has been shown to be particularly true among subjects who have diseases or medical conditions that would benefit from quitting.

In a smoking abstinence group, compliance to abstinence is, in theory, relatively easy to monitor by verifying the absence of nicotine and its metabolites in saliva or urine or absence of exhaled carbon monoxide (COex), for example. Typically, smoking abstinence is checked via (1) self-reporting of tobacco/nicotine-containing product use; (2) a carbon monoxide (CO) breath test (≤10 ppm); or (3) a urine dipstick cotinine test (<100 ng/mL). However, as NRT is typically provided to help smokers maintain abstinence, nicotine verification is often not applicable. An alternative is postvisit chemical verification of NEQ or some of the nicotine metabolites that are commonly measured by the liquid chromatography—mass spectrometry method (Society for Research on Nicotine and Tobacco Subcommittee on Biochemical Verification et al., 2002). Such a methodology offers better sensitivity and accuracy for nicotine exposure detection. Given the linear relationship between nicotine exposure and the number of cigarettes smoked, it offers the advantage of detecting cigarette smoking and estimating its intensity. Usually, the threshold used to discriminate a smoker from a nonsmoker is 50 ng/mL for urinary free cotinine concentration. Using BoExps to HPHCs other than nicotine, such as COex, for example, is challenging, as (1) most of the BoExps have a short half-life and may fail to reveal smoking that occurred a few days earlier, (2) have sources other than cigarettes that can potentially confound the results, and (3) can be quite costly and time-consuming to measure.

Assessing compliance to ENDP use, including EHTPs, is even more challenging than confirming smoking abstinence, as measurement of nicotine and/or its metabolites does not allow discrimination between cigarette smoking and ENDP use. Considering that ENDPs are noncombustible products (both EHTPs and EVPs), BoExps that enable specific detection of combustible tobacco product use are necessary. Therefore, there is great interest in validating one or more BoExps that are qualified to estimate the intensity of concomitant cigarette smoking and ENDP use. In the context of harm reduction assessment, such tools would enable identification of dual users of ENDPs and cigarettes versus complete switchers to ENDP. This is necessary to accurately estimate the relative risk and harm reduction of an ENDP when used predominantly/exclusively in comparison with cigarettes. Some BoExps have shown promise with regard to their specificity to combustible tobacco; but, they are still under investigation, and no consensus exists yet within the scientific community. The BoExps explored include CEMA, total NNAL, and N-(2-cyanoethyl)valine hemoglobin adducts (CEVal), with half-lives of <1 day, 10−18 days, and 90−120 days, respectively. BoExps with long half-lives offer the advantage of detecting cigarette smoking retrospectively over longer time periods than BoExps with short half-lives. Cutoffs to be applied should be selected on the basis of sound scientific evidence showing that they can discriminate smokers from nonsmokers.

Typically, total NNAL, which has a described half-life of 10−18 days and is specific for exposure to tobacco smoke, could be used to detect cigarette use several weeks after cessation or switching to an ENDP (Goniewicz et al., 2009). A publication in 2012 used a cutoff of >75.9 pg/mL for urinary total NNAL concentration to discriminate smokers from nonsmokers (Berg et al., 2012). Such an approach could also be considered in the context of understanding the level of dual use during switching to ENDP in clinical studies.

Another BoExp being investigated by PMI is CEMA, an acrylonitrile metabolite found in the urine of smokers, which is also quite specific for tobacco exposure in the general population. Despite a relatively short half-life of around 8 h (Jakubowski et al., 1987), CEMA levels display a dose-dependent relationship with the number of cigarettes smoked and would be amenable for testing in spot urine. Creatinine-adjusted CEMA with a cutoff of <40 ng/mg creatinine was derived in an initial exploratory population PK approach that described the levels of CEMA following use of cigarettes

or an EHTP (Claussen et al., 2019). This cutoff value should distinguish subjects who mostly used THS (mainly adherent) and those who also smoked cigarettes.

CEVal, another BoExp of interest, has the longest half-life, based on the red blood cell life cycle, which is between 90 and 120 days in healthy individuals (Forster et al., 2018). This marker has been shown to display a dose-dependent relationship with the number of cigarettes smoked (Schettgen et al., 2002).

To date, there is no consensus on how to best discriminate dual users from complete quitters or complete switchers. But, this will become more and more important in the context of ENDP assessment, especially when estimating their potential to reduce risk.

17.3 EXAMPLE CLINICAL ASSESSMENT PROGRAM

At the time of writing, very few ENDPs have been thoroughly assessed in large clinical programs. The purpose of this section, therefore, is to describe the clinical program developed by PMI to assess the THS, which is an ENDP (Smith et al., 2016) (Chapter 2). While this program has been developed for THS, it is generally applicable to most other ENDPs. The clinical program involves a step-by-step assessment that is intended to cover multiple populations (race and ethnicities) and a diversity of healthy adult smokers in term of age, sex, smoking history, and socioeconomic status (Table 17.6):

- Four crossover PK/PD studies were conducted to compare the nicotine uptake profile (amount and speed of absorption) following single use of THS or cigarettes after a 1-day wash out period. As the route of absorption of nicotine (inhalation) is similar with both products, the nicotine absorption profile was expected to be comparable (Brossard et al., 2017; Marchand et al., 2017; Picavet et al., 2015). NRTs (nasal spray or gum, depending on the study type) were used as additional comparators.
- Four randomized, controlled, open-label, 3-arm parallel-group reduced exposure studies were conducted to determine the degree of HPHC exposure reduction in smokers who switched to THS (menthol or nonmenthol variants) and those who continued to smoke their own cigarettes. These studies included a smoking abstinence arm to compare the effects of switching to those of cessation on HPHC exposure.
  - ○ Two studies were conducted in a confined clinical setting in the EU (ZRHR-EXC-03-EU)

TABLE 17.6
Clinical assessment program for THS.

Study code/Clinicaltrials.gov ID	Study type	Investigational product	Comparators	Duration of exposure
ZRHR-PK-01-EU NCT01967732	PK/PD	THS	CC; NRT (NNS)	Single use
ZRHR-PK-02-JP NCT01959607	PK/PD	THS	CC, NRT (nicotine gum)	Single use
ZRHM-PK-05-JP NCT01967706	PK/PD	mTHS	mCC, NRT (nicotine gum)	Single use
ZRHM-PK-06-US NCT01967719	PK/PD	mTHS	mCC, NRT (NNS)	Single use
ZRHR-REXC-03-EU NCT01959932	Reduced exposure	THS	CC; SA	5 days ad libitum use in confinement
ZRHR-REXC-04-JP NCT01970982	Reduced exposure	THS	CC, SA	5 days ad libitum use in confinement
ZRHM-REXA-07-JP NCT01970995	Reduced exposure	mTHS	mCC, SA	90 days ad libitum use (5 days in confinement and 85 days ambulatory)
ZRHM-REXA-08-US NCT01989156	Reduced exposure	mTHS	mCC; SA	90 days ad libitum use (5 days in confinement and 86 days ambulatory)
ZRHR-ERS-09-US NCT02396381	Exposure response	THS	CC	26 weeks ad libitum use (ambulatory)

CC, cigarette; EU, European Union; ID, identification; JP, Japan; mCC, mentholated cigarette; mTHS, menthol version of THS; NNS, nicotine nasal spray; NRT, nicotine replacement therapy; PD, pharmacodynamics; PK, pharmacokinetics; SA, smoking abstinence; THS, Tobacco Heating System 2.2; US, United States.

(Haziza et al., 2016b, 2017) and Japan (ZRHR-REXC-04-JP) (Haziza et al., 2016a). Both included 2 days of a baseline period (cigarette smoking for all subjects), followed by a 5-day randomized exposure period according to product/regimen allocation. These confinement studies, with strict surveillance of product use, allowed us to determine the maximum effect of switching and cessation on the reduction of HPHC exposure.

O Two studies were conducted with THS in Japan (ZRHM-REXA-07-JP) (Lüdicke et al., 2018b) and the US (ZRHM-REXA-08-US) (Haziza et al., 2019) over 3 months, with 2 days of a baseline period, an initial 5 days of exposure in a confined clinical setting, followed by 85 days in an ambulatory setting. The purpose of the additional 85 days was to demonstrate whether the reduction in HPHC exposure observed in confinement would be sustained over a longer period in a near real-world setting in the presence of confounding factors that are known to potentially influence the levels of some BoExps. Furthermore, these two studies were long enough to assess the initial changes in some of the BoPHs that have been shown to be reversible within 2 weeks–3 months (Haziza et al., 2020; Lüdicke et al., 2018a).

• A 6-month, randomized, controlled, open-label, 2-arm parallel-group, multicenter exposure response study was conducted in an ambulatory setting in the US (ZRHR-ERS-09-US) (Ansari et al., 2018; Lüdicke et al., 2019) in smokers who were asked to switch to THS and smokers who continued to smoke their own cigarettes. The main goal of this study was to demonstrate favorable changes in a core set of BoPHs, as presented in Table 17.5, that are indicative of multiple key pathways underlying the development of smoking-related diseases and may be used as indicators of future risk. Furthermore, to establish the effect of smoking cessation on the reversibility of the same core set of BoPHs, PMI conducted a 1-year multiregional continuous smoking abstinence study (NCT02432729) in the US, Japan, and Europe (Tran et al., 2019) in healthy smokers willing to quit smoking. This study will enable comparison of the effects of switching to ENDPs in general, and THS in particular, with those of smoking cessation on these BoPHs.

All clinical studies were approved by an institutional ethics committee/institutional review board (IRB) and, after approval, conducted in accordance with the principles of ICH/GCP (International Council for Harmonisation of Technical Requirements for Pharmaceuticals for Human Use/Good clinical practice) guidelines and registered on www.clinicaltrials.gov (a resource provided by the US National Library of Medicine).

17.4 CLINICAL NICOTINE PK ASSESSMENT OF ENDPS

17.4.1 PK Studies on EHTPs—PMI Studies

17.4.1.1 General design, population, and methods

The full names of these studies are provided in Table 17.6 but, for simplification purposes, are abbreviated herein as PK-01-EU, PK-02-JP, PK-05-JP, and PK-06-US. These crossover studies evaluated nicotine uptake and rate and extent of nicotine absorption following single use of cigarettes, THS, or NRTs (used

as a reference product) (Table 17.6). Crossover studies offer the advantage of minimizing the influence of confounding covariates, because each crossover subject serves as his/her own control. Subjective effects—such as urge to smoke, measures related to reinforcing or aversive effects, and sensory and satisfactory product experiences (some important components of long-term acceptance of the product during the switching process)—were part of the assessment. Safety was monitored during the studies.

Japanese populations were enrolled in the PK-02-JP and PK-05-JP studies, a White population in the PK-01-EU study, and White and Black populations in the PK-06-US study. All studies included subjects between 21 and 22 and 65 years of age. This diversity in populations made it possible to cover known polymorphisms in *CYP2A6* (e.g., in the Japanese) that may result in differences in nicotine metabolism and among age groups. Subjects were stratified on the basis of the ISO (International Organization for Standardization) nicotine level of the preferred brand of cigarettes they smoked at admission. The ISO nicotine levels were ≤ 0.6 mg and >0.6 to ≤ 1 mg for the PK-01-EU, PK-02-JP, and PK-05-JP studies and ≤ 1.0 mg and >1.0 mg for the PK-06-US study. The baseline demographic characteristics for the four PK studies are summarized in Fig. 17.1.

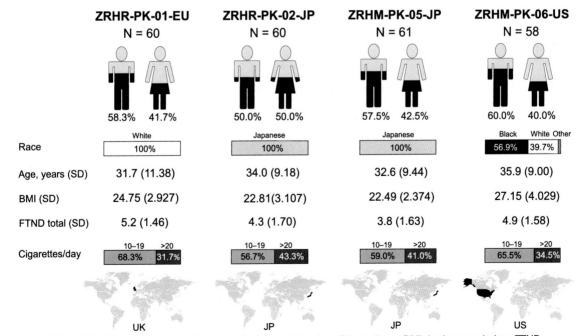

FIG. 17.1 Baseline demographic characteristics of the four PK studies. *BMI*, body mass index; *FTND*, Fagerström test for nicotine dependence; *SD*, standard deviation.

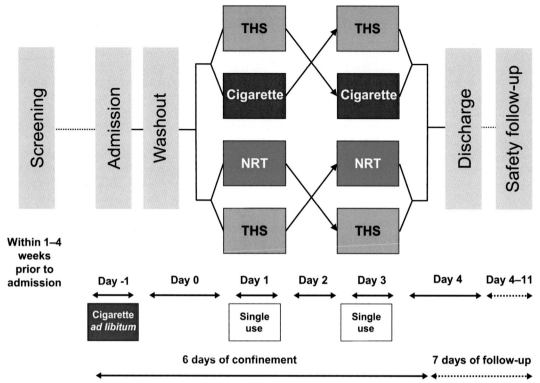

FIG. 17.2 Study flow chart of the four PK studies. *NRT*, nicotine replacement therapy; *THS*, Tobacco Heating System 2.2.

The overall study design of the four PK studies is presented in Fig. 17.2.

The confinement period consisted of two periods (Period 1 and Period 2), each comprising at least one 24-h nicotine washout (nicotine abstinence) and 1 day of single product use. The subjects were randomized into one of four sequences:

- Sequence 1: THS → cigarette
- Sequence 2: cigarette → THS
- Sequence 3: THS → NRT
- Sequence 4: NRT → THS

The washout period was considered long enough for nicotine, with a half-life of approximately 2 h. In all four studies, the subjects were randomized to ensure that men and women were properly represented (at least 40% of the study population for each sex).

The study prohibited the use of any drugs that could influence nicotine metabolism. Female subjects were not allowed to use hormonal contraception containing estrogens or hormone replacement therapy. To minimize any impact of diet on the nicotine measurements, a restricted diet was used, and extensive exercise was not allowed.

During single use of cigarettes and THS, smokers used their allocated products according to their own puffing behavior to allow a more realistic evaluation of how the product is used. Smokers can modulate their nicotine intake by controlling the way they use the product, including the duration and volume of puffs or depth/intensity of inhalation. Requesting the users to use the products according to a fixed regimen with a set number of puffs and intervals between puffs might have resulted in a decreased intra- and/or inter-subject variability; but, the large sample size allowed adequate precision (between 15% and 26%) of the C_{max} and area under the curve (AUC) (Table 17.7). The NRTs were used as per label.

In order to verify the appropriateness of the study design and accuracy of the related outcomes, THS and cigarettes were compared to NRTs (nicotine nasal spray [NNS] and nicotine gum), as the nicotine PK parameters for these NRTs are well described in the literature. The nicotine PK profile of THS was expected to be comparable to that of cigarettes, considering that nicotine is inhaled with both products. According to the literature, the nicotine PK profile of NNS is the closest to that of

TABLE 17.7

THS versus cigarette: Single product use noncompartmental PK analysis, with 95% confidence intervals for the ratio of means.

Variable	Study	THS geometric mean	Cigarettes geometric mean	THS: Cigarette ratio	95% CI lower limit	95% CI upper limit	Precision (%)
C_{max} (ng/mL)	PK-01-EU	9.62	12.42	77.43	62.69	95.63	18.20
	PK-02-JP	14.30	13.82	103.50	84.94	126.11	22.61
	PK-05-JP	10.70	12.09	88.47	68.64	114.03	25.55
	PK-06-US	7.40	13.08	56.57	44.21	72.39	15.81
$AUC_{(0-last)}$ (h × ng/mL)	PK-01-EU	15.10	20.28	74.47	61.52	90.14	15.67
	PK-02-JP	23.75	24.66	96.34	85.10	109.07	12.72
	PK-05-JP	23.99	24.45	98.13	80.61	119.46	21.33
	PK-06-US	16.53	29.71	55.64	43.30	71.50	15.86

AUC, area under the curve; *CI*, confidence interval; C_{max}, maximum concentration; *EU*, European Union; *JP*, Japan; *PK*, pharmacokinetics; *THS*, Tobacco Heating System 2.2; *US*, United States.

cigarettes, with a comparable time to maximum nicotine concentration (T_{max}), while nicotine gum has a longer time.

To evaluate the concentration—time profile of plasma nicotine, multiple blood samples were collected 24 h before and after single product use. CYP2A6 activity was measured as a baseline characteristic. Subjective effects (PD) were evaluated by means of two self-reported questionnaires, the QSU-brief (administered at multiple instances over 12 h) and the mCEQ. The latter questionnaire was only administered following THS and cigarette use between 8.00 and 11.00 p.m. on the day of product use.

Statistical analyses for evaluating nicotine PK parameters were performed in accordance with the FDA 2001 recommendations for nonreplicated crossover 2 × 2 study designs. In compliance with these guidelines, the general linear model procedure was used for analysis. The model included factors accounting for sequence, subjects nested in sequences, period, and exposure (FDA (Food and Drug Administration), 2001). Subjective effects were compared by using a mixed-effects model, including terms for product, sequence, period, and subject nested within sequence as a random effect, in accordance with the recommendation for assessment of tobacco craving and withdrawal (Shiffman et al., 2004).

17.4.1.2 PK results across studies
The plasma nicotine concentration—time profiles (up to 120 min) following single use of THS and cigarettes in all four studies (PK-01-EU, PK-02-JP, PK-05-JP, and PK-06-US) are shown in Fig. 17.3. The overall shape of the mean nicotine concentration—time curves was similar

for THS and cigarettes across all studies, but especially so in the studies conducted in Japanese populations (PK-02 and PK-05). In the PK-06 study, the concentration of nicotine was generally lower after single use of THS than after cigarette use.

The C_{max} and amount of nicotine absorbed ($AUC_{(0-last)}$)—calculated by noncompartmental analysis—were comparable between THS and cigarettes in PK-02-JP and PK-05-JP (THS:cigarette ratio for $AUC_{(0-last)}$, 96.3% and 98.1%, respectively) (Table 17.7) but lower after single use of THS than after single cigarette use in PK-01-EU and in PK-06-US.

The C_{max} and $AUC_{(0-last)}$ calculated by noncompartmental analysis were higher for THS than for NNS in PK-01-EU and PK-06-US (THS:NNS ratio of $AUC_{(0-last)}$, 222.9% and 178.8%, respectively) (Table 17.8). The time to reach C_{max} was shorter (0.8—1.2 min) with THS than with NNS. The $AUC_{(0-last)}$ was higher for NRT gum than THS in PK-05-JP, while there was little difference in C_{max} between the two products. In contrast, the $AUC_{(0-last)}$ was 20% lower for the NRT gum than for THS in PK-02-JP. There was considerable variability in the PK parameters of the nicotine gum, which is in line with published reports (Lunell and Curvall, 2011; Lunell and Lunell, 2005).

17.4.1.3 PD results across studies
17.4.1.3.1 QSU-brief results. The urge-to-smoke profiles were similar across studies for THS and cigarettes (Fig. 17.4), with a maximum reduction in urge to smoke from baseline observed ~15—20 min after single product use, followed by a progressive return to the baseline value. The overall total scores

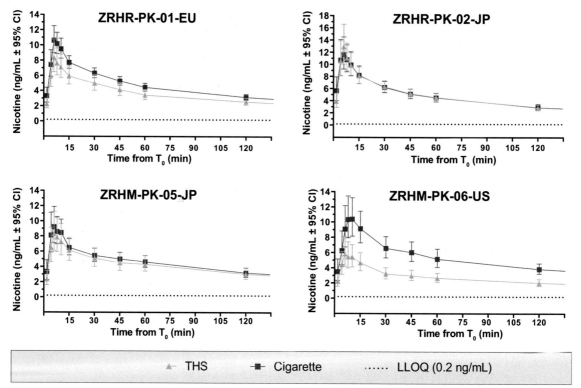

FIG. 17.3 Geometric mean nicotine plasma concentration (ng/mL) on single use days in the four PK studies (THS vs. cigarettes).   *CI*, confidence interval; *LLOQ*, lower limit of quantification; *THS*, Tobacco Heating System 2.2.

TABLE 17.8
THS versus NRT: Single product use noncompartmental PK analysis, with 95% confidence intervals for the ratio of means.

Variable	Study	THS geometric mean	NRTs geometric mean	THS:NRT ratio	95% CI lower limit	95% CI upper limit	Precision (%)
C_{max} (ng/mL)	PK-01-EU[a]	10.52	3.51	299.96	200.74	448.22	61.75
	PK-02-JP[b]	11.53	4.80	240.23	130.60	441.90	105.08
	PK-05-JP[b]	7.64	7.52	101.63	62.21	166.04	78.75
	PK-06-US[a]	8.40	3.23	259.75	168.00	401.60	65.18
$AUC_{(0-last)}$ (ng.h/mL)	PK-01-EU[a]	17.87	8.02	222.90	154.60	321.39	55.46
	PK-02-JP[b]	18.92	14.88	127.15	77.26	209.24	80.22
	PK-05-JP[b]	15.61	27.94	55.87	38.36	81.36	57.19
	PK-06-US[a]	15.59	8.72	178.78	106.45	300.25	80.66

AUC, area under the curve; *CI*, confidence interval; *C_{max}*, maximum concentration; *EU*, European Union; *JP*, Japan; *NNS*, nasal nicotine spray; *NRT*, nicotine replacement therapy; *PK*, pharmacokinetics; *THS*, Tobacco Heating System 2.2; *US*, United States.
[a] NNS.
[b] Gum.

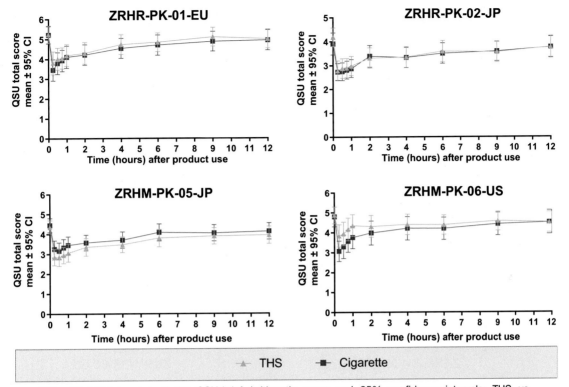

FIG. 17.4 Total score of the QSU-brief (arithmetic mean and 95% confidence intervals; THS vs. cigarettes). *CI*, confidence interval; *QSU*, Questionnaire of Smoking Urges; *THS*, Tobacco Heating System 2.2.

TABLE 17.9
Analysis of urge to smoke after single use, by study—THS versus cigarettes.

QSU-b total score	ZRHR-PK-01-EU (N = 42)	ZRHR-PK-02-JP (N = 42)	ZRHM-PK-05-JP (N = 43)	ZRHM-PK-06-US (N = 41)
THS	4.47 (3.37, 5.57)	3.24 (2.49, 3.98)	3.36 (2.74, 3.97)	4.28 (3.69, 4.87)
CC	4.30 (3.20, 5.40)	3.19 (2.45, 3.94)	3.64 (3.02, 4.26)	3.91 (3.32, 4.50)
THS-CC	0.17 (−0.93, 1.26)	0.04 (−0.70, 0.79)	−0.28 (−0.79, 0.22)	0.37 (−0.02, 0.77)

Means (95% CI) are the adjusted least squares means and 95% confidence intervals from an ANOVA model (overall time points). *CC*, cigarettes; *QSU-b*, Questionnaire of Smoking Urges, brief version; *THS*, Tobacco Heating System 2.2.

were comparable among THS, cigarettes, and NRT (NNS or gum) across all studies (Tables 17.9 and Table 17.10).

In conclusion, THS can reduce the urge to smoke relative to cigarettes and NNS or NRT gum.

17.4.1.3.2 mCEQ results. All mCEQ domains scored slightly lower for THS than cigarettes (Fig. 17.5), with the exception of aversion, where the effects of THS and cigarettes were comparable.

The craving reduction score for THS was close to that for cigarettes in the two Japanese studies (PK-02-JP and PK-05-JP) but lower in the other studies, particularly in PK-06-US, where the difference between THS and cigarettes was greater than 1 point.

The enjoyment of respiratory tract sensation and psychological reward domain scores were slightly higher for cigarettes than THS, with the greatest differences seen in PK-01-EU and PK-06-US (but with a difference <1).

TABLE 17.10

Analysis of urge to smoke after single use, by study—THS versus NRT.

QSU-b total score	ZRHR-PK-01-EU (N = 18)	ZRHR-PK-02-JP (N = 18)	ZRHM-PK-05-JP (N = 18)	ZRHM-PK-06-US (N = 17)
THS	3.92 (2.55, 5.28)	3.00 (2.13, 3.87)	3.33 (2.35, 4.31)	3.34 (2.64, 4.05)
NRT	4.07 (2.70, 5.44)	3.20 (2.33, 4.07)	3.66 (2.69, 4.64)	3.70 (2.99, 4.40)
THS-NRT	−0.15 (−1.35, 1.05)	−0.20(−0.87, 0.48)	−0.34 (−0.87, 0.19)	−0.35 (−0.79, 0.09)

Means (95% CI) are the adjusted least squares means and 95% confidence intervals from an ANCOVA model (overall time points). *NRT*, nicotine replacement therapy; *QSU-b*, Questionnaire of Smoking Urges, brief version; *THS*, Tobacco Heating System 2.2.

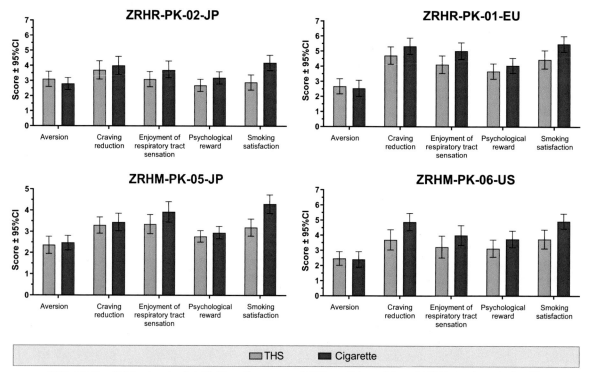

FIG. 17.5 mCEQ subscales brief (arithmetic mean and 95% confidence intervals; THS vs. cigarettes). *CI*, confidence interval; *mCEQ*, modified Cigarette Evaluation Questionnaire; *THS*, Tobacco Heating System 2.2.

The smoking satisfaction score was higher for cigarettes than THS, with the THS—cigarettes differences ranging from 1.0 to 1.3 points.

In conclusion, the reinforcing and aversive effects after THS use were reduced to a lesser extent than after smoking a cigarette, with the exception that both products had a comparable effect on aversion. The differences in craving reduction between THS and cigarettes were lower in the Japanese studies than in the non-Japanese studies. No relevant differences were observed in the other parameters among the studies.

17.4.2 PK Studies on e-Cigarettes

While NRTs deliver nicotine rather slowly and with a PK profile that does not resemble that of cigarettes (Bullen et al., 2010; Digard et al., 2013), e-cigarettes are much closer to cigarettes in terms of both C_{max} and T_{max} (Caldwell et al., 2012; Hajek et al., 2014; Helen et al., 2016; Schroeder and Hoffman, 2014). There are, however, several factors that can affect these parameters, including e-cigarette puffing behavior and nicotine concentration in the e-liquid.

17.4.2.1 E-cigarette puffing topography

A user's puffing behavior, known as puffing topography, affects the composition of e-cigarette emissions (Cheng, 2014; Evans and Hoffman, 2014; Farsalinos et al., 2013; Sleiman et al., 2016). While e-cigarette nicotine delivery can, in some cases, exceed that of cigarettes (Ramoa et al., 2016), the volume of inhaled e-cigarette vapor needed to achieve a comparable nicotine intake can be up to four times that of smoke from a single cigarette (Ramoa et al., 2016). Therefore, information on e-cigarette puffing topography as well as its variability among different e-cigarette models and users can provide insights into nicotine uptake. In addition, topography data, which have been well documented for cigarettes (De Jesus et al., 2013), are needed to understand the baseline characteristics pertaining to e-cigarette use. For instance, Behar and colleagues evaluated the e-cigarette puffing topography parameters for two e-cigarettes in 16 male and 4 female subjects (Behar et al., 2015). The study showed that the puffing topography varied significantly with the type of e-cigarette used. All parameters, with the exception of total puff count, were significantly different between the two brands tested, which is likely because of differences in product performance. There were also large variations in puffing topography among users, which is consistent with the high variability among individuals smoking cigarettes (Hammond et al., 2005).

Importantly, switching from cigarette smoking to e-cigarette use requires an adaptation period, during which the original cigarette puffing topography will transition to a new e-cigarette puffing topography. In an observational nonblinded study (Guerrero-Cignarella et al., 2018) where active cigarette smokers were asked to replace their cigarette with an e-cigarette over a 4-week period, followed by exclusive e-cigarette use for an additional 12 weeks, the data revealed that the topography of smokers who adhered to exclusive e-cigarette use reflected progressive and dynamic device adaptation over weeks in order to maintain baseline cotinine levels. Subjects who used the e-cigarette for the complete study period had significantly longer durations per puff and overall inhalation time. As puffing topography affects nicotine delivery, nicotine PK will also be affected by product familiarity (Fearon et al., 2018). This relationship was, for instance, investigated by Fearon et al. (2017), who measured the nicotine PK in participants who used e-cigarettes under different puffing regimens (Study 1). The authors then compared the effects of product familiarity on nicotine PK in smokers who were familiar with, but not current users of, e-cigarettes with that in accustomed e-cigarette users who were occasional cigarette smokers (Study 2).

Study 1 was a part-randomized, part-blinded, crossover study in 24 healthy male (n = 17) and female (n = 7) volunteer cigarette smokers. This study showed that nicotine absorption was lower in cigarette smokers using an e-cigarette than in those smoking a cigarette under both controlled and ad libitum use (Fig. 17.6). This study also showed that the urge to smoke was reduced to a lesser extent in participants who used the e-cigarette than in those who smoked cigarettes.

Study 2 was a part-randomized, open-label, crossover study in 18 healthy male and female volunteers who were accustomed and regular users of e-cigarettes and occasionally smoked cigarettes. While

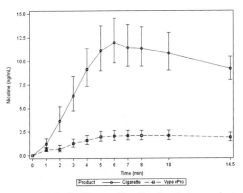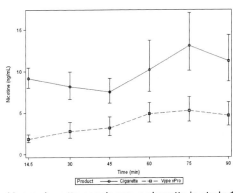

FIG. 17.6 Left: Plasma Nicotine levels in smokers smoking a cigarette or using an e-cigarette in study 1. Right: Nicotine levels in smokers smoking a cigarette or using an e-cigarette ad libitum in study 1. (*Circles*, cigarettes; *Squares*, e-cigarettes. Data are Geometric Means $\pm$ 95% Cnfidence Intervals for 23–24 participants in each case). (Figures 1 and 2 from Fearon IM, Eldridge A, Gale N, Shepperd CJ, McEwan M, Camacho OM, Nides M, McAdam K, Proctor CJ. E-cigarette nicotine delivery: data and learnings from pharmacokinetic studies. Am J Health Behav. 2017; 41(1):16–32.)

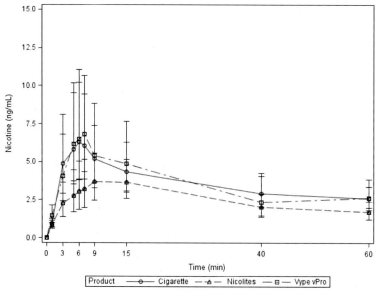

FIG. 17.7 Plasma nicotine evels in e-cigarette users smoking a cigarette or using one of two different e-cigarettes in study 2. (*Circles*, cigarettes; *Squares* and *Triangles*, e-cigarettes. Data are geometric means ± 95% confidence intervals for 23−24 participants in each case). (Figure 4 from Fearon IM, Eldridge A, Gale N, Shepperd CJ, McEwan M, Camacho OM, Nides M, McAdam K, Proctor CJ. E-cigarette nicotine delivery: data and learnings from pharmacokinetic studies. Am J Health Behav. 2017; 41(1):16−32.)

this study found that e-cigarettes were effective at delivering nicotine, the predominant finding was that the magnitude of nicotine absorption was far greater in accustomed users during ad libitum puffing than in smokers who did not use e-cigarettes (Fig. 17.7). Study 2 also showed that nicotine absorption from a newer generation e-cigarette was similar to that from cigarettes with respect to C_{max} and AUC, which is in general agreement with the findings of an earlier study (Ramoa et al., 2016).

17.4.2.2 Nicotine concentration in e-liquids

Nicotine uptake is affected by the nicotine concentration in the aerosol, which depends on both the nicotine concentration in the e-liquid and the device technology. However, to date, there have been very few studies that have compared the effects of nicotine concentrations and formulations on nicotine PK. One such study was a randomized, open-label, six-period crossover study aimed at comparing nicotine uptake from two e-cigarette device platforms (a replaceable pod system and an open refillable clearomizer) with varying concentrations of nicotine lactate or freebase nicotine, relative to cigarettes (O'Connell et al., 2019). The study involved 15 healthy American smokers aged 21−65 years and had plasma nicotine PK parameter assessment as the primary outcome measure. This study showed that nicotine is rapidly delivered to systemic circulation, with plasma PK profiles consistent with pulmonary absorption. In all cases, however, the nicotine absorption was lower than that obtained with a cigarette.

Importantly, the study showed that nicotine absorption was correlated with the nicotine concentration in the e-liquid/aerosol, with the notable exception of the open refillable system. This system, while having the highest nicotine concentration among all tested e-cigarettes, delivered far less aerosol per puff than the replaceable pod system. Furthermore, the C_{max} for the product with freebase nicotine was lower than that for the product with the same level of nicotine lactate. In all cases, the T_{max} values for the e-cigarettes were comparable with that obtained for the cigarette, which is in line with previously published data (Benowitz et al., 2009) (Table 17.11). In this study, the urge to smoke was consistently reduced as a function of nicotine uptake (O'Connell et al., 2019).

A recently published crossover within-subject study aimed to establish the PK profile of an e-cigarette with a high e-liquid nicotine concentration (59 mg/mL) and compare this with the PK profile of cigarettes and e-cigarettes with lower e-liquid nicotine concentrations (<20 mg/mL) (Hajek et al., 2020). The study enrolled

TABLE 17.11
Summary of pharmacokinetic parameters by investigational product type.

	Cigarette	E-cigarette 40 mg nicotine lactate	E-cigarette 25 mg nicotine lactate	E-cigarette 16 mg nicotine lactate	E-cigarette 25 mg freebase nicotine	E-cigarette 48 mg nicotine lactate
Technology	Combustible	Replaceable pod system	Replaceable pod system	Replaceable pod system	Replaceable pod system	Open refillable clearomizer
Aerosol per puff	NA	7–8 mg	7–8 mg	7–8 mg	7–8 mg	2–3 mg
C_{max} (ng/mL)	17.81 (49.6)	10.27 (83.6)	7.58 (80.6)[a]	6.51 (76.5)[b]	5.048 (49.9)[b]	4.85 (108.3)[b]
T_{max}, median (range) (min)	8.05 (5.0–15.1)	7.9 (2.0–15.0)	6.0 (4.6–16.8)	7.0 (4.0–15.0)	8.0 (2.3–15.1)	6.91 (2.4–15.0)
AUC_{0-30} (ng.Min/mL)	324.9 (35.8)	190.7 (71.8)	125.2 (53.4)[b]	118.5 (60.8)[b]	98.99 (35.8)[b]	84.84 (89.8)[b]

All values are geometric means and geometric coefficients of variation (%CV) unless stated otherwise. AUC_{0-30}, area under the concentration–time curve from time zero to the last quantifiable concentration (30 min); C_{max}, maximum plasma nicotine concentration; *NA*, not available; T_{max}, time to maximum nicotine concentration.

[a] $P < .01$.
[b] $P < .001$.

Data from O'Connell G, Pritchard JD, Prue C, Thompson J, Verron T, Graff D, Walele T. A randomized, open-label, crossover clinical study to evaluate the pharmacokinetic profiles of cigarettes and e-cigarettes with nicotine salt formulations in US adult smokers. Intern Emerg Med. 2019; 14(6):853–61.

20 "dual users" (who vaped daily and occasionally used cigarettes). The results showed that the high-nicotine e-cigarette led to similar nicotine uptake as a cigarette when used ad libitum for 5 min after overnight abstinence. Although, in this study, the high-nicotine e-cigarette had a slightly shorter T_{max} than the cigarette, the difference was not considered significant because of the variability of T_{max}. Accordingly, use of the high-nicotine e-cigarette led to a similar reduction in urge to smoke as cigarette smoking. Furthermore, this study showed that use of e-cigarettes with lower nicotine concentrations in the e-liquid led to much lower C_{max} but similar T_{max} values (Hajek et al., 2020).

Finally, St Helen and colleagues reported a two-armed, counterbalanced crossover study involving 28 male and 8 female dual users. In this study, subjects used their usual brand of cigarette and e-cigarette during standardized sessions over a 2-week period (St Helen et al., 2020). The data showed that, compared with cigarette smoking, e-cigarette use led to lower C_{max} values (20.2 ± 11.1 and 6.15 ± 5.5 ng/mL respectively) and that the T_{max} was longer during e-cigarette use (6.5 ± 5.4 min) than cigarette smoking (2.7 ± 2.4 min). On average, the plasma nicotine C_{max} was 5.4 times higher with cigarettes than e-cigarettes.

Furthermore, comparison of different e-cigarette types showed that cig-a-like and fixed-power tank users had lower C_{max} values than variable-power tank users.

Nicotine PK parameters were also assessed with a prototype novel tobacco vapor product consisting of a cartridge with a heater and liquid and a capsule filled with a tobacco blend (Yuki et al., 2017). This hybrid product (Chapter 2) generates a nicotine-free vapor by electrically heating a liquid (containing glycerin, propylene glycol, and water, but neither nicotine nor flavors). The vapor then passes through the tobacco capsule, where evaporated constituents from a tobacco blend (including nicotine and flavors) pass into the inhaled vapor. This study was an open-label, two-sequence, two-period, randomized crossover design to investigate the PK of nicotine following use of the prototype product in comparison with smoking of a commercially available cigarette (1 mg tar and 0.1 mg nicotine). The subjects were 24 adult male smokers ranging in age from 21 to 65 years. This study showed that the nicotine PK following use of the novel product were not markedly different from those obtained following cigarette use, although the prototype product provided less nicotine following a controlled single use (Yuki et al., 2017).

17.5 CLINICAL REDUCED EXPOSURE ASSESSMENT OF ENDPS

A number of studies have assessed the reduction in HPHC exposure when switching from cigarette smoking to using ENDP, smokeless tobacco products, or NRTs. The typical design that most studies have applied is a confined setting—with smokers switching to the test product or continuing to smoke cigarettes— often with the addition of a smoking abstinence arm. The exposure period in confinement varied from 3 (Stepanov et al., 2009) to 8 days (Frost-Pineda et al., 2008; Tricker et al., 2012a, 2012b, 2012d) in earlier studies but is now typically 5 days (Gale et al., 2018; Gale et al., 2017; Haziza et al., 2019; Haziza et al., 2016a; Haziza et al., 2016b; Haziza et al., 2017; Jay et al., 2019; Krautter et al., 2015; Lüdicke et al., 2018b; O'Connell et al., 2016; Tricker et al., 2012c). This is mainly because most of the BoExps exhibit a half-life of <1 day, with the exception of total NNAL. A 5-day washout is considered sufficient for estimating the maximum reduction in the BoExps under investigation. Some studies have covered longer exposure periods in an ambulatory setting, lasting from 30 days (Martin Leroy et al., 2012; Sakaguchi et al., 2014) or 90 days (Haziza et al., 2019; Lüdicke et al., 2018b) to up to 24 weeks (Sarkar et al., 2008) or 6 months (Lüdicke et al., 2019). This type of study offers three advantages:

1. Helps evaluate the maximum reduction in BoExps with longer half-lives, such as total NNAL.
2. Helps evaluate the reduction in exposure in a realistic setting where confounding variables may have an effect on the level of BoExps (e.g., diet, passive exposure, and social environment).
3. Given the duration of the ambulatory exposure period, the study is long enough for assessing the initial changes in some of the BoPHs that have been shown to be reversible within 2 weeks—3 months.

Typically, these studies have involved urine collection over 24 h for assessing the levels of BoExps; but, this is likely to become operationally difficult in longer-term studies when no confinement is planned. Spot urine collection will, therefore, become increasingly common. However, interpretation of those data will be more complex when considering potential dual use of the test product and cigarettes (i.e., noncompliance) and the rates of urine excretion, which can vary during the day and among subjects.

17.5.1 Clinical Reduced Exposure Studies on EHTPs—PMI Studies

17.5.1.1 General design, population, and methods

PMI conducted four clinical studies designed to compare the effects of switching to THS with those of continued cigarette smoking and smoking abstinence on exposure to cigarette smoke toxicants (Table 17.6). These studies were also designed to determine whether THS has the potential to be an acceptable alternative to cigarettes for smokers who did not intend to quit smoking.

The full names of these studies are provided in Table 17.6; but, for simplification, they are herein referred to as REXC-03-EU, REXC-04-JP, REXA-07-JP, and REXA-08-US. The REXC-03-EU and REXC-04-JP studies involved a 2-day baseline period, followed by 5 days of exposure in confinement, where switching from cigarette smoking to THS use was compared with cigarette smoking and smoking abstinence. The REXA-07-JP and REXA-08-US studies also included a confinement period (a 2-day baseline period, followed by a 5-day exposure period) but were extended with an ambulatory period of 85—86 days (for a total duration of ~3 months). They also compared switching from cigarette smoking to THS use with cigarette smoking and smoking abstinence.

The study populations were healthy adult smokers who self-reported the use of at least 10 commercially available cigarettes per day for the last 3 years prior to enrollment in the study and did not plan to quit smoking in the next 3 months. The study participants were randomized into three study groups:

• Adult smokers who continued to smoke cigarettes,
• Adult smokers who switched to smoking abstinence, and
• Adult smokers who switched from cigarettes to THS.

In all four studies, the subjects were randomized so as to ensure that men and women were properly represented (at least 40% of the study population for each sex). The female subjects needed a confirmed negative pregnancy test and had to use effective methods of contraception. Only subjects between 21—23 and 65 years of age were included. Japanese populations were enrolled in REXC-04-JP and REXA-07-JP and a Caucasian population in REXC-03-EU; the REXA-08-US study was conducted in White and Black or African-American subjects. The baseline demographic characteristics of the four studies are presented in Fig. 17.8.

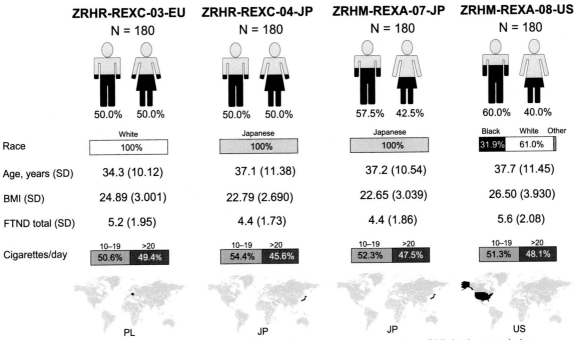

FIG. 17.8 Baseline demographic characteristics of the four exposure studies. *BMI*, body mass index; *FTND*, Fagerström test for nicotine dependence; *SD*, standard deviation.

The flowchart of the REXA-07-JP study is presented in Fig. 17.9. The REXA-08-US study followed the same design as REXA-07-JP, while REXC-03-EU and REXC-04-JP ended after the confinement phase.

Diet restrictions (based on foods/beverages known to potentially affect one or several endpoints in the studies) were imposed during the confinement period in all four studies, while no restrictions were applied during the ambulatory phase of the REXA studies.

The main specific objectives of these four studies were

- To demonstrate the reduction in S-PMA, 3-HPMA, monohydroxybutenylmercapturic acid (MHBMA), and COHb levels after 5 days of exposure in confinement, as a primary objective,
- To demonstrate the reduction in total NNAL levels in an ambulatory setting after 3 months of exposure, as a primary objective,
- To determine the reduction in other BoExps (listed in Table 17.3) in confinement setting and ambulatory settings,
- To assess the change in CYP1A2 enzymatic activity,
- To determine the exposure to nicotine by measuring its urinary metabolites (free nicotine, nicotine glucuronide, free cotinine, cotinine glucuronide, free *trans*-

3'-hydroxycotinine, and *trans*-3'-hydroxycotinine glucuronide,
- To monitor selected BoPHs,
- To monitor safety.

Subjective effects, such as urge to smoke and measures related to reinforcing or aversive effects, were part of the assessment. In all four reduced exposure studies, the pattern of withdrawal symptoms experienced during the study period was evaluated by administration of the MNWS questionnaire at each visit. The trend of urge to smoke over time was evaluated by administration of the QSU-brief questionnaire at each visit. The mCEQ, which assesses both the reinforcing and aversive effects of smoking, was also administered at each visit in all clinical studies as a measure of product acceptance.

Exposure was assessed by measuring a set of BoExps to HPHCs. NEQ was used to evaluate nicotine exposure following ad libitum product use in our reduced exposure studies. Adult smokers used THS without restriction (ad libitum), but dual use of cigarettes and THS was not allowed during the confinement period and discouraged during the ambulatory period of the study. The levels of BoExps and NEQ were measured in urine samples collected over 24 h.

HPT was also assessed in these studies. HPT assesses each user's unique way of using a product and

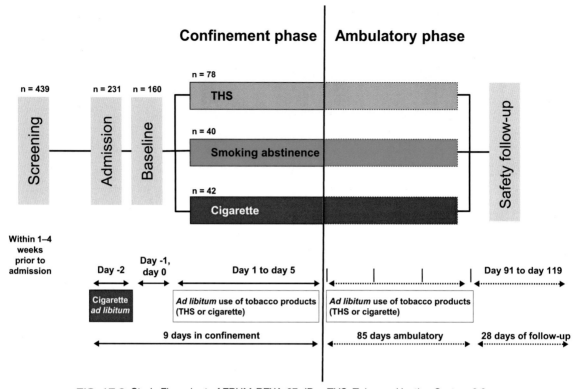

FIG. 17.9 Study Flow chart of ZRHM-REXA-07-JP. *THS*, Tobacco Heating System 2.2.

constitutes an established research tool in smoking behavior research for assessing individual product use patterns on a per-single-use basis. Total puff volume—the sum of the volume of all puffs taken during the cigarette smoking or THS use experience—is a key measure for quantifying mouth-level exposure to cigarette smoke or THS aerosol. By considering additional parameters such as product use duration, puff volume, and number of puffs, HPT allows evaluation of changes in product use behavior when switching from one product to another (e.g., subjects' own brand of cigarettes to THS).

Chronic inhalation of cigarette smoke, and especially inhalation of constituents such as aromatic amines and PAHs, leads to activation of the hepatic xenobiotic enzyme CYP1A2. Importantly, many xenobiotic substances, including caffeine and antidepressants, as well as some analgesics, antiinflammatory, and other drugs are metabolized by CYP1A2. It has been shown that drugs that are primarily metabolized by CYP1A2 will have faster systemic clearance as a result of enzyme induction in smokers (Anderson and Chan, 2016), while smoking cessation will reverse the hepatic enzyme's

levels to normal (MacLeod et al., 1997). This leads to markedly augmented plasma drug concentrations in patients whose dose was established while the patient was a smoker (Faber and Fuhr, 2004). Determining the extent to which smoking cessation could alter the PK of existing drug regimens is, therefore, essential for smokers who want to quit and are receiving medications metabolized by CYP1A2 (Anderson and Chan, 2016). As the turnover time of CYP1A2 is just under 2 days, a clinically significant effect can be detected within a week of smoking cessation. Empirical dose reduction may be necessary within 2–3 days after smoking cessation (Faber and Fuhr, 2004). In patients taking drugs with narrow therapeutic indices, close monitoring of clinical symptoms for adverse events is necessary within the first week of smoking cessation. Therapeutic drug monitoring, if available and clinically feasible, should be performed (Anderson and Chan, 2016). For these reasons, the four reduced exposure studies—REXC-03-EU, REXC-04-JP, REXA-07-JP, and REXA-08-US—evaluated CYP1A2 activity by measuring the molar metabolic ratio of paraxanthine (PX)/caffeine (CAF) in plasma at baseline and on days 5 and 90 in the 90-day studies.

This combination of studies allowed comparison, in different study populations, of (1) the HPHC exposure reduction achieved by switching to THS and mTHS relative to cigarette smoking, (2) the exposure reduction achieved by switching to mTHS relative to smoking abstinence, and (3) the product use and subjective effects in switchers compared with cigarette smokers.

Only the most relevant features and outcomes of the reduced exposure assessment in the four studies on healthy smokers are reported here. More details can be found in the synopses of the individual studies reported on the FDA website (Section 6.2.1.2) (FDA (Food and Drug Administration), 2017).

17.5.1.2 Product adherence
For interpretation of results, it is necessary to consider adaptation to the product during the switching process. In switching studies such as these, it is not feasible to expect full adherence to the product over time because of the following facts: (1) subjects are required to switch to a new product with characteristics different from those of their preferred brand of cigarettes; (2) communication on potential benefits of the product that may encourage switching is not possible; and (3) according to previous clinical studies and market data, dual use of cigarettes and THS is possible. Therefore, it is important to understand how many cigarettes are smoked concomitantly with THS.

In our reduced exposure studies, product consumption during the study was measured as the number of cigarettes or THS tobacco sticks used per day by the subjects. During the confinement period, compliance in all study arms was ensured by strict dispensation of the products (product-by-product). During the ambulatory period, subjects in the THS arm were provided a sufficient number of THS tobacco sticks to cover their estimated needs. Upon request from the subject, additional visits were organized to provide an extra number of THS tobacco sticks if needed. Consumption was recorded by the study site staff when the subjects were confined or, otherwise, self-reported by the subjects in a diary (paper or electronic) on a stick-by-stick basis when in ambulatory or "home-use" settings. During the ambulatory period, subjects in the three study arms self-reported the number of products used (e.g., cigarette, THS tobacco sticks, or any other tobacco-/ nicotine-containing products, including NRTs) daily in a product use electronic diary, which served as a compliance tool in the three arms.

In addition, in the smoking abstinence arm, compliance was chemically verified by a COex breath test both during confinement and at each ambulatory visit. The

cutoff point for the CO breath test value for distinguishing cigarette smoking versus smoking abstinence was 10 ppm (Society for Research on Nicotine and Tobacco Subcommittee on Biochemical Verification et al., 2002).

17.5.1.3 Statistical approach and sample size
The sample size for all studies was calculated to demonstrate a reduction in exposure to selected HPHCs. The per-protocol set was the primary analysis population for BoExps and questionnaire assessments. To be a part of the per-protocol population, subjects in the smoking abstinence and THS arms were allowed no more than 0.5 uses of any tobacco or nicotine-containing product per day, on average, and no more than two uses on a single day.

The urinary BoExps tested for the primary objective were adjusted for creatinine. The BoExp levels included in the primary objective were log-transformed prior to analysis. An analysis of covariance (ANCOVA) model was used, with terms for the log-transformed baseline value, stratification factors, and randomization arm. The least squares (LS) means, estimate of the difference, and its 2-sided 95% confidence intervals (CI) were back-transformed. The geometric LS means for each randomization arm, along with the ratio (THS:cigarette), two-sided 95% CI, and one-sided P value were reported.

17.5.1.4 Reduced exposure studies: results across studies during the confinement period (REXC and REXA)
All four exposure studies demonstrated that smokers who switched to THS or smoking abstinence had decreased levels of exposure to the measured HPHCs. The time course of the decrease in S-PMA, MHBMA, 3-HPMA, and COHb levels—tested as part of the primary objective—in the 5-day exposure study in the EU (REXC-03-EU) is shown in Fig. 17.10 (geometric means). The drop in exposure levels to HPHCs with THS use was rapid and of a magnitude that approached the reductions seen in the group that had abstained from smoking during the same period.

Similar patterns of change were seen in CEMA, 4-aminobiphenyl (4-ABP), total 3-hydroxybenzo[a]pyrene (3-OH-B[a]P), 3-HMPMA, 2-hydroxyethylmercapturic acid (HEMA), 1-aminonaphthalene (1-NA), 2-aminonaphthalene (2-NA), total NNAL, total NNN, o-toluidine, and total 1-OHP levels. The reductions in BoExp levels were of a similar magnitude in the THS and smoking abstinence groups. S-BMA levels did not show any difference across the study arms. These data are shown

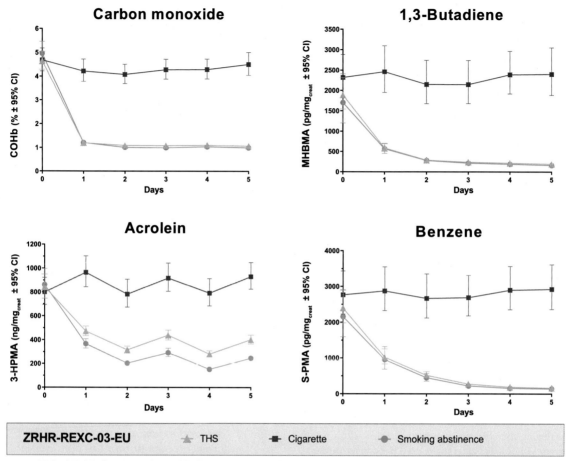

FIG. 17.10 Concentrations of BoExps to four HPHCs at baseline and over 5 days of ad libitum use of THS and cigarettes and smoking abstinence in the REXC-03-EU study. *3-HPMA*, 3-hydroxypropylmercapturic acid; *BoExp*, biomarker of exposure; *CI*, confidence interval; *COHb*, carboxyhemoglobin; *HPHC*, harmful and potentially harmful constituents of tobacco smoke, *MHBMA*, monohydroxybutenylmercapturic acid; *S-PMA*, S-phenylmercapturic acid; *THS*, Tobacco Heating System 2.2.

for the REXC-03-EU study in Fig. 17.11 (geometric means).

The results following the first 5 days in confinement were comparable across the REXC and REXA studies. The four BoExps tested for the primary objective—S-PMA, MHBMA, 3-HPMA, and COHb—were significantly reduced in both the THS and smoking abstinence groups and by a similar magnitude (Table 17.12, calculated as geometric means). All other BoExps also showed comparable reductions among the studies, except S-BMA, a marker for toluene, which proved to be not fit for purpose, as it could not distinguish smoking abstinent subjects from smokers. The reductions were generally more than 50%, but could be up to 97% for certain BoExps.

17.5.1.5 Reduced exposure studies in an ambulatory setting (REXA)

The results of the first 5-day exposure are presented in the previous section, as these data were obtained in confinement, as in the REXC studies. However, the profiles of the BoExp levels over time in the REXA-08-US study also show the confinement period results (first 5 days) (Figs. 17.12 and 17.13; geometric means).

The baseline demographic data were balanced across the studies (e.g., sex, race, age, body mass index, nicotine dependence, and smoking intensity) (Fig. 17.8). The results over 3 months were also consistent between the two REXA studies conducted in an ambulatory setting. Fig. 17.12 shows the results of the REXA-08-

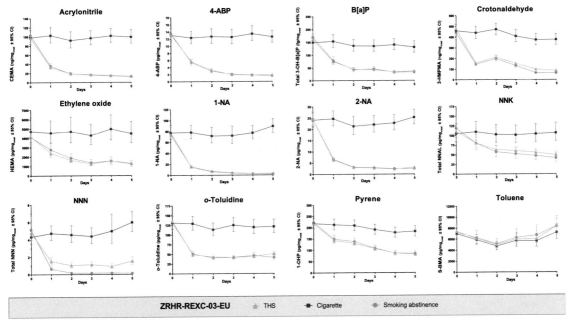

FIG. 17.11 Concentrations of BoExps to 12 HPHCs at baseline and over 5 days of ad libitum use of THS and cigarettes and smoking abstinence in the REXC-03-EU study. *1-NA*, 1-aminonaphthalene; *1-OHP*, total 1-hydroxypyrene; *2-NA*, 2-aminonaphthalene; *3-HMPMA*, 3-hydroxy-1-methylpropyl-mercapturic acid; *3-OH-B[a]P*, 3-hydroxybenzo[a]pyrene; *4-ABP*, 4-aminobiphenyl; *B[a]P*, benzo[a]pyrene; *BoExp*, biomarker of exposure; *CEMA*, 2-cyanoethylmercapturic acid; *CI*, confidence interval; *creat*, creatinine; *HEMA*, 2-hydroxyethylmercapturic acid; *HPHC*, harmful and potentially harmful constituents of tobacco smoke; *NNAL*, 4-(methylnitrosamino)-1-(3-pyridyl)-1-butanol; *NNK*, 4-methylnitrosamino-1-(3-pyridyl)-1-butanone; *NNN*, N-nitrosonornicotine; *S-BMA*, S-benzylmercapturic acid; *THS*, Tobacco Heating System 2.2.

US study, with the five BoExps measured as primary endpoints showing comparable dose–response curves in the THS switching and smoking abstinence groups. Both the mTHS and smoking abstinence groups had a significant reduction in BoExps relative to the smoking group.

Similar patterns of change were seen in CEMA, 4-ABP, total 3-OH-B[a]P, 3-HMPMA, HEMA, 1-NA, 2-NA, total NNAL, total NNN, o-toluidine, and total 1-OHP levels throughout the studies. The reductions in BoExp levels were of a similar magnitude in the THS and smoking abstinence groups. As in the other studies, S-BMA levels did not show any difference across the study arms. These data are shown for the REXA-08-US study in Fig. 17.13 (geometric means).

These findings reinforce the overall theme that switching to THS results in a reduced exposure to HPHCs that is similar to smoking abstinence.

All four BoExps measured as primary endpoints on day 5 were still significantly reduced in both the THS and smoking abstinence groups and by a similar magnitude on day 90. The total NNAL levels measured as a primary endpoint on day 5 had decreased even further on day 90 (56% on day 5 vs. ~75% on day 90) (Table 17.13, calculated as geometric means). Except S-BMA, the other BoExps also showed sustained reductions between day 5 and day 90, with values that were generally slightly less on day 90 than on day 5, likely reflecting the ambulatory conditions, where no restrictions could be imposed. The reductions varied from slightly less than 50% to more than 90%.

In summary, the clinical studies demonstrated a consistent reduction in BoExps in smokers who switched to THS and smoking abstinence. These changes were evident as early as 5 days following the switch and were preserved throughout the 90-day duration of the REXA studies. The reductions seen in the THS group were similar in both magnitude and direction to those seen upon smoking abstinence. This is plausible, given that THS aerosol contains HPHC levels that are reduced by over 90% relative to cigarette smoke.

TABLE 17.12

Summary of the reduced exposure study results: BoExp (100—[THS:CC] ratio and 100—[SA:CC] ratio in %) on day 5.

BoExp	HPHC	Comparison	REXC-03-EU Reduction (%) (95% CI)	REXC-04-JP Reduction (%) (95% CI)	REXA-07-JP Reduction (%) (95% CI)	REXA-08-US Reduction (%) (95% CI)
COHb (%)	CO	THS:CC	−77% (−75.0, −78.0)	−53% (−49.9, −55.7)	−55% (−57.9, −52)	−62% (−65.8, −57.5)
		SA:CC	−78.32% (−79.9, −76.7)	−53.85% (−57.0, −50.4)	−54.74% (−58.0, −51.2)	−60.80% (−65.9, −54.9)
MHBMA (pg/mg creat)	1,3-Butadiene	THS:CC	−92% (−89.8, −93.1)	−77% (−81.6, −71.1)	−87% (−89, −83.4)	−87% (−90.7, −83)
		SA:CC	−92.7% (−94.2, −90.9)	−80.1% (−84.7, −74)	−86.5% (−89.3, −82.8)	−89.2% (−92.7, −84.2)
3-HPMA (ng/mg creat)	Acrolein	THS:CC	−58% (−54.1, −62.2)	−47% (−54.3, −38.8)	−49% (−55.1, −42.8)	−54% (−60.8, −46.6)
		SA:CC	−74.7% (−77.4, −71.6)	−65.4% (−70.8, −58.9)	−69.5% (−73.5, −64.9)	−75.0% (−79.5, −69.4)
S-PMA (pg/mg creat)	Benzene	THS:CC	−94% (−93.1, −94.8)	−84% (−86.9, −81.2)	−89% (−90.7, −87)	−87% (−90.5, −83.4)
		SA:CC	−94% (−95.2, −93.4)	−86% (−89.1, −83.4)	−90% (−92.1, −88.3)	−88% (−91.4, −82.5)
1-OHP (pg/mg creat)	Pyrene	THS:CC	−56% (−50.7, −60.1)	−54% (−58.7, −47.8)	−61% (−65.2, −55.9)	−52% (−57.9, −45)
		SA:CC	−54% (−59.4, −48.1)	−56% (−61.3, −49.1)	−64% (−68.8, −59.1)	−64% (−61.4, −45.6)
Total NNN (pg/mg creat)	NNN	THS:CC	−76% (−67.3, −82.2)	−70% (−76.3, −61.9)	−73% (−78.3, −64.5)	−86% (−57.9, −45)
		SA:CC	−98% (−98.3, −96.5)	−96% (−97, −94.8)	−97% (−97.3, −95.6)	−98% (−98.6, −96.9)
4-ABP (pg/mg creat)	4-ABP	THS:CC	−85% (−87.1, −82.7)	−82% (−84.7, −78.3)	−80% (−82.9, −76.4)	−81% (−85.1, −75)
		SA:CC	−87% (−89.4, −85)	−82% (−85.7, −78.5)	−77% (−80.7, −71.9)	−84% (−88.6, −77.6)
1-NA (pg/mg creat)	1-NA	THS:CC	−96% (−96.9, −95.6)	−96% (−96.2, −94.8)	−94% (−95.1, −93.4)	−96% (−96.7, −94.8)
		SA:CC	−97% (−97.6, −96.5)	−95% (−96.4, −94.9)	−95% (−95.4, −93.6)	−96% (−97.4, −95.2)
2-NA (pg/mg creat)	2-NA	THS:CC	−88% (−89.9, −86.8)	−82% (−85.3, −78.9)	−86% (−88.0, −84.5)	−87% (−89.5, −83.6)
		SA:CC	−90% (−91.5, −88.4)	−83% (−86.3, −79.1)	−85% (−87.1, −82.8)	−88% (−91, −83.9)
Total NNAL (pg/mg creat)	NNK	THS:CC	−56% (−60.7, −51.8)	−51% (−58.1, −42.7)	−56% (−60.4, −51.8)	−56% (−63.1, −48.0)
		SA:CC	−66% (−69.6, −61.5)	−62% (−68.7, −55)	−63% (−67.4, −59.1)	−56% (−64.9, −45.4)
o-tol (pg/mg creat)	o-toluidine	THS:CC	−56% (−64.0, −51.7)	−49% (−57.7, −39.6)	−56% (−63.7, −47.2)	−51% (−60.3, −40.2)
		SA:CC	−66% (−71, −59.2)	−50% (−59.1, −37.9)	−57% (−65.6, −47.2)	−62% (−71, −50.7)
CEMA (pg/mg creat)	Acrylonitrile	THS:CC	−87% (−88.4, −85.1)	−79% (−81.9, −75.1)	−82% (−83.8, −79.4)	−83% (−85.6, −79.5)
		SA:CC	−88% (−89.6, −86.0)	−82% (−84.9, −78.1)	−83% (−85.2, −80.4)	−84% (−87.0, −79.6)
HEMA (pg/mg creat)	Ethylene oxide	THS:CC	−88% (−72.9, −62.2)	−51% (−60.5, −45.3)	−50% (−55.9, −43)	−61% (−68.8, −50.8)

TABLE 17.12
Summary of the reduced exposure study results: BoExp (100—[THS:CC] ratio and 100—[SA:CC] ratio in %) on day 5.—cont'd

BoExp	HPHC	Comparison	REXC-03-EU Reduction (%) (95% CI)	REXC-04-JP Reduction (%) (95% CI)	REXA-07-JP Reduction (%) (95% CI)	REXA-08-US Reduction (%) (95% CI)
		SA:CC	−70% (−75.1, −63.4)	−60% (−67.2, −52.1)	−51% (−57.7, −43)	−63% (−72.1, −49.8)
3-OH-B[a]P (fg/mg creat)	B[a]P	THS:CC	−73% (−76.8, −67.5)	−70% (−75.2, −63.8)	−73% (−76.8, −68.1)	−71% (−76.9, −63.8)
		SA:CC	−75% (−79.7, −70.1)	−75% (−80.2, −69.2)	−75% (−79.6, −70.4)	−81% (−85.9, −74.5)
HMPMA (ng/mg creat)	Crotonaldehyde	THS:CC	−77% (−79.9, −74.7)	−62% (−68.4, −55.0)	−57% (−62.3, −59.9)	−62% (−69.3, −52.4)
		SA:CC	−83% (−85.1, −80.6)	−69% (−74.9, −61.9)	−61% (−66.2, −54.3)	−68% (−76.2, −58.0)

1-NA, 1-aminonaphthalene; *1-OHP*, total 1-hydroxypyrene; *2-NA*, 2-aminonaphthalene; *3-HMPMA*, 3-hydroxy-1-methylpropyl-mercapturic acid; *3-HPMA*, 3-hydroxypropylmercapturic acid; *3-OH-B[a]P*, 3-hydroxybenzo[a]pyrene; *4-ABP*, 4-aminobiphenyl; *B[a]P*, benzo[a]pyrene; *BoExp*, biomarker of exposure; *CC*, cigarettes; *CEMA*, 2-cyanoethylmercapturic acid; *CI*, confidence interval; *COHb*, carboxyhemoglobin; *creat*, creatinine; *HEMA*, 2-hydroxyethylmercapturic acid; *HPHC*, harmful and potentially harmful constituents of tobacco smoke; *MHBMA*, monohydroxybutenylmercapturic acid; *NNAL*, 4-(methylnitrosamino)-1-(3-pyridyl)-1-butanol; *NNK*, 4-methylnitrosamino-1-(3-pyridyl)-1-butanone; *NNN*, N-nitrosonornicotine; *o-tol*, o-toluidine; *SA*, smoking abstinence; *S-BMA*, S-benzylmercapturic acid; *S-PMA*, S-phenylmercapturic acid; *THS*, Tobacco Heating System 2.2.

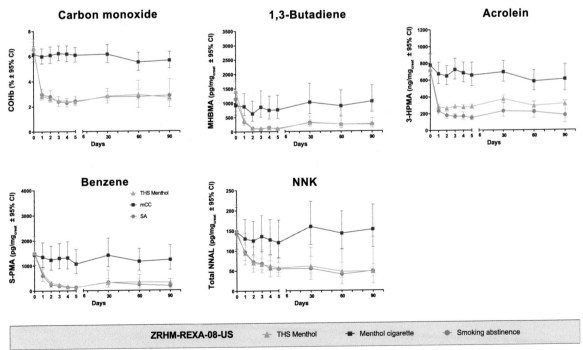

FIG. 17.12 Concentrations of BoExps to 5 HPHCs at baseline and over 90 days of ad libitum use of THS and cigarettes and smoking abstinence (including 5 days in confinement) in the REXA-08-US study. *3-HPMA*, 3-hydroxypropylmercapturic acid; *BoExp*, biomarker of exposure; *CI*, confidence interval; *COHb*, carboxyhemoglobin; *creat*, creatinine; *HPHC*, harmful and potentially harmful constituents of tobacco smoke; *MHBMA*, monohydroxy-butenylmercapturic acid; *NNAL*, 4-(methylnitrosamino)-1-(3-pyridyl)-1-butanol; *NNK*, 4-methylnitrosamino-1-(3-pyridyl)-1-butanone; *S-PMA*, S-phenylmercapturic acid; *THS*, Tobacco Heating System 2.2.

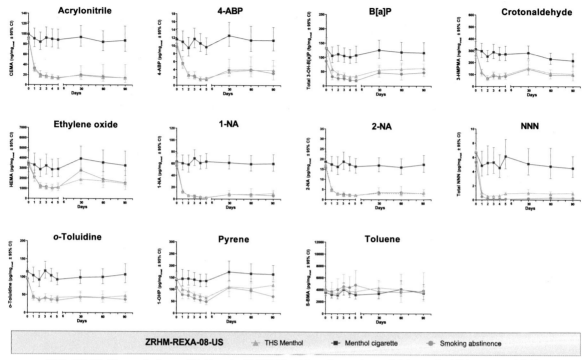

FIG. 17.13 Concentrations of BoExps to 11 HPHCs at baseline and over 90 days of ad libitum use of THS and cigarettes and smoking abstinence (including 5 days in confinement) in the REXA-08-US study. *1-NA*, 1-aminonaphthalene; *1-OHP*, total 1-hydroxypyrene; *2-NA*, 2-aminonaphthalene; *3-HMPMA*, 3-hydroxy-1-methylpropyl-mercapturic acid; *3-OH-B[a]P*, 3-hydroxybenzo[a]pyrene; *4-ABP*, 4-aminobiphenyl; *B[a]P*, benzo[a]pyrene; *BoExp*, biomarker of exposure; *CEMA*, 2-cyanoethylmercapturic acid; *CI*, confidence interval; *creat*, creatinine; *HEMA*, 2-hydroxyethylmercapturic acid; *HPHC*, harmful and potentially harmful constituents of tobacco smoke; *NNN*, N-nitrosonornicotine; *S-BMA*, S-benzylmercapturic acid; *THS*, Tobacco Heating System 2.2.

17.5.1.6 CYP1A2 activity across reduced exposure studies

The profiles of CYP1A2 activity across the studies are presented in Fig. 17.14, and the values are presented in Table 17.14.

In all studies, the profiles of CYP1A2 activity in the THS arms showed a decrease comparable to that in the smoking abstinence arms (Fig. 17.14). The maximum decrease was observed as early as on 5 days, and the enzyme activity then remained stable until day 90 in the REXA-07-JP and REXA-08-US studies. In contrast, CYP1A2 activity in the cigarette arms remained consistently higher than that in the other arms, except in REXA-08-US, where a decrease was observed on day 90 to levels comparable to those in the other arms. This might be attributable to the high variability observed in this study, as there is no other plausible explanation for this drop.

During the confinement period, the differences in CYP1A2 activity between the THS and cigarette arms were −33.60% and −21.65% in the REXC-03-EU and REXC-04-JP studies, respectively. The corresponding reductions (in percentage) in the REXA-07-EU and REXA-08-US studies were −28.04% and −36.48%, respectively (Table 17.14); these reductions were largely maintained on day 90 (−30.91% and −21.43%, respectively). The differences between the THS and smoking abstinent arms, on the other hand, were comparable across studies and over time.

Because switching to THS reverses the smoking-induced increase in CYP1A2 levels to those comparable to what is observed when smokers quit (Haziza et al., 2016a, 2016b; Lüdicke et al., 2018b), it might be necessary to reduce the dosing of certain drugs metabolized by CYP1A2 when switching to THS. Close monitoring of patients taking drugs with narrow therapeutic indices

TABLE 17.13

Summary of the reduced exposure study results: BoExp (100—[THS:CC] ratio and 100—[THS:SA] ratio in %] on day 90.

BoExp	HPHC	Comparison	ZRHM-REXA-07-JP Reduction (%) (95% CI)	ZRHM-REXA-08-US Reduction (%) (95% CI)
COHb (%)	CO	THS:CC	−48% (−51.9, −44.4)	−53% (−60.3, −45)
		THS:SA	−3% (−10, 4.7)	−10% (−30.1, 17.2)
		SA:CC	−47% (−51.0, −42)	−48% (−60.4, −32.6)
MHBMA (pg/mg creat)	1,3-Butadiene	THS:CC	−81% (−85.3, −75.4)	−81% (−87.2, −73.3)
		THS:SA	1% (−22.3, 32.2)	−35% (−63.1, 13.7)
		SA:CC	−81% (−86.1, −74.7)	−71% (−83.8, −49.4)
3-HPMA (ng/mg creat)	Acrolein	THS:CC	−46% (−53.1, −37.7)	−48% (−59.2, −33.7)
		THS:SA	39% (19.7, 60.3)	47% (1.2, 114.5)
		SA:CC	−61% (−66.8, −54.0)	−65% (−76.1, −47.9)
S-PMA (pg/mg creat)	Benzene	THS:CC	−87% (−90.1, −83.4)	−78% (−86.5, −63.9)
		THS:SA	−1% (−24.3, 28.9)	18% (−44.7, 149.6)
		SA:CC	−87% (−90.4, −82.6)	−81% (−91.4, −59.0)
1-OHP (pg/mg creat)	Pyrene	THS:CC	−48% (−55.2, −39.6)	−34% (−47.3, −16.2)
		THS:SA	−5% (−18.7, 10.5)	15% (−20.2, 64.9)
		SA:CC	−45% (−53.8, −34.8)	−42% (−59.8, −16.5)
Total NNN (pg/mg creat)	NNN	THS:CC	−71% (−78.5, −60.0)	−82% (−87.7, −74.3)
		THS:SA	389% (254.6, 573.1)	169% (53.1, 371.0)
		SA:CC	−94% (−95.8, −91.4)	−93% (−96.3, −88.2)
4-ABP (pg/mg creat)	4-ABP	THS:CC	−79% (−83, −74.1)	−72% (−80.5, −58.4)
		THS:SA	−14% (−31, 6.6)	2% (−43.2, 81.9)
		SA:CC	−76% (−80.8, −68.8)	−72% (−84.6, −48.9)
1-NA (pg/mg creat)	1-NA	THS:CC	−94% (−95.3, −91.8)	−86% (−90.5, −78.4)
		THS:SA	−19% (−39.1, 8.5)	34% (−28.9, 152.3)
		SA:CC	−92% (−94.4, −89.5)	−89% (−94.5, −79.5)
2-NA (pg/mg creat)	2-NA	THS:CC	−85% (−87.0, −81.6)	−84% (−88.1, −78.3)
		THS:SA	−15% (−28.7, 2.5)	−16% (−47.4, 33)
		SA:CC	−82% (−85.2, −77.9)	−81% (−88.1, −69.0)
Total NNAL (pg/mg creat)	NNK	THS:CC	−77% (−82.6, −68.9)	−74% (−24.8, 60.4)
		THS:SA	51% (11.6, 103.9)	−24% (−50.6, 57.2)
		SA:CC	−85% (−89.0, −78.4)	−65% (−82.1, −32.5)
o-tol (pg/mg creat)	o-toluidine	THS:CC	−41% (−58, −16.7)	−57% (−82.7, −59.7)
		THS:SA	−13% (−38, 22.8)	12% (−60.1, 44.6)
		SA:CC	−32% (−54.1, 0.3)	−61% (−76.1, −37.6)
CEMA (pg/mg creat)	Acrylonitrile	THS:CC	−91% (−93.0, −88.0)	−86% (−68, −41.5)
		THS:SA	−8% (−30.4, 21.3)	−18% (−29.2, 77.4)
		SA:CC	−90% (−92.7, −86.4)	−83% (−91.6, −63.9)
HEMA (pg/mg creat)	Ethylene oxide	THS:CC	−55% (−62.8, −45.6)	−62% (−91, −77.3)
		THS:SA	2% (−16.2, 24.2)	−22% (−59.4, 66.2)
		SA:CC	−56% (−64.6, −45.1)	50% (−69.5, −19.7)
3-OH-B[a]P (fg/mg creat)	B[a]P	THS:CC	−67% (−74.1, −57.9)	−57% (−71.7, −47.6)
		THS:SA	−4% (−25.4, 23.4)	−7% (−51.9, 24.1)
		SA:CC	−66% (−74.0, −54.5)	−53% (−71.5, −23.7)
HMPMA (ng/mg creat)	Crotonaldehyde	THS:CC	−50% (−57, −41.1)	−50% (−68.5, −40.4)
		THS:SA	−4% (−18.5, 12.9)	2% (−42.9, 51.2)
		SA:CC	−48% (−56.3, −37.1)	−52% (−69.2, −23.8)

1-NA, 1-aminonaphthalene; *1-OHP*, total 1-hydroxypyrene; *2-NA*, 2-aminonaphthalene; *3-HPMA*, 3-hydroxy-1-methylpropyl-mercapturic acid; *3-HPMA*, 3-hydroxypropylmercapturic acid; *3-OH-B[a]P*, 3-hydroxybenzo[a]pyrene; *4-ABP*, 4-aminobiphenyl; *B[a]P*, benzo[a]pyrene; *BoExp*, biomarker of exposure; *CC*, cigarettes; *CEMA*, 2-cyanoethylmercapturic acid; *CI*, confidence interval; *COHb*, carboxyhemoglobin; *creat*, creatinine; *HEMA*, 2-hydroxyethylmercapturic acid; *HPHC*, harmful and potentially harmful constituents of tobacco smoke; *MHBMA*, monohydroxybutenylmercapturic acid; *NNAL*, 4-(methylnitrosamino)-1-(3-pyridyl)-1-butanol; *NNK*, 4-methylnitrosamino-1-(3-pyridyl)-1-butanone; *NNN*, N-nitrosonornicotine; *o-tol*, *o*-toluidine; *SA*, smoking abstinence; *S-BMA*, S-benzylmercapturic acid; *S-PMA, S*-phenylmercapturic acid; *THS*, Tobacco Heating System 2.2.

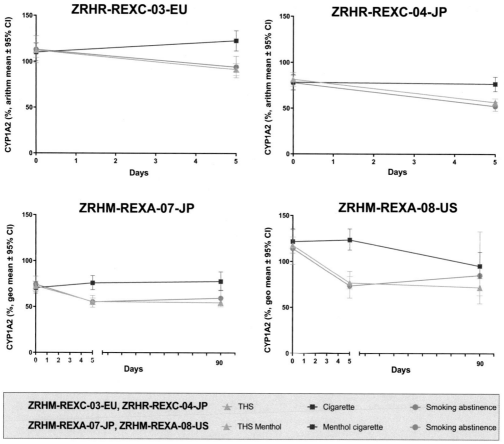

FIG. 17.14 CYP1A2 activity in reduced exposure studies. *Arithm*, arithmetic; *CI*, confidence interval; *CYP*, cytochrome P450; *geo*, geometric; *THS*, Tobacco Heating System 2.2.

is necessary during the first weeks of switching to such ENDPs.

17.5.1.7 Product use behavior

This section describes the assessment of product use behavior, including nicotine uptake, level of consumption, and HPT.

17.5.1.7.1 Nicotine uptake and product use. The profiles of NEQ in the four studies are shown in Fig. 17.15. In parallel, daily product use was recorded by the study site staff during the confinement period and by the subjects themselves during the ambulatory period (self-reporting). The profiles of daily consumption of THS and cigarette in the four studies are shown in Fig. 17.16.

These data clearly show that, at baseline, the levels of NEQ depend largely on the amount of product used per day, with subjects in Poland exhibiting the highest levels of NEQ and product use throughout the study. This is in line with the fact that the Polish population has been shown to have a high prevalence of heavy smokers (Jassem et al., 2014). Conversely, subjects in Japan had consistently lower levels of NEQ and product use.

The NEQ concentrations were comparable between the THS and cigarette arms within the studies and remained close to baseline values, except for a decrease in the THS arm of REXA-08-US during the confinement period, which could be indicative of some difficulty in adapting to the product (Fig. 17.15). Cigarette consumption in the cigarette arms throughout each study remained largely unchanged. Because no cigarette use was allowed in the smoking abstinence arms during the confinement period, all NEQ levels decreased consistently, reaching the lowest after 5 days. In the

TABLE 17.14
Summary of CYP1A2 activity across studies, including differences and reductions (100—[THS:CC] ratio and 100—[THS:SA] ratio in %).

	Group	ZRHR-REXC-03-EU [LS means and (95% CI)]	ZRHR-REXC-04-JP [LS means and (95% CI)]	ZRHM-REXA-07-JP [Geo means and (95% CI)]	ZRHM-REXA-08-US [Geo means and (95% CI)]
Baseline	CC	110.26 (100.69, 119.83)	78.21 (69.82, 86.60)	70.45 (64.48, 76.97)	121.60 (109.16, 135.46)
	THS	112.43 (104.41, 120.44)	81.32 (73.88, 88.76)	72.43 (67.46, 77.77)	117.60 (109.21, 126.63)
	SA	113.14 (98.40, 127.88)	77.59 (69.57, 85.62)	74.18 (66.13, 83.21)	114.03 (96.68, 134.49)
Day 5	CC	123.01 (112.07, 133.95)	76.50 (68.68, 84.31)	75.84 (68.41, 84.07)	123.55 (112.66, 135.50)
	THS	91.71 (85.18, 98.24)	56.56 (52.34, 60.78)	55.62 (52.02, 59.47)	76.70 (70.33, 83.64)
	SA	94.45 (82.59, 106.31)	52.25 (47.40, 57.11)	55.34 (49.35, 62.05)	73.44 (60.32, 89.40)
	THS—CC	−33.60 (−40.59, −26.61)	−21.65 (−25.49, −17.81)	NA	NA
	THS—SA	−1.99 (−9.10, 5.12)	2.29 (−1.62, 6.19)	NA	NA
	THS:CC ratio	NA	NA	−28.04 (−32.88, −22.84)	−36.48 (30.83, 41.66)
	THS:SA ratio	NA	NA	2.43 (−4.62, 10.00)	1.54 (−7.86, 11.89)
Day 90	CC	NA	NA	77.67 (68.27, 88.37)	95.14 (81.90, 110.51)
	THS	NA	NA	54.57 (50.23, 59.28)	71.82 (63.16, 81.68)
	SA	NA	NA	59.51 (52.28, 67.74)	85.02 (54.41, 132.83)
	THS:CC ratio	NA	NA	−30.91 (−38.55, −22.32)	−21.43 (−33.64, −6.98)
	THS: SA ratio	NA	NA	−7.52 (−18.05, 4.35)	5.34 (−19.51, 37.86)

CC, cigarettes, *CI*, confidence interval; *CYP*, cytochrome P450; *LS*, least squares; *NA*, not available; *SA*, smoking abstinence; *THS*, Tobacco Heating System 2.2.

two REXA studies, the levels of urinary NEQ concentrations were generally maintained on day 90 and comparable in the THS and cigarette arms. The NEQ levels in the THS arms indicate that the subjects were able to adapt to THS use, thereby getting exposed to comparable levels of nicotine as they would have if they were still smoking cigarettes. In contrast to the smoking abstinence arm in the REXA-07-JP study, where the NEQ levels during the ambulatory period remained within the same range as those observed during the confinement period, the levels of NEQ in the smoking abstinence arm of the REXA-08-US study increased slightly during the transition from confinement to ambulatory settings. Nevertheless, at the end of the ambulatory period on day 90, the NEQ levels were still largely lower.

An initial decrease in product consumption was observed in the THS arm during the confinement period in the REXC-4-JP study, while the THS arms in REXC-03-EU and REXA-08-US showed an increase in product consumption. During the ambulatory period, THS tobacco stick consumption initially decreased in both studies, but then returned to levels comparable to the baseline.

During the ambulatory period, compliance to the product/regimen allocation in the REXA-07-JP study was particularly high in all three arms, while the compliance in the smoking abstinence group of the REXA-08-US study was poor (7—9 of 41 subjects).

In summary, nicotine exposure and product use varied across studies, but the profiles of urinary NEQ and amount of daily product use in the four studies mostly remained comparable between the THS and cigarette arms, indicating that THS delivers nicotine to the users at levels comparable to those delivered by cigarettes.

17.5.1.7.2 Human puffing topography. A total of 18 parameters were recorded by using the HPT SODIM

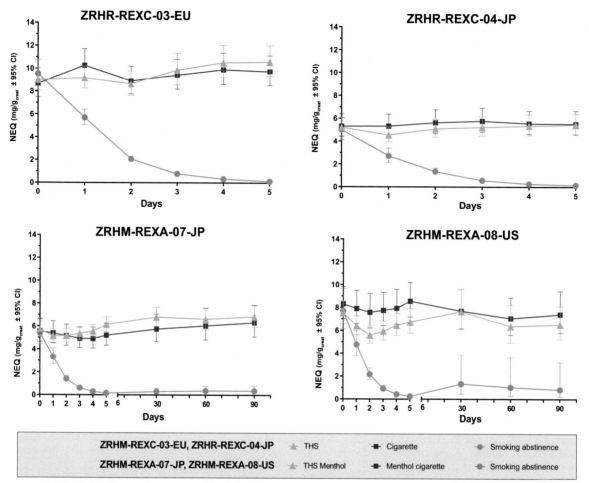

FIG. 17.15 Geometric means and 95% CIs of urinary NEQ concentrations (mg/g creat) during the course of the four reduced exposure studies. *CI*, confidence interval; *creat*, creatinine; *NEQ*, nicotine equivalent; *THS*, Tobacco Heating System 2.2.

device, model SPA/M (SODIM Instrumentation, Fleury les Aubrais, France). Of these, seven parameters are reported here, including 3 at the puff level (average puff volume, puff duration, and pressure drop; Table 17.15) and 4 at the product use level (total puff volume, total number of puffs, total smoking duration, and puff frequency; Table 17.16). These seven parameters were selected because they reflect how the users changed or adapted their puffing at an average puff level (i.e., by changing the puffing duration and inhaled volume) while, at the same time, undergoing a full product use experience (i.e., at the product use level, by changing the puffing frequency). The other parameters either were correlated to the selected parameters (e.g., pressure drop was correlated to flow and resistance) or were

technical parameters (e.g., work) describing the intrinsic properties of THS. HPT parameters were assessed on day 1 and day 4 of the confinement period and additionally on day 90 of the two 90-day studies.

17.5.1.7.2.1 Per-puff parameters. Fig. 17.17 shows graphical representations of the geometric values of the per-puff parameters throughout the study duration for all studies.

17.5.1.7.2.1.1 Average puff volume. There were variations across the studies in how subjects switching to THS changed their puffing topography, particularly in the HPT parameter average puff volume (Fig. 17.17).

The THS:cigarette ratios for average puff volume on day 4 in REXC-03-EU and REXA-08-US were 106%

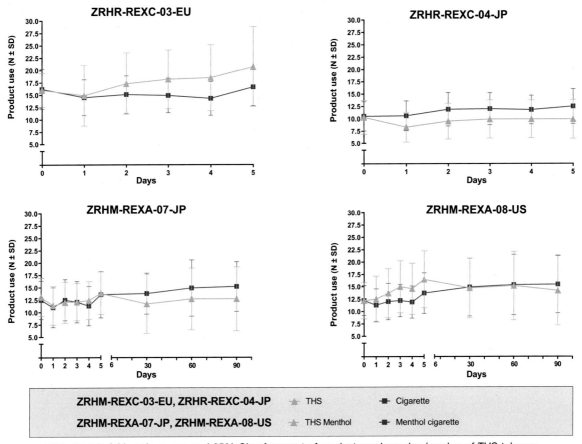

FIG. 17.16 Arithmetic means and 95% CIs of amount of product used per day (number of THS tobacco sticks or cigarettes) during the course of the four reduced exposure studies.   *CI*, confidence interval; *creat*, creatinine; *N*, number; *SD*, standard deviation; *THS*, Tobacco Heating System 2.2.

and 113%, respectively, while those in REXC-04-JP and REXA-07-JP were 85% and 91%, respectively (Table 17.17).

During the ambulatory period in REXA-07-JP and REXA-08-US, the THS:cigarette ratios for average puff volume were at 81% and 98% on day 90, respectively, indicating a small decrease during the ambulatory period in the US study relative to the confinement period.

In conclusion, the average puff volume for THS varied among the different populations, with comparable values to the baseline and cigarette arm in ZRHR-REXC-03-EU and a decreased volume from baseline for THS in Japan. In the US, the values for THS during most of the study period were higher than the baseline values as well as the values in the cigarette arm; these values returned close to baseline levels at the end of the ambulatory period. This suggests different patterns of adaptation to THS across the populations, with a

reduction in average puff volume in Japan and a stable puff volume in the non-Japanese regions. Adaptation to THS in Japan (REXA-07-JP) seemed faster than that in the US.

17.5.1.7.2.1.2 Average puff duration. When using a novel tobacco product, it is expected that users might change their puffing behavior to adapt to the intrinsic properties of the new product, such as altering their normal puffing duration. Average puff duration was another parameter that differed across the four studies (Fig. 17.17).

The THS:cigarette ratios for average puff duration on day 4 in REXC-03-EU and REXA-08-US were 132% and 124%, respectively, while those in REXC-04-JP and REXA-07-JP were 102% and 117%, respectively (Table 17.18).

During the ambulatory period in REXA-07-JP and REXA-08-US, the THS:cigarette ratios for average puff

TABLE 17.15
Human puffing topography—Per-puff parameters.

Description	Variable	Unit
Average puff volume	Vi	mL
Average puff duration	Di	s
Average pressure drop	Pmi	mmWG

mmWg, millimeters, water gauge, or mmH$_2$O.

TABLE 17.16
Human puffing topography—Per-product use.

Description	Variable	Formula	Unit
Total number of puffs	NPC	$\sum Ni$	
Total puff volume	TVOL	$\sum Vi$	mL
Total smoking duration	TDFi	$\sum DFi$	s
Puff frequency	PFeq	NPC/(TDFi/60)	

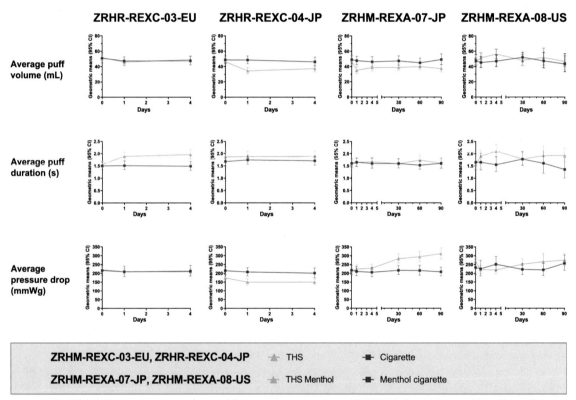

FIG. 17.17 Geometric means of per-puff topography parameters with 95% CIs by study arm at baseline and on day 1, day 4, day 30, day 60, and day 90 in ZRHR-REXC-03-EU, ZRHR-REXC-04-JP, ZRHM-REXA-07-JP, and ZRHM-REXA-08-US. *CI*, confidence interval; *THS*, Tobacco Heating System 2.2.

duration were at 114% and 116% on day 90, respectively, which confirmed the trend toward an increase in puff duration with THS.

In conclusion, in the Japanese studies, the average puff duration with THS was comparable to that at baseline and in the cigarette arm, particularly when considering the profile over time; in contrast, the puffing duration with THS in the Polish study was increased relative to the baseline and cigarette arm. In the US study, the puffing duration was variable, although the values for THS remained higher than those for cigarettes.

17.5.1.7.2.1.3 Average pressure drop. Change in pressure drop, an indicator of resistance to draw (how easy or difficult it is to draw a puff), is generally linked to the

TABLE 17.17
Average puff volume during the course of the four reduced exposure studies (mL, geometric means).

			ZRHR-REXC-03-EU	ZRHR-REXC-04-JP	ZRHM-REXA-07-JP	ZRHM-REXA-08-US
Baseline	CC	Mean	51.04	48.69	49.11	47.74
		95% CI	(44.85, 58.07)	(44.01, 53.87)	(43.95, 54.88)	(40.86, 55.77)
	THS	Mean	51.73	46.28	47.68	46.83
		95% CI	(48.16, 55.56)	(42.17, 50.8)	(42.46, 53.54)	(42.78, 51.25)
Day 4	CC	Mean	47.55	46.28	46.38	47.26
		95% CI	(42.31, 53.43)	(40.82, 52.46)	(40.56, 53.04)	(40.21, 55.55)
	THS	Mean	49.33	37.41	38.85	56.45
		95% CI	(45.02, 54.06)	(33.27, 42.07)	(34.25, 44.07)	(50.72, 62.82)
	THS:CC ratio (%)	Mean	105.50	85.45	91.44	112.64
		95% CI	(95.55, 116.48)	(75.93, 96.16)	(76.27, 109.63)	(96.03, 132.11)
Day 90	CC	Mean	NA	NA	49.33	43.59
		95% CI	NA	NA	(42.94, 56.68)	(33.27, 57.11)
	THS	Mean	NA	NA	37.50	46.75
		95% CI	NA	NA	(33.15, 42.42)	(40.34, 54.18)
	THS:CC ratio (%)	Mean			80.62	97.55
		95% CI			(69.91, 92.98)	(73.62, 129.25)

CC, cigarettes, CI, confidence interval; THS, Tobacco Heating System 2.2.

level of ventilation in the cigarette filter, which influences smoke yield and puffing behavior. An increase in pressure drop reflects the increased work required of the user to draw a puff from a product. Pressure drop is also related to the flow rate of aerosol through the mouthpiece of the HPT SODIM device. Average pressure drop was also a parameter that varied across the four studies (Fig. 17.17).

The THS:cigarette ratios for average pressure drop on day 4 in REXC-03-EU and REXA-08-US were 94% and 88%, respectively, while those in REXC-04-JP and REXA-07-JP were 90% and 112%, respectively (Table 17.19).

During the ambulatory period in REXA-07-JP and REXA-08-US, the THS:cigarette ratios for average puff duration were at 146% and 98% on day 90, respectively, which confirmed the trend toward increase in puff duration with THS.

In conclusion, the average pressure drop was stable overall and comparable in the THS and cigarette arms of each study during the study period, with the exception of a relative increase in average pressure drop with THS relative to cigarettes in REXA-07-JP

throughout the study period. The baseline values varied markedly among the four studies.

17.5.1.7.2.2 Per-product parameters. Fig. 17.18 shows graphical representations of the per-product parameters throughout the study duration for all studies.

The HPT parameter total number of puffs is a key parameter in a subject's individual puffing profile and one of the parameters most often affected when smokers adjust their puffing behavior after switching to a new product. In THS, the system limits the product use experience to a maximum of 6 min or 14 puffs, whichever comes first. The HPT SODIM device used for HPT assessment in PMI studies, however, is more sensitive in puff detection than the THS puff sensor and is, therefore, able to detect multipuffs (i.e., continuous puffing with varying intensity, such as intense puffing followed by continuous shallow puffing and intense puffing again). Therefore, the number of puffs can exceed the THS device limitation of 14 noncontiguous puffs.

The total number of puffs changed very little across the studies, with an overall slight increase in the

TABLE 17.18
Average puff duration during the course of the four reduced exposure studies (seconds, geometric means).

			ZRHR-REXC-03-EU	ZRHR-REXC-04-JP	ZRHM-REXA-07-JP	ZRHM-REXA-08-US
Baseline	CC	Mean	1.50	1.68	1.61	1.65
		95% CI	(1.35, 1.67)	(1.51, 1.86)	(1.45, 1.79)	(1.34, 2.01)
	THS	Mean	1.57	1.87	1.55	1.55
		95% CI	(1.44, 1.70)	(1.70, 2.05)	(1.39, 1.74)	(1.42, 1.70)
Day 4	CC	Mean	1.49	1.71	1.60	1.55
		95% CI	(1.32, 1.68)	(1.53, 1.91)	(1.41, 1.82)	(1.28, 1.88)
	THS	Mean	1.96	1.89	1.67	2.10
		95% CI	(1.78, 2.16)	(1.70, 2.1)	(1.50, 1.85)	(1.86, 2.37)
	THS:CC ratio (%)	Mean	132.25	102.64	116.65	124.27
		95% CI	(120.24, 145.46)	(93.42, 112.78)	(106.55, 127.71)	(109.32, 141.26)
Day 90	CC	Mean	NA	NA	1.61	1.36
		95% CI	NA	NA	(1.41, 1.82)	(1.01, 1.84)
	THS	Mean	NA	NA	1.61	1.93
		95% CI	NA	NA	(1.42, 1.82)	(1.68, 2.23)
	THS:CC ratio (%)	Mean	NA	NA	114.00	115.61
		95% CI	NA	NA	(100.50, 129.32)	(94.74, 141.08)

CC, cigarettes; *CI*, confidence interval; *THS*, Tobacco Heating System 2.2.

number of puffs in the THS arm, except in the REXC-03-EU study (Fig. 17.18).

The THS:cigarette ratios for total number of puffs on day 4 were 118%, 105%, and 115% in REXC-04-JP, REXA-07-JP, and REXA-08-US, respectively, and 97% in REXC-03-EU (Table 17.20).

During the ambulatory period in REXA-07-JP and REXA-08-US, the THS:cigarette ratios for average puff duration were 123% and 121% on day 90, respectively, which confirmed the trend toward increase in total number of puffs with THS.

In conclusion, the total number of puffs drawn increased when the smokers switched to THS. Except in REXC-03-EU, the values for THS were higher than those for cigarettes across the studies. The geometric mean values for total number of puffs exceeded the intrinsic limitation of the system (14 puffs), which suggests that users were adapting their puffing behavior by using a multipuff technique (i.e., not completely stopping inhalation between puffs). This is supported by the results of evaluation of individual profiles, which showed the presence of multiple peaks in some individual puffs.

17.5.1.7.2.2.1 Total puff volume. The HPT parameter total puff volume, expressed in mL, is a measure that estimates the subjects' exposure to a product (cigarettes and THS) at the mouth level.

Total puff volume profiles varied across the studies, with an overall stable profile in REXC-03-EU, a decrease in the THS arms during the confinement period in the two Japanese studies, and a marked continuous increase in the THS arm in REXA-08-US throughout the study period (Fig. 17.18).

The THS:cigarette ratios for total puff volume on day 4 in REXC-03-EU, REXC-04-JP, and REXA-07-JP were 105%, 99%, and 95%, respectively, while that in REXA-08-US was 130% (Table 17.21).

During the ambulatory period in REXA-07-JP and REXA-08-US, the THS:cigarette ratios for total puff volume were 99% and 120% on day 90, respectively, which confirmed an increase in total puff volume with THS in the US study.

TABLE 17.19

Average pressure drop during the course of the four reduced exposure studies (mmWg, geometric means).

			ZRHR-REXC-03-EU	ZRHR-REXC-04-JP	ZRHM-REXA-07-JP	ZRHM-REXA-08-US
Baseline	CC	Mean	215.90	214.74	217.68	232.81
		95% CI	(188.83, 246.85)	(194.16, 237.49)	(194.03, 244.23)	(194.19, 279.11)
	THS	Mean	220.78	174.33	211.15	266.31
		95% CI	(203.97, 238.96)	(155.47, 195.47)	(191.87, 232.36)	(243.19, 291.64)
Day 4	CC	Mean	212.23	201.18	206.12	251.74
		95% CI	(184.45, 244.19)	(175.47, 230.64)	(181.36, 234.26)	(214.14, 295.94)
	THS	Mean	208.48	150.26	229.35	219.38
		95% CI	(192.11, 226.23)	(133.97, 168.52)	(208.79, 251.93)	(198.27, 242.74)
	THS:CC ratio (%)	Mean	93.74	90.47	111.56	88.03
		95% CI	(83.72, 104.95)	(81.40, 100.55)	(102.45, 121.48)	(78.24, 99.04)
Day 90	CC	Mean	NA	NA	208.67	256.99
		95% CI	NA	NA	(185.38, 234.89)	(217.02, 304.32)
	THS	Mean	NA	NA	312.11	275.48
		95% CI	NA	NA	(281.80, 345.68)	(243.63, 311.50)
	THS:CC ratio (%)	Mean	NA	NA	145.98	97.94
		95% CI	NA	NA	(128.09, 166.37)	(78.78, 121.77)

CC, cigarettes; CI, confidence interval; mmWg, millimeters water gauge, or mmH$_2$O; THS, Tobacco Heating System 2.2.

In conclusion, in the Japanese studies, the total puff volume for THS decreased from the beginning of the confinement period but increased afterward, reaching levels comparable to those for cigarettes; however, the values remained generally lower than the baseline values throughout the study. In contrast, the total puff volumes remained stable in the European study (REXC-03-EU) and increased in the US study (REXA-08-US) from day 1 onwards, remaining at consistently higher levels than those at baseline and in the cigarette arm.

17.5.1.7.2.2.2 Total smoking duration. The HPT parameter total smoking duration, expressed in seconds, is a measure that estimates the subjects' duration of a product use experience, from the time of the first puff to the time of the last. In THS, the system limits the product use experience to a maximum of 6 min or 14 puffs, whichever comes first.

The total smoking duration profiles varied across the studies, with an overall relatively stable profile in the Japanese studies, where the total smoking duration with THS was slightly lower than that with cigarettes (REXC-04-JP and REXA-07-JP). In contrast, there was a more obvious decrease in total smoking duration in the THS groups during the confinement period in REXC-03-EU and REXA-08-US. This decrease was maintained throughout the ambulatory period in REXA-08-US (Fig. 17.18). The total smoking duration at baseline was markedly higher in REXA-08-US than in the other studies and remained higher over the study duration in the THS and cigarette arms in comparison with the remaining studies.

In REXC-03-EU, REXC-04-JP, REXA-07-JP, and REXA-08-US, the THS:cigarette ratios for total smoking duration were 78%, 93%, 91%, and 80% on day 4, respectively (Table 17.22).

During the ambulatory period in REXA-07-JP and REXA-08-US, the THS:cigarette ratios for total puff volume were 98% and 68% on day 90, respectively, which confirmed an increase in total puff volume with THS in the US study.

In conclusion, the total smoking duration was overall shorter with THS than with cigarettes, with a more pronounced decrease in the non-Japanese studies (REXC-03-EU and REXA-08-US). This reduction with THS might have been due to the intrinsic limitation

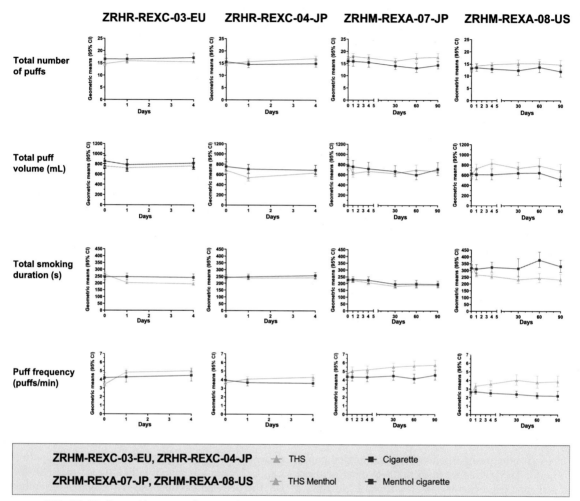

FIG. 17.18 Geometric means of per-product topography parameters with 95% CIs by study arm at baseline and on day 1, day 4, day 30, day 60, and day 90 in ZRHR-REXC-03-EU, ZRHR-REXC-04-JP, ZRHM-REXA-07-JP, and ZRHM-REXA-08-US. *CI*, confidence interval; *THS*, Tobacco Heating System 2.2.

of the THS system (maximum of 14 puffs or 6 min of product use, whichever comes first).

17.5.1.7.2.2.3 Puff frequency. Puff frequency is defined as the total number of puffs divided by the total smoking duration and offers an estimate of how often, on average, a subject takes a puff from a tobacco product during a defined period of time (puffs/min).

In all four studies, subjects who switched to THS had already increased their puff frequency on day 1, when they began to use THS, and stabilized by day 4 (Fig. 17.18). The puff frequency was higher for THS than for cigarettes, for which it remained stable overall throughout the studies. During the ambulatory period in REXA-07-JP and REXA-08-US, the puff frequency increased from day 4 to day 30 for THS, before stabilizing from day 30 onwards.

On day 4, the largest increases in puff frequency were observed in REXC-03-EU, REXC-04-JP, and REXA-08-US, with the THS:cigarette ratios being 132%, 127%, and 139%, respectively (Table 17.23).

During the ambulatory period in REXA-07-JP and REXA-08-US, the THS:cigarette ratios for total puff volume were 122% and 174% on day 90, respectively, which confirmed an increase in puff frequency with THS relative to cigarettes.

In conclusion, when subjects switched to THS, the puff frequency increased in all studies from day 1 until day 30, before stabilizing through day 90.

17.5.1.7.2.3 General conclusions on HPT. In summary, THS users took more puffs from THS than from cigarettes, at a higher frequency and for shorter total duration of use. The total puff volume was variable,

TABLE 17.20
Total number of puffs during the course of the four reduced exposure studies (number, geometric means).

			ZRHR-REXC-03-EU	ZRHR-REXC-04-JP	ZRHM-REXA-07-JP	ZRHM-REXA-08-US
Baseline	CC	Mean	16.62	15.55	15.98	13.14
		95% CI	(15.02, 18.39)	(14.22, 17.00)	(14.29, 17.87)	(11.65, 14.81)
	THS	Mean	14.66	14.72	17.27	12.84
		95% CI	(13.73, 15.66)	(13.70, 15.82)	(15.66, 19.03)	(11.92, 13.84)
Day 4	CC	Mean	17.20	14.89	15.49	12.88
		95% CI	(15.53, 19.05)	(13.56, 16.35)	(13.59, 17.66)	(11.45, 14.48)
	THS	Mean	15.54	16.97	17.31	14.78
		95% CI	(14.95, 16.16)	(15.96, 18.05)	(16.06, 18.66)	(14.00, 15.61)
	THS:CC ratio (%)	Mean	97.14	118.57	104.96	115.49
		95% CI	(89.42, 105.53)	(109.35, 128.57)	(90.58, 121.63)	(104.74, 127.33)
Day 90	CC	Mean	NA	NA	14.35	11.84
		95% CI	NA	NA	(12.90, 15.95)	(9.73, 14.42)
	THS	Mean	NA	NA	17.65	14.67
		95% CI	NA	NA	(16.17, 19.27)	(12.96, 16.61)
	THS:CC ratio (%)	Mean	NA	NA	122.76	121.01
		95% CI	NA	NA	(108.71, 138.63)	(92.51, 158.27)

CC, cigarettes; CI, confidence interval; THS, Tobacco Heating System 2.2.

with an increase over time observed in the US, a stable volume in Europe, and an initial decrease in the Japanese studies. No relevant changes were observed in subjects who continued to use their cigarettes.

Taken together, the results from the "at the puff level" and "at the product use experience level" analyses indicate that smokers switching from cigarettes to THS adapted their puffing behaviors. The changes in average and total puff volume varied among the studies, as did their effects on other parameters; but, a general trend for longer and more frequent puffs with a shorter total puff duration was observed for THS in comparison with cigarettes in all studies.

It is likely that differences in product satisfaction, ritual, sensorial experience, and taste caused the observed adaptation. The limit of 14 puffs or a maximum of 6 min for THS use might also have played a role.

17.5.1.7.3 Product acceptance—subjective effects
17.5.1.7.3.1 QSU-brief. The QSU-brief is the most widely used self-reported questionnaire for measuring

urge to smoke (refer to Section 17.2.1.3.2). In the context of the confinement studies, Fig. 17.19 shows graphical representations of the arithmetic mean values of the total QSU-brief scores.

During the confinement period, the total urge-to-smoke score for THS was stable and comparable to that of cigarettes (THS:cigarettes difference, −0.4 to 0.0 on day 5) across all studies and remained stable during the ambulatory period in REXA-07-JP and REXA-08-US, with slightly higher values for THS than cigarettes (THS:cigarettes differences, 0.32 and 0.4, respectively).

During the confinement period, the scores in the smoking abstinence arms were higher than those in the THS arms in REXC-03-EU and REXA-07-JP (difference, −1.6 and −1.4, respectively) but closer to the scores in the THS arms in REXC-04-JP and REXA-08-US (difference, −0.5 and −0.3, respectively). The values in the smoking abstinence arms continuously decreased from the end of the confinement (day 5) until the last day of the ambulatory period (THS—SA difference on day 90, 1.1 and 1.3).

TABLE 17.21

Total puff volume during the course of the four reduced exposure studies (mL, geometric means).

			ZRHR-REXC-03-EU	ZRHR-REXC-04-JP	ZRHM-REXA-07-JP	ZRHM-REXA-08-US
Baseline	CC	Mean	854.47	754.47	779.13	627.44
		95% CI	(756.87, 964.65)	(673.60, 845.05)	(677.44, 896.10)	(526.81, 747.29)
	THS	Mean	756.88	680.12	820.93	600.85
		95% CI	(713.79, 802.58)	(619.40, 746.78)	(725.60, 928.77)	(545.59, 661.70)
Day 4	CC	Mean	816.01	687.67	716.49	609.10
		95% CI	(730.21, 911.90)	(603.42, 783.68)	(606.54, 846.36)	(511.39, 725.48)
	THS	Mean	762.44	632.03	667.14	832.89
		95% CI	(699.70, 830.81)	(566.85, 704.71)	(578.59, 769.25)	(759.45, 913.43)
	THS:CC ratio (%)	Mean	105.26	99.24	95.11	130.10
		95% CI	(92.59, 119.65)	(85.90, 114.64)	(71.93, 125.76)	(108.82, 155.54)
Day 90	CC	Mean	NA	NA	707.20	516.65
		95% CI	NA	NA	(592.92, 843.52)	(383.35, 696.30)
	THS	Mean	NA	NA	663.21	685.37
		95% CI	NA	NA	(589.77, 745.79)	(571.73, 821.59)
	THS:CC ratio (%)	Mean	NA	NA	99.36	119.98
		95% CI	NA	NA	(84.98, 116.16)	(80.26, 179.37)

CC, cigarettes; CI, confidence interval; THS, Tobacco Heating System 2.2.

In conclusion, the effects on urge to smoke were stable and comparable between THS and cigarettes. The values in the smoking abstinence arms were higher than those in the THS arms during the confinement period, before decreasing continuously during the ambulatory period and reaching values lower than those in the THS and cigarette arms.

17.5.1.7.3.2 mCEQ. The mCEQ was employed in all studies to assess product evaluation (refer to Section 17.2.1.3.3). An example of the profiles of the individual scores of the mCEQ subscales (i.e., smoking satisfaction, craving reduction, enjoyment of respiratory tract sensation, psychological reward, and aversion) throughout the study is shown for REXA-08-US in Fig. 17.20 (arithmetic means). Graphical representations of the mCEQ subscale scores for THS and cigarettes at day 5 are presented in Fig. 17.21 and those at day 90 in Fig. 17.22 (arithmetic means).

During confinement in REXA-08-US, the subscale scores for THS showed a general trend for reduction on day 1, before stabilizing from day 2 to day 5 (Fig. 17.20). The different subscale scores then remained relatively stable throughout the study, with the scores for THS remaining lower than those for cigarettes. The aversion scores for THS were slightly higher than those for cigarettes during confinement, after which they remained fairly comparable to the cigarette scores during the ambulatory period.

On day 5 (Fig. 17.21), for all the parameters except aversion, the highest differences between THS and cigarettes were systematically reported in REXC-03-EU and the lowest in REXC-04-JP and REXA-07-JP. In the Japanese studies, craving reduction, enjoyment of respiratory tract sensation, psychological reward, and smoking satisfaction with THS were lower but close to those with cigarettes, with the differences being less than −0.7. The REXA-08-US scores for these domains were close to those of REXC-03-EU, while the differences in craving reduction and enjoyment of respiratory tract sensation were ≥1 between THS and cigarettes.

In REXA-07-JP, the scores for all domains on day 90 were comparable between THS and cigarettes (Fig. 17.21). In REXA-08-US, the aversion scores on day 90 remained comparable to those in the

TABLE 17.22
Total smoking duration during the course of the four reduced exposure studies (seconds, geometric means).

			ZRHR-REXC-03-EU	ZRHR-REXC-04-JP	ZRHM-REXA-07-JP	ZRHM-REXA-08-US
Baseline	CC	Mean	245.71	242.77	226.51	315.71
		95% CI	(223.60, 270.01)	(225.78, 261.05)	(205.70, 249.42)	(289.25, 344.60)
	THS	Mean	263.75	249.00	225.91	342.09
		95% CI	(249.49, 278.82)	(237.62, 260.92)	(208.55, 244.71)	(318.91, 366.95)
Day 4	CC	Mean	242.49	258.18	223.77	322.16
		95% CI	(220.00, 267.29)	(237.30, 280.90)	(198.99, 251.64)	(287.77, 360.66)
	THS	Mean	194.09	242.98	205.59	255.75
		95% CI	(182.94, 205.93)	(230.56, 256.08)	(189.65, 222.88)	(238.34, 274.43)
	THS:CC ratio (%)	Mean	77.64	92.91	91.09	80.43
		95% CI	(69.77, 86.41)	(85.22, 101.29)	(76.28, 108.77)	(70.30, 92.03)
Day 90	CC	Mean	NA	NA	194.62	329.70
		95% CI	NA	NA	(172.40, 219.70)	(288.08, 377.33)
	THS	Mean	NA	NA	188.07	231.07
		95% CI	NA	NA	(168.29, 210.19)	(196.81, 271.31)
	THS:CC ratio (%)	Mean	NA	NA	97.50	67.77
		95% CI	NA	NA	(82.55, 115.16)	(47.68, 96.33)

CC, cigarettes; *CI*, confidence interval; *THS*, Tobacco Heating System 2.2.

confinement period, while the differences between THS and cigarettes decreased over time, with the differences being ≤1 for all other domains.

In conclusion, no differences in aversion were observed between THS and cigarettes across the studies. For the other domains, regional differences were observed, with the scores being comparable between THS and cigarettes in REXC-04-JP and REXA-07-JP.

17.5.1.7.3.3 MNWS-R. The MNWS-R is a valid and reliable scale of craving and withdrawal symptoms. In our four studies, subjects were asked to rate items for the previous 24 h on a scale ranging from 0 to 4 (where 0 = none, 1 = slight, 2 = mild, 3 = moderate, and 4 = severe), and the total score was calculated by summing up the results of the first nine responses on the MNWS questionnaire.

Graphical representations of the arithmetic values are presented in Fig. 17.23.

The MNWS-R total score was not calculated in either REXC study. The results were instead assessed by means of MNWS total scores 1 and 2. In REXC-03-EU, total score

1 was slightly higher for THS than cigarettes at baseline and remained stable throughout the confinement period. In the smoking abstinence arm, total score 1 increased markedly from baseline to day 2 and then progressively returned toward the baseline value. The profile of MNWS-R total score 2 was comparable to that of MNWS-R total score 1 in the three study arms (not shown). The effects in REXC-04-JP were consistent with those in REXC-03-EU, with comparable values between THS and cigarettes. In REXC-04-JP, total score 2 on day 2 in the SA arm showed a more moderate increase than that in REXC-03-EU, before continuously decreasing toward baseline values. The profile of MNWS-R total score 2 was comparable with that of MNWS-R total score 1 for the three study arms (data not shown).

During the confinement period in REXA-07-JP and REXA-08-US, the MNWS-R total scores at baseline were higher for THS than cigarettes. These values remained stable between day 1 and day 5 for both products in REXA-07-JP. In REXA-08-US, the MNWS-R total score in the THS arm declined from baseline to day 1

TABLE 17.23
Puff frequency during the course of the four reduced exposure studies (puffs/min, geometric means).

			ZRHR-REXC-03-EU	ZRHR-REXC-04-JP	ZRHM-REXA-07-JP	ZRHM-REXA-08-US
Baseline	CC	Mean	4.19	3.94	4.36	2.60
		95% CI	(3.68, 4.78)	(3.59, 4.33)	(3.96, 4.79)	(2.34, 2.90)
	THS	Mean	3.43	3.64	4.70	2.38
		95% CI	(3.16, 3.71)	(3.40, 3.89)	(4.29, 5.15)	(2.13, 2.66)
Day 4	CC	Mean	4.47	3.60	4.32	2.50
		95% CI	(3.82, 5.24)	(3.25, 3.99)	(3.80, 4.92)	(2.17, 2.89)
	THS	Mean	5.01	4.30	5.19	3.58
		95% CI	(4.67, 5.37)	(4.00, 4.63)	(4.77, 5.64)	(3.23, 3.96)
	THS:CC ratio (%)	Mean	132.33	126.61	106.93	138.65
		95% CI	(118.25, 148.09)	(114.73, 139.72)	(96.65, 118.31)	(115.68, 166.18)
Day 90	CC	Mean	NA	NA	4.57	2.19
		95% CI	NA	NA	(4.02, 5.19)	(1.74, 2.76)
	THS	Mean	NA	NA	5.73	3.87
		95% CI	NA	NA	(5.17, 6.34)	(3.30, 4.54)
	THS:CC ratio (%)	Mean	NA	NA	121.95	174.02
		95% CI	NA	NA	(103.78, 143.30)	(120.77, 250.74)

CC, cigarettes; *CI*, confidence interval; *THS*, Tobacco Heating System 2.2.

and then remained stable until day 5. These values were overall comparable to or only slightly lower than those observed in the cigarette arm.

During the ambulatory period, from day 30 to day 90, the MNWS-R total score profiles were largely comparable between THS and cigarettes in REXA-07-JP, despite the values for THS being slightly higher than those for cigarettes. In REXA-08-US, the scores for THS and cigarettes were stable but lower than those in the confinement period; the scores for cigarettes, however, remained generally higher than those for THS.

In the smoking abstinence arms, the values increased markedly between baseline and day 1, before declining, with the values returning to baseline by day 4 in REXA-08-US or close to baseline on day 5 in REXA-07-JP. During the ambulatory period, the scores continuously decreased in the SA arms of both studies, with the scores on day 90 being lower than those in the THS and cigarette arms.

In conclusion, the effects on withdrawal symptoms were comparable between THS and cigarettes, while the withdrawal scores in the smoking abstinence arm increased markedly between baseline and day 1, before progressively decreasing throughout the study and reaching values lower than baseline by day 90.

17.5.2 Clinical Reduced Exposure Studies on EHTPs—Other Studies

Only very few clinical reduced exposure studies have been conducted with other EHTPs.

First, three studies assessed the reduction in CO exposure following switching from cigarette smoking to EHTP use. These short-term (Adriaens et al., 2018; Caponnetto et al., 2018) and longer-term (Beatrice and Massaro, 2019) studies confirmed that switching completely from cigarette smoking to THS use reduces CO exposure to levels approaching those following smoking abstinence. Two of these studies also showed that this change is similar to that induced by switching to an e-cigarette (Adriaens et al., 2018; Beatrice and Massaro, 2019).

Second, a study compared the exposure reduction to HPHCs induced by switching from cigarette smoking to

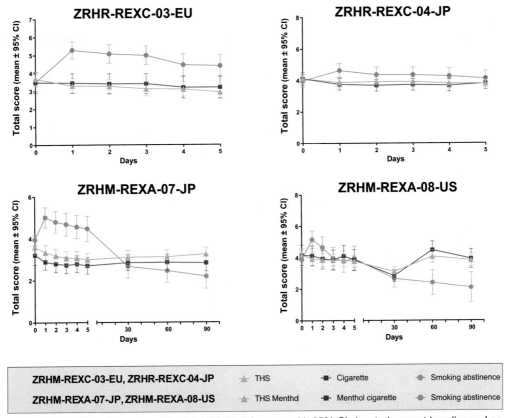

FIG. 17.19 Arithmetic means of the total QSU-brief scores with 95% CIs by study arm at baseline and on days 1–5, day 30, day 60, and day 90 in ZRHR-REXC-03-EU, ZRHR-REXC-04-JP, ZRHM-REXA-07-JP, and ZRHM-REXA-08-US. *CI*, confidence interval; *QSU*, Questionnaire of Smoking Urges; *THS*, Tobacco Heating System 2.2.

two different EHTPs and cessation (Gale et al., 2018). This 5-day clinical reduced exposure study conducted in a confined setting in Japan confirmed the results of the PMI studies and demonstrated that switching completely from cigarette smoking to any of the tested EHTPs led to an exposure reduction approaching that caused by smoking abstinence.

17.5.3 Clinical Reduced Exposure Studies on EVPs—Other Studies

There are a limited number of randomized clinical reduced exposure studies that have been conducted and published on ENDPs other than EHTPs (O'Connell et al., 2016; Yuki et al., 2018). These switching studies were conducted in a confined setting, with an exposure phase that lasted 5 days. Both studies showed that the BoExps to the selected HPHCs were significantly reduced among smokers who completely switched to

an e-cigarette (O'Connell et al., 2016) or a hybrid product (Yuki et al., 2018) (see Chapter 2). These exposure reductions were similar to those observed in the respective smoking abstinence groups. One of the studies (O'Connell et al., 2016) also demonstrated that dual users displayed a more limited reduction in BoExps, which is expected. A 2-week ambulatory study further confirmed that smokers who switched to an e-cigarette displayed a substantial reduction in the BoExps to HPHCs (Goniewicz et al., 2017).

A cross-sectional analysis of urinary BoExps to tobacco-related toxicants further confirmed that e-cigarette-only users had a significantly lower level of exposure to HPHCs than dual users and cigarette smokers. Furthermore, this study also confirmed that e-cigarette-only users have a level of exposure to tobacco-related toxicants that approaches that of non-smokers (Goniewicz et al., 2018).

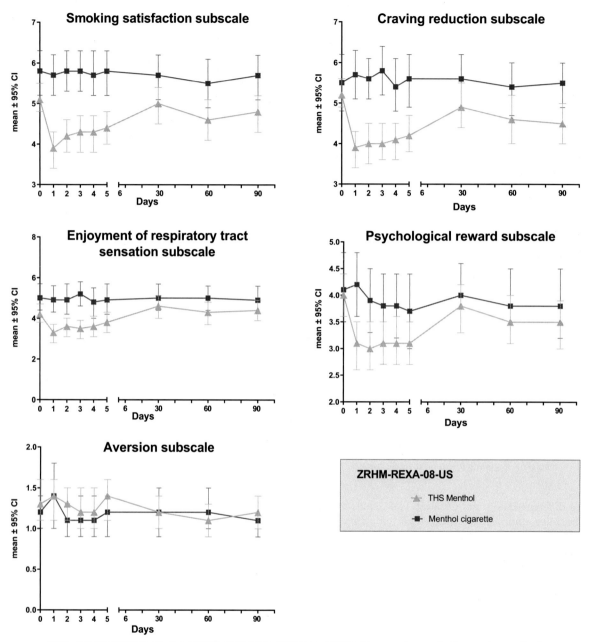

FIG. 17.20 Profiles of the mCEQ subscales (smoking satisfaction, craving reduction, enjoyment of respiratory tract sensation, psychological reward, and aversion) in ZRHM-REXA-08-US throughout the study. *CI*, confidence interval; *mCEQ*, modified Cigarette Evaluation Questionnaire; *THS*, Tobacco Heating System 2.2.

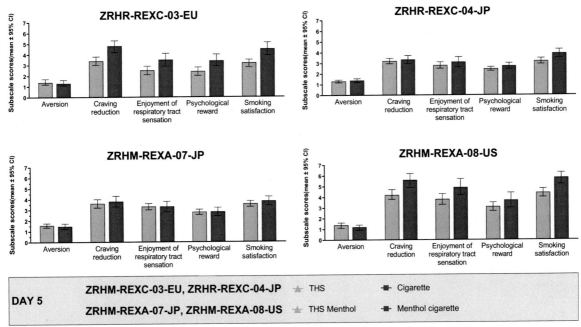

FIG. 17.21 mCEQ subscales on day 5 in ZRHR-REXC-03-EU, ZRHR-REXC-04-JP, ZRHM-REXA-07-JP, and ZRHM-REXA-08-US. *CI*, confidence interval; *mCEQ*, modified Cigarette Evaluation Questionnaire; *THS*, Tobacco Heating System 2.2.

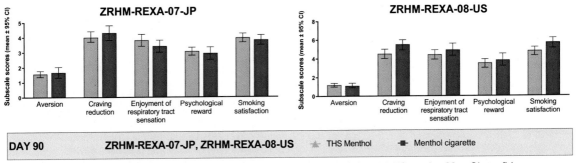

FIG. 17.22 mCEQ subscales in ZRHM-REXA-07-JP and ZRHM-REXA-08-US, at day 90. *CI*, confidence interval; *mCEQ*, modified Cigarette Evaluation Questionnaire; *THS*, Tobacco Heating System 2.2.

A recent study has shown that short-term use of first-generation e-cigarettes leads to lower levels of exposure to the most volatile organic compounds (VOCs), with the exception of xylene, *N,N*-dimethylformamide, and acrylonitrile, the metabolite levels of which were higher in the urine of short-term e-cigarette users than nontobacco users (Lorkiewicz et al., 2018). Some e-cigarettes have been shown to expose users to VOCs such as acrylamide, benzene, and propylene oxide, which may pose health risks to users (St Helen et al., 2020). In another

cross-sectional study (Wang et al., 2019), for all BoExps examined, cigarette users had the highest levels among all tobacco product users. The study also found that urinary levels of 2-hydroxyfluorene, 3-hydroxyfluorene, and $\sum$2,3-hydroxyphenanthrene were significantly higher in smokeless tobacco users than in e-cigarette users; but, 3-hydroxyfluorene and 1-hydroxypyrene levels were significantly higher in e-cigarette and smokeless cigarette users than in never users.

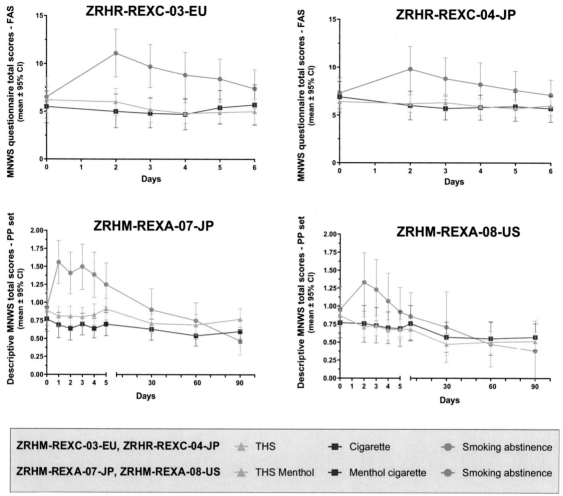

FIG. 17.23 Arithmetic means of MNWS-total score 1 (REXC) and the MNWS-R withdrawal score (REXA) with 95% CIs in at baseline and on days 2–6, day 30, day 60, and day 90 in ZRHR-REXC-03-EU, ZRHR-REXC-04-JP, ZRHM-REXA-07-JP, and ZRHM-REXA-08-US. *CI*, confidence interval; *FAS*, full analysis set; *MNWS*, Minnesota Nicotine Withdrawal Scale; *PP*, per-protocol; *THS*, Tobacco Heating System 2.2.

17.6 CLINICAL EXPOSURE RESPONSE ASSESSMENT OF ENDPS

17.6.1 Clinical Studies on EHTPs—PMI Studies

The clinical assessment program for THS consisted of several mid- to long-term studies and posthoc analyses.

First, two 90-day studies (REXA-07-JP and REXA-08-US) were conducted in Japan and the US (Fig. 17.24) with the primary goal of assessing the magnitude of toxicant exposure reduction in smokers who either switched to THS or remained abstinent from smoking (see Section 17.5). The eight selected BoPHs were, however, also measured in these studies to gain preliminary

insights into the magnitude of the effects and related variability that switching to THS would have on these BoPHs.

Second, to assess the effects of cessation on the BoPHs included in the 90-day reduced exposure studies, a 12-month smoking cessation study (SA-SCR-01) (Fig. 17.24) was conducted in smokers willing to quit smoking. This study was designed to contextualize the effects of switching to THS in particular and ENDPs in general with the effects of cessation on the selected BoPHs.

Third, a 6-month exposure response study (ERS-09-US) was conducted to demonstrate the favorable

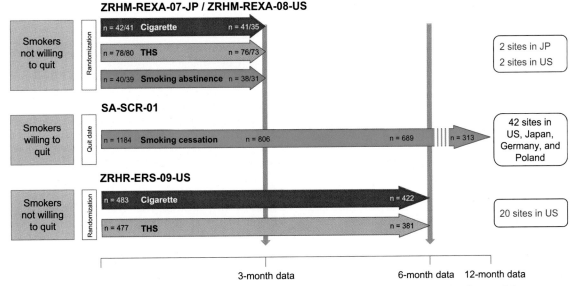

FIG. 17.24 Studies conducted to assess the THS risk profile. *THS,* Tobacco Heating System 2.2.

effects of switching from cigarette smoking to THS use on the eight BoPHs (Fig. 17.24). This study was sufficiently powered, according to the preliminary data of the two 90-day studies and the findings in the literature. The goal of ERS-09-US was to determine whether switching to THS instead of continuing to smoke cigarettes had a statistically significant favorable impact on at least five of the eight selected BoPHs, with all eight BoPHs showing changes in the direction of smoking cessation.

Bearing in mind that the trajectories and extent of changes in BoPHs and BoExps following complete switching to THS should be as close as possible to those of cessation in order to achieve a reduction in risk and harm, the data from ERS-09-US can be further compared with the data from the subjects who stopped smoking for 6 months in the SA-SCR-01 study. A smoking abstinence arm could have been added to the ERS-09-US study. However, cessation arms are complex to follow because of multiple failures in quitting among subjects and the necessity for chemical verification of whether the subjects have completely stopped smoking. In addition, for ethical reasons, ERS-09-US enrolled smokers who were not willing to quit; therefore, the likelihood of enrolling a sufficient number of smokers who would complete the study while remaining abstinent would have been low, as it is well established that the success rate of quitting smoking is higher in smokers willing to quit upfront than in smokers unwilling to quit. This smoking cessation study was, thus,

conducted separately and can, in the future, serve as a smoking cessation benchmark for future PMI studies.

17.6.1.1 Favorable biological effects of switching to THS after 3 months—PMI study

17.6.1.1.1 General design, population, and methods. In addition to being used for assessing reduced exposure to smoke toxicants when switching to THS [see Section 17.5.1.1], the BoPHs selected as part of PMI's risk assessment framework were monitored in the two 90-day reduced exposure studies (REXA-07-JP and REXA-08-US). The BoPHs were monitored to gain early insights into their magnitude of change and variability following switching to THS or smoking abstinence. The levels of BoPHs were measured at baseline and on day 90 (see Section 17.5.1.1 for design and more detailed information). Adherence was estimated as described in Section 17.5.1.2.

17.6.1.1.2 Statistical approach. The sample sizes for both studies were calculated to demonstrate the reduction in exposure to selected HPHCs (see Section 17.5.1.3); therefore, the study was not powered to demonstrate the changes in BoPH levels. The results obtained on BoPHs were descriptive in nature.

The BoPHs were analyzed on the basis of distribution of the data; those that were not normally distributed were log-transformed (base e) prior to analysis. A generalized linear model—analysis of covariance (ANCOVA) (Snedecor and Cochran, 1989)—was applied to the BoPH data on day 90, with the study arm as a factor adjusting for baseline value, sex, and average daily cigarette consumption over the last 4 weeks, as reported during screening. Estimates of differences from the model when the data were log-transformed were back-transformed (exponentiated) to calculate the LS mean ratios of the BoPH levels in the THS arm compared with those in the cigarette or smoking abstinence arms.

17.6.1.1.3 Key BoPHs findings from the REXA studies.
The key study results on reduced exposure to HPHCs after 3 months of switching and abstinence are presented in Section 17.5.1.5. Three-months of switching to THS and smoking abstinence led to initial favorable changes in BoPHs similar to those described in the literature for smoking cessation (Table 17.24).

To understand the relevance of the changes in BoPHs following switching from cigarette smoking to THS use, the results have to be compared with the changes observed following 3 months of smoking abstinence. Although the changes following smoking abstinence were small, they can certainly be considered relevant because smoking cessation is known to lead to a reduction in smoking-related disease. These early results suggest that the exposure reduction achieved by switching to THS may lead to positive changes in key BoPHs. Therefore, switching to THS may translate into reduced risk and harm of smoking-related diseases.

17.6.1.1.4 Conclusions.
The changes observed 3 months after switching to THS were comparable to, and in the same direction as, those following 3 months of abstinence. These changes were also of a similar magnitude. However, considering that these studies were not designed to demonstrate changes in BoPHs, the sample size and duration of these studies

TABLE 17.24
Analysis of changes in the eight selected BoPHs between the THS use and cigarette smoking categories on day 90.

BoPH		ZRHR-REXA-07-JP		ZRHM-REXA-08-US	
8-epi-PGF2α	THS:CC % reduction	12.71% ↓ (2.55, 21.81)	THS:CC % reduction	13.46% ↓ (−1.95, 23.61)	
	SA:CC %reduction	5.92% ↓ (6.80; 17.13)	SA:CC % reduction	8.51% ↓ (−11.79; 25.13)	
11-DTX-B2	THS:CC % reduction	8.98% ↓ (−2.93, 19.52)	THS:CC % reduction	3.56% ↓ (−23.31, 24.57)	
	SA:CC %reduction	19.37% ↓ (−7.04; 30.07)	SA:CC % reduction	7.15% ↓ (−38.30; 37.68)	
FEV$_1$	Diff THS−CC	1.91 %pred ↑ (−0.14, 3.97)	Diff THS−CC	0.53 %pred ↑ (−2.79; 3.85)	
	Diff SA−CC	1.94 %pred ↑ (−0.43; 4.31)	Diff SA−CC	2.05 %pred ↑ (−3.36; 7.36)	
HDL-C	Diff THS−CC	4.53 mg/dL ↑ (1.17, 7.88)	Diff THS−CC	1.4 mg/dL ↑ (−2.3, 5.0)	
	Diff SA−CC	6.40 mg/dL ↑ (2.51; 10.21)	Diff SA−CC	0.03 mg/dL ↑ (−5.77; 5.84)	
WBC	Diff THS−CC	−0.57 Gl/L ↓ (−1.04, −0.10)	Diff THS−CC	0.17 Gl/L (−0.47, 0.81)	
	Diff SA−CC	−0.40 Gl/L ↓ (−0.94; 0.14)	Diff SA−CC	−0.94 Gl/L ↓ (−2.01; 0.13)	
sICAM-1	THS:CC % reduction	8.72% ↓ (2.05, 14.94)	THS:CC % reduction	10.59% ↓ (4.03, 16.71)	
	SA:CC %reduction	10.87% ↓ (3.36; 17.79)	SA:CC % reduction	9.90% ↓ (−1.07; 19.69)	
COHb	THS:CC % reduction	48.2% ↓ (44.4, 51.9)	THS:CC % reduction	53.2% ↓ (45.0, 60.2)	
	SA:CC %reduction	46.7% ↓ (42.0, 51.0)	SA:CC % reduction	48.3% ↓ (32.6, 60.4)	
Total NNAL	THS:CC % reduction	76.7% ↓ (68.8, 82.7)	THS:CC % reduction	73.6% ↓ (59.7, 82.7)	
	SA:CC %reduction	84.6% ↓ (78.4, 89.0)	SA:CC % reduction	65.2% ↓ (32.4, 82.2)	

11-DTX-B2, 11-dehydrothromboxane B2; *1THS*, Tobacco Heating System 2.2; *8-epi-PGF2α*, 8-epi-prostaglandin F2α; *BoPH*, biomarker of potential harm; *CC*, cigarettes; *COHb*, carboxyhemoglobin; *FEV$_1$*, forced expiratory volume in 1 s; *HDL-C*, high-density lipoprotein cholesterol; *NNAL*, 4-(methylnitrosamino)-1-(3-pyridyl)-1-butanol; *SA*, smoking abstinence; *sICAM-1*, soluble intercellular adhesion molecule; *WBC*, white blood cells.

TABLE 17.25
Changes from baseline in the eight BoPHs at 6 and 12 months after the subjects completely quit smoking cigarettes.

Mechanism	BoPH	CHANGE (SD) FROM BASELINE (CV%) 95% CI	
		Month 6	Month 12
Lipid metabolism	HDL-C (mg/dL)	1.6 (9.73) 0.646, 2.55	0.856 (10.4) −0.285, 2
Inflammation	WBC count (GI/L)	−0.629 (1.48) −0.768, −0.491	−0.545 (1.68) −0.721, −0.37
Platelet function	11-DTXB2 concentration adjusted for creatinine[a]	−24.9 (65.7) −29, −20.5	−22.2 (66.8) −27, −17
Oxidative stress	8-epi-PGF2α concentration adjusted for creatinine[a]	−16.2 (45.3) −19.5, −12.7	−18.8 (45.8) −22.4, −15
Endothelial dysfunction	sICAM-1[a]	−11.8 (20.5) −13.5, −10.1	−13.2 (24.2) −15.4, −11
Acute cardiovascular effect	COHb[a]	−73.7 (138) −76.3, −70.8	−71.5 (157) −74.7, −67.8
Lung function	FEV$_1$[b]	−0.0496 (0.242) −0.0731, −0.0261	−0.0491 (0.238) −0.0755, −0.0227
Genotoxicity	Total NNAL[a]	−95.4 (209) −96, −94.8	−95.9 (205) −96.5, −95.4

11-DTX-B2, 11-dehydrothromboxane B2; *1THS*, Tobacco Heating System 2.2; *8-epi-PGF2α*, 8-epi-prostaglandin F2α; *BoPH*, biomarker of potential harm; *CC*, cigarettes; *COHb*, carboxyhemoglobin; *FEV$_1$*, forced expiratory volume in 1 s; *HDL-C*, high-density lipoprotein cholesterol; *NNAL*, 4-(methylnitrosamino)-1-(3-pyridyl)-1-butanol; *SA*, smoking abstinence; *sICAM-1*, soluble intercellular adhesion molecule; *WBC*, white blood cells.
[a] Corresponds to relative change from baseline.
[b] Postbronchodilator.

were too limited. Thus, these data needed to be further substantiated in a longer-term exposure response study.

17.6.1.2 Favorable biological effects of smoking cessation—PMI study

17.6.1.2.1 Study design, population, and methods.
SA-SCR-01 was a multicenter, multiregional (US, Europe, and Japan) smoking cessation study conducted with healthy adult smokers planning to quit smoking within the next 30 days and willing to continuously abstain from smoking during a 1-year period in an ambulatory setting.

The overall study design of SA-SCR-01 is described in Fig. 17.25 (Tran et al., 2019). From the actual quit date (AQD) onwards, strict abstinence was required from all tobacco- or nicotine-containing products (including electronic cigarettes) other than NRTs. From the AQD, the subjects were asked to return to the study site after 1 and 2 weeks and then on a monthly basis. Counseling and behavioral support were provided throughout the study and upon the subjects' request. Additionally, NRT

was provided at the subjects' request and used for up to 3 months, as per country label. The 3-, 6-, and 12-month visits corresponded to on-site full assessment visits, where 24-h urine and blood samples were collected for analysis of BoExps and BoPHs, while the other visits were organized for safety purposes and follow-up of the subjects' adherence to smoking cessation.

Subjects who were not continuously abstinent from smoking or using any nicotine-containing product (including electronic cigarettes), other than NRT, after AQD were discontinued from the study.

17.6.1.2.2 Adherence to smoking abstinence.
Continuous adherence to smoking abstinence was verified by using multiple tools, including CO breath test, nicotine dipstick test, measurement of NEQ and total NNAL levels, and self-reported product use.

17.6.1.2.3 Statistical approach.
Descriptive statistics for BoExps and BoPHs were calculated at baseline, month 3, month 6, and month 12 for subjects who were continuously abstinent from smoking throughout

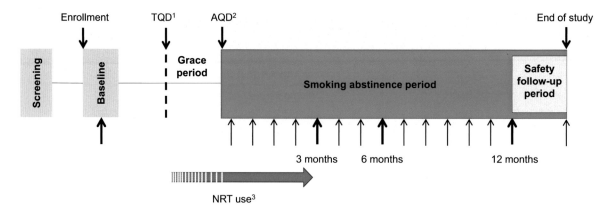

[1] Target quit date (TQD) is within 1–14 days of checkout of V2
[2] Actual quit date (AQD) is within 14 days of TQD (grace period with occasional CC use)
[3] Smoking abstinence (SA)
[4] Use of NRT is only allowed for up to 3 months (+2 weeks) after the start date of NRT. NRT may be started at any time between the TQD and 1 week after the AQD

FIG. 17.25 Smoking cessation study design.[1] TQD was within 1–14 days of checkout of V2. [2] AQD was within 14 days of TQD (grace period with occasional CC use). [3] Use of NRT was only allowed for up to 3 months after the start date of NRT. NRT could be started at any time between the TQD and 1 week after the AQD.   *AQD*, actual quit date; *CC*, cigarettes, *CO*, carbon monoxide; *NRT*, nicotine replacement therapy; *TQD*, target quit date; *V*, visit.

the study. The summaries included changes and relative percentage changes from baseline.

Analyses were conducted on the population defined as continuously abstinent at 3 months from the AQD. This population analysis included all enrolled subjects with at least one evaluable BoPH, BoExp, or questionnaire assessment after the AQD.

17.6.1.2.4 Key findings of the SA-SCR-01 study. The baseline demographic data were overall balanced across the regions (e.g., sex, body mass index, smoking intensity, race, and ethnicity) (Fig. 17.26).

Overall, the key study results after 12 months of smoking cessation were as follows:

(1) Of the 1184 enrolled subjects, 720 remained abstinent from smoking from the AQD to month 3, 450 to month 6, and 358 to month 12, according to data from predefined adherence tools (Section 17.6.1.2.2). The continuous abstinence rate was high until month 5 and decreased at month 6 because of the implementation of more rigorous and sensitive adherence tools (Fig. 17.27).

(2) After the subjects quit smoking completely, the eight BoPHs considered for coprimary endpoints in studies with THS changed in the expected direction (Table 17.25 and Fig. 17.28).

(3) Exposure to various HPHCs was reduced by 54.5% −97.9% at 12 months after the subject completely

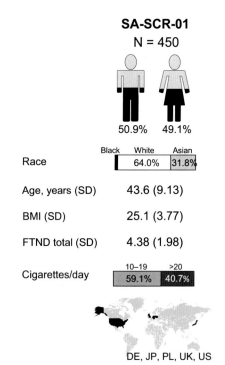

FIG. 17.26 Main baseline characteristics of the subjects in the SA-SCR-01 study.   *BMI*, body mass index; *FTND*, Fagerström test for nicotine dependence; *SD*, standard deviation.

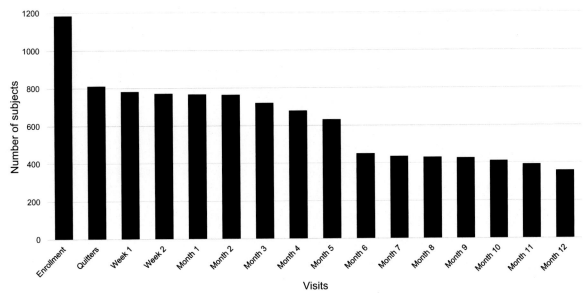

FIG. 17.27 Number of subjects who were continuously abstinent from smoking at each visit.

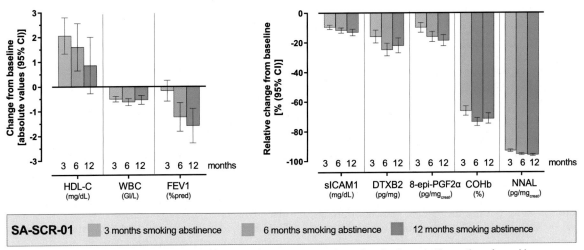

FIG. 17.28 Graphical representation of change from baseline after 3, 6, and 12 months of smoking cessation. *11-DTX-B2*, 11-dehydrothromboxane B2; *1THS*, Tobacco Heating System 2.2; *8-epi-PGF2α*, 8-epi-prostaglandin F2α; *BoPH*, biomarker of potential harm; *CC*, cigarettes; *COHb*, carboxyhemoglobin; *FEV₁*, forced expiratory volume in 1 s; *HDL-C*, high-density lipoprotein cholesterol; *NNAL*, 4-(methylnitrosamino)-1-(3-pyridyl)-1-butanol; *SA*, smoking abstinence; *sICAM-1*, soluble intercellular adhesion molecule; *WBC*, white blood cells.

quit smoking (Fig. 17.29). Similar reductions had already been observed after 3 and 6 months. The reductions in NEQ levels reached 99% at both 6 and 12 months.

Favorable changes were observed in (1) lipid metabolism, as indicated by an increase in HDL-C and apolipoprotein A1 (Apo A1) levels; (2) inflammatory state, as indicated by a decrease in WBC count; (3) platelet activation, as indicated by a decrease in 11-DTXB2 levels; (4) oxidative stress, as indicated by a decrease in 8-epi-PGF2α levels; and (5) endothelial function, as indicated by a decrease in sICAM-1 levels. All

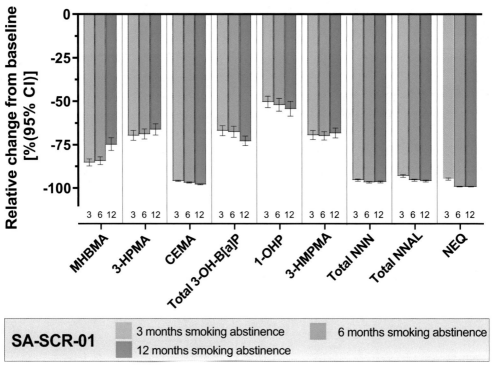

FIG. 17.29 BoExps to HPHCs. *1-OHP*, total 1-hydroxypyrene; *3-HMPMA*, 3-hydroxy-1-methylpropyl-mercapturic acid; *3-HPMA*, 3-hydroxypropylmercapturic acid; *3-OH-B[a]P*, 3-hydroxybenzo[a]pyrene; *BoExp*, biomarker of exposure; *CI*, confidence interval; *CEMA*, 2-cyanoethylmercapturic acid; *MHBMA*, monohydroxybutenylmercapturic acid; *NNN*, N-nitrosonornicotine; *NEQ*, nicotine equivalent.

these favorable changes were observed as early as 3 months after smoking cessation. The magnitudes of the changes were sustained and, in some cases, even increased with time up to 12 months, except in the case of HDL-C, for which the magnitude of favorable change decreased after 12 months of smoking cessation. In addition, smoking cessation resulted in a marked reduction in all BoExps, including a reduction in NEQ level by 99% from baseline at months 6 and 12, thus confirming continuous abstinence from smoking during the study. This was the first study to describe the changes induced by smoking cessation in a broad set of smoking-associated BoPHs and BoExps across multiple geographic regions.

These findings are overall consistent with published data on the effects of smoking cigarettes and benefits of smoking cessation. In general, cigarette smoking results in an alteration in lipid metabolism, reflected by a decrease in HDL-C levels, while smoking cessation reverses these changes (Andrikoula and McDowell, 2008; Lu et al., 2011).

17.6.1.2.5 Conclusions. The magnitudes of the favorable changes induced by smoking cessation provide

insights into how these smoking-associated BoPHs and the mechanistic pathways they represent are linked to the harm and disease risk reduction associated with smoking cessation. Considering that, from an epidemiological point of view, the risk of disease in smokers can return to the level of that in nonsmokers upon quitting cigarettes, this study provides evidence of short-term effects that occur upon smoking cessation. These effects are likely involved in the attenuation of long-term disease risk.

This study confirmed the favorable response to smoking cessation of the eight BoPHs that were preselected (Section 17.2.3.2) for assessing the reduced risk profile of ENDPs. The study determined the magnitude of the changes associated with smoking cessation and will serve to benchmark the effects of switching from cigarettes to ENDP use against the gold standard of smoking cessation as outlined in Chapter 3.

17.6.1.3 Favorable biological effects of switching from cigarettes to EHTPs at 6 months—PMI study.

17.6.1.3.1 Study design, population, and methods. The ERS-09-US study was a 6-month randomized, controlled, two-arm study in an

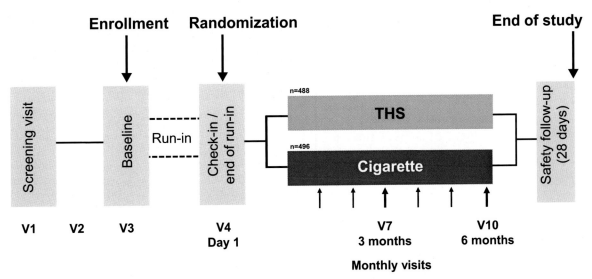

FIG. 17.30 ERS-09-US study flow chart. *THS*, Tobacco Heating System 2.2; *V*, visit.

ambulatory setting. The study enrolled adult healthy smokers who were not willing to quit smoking. After a run-in period (familiarization with THS), a total of 984 subjects were randomized into two groups:

(1) One group of subjects who continued to smoke their own preferred brand(s) of cigarette ad libitum (496 participants) and

(2) Another group of subjects who switched to ad libitum use of THS (488 participants).

The primary objective of the study was to demonstrate that switching from cigarette smoking to THS use has a positive and meaningful impact on the eight coprimary BoPHs of the risk assessment framework (Section 17.2.3.2) compared with continuing to smoke cigarettes. To establish risk modification relative to cigarettes, five of the eight endpoints had to display statistically significant changes between the two groups, and all BoPHs had to show positive changes—in other words, change in the direction of cessation. The design of the study is summarized in Fig. 17.30. Blood and 24-h urine samples were collected for assessment of BoExps and BoPHs during main visits V7 and V10 (i.e., 3 and 6 months).

17.6.1.3.2 Product adherence and product use categories.
As described in Section 17.5.1.2, it is important to estimate the numbers of each product (both THS and cigarette) that were used over the investigational period in a switching study to enable accurate interpretation of the results. In this study, product consumption was self-reported by the subjects daily over the 6-month period.

Each subject was then classified according to predefined product use categories postrandomization estimated over the entire study period (Table 17.26).

17.6.1.3.3 Statistical approach.
The primary analysis was performed on the "as exposed" population in accordance with the product use categories described in Section 17.6.1.3.2. The sample size was thus estimated to meet the primary objective. The test-wise power of each BoPH was calculated on the basis of reported changes induced by smoking cessation and by assuming preserved effects of cessation when switching to THS. The Hailperin–Rüger statistical approach (Hailperin, 1965; Rüger, 1978) was chosen for testing the BoPH risk assessment framework. This method is an extension of the Bonferroni method which preserves the study-wise α level by requiring that any subset of an endpoint be found to be statistically significant out of a set of coprimary endpoints. The overall study-wise type I error was set at a level of 5%. Each primary endpoint was tested by using a one-sided type I error of 1.5625%, with the changes in at least five coprimary endpoints required to be statistically significant. The decision not to use a composite endpoint was taken because the data for weighing the contribution of each BoPH to smoking-attributable disease development were lacking.

17.6.1.3.4 Key findings of the ERS-09-US study.
The distribution of randomized subjects per product use category is described in Table 17.27.

TABLE 17.26
Actual product use categories.

Category	General Description
THS use	≥1 THS or CC and ≥70% THS use over the entire analysis period and ≥70% THS use on ≥50% of the days in the analysis period.
Dual use	≥1 THS or CC and 1% ≤ THS <70% over the entire analysis period or THS use and CC use on <50% of the days.
CC use	≥1 THS or CC and <1% THS over the entire analysis period and <1% THS on ≥ 50% of the days in the analysis period.
Other use	General category encompassing subjects with missing product use, subjects using e-cigarettes or other tobacco products, subjects who quit, or subjects who switched across different use patterns between consecutive analysis periods.

CC, cigarettes; THS, Tobacco Heating System 2.2.

TABLE 17.27
Distribution of randomized subjects by product use categories (FAS-EX).

		PRODUCT USE	
Category	Description	THS arm: n (%)	Cigarette arm: n (%)
THS use	>70% use and more than 50% of days THS use	245 (59.2)	0
Dual use	<70% use or less than 50% of days	142 (34.3)	0
Cigarette use	<1% THS use	3 (0.7)	425 (95.9)
Other use	E-cigarette, quitters, other products	24 (5.8)	18 (4.1)

FAS-EX, full analysis set as exposed; n, number; THS, Tobacco Heating System 2.2.

TABLE 17.28
Primary comparative analysis of the selected eight coprimary endpoints between the THS use and CC use categories at month 6.

Endpoint	Change from CC use	LS mean difference, relative reduction	96.875% CI	1-sided P value
HDL-C	Difference	3.09 mg/dL	1.10, 5.09	<0.001[a]
WBC	Difference	−0.420 GI/L	−0.717, −0.123	0.001[a]
sICAM-1	%Reduction	2.86%	−0.426, 6.04	0.030
11-DTX-B$_2$	%Reduction	4.74%	−7.50, 15.6	0.193
8-epi-PGF$_{2\alpha}$	%Reduction	6.80%	−0.216, 13.3	0.018
COHb	%Reduction	32.2%	24.5, 39.0	<0.001[a]
FEV$_1$ %pred	Difference	1.28 %pred	0.145, 2.42	0.008[a]
Total NNAL	%Reduction	43.5%	33.7, 51.9	<0.001[a]

11-DTX-B2, 11-dehydrothromboxane B2; 1THS, Tobacco Heating System 2.2; 8-epi-PGF2α, 8-epi-prostaglandin F2α; BoPH, biomarker of potential harm; CC, cigarettes; COHb, carboxyhemoglobin; FEV$_1$, forced expiratory volume in 1 s; HDL-C, high-density lipoprotein cholesterol; NNAL, 4-(methylnitrosamino)-1-(3-pyridyl)-1-butanol; SA, smoking abstinence; sICAM-1, soluble intercellular adhesion molecule; WBC, white blood cells.
[a] Denotes significant P value at the 1.5625% level following test multiplicity adjustment by using the Hailperin–Rüger approach.

In the population of analysis "as exposed" post-randomization, the 428 participants in the cigarette-use group smoked 16.8 ± 6.8 cigarettes per day, on average. The average daily consumption of the 142 participants in the dual-use group was 7.6 ± 5.2 THS tobacco sticks and

10.0 ± 5.9 cigarettes. The average daily consumption of the 245 participants in the THS use group was 16.5 ± 8.9 THS tobacco sticks and 2.0 ± 2.4 cigarettes.

The baseline demographic data were balanced across product use categories (e.g., body mass index, smoking intensity, race, and ethnicity), with a higher proportion of men than women present in the groups (Fig. 17.31).

Overall, the key study results after the 6-month investigational period were as follows:

(1) The primary objective was met, with the study demonstrating that five of the eight coprimary BoPHs were favorably and statistically significantly different in smokers switching to THS than in those continuing to smoke. All coprimary BoPHs shifted in the same direction as those in smoking cessation, as reported in the literature (Table 17.28 and Fig. 17.32). Favorable changes were also observed in some BoPHs in dual users, but to a much lesser extent than in THS users.

(2) In THS users, exposure to seven HPHCs was reduced by 21%–52% after 3 months and 16% –49% after 6 months. In dual users, these reductions ranged from 1% to 16% and 3%–13% after 3 and 6 months, respectively (Fig. 17.33). This emphasizes the importance of subjects adhering to product use to obtain the maximum benefit from switching.

In subjects classified in the THS use category, the reductions at 3 and 6 months were less pronounced than those measured in the 90-day reduced exposure studies (REXA-07-JP and REXA-08-US) [Section 17.5.1.5]. This is likely due to the difference in the definition of the intensity of cigarette smoking concomitant to THS use between the two types of studies. In the THS use category defined as per ERS-09-US, the subjects were allowed to smoke cigarettes to a maximum of 30% cigarette use. In the REXA studies, the intensity of cigarette smoking was more restrictive in the THS group (no more than 0.5 cigarettes per day, on average, over 1 month and no more than two cigarettes on a single day in the two 90-days studies).

Switching to THS use favorably modified the trajectory of the eight BoPHs in the direction of smoking cessation. Of note, THS switching had a favorable effect on FEV_1, indicating a smaller decline in lung function in subjects who switched to THS than in those who continued to smoke. The magnitude of effect on BoPHs was largely attenuated in the dual-use category, relative to the THS-use category, as was expected because of the higher degree of cigarette smoking in this category.

Together with the decrease in exposure to various carcinogenic HPHCs measured in REXA-07-JP and REXA-08-US—including NNK (BoExp: total NNAL), 1–3 butadiene (BoExp: MHBMA), crotonaldehyde (BoExp: 3-HMPMA), benzene (BoExp: S-PMA), aromatic amines (BoExps: 1-aminonaphtalene, 2-aminonaphtalene, 4-aminobiphenyl, and o-toluidine), and benzo[a] pyrene (BoExp: benzo[a]pyrene)—and the decrease in total NNAL level observed in THS users over 6 months in the ERS-09-US study, it is likely that the risk of cancer in smokers might be decreased by using THS, even though data are lacking to formally predict this at this stage. It is worth noting that total NNAL was reported to be associated with the incidence of lung cancer in humans (Yuan et al., 2014).

Additionally, the following short-term health benefits when switching to THS were observed:

- The number of individuals who reported a regular need to cough after 6 months of THS use was significantly lower compared with the corresponding number among individuals who continued smoking (Table 17.29). This health outcome was not observed in dual-users.
- In addition, in contrast to smoking cessation, which is associated with weight gain of about 1 kg per month for the first 3 months of smoking cessation (Aubin et al., 2012), no such increase in weight was observed when switching to THS (not shown).

17.6.1.3.5 Additional analyses
17.6.1.3.5.1 Results. Interestingly, the ERS-09-US study showed favorable changes in eight BoPHs, although the subjects classified in the THS use category were concomitantly using up to 30% cigarettes (with a self-reported average cigarette consumption of 2.0 ± 2.4 cigarettes per day).

The limitations of self-reported nicotine product use in smoking cessation studies are known and can be mitigated by biochemical verification of smoking status. Scheuermann et al. reported that, in the US, high rates (40%) of recently hospitalized smokers in smoking cessation trials failed the biochemical verification of their self-reported abstinence (Scheuermann et al., 2017). Furthermore, a retrospective analysis of three studies showed that cigarette counts, but not self-reported cigarette numbers per day, were significantly associated with exposure to smoke toxicants (Blank et al., 2016).

With this context, a posthoc analysis of the ERS-09-US study data was conducted to explore whether objective biochemical verification for detecting the intensity of concomitant cigarette smoking in the THS use category could provide more granularity on the BoPH response. To that end, the distribution of the quartile levels of CEMA—a BoExp to acrylonitrile, known to show a linear relationship with the number of cigarettes smoked—was evaluated in the THS use category (with quartile 1 having the lowest and quartile 4 the highest levels) as a function of BoPH

ZRHR-ERS-09-US

N = 857

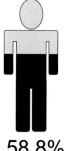 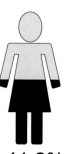

58.8%   41.2%

	Black	White	Other
Race	17.6%	79.2%	

Age, years (SD)   44.6 (9.55)

BMI (SD)   27.0 (4.18)

FTND total (SD)   5.78 (2.07)

	10–19	>20
Cigarettes/day	44.0%	56.0%

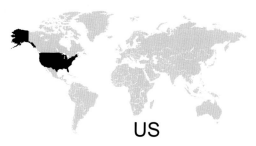

US

FIG. 17.31 Main baseline characteristics of the subjects in ZRHR-ERS-09-US (as-exposed set). *BMI*, body mass index; *FTND*, Fagerström test for nicotine dependence; *SD*, standard deviation.

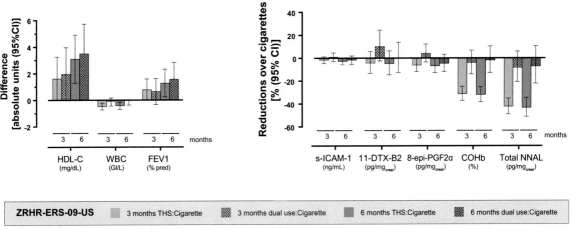

FIG. 17.32 Differences and reductions in the eight selected coprimary endpoints between THS use and cigarette use and between dual use and cigarette use at month 3 and month 6. *11-DTX-B2*, 11-dehydrothromboxane B2; *1THS*, Tobacco Heating System 2.2; *8-epi-PGF2α*, 8-epi-prostaglandin F2α; *BoPH*, biomarker of potential harm; *CC*, cigarettes; *COHb*, carboxyhemoglobin; *FEV₁*, forced expiratory volume in 1 s; *HDL-C*, high-density lipoprotein cholesterol; *NNAL*, 4-(methylnitrosamino)-1-(3-pyridyl)-1-butanol; *SA*, smoking abstinence; *sICAM-1*, soluble intercellular adhesion molecule; *WBC*, white blood cells. **$P < .001$; *$P < .015625$.

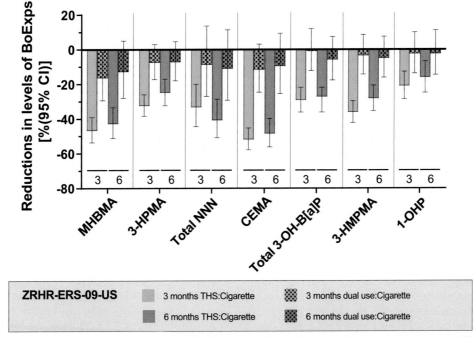

FIG. 17.33 Relative reductions in levels of BoExps at 3 and 6 months according to actual product use (FAS-EX). *1-OHP*, total 1-hydroxypyrene; *3-HMPMA*, 3-hydroxy-1-methylpropyl-mercapturic acid; *3-HPMA*, 3-hydroxypropylmercapturic acid; *3-OH-B[a]P*, 3-hydroxybenzo[a]pyrene; *BoExp*, biomarker of exposure; *CI*, confidence interval; *CEMA*, 2-cyanoethylmercapturic acid; *FAS-EX*, full analysis set as exposed; *MHBMA*, monohydroxybutenylmercapturic acid; *NNN*, N-nitrosonornicotine; *THS*, Tobacco Heating System 2.2.

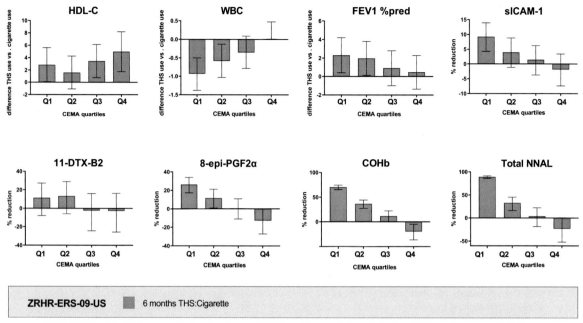

FIG. 17.34 Model-based effect estimates and 95% confidence intervals in the eight coprimary endpoints at month 6, presented per CEMA quartile in the THS use category.   *11-DTX-B2*, 11-dehydrothromboxane B2; *8-epi PGF2α*, 8-epi prostaglandin F2α; *CEMA*, 2-cyanoethylmercapturic acid; *COHb*, carboxyhemoglobin; *FEV₁*, forced expiratory volume in 1 s; *HDL-C*, high-density lipoprotein cholesterol; *NNAL*, 4-(methylnitrosamino)-1-(3-pyridyl)-1-butanol; *pred*, predicted; *sICAM-1*, soluble intercellular adhesion molecule 1; *THS*, Tobacco Heating System 2.2; *WBC*, white blood cells.

response at month 6. Acrylonitrile is generated at temperatures of 500–800°C and thus reduced by >99% in the THS aerosol relative to the smoke of the 3R4F reference cigarette (Schaller et al., 2016). Therefore, CEMA, the biomarker for acrylonitrile exposure, can be used to distinguish cigarette smoking from THS use (Rodgman and Perfetti, 2013). It was expected that the favorable effects on the eight coprimary BoPHs would be more pronounced with lower levels of CEMA.

Overall, the key results of the posthoc analysis were as follows:

(1) The eight coprimary endpoints at month 6 by CEMA quartiles showed an inverse dose–response relationship between the degree of smoking and overall magnitude of favorable changes in BoPHs. The comparisons between THS use and cigarette smoking for each BoPH are reported in Table 17.30 for the first quartile of CEMA. A graphical representation of all BoPHs as a function of CEMA quartile is shown in Fig. 17.34.

The results of the posthoc analysis show that, for seven of the eight coprimary endpoints, the

favorable changes were more pronounced as a function of decreased CEMA levels. This was the case for COHb, 8-epi-PGF-2α, 11-DTX-B2, sICAM-1, total NNAL, WBC, and FEV1%pred. The HDL-C levels were unexpectedly higher in the third and fourth quartiles than in the first and second quartiles. The apparent trend was, however, not flat across the quartiles, and the accuracy of the HDL-C estimates is relatively low compared to the estimates of the other endpoints. The group with the lowest CEMA levels consisted of about 23% (n = 56) of the 245 subjects in the THS use category. On the basis of the CEMA levels observed in this group (10.7 ± 9.77 ng/mg$_{creat}$) and upon comparison with the CEMA levels observed in the THS group on day 90 in the 3-month reduced exposure clinical study in the US (REXA-08-US) (24.62 ± 26.891 ng/mg$_{creat}$), these 23% of the subjects can be assumed to have switched completely to THS (i.e., above 95% product use). The analysis, using objective biochemical verification of concomitant cigarette use, allowed elucidation of the dose–response relationship between degrees of concomitant

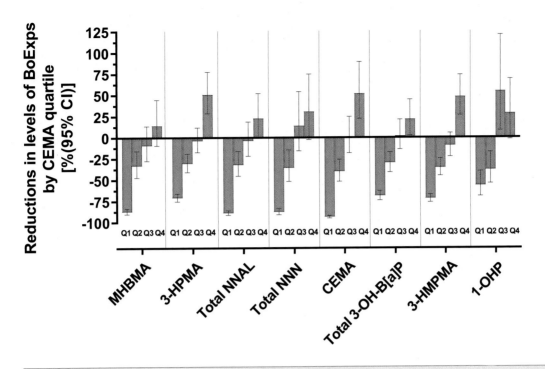

ZRHR-ERS-09-US   6 months THS:Cigarette

FIG. 17.35 Reductions in levels of urinary BoExps in THS users classified per CEMA quartile at month 6. *1-OHP*, total 1-hydroxypyrene; *3-HMPMA*, 3-hydroxy-1-methylpropyl-mercapturic acid; *3-HPMA*, 3-hydroxypropylmercapturic acid; *3-OH-B[a]P*, 3-hydroxybenzo[a]pyrene; *BoExp*, biomarker of exposure; *CI*, confidence interval; *CEMA*, 2-cyanoethylmercapturic acid; *MHBMA*, monohydroxybutenylmercapturic acid; *NNN*, N-nitrosonornicotine; *THS*, Tobacco Heating System 2.2.

TABLE 17.29
Proportion of subjects who reported a regular need to cough at 6 months.

	THS use LS mean (95%CI)	CC LS mean (95% CI)	Dual use LS mean (95%CI)	Odds ratio THS use/CC use LS mean (95%CI)	Odds ratio dual use/CC use LS mean (95%CI)
Proportion of subjects reporting regular need to cough at 6 months (%)	20.8 (14.7, 28.6)	30.7 (24.6, 37.5)	28.7 (20.3, 39.0)	0.593 (0.377, 0.932) $P = .024^*$	0.911 (0.554, 1.50) $P = .712$

CC, cigarettes; *CI*, confidence interval; *LS*, least squares; *THS*, Tobacco Heating System 2.2.

product use. It also strengthens the validity of the selected coprimary BoPHs and reinforces their role as intermediate endpoints for assessing the health risk associated with new tobacco products in a premarket setting until long-term data can be obtained when such products are commercialized.

(2) In THS users, the reductions in all BoExp relative to subjects who continued smoking were, as expected, much higher in the lowest quartile of CEMA (Fig. 17.35).

The reductions in BoExps in the THS arm versus the cigarette arm were much more pronounced in subjects

TABLE 17.30
Primary comparative analysis of the selected eight coprimary endpoints between the THS use and CC use categories at month 6.

Endpoint	Change from CC use	LS mean difference relative reduction	95% CI	LS mean difference relative reduction	95% CI
		Primary analysis		Posthoc analysis—1st quartile CEMA	
HDL-C	Difference	3.09 mg/dL	1.10, 5.09	2.84 mg/dL	0.08, 5.61
WBC	Difference	−0.420 GI/L	−0.717, −0.123	−0.93 GI/L	−1.38, −0.5
sICAM-1	%Reduction	2.86%	−0.426, 6.04	9.24%	4.30, 13.9
11-DTX-B$_2$	%Reduction	4.74%	−7.50, 15.6	11.3%	−8.00, 27.2
8-epi-PGF$_{2\alpha}$	%Reduction	6.80%	−0.216, 13.3	26.2%	17.3, 34.1
Total NNAL	%Reduction	56.5%	48.1, 66.30	89.0%	86.1, 91.3
COHb	%Reduction	32.2%	24.5, 39.0	70.2%	65.4, 74.4
FEV$_1$	Difference	1.28 %pred	0.145, 2.42	2.3%	0.40, 4.20

1-DTX-B2, 11-dehydrothromboxane B2; *THS*, Tobacco Heating System 2.2; *8-epi-PGF2α*, 8-epi-prostaglandin F2α; *BoPH*, biomarker of potential harm; *CC*, cigarettes; *COHb*, carboxyhemoglobin; *FEV$_1$*, forced expiratory volume in 1 s; *HDL-C*, high-density lipoprotein cholesterol; *NNAL*, 4-(methylnitrosamino)-1-(3-pyridyl)-1-butanol; *SA*, smoking abstinence; *sICAM-1*, soluble intercellular adhesion molecule; *WBC*, white blood cells.

who had low levels of urinary CEMA (first quartile) than in those who had high levels of urinary CEMA, with reductions ranging from −45% to −85% in the first quartile and −1% to +37% in subjects with the highest levels of urinary CEMA (fourth quartile).

17.6.1.3.5.2 Conclusions on the additional analyses. Importantly, this posthoc analysis—based on objective biochemical evaluation of cigarette smoke exposure on the basis of the CEMA distribution levels in the THS use group—showed that there is an inverse dose—effect relationship between the degree of smoking and overall magnitude of favorable changes in BoPHs. The degrees of exposure reduction and favorable changes in BoPHs are thus maximized upon complete switching, that is, abandoning cigarettes completely.

17.6.1.3.6 Conclusions. Altogether, the changes observed in this 6-month study indicate that switching completely from smoking cigarettes to THS use could have benefits from cardiovascular, respiratory, and cancer perspectives, as indicated by the favorable changes observed in the BoPHs covering the main pathways underlying disease development.

Switching to THS impacted lipid metabolism favorably, as smoking cessation does, with a significant increase in the levels of HDL-C. Similar to what has been reported for smoking cessation (Lee et al., 2014; Lowe et al., 2009; Oguogho et al., 2000; Tonstad and Cowan, 2009), oxidative stress and inflammation were reduced upon switching to THS use, as reflected by the significant reduction in WBC counts and 8-epi-PGF2α levels (Eliasson et al., 2001; Hammett et al., 2007; Pilz et al., 2000; U.S. Department of Health and Human Services, 2010). Only slight changes were observed in vascular function (clotting, thrombosis, and endothelial function) in general, with trends of reduction in sICAM-1 and 11-DTX-B2 levels that were more pronounced in the THS use group than in the dual use group. These findings mirror the data reported when subjects stop smoking, with a decrease in the levels of 11-DTX-B2 (Rangemark et al., 1993) and sICAM-1 (Scott et al., 2000).

This was the first clinical study to demonstrate favorable positive biological impacts on multiple pathophysiological mechanistic pathways involved in the development of smoking-related diseases, following switching from smoking to an EHTP versus continued cigarette smoking over a 6-month period of product use.

17.6.2 Clinical studies on EHTPs — Other studies

In addition to PMI, BAT and Japan Tobacco International (JTI) are major players in the field of EHTPs.

BAT has taken a clinical assessment approach for their EHTP that is comparable to the one followed by PMI. They have published two papers, in 2019 (Newland et al., 2019) and 2020 (Camacho et al., 2020), describing a 1-year study in the United Kingdom, which should be now almost complete. They planned to enroll up to 280 participants who did not intend to quit smoking and randomize them to a continued combustible smoking group (arm A; up to n = 80) or to a group that would use BAT's commercially available EHTP (arm B; n = 200). Furthermore, they planned to enroll up to 190 participants with a high intent to quit smoking in a smoking cessation group (arm D) and 40 never-smokers in a control group (arm E). Their primary objective is to "quantitatively assess differences in primary study endpoints at 90, 180, and 360 days between subjects who continue to smoke conventional cigarettes and subjects who switch to a tobacco heating product (THP)," and their selected endpoints are total NNAL, 8-epi-PGF-2α, and augmentation index, which is a physiological measure of systemic arterial stiffness. In their analyses, they plan to test CEVal as a marker of compliance in the EHTP arm by using a stepwise merging method starting with the lower category of CEVal levels; this category will be merged with the next category until the minimum number of 30 subjects is reached (Camacho et al., 2020).

The study was initiated in February 2018 and planned to be completed in early 2020; thus, data may be expected to be released by the beginning of 2021.

JTI has recently released data from a clinical study, in which seven BoPHs linked to smoking-related diseases were measured in 259 hybrid tobacco product users, 100 cigarette smokers, and 100 never-smokers (Japan Tobacco Inc., 2020). This study was conducted after approval from the IRB of each site.

The selected BoPHs were the same as the eight BoPHs PMI had selected for the ERS-09-US study, except for total NNAL, which was not measured as part of JTI's main assessments. Not all the study details were released, preventing a proper understanding of the study design and statistical approach, but it appears that the study duration was likely to have been 3 months.

There is no mention of statistical significance in the changes in the BoPHs; however, at the end of the study, it appears that most BoPHs were reaching levels comparable with those in never-smokers.

17.7 OVERALL CONCLUSIONS

The clinical assessment of ENDPs is designed to assess the disease risk reduction potential of ENDPs and their ability to protect public health from the harms caused by cigarette smoking (Chapter 1). As depicted by the THR equation (Chapter 1), to achieve this objective, an ENDP must not only reduce the risk of developing smoking-related diseases among smokers who switch to it but also be an acceptable long-term alternative to cigarettes for current smokers, while not attracting unintended audiences, as described in Chapter 1. While the clinical assessment of ENDPs addresses the risk to the individual, it can also provide important insights into product acceptance. This includes parameters such as the nicotine absorption profile, ENDP safety and tolerability, product use patterns during the switching process, as well as self-reported outcomes (e.g., sensory experience, urge-to-smoke a cigarette, withdrawal symptoms, and perceived risk) related to ENDP use by smokers.

The central tenet of THR is that ENDPs emit a significantly lower level of toxicants than cigarettes (Chapters 4, 6 and 7) and, hence, switching from cigarette smoking to ENDP use should lead to a significant reduction in exposure to cigarette smoke toxicants; this is the first causal link of the CELSD (Chapter 3). The substantial overall reduction in toxicant exposure of smokers who switched to ENDP use has been demonstrated in clinical reduced exposure studies across a variety of ENDPs. Furthermore, this substantial drop in toxicant exposure approached that observed in smokers who abstained from smoking during the same investigational period.

According to the principle of toxicology, a reduction in toxicant exposure should lead to reduced adverse effects in the subsequent events along the CELSD. A 6-month clinical exposure response study has confirmed this, as BoPHs have displayed positive changes, i.e., in the direction of cessation, upon switching from cigarette smoking to the use of THS. Importantly, this study also showed that the positive changes in BoPHs are in a dose—response relationship with the degree of concurrent cigarette and THS use; the most positive changes were achieved by the study participants who switched completely to THS. This observation parallels the results of the nonclinical studies summarized earlier (Chapters 13—15).

While long-term disease risk reduction and epidemiological studies (Chapter 21) are still outstanding, the totality of the available evidence shows that ENDPs have the potential to reduce the risk of smoking-related disease and, thereby, reduce the harm caused by cigarette smoking.

REFERENCES

Adriaens, K., Gucht, D.V., Baeyens, F., 2018. IQOS(TM) vs. e-cigarette vs. tobacco cigarette: a direct comparison of short-term effects after overnight-abstinence. Int. J. Environ. Res. Publ. Health 15 (12).

Anderson, G.D., Chan, L.N., 2016. Pharmacokinetic drug interactions with tobacco, cannabinoids and smoking cessation products. Clin. Pharmacokinet. 55 (11), 1353–1368.

Andrikoula, M., McDowell, I.F.W., 2008. The contribution of ApoB and ApoA1 measurements to cardiovascular risk assessment. Diabetes Obes. Metabol. 10 (4), 271–278.

Ansari, S.M., Lama, N., Blanc, N., Skiada, D., Ancerewicz, J., Picavet, P., et al., 2018. Evaluation of biological and functional changes in healthy smokers after switching from cigarettes to Tobacco Heating System (THS) 2.2 for 6 months. In: Oral Presentation at the Fifth Global Forum on Nicotine, Warsaw, Poland. Available from: https://www.pmiscience.com/resources/docs/default-source/gfn-2018/evaluation-of-biological-and-functional-changes.pdf?sfvrsn=1adfc006_2. (Accessed 27 August 2018).

Asmat, U., Abad, K., Ismail, K., 2016. Diabetes mellitus and oxidative stress - a concise review. Saudi Pharmaceut. J. 24, 547–553.

Aubin, H.J., Farley, A., Lycett, D., Lahmek, P., Aveyard, P., 2012. Weight gain in smokers after quitting cigarettes: meta-analysis. Br. Med. J. 345, e4439.

Beatrice, F., Massaro, G., 2019. Exhaled carbon monoxide levels in forty resistant to cessation male smokers after six months of full switch to electronic cigarettes (e-cigs) or to a Tobacco Heating Systems (THS). Int. J. Environ. Res. Publ. Health 16 (20).

Behar, R.Z., Hua, M., Talbot, P., 2015. Puffing topography and nicotine intake of electronic cigarette users. PloS One 10 (2), e0117222.

Belushkin, M., Tafin Djoko, D., Esposito, M., Korneliou, A., Jeannet, C., Lazzerini, M., et al., 2019. Selected harmful and potentially harmful constituents levels in commercial e-cigarettes. Chem. Res. Toxicol. https://doi.org/10.1021/acs.chemrestox.9b00470. Epub ahead of print 2019/12/21.

Benowitz, N.L., Hukkanen, J., Jacob 3rd, P., 2009. Nicotine chemistry, metabolism, kinetics and biomarkers. Handb. Exp. Pharmacol. 192, 29–60. https://doi.org/10.1007/978-3-540-69248-5_2. Epub ahead of print 2009/02/03.

Benowitz, N.L., Jacob 3rd, P., 1993. Nicotine and cotinine elimination pharmacokinetics in smokers and nonsmokers. Clin. Pharmacol. Therapeut. 53 (3), 316–323.

Benowitz, N.L., Jacob 3rd, P., 1994. Metabolism of nicotine to cotinine studied by a dual stable isotope method. Clin. Pharmacol. Therapeut. 56 (5), 483–493.

Benowitz, N.L., Jacob 3rd, P., 2000. Effects of cigarette smoking and carbon monoxide on nicotine and cotinine metabolism. Clin. Pharmacol. Therapeut. 67, 653–659.

Benowitz, N.L., Jacob 3rd, P., Fong, I., Gupta, S., 1994. Nicotine metabolic profile in man: comparison of cigarette smoking and transdermal nicotine. J. Pharmacol. Exp. Therapeut. 268 (1), 296–303.

Benowitz, N.L., Lessov-Schlaggar, C.N., Swan, G.E., Jacob 3rd, P., 2006. Female sex and oral contraceptive use accelerate nicotine metabolism. Clin. Pharmacol. Therapeut. 79 (5), 480–488.

Benowitz, N.L., Perez-Stable, E.J., Fong, I., Modin, G., Herrera, B., Jacob 3rd, P., 1999. Ethnic differences in N-glucuronidation of nicotine and cotinine. J. Pharmacol. Exp. Therapeut. 291, 1196–1203.

Benowitz, N.L., Perez-Stable, E.J., Herrera, B., Jacob 3rd, P., 2002. Slower metabolism and reduced intake of nicotine from cigarette smoking in Chinese-Americans. J. Natl. Cancer Inst. 94 (2), 108–115.

Berg, C., Schauer, G.L., Ahluwalia, J.S., Benowitz, N., 2012. Correlates of NNAL levels among nondaily and daily smokers in the college student population. Curr. Biomark. Find. 2, 87–94.

Blank, M.D., Breland, A.B., Enlow, P.T., Duncan, C., Metzger, A., Cobb, C.O., 2016. Measurement of smoking behavior: comparison of self-reports, returned cigarette butts, and toxicant levels. Exp. Clin. Psychopharmacol 24 (5), 348–355.

Bozinoff, N., Le Foll, B., 2018. Understanding the implications of the biobehavioral basis of nicotine addiction and its impact on the efficacy of treatment. Expet Rev. Respir. Med. 12 (9), 793–804.

Breland, A.B., Buchhalter, A.R., Evans, S.E., Eissenberg, T., 2002. Evaluating acute effects of potential reduced-exposure products for smokers: clinical laboratory methodology. Nicotine Tob. Res. 4 (Suppl. 2), S131–S140.

Brossard, P., Weitkunat, R., Poux, V., Lama, N., Haziza, C., Picavet, P., et al., 2017. Nicotine pharmacokinetic profiles of the Tobacco Heating System 2.2, cigarettes and nicotine gum in Japanese smokers. Regul. Toxicol. Pharmacol. 89, 193–199.

Bullen, C., McRobbie, H., Thornley, S., Glover, M., Lin, R., Laugesen, M., 2010. Effect of an electronic nicotine delivery device (e cigarette) on desire to smoke and withdrawal, user preferences and nicotine delivery: randomised cross-over trial. Tobac. Contr. 19 (2), 98–103.

Byrd, G.D., Chang, K.M., Greene, J.M., deBethizy, J.D., 1992. Evidence for urinary excretion of glucuronide conjugates of nicotine, cotinine, and trans-3'-hydroxycotinine in smokers. Drug Metabol. Dispos. 20 (2), 192–197.

Cagle, P.T., Allen, T.C., Olsen, R.J., 2013. Lung cancer biomarkers: present status and future developments. Arch. Pathol. Lab Med. 137 (9), 1191–1198.

Caldwell, B., Sumner, W., Crane, J., 2012. A systematic review of nicotine by inhalation: is there a role for the inhaled route? Nicotine Tob. Res. 14 (10), 1127–1139.

Camacho, O.M., Hedge, A., Lowe, F., Newland, N., Gale, N., McEwan, M., et al., 2020. Statistical analysis plan for "A randomised, controlled study to evaluate the effects of switching from cigarette smoking to using a tobacco heating product on health effect indicators in healthy subjects". Contem. Clin. Trials Commun. 17, 100535.

Caponnetto, P., Maglia, M., Prosperini, G., Busa, B., Polosa, R., 2018. Carbon monoxide levels after inhalation from new generation heated tobacco products. Respir. Res. 19 (1), 164.

Cappelleri, J.C., Bushmakin, A.G., Baker, C.L., Merikle, E., Olufade, A.O., Gilbert, D.G., 2007. Confirmatory factor analyses and reliability of the modified cigarette evaluation questionnaire. Addict. Behav. 32, 912–923.

Caraballo, R.S., Giovino, G.A., Pechacek, T.F., Mowery, P.D., Richter, P.A., Strauss, W.J., et al., 1998. Racial and ethnic differences in serum cotinine levels of cigarette smokers: third National Health and Nutrition Examination Survey, 1988-1991. JAMA, J. Am. Med. Assoc. 280 (2), 135–139.

Carter, B.D., Abnet, C.C., Feskanich, D., Freedman, N.D., Hartge, P., Lewis, C.E., et al., 2015. Smoking and mortality–Beyond established causes. New England J. Med. 372 (7), 631–640. https://doi.org/10.1056/NEJMsa1407211.

Ceriello, A., Motz, E., 2004. Is oxidative stress the pathogenic mechanism underlying insulin resistance, diabetes, and cardiovascular disease? The common soil hypothesis revisited. Arterioscler. Thromb. Vasc. Biol. 24 (5), 816–823.

Chang, C.M., Cheng, Y.C., Cho, T.M., Mishina, E.V., Del Valle-Pinero, A.Y., van Bemmel, D.M., et al., 2019. Biomarkers of potential harm: summary of an FDA-sponsored public workshop. Nicotine Tob. Res. 21 (1), 3–13.

Chen, Z.-H., Kim, H.P., Sciurba, F.C., Lee, S.-J., Feghali-Bostwick, C., Stolz, D.B., et al., 2008. Egr-1 regulates autophagy in cigarette smoke-induced chronic obstructive pulmonary disease. PloS One 3 (10), e3316.

Cheng, T., 2014. Chemical evaluation of electronic cigarettes. Tobac. Contr. 23 (Suppl. 2), ii11–17.

Claussen, A., Donelli, A., Copalu, W., Lama, N., Weitkunat, R., Haziza, C., et al., 2019. Exploring discriminant capacity of urinary CEMA as combustion marker in tobacco users - a population pharmacokinetic approach. In: Poster Presented at the Society for Research on Nicotine and Tobacco Meeting, San Francisco, CA, USA. Available from: https://www.pmiscience.com/library/publication/exploring-discriminant-capacity-of-urinary-cema-as-combustion-marker-in-tobacco-users. (Accessed 22 March 2019).

Cobb, C.O., Weaver, M.F., Eissenberg, T., 2010. Evaluating the acute effects of oral, non-combustible potential reduced exposure products marketed to smokers. Tobac. Contr. 19 (5), 367–373.

Cox, L.S., Tiffany, S.T., Christen, A.G., 2001. Evaluation of the brief questionnaire of smoking urges (QSU-brief) in laboratory and clinical settings. Nicotine Tob. Res. 3, 7–16.

De Jesus, S., Hsin, A., Faulkner, G., Prapavessis, H., 2013. A systematic review and analysis of data reduction techniques for the CReSS smoking topography device. J. Smok. Cessat. 10, 1–17.

Dempsey, D., Tutka, P., Jacob 3rd, P., Allen, F., Schoedel, K., Tyndale, R.F., et al., 2004. Nicotine metabolite ratio as an index of cytochrome P450 2A6 metabolic activity. Clin. Pharmacol. Therapeut. 76 (1), 64–72.

Dempsey, D.A., St Helen, G., Jacob 3rd, P., Tyndale, R.F., Benowitz, N.L., 2013. Genetic and pharmacokinetic determinants of response to transdermal nicotine in white, black, and Asian nonsmokers. Clin. Pharmacol. Therapeut. 94 (6), 687–694.

Denton, T.T., Zhang, X., Cashman, J.R., 2004. Nicotine-related alkaloids and metabolites as inhibitors of human cytochrome P-450 2A6. Biochem. Pharmacol. 67 (4), 751–756.

Digard, H., Proctor, C., Kulasekaran, A., Malmqvist, U., Richter, A., 2013. Determination of nicotine absorption from multiple tobacco products and nicotine gum. Nicotine Tob. Res. 15 (1), 255–261.

Doll, R., Peto, R., 1981. The causes of cancer: quantitative estimates of avoidable risks of cancer in the United States today. J. Natl. Cancer Inst. 66 (6), 1191–1308.

Domino, E.F., Kadoya, C., Matsuoka, S., Ni, L., Fedewa, K.S., 2003. Comparative American and Japanese tobacco smoke uptake parameters after overnight tobacco deprivation. Prog. Neuro Psychopharmacol. Biol. Psychiatr. 27 (6), 973–984.

Doyle, T.J., Pinto-Plata, V., Morse, D., Celli, B.R., Rosas, I.O., 2012. The expanding role of biomarkers in the assessment of smoking-related parenchymal lung diseases. Chest 142 (4), 1027–1034.

Eliasson, B., Hjalmarson, A., Kruse, E., Landfeldt, B., Westin, A., 2001. Effect of smoking reduction and cessation on cardiovascular risk factors. Nicotine Tob. Res. 3 (3), 249–255.

EMA (European Medicines Agency), 2008. Guideline on the Development of Medicinal Products for the Treatment of Smoking (CHMP/EWP/369963/05).

English, P.B., Eskenazi, B., Christianson, R.E., 1994. Black-White differences in serum cotinine levels among pregnant women and subsequent effects on infant birthweight. Am. J. Publ. Health 84 (9).

Ersoz, G., Ersoz, S., 2003. Changes in portal blood flow following acute exercise in liver transplant recipients. Transplant. Proc. 35 (4), 1456–1457.

Evans, S.E., Hoffman, A.C., 2014. Electronic cigarettes: abuse liability, topography and subjective effects. Tobac. Contr. 23 (Suppl. 2), ii23–29.

Faber, M.S., Fuhr, U., 2004. Time response of cytochrome P450 1A2 activity on cessation of heavy smoking. Clin. Pharmacol. Therapeut. 76 (2), 178–184.

Farsalinos, K.E., Romagna, G., Tsiapras, D., Kyrzopoulos, S., Voudris, V., 2013. Evaluation of electronic cigarette use (vaping) topography and estimation of liquid consumption: implications for research protocol standards definition and for public health authorities' regulation. Int. J. Environ. Res. Publ. Health 10 (6), 2500–2514.

FDA (Food and Drug Administration), 2001. Guidance for Industry - Bioanalytical Method Validation.

FDA (Food and Drug Administration), 2012. Guidance for Industry - Reporting Harmful and Potentially Harmful Constituents in Tobacco Products and Tobacco Smoke Under Section 904(a)(3) of the Federal Food, Drug, and Cosmetic Act - Draft Guidance.

FDA (Food and Drug Administration), 2017. Philip Morris Products S.A. Modified Risk Tobacco Product (MRTP)

Applications - Module 6: Summaries of All Research Findings. Available from: https://www.fda.gov/tobacco-products/advertising-and-promotion/philip-morris-products-sa-modified-risk-tobacco-product-mrtp-applications#6. (Accessed 26 February 2020).

FDA (Food and Drug Administration), 2019. Guidance for Industry - Premarket Tobacco Product Applications for Electronic Nicotine Delivery Systems. Available from: https://www.fda.gov/media/127853/download. (Accessed 27 September 2019).

Fearon, I.M., Eldridge, A., Gale, N., Shepperd, C.J., McEwan, M., Camacho, O.M., et al., 2017. E-cigarette nicotine delivery: data and learnings from pharmacokinetic studies. Am. J. Health Behav. 41 (1), 16–32.

Fearon, I.M., Eldridge, A.C., Gale, N., McEwan, M., Stiles, M.F., Round, E.K., 2018. Nicotine pharmacokinetics of electronic cigarettes: a review of the literature. Regul. Toxicol. Pharmacol. 100, 25–34.

Fearon, I.M., Phillips, G., Carr, T., Taylor, M., Breheny, D., Faux, S.P., 2011. The role of oxidative stress in smoking-related diseases. Mini-Reviews Org. Chem. 8 (4), 360–371.

Federico, A., Morgillo, F., Tuccillo, C., Ciardiello, F., Loguercio, C., 2007. Chronic inflammation and oxidative stress in human carcinogenesis. Int. J. Canc. 121 (11), 2381–2386.

Forster, M., Fiebelkorn, S., Yurteri, C., Mariner, D., Liu, C., Wright, C., et al., 2018. Assessment of novel tobacco heating product THP1.0. Part 3: comprehensive chemical characterisation of harmful and potentially harmful aerosol emissions. Regul. Toxicol. Pharmacol. 93, 14–33. https://doi.org/10.1016/j.yrtph.2017.10.006. 29080848.

Frost-Pineda, K., Zedler, B.K., Oliveri, D., Feng, S., Liang, Q., Roethig, H.J., 2008. Short-term clinical exposure evaluation of a third-generation Electrically Heated Cigarette Smoking System (EHCSS) in adult smokers. Regul. Toxicol. Pharmacol. 52, 104–110.

Gale, N., McEwan, M., Eldridge, A.C., Fearon, I.M., Sherwood, N., Bowen, E., et al., 2018. Changes in biomarkers of exposure on switching from a conventional cigarette to tobacco heating products: a randomized, controlled study in healthy Japanese subjects. Nicotine Tob. Res. https://doi.org/10.1093/ntr/nty104. Epub ahead of print 2018/06/19.

Gale, N., McEwan, M., Eldridge, A.C., Sherwood, N., Bowen, E., McDermott, S., et al., 2017. A randomised, controlled, two-Centre open-label study in healthy Japanese subjects to evaluate the effect on biomarkers of exposure of switching from a conventional cigarette to a tobacco heating product. BMC Publ. Health 17 (1), 673.

Gaur, S., Agnihotri, R., 2019. Health effects of trace metals in electronic cigarette aerosols-a systematic review. Biol. Trace Elem. Res. 188 (2), 295–315.

Global Initiative for Chronic Obstructive Lung Disease (GOLD), 2020. Global Strategy for the Diagnosis, Management, and Prevention of Chronic Obstructive Lung Disease: The GOLD Science Committee Report 2020. Available from: https://goldcopd.org/gold-reports/. (Accessed 18 April 2020).

Goniewicz, M.L., Gawron, M., Smith, D.M., Peng, M., Jacob 3rd, P., Benowitz, N.L., 2017. Exposure to nicotine and selected toxicants in cigarette smokers who switched to electronic cigarettes: a longitudinal within-subjects observational study. Nicotine Tob. Res. 19 (2), 160–167.

Goniewicz, M.L., Havel, C.M., Peng, M.W., Jacob 3rd, P., Dempsey, D., Yu, L., et al., 2009. Elimination kinetics of the tobacco-specific biomarker and lung carcinogen 4-(methylnitrosamino)-1-(3-pyridyl)-1-butanol. Canc. Epidemiol. Biomarkers Prev. 18 (12), 3421–3425.

Goniewicz, M.L., Smith, D.M., Edwards, K.C., Blount, B.C., Caldwell, K.L., Feng, J., et al., 2018. Comparison of nicotine and toxicant exposure in users of electronic cigarettes and combustible cigarettes. JAMA Network Open 1 (8), e185937.

Gries, J.M., Benowitz, N., Verotta, D., 1996. Chronopharmacokinetics of nicotine. Clin. Pharmacol. Therapeut. 60 (4), 385–395.

Guerrero-Cignarella, A., Luna Diaz, L.V., Balestrini, K., Holt, G., Mirsaeidi, M., Calderon-Candelario, R., et al., 2018. Differences in vaping topography in relation to adherence to exclusive electronic cigarette use in veterans. PloS One 13 (4), e0195896.

Hailperin, R., 1965. Best possible inequalities for the probability of a logical function of events. Am. Math. Mon. 72 (4), 343–359.

Hajek, P., Goniewicz, M.L., Phillips, A., Myers Smith, K., West, O., McRobbie, H., 2014. Nicotine intake from electronic cigarettes on initial use and after 4 weeks of regular use. Nicotine Tob. Res. https://doi.org/10.1093/ntr/ntu153. Epub ahead of print 2014/08/15.

Hajek, P., Pittaccio, K., Pesola, F., Myers Smith, K., Phillips-Waller, A., Przulj, D., 2020. Nicotine delivery and users' reactions to Juul compared with cigarettes and other e-cigarette products. Addiction 115 (6), 1141–1148.

Halliwell, B., 2007. Oxidative stress and cancer: have we moved forward? Biochem. J. 401 (1), 1–11.

Hammett, C.J., Prapavessis, H., Baldi, J.C., Ameratunga, R., Schoenbeck, U., Varo, N., et al., 2007. Variation in blood levels of inflammatory markers related and unrelated to smoking cessation in women. Prev. Cardiol. 10 (2), 68–75.

Hammond, D., Fong, G.T., Cummings, K.M., Hyland, A., 2005. Smoking topography, brand switching, and nicotine delivery: results from an in vivo study. Canc. Epidemiol. Biomarkers Prev. 14 (6), 1370–1375.

Hanson, K., O'Connor, R., Hatsukami, D., 2009. Measures for assessing subjective effects of potential reduced-exposure products. Canc. Epidemiol. Biomarkers Prev. 18 (12), 3209–3224.

Harris, J.E., Thun, M.J., Mondul, A.M., E, C.E., 2004. Cigarette tar yields in relation to mortality from lung cancer in the cancer prevention study II prospective cohort, 1982-8. Br. Med. J. 328 (7431), 72.

Harrison, D., Griendling, K.K., Landmesser, U., Hornig, B., Drexler, H., 2003. Role of oxidative stress in atherosclerosis. Am. J. Cardiol. 91 (3), 7–11.

Haziza, C., de La Bourdonnaye, G., Donelli, A., Poux, V., Skiada, D., Weitkunat, R., et al., 2019. Reduction in exposure to selected Harmful and Potentially Harmful Constituents approaching those observed upon smoking abstinence in smokers switching to the menthol Tobacco Heating System 2.2 for three months (part 1). Nicotine Tob. Res. https://doi.org/10.1093/ntr/ntz013. Epub ahead of print 2019/02/06.

Haziza, C., de La Bourdonnaye, G., Donelli, A., Skiada, D., Poux, V., Weitkunat, R., et al., 2020. Favorable changes in biomarkers of potential harm to reduce the adverse health effects of smoking in smokers switching to the menthol tobacco heating system 2.2 for three months (Part 2). Nicotine Tob. Res. 22 (4), 549—559.

Haziza, C., de La Bourdonnaye, G., Merlet, S., Benzimra, M., Ancerewicz, J., Donelli, A., et al., 2016. Assessment of the reduction in levels of exposure to harmful and potentially harmful constituents in Japanese subjects using a novel tobacco heating system compared with conventional cigarettes and smoking abstinence: a randomized controlled study in confinement. Regul. Toxicol. Pharmacol. 81, 489—499.

Haziza, C., de La Bourdonnaye, G., Skiada, D., Ancerewicz, J., Baker, G., Picavet, P., et al., 2016. Evaluation of the Tobacco Heating System 2.2. Part 8: 5-day randomized reduced exposure clinical study in Poland. Regul. Toxicol. Pharmacol. (Suppl. 2), S139—S150. Available from: http://www.sciencedirect.com/science/article/pii/S0273230016303312. (Accessed 3 May 2017).

Haziza, C., de La Bourdonnaye, G., Skiada, D., Ancerewicz, J., Baker, G., Picavet, P., et al., 2017. Biomarker of exposure level data set in smokers switching from conventional cigarettes to Tobacco Heating System 2.2, continuing smoking or abstaining from smoking for 5 days. Data Brief 10, 283—293.

Health Canada, 2013. Consolidation - Tobacco Reporting Regulations. DORS/2000-273.

Health Canada, Modified, 2011. Tobacco Reporting Regulations. Available from: http://www.hc-sc.gc.ca/hc-ps/tobac-tabac/legislation/reg/indust/method/index-eng.php#main. (Accessed 21 May 2014).

Helen, G.S., Ross, K.C., Dempsey, D.A., Havel, C.M., Jacob, P., Benowitz, N.L., 2016. Nicotine delivery and vaping behavior during ad libitum E-cigarette access. Tobacco Regul. Sci. 2 (4), 363—376.

Hengstermann, A., Müller, T., 2008. Endoplasmic reticulum stress induced by aqueous extracts of cigarette smoke in 3T3 cells activates the unfolded-protein-response-dependent PERK pathway of cell survival. Free Radic. Biol. Med. 44 (6), 1097—1107.

Higashi, E., Fukami, T., Itoh, M., Kyo, S., Inoue, M., Yokoi, T., et al., 2007. Human CYP2A6 is induced by estrogen via estrogen receptor. Drug Metabol. Dispos. 35 (10), 1935—1941.

Hill, A.B., 1965. The environment and disease: association or causation? Proc. Roy. Soc. Med. 58 (5), 295—300.

Hoeng, J., Maeder, S., Vanscheeuwijck, P., Peitsch, M.C., 2019. Assessing the lung cancer risk reduction potential of candidate modified risk tobacco products. Internal and Emergency Medicine 14 (6), 821—834. https://doi.org/10.1007/s11739-019-02045-z.

Hoffmann, D., Wynder, E.L., 1986. Chemical constituents and bioactivity of tobacco smoke. IARC (Int. Agency Res. Cancer) Sci. Publ. 74, 145—165. Epub ahead of print 1986/01/01.

Hughes, J.R., Hatsukami, D., 1986. Signs and symptoms of tobacco withdrawal. Arch. Gen. Psychiatr. 43 (3), 289—294.

Hughes, J.R., Hatsukami, D., 2012. Background on the Minnesota Withdrawal Scale-Revised (MNWS-R). Available from: http://www.uvm.edu/medicine/behaviorandhealth/documents/Background_8_2012.pdf. (Accessed 11 July 2016).

Hukkanen, J., Jacob 3rd, P., Benowitz, N.L., 2005. Metabolism and disposition kinetics of nicotine. Pharmacol. Rev. 57 (1), 79—115.

Hukkanen, J., Jacob 3rd, P., Benowitz, N.L., 2006. Effect of grapefruit juice on cytochrome P450 2A6 and nicotine renal clearance. Clin. Pharmacol. Therapeut. 80 (5), 522—530.

Hwang, J.W., Chung, S., Sundar, I.K., Yao, H., Arunachalam, G., McBurney, M.W., et al., 2010. Cigarette smoke-induced autophagy is regulated by SIRT1-PARP-1-dependent mechanism: implication in pathogenesis of COPD. Arch. Biochem. Biophys. 500 (2), 203—209.

IARC (International Agency for Research on Cancer), 2008. Measuring tobacco use behaviours. In: IARC Handbook of Cancer Prevention: Methods for Evaluating Tobacco Control Policies, pp. 75—105.

IOM (Institute of Medicine), 2012. Scientific Standards for Studies on Modified Risk Tobacco Products. The National Academies Press, Washington, DC, ISBN 978-0-309-22398-0.

Jakubowski, M., Linhart, I., Pielas, G., Kopecky, J., 1987. 2-Cyanoethylmercapturic acid (CEMA) in the urine as a possible indicator of exposure to acrylonitrile. Br. J. Ind. Med. 44 (12), 834—840.

Japan Tobacco Inc, 2020. Press Release - Clinical Study Shows Biomarker of Potential Harm Measured in Ploom TECH Users is Close to Never-Smokers. Available from: https://www.jt.com/media/news/2020/pdf/20200326_E01.pdf. (Accessed 15 April 2020).

Jassem, J., Przewozniak, K., Zatonski, W., 2014. Tobacco control in Poland-successes and challenges. Transl. Lung Cancer Res. 3 (5), 280—285.

Jay, J., Pfaunmiller, E.L., Huang, N.J., Cohen, G., Graff, D., 2019. 5-Day changes in biomarkers of exposure among adult smokers after completely wwitching from combustible cigarettes to a nicotine-salt pod system. Nicotine Tob. Res. https://doi.org/10.1093/ntr/ntz206. Epub ahead of print 2019/11/07.

Johnstone, E., Benowitz, N., Cargill, A., Jacob, R., Hinks, L., Day, I., et al., 2006. Determinants of the rate of nicotine metabolism and effects on smoking behavior. Clin. Pharmacol. Therapeut. 80 (4), 319—330.

Kandel, D.B., Hu, M.C., Schaffran, C., Udry, J.R., Benowitz, N.L., 2007. Urine nicotine metabolites and smoking behavior in a nultiracial/multiethnic national sample of young adults. Am. J. Epidemiol. 165 (8), 901—910.

Keaney, J.F., Larson, M.G., Vasan, R.S., Wilson, P.W.F., Lipinska, I., Corey, D., et al., 2003. Obesity and systemic oxidative stress clinical correlates of oxidative stress in the Framingham Study. Arterioscler. Thromb. Vasc. Biol. 23 (3), 434—439.

Krautter, G.R., Chen, P.X., Borgerding, M.F., 2015. Consumption patterns and biomarkers of exposure in cigarette smokers switched to Snus, various dissolvable tobacco products, Dual use, or tobacco abstinence. Regul. Toxicol. Pharmacol. 71 (2), 186—197.

Le Gal, A., 2003. Diversity of selective environmental substrates for human cytochrome P450 2A6: alkoxyethers, nicotine, coumarin, N-nitrosodiethylamine, and N-nitrosobenzylmethylamine. Toxicol. Lett. 144 (1), 77—91.

Lee, B.L., Jacob 3rd, P., Jarvik, M.E., Benowitz, N.L., 1989. Food and nicotine metabolism. Pharmacol., Biochem. Behav. 33, 621—625.

Lee, P.N., Forey, B.A., Fry, J.S., Thornton, A.J., Coombs, K.J., 2014. The Effect of Quitting Smoking on White Blood Cell Count - A Review Based on Within-Subject Changes [Internet]. Available from: http://www.pnlee.co.uk/documents/refs/lee2014D.pdf. (Accessed 15 May 2014).

Lenz, T.L., Gillespie, N., 2011. Transdermal patch drug delivery interactions with exercise. Sports Med. 41 (3), 177—183.

Lerman, C., Tyndale, R., Patterson, F., Wileyto, E.P., Shields, P.G., Pinto, A., et al., 2006. Nicotine metabolite ratio predicts efficacy of transdermal nicotine for smoking cessation. Clin. Pharmacol. Therapeut. 79 (6), 600—608.

Libby, P., Ridker, P.M., Maseri, A., 2002. Inflammation and atherosclerosis. Circulation 105 (9), 1135—1143.

Lorkiewicz, P., Riggs, D.W., Keith, R.J., Conklin, D.J., Xie, Z., Sutaria, S., et al., 2018. Comparison of urinary biomarkers of exposure in humans using electronic cigarettes, combustible cigarettes, and smokeless tobacco. Nicotine Tob. Res. https://doi.org/10.1093/ntr/nty089. Epub ahead of print 2018/06/06.

Lowe, F.J., Gregg, E.O., McEwan, M., 2009. Evaluation of biomarkers of exposure and potential harm in smokers, former smokers and never-smokers. Clin. Chem. Lab. Med. 47 (3), 311—320.

Lu, M., Lu, Q., Zhang, Y., Tian, G., 2011. ApoB/ApoA1 is an effective predictor of coronary heart disease risk in overweight and obesity. J. Biomed. Res. 25 (4), 266—273.

Lüdicke, F., Ansari, S.M., Lama, N., Blanc, N., Bosilkovska, M., Donelli, A., et al., 2019. Effects of switching to a heat-not-burn tobacco product on biologically relevant biomarkers to assess a candidate modified risk tobacco product: a randomized trial. Canc. Epidemiol. Biomarkers Prev. 28 (11), 1934—1943.

Lüdicke, F., Picavet, P., Baker, G., Haziza, C., Poux, V., Lama, N., et al., 2018. Effects of switching to the Menthol Tobacco Heating System 2.2, smoking abstinence, or continued cigarette smoking on clinically relevant risk markers: a randomized, controlled, open-label, multicenter study in sequential confinement and ambulatory settings (Part 2). Nicotine Tob. Res. 20 (2), 173—182.

Lüdicke, F., Picavet, P., Baker, G., Haziza, C., Poux, V., Lama, N., et al., 2018. Effects of switching to the Tobacco

Heating System 2.2 menthol, smoking abstinence, or continued cigarette smoking on biomarkers of exposure: a randomized, controlled, open-label, multicenter study in sequential confinement and ambulatory settings (Part 1). Nicotine Tob. Res. 20 (2), 161—172.

Lunell, E., Curvall, M., 2011. Nicotine delivery and subjective effects of Swedish portion snus compared with 4 mg nicotine polacrilex chewing gum. Nicotine Tob. Res. 13 (7), 573—578.

Lunell, E., Lunell, M., 2005. Steady-state nicotine plasma levels following use of four different types of Swedish snus compared with 2-mg Nicorette chewing gum: a crossover study. Nicotine Tob. Res. 7 (3), 397—403.

MacDougall, J.M., Fandrick, K., Zhang, X., Serafin, S.V., Cashman, J.R., 2003. Inhibition of human liver microsomal (S)-nicotine oxidation by (-)-menthol and analogues. Chem. Res. Toxicol. 16 (8), 988—993.

MacLeod, S., Sinha, R., Kadlubar, F.F., Lang, N.P., 1997. Polymorphisms of CYP1A1 and GSTM1 influence the in vivo function of CYP1A2. Mutat. Res. 376 (1—2), 135—142.

Madamanchi, N.R., Vendrov, A., Runge, M.S., 2005. Oxidative stress and vascular disease. Arterioscler. Thromb. Vasc. Biol. 25 (1), 29—38.

Malaiyandi, V., Goodz, S.D., Sellers, E.M., Tyndale, R.F., 2006. CYP2A6 genotype, phenotype, and the use of nicotine metabolites as biomarkers during ad libitum smoking. Canc. Epidemiol. Biomarkers Prev. 10, 1812—1819.

Marchand, M., Brossard, P., Merdjan, H., Lama, N., Weitkunat, R., Lüdicke, F., 2017. Nicotine population pharmacokinetics in healthy adult smokers: a retrospective analysis. Eur. J. Drug Metab. Pharmacokinet. https://doi.org/10.1007/s13318-017-0405-2. Epub ahead of print 2017/03/12.

Martin Leroy, C., Jarus-Dziedzic, K., Ancerewicz, J., Lindner, D., Kulesza, A., Magnette, J., 2012. Reduced exposure evaluation of an Electrically Heated Cigarette Smoking System. Part 7: a one-month, randomized, ambulatory, controlled clinical study in Poland. Regul. Toxicol. Pharmacol. 64 (2 Suppl. l), S74—S84.

Messina, E.S., Tyndale, R.F., Sellers, E.M., 1997. A major role for CYP2A6 in nicotine C-oxidation by human liver microsomes. J. Pharmacol. Exp. Therapeut. 282, 608—1614.

Molander, L., Hansson, A., Lunell, E., 2001. Pharmacokinetics of nicotine in healthy elderly people. Clin. Pharmacol. Therapeut. 69 (1), 57—65.

Nakajima, M., Yamamoto, T., Nunoya, K., Yokoi, T., Nagashima, K., Inoue, K., et al., 1996. Characterization of CYP2A6 involved in 3'-hydroxylation of cotinine in human liver microsomes. J. Pharmacol. Exp. Therapeut. 277 (2), 1010—1015.

Nakajima, M., Yamamoto, T., Nunoya, K., Yokoi, T., Nagashima, K., Inoue, K., et al., 1996. Role of human cytochrome P4502A6 in C-oxidation of nicotine. Drug Metabol. Dispos. 24 (11), 1212—1217.

Newland, N., Lowe, F.J., Camacho, O.M., McEwan, M., Gale, N., Ebajemito, J., et al., 2019. Evaluating the effects of switching from cigarette smoking to using a heated tobacco product on health effect indicators in healthy subjects: study protocol for a randomized controlled trial. Inter. Emergen. Med. https://doi.org/10.1007/s11739-019-02090-8. Epub ahead of print 2019/05/03.

Nozaki, T., Sugiyama, S., Koga, H., Sugamura, K., Ohba, K., Matsuzawa, Y., et al., 2009. Significance of a multiple biomarkers strategy including endothelial dysfunction to improve risk stratification for cardiovascular events in patients at high risk for coronary heart disease. J. Am. Coll. Cardiol. 54 (7), 601–608.

O'Connell, G., Graff, D.W., D'Ruiz, C.D., 2016. Reductions in biomarkers of exposure (BoE) to harmful or potentially harmful constituents (HPHCs) following partial or complete substitution of cigarettes with electronic cigarettes in adult smokers. Toxicol. Mech. Method. 26 (6), 443–454.

O'Connell, G., Pritchard, J.D., Prue, C., Thompson, J., Verron, T., Graff, D., et al., 2019. A randomised, open-label, cross-over clinical study to evaluate the pharmacokinetic profiles of cigarettes and e-cigarettes with nicotine salt formulations in US adult smokers. Inter. Emergen. Med. 14 (6), 853–861.

Oguogho, A., Lupattelli, G., Palumbo, B., Sinzinger, H., 2000. Isoprostanes quickly normalize after quitting cigarette smoking in healthy adults. Vasa 29 (2), 103–105.

Patterson, F., Schnoll, R.A., Wileyto, E.P., Pinto, A., Epstein, L.H., Shields, P.G., et al., 2008. Toward personalized therapy for smoking cessation: a randomized placebo-controlled trial of Bupropion. Clin. Pharmacol. Therapeut. 84 (3), 320–325.

Peck, M.J., Sanders, E.B., Scherer, G., Ludicke, F., Weitkunat, R., 2018. Review of biomarkers to assess the effects of switching from cigarettes to modified risk tobacco products. Biomarkers. https://doi.org/10.1080/1354750x.2017.1419284.1-32. Epub ahead of print 2018/01/04.

Pérez-Stable, E.J., Herrera, B., Jacob 3rd, P., Benowitz, N.L., 1998. Nicotine metabolism and intake in black and white smokers. JAMA, J. Am. Med. Assoc. 280 (2), 152–156.

Picavet, P., Haziza, C., Lama, N., Weitkunat, R., Ludicke, F., 2015. Comparison of the pharmacokinetics of nicotine following single and ad libitum use of a Tobacco Heating System or Combustible Cigarettes. Nicotine Tob. Res. https://doi.org/10.1093/ntr/ntv220.1-7. Epub ahead of print 2015/10/07.

Pilz, H., Oguogho, A., Chehne, F., Lupattelli, G., Palumbo, B., Sinzinger, H., 2000. Quitting cigarette smoking results in a fast improvement of in vivo oxidation injury (determined via plasma, serum and urinary isoprostane). Thromb. Res. 99 (3), 209–221.

R, D., R, P., Boreham, J., Sutherland, I., 2004. Mortality in relation to smoking: 50 years' observations on male British doctors. Br. Med. J. 328 (7455), 1519.

Ramoa, C.P., Hiler, M.M., Spindle, T.R., Lopez, A.A., Karaoghlanian, N., Lipato, T., et al., 2016. Electronic cigarette nicotine delivery can exceed that of combustible cigarettes: a preliminary report. Tobac. Contr. 25 (e1), e6–9.

Rangemark, C., Ciabattoni, G., Wennmalm, A., 1993. Excretion of thromboxane metabolites in healthy women after cessation of smoking. Arterioscler. Thromb. 13 (6), 777–782.

Raunio, H., Rautio, A., Gullsten, H., Pelkonen, O., 2001. Polymorphisms of CYP2A6 and its practical consequences. Br. J. Clin. Pharmacol. 52 (4), 357–363.

Rodgman, A., Perfetti, T.A., 2013. The Chemical Components of Tobacco and Tobacco Smoke. CRC Press, Taylor & Francis Inc (United States).

Rodriguez-Porcel, M., Lerman, A., Best, P.J., Krier, J.D., Napoli, C., Lerman, L.O., 2001. Hypercholesterolemia impairs myocardial perfusion and permeability: role of oxidative stress and endogenous scavenging activity. J. Am. Coll. Cardiol. 37 (2), 608–615.

Roemer, E., Schramke, H., Weiler, H., Buettner, A., Kausche, S., Weber, S., et al., 2012. Mainstream smoke chemistry and in vitro and in vivo toxicity of the reference cigarettes 3R4F and 2R4F. Beiträge zur Tabakforschung Int. 25 (1), 316–335.

Roemer, E., Stabbert, R., Rustemeier, K., Veltel, D.J., Meisgen, T.J., Reininghaus, W., et al., 2004. Chemical composition, cytotoxicity and mutagenicity of smoke from US commercial and reference cigarettes smoked under two sets of machine smoking conditions. Toxicology 195 (1), 31–52.

Rose, J.E., Mukhin, A.G., Lokitz, S.J., Turkington, T.G., Herskovic, J., Behm, F.M., et al., 2010. Kinetics of brain nicotine accumulation in dependent and nondependent smokers assessed with PET and cigarettes containing 11C-nicotine. Proc. Natl. Acad. Sci. U. S. A. 107 (11), 5190–5195.

Rosenberg, H., 2009. Clinical and laboratory assessment of the subjective experience of drug craving. Clin. Psychol. Rev. 29, 519–534.

Ross, R., 1999. Atherosclerosis - an inflammatory disease. N. Engl. J. Med. 340 (2), 115–126.

Rüger, B., 1978. [Das maximale Signifikanzniveau des Tests: "Lehne H_0 ab, wenn k unter n gegebenen Tests zur Ablehnung führen"] German. Metrika 25, 171–178.

Runkel, M., Bourian, M., Tegtmeier, M., Legrum, W., 1997. The character of inhibition of the metabolism of 1,2-benzopyrone (coumarin) by grapefruit juice in human. Eur. J. Clin. Pharmacol. 53, 265–269.

Rupprecht, L.E., Smith, T.T., Schassburger, R.L., Buffalari, D.M., Sved, A.F., Donny, E.C., 2015. Behavioral mechanisms underlying nicotine reinforcement. Curr Top Behav Neurosci 24, 19–53.

Sakaguchi, C., Kakehi, A., Minami, N., Kikuchi, A., Futamura, Y., 2014. Exposure evaluation of adult male Japanese smokers switched to a heated cigarette in a controlled clinical setting. Regul. Toxicol. Pharmacol. 69 (3), 338–347.

Sarkar, M., Kapur, S., Frost-Pineda, K., Feng, S., Wang, J., Liang, Q., et al., 2008. Evaluation of biomarkers of exposure to selected cigarette smoke constituents in adult smokers switched to carbon-filtered cigarettes in short-term and long-term clinical studies. Nicotine Tob. Res. 10 (12), 1761–1772.

Schaller, J.P., Keller, D., Poget, L., Pratte, P., Kaelin, E., McHugh, D., et al., 2016. Evaluation of the Tobacco Heating System 2.2. Part 2: chemical composition, genotoxicity, cytotoxicity, and physical properties of the aerosol. Regul. Toxicol. Pharmacol. (Suppl. 2), S27–S47. Available from: http://www.sciencedirect.com/science/article/pii/S027323 0016302902. (Accessed 3 May 2017).

Scherer, G., 2018. Suitability of biomarkers of biological effects (BOBEs) for assessing the likelihood of reducing the tobacco related disease risk by new and innovative tobacco products: a literature review. Regul. Toxicol. Pharmacol. 94, 203–233.

Schettgen, T., Broding, H.C., Angerer, J., Drexler, H., 2002. Hemoglobin adducts of ethylene oxide, propylene oxide, acrylonitrile and acrylamide-biomarkers in occupational and environmental medicine. Toxicol. Lett. 134 (1–3), 65–70.

Scheuermann, T.S., Richter, K.P., Rigotti, N.A., Cummins, S.E., Harrington, K.F., Sherman, S.E., et al., 2017. Accuracy of self-reported smoking abstinence in clinical trials of hospital-initiated smoking interventions. Addiction 112 (12), 2227–2236.

Schoedel, K.A., Sellers, E.M., Palmour, R., Tyndale, R.F., 2003. Down-regulation of hepatic nicotine metabolism and a CYP2A6-like enzyme in African green monkeys after long-term nicotine administration. Mol. Pharmacol. 63 (1), 96–104.

Schroeder, M.J., Hoffman, A.C., 2014. Electronic cigarettes and nicotine clinical pharmacology. Tobac. Contr. 23 (Suppl. 2), ii30–35.

Scott, D.A., Stapleton, J.A., Wilson, R.F., Sutherland, G., Palmer, R.M., Coward, P.Y., et al., 2000. Dramatic decline in circulating intercellular adhesion molecule-1 concentration on quitting tobacco smoking. Blood Cell Mol. Dis. 26 (3), 255–258.

Shiffman, S., West, R.J., Gilbert, D.G., 2004. Recommendation for the assessment of tobacco craving and withdrawal in smoking cessation trials. Nicotine Tob. Res. 6 (4), 599–614.

Sleiman, M., Logue, J.M., Montesinos, V.N., Russell, M.L., Litter, M.I., Gundel, L.A., et al., 2016. Emissions from electronic cigarettes: key parameters affecting the release of harmful chemicals. Environ. Sci. Technol. 50 (17), 9644–9651.

Smith, M.R., Clark, B., Ludicke, F., Schaller, J.P., Vanscheeuwijck, P., Hoeng, J., et al., 2016. Evaluation of the Tobacco Heating System 2.2. Part 1: description of the system and the scientific assessment program. Regul. Toxicol. Pharmacol. (Suppl. 2), S17–S26. Available from: http://www.sciencedirect.com/science/article/pii/S027323 0016301891. (Accessed 3 May 2017).

Snedecor, G.W., Cochran, W.G., 1989. Analyis of variance: the random effects model. In: Statistical Methods, eighth ed. Iowa State Univ Press, Iowa, pp. 237–253.

Society for Research on Nicotine and Tobacco Subcommittee on Biochemical Verification, Benowitz, N.L., J. III, P., Ahijevych, K., Jarvis, M.J., Hall, S., et al., 2002. Biochemical verification of tobacco use and cessation. Nicotine Tob. Res. 4, 149–159.

St Helen, G., Liakoni, E., Nardone, N., Addo, N., Jacob 3rd, P., Benowitz, N.L., 2020. Comparison of systemic exposure to toxic and/or carcinogenic volatile organic compounds (VOC) during vaping, smoking, and abstention. Canc. Prev. Res. 13 (2), 153–162.

Stepanov, I., Carmella, S.G., Briggs, A., Hertsgaard, L., Lindgren, B., Hatsukami, D., et al., 2009. Presence of the carcinogen N'-nitrosonornicotine in the urine of some users of oral nicotine replacement therapy products. Canc. Res. 69 (21), 8236–8240.

Storz, P., 2005. Reactive oxygen species in tumor progression. Front. Biosci. 10, 1881–1896.

Strasser, A.A., Ashare, R.L., Kaufman, M., Tang, K.Z., Mesaros, A.C., Blair, I.A., 2013. The effect of menthol on cigarette smoking behaviors, biomarkers and subjective responses. Canc. Epidemiol. Biomarkers Prev. https://doi.org/10.1158/1055-9965.EPI-12-1097. Epub ahead of print 18 January 2013.

Tiffany, S.T., Drobes, D.J., 1991. The development and initial validation of a questionnaire on smoking urges. Br. J. Addict. 86, 1467–1476.

Tobacco Products Scientific Advisory Committee (TPSAC), 2011. Menthol Cigarettes and Public Health: Review of the Scientific Evidence and Recommendations. Available from: http://www.fda.gov/downloads/AdvisoryCommittees/Com mitteesMeetingMaterials/TobaccoProductsScientificAdvisory Committee/UCM269697.pdf.

Tonstad, S., Cowan, J.L., 2009. C-reactive protein as a predictor of disease in smokers and former smokers: a review. Int. J. Clin. Pract. 63 (11), 1634–1641.

Tran, C.T., Felber Medlin, L., Lama, N., Taranu, B., Ng, W., Haziza, C., et al., 2019. Biological and functional changes in healthy adult smokers who are continuously abstinent from smoking for one year: protocol for a prospective, observational, multicenter cohort study. JMIR Res. Protoc. 8 (6), e12138.

Tricker, A.R., 2006. Biomarkers derived from nicotine and its metabolites: a review. Beiträge zur Tabakforschung Int. 22, 147–175.

Tricker, A.R., Jang, I.J., Martin Leroy, C., Lindner, D., Dempsey, R., 2012. Reduced exposure evaluation of an electrically heated cigarette smoking system. Part 4: eight-day randomized clinical trial in Korea. Regul. Toxicol. Pharmacol. 64 (2 Suppl. l), S45–S53.

Tricker, A.R., Kanada, S., Takada, K., Leroy, C.M., Lindner, D., Schorp, M.K., et al., 2012. Reduced exposure evaluation of an electrically heated cigarette smoking system. Part 5: 8-day randomized clinical trial in Japan. Regul. Toxicol. Pharmacol. 64 (2), S54–S63.

Tricker, A.R., Kanada, S., Takada, K., Martin Leroy, C., Lindner, D., Schorp, M.K., et al., 2012. Reduced exposure evaluation of an Electrically Heated Cigarette Smoking System. Part 6: 6-day randomized clinical trial of a menthol cigarette in Japan. Regul. Toxicol. Pharmacol. 64 (2 Suppl. l), S64–S73.

Tricker, A.R., Stewart, A.J., Leroy, C.M., Lindner, D., Schorp, M.K., Dempsey, R., 2012. Reduced exposure evaluation of an Electrically Heated Cigarette Smoking System. Part 3: eight-day randomized clinical trial in the UK. Regul. Toxicol. Pharmacol. 64, S35–S44.

U.S. Department of Health and Human Services, 2010. How Tobacco Smoke Causes Disease: The Biology and Behavioral Basis for Smoking-Attributable Disease: a Report of the Surgeon General. U.S. Department of Health and Human Services, Centers for Disease Control and Prevention, National Center for Chronic Disease Prevention and Health Promotion, Office on Smoking and Health, Atlanta, GA.

U.S. Department of Health and Human Services and FDA (Food and Drug Administration), 2012. [Docket No. FDA-2012-N-0143]: harmful and potentially harmful constituents in tobacco products and tobacco smoke; established list. Fed. Regist. 77 (64), 20034–20037.

Viegi, G., Sherrill, D.L., Carrozzi, L., Di Pede, F., Baldacci, S., Pistelli, F., et al., 2001. An 8-year follow-up of carbon monoxide diffusing capacity in a general population sample of northern Italy. CHEST Journal 120 (1), 74–80.

Vu, A.T., Taylor, K.M., Holman, M.R., Ding, Y.S., Hearn, B., Watson, C.H., 2015. Polycyclic aromatic hydrocarbons in the mainstream smoke of popular U.S. cigarettes. Chem. Res. Toxicol. 28 (8), 1616–1626.

Wagenknecht, L.E., Cutter, G.R., Haley, N.J., Sidney, S., Manolio, T.A., Hughes, G.H., et al., 1990. Racial differences in serum cotinine levels among smokers in the coronary artery risk development in (young) adults Study. Am. J. Publ. Health 80, 1053–1056.

Wakai, K., Inoue, M., Mizoue, T., Tanaka, K., Tsuji, I., Nagata, C., et al., 2006. Tobacco smoking and lung cancer risk: an evaluation based on a systematic review of epidemiological evidence among the Japanese population. Jpn. J. Clin. Oncol. 36 (5), 309–324.

Wang, T.J., Gona, P., Larson, M.G., Tofler, G.H., Levy, D., Newton-Cheh, C., et al., 2006. Multiple biomarkers for the prediction of first major cardiovascular events and death. N. Engl. J. Med. 355 (25), 2631–2639.

Wang, Y., Wong, L.Y., Meng, L., Pittman, E.N., Trinidad, D.A., Hubbard, K.L., et al., 2019. Urinary concentrations of monohydroxylated polycyclic aromatic hydrocarbons in adults from the U.S. Population Assessment of Tobacco and Health (PATH) Study Wave 1 (2013-2014). Environ. Int. 123, 201–208.

Watson, A., Joyce, H., Hopper, L., Pride, N., 1993. Influence of smoking habits on change in carbon monoxide transfer factor over 10 years in middle aged men. Thorax 48 (2), 119–124.

West, R., Ussher, M., Evans, M., Rashid, M., 2006. Assessing DSM-IV nicotine withdrawal symptoms: a comparison and evaluation of five different scales. Psychopharmacology 184, 619–627.

WHO Study Group, Ashley, D.L., Ayo-Yusuf, O.A., Boobis, A.R., da Costa e Silva, V.L., Djordjevic, M.V., et al., 2015. WHO Study Group on Tobacco Product Regulation - Report on the Scientific Basis of Tobacco Product Regulations: Fifth Report of a WHO Study Group.

WHO Study Group, Ashley, D.L., Burns, D., Djordjevic, M., Dybing, E., Gray, N., et al., 2008. The Scientific Basis of Tobacco Product Regulation: Second Report of a WHO Study Group, pp. 1–277. World Health Organization Technical Report Series. Epub ahead of print 2008/01/01.(951).

Yuan, J.M., Butler, L.M., Stepanov, I., Hecht, S.S., 2014. Urinary tobacco smoke-constituent biomarkers for assessing risk of lung cancer. Canc. Res. 74 (2), 401–411.

Yuki, D., Sakaguchi, C., Kikuchi, A., Futamura, Y., 2017. Pharmacokinetics of nicotine following the controlled use of a prototype novel tobacco vapor product. Regul. Toxicol. Pharmacol. 87, 30–35.

Yuki, D., Takeshige, Y., Nakaya, K., Futamura, Y., 2018. Assessment of the exposure to harmful and potentially harmful constituents in healthy Japanese smokers using a novel tobacco vapor product compared with conventional cigarettes and smoking abstinence. Regul. Toxicol. Pharmacol. 96, 127–134.

Zhang, H., Cai, B., 2003. The impact of tobacco on lung health in China. Respirology 8 (1), 17–21.

Zhang, W., Kilicarslan, T., Tyndale, R.F., Sellers, E.M., 2001. Evaluation of methoxalen, tranylcypromine, and tryptamine as specific and selective CYP2A6 inhibitors in vitro. Drug Metabol. Dispos. 26 (6), 897–902.

CHAPTER 18

Smoking-Related Disease Risk Reduction Potential of ENDPs

JULIA HOENG • JUSTYNA SZOSTAK • STÉPHANIE BOUÉ • CHRISTELLE HAZIZA • MANUEL C. PEITSCH

18.1 INTRODUCTION

Cigarette smoking is one of the leading preventable causes of human morbidity and mortality, causing serious diseases such as cardiovascular diseases (CVDs), chronic obstructive pulmonary disease (COPD), and lung cancer. The vast majority of smoking-related diseases are caused by the toxicants[1] present in cigarette smoke (Farsalinos and Le Houezec, 2015), which are mostly formed during the combustion of tobacco.[2] The United States (US) Surgeon General has stated that the "burden of death and disease from tobacco use in the United States is overwhelmingly caused by cigarettes and other combusted tobacco products" (National Center for Chronic Disease Prevention and Health Promotion (US) Office on Smoking and Health, 2014). Nicotine—while addictive, not risk-free, and an important factor of why people smoke—is not the primary cause of diseases (Benowitz, 2010; National Center for Chronic Disease Prevention and Health Promotion (US) Office on Smoking and Health, 2014; Tobacco Advisory Group of the Royal College of Physicians, 2016).

For decades, the efforts to reduce the harm caused by smoking have been focused on preventing smoking initiation and promoting smoking cessation (Surgeon General, 2010; Zhu et al., 2012). More recently, tobacco harm reduction (THR) has emerged as a third complementary approach that can help to reduce the adverse effects of smoking (Ashley et al., 2008) (Chapter 1). THR is based on switching smokers who would otherwise continue smoking to less harmful products that emit significantly lower levels of toxicants while providing levels of nicotine comparable to those of cigarettes (Smith et al., 2016; Tobacco Advisory Group of the Royal College of Physicians, 2016). As noted by McNeil (2012), "Since nicotine itself is not a highly hazardous drug, encouraging smokers to obtain nicotine from sources that do not involve tobacco combustion is a potential means to reduce the morbidity and mortality they sustain, without the need to overcome their addiction to nicotine." This new approach complements those aimed at reducing smoking prevalence and aims to provide smokers who will not quit with novel tobacco- or nicotine-containing products that are substantially less toxic than cigarettes (Fig. 18.1).

Electronic nicotine delivery products (ENDPs) are products designed to avoid combustion and, thereby, significantly reduce the emission of toxicants while delivering satisfying levels of nicotine, sensory satisfaction, and a ritual close to that of cigarettes. ENDPs that deliver nicotine-containing aerosol are based primarily on two technologies (Chapter 2). First, e-vapor products (EVPs) (a.k.a. e-cigarettes) generate the aerosol from a flavored e-liquid with a heating element consisting of a coil around a wick. Generally, e-liquids are mixtures of constituents such as vegetable glycerin (VG), propylene glycol, water, nicotine, and flavors. Second, electrically heated tobacco products (EHTPs) heat a tobacco substrate at temperatures well below that needed for combustion by using an electronically controlled heating element. This leads to formation of an aerosol consisting mainly of the water, VG, nicotine, and flavors contained in the tobacco substrate. Both technologies deliver various levels of nicotine, which is addictive, as well as low levels of certain toxicants because of the limited thermal degradation of the heated substrates. Furthermore, ENDPs deliver flavor ingredients, both natural and artificial, some of which might not be completely safe. Therefore, ENDPs are not risk-free.

---

[1] General term including harmful and potentially harmful constituents, free radicals, and carbon-based nanoparticles.
[2] While most toxicants are formed by combustion processes, tobacco-specific nitrosamines are released from the tobacco.

Toxicological Evaluation of Electronic Nicotine Delivery Products. https://doi.org/10.1016/B978-0-12-820490-0.00023-7

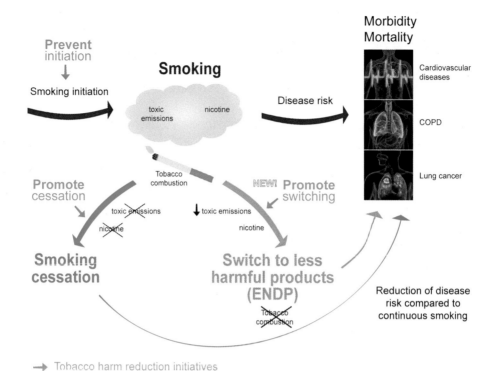

FIG. 18.1 **Tobacco harm reduction.** To accelerate the reduction in smoking-related morbidity and mortality caused by smoking that is already achieved by preventing smoking initiation and promoting smoking cessation, tobacco harm reduction includes a new approach—promoting switching to less harmful products—that is designed to complement the other two more established approaches and is targeted at current smokers who would otherwise continue smoking. *COPD*, chronic obstructive pulmonary disease; *ENDP*, electronic nicotine delivery product.

As outlined in Chapter 3, assessing the smoking-related disease risk reduction potential of ENDPs is hampered by (i) the latency of disease manifestations in smokers (decades of smoking), (ii) the slow reduction in excess risk upon cessation and, a fortiori, upon switching from cigarette smoking to the use of ENDPs, and (iii) the dearth of clinical risk markers that are predictive of future disease development. It is, therefore, likely that only long-term epidemiological data will provide definitive answers to this question and allow to verify that an ENDP reduces the risk of smoking-related disease, and to quantify the reduction in excess disease risk associated with an ENDP. However, to enable epidemiological studies, the ENDP would need to be available in the market and used exclusively by a large portion of current smokers, which is clearly impossible before a product is launched. In this context, we propose that a mechanism-based approach represents a solid alternative for showing that switching completely to an ENDP is likely to significantly reduce

the risk of smoking-related disease in a premarket setting. This approach is based on the previously described causal chain of events linking smoking to disease (CELSD) (Smith et al., 2016) (Chapter 3) (Fig. 18.2), the "assessment framework for ENDPs" (Chapter 3) and leverages the principles of systems toxicology (Sturla et al., 2014) (Chapters 3 and 9) and its predictive power (Chapter 3).

The aim of this chapter is to review the available scientific evidence to evaluate whether ENDPs have the potential to significantly reduce harm and the risk of tobacco-related disease to smokers who switch to them completely. While in previous chapters we have reviewed the available evidence[3] regarding toxicant emissions (Chapters 4, 6, 7), in vitro and in vivo toxicologically (Chapters 13–15), human toxicant exposure

---

[3]In general, comparing ENDP aerosols with cigarette smoke or ENDP use with cigarette smoking. When feasible, smoking cessation was included as the second comparator.

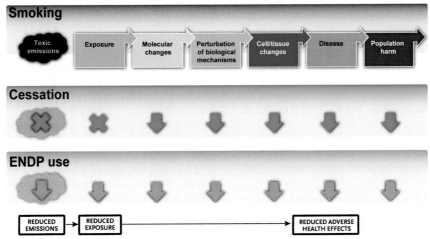

FIG. 18.2 The causal chain of events linking smoking to disease. Top row, Smoking: CELSD. Smoking leads to inhalation of toxicants, which leads to exposure of the body to toxicants, which, in turn, leads to molecular changes in the body that perturb biological mechanisms. These perturbations are the cause of cell and tissue changes that lead to disease and, by extension, population harm. Middle row, Cessation: Smoking cessation is effectively the elimination of the first step in the CELSD and the gold standard in THR. Therefore, all subsequent steps in the causal chain of events are reduced (downward arrows for each event in the CELSD). Bottom row, ENDP use: Switching to ENDPs with significantly reduced toxic emissions (relative to cigarettes) will also lead to a reduction in toxicant exposure. Consequently, all following steps in the causal chain of events, including adverse health effects and population harm, will be reduced (downward arrows for each event in the CELSD). CELSD, causal chain of events linking smoking to disease; ENDP, electronic nicotine delivery product; THR, tobacco harm reduction.

and effects on clinical biomarkers of potential harm (BoPHs) (Chapter 17), here we review this evidence focusing on the causal relationship between the events along the CELSD (Fig. 18.2) and their implications for the disease risk reduction potential of ENDPs.

18.2 THE FUNDAMENTAL PRINCIPLE OF HARM REDUCTION

As outlined in Chapter 3, the fundamental principle of toxicology is that the degree of exposure to toxicants determines the nature and degree of adverse health effects. Therefore, the central tenet of THR is that ENDPs must emit significantly lower levels of toxicants than cigarettes. Therefore, as outlined in Chapter 2, the fundamental design objective of ENDPs is to reduce and even eliminate the emission of toxicants while maintaining a satisfactory level of nicotine delivery and product features that enable smokers to switch completely to ENDPs.

18.2.1 Reduced Emission of Toxicants
The US Food and Drug Administration (FDA) has established a list of 93 known harmful and potentially

harmful constituents (HPHCs) found in tobacco products and tobacco smoke (Center for Tobacco Products, 2019). This list contains carcinogens, respiratory toxicants, cardiovascular toxicants, and reproductive and developmental toxicants as well as addictive substances: 79 of these HPHCs are classified as carcinogens, while, of the 14 noncarcinogenic compounds, 9 are respiratory toxicants, 4 are cardiovascular toxicants, and 3 are reproductive and developmental toxicants.

As outlined in Chapter 3 and extensively described in Chapters 4, 6, and 7, the reduction of toxicant emissions by ENDPs can be assessed by a combination of analytical chemistry methods for comparing the composition of the ENDP aerosol with that of cigarette smoke. Studies aimed at comparing the composition of heated tobacco product aerosols with that of cigarette smoke showed that EHTPs emit on average > 90% lower levels of HPHCs than cigarettes (Bekki et al., 2017; Breheny et al., 2019; Farsalinos et al., 2018; Forster et al., 2018; Jaccard et al., 2019; Li et al., 2018; Mallock et al., 2018; Schaller et al., 2016, 2019a,b; Takahashi et al., 2019). While there are only a few available EHTPs, there are numerous commercially available EVPs with different design principles, as outlined in

Chapter 2. Despite this broad diversity, numerous studies have shown that EVPs emit overall significantly lower levels of HPHCs than cigarettes, depending on product design, puffing regimen, and power settings (Bekki et al., 2017; Belushkin et al., 2020; Geiss et al., 2016; Gillman et al., 2016; Goniewicz et al., 2014; Laugesen, 2015; Ogunwale et al., 2017; Sleiman et al., 2016; Tayyarah and Long, 2014; Uchiyama et al., 2016). A recent study showed that emissions of benzene, 1,3-butadiene, and benzo[a]pyrene by commercially available EVPs were generally not quantifiable (Belushkin et al., 2020), while the emission of carbonyls is highly variable. Importantly, closed-system EVPs emit significantly lower levels of carbonyls than open systems and cigarettes (Belushkin et al., 2020).

While HPHCs—including (i) the tobacco-specific nitrosamines (TSNAs), N-nitrosonornicotine (NNN), and 4-(methylnitrosamino)-1-(3-pyridyl)-1-butanone (NNK), (ii) polycyclic aromatic hydrocarbons (PAHs), and (iii) carbonyls—have been the main classes of HPHCs targeted for reduction in ENDP aerosols, the absence of combustion in ENDPs also results in the reduction of other substances of toxicological concern. For instance, it has been shown that, in contrast to cigarettes, the Tobacco Heating Systems 2.2 (THS) and an EVP do not emit quantifiable levels of solid carbon-based nanoparticles (cbNPs) (Pratte et al., 2017) (Chapter 7) and that both heated tobacco products and EVPs emit 95%—99% lower levels of organic radicals than cigarettes (Bitzer et al., 2020; Pryor et al., 1990; Shein and Jeschke, 2019) (Chapter 7).

18.2.2 Reduced Exposure to Toxicants

The significantly reduced emission of HPHCs and other substances of toxicological concern by ENDPs should lead to an equally significant reduction in exposure to these substances in human subjects who switch from cigarette smoking to ENDP use in clinical studies. This is the second event in the CELSD (Fig. 18.2). Ideally, these levels of exposure reduction should approach those observed in study subjects who abstain from smoking for the duration of the study, as this is the maximum achievable reduction in HPHC exposure.

Over the past few years, several clinical reduced exposure studies were conducted with either EHTPs or EVPs (Chapter 17). In these studies, biomarkers of exposure (BoExps) to key HPHCs were measured in the blood and urine of study participants. The studies were designed to compare the levels of these BoExps in study subjects who switched to an ENDP with the levels in subjects who continued to smoke their own brand of cigarettes and, in many cases, with the levels

in study participants who abstained from smoking for the duration of the study. Collectively, these studies have demonstrated that the levels of BoExps to HPHCs are reduced upon complete switching from cigarette smoking to ENDP use (Gale et al., 2019; Goniewicz et al., 2017; Haziza et al., 2016, 2019a; Lüdicke et al., 2018a; O'Connell et al., 2016; Yuki et al., 2018). Studies that also included a smoking abstinence arm showed that the degree of exposure reduction among complete switchers approached that among participants who abstained from smoking for the duration of the study, while dual use with cigarettes had, as expected, a lower effect of exposure reduction (O'Connell et al., 2016) (Chapter 17). Furthermore, these clinical studies also confirmed the observation that animals first exposed to cigarette smoke before being exposed to the aerosol of an electronically heated tobacco product display a reduction in BoExps similar to that in animals switched from cigarette smoke to air exposure (Phillips et al., 2016).

It has been shown that cigarette smoking causes changes in gene expression in the whole blood transcriptome (Beane et al., 2007; Beineke et al., 2012; Spira et al., 2004). The vast majority of these changes are also reversible upon smoking cessation (Vink et al., 2017). It was, therefore, possible to develop a gene expression signature from whole blood transcriptomics data that distinguishes smokers from former- and never-smokers (Beineke et al., 2012; Belcastro et al., 2018; Martin et al., 2015, 2020). The mechanistic meaning of these gene expression changes is still under investigation; yet, it appears that they occur in pathways involved in immune response, blood coagulation, and other cellular processes (Vink et al., 2017). While this research might yield novel and valuable BoPHs in the future, these gene expression changes, and associated signatures, are biomarkers of effect that can be used to assess changes in cigarette smoke exposure. Such a gene expression signature can, therefore, be used to study the effects of switching from cigarette smoking to ENDP use and smoking abstinence in clinical studies (Martin et al., 2020; Poussin et al., 2017). In clinical studies, the effects of switching to THS and smoking abstinence on a previously identified gene expression signature (Martin et al., 2015) were visible after only 5 days (Martin et al., 2016; Poussin et al., 2017) and confirmed that the effects of switching from cigarette smoking to THS use approached the effects of smoking abstinence in two 90-day clinical reduced exposure studies (Martin et al., 2019). Moreover, such a gene expression signature can also be applied to mouse whole blood transcriptomics data (Belcastro et al.,

2018; Martin et al., 2015) and was shown to distinguish cigarette smoke—exposed mice from mice that were exposed to fresh air or THS aerosol. This gene expression signature was also able to clearly distinguish cigarette smoke—exposed mice from mice that were first exposed to cigarette smoke and then switched to either THS aerosol or fresh air exposure (Belcastro et al., 2018; Poussin et al., 2017). These studies showed that the effects of switching to THS were very similar to those of smoking abstinence and cessation in both humans and mice.

As outlined above, it has been shown that ENDPs do not emit quantifiable levels of solid cbNPs (Pratte et al., 2017, 2019) (Chapter 7), which are a hallmark of incomplete combustion (Lighty et al., 2000). As the exposure to these cbNPs cannot be easily measured in clinical studies, we leveraged our long-term in vivo studies to assess their deposition in the lungs. For instance, in a recent 6-month e-liquid inhalation study conducted in mice, we observed that the lungs of mice exposed to cigarette smoke had a dark color, while those of mice exposed to aerosol from an e-liquid were of the same light color as the lungs of fresh air—exposed mice (Fig. 18.3). Similar observations were made for lungs exposed to the aerosol from an EHTP. While there are many chromogenic substances in cigarette smoke, it is most likely that the discoloration of mouse lungs is due, at least in part, to the deposition of cbNPs.

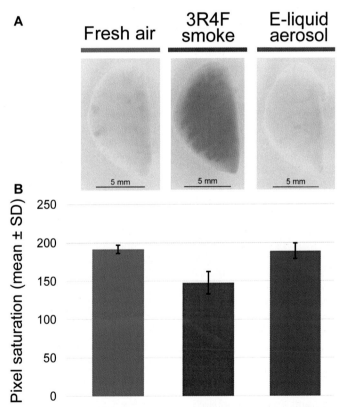

FIG. 18.3 Lung discoloration caused by cigarette smoke and e-vapor exposure. **(A)** Mice were exposed for 3 h/day, 5 days/week, for 6 months to fresh air, smoke of the 3R4F reference cigarette, or aerosol of a flavored e-liquid composed of 66.7% PG, 28.5% VG, 4.8% nicotine, and 0.12% of a flavor mixture. The concentration of nicotine was 36.7 μg/L in the test atmosphere. The lungs were flushed with PBS to collect bronchoalveolar lavage fluid. The flushed left lungs were imaged under immersion in PBS. **(B)** Mean pixel saturation of the lungs determined by using the Visiopharm image analysis software; pixel saturation ranges from 0 (black) to 255 (white). *PBS*, phosphate-buffered saline; *PG*, propylene glycol; *SD*, standard deviation; *VG*, vegetable glycerin. (Adapted from Hoeng, J., Maeder, S., Vanscheeuwijck, P., Peitsch, M.C., 2019. Assessing the lung cancer risk reduction potential of candidate modified risk tobacco products. Intern. Emerg. Med. 14, 821—834. https://doi.org/10.1007/s11739-019-02045-z.)

Finally, it has been reported that cigarette smoke, but not ENDP aerosols, causes significant discoloration of composite resin (used for dental fillings) as well as dentin and enamel in vitro (Dalrymple et al., 2018; Zanetti et al., 2019; Zhao et al., 2019a, b; Zhao et al., 2017, 2020a, b). These differences in discoloration further show that ENDP use leads to lower toxicant exposure than cigarette smoking.

18.3 IMPLICATIONS FOR LUNG CANCER

Smoking is the major cause of lung cancer, and this risk increases with the number of cigarettes smoked and the duration of smoking (Doll and Peto, 1978; Flanders et al., 2003; Knoke et al., 2004; Surgeon General, 2010). It is also known that the risk of lung cancer decreases upon cessation (Carter et al., 2015; Choi et al., 2018; Zha et al., 2019), with a slow decline in excess risk (approximately 50% excess risk reduction 10 years after quitting) (Fry et al., 2013). This decrease in lung cancer risk upon smoking cessation is due to the discontinuation of exposure to the toxicants contained in cigarette smoke.

As outlined in the introduction and Chapter 3, assessing the lung cancer risk reduction potential of ENDPs before or soon after they are introduced into the market is hampered by (i) the dearth of clinical risk markers that are predictive of future lung cancer development, (ii) the latency of lung cancer manifestation (decades of smoking), and (iii) the slow reduction in excess risk upon smoking cessation and, a fortiori, upon switching to an ENDP. In this context, we have proposed that a mechanism-based approach represents a scientifically robust alternative for showing that switching to an ENDP is likely to significantly reduce the risk of lung cancer (Hoeng et al., 2019). This approach is based on the previously described CELSD (Fig. 18.2) (Chapter 3) (Smith et al., 2016) and leverages the principles of systems toxicology (Chapters 3 and 9) (Sturla et al., 2014).

18.3.1 Three-Questions Approach

Smoking-related lung cancer is caused by chronic exposure to the carcinogenic toxicants found in tobacco smoke. These substances trigger the key pathways that lead to cancer. Carcinogenic toxicants contained in cigarette smoke, such as TSNA, PAHs, free radicals (including reactive oxygen species [ROS] and reactive nitrogen species [RNS]), and various aldehydes, will cause genetic damage that can lead to the loss of normal cellular growth control mechanisms and cell proliferation (Abbas et al., 2013; Hecht, 2012; Jorgensen et al., 2010; Zhao et al.,

2009). The toxicants in cigarette smoke also cause chronic inflammation (Grivennikov et al., 2010; Kuschner et al., 1996; Lee et al., 2012; Song et al., 2020; Yang et al., 2011), which promotes tumor formation (Coussens and Werb, 2002; Durham and Adcock, 2015; Parris et al., 2019). The 2010 US Surgeon General's Report, *How Tobacco Smoke Causes Disease: The Biology and Behavioral Basis for Smoking-Attributable Disease*, identifies inflammation and oxidative stress, among others, as key mechanisms underlying all major smoking-related diseases (Surgeon General, 2010).

In 2001, Balkwill and Mantovani hypothesized that "if *genetic damage* is the match that lights the fire of cancer, some types of *inflammation* may provide the fuel that feeds the flames" (Balkwill and Mantovani, 2001). This hypothesis is consistent with the two characteristics, "genome instability and mutation" and "tumor-promoting inflammation," that enable the acquisition of the hallmarks of cancer defined by Hanahan and Weinberg (2011). This provides us with a mechanistic framework for developing an approach for assessing ENDPs for their potential to reduce the risk of lung cancer. This approach is based on three important questions that can be answered long before epidemiological data are available, by using a combination of nonclinical and clinical studies (Fig. 18.4):

- Does switching from cigarettes to the ENDP reduce genetic damage?
- Does switching from cigarettes to the ENDP reduce inflammation?
- Does switching from cigarettes to the ENDP reduce the risk of lung cancer?

On the basis of the hypothesis of Balkwill and Mantovani, a positive answer to the first two questions should lead to a positive answer to the third question. A positive answer to all three questions would indicate that switching completely from cigarette smoking to ENDP use will likely reduce the risk of lung cancer.

18.3.1.1 Question 1: does switching from cigarettes to ENDPs reduce genetic damage?

Cigarette smoke contains many carcinogenic toxicants, including carcinogens, free radicals, and ROS/RNS-inducing agents. Cigarette smoking leads to the uptake of these carcinogenic toxicants, many of which can bind DNA directly, or after activation through enzymatic pathways (Penning, 2014), to form DNA adducts. DNA can also be altered by oxidative damage induced by free radicals such as the ROS and RNS contained in cigarette smoke or those formed endogenously by cells exposed to cigarette smoke constituents (Faux et al., 2009; Helfinger

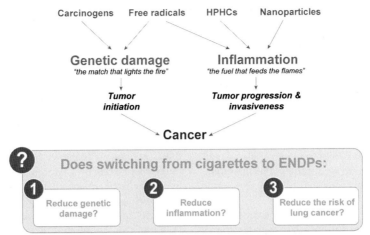

FIG. 18.4 Approach for assessing the lung cancer risk reduction potential of ENDPs based on the hypothesis of Balkwill and Mantonvani: "if genetic damage is the match that lights the fire of cancer, some types of inflammation may provide the fuel that feeds the flames." Carcinogenic toxicants include carcinogens, free radicals, and ROS/RNS-inducing agents. *ENDP*, electronic nicotine delivery product; *HPHC*, harmful and potentially harmful constituents; *RNS*, reactive nitrogen species; *ROS*, reactive oxygen species. (Adapted from Hoeng, J., Maeder, S., Vanscheeuwijck, P., Peitsch, M.C., 2019. Assessing the lung cancer risk reduction potential of candidate modified risk tobacco products. Intern. Emerg. Med. 14, 821–834. https://doi.org/10.1007/s11739-019-02045-z.)

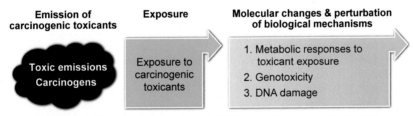

FIG. 18.5 The causal chain of events linking smoking to genetic damage.

and Schröder, 2018; Kawanishi et al., 2017; Valavanidis et al., 2013). DNA damage triggers complex surveillance and repair systems of the cell (Jorgensen et al., 2010; Zhao et al., 2009). Because this repair system is not error-free, DNA strand breaks and erroneous base substitutions may occur and accumulate, eventually leading to genomic instability. In most cases, these errors lead to cellular dysfunction or programmed cell death. However, in some cases, these errors can lead to activating mutations in oncogenes, growth factors, and their receptors or inactivating mutations in tumor suppressors, leading to changes in cellular function. These changes can generate neoplastic cell populations with the potential to form tumors, for instance, in a tumor-promoting chronically inflamed tissue environment (Abbas et al., 2013; Sethi et al., 2012).

To answer this question, let us consider the causal chain of events linking smoking to genetic damage (Fig. 18.5). This causal chain also means that a

reduction in emission of carcinogenic toxicants should lead to a reduction in exposure to these toxicants, which, in turn, should lead to a reduction in the metabolic responses to these toxicants, a reduction in genotoxicity, and, hence, a reduction in DNA damage.

A combination of aerosol chemistry, nonclinical studies, and clinical studies can be used to gather evidence for each step in this causal chain of events. The key results of such studies are summarized hereafter.

18.3.1.1.1 Reduced exposure to carcinogenic toxicants.
As outlined above, the reduced emission of toxicants (Chapters 4, 6, 7) leads to a coherent reduction in exposure to toxicants in human subjects who switch completely from cigarette smoking to ENDP use (Chapter 17). Importantly, as carcinogenic toxicants are significantly reduced (>95%) in the aerosols of ENDPs relative to cigarette smoke, exposure to this class of toxicants is also significantly reduced, to a

level approaching the reduction caused by smoking abstinence (Chapter 17). Furthermore, and as a direct consequence of this reduction in exposure to carcinogens, switching from cigarette smoking to ENDP use also leads to a significant reduction in urinary genotoxicity (a biomarker of total genotoxic exposure) relative to continued smoking, approaching the urinary genotoxicity observed upon smoking abstinence in human clinical studies (Haziza et al., 2016, 2019a; Lüdicke et al., 2018a). Finally, this reduction in exposure to carcinogens was also observed in both in vitro (Iskandar et al., 2017a, 2019a, b) and in vivo studies (Phillips et al., 2016, 2019a, b; Szostak et al., 2020a, b).

18.3.1.1.2 Linking reduced carcinogen exposure to cancer risk reduction. Using an approach based on the inhalation unit risks of the most important carcinogenic toxicants in cigarette smoke, Stephens compared the cancer potencies of various ENDP emissions and their lifetime cancer risks on the basis of daily product consumption estimates (Stephens, 2017). These analyses allowed translation of aerosol chemistry results into a continuum of lifetime cancer risks, as represented in Fig. 18.6.

The two most abundant TSNAs, NNN and NNK, have been linked epidemiologically to cancer (Hecht et al., 2013; Stepanov et al., 2014). Indeed, studies such as the Shanghai Cohort Study (Hecht et al., 2013), the Singapore Chinese Health Study (Yuan et al., 2017), and the Prostate, Lung, Colorectal, and Ovarian Cancer Screening Trial (Church et al., 2009) have reported a significant relationship between (i) total 4-(methylnitrosamino)-1-(3-pyridyl)-1-

butanol (tNNAL) and lung cancer and (ii) total *N*-nitrosonornicotine (tNNN) and esophageal cancer (Hecht et al., 2013). Hecht and colleagues reported odds ratios (ORs) of 1.89–2.6 for lung cancer depending on the level of tNNAL (BoExp to NNK) as well as ORs of 3.99–17 for esophageal cancer, again, depending on the levels to tNNN. As the emission of TSNAs is markedly reduced in ENDP aerosols (Chapter 4), smokers who switch completely from cigarette smoking to ENDP use will be exposed to markedly lower levels of these carcinogens (Chapter 17), which also contributes to the reduced lifetime cancer risks of ENDPs described by Stephens (Stephens, 2017).

Taken together, these studies and analyses, which de facto incorporate the principle of epidemiology (Chapter 3), show that a significant reduction in carcinogen emission and, consequently, exposure should lead to a reduced risk of cancer, which follows the principle of toxicology (Chapter 3). This finding will be further substantiated by comparing the biological effects of ENDP aerosols with those of cigarette smoke.

18.3.1.1.3 Reduced metabolic responses to carcinogenic toxicants exposure. A significant reduction in exposure to carcinogens (including PAHs), free radicals (including ROS and RNS), and other oxidative stressors (such as aldehydes) should lead to a significant reduction in the activation of xenobiotic metabolism and oxidative stress responses.

The activation and/or upregulation of many xenobiotic metabolism enzymes is driven by exposure to chemicals that can serve as substrates. The PAHs contained in

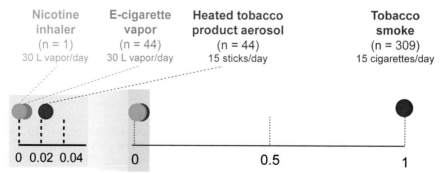

Mean lifetime cancer risk relative to tobacco smoke

FIG. 18.6 Mean lifetime cancer risk of ENDP aerosols expressed as ratio to cigarette smoke. The heated tobacco product was an electrically heated tobacco heating system. *ENDP*, electronic nicotine delivery product. (Adapted from Stephens, W.E., 2017. Comparing the cancer potencies of emissions from vapourised nicotine products including e-cigarettes with those of tobacco smoke. Tob. Control. https://doi.org/10.1136/tobaccocontrol-2017-053808.)

smoke, such as benzo[*a*]pyrene, drive the upregulation of enzymes belonging to the cytochrome P450 1A (CYP1A) and 1B (CYP1B) families. Therefore, members of these families are useful markers of exposure response. In particular, CYP1A2, which is important for elimination of environmental chemicals, is strongly induced by PAHs. A reduction in PAH exposure should, therefore, lead to a reduction in CYP1A and CYP1B gene expression, protein abundance, and enzymatic activity.

Oxidative stress results from an imbalance between the levels of oxidants and antioxidants. This imbalance allows ROS and other reactive species contained in cigarette smoke, or generated endogenously, to act directly on cellular components, damaging lipids, proteins, and DNA. Glutathione (GSH) is a potent and essential intracellular free radical-scavenging and oxidant-detoxification agent. For instance, ROS oxidizes GSH to GSH disulfide (GSSG), while other HPHCs contained in cigarette smoke, such as acrolein (Gonzalez-Suarez et al., 2014), will bind to GSH via other mechanisms. Taken together, these oxidant detoxification mechanisms will lead to depletion of the GSH pool if the oxidant exposure is greater than the ability of the cell to produce and recycle oxidized GSH. In an attempt to counteract this depletion, cells exposed to cigarette smoke will increase the expression of enzymes involved in the biosynthesis of new GSH (glutathione—cysteine ligase modifier and catalytic subunits [GCLM and GCLC]) and the recycling of GSSG to GSH (glutathione-disulfide reductase [GSR]). A reduction in exposure to free radicals and other oxidative stressors should, therefore, lead to a reduction in GSH depletion and a concomitant reduction in the expression of oxidative stress response genes, including those involved in maintaining the GSH pool.

In clinical and in vivo studies, one can assess the effect of switching from cigarette smoking to ENDP use on exposure responses by measuring biomarkers indicative of these mechanisms. For example, one can measure the plasma level of CYP1A2 enzyme activity (van der Plas et al., 2020). Clinical studies with THS showed that both smoking abstinence and switching from cigarette smoking to THS use reduced the plasma level of CYP1A2 enzyme activity to a similar extent (Haziza et al., 2016, 2019a; Lüdicke et al., 2018a). Similarly, exposure to cigarette smoke induced both gene and protein expression of hepatic CYP1A2 in mice, while exposure to THS aerosol did not (Lo Sasso et al., 2016b). Furthermore switching mice from cigarette smoke to THS aerosol exposure led to a similar reduction in CYP1A2 expression than cessation.

The level of oxidative stress can be assessed in both clinical and nonclinical in vivo studies by measuring

specific biomarkers. For instance, urinary biomarkers such as 8-epi-prostaglandin F2α (Lüdicke et al., 2018b), malondialdehyde, and 4-hydroxynonenal (Phillips et al., 2016; Szostak et al., 2020b) were significantly reduced in study subjects exposed to ENDP aerosols relative to those exposed to cigarette smoke.

Differences in xenobiotic metabolism and oxidative stress responses can also be assessed in human organotypic airway epithelial tissue cultures grown at the air—liquid interface. For instance, it has been shown that the effects of cigarette smoke exposure of these cultures mirror many of the gene expression changes induced by smoking in human airway biopsy samples (Mathis et al., 2013). In these cultures, ENDP aerosol exposure caused a reduced and more transient expression of genes related to xenobiotic metabolism (e.g., *CYP1A1*, *CYP1B1*, *AKR1B/1C*, and *ALDH3A1*) and oxidative stress (e.g., *NQO1*, *TXNRD1*, *GCLM/C*, *GSR*, and *SRXN1*) than cigarette smoke (Haswell et al., 2017, 2018; Iskandar et al., 2017a). Importantly, these genes were expressed at significantly lower levels in the bronchial cells of study participants who switched to EVPs than in those who smoked cigarettes (Song et al., 2020), further confirming the lower impact of ENDP aerosols on xenobiotic metabolism and oxidative stress. Furthermore, as a consequence of the significantly lower effect of ENDP aerosols than cigarette smoke on oxidative stress, the aerosol of ENDPs should also have a lower effect on the intracellular GSH pool and ROS generation than cigarette smoke. These toxicity endpoints can be assessed in normal human bronchial epithelial cell cultures by high-content screening (HCS) (Gonzalez-Suarez et al., 2014). Such HCS studies have consistently shown that ENDP aerosols have a significantly reduced effect on the intracellular GHS pool and ROS formation relative to cigarette smoke (Gonzalez-Suarez et al., 2016; Iskandar et al., 2019b; Taylor et al., 2018).

18.3.1.1.4 Reduced genotoxicity. As a direct consequence of the reduction in carcinogenic toxicant emissions and, therefore, exposure, ENDP aerosols displayed significantly reduced mutagenicity and genotoxicity in standard cell-based assays, such as the Ames, in vitro micronucleus, and mouse lymphoma assays (Schaller et al., 2016; Taylor et al., 2018) (Chapter 13).

18.3.1.1.5 Reduced DNA damage. To confirm the reduced genotoxicity of an ENDP aerosol relative to cigarette smoke, the biological response to DNA damage can be measured in vitro. For instance, the extent of DNA double-strand breaks is reflected by the increase in γH2AX, an early step in the DNA damage response (DDR) machinery (Nakamura et al., 2010). An assay measuring the abundance of γH2AX in human bronchial epithelial cells was, therefore, used to show that the extent of DNA double-strand breaks caused by the ENDP aerosol is lower than that caused by cigarette smoke (Gonzalez-Suarez et al., 2016; Taylor et al., 2018). Furthermore, in vitro and in vivo studies allow measurement of the relative expression levels of genes involved in the DDR machinery and provide further confirmation that ENDP aerosols cause less DNA damage than cigarette smoke in exposed tissues (Haswell et al., 2017, 2018; Iskandar et al., 2017a; Phillips et al., 2016).

Taken together, the available study results showed a significant reduction in all steps of the causal chain of events linking smoking to genetic damage, which demonstrates that ENDPs cause less genetic damage than cigarette smoke (Fig. 18.5). This indicates that ENDP aerosols are less likely to cause tumor initiation than cigarette smoke.

18.3.1.2 Question 2: does switching from cigarettes to ENDPs reduce inflammation?

Many cancers arise in areas of chronic inflammation, which plays a major role in tumor invasion, progression, and metastasis, largely through cytokine-mediated activation of mechanisms involved in tissue repair, cell proliferation, and angiogenesis (Apte et al., 2006; Coussens and Werb, 2002; Grivennikov et al., 2010; Mantovani, 2010; Porta et al., 2009). Furthermore, inflammation might also contribute to tumor initiation, because activated inflammatory cells can induce the formation of ROS and RNS, which can induce genetic damage (Coussens and Werb, 2002; Grivennikov et al., 2010). Consequently, a reduction in inflammation should be accompanied by a reduction in cancer risk, which is confirmed by recent observations that reducing inflammation (e.g., through chronic use of nonsteroidal antiinflammatory drugs) can reduce the mortality of colorectal cancer and lung cancer. Recent trials with antiinflammatory treatments of COPD and CVD patients demonstrate an attenuation of the risk of developing lung cancer as a comorbidity (Lee et al., 2013; Ridker et al., 2017).

Inflammation is of particular pathophysiological relevance to lung diseases and cancer, as chronic bronchitis triggered by asbestos, silica, smoke, and other inhaled toxins results in a persistent inflammatory response, which significantly increases the risk for lung cancer (O'Callaghan et al., 2010; Walser et al.,

2008). This is also supported by the fact that lung cancer is a frequent comorbidity of COPD, a major inflammatory lung disease caused by smoke exposure. Indeed, COPD stages 1 and 2 and the presence of emphysema were shown to be among the strongest independent risk factors for lung cancer, with respective hazard ratios of 1.4 and 3.5 in the Pittsburgh Lung Screening Study cohort (de-Torres et al., 2015; Durham and Adcock, 2015). This is not surprising, as COPD and lung cancer share several underlying disease mechanisms, such as oxidative stress and inflammation (Walser et al., 2008).

Smoke-induced lung inflammation is triggered by particulate matter and, in part, by aldehyde exposure, which leads to increased levels of, for example, interleukin 8 (IL-8) and monocyte chemoattractant protein 1 (MCP-1) in both mouse and human lungs (Kuschner et al., 1996; Moretto et al., 2009; van der Toorn et al., 2013). It is also recognized that smoke exposure leads to activation of the Nod-like receptor protein 3 (NLRP3) inflammasome (Eltom et al., 2014), with consequent local generation of active interleukin 1β (IL-1β), a process that induces inflammation and, thereby, can lead to both chronic fibrosis and cancer in mice (Dostert et al., 2008; Gasse et al., 2007). In 1996, Kuschner and colleagues showed that the concentrations of macrophages, neutrophils, IL-1β, and IL-8 are elevated in the pulmonary microenvironment of smokers in a dose-dependent manner (Kuschner et al., 1996). This was recently confirmed by Song et al. (2020). It has long been known that, in mice, inflammasome activation and IL-1β accelerate tumor invasiveness, growth, and metastatic spread (Voronov et al., 2003). For example, in a previous study in IL-1β-deficient mice, neither local tumors nor lung metastases developed after localized or intravenous inoculation with melanoma cell lines, which suggests that IL-1β-induced inflammation participates in the invasiveness of already existing tumor cells (Voronov et al., 2003). This observation, made in an animal model, was recently confirmed by the results of the Canakinumab Anti-inflammatory Thrombosis Outcomes Study in patients with a history of myocardial infarction (Ridker et al., 2017). Treatment with canakinumab, a monoclonal antibody against IL-1β, led to a dose-dependent reduction in the concentrations of the inflammation markers high-sensitivity C-reactive protein and interleukin 6 (IL-6) as well as a reduction in lung cancer incidence and mortality. Taken together, these observations demonstrate that chronic activation of the NLRP3 inflammasome, and the resulting inflammation, also play a role in promoting lung cancer.

To answer this question, let us consider the causal chain of events linking smoking to lung inflammation (Fig. 18.7). This causal chain also means that a reduction in emission of toxicants should lead to a reduction in exposure to these toxicants, which, in turn, should lead to a reduction in lung inflammation.

A combination of aerosol chemistry, nonclinical studies, and clinical studies can be used to gather evidence for each step in this causal chain of events. The key results of such studies are summarized hereafter.

18.3.1.2.1 Reduced exposure to toxicants. Above, we have summarized the data showing that ENDPs emit significantly lower levels of HPHCs than cigarettes and that this leads to a concomitant and significant reduction in exposure to HPHCs across in vitro, in vivo, and clinical studies. Importantly, the degree of exposure reduction in study subjects who switched from cigarette smoke to ENDP aerosol exposure approached that caused by smoking abstinence (the maximum achievable degree of reduction) in both clinical and in vivo studies.

We have also summarized the evidence showing that the absence of quantifiable cbNPs in ENDP aerosols leads to a reduction in exposure to these particles (Chapter 7). In cigarettes, these particles are generated by incomplete combustion of tobacco (Fariss et al., 2013; Lighty et al., 2000), which is consistent with the processes involved in soot formation during combustion. These cbNPs consist, at least in part, of humic-like substances (Fariss et al., 2013) and PAHs (Lindner et al., 2017) surrounding a core of elemental carbon. A significant reduction in exposure to cbNPs is important in the context of switching from cigarette smoking to ENDP use, because these particles are highly likely to cause adverse health effects and contribute to lung injury beyond the known carcinogenicity of PAHs. Numerous in vivo and in vitro studies have shown that nanoparticles, across a very wide range of sizes, shapes, and compositions, cause pulmonary inflammation (Braakhuis et al., 2014; Sahu et al., 2014; Stoeger et al., 2006). It has also been shown that human exposure to nanoscale carbon black leads to an increase in proinflammatory cytokine levels and a reduction in pulmonary function (Zhang et al., 2014).

Lung exposure to fine particulate matter, such as monosodium urate crystals, asbestos, and crystalline silica, results in persistent inflammation, mediated primarily by the NLRP3 inflammasome (Ather et al., 2014). Similarly, mouse lung exposure to carbon black nanoparticles causes activation of the NLRP3 inflammasome, which leads to lung injury and emphysema (You et al., 2015). This is consistent with previous observations that cbNP exposure leads to increased levels of IL-1β in mice (Stoeger et al., 2006) and humans (Zhang et al., 2014). It has also been shown that cbNPs accumulate in antigen-presenting dendritic cells derived from emphysematous lung tissues of smokers (You et al., 2015) and that cigarette smoke triggers the NLRP3 inflammasome (Eltom et al., 2014), which is again consistent with the observation that IL-1β levels are elevated in smokers' lungs (Kuschner et al., 1996; Song et al., 2020).

Taken together, these lines of evidence suggest that cbNPs might participate in the proinflammatory effect of cigarette smoke and that their absence from ENDP aerosol will contribute, together with the overall reduction in HPHCs, to a reduction in lung inflammation in smokers who switch completely from cigarette smoking to ENDP use.

18.3.1.2.2 Reduced lung inflammation. The reduced exposure to toxicants should then lead to a reduction in lung inflammation. The extent of lung inflammation can be readily measured in studies conducted with animal models of disease, but requires invasive methods in humans (Kuschner et al., 1996; Song et al., 2020). Such studies should confirm that cigarette smoke exposure causes lung inflammation (positive control), while ENDP aerosols should have a very limited effect on this mechanism. Furthermore, a study design that includes both an ENDP switching and a cessation arm (exposure to cigarette smoke for a few months followed by exposure to either ENDP aerosol or fresh air for

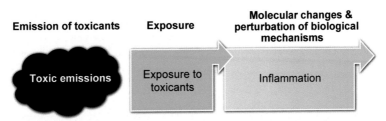

Emission of toxicants   **Exposure**   **Molecular changes & perturbation of biological mechanisms**

Toxic emissions   Exposure to toxicants   Inflammation

FIG. 18.7 The causal chain of events linking smoking to lung inflammation.

several months) is essential for assessing (i) the effects of a change in exposure that mimics the intended use of ENDPs (i.e., switching current smokers) and (ii) how this compares with the effects of smoking cessation. In such studies, the extent of lung inflammation can be assessed by bronchoalveolar lavage fluid (BALF) analysis (quantification of inflammatory cells, such as neutrophils and macrophages, and molecular markers, such as cytokines and chemokines), histopathological evaluation (assessment of lung infiltration by inflammatory cells, such as neutrophils and pigmented macrophages), and lung gene and protein expression analysis.

In all our rodent studies, smoke exposure caused pronounced lung inflammation, as evidenced by a broad range of inflammation markers measured in the BALF of the animals (Oviedo et al., 2016; Phillips et al., 2016; Wong et al., 2016, Wong et al., 2020). In contrast, exposure to the aerosol of THS had only limited effects on this mechanism. A very similar observation was made when C57Bl/6J mice were exposed to flavored and unflavored e-liquid aerosols (Lee et al., 2018; Madison et al., 2019). Furthermore, a switching study conducted in Apolipoprotein E-deficient (Apoe$^{-/-}$) mice showed that cigarette smoke–induced lung inflammation increased rapidly and was maintained for the duration of the study (Phillips et al., 2016). In contrast, exposure to THS aerosol only caused

minimal inflammation (Fig. 18.8), and switching to THS aerosol exposure following 2 months of smoke exposure led to a rapid reduction in inflammation that approached the reduction observed in the cessation group (Fig. 18.8) (Phillips et al., 2016).

Several lung inflammation markers have been reported to be increased in smokers (neutrophils, macrophages, IL-1β, IL-8, IL-6, and MCP-1) (Kuschner et al., 1996; Song et al., 2020). It is of particular interest that these markers were also increased by exposure to cigarette smoke, but not by exposure to ENDP aerosols, in mouse models of disease (Lee et al., 2018; Phillips et al., 2016; Wong et al., 2020) (Fig. 18.9). Furthermore, switching from cigarette smoke exposure to either THS aerosol or fresh air (to mimic smoking cessation) reduced the levels of these inflammatory markers (Phillips et al., 2016). This confirms not only that mouse models can be relevant to key aspects of human biology (Chapter 10) but also that the NLRP3 inflammasome is activated by smoke exposure in both mice and humans and might play a central role in the inflammatory processes involved in promoting lung tumors (Ridker et al., 2017; Voronov et al., 2003).

The effects of cigarette smoke and ENDP aerosol on lung inflammation can also be assessed in vitro (Haswell et al., 2017, 2018; Iskandar et al., 2017a) by using both gene expression and protein abundance measurements. Studies conducted in human organotypic airway

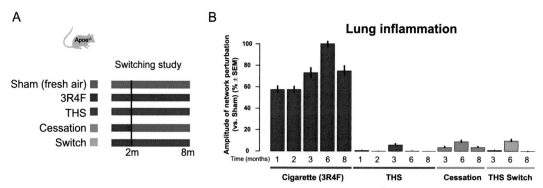

FIG. 18.8 Lung inflammation relative to air exposure in the 8-month Apoe$^{-/-}$ mouse switching study. **(A)** Study design. Exposure conditions: Sham, fresh air for 8 months; 3R4F, cigarette smoke for 8 months; THS, THS aerosol for 8 months; Cessation, fresh air for 6 months following 2 months of 3R4F cigarette smoke exposure; Switch, THS aerosol for 6 months following 2 months of 3R4F cigarette smoke exposure. Exposure, fresh air or 29.9 μg/L nicotine in the test atmosphere, 3 h/day, 5 days/week for up to 8 months. (B) Perturbation of the networks recapitulating lung inflammation in the Apoe-/- switching study with THS. *SEM*, standard error of the mean; *THS*, tobacco heating system. (Adapted from Phillips, B., Veljkovic, E., Boué, S., Schlage, W.K., Vuillaume, G., Martin, F., Titz, B., Leroy, P., Buettner, A., Elamin, A., Oviedo, A., Cabanski, M., De León, H., Guedj, E., Schneider, T., Talikka, M., Ivanov, N.V., Vanscheeuwijck, P., Peitsch, M.C., Hoeng, J., 2016. An 8-month systems toxicology inhalation/cessation study in Apoe$^{-/-}$ mice to investigate cardiovascular and respiratory exposure effects of a candidate modified risk tobacco product, THS 2.2, compared with conventional cigarettes. Toxicol. Sci. 149, 411–432. https://doi.org/10.1093/toxsci/kfv243.)

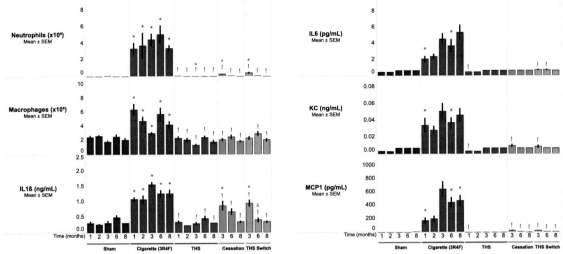

FIG. 18.9 Number of neutrophils and macrophages in BALF and concentrations of IL-1β, KC, IL-6, and MCP-1 at months 1, 2, 3, 6, and 8. Each graph shows the data for sham-exposed (blue), cigarette smoke—exposed (red), and THS aerosol—exposed (purple) animals. Animals exposed under a cessation and switching exposure protocol are depicted in green and orange, respectively. KC is the mouse orthologue of human IL-8. Study design and exposure conditions are described in Fig. 18.8. *, $P < .05$ versus sham (fresh air); !, $P < .05$ versus 3R4F; and, $P < .05$ versus cessation. *BALF*, bronchoalveolar lavage fluid; *IL-1β*, interleukin 1β; *IL-6*, interleukin 6; *KC*, murine chemokines KC; *MCP-1*, monocyte chemoattractant protein 1; *SEM*, standard error of the mean; *THS*, tobacco heating system.

epithelial tissue cultures grown at the air—liquid interface showed that cigarette smoke also induced the expression of several inflammation markers, including IL-1β. In contrast, ENDP aerosols applied at equivalent nicotine concentrations had little or no effect on these markers (Haswell et al., 2017, 2018; Iskandar et al., 2017).

This was further confirmed by a 40-day repeated exposure study conducted in human organotypic bronchial epithelial tissue cultures (Ito et al., 2020). This study showed that exposure to total particulate matter of cigarette smoke caused cumulative inflammatory and other biological perturbations, while exposure to the aerosol of a hybrid ENDP (Chapter 2) had negligible effects (Ito et al., 2020). This in vitro study, which included both switching and cessation arms, also showed that the effects of switching to a hybrid ENDP are similar to those of cessation (Ito et al., 2020).

Finally, one can also assess the immune cell responses to ENDP aerosol exposure by using cell lines or primary cells and compare them with those caused by cigarette smoke. These studies have shown that immune cell responses are less affected by ENDP aerosols than cigarette smoke, especially regarding their release of chemokines and cytokines such as IL-8 and tumor

necrosis factor alpha (TNFα) (Poussin et al., 2016; Ween et al., 2017).

In clinical studies, direct quantification of lung inflammation is difficult, as it involves invasive procedures such as BALF collection (Kuschner et al., 1996; Song et al., 2020). It has been also suggested that the small positive changes in lung function and respiratory symptoms observed in smokers who switched to an ENDP for 6—12 months may be a reasonable proxy for reduction in lung inflammation. In clinical studies conducted with ENDPs, lung function improved slightly over 6 months to 1 year, while the incidence of cough/phlegm and shortness of breath decreased substantially (Cibella et al., 2016; Lüdicke et al., 2019). Importantly, the positive changes in forced expiratory volume in 1 s (FEV$_1$) increased with decreasing dual-use with cigarettes (Lüdicke et al., 2019) (Chapter 17). The results of these studies indicate that ENDP aerosols cause less lung inflammation than cigarette smoke and further strengthen the results obtained in animal models and human organotypic tissue cultures of the respiratory tract.

Taken together, the available study results showed a significant reduction in all steps of the causal chain of events linking smoking to lung inflammation, which demonstrates that ENDPs cause less lung inflammation than cigarette smoke (Fig. 18.8). This would indicate that ENDP aerosols are less likely to cause tumor initiation, progression, and invasiveness than cigarette smoke.

18.3.1.3 Question 3: does switching from cigarettes to an ENDP reduce the risk of lung cancer?

ENDP aerosols with significantly reduced effects on both key mechanisms involved in cancer causation hypothesized by Balkwill and Mantovani (genetic damage and inflammation) (Balkwill and Mantovani, 2001) would be reasonably expected to also reduce the risk of lung cancer relative to cigarette smoking. To confirm this, two complementary nonclinical approaches can be adopted in the absence of long-term epidemiological data.

First, in vitro studies can be conducted in cell lines to assess the relative effects of cigarette smoke and ENDP aerosols on cellular and molecular endpoints linked to carcinogenesis. For instance, a Bhas 42 cell (mouse fibroblast—derived) transformation assay was used to show that the aerosols of ENDPs cause significantly less cell transformation than cigarette smoke (Breheny et al., 2017; Taylor et al., 2018). Similarly, long-term exposure (up to 12 weeks) of human bronchial epithelial BEAS-2B cells showed that the functional and molecular changes linked to lung carcinogenesis are less pronounced following ENDP aerosol than cigarette smoke exposure (van der Toorn et al., 2018).

Second, in vivo carcinogenesis studies, such as 18-month chronic inhalation studies, can be conducted in A/J mice to compare the effects of ENDP aerosol and cigarette smoke on lung tumor incidence and multiplicity (Chapter 15). The A/J mouse is highly susceptible to lung tumor development and has been widely used in carcinogenicity testing. These inbred mice often develop spontaneous benign tumors in the lungs (adenomas) that may, on occasion, progress to cancerous lesions (adenocarcinomas). The A/J mouse strain is highly sensitive to toxicants/compounds that are carcinogenic, and exposure to these carcinogenic materials causes an increase in the number of animals that develop both adenomas and adenocarcinomas (incidence). In addition, a hallmark of carcinogen exposure in these mice is the occurrence of multiple lung tumors in any given animal (multiplicity) (Witschi, 2005). A/J mouse inhalation studies performed with cigarette smoke have shown that exposure to smoke leads to lung tumors (Stinn et al., 2013a). While such studies are complex and require the use of mice, they enable a comprehensive nonclinical systems toxicology—based evaluation of all causally linked events linking smoking

to disease (Smith et al., 2016; Sturla et al., 2014) (Chapter 9). This means that, in the same study, one can evaluate lung inflammation (BALF analysis, gene and protein expression analysis, and histopathological analyses), emphysematous changes (histopathological analysis), lung function, and lung carcinogenesis (histopathological analysis) together with carcinogen exposure (BoExps and metabolic responses to carcinogen exposure [gene and protein expression analysis]) and response to DNA damage on the basis of gene expression data. This allows a coherent and integrated depiction of the biological effects of an ENDP aerosol in comparison with those of cigarette smoke.

To compare the tumorigenesis of cigarette smoke with that of an ENDP aerosol, we conducted an 18-month A/J mouse inhalation study to evaluate the difference in tumor incidence and multiplicity[4] caused by 3R4F reference cigarette smoke and THS aerosol (Wong et al., 2020) (Chapter 15). This model was previously established in our laboratory and shows a dose-dependent increase in lung adenocarcinomas upon cigarette smoke exposure (Stinn et al., 2013a). Briefly, female A/J mice were exposed for 6 h/day, 5 days/week for 18 months to fresh air (sham), 3R4F smoke at 13.4 μg/L nicotine, or THS aerosol at three concentrations of nicotine: 6.7, 13.4, or 26.8 μg/L.[5] The medium concentration of THS aerosol was set to match that of 3R4F smoke. Furthermore, male mice were exposed to either fresh air (sham) or THS aerosol at 26.8 μg/L.

The study results show that, at the end of the life-long exposure period, a greater number (incidence) of A/J mice exposed to 3R4F smoke had lung adenomas and carcinomas than mice exposed to fresh air (Fig. 18.10). In contrast, mice exposed to THS aerosol did not show an increase in tumor incidence relative to those exposed to fresh air. Furthermore, mice exposed to 3R4F smoke had more lesions and tumors per mouse than those exposed to fresh air (multiplicity) (Fig. 18.11),[6] while mice exposed to THS aerosol did not show an increase in tumor multiplicity relative to those exposed to fresh air.

---

[4]Tumor *incidence* refers to the number of animals with tumors, while tumor *multiplicity* refers to number of tumors per animal having at least one tumor.

[5]The human equivalent exposure to the high concentration corresponds to 56 cig/day for 60 kg body weight.

[6]The A/J mouse strain is very tumor-sensitive in contrast to most other mouse strains and, therefore, has a high background incidence. Tumor multiplicity, which provides a better dynamic range, is reproducible between assays (Witschi, 2005).

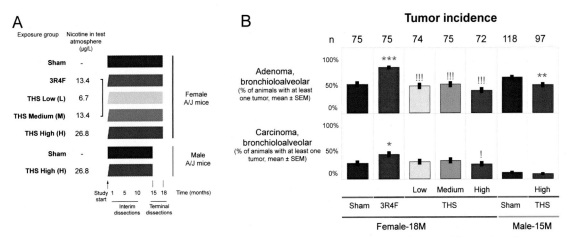

FIG. 18.10 **Lung tumor incidence in the A/J mouse study with THS.** **(A)** Study design. The medium dose of THS 2.2 corresponds to the dose of 3R4F in terms of nicotine. Exposure conditions: 6 h/day, 5 days/week for up to 18 months. **(B)** Incidence of lung adenoma and carcinoma in A/J mouse lungs at the end of the study. *, $P < .05$; **, $P < .01$; ***, $P < .001$ versus sham (fresh air); !, $P < .05$, !!, $P < .01$, !!!, $P < .001$ versus 3R4F. *n*, number of animals per group at terminal dissection; *3R4F*, reference cigarette; *SEM*, standard error of the mean; *THS*, Tobacco Heating System.

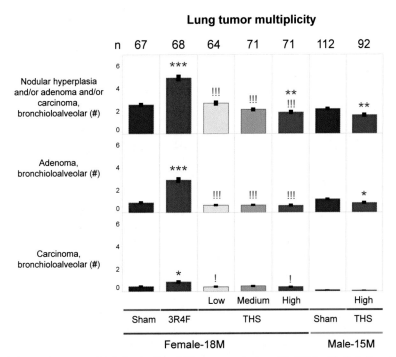

FIG. 18.11 **Lung tumor multiplicity in the A/J mouse study with THS.** Multiplicity of all lesions (hyperplasia and neoplasia), lung adenoma, and carcinoma in A/J mouse lungs at the end of the study. Study design and exposure conditions are described in Fig. 18.10. *, $P < .05$; **, $P < .01$, ***, $P < .001$ versus sham (fresh air); !, $P < .05$; !!, $P < .01$; !!!, $P < .001$ versus 3R4F. *n*, number of animals per group at terminal dissection; *3R4F*, reference cigarette; *THS*, Tobacco Heating System.

This study also showed that, while cigarette smoke caused significant genetic damage and lung inflammation, THS aerosol caused only minor changes in all related endpoints (BALF, gene and protein expression, and histopathological endpoints), further confirming that ENDPs do not trigger these two fundamental mechanisms involved in lung tumorigenesis.

18.3.1.4 Summary and conclusions for lung cancer

The totality of the available evidence shows that exposure to ENDP aerosols instead of cigarette smoke leads to a reduction in genetic damage, lung inflammation, and tumorigenesis. These reductions are consistent across all animal and human experimental models and are due to the reduced exposure to HPHCs, free radicals, and cbNPs. Furthermore, human subjects who switched from cigarette smoking to ENDP use showed reduced exposure to carcinogenic toxicants to levels that approached those in subjects who abstained from smoking for the duration of the clinical studies. Finally, clinical studies showed that switching completely from cigarette smoking to ENDP use slightly improved lung function and substantially decreased the incidence of cough/phlegm and shortness of breath within 6 months to a year. Therefore, switching completely from cigarette smoking to ENDP use is likely to reduce the risk of lung cancer.

18.4 IMPLICATIONS FOR OTHER SMOKING-INDUCED CANCERS

Cigarette smoking causes not only lung cancer but also a large number of other malignancies, while smoking cessation clearly correlates with an overall reduction in relative cancer risk (Carter et al., 2015). It is, therefore, important to understand whether switching from cigarette smoking to ENDP use can also reduce the risk of other malignancies. While epidemiological data provide the primary link between smoking and cancer, smoking behavior data are generally not sufficiently precise to enable a detailed analysis linking exposure to HPHCs with the relative risk of cancer, even though it has been shown recently that changes in smoking intensity (number of cigarettes per day) over the course of a lifetime have an influence on the risk of cancer and all causes of mortality (Inoue-Choi et al., 2019). To address this question, we conducted a simple analysis of the relative risk of different malignancies by mapping them to the relative exposure of the affected organs to HPHCs.

18.4.1 Epidemiological Link Between Relative Risk of Cancer and Toxicant Exposure

Cigarette smoke exposure occurs through three different routes. First and foremost, smoke is inhaled and, therefore, the oral cavity, nose, respiratory tract, and lungs are directly exposed to whole smoke. Second, smoke deposits in the oral cavity and the resulting condensates are swallowed and follow the route of the digestive tract. Finally, smoke constituents enter the bloodstream, mainly through the lungs, and are metabolized in the liver and other locations. These metabolic products, as well as nonmetabolized constituents, will reach every organ system. Therefore, it is not surprising that many organ systems are affected by smoking and that malignancies occur in locations that are not directly exposed to cigarette smoke.

We have classified the relative risk of mortality from cancer (RR-MC) caused by smoking and cessation according to both cancer site and primary type of exposure (i.e., *"direct smoke exposure," "smoke condensate exposure,"* and *"smoke constituent and metabolite exposure"*) (Table 18.1). For instance, the respiratory tract is directly exposed to smoke, while the digestive tract is exposed to "swallowed smoke condensate," and the urinary tract is exposed to both smoke constituents and their metabolites. This reveals a striking correlation between the type of exposure and RR-MC.

While the information in Table 18.1 shows the obvious, namely that the highest RR-MC correlates with the sites of direct exposure to cigarette smoke in the respiratory tract, it also shows that the esophagus, liver, and urinary bladder have higher RR-MCs than other sites. In the digestive tract, the esophagus and stomach[8] will likely be exposed to higher concentrations of smoke condensate than the colorectum, which correlates with a lower RR-MC. The liver, which metabolizes smoke constituents and metabolically activates procarcinogens such as PAHs or TSNAs, shows a higher RR-MC than the pancreas and prostate. Finally, the urinary bladder concentrates both smoke constituents and their carcinogenic metabolites and, therefore, displays a higher RR-MC than the kidney and renal pelvis. Taken together, these observations suggest that there is a direct correlation between local HPHC dose and RR-MC. In all cases, the RR-MC is lower in quitters than in smokers (Table 18.1).

---

[8]The stomach might also be more resistant to smoke condensate-induced carcinogenesis than the esophagus.

TABLE 18.1
Relative Risk of Cancer Mortality in Smokers and Quitters by Exposure Site and Type[7].

Organ System	Cancer Site	Direct Smoke Exposure	Smoke Condensate Exposure	Smoke Constituent and Metabolite Exposure	
				High Concentration	**Low Concentration**
Respiratory	Lips and oral cavity (C00—C14)[a]	5.7 (1.7)			
	Larynx (C32)	13.9 (2.4)[b]			
	Trachea, lungs, and bronchus (C33—C34)	25.3 (6.8)[c]			
Digestive	Esophagus (C15)		3.9 (2.6)		
	Stomach (C16)		1.9 (1.5)		
	Colorectum (C18—C20)		1.4 (1.2)		
Urinary	Urinary bladder (C67)			3.9 (2.4)	
	Kidney and renal pelvis (C64—C66)				1.8 (1.5)
Bone marrow	Acute myeloid leukemia (C92.0)				1.9 (1.4)
	Other leukemias (C92.1—C95)				2.1 (1.3)
Other	Liver (C22)			2.3 (1.5)	
	Pancreas (C25)				1.6 (1)
	Prostate (C61)				1.4 (1)

[a] ICD-10 codes.
[b] Relative risk in smokers and quitters in parenthesis.
[c] Relative risk of COPD is 27.8 (7.5)[b].

18.4.2 Summary and Conclusions for Other Cancers

The obvious question is whether switching from smoking to ENDP use will lead to a reduction in cancer risk beyond that of lung cancer. As described above, switching from cigarette smoking to ENDP use leads to a reduction in exposure to carcinogenic toxicants that approaches the exposure reduction achieved by smoking abstinence. We have also shown that switching to THS reverses the level of CYP1A2 (produced by the liver) to similar levels than abstinence in humans and cessation in mice. Finally, the results of the urinary Ames tests conducted in the context of clinical reduced exposure studies support the conclusion

that smokers who switch completely to this ENDP are exposed to significantly lower levels of carcinogenic toxicants. Taken together, these lines of evidence indicate that switching completely from smoking to ENDP use is likely to also reduce the risk of cancer at sites other than the respiratory tract.

18.5 IMPLICATIONS FOR CHRONIC OBSTRUCTIVE PULMONARY DISEASE

Chronic exposure of the lungs to cigarette smoke, which is a major risk factor for COPD, results in oxidative stress and inflammation. Oxidative stress and chronic inflammation, in turn, cause changes in alveolar and airway tissues. Cigarette smoke can trigger and enhance pulmonary inflammation via several distinct yet partially overlapping mechanisms involving many different cell types. Over time, persistence of these mechanisms in the lungs leads to goblet cell

[7]Adapted from Carter et al. (2015): Supplementary Appendix D. Relative Risks (RR) of death from all causes of death accounting for at least 20 deaths in current smokers in men aged 55 years of age or older. NIH-AARP, CPS-II Nutrition Cohort, and Health Professionals Follow-up Study, 2000—11.

metaplasia/hyperplasia, mucus hypersecretion, airway remodeling, and alveolar destruction, that are characteristics of COPD (Barnes, 2004; Rogers, 2007). These changes have an adverse impact on the overall pulmonary structure and function, leading to COPD.

To assess the COPD risk reduction potential of ENDPs, one can again use the CELSD as a guide for the integrative evaluation of studies.

As outlined in the section on lung cancer, ENDPs emit on average > 90% lower levels of HPHCs than cigarettes and extremely low levels of free radicals and no cbNPs. This leads to a significant reduction in exposure to HPHCs in human subjects who switch from cigarette smoking to ENDP use and across all experimental biological systems. This, in turn, leads to a reduction in the molecular changes and mechanistic perturbations linked to oxidative stress and inflammation across all biological systems, as outlined above. According to the CELSD, these reductions should also lead to a reduction in tissue damage and lung function loss. To complete the assessment of the COPD risk reduction potential of ENDPs, we now address the following important questions in both in vivo nonclinical and clinical studies:

- Does switching from cigarette smoking to ENDP use reduce tissue damage?
- Consequently, does switching from cigarette smoking to ENDP use reduce lung function loss?

A positive answer to these two questions would indicate that switching completely from cigarette smoking to ENDP use will likely reduce the risk of COPD.

18.5.1 Animal Models of Emphysema

Many cellular and molecular mechanisms involved in the pathogenesis of human COPD are also observed in murine pulmonary emphysema models (Brusselle et al., 2006). Several features are shared between human early-stage disease and mouse disease development, which primarily recapitulates the emphysema component (Churg et al., 2011). Lesions in mice caused by chronic cigarette smoke exposure resemble mild centrilobular human emphysema, both morphologically and physiologically (Churg et al., 2008). Small airway remodeling, an important cause of airflow obstruction in cigarette smokers with COPD (Hogg et al., 2004), was also observed in cigarette smoke–exposed mice (Churg et al., 2008). In addition, exposure activates the innate immune response cascade in mice, leading to protease/antiprotease imbalances in lung tissue and eventually to alveolar destruction, suggesting that murine models can also replicate these features of human COPD (Yoshida and Tuder, 2007). Finally, as observed in humans, the small airways of cigarette smoke–

exposed C57BL/6 mice exhibit persistent upregulation of type I procollagen and profibrotic cytokine gene expression, which is expected to contribute to airway remodeling (Churg et al., 2006).

Previous studies have shown that chronic exposure of mice to cigarette smoke results in reduced lung function, sustained pulmonary inflammation, and emphysema with features resembling those underlying the pathophysiology of human COPD (Awji et al., 2015; Churg et al., 2009; Phillips et al., 2015; Stinn et al., 2013b).

To date, only very few studies have been conducted with ENDPs in animal models of COPD (Phillips et al., 2016, 2019a, 2019b). The animal model used is the Apoe$^{-/-}$ mouse, which is derived from the C57BL/6 strain (Chapter 15).

18.5.1.1 Apoe$^{-/-}$ mouse switching study

Apoe$^{-/-}$ mice are commonly used as a model for atherogenesis (Veniant et al., 2001) and have been valuable tools for investigating smoking-related atherosclerosis (Boue et al., 2012; Lietz et al., 2013; Lo Sasso et al., 2016b). This mouse model has also been used to study cigarette smoke–induced lung inflammation and emphysema (Arunachalam et al., 2010; Boue et al., 2013; Lo Sasso et al., 2016a). We conducted an 8-month exposure study in Apoe$^{-/-}$ mice to compare the effects of THS aerosol exposure with those of 3R4F reference cigarette smoke exposure on the development and progression of emphysema and formation of atherosclerotic plaque (Phillips et al., 2016). This study allowed us to compare the effects of these exposures on the full CELSD from molecular changes through biological network perturbations and cellular and tissue changes to lung function changes. Furthermore, in this study, we also compared the effects of switching from cigarette smoke to THS aerosol exposure with the effects of smoking cessation (Phillips et al., 2016).

18.5.1.1.1 Reduced molecular changes and biological network perturbations by THS. Most inflammatory mediators measured in BALF were significantly elevated in 3R4F smoke–exposed animals, showing a rapid increase following 1 month of exposure (Phillips et al., 2016). However, inflammatory mediator and proteolytic enzyme concentrations (Fig. 18.12) in the BALF of THS aerosol–exposed mice were very similar to those in sham-exposed animals. Furthermore, animals switched from cigarette smoke to THS aerosol exposure or smoking cessation showed attenuation of these changes to almost normal values (Phillips et al.,

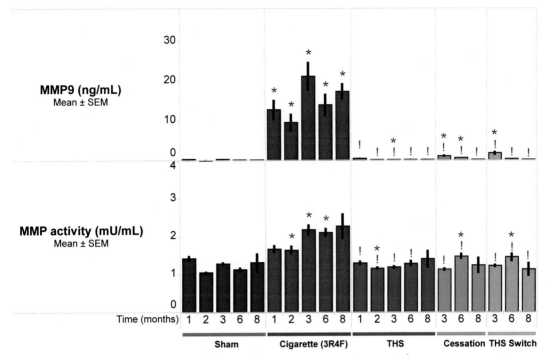

FIG. 18.12 MMP-9 protein concentrations and MMP activity in BALF in the Apoe$^{-/-}$ mouse switching study. The graphs show the data for fresh air-exposed (blue), cigarette smoke–exposed (red), and THS-exposed (purple) animals. Animals exposed under the cessation and switching exposure protocols are depicted in green and orange, respectively. Study design and exposure conditions are described in Fig. 18.8. *, $P < .05$ versus sham (fresh air); !, $P < .05$ versus 3R4F. BALF, bronchoalveolar lavage fluid; MMP, matrix metalloproteinase; SEM, standard error of the mean; THS, tobacco heating system. (Adapted from Phillips, B., Veljkovic, E., Boué, S., Schlage, W.K., Vuillaume, G., Martin, F., Titz, B., Leroy, P., Buettner, A., Elamin, A., Oviedo, A., Cabanski, M., De León, H., Guedj, E., Schneider, T., Talikka, M., Ivanov, N.V., Vanscheeuwijck, P., Peitsch, M.C., Hoeng, J., 2016. An 8-month systems toxicology inhalation/cessation study in Apoe$^{-/-}$ mice to investigate cardiovascular and respiratory exposure effects of a candidate modified risk tobacco product, THS 2.2, compared with conventional cigarettes. Toxicol. Sci. 149, 411–432. https://doi.org/10.1093/toxsci/kfv243.)

2016). Analysis of the lung proteome across all study groups showed a pattern that was entirely consistent with these observations (Phillips et al., 2016).

Using a systems toxicology approach (Chapter 9), we analyzed the biological network perturbations underlying the toxicological impact of 3R4F smoke exposure. This analysis encompassed a very broad range of mechanisms, including Inflammation (Fig. 18.8), Cell Stress, Cell Proliferation, Cell Fate and Apoptosis, and Tissue Repair and Angiogenesis. 3R4F smoke exposure caused a sustained and generalized activation of all these mechanisms (Phillips et al., 2016). While most of the networks affected by the initial 3R4F smoke exposure remained perturbed throughout the cessation period, the extent of these perturbations was

significantly attenuated. In contrast, the lungs of animals exposed from the beginning to THS aerosol exhibited only a few significant network perturbations. Furthermore, the effects of switching from 3R4F smoke to THS aerosol exposure were similar to those of cessation. These results show that the overall biological impact of THS on the lungs is very low compared to that of 3R4F and that the effects switching to THS aerosol exposure approach those of cessation.

18.5.1.1.2 Reduced cellular and tissue changes by THS. The total number of free lung cells in BALF increased and remained elevated in the 3R4F smoke–exposed animals, primarily because of infiltration

of neutrophils. In contrast, prolonged exposure to the THS aerosol had no effect on free lung cell count. Both cessation and switching to THS aerosol exposure resulted in a rapid decline in the number of free lung cells, nearly reaching those already seen in sham or THS aerosol–exposed mice after 1 month (Phillips et al., 2016). Histopathological evaluation of respiratory tract organs, at multiple time points, showed typical cigarette smoke exposure–related changes, including adaptive changes of epithelia (nasal, laryngeal, and tracheal), infiltration of inflammatory cells, and emphysematous lesions, which were expressed in terms of destructive index and emphysema score (Fig. 18.13). The degree of inflammation and inflammatory cell infiltrates was much reduced in THS aerosol–exposed animals, and, importantly, the THS aerosol–exposed lungs were indistinguishable from sham-exposed lungs in terms of histological appearance. Both cessation and switching to THS

aerosol exposure resulted in very similar histopathological findings (Fig. 18.13) (Phillips et al., 2016).

18.5.1.1.3 Reduced lung function loss by THS.
3R4F smoke exposure led to a gradual reduction in lung function, as determined by pressure–volume (PV) loop measurement (increased lung volume at a given pressure indicates loss of lung function) (Fig. 18.14).

In contrast, there was no significant effect of THS aerosol exposure on lung function relative to sham exposure at any time point. Switching and cessation resulted in stabilization of the values, while continued 3R4F smoke exposure led to further decline in lung function (Phillips et al., 2016). These functional measurements corroborate the histological observations outlined above.

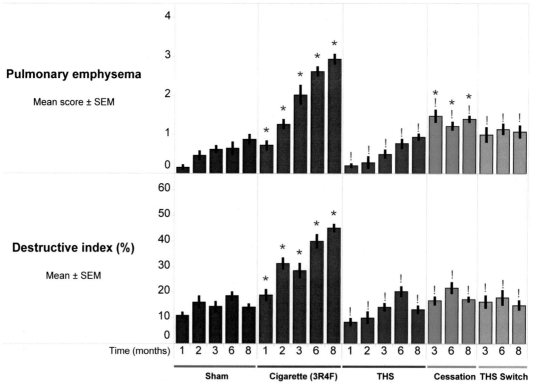

FIG. 18.13 Lung destructive index and emphysema scores in the Apoe$^{-/-}$ mouse switching study. Study design and exposure conditions are described in Fig. 18.8. *, $P < .05$ versus sham (fresh air); !, $P < .05$ versus 3R4F. SEM, standard error of the mean; THS, Tobacco Heating System. (Adapted from Phillips, B., Veljkovic, E., Boué, S., Schlage, W.K., Vuillaume, G., Martin, F., Titz, B., Leroy, P., Buettner, A., Elamin, A., Oviedo, A., Cabanski, M., De León, H., Guedj, E., Schneider, T., Talikka, M., Ivanov, N.V., Vanscheeuwijck, P., Peitsch, M.C., Hoeng, J., 2016. An 8-month systems toxicology inhalation/cessation study in Apoe$^{-/-}$ mice to investigate cardiovascular and respiratory exposure effects of a candidate modified risk tobacco product, THS 2.2, compared with conventional cigarettes. Toxicol. Sci. 149, 411–432 https://doi.org/10.1093/toxooi/kfv240.)

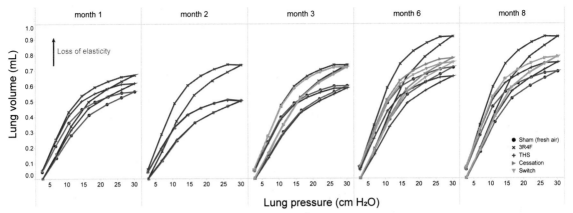

FIG. 18.14 Lung function measurements in the Apoe$^{-/-}$ mouse switching study. The pressure—volume graphs show the data for sham-exposed (blue), cigarette smoke—exposed (red), and THS-exposed (purple) animals. Animals exposed under the cessation and switching exposure protocols are depicted in green and orange, respectively. Study design and exposure conditions are described in Fig. 18.8. *Ppl(H_2O)*, pressure in cm H_2O; *3R4F*, reference cigarette; *Vpl (mL)*, lung volume in mL at a given pressure; *THS*, Tobacco Heating System. (Adapted from Phillips, B., Veljkovic, E., Boué, S., Schlage, W.K., Vuillaume, G., Martin, F., Titz, B., Leroy, P., Buettner, A., Elamin, A., Oviedo, A., Cabanski, M., De León, H., Guedj, E., Schneider, T., Talikka, M., Ivanov, N.V., Vanscheeuwijck, P., Peitsch, M.C., Hoeng, J., 2016. An 8-month systems toxicology inhalation/cessation study in Apoe$^{-/-}$ mice to investigate cardiovascular and respiratory exposure effects of a candidate modified risk tobacco product, THS 2.2, compared with conventional cigarettes. Toxicol. Sci. 149, 411—432. https://doi.org/10.1093/toxsci/kfv243.)

In conclusion, the results from the 8-month Apoe$^{-/-}$ mouse switching study provide very strong and consistent evidence that, relative to 3R4F smoke, THS aerosol has a significantly reduced adverse biological impact on the lungs at the molecular, cellular, tissue, and functional levels. Moreover, the study results show that smoke-exposed animals switched to either THS aerosol or smoking cessation present very similar global recovery of the broad molecular changes, multifaceted biological network perturbations, and cellular changes induced by smoke exposure. Importantly, the tissue and functional changes induced by the initial smoke exposure did not progress further following switching to THS aerosol or air exposure.

18.5.1.2 A/J mouse inhalation study

The results of the A/J mouse inhalation study described under Section 18.3.1.3 have shown that, relative to cigarette smoke, THS aerosol had a substantially reduced impact on lung inflammation at months 1 and 5 (Figs. 18.15 and 18.16) as well as on histopathological changes in the lungs at months 5, 10, and 18 (Fig. 18.17) (Titz et al., 2020; Wong et al., 2020) (Chapter 15).

Importantly, cigarette smoke and cbNPs were shown to trigger the production of IL-1β, IL-18, IL-6, KC, MMP-9, and IL-17A in mice. These markers have been linked to development of emphysema (Liang et al., 2018; You

et al., 2015). In the A/J mouse study, these inflammatory markers were also significantly increased in the BALF of 3R4F smoke—exposed mice but not in that of THS aerosol—exposed mice (Fig. 18.16).

These findings are in direct correlation with the observation that THS aerosol—exposed animals did not experience a significant effect on lung function (PV loops) relative to sham-exposed mice at either time point of evaluation (1 or 5 months), irrespective of the exposure dose (Fig. 18.18). These results furthermore corroborate our findings in the Apoe$^{-/-}$ mouse switching study (Fig. 18.14) (Phillips et al., 2016).

In conclusion, the results from the A/J mouse study are consistent with those of the Apoe$^{-/-}$ switching study described above and provide very strong and consistent evidence that THS aerosol has a significantly reduced adverse biological impact on the lungs at the molecular, cellular, tissue, and functional levels relative to 3R4F smoke.

18.5.2 Improved Clinical Endpoints Associated with COPD Risk

As outlined in Section 18.3.1.2.2, in smokers who switched to ENDP use, lung function improved slightly over 6 months to 1 year, while the incidence of cough/phlegm and shortness of breath decreased substantially (Cibella et al., 2016; Lüdicke et al., 2019; Sharman and Nurmagambetov, 2020). Importantly, the positive

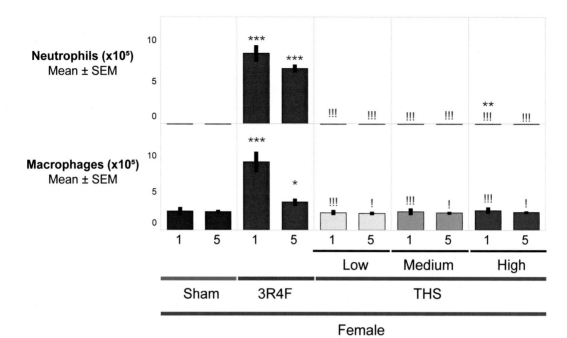

FIG. 18.15 Quantification of free lung cells in female A/J mouse BALF at months 1 and 5. Exposure conditions are described in Fig. 18.10. *, $P < .05$; **, $P < .01$; and ***, $P < .001$ versus sham (fresh air); !, $P < .05$; !!, $P < .01$, and !!!, $P < .001$ versus 3R4F. BALF, bronchoalveolar lavage fluid; 3R4F, reference cigarette; SEM, standard error of the mean; THS, tobacco heating system. (Adapted from Wong, E., Luettich, K., Krishnan, S., Wong, S.K., Lim, S.K., Yeo, D., Büttner, A., Leroy, P., Vuillaume, G., Boué, S., Hoeng, J., Vanscheeuwijck, P., Peitsch, M.C., 2020. Reduced chronic toxicity and carcinogenicity in A/J mice in response to life-time exposure to aerosol from a heated tobacco product compared with cigarette smoke. Toxicol. Sci. (in press).)

changes in FEV$_1$ increased with decreasing dual use with cigarettes (Lüdicke et al., 2019) (Chapter 17). The results of these studies indicate that ENDP aerosols cause less lung inflammation than cigarette smoke and further strengthen the results obtained in animal models and human organotypic tissue cultures of the respiratory tract. Furthermore, a recent 5-year study showed that COPD patients who switched to EVPs had a significant reduction in the number of COPD exacerbations as well as an improvement in lung function compared with those who continued to smoke (Polosa et al., 2020a).

Cigarette smoking leads to impaired nasal and bronchial epithelia cilia function and hence reduced mucociliary clearance (Baby et al., 2014; Polosa et al., 2020b; Stanley et al., 1986). This impairment has been associated with COPD (Koblizek et al., 2011; Perotin et al., 2018; Yaghi et al., 2012). In contrast to cigarette smoke, ENDP aerosols have a strongly reduced effect on cilia function (Iskandar et al., 2017a, b, 2019a), and switching completely from cigarette smoking to ENDP use restores mucociliary clearance to levels similar to those following smoking cessation (Polosa et al., 2020b).

18.5.3 Summary and Conclusions for COPD

The totality of available evidence shows that exposure to ENDP aerosols instead of cigarette smoke leads to a reduction in lung inflammation relative to cigarette smoke. These reductions are consistent across all animal and human experimental models and are due to their reduced exposure to the broad spectrum of toxicants emitted by cigarettes. Furthermore, human subjects who switched from cigarette smoking to ENDP use showed reduced exposure to toxicants to levels that approached those in subjects who abstained from smoking for the duration of the clinical studies. Finally, the clinical studies showed that switching completely from cigarette smoking to ENDP use slightly improved lung function and substantially decreased the incidence of cough/phlegm and shortness of breath within 6 months to 1 year. Furthermore, ENDP aerosols have a significantly lower effect than cigarettes smoke on respiratory epithelia cilia function in vitro and mucociliary clearance in clinical study subjects. Therefore, switching completely from cigarette smoking to ENDP use is likely to reduce the risk of COPD.

	Female (1M)				Female (5M)			
	3R4F	THS L	THS M	THS H	3R4F	THS L	THS M	THS H
Apo A-I (µg/mL)	1.57 **	0.82 !	0.51 !!!	0.60 !!!				
CRP Mouse (µg/mL)	1.95 **	1.00 !!	1.00 !!	1.00 !!	1.65 *	1.00	1.18	1.00 !
Eotaxin (pg/mL)	5.15 **	0.88 !!!	0.94 !!!	0.75 !!!	7.45 ***	1.46 !!!	1.64 !!!	1.39 !!!
EGF Mouse (pg/mL)	4.40 ***	1.00 !!!	1.00 !!!	1.00 !!!	7.43 ***	0.50 !!!	0.70 !!!	0.74 !!!
Fibrinogen (mg/mL)	5.24 ***	0.86 !!!	0.91 !!!	0.85 !!!	3.79 ***	0.97 !!!	1.78 * !!	1.15 !!!
FGF-9 (ng/mL)	1.62 *	1.00 !	1.00 !	1.00 !	1.55	1.00	1.00	1.00
FGF-basic (ng/mL)	1.41	1.00	1.00	1.00	1.52 *	0.74 !!	1.17	0.81 !
GCP-2 Mouse (ng/mL)	2.54 ***	0.78 !!!	0.70 * !!!	0.76 !!!	2.63 ***	1.08 !!!	0.75 !!!	0.76 !!!
GM-CSF (pg/mL)	6.28 ***	1.00 !!!	1.00 !!!	1.00 !!!	2.59 ***	1.00	1.00 !!!	1.00
GH (ng/mL)	1.00	1.00	1.00	1.00	1.00	1.13	1.00	1.00
KC/GRO (ng/mL)	68.39 ***	1.19 !!!	1.00 !!!	1.00 !!!	20.23 ***	1.14 !!!	1.00 !!!	1.00 !!!
Haptoglobin (µg/mL)	1.00	0.98 !	0.98 !!	0.99 !	1.41 **	1.38 !!	1.38 !!	1.38 !!
IgA (µg/mL)	24.86 ***	0.82	5.35 !!	0.67	247.45 ***	1.71 !!!	1.83 !!!	1.57 !!!
Insulin (uIU/mL)	1.08	1.28	0.78	1.17	1.37 *	1.43	1.95 !	1.76
IFN-gamma (pg/mL)	1.00	1.00	1.00	1.00	1.00	1.00	1.00	1.00
IP-10 (pg/mL)	30.47 ***	1.00 !!!	1.00 !!!	1.11 !!!	6.01 ***	1.00 !!!	1.00 !!!	1.11 !!!
IL-1 alpha (pg/mL)	13.71 ***	1.00 !!!	1.00 !!!	1.00 !!!	18.64 ***	1.00 !!!	1.00 !!!	1.00 !!!
IL-1 beta (ng/mL)	3.01 ***	1.00 !!!	1.00 !!!	1.00 !!!	4.47 ***	1.51 !!!	1.51 !!!	1.51 !!!
IL-2 (pg/mL)	1.10	1.00	1.00	1.00	1.00	1.00	1.00	1.00
IL-3 (pg/mL)	1.23	1.00	1.00	1.00	1.12	1.00	1.00	1.00
IL-4 (pg/mL)	1.87 **	1.21 !	1.11 !	1.10 !	1.13	1.00	1.11	1.00
IL-5 (ng/mL)	1.00	1.00	1.00	1.00	0.71	0.71	0.71	0.79
IL-6 (pg/mL)	8.97 ***	1.27 !!!	1.22 !!!	1.00 !!!	6.33 ***	1.00 !!!	1.14 !!!	1.00 !!!
IL-7 (pg/mL)	2.96 ***	1.10 !!!	1.00 !!!	1.00 !!!	3.08 ***	1.00 !!!	1.00 !!!	1.00 !!!
IL-10 (pg/mL)	1.24	1.00	1.00	1.00	1.00	1.00	1.00	1.00
IL-11 (pg/mL)	2.33 ***	1.00 !!!	1.00 !!!	1.00 !!!	2.24 ***	1.00 !!	1.00 !!	1.00 !!
IL-12p70 (ng/mL)	1.12	1.00	1.00	1.00	1.00	1.00	1.00	1.00
IL-17A (pg/mL)	2.39	1.04	0.88 !	0.88 !	2.00 *	0.99	1.16	0.88 !
IL-18 (ng/mL)	7.48 ***	1.00 !!!	1.00 !!!	1.00 !!!	4.39 ***	1.23 !!!	1.49 !!!	1.27 !!!
Leptin (ng/mL)	0.92	0.76	0.88	0.89	0.98 *	0.89 *	1.25	1.02
LIF (pg/mL)	5.97 ***	1.02 !!!	0.88 !!!	0.86 !!!	1.96 ***	0.47 !!!	0.42 !!!	0.46 !!!
M-CSF-1 (ng/mL)	7.28 ***	1.08 !!!	1.08 !!!	1.11 !!!	6.28 ***	1.12 !!!	0.99 !!!	1.02 !!!
MIP-1 alpha (ng/mL)	7.83 ***	1.00 !!!	1.00 !!!	1.00 !!!	13.13 ***	0.90 !!!	0.90 !!!	0.90 !!!
MIP-1 beta (pg/mL)	84.48 ***	1.04 !!!	0.99 !!!	1.08 !!!	105.13 **	0.83 !!!	1.17 !!!	0.78 !!!
MIP-1 gamma (ng/m..)	17.53 ***	1.06 !!!	1.08 !!!	0.93 !!!	13.53 ***	0.91 !!!	1.05 !!!	1.13 !!!
MIP-2 (pg/mL)	6.43 ***	0.95 !!!	1.03 !!	1.14	3.51 ***	1.11 !!	1.03 !!	0.93 !!
MIP-3 beta (pg/mL)	4.72 ***	0.92 !!!	0.88 !!!	0.88 !!!	1.96 ***	0.53 !!!	0.47 !!!	0.48 !!!
MDC (pg/mL)	20.19 ***	1.02 !!!	1.03 !!!	0.93 !!!	8.41 ***	0.82 !!!	0.85 !!!	0.81 !!!
MMP-9 (ng/mL)	181.07 ***	0.51 !!!	0.89 !!!	0.47 !!!	101.99 ***	2.41 !!!	1.40 !!!	1.24 !!!
MCP-1 (pg/mL)	1,498.25 ***	1.00 !!!	1.79 !!!	1.00 !!!	1,829.75 ***	4.92 !!!	3.90 !!!	3.35 !!!
MCP-3 (pg/mL)	350.26 ***	1.00 !!!	1.51 !!!	1.00 !!!	341.48 ***	1.84 !!!	2.04 !!	1.36 !!!
MCP-5 (pg/mL)	70.67 ***	1.00 !!!	1.00 !!!	1.00 !!!	29.25 ***	1.00 !!!	1.00 !!!	1.00 !!!
Myoglobin (ng/mL)	0.84	1.61	1.13	1.39	4.04	2.24	2.60 *	7.14
OSM (ng/mL)	6.39 ***	1.00 !!!	1.00 !!!	1.00 !!!	6.26 ***	1.00 !!!	1.00 !!!	1.00 !!!
PAI-1 (ng/mL)	5.00 ***	1.03 !!!	1.00 !!	1.01 !!!	5.46 ***	1.27 !!!	1.31 !!!	1.35 !!!
Resistin (ng/mL)	1.30 *	0.95 !	0.98	1.17	1.48	1.22	1.27	1.19
SAP (µg/mL)	1.37	1.00	1.00	1.00	1.94 **	1.00 !	1.18 !	1.00 !!
SCF (pg/mL)	7.42 ***	1.10 !!!	0.86 !!!	0.90 !!!	8.09 ***	1.21 !!!	1.08 !!!	0.88 * !!!
Thrombopoietin (ng/mL)	5.01 ***	1.00 !!!	1.00 !!!	1.00 !!!	2.50 ***	0.54 !!!	0.62 !!!	0.62 !!!
TIMP-1 Mouse (ng/mL)	10.79 **	1.12 !!!	1.14 !!!	1.09 !!	7.04 ***	1.19 !!!	1.28 !!!	1.10 !!!
TNF-alpha (ng/mL)	7.37 ***	1.39 !!!	1.00 !!!	1.00 !!!	7.97 ***	1.14 !!!	1.33 !!!	1.00 !!!
VCAM-1 (ng/mL)	11.16 ***	1.31 ** !!!	1.45 !!!	1.02 !!!	22.84 ***	1.96 !!!	1.96 !!!	1.99 !!!
VEGF-A (pg/mL)	8.84 ***	1.06 !!!	0.98 !!!	1.20 !!!	4.76 ***	1.33 !!!	1.24 !!!	1.19 !!!
vWF (ng/mL)	4.76 ***	0.83 !!!	0.80 !!	0.80 !!!	3.42 ***	0.77 !!!	0.79 !!!	0.66 !!!
MMP activity (mU/mL)	1.28	1.19	0.94	0.86	4.68 ***	1.15 !!!	1.15 !!!	0.97 !!!

FIG. 18.16 Quantification of soluble markers in female A/J mouse bronchoalveolar lavage fluid at months 1 and 5. Values shown are average concentrations of each marker per exposure group. *, $P < .05$; **, $P < .01$; and ***, $P < .001$ versus sham (fresh air); !, $P < .05$; !!, $P < .01$; and !!!, $P < .001$ versus 3R4F. Exposure conditions are described in the legend of Fig. 18.10. *3R4F*, reference cigarette; *THS*, tobacco heating system.

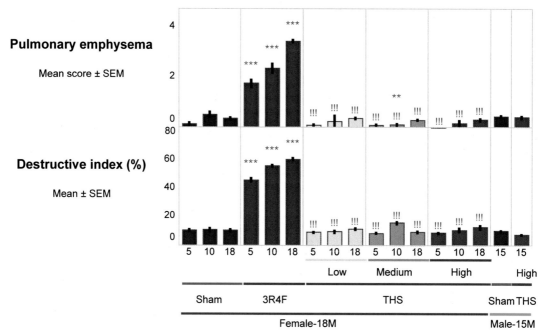

FIG. 18.17 Lung destructive index and emphysema scores in the A/J mouse study at months 1, 5, and 18. Exposure conditions are described in the legend of Fig. 18.10. ***, $P < .001$; **, $P < .01$ versus fresh Air; !!!, $P < .001$ versus 3R4F. 3R4F reference cigarette; *SEM*, standard error of the mean; *THS*, tobacco heating system. (Adapted from Wong, E., Luettich, K., Krishnan, S., Wong, S.K., Lim, S.K., Yeo, D., Büttner, A., Leroy, P., Vuillaume, G., Boué, S., Hoeng, J., Vanscheeuwijck, P., Peitsch, M.C., 2020. Reduced chronic toxicity and carcinogenicity in A/J mice in response to life-time exposure to aerosol from a heated tobacco product compared with cigarette smoke. Toxicol. Sci. (in press).)

18.6 IMPLICATIONS FOR CARDIOVASCULAR DISEASE

Cigarette smoking is a major risk factor for development of CVD (Ambrose and Barua, 2004; Messner and Bernhard, 2014). Several discrete steps in the CELSD have been described previously (Ambrose and Barua, 2004; Csordas and Bernhard, 2013). Cigarette smoke contains toxicants that cross the alveolar barrier into the blood stream and elicit systemic oxidative stress and inflammatory responses that can lead to an abnormal lipid profile and affect normal vascular functions. These changes predispose smokers to the development and progression of atherosclerosis (Fig. 18.19), leading to various types of CVDs, such as ischemic heart disease, cerebrovascular disease, peripheral artery disease, and aortic aneurysm (Ambrose and Barua, 2004).

This section summarizes the results of in vitro, in vivo, and clinical studies that, taken together, show the CVD risk reduction potential of switching from cigarette smoking to ENDP use.

As outlined in the section on lung cancer, ENDPs emit on average > 90% lower levels of HPHCs than cigarette smoke and extremely low levels of free radicals and cbNPs. This leads to a significant reduction in exposure to HPHCs, including those classified as cardiovascular toxicants by the FDA (Center for Tobacco Products, 2019), in human subjects who switch from cigarette smoking to ENDP use and across all experimental biological systems. This, in turn, leads to a reduction in the molecular changes and mechanistic perturbations linked to oxidative stress and inflammation across all biological systems, as outlined above. According to the CELSD, these reductions should also lead to a reduction in tissue damage and CVD manifestations, including atherosclerotic plaque growth.

Carbon monoxide (CO) is a key cardiovascular toxicant of cigarette smoke produced by the incomplete combustion of tobacco. In contrast to cigarettes, ENDPs emit no or only very low levels of CO (Chapter 4) because of the absence of combustion in these products (Cozzani et al., 2020). The binding of CO to hemoglobin leads to the formation of carboxyhemoglobin (COHb) and results in the reduced oxygen—binding capacity of hemoglobin and, hence, reduced oxygen transport to peripheral tissues. CO induced adverse effects on the cardiovascular system have been shown in a

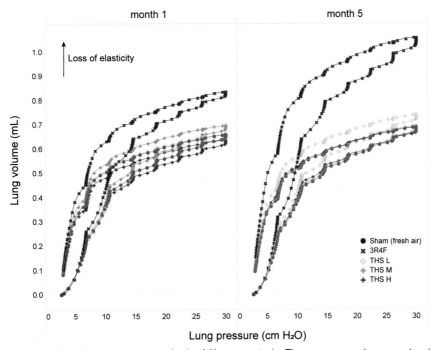

FIG. 18.18 Lung function measurements in the A/J mouse study. The pressure–volume graphs show the data for sham-exposed animals (blue), cigarette smoke–exposed animals (red), and animals exposed to three doses of THS aerosol (purple). Exposure conditions are described in the legend of Fig. 18.10. *H*, high; *L*, low; *M*, medium; *Ppl (H₂O)*, pressure in cm H₂O; *THS*, tobacco heating system; *Vpl (mL)*, lung volume in mL at a given pressure. 3R4F reference cigarette. (Adapted from Wong, E., Luettich, K., Krishnan, S., Wong, S.K., Lim, S.K., Yeo, D., Büttner, A., Leroy, P., Vuillaume, G., Boué, S., Hoeng, J., Vanscheeuwijck, P., Peitsch, M.C., 2020. Reduced chronic toxicity and carcinogenicity in A/J mice in response to life-time exposure to aerosol from a heated tobacco product compared with cigarette smoke. Toxicol. Sci. (in press).)

series of controlled human exposure studies in individuals with CVD. Moreover, the results of studies on chronic environmental exposure to CO are consistent with those of the controlled human exposure studies, showing a positive association between ambient CO exposure and hospital admissions for CVDs, including ischemic heart disease and congestive heart failure (Bell et al., 2009; Silkoff et al., 2006). Furthermore, acute elevation of blood COHb level impairs exercise performance and aggravates symptoms in patients with ischemic heart disease (Adams et al., 1988; Allred et al., 1989). Cigarette smoking is known to elevate both respiratory and blood CO levels, and the levels of COHb correlate with CVD risk in nonsmokers and smokers (Hedblad et al., 2006, 2005). In contrast, switching from cigarette smoking to ENDP use leads to a marked reduction in CO exposure, as evidenced by the exhaled CO (Adriaens et al., 2018; Beatrice and Massaro, 2019; Caponnetto et al., 2018) and blood COHb measurements in clinical studies (Beatrice and

Massaro, 2019) (Chapter 17). It is, therefore, highly likely that completely switching from cigarette smoking to ENDPs will reduce the risk of the acute effects linked to CO in cigarette smoke.

To complete the assessment of the CVD risk reduction potential of ENDPs, we now address the following important questions across in vitro and in vivo nonclinical as well as clinical studies:

- Does switching from cigarette smoking to ENDP use reduce oxidative stress and inflammation?
- Does switching from cigarette smoking to ENDP use reduce endothelial dysfunction?
- Does switching from cigarette smoking to ENDP use improve the proatherogenic lipid profile?
- Consequently, does switching from cigarette smoking to ENDP use reduce the progression of atherosclerotic plaque?

A positive answer to these questions would indicate that switching completely from cigarette smoking to ENDP use will likely reduce the risk of CVD.

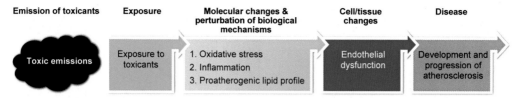

FIG. 18.19 The causal chain of events linking smoking to cardiovascular disease. (Adapted from Ambrose, J.A., Barua, R.S., 2004. The pathophysiology of cigarette smoking and cardiovascular disease: an update. J. Am. Coll. Cardiol. 43, 1731–1737. https://doi.org/10.1016/j.jacc.2003.12.047.)

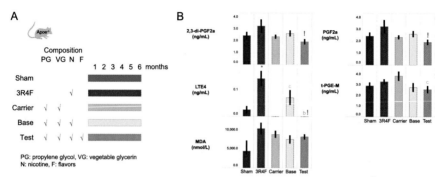

FIG. 18.20 **Urinary biomarkers of oxidative stress and inflammation in Apoe$^{-/-}$ mice exposed to cigarette smoke and e-vapor aerosols.** **(A)** Study design. Exposure conditions: fresh air or 36 μg nicotine/L in the test atmosphere for 3 h/day, 5 days/week for up to 6 months, Carrier aerosol was matched on the basis of PG/VG levels. **(B)** Urinary biomarkers of oxidative stress and inflammation. *, $P < .05$ versus sham; !, $P < .05$ versus test; c, $P < .05$ versus carrier; b, $P < .05$ versus base (n = 8). *LTE4*, leukotriene E4; *MDA*, malondialdehyde; *PG*, propylene glycol; *PGF2a*, prostaglandin F2α; *3R4F*, reference cigarette; *t-PGE-M*, tetranor-prostaglandin E-M; *VG*, vegetable glycerin. (Adapted from Szostak, J., Wong, E.T., Titz, B., Lee, T., Wong, S.K., Low, T., Lee, K.M., Zhang, J., Kumar, A., Schlage, W.K., Guedj, E., Phillips, B., Leroy, P., Buettner, A., Xiang, Y., Martin, F., Sewer, A., Kuczaj, A., Ivanov, N.V., Luettich, K., Vanscheeuwijck, P., Peitsch, M.C., Hoeng, J., 2020b. A 6-month systems toxicology inhalation study in ApoE$^{-/-}$ mice demonstrates reduced cardiovascular effects of E-vapor aerosols compared to cigarette smoke. Am. J. Physiol. Heart Circ. Physiol. https://doi.org/10.1152/ajpheart.00613.2019.)

18.6.1 Does Switching From Cigarette Smoking to ENDP Use Reduce Oxidative Stress and Inflammation?

Cigarette smoke is known to affect endothelial function (Rahman and Laher, 2007; Winkelmann et al., 2009) and increase the adhesion of circulating monocytes to the endothelium, an early event in the development of atherosclerosis (Kalra et al., 1994). This phenomenon is driven by oxidative stress and vascular inflammation (Poussin et al., 2014, 2015).

Studies designed for comparing the effects of ENDP aerosols with those of cigarette smoke on systemic oxidative stress and vascular inflammation were conducted in in vitro, in vivo, and clinical settings.

In vitro studies have shown that exposure to ENDP aerosol causes significantly less oxidative stress and inflammation in endothelial cells than exposure to cigarette smoke (Anderson et al., 2016; Poussin et al., 2016; van der Toorn et al., 2015) (Chapter 13). In vivo

inhalation studies conducted in Apoe$^{-/-}$ mice showed that animals exposed to ENDP aerosols had significantly lower levels of urinary biomarkers of oxidative stress than mice exposed to cigarette smoke (Phillips et al., 2016; Szostak et al., 2020b) (Chapter 15). This is exemplified in Fig. 18.20 by the results of the study conducted with e-liquid aerosols (Szostak et al., 2020b).

Furthermore, switching from cigarette smoking to THS use for 3–6 months led to positive changes in both oxidative stress and inflammatory markers in human subjects (Haziza et al., 2019a; Lüdicke et al., 2018b, 2019). Importantly, these changes were more pronounced in THS users who switched completely than in those who used both THS and cigarettes (Lüdicke et al., 2019) (Chapter 17). These findings are also supported by the results of a study that compared the acute effects of cigarettes and ENDPs on oxidative stress, antioxidant reserves, and other cardiovascular endpoints (Biondi-Zoccai et al., 2019). This study aimed to investigate the acute effects of single use of THS, EVPs, and cigarettes in healthy smokers in a randomized, controlled, crossover trial in 20 smokers allocated to different cycles of THS, EVP, and cigarette use. All participants used all types of products, with an intercycle washout of 1 week. The endpoints were oxidative stress, antioxidant reserves, platelet activation, flow-mediated dilation (FMD), blood pressure (BP), and satisfaction scores. The study reported that single use of any product led to an adverse impact on oxidative stress, antioxidant reserves, platelet function, FMD, and BP. However, the ENDPs had less impact than cigarettes on soluble Nox2-derived peptide, 8-iso-prostaglandin F2α-III, and vitamin E levels, FMD, H_2O_2 breakdown activity, soluble CD40 ligand levels, and soluble P-selectin levels. ENDP use also had a lower effect on BP than cigarette smoking.

18.6.2 Does Switching from Cigarette Smoking to ENDP Use Reduce Endothelial Dysfunction?

18.6.2.1 Endothelial cells: molecular and cellular changes

Cigarette smoke is known to increase the adhesion of circulating monocytes to the endothelium, which is an early event in the development of atherosclerosis (Kalra et al., 1994). The effects of ENDP aerosol and cigarette smoke on endothelial cells can be compared in vitro by measuring the adhesion of monocytic cells to arterial endothelial cells. The key mechanism involved in this adhesion process is the increased expression of surface-bound adhesion molecules on endothelial cells, induced by the TNFα secreted by the cigarette smoke−exposed monocytic cells (Poussin et al., 2014, 2015). In such previous studies conducted with human cells, the aerosol of THS caused significantly less monocyte adhesion to endothelial cells than cigarette smoke (Poussin et al., 2016, 2020). Similarly, the aerosol of THS had a significantly lower effect on transendothelial monocyte migration than cigarette smoke (van der Toorn et al., 2015). Furthermore, in a model of wound healing, endothelial cell migration was significantly less affected by an ENDP aerosol than by cigarette smoke (Taylor et al., 2017), which also indicates that ENDP aerosols have a lower impact on endothelial cells than cigarette smoke. In human subjects, switching from cigarette smoking to THS use for 3−6 months led to positive changes in circulating soluble intercellular adhesion molecule-1 levels, a marker of vascular inflammation (Haziza et al., 2019b; Lüdicke et al.,

2018b, 2019). Importantly, these changes were more pronounced in THS users who switched completely than in those who used both THS and cigarettes (Lüdicke et al., 2019) (Chapter 17).

18.6.2.2 Endothelium: physiological changes

Chronic smoking causes alterations in vasomotor function, or endothelial dysfunction (ED), which are the earliest detectable changes in vascular physiology and health associated with atherosclerosis (Rahman and Laher, 2007). ED has consistently been shown to be associated with cardiovascular risk and long-term outcomes (Inaba et al., 2010; Ras et al., 2013; Willum-Hansen et al., 2006). Several epidemiological studies, including ones in healthy subjects, hypertensive subjects, and diabetic and renal disease patients, have documented that smokers have a lower FMD and higher BP than non-smokers (Barbato et al., 2019; Celermajer et al., 1993; Miyata et al., 2015; Orth, 2004; Rodriguez-Portelles and Rodriguez-Leyva, 2019; Sultana et al., 2019). While smoking has been shown to also affect pulse wave velocity (PWV) in a number of relatively small and/or acute studies (Mahmud and Feely, 2003; Schmidt et al., 2019), this effect could not be confirmed in large-cohort studies that lasted 3 years (Schmidt et al., 2019).

A recent clinical study showed that switching from cigarette smoking to EVP use improved FMD after 1 month and that subjects who complied best with switching to EVPs demonstrated the greatest improvement (George et al., 2019). There was also a reduction in systolic BP among smokers who switched to EVPs, with the most significant reduction being among those who switched to nicotine-free EVPs (George et al., 2019). Furthermore, smokers who smoked ≤20 pack-years and switched to EVPs displayed an improvement in PWV (vascular stiffness) after 1 month, whereas those smoking >20 pack-years did not (George et al., 2019). This finding is interesting, as changes in PWV did not seem to correlate well with long-term smoking status in the above-mentioned large-cohort study (Schmidt et al., 2019); rather, they reflect the acute effects of cigarette smoking, ENDP use, and nicotine exposure (Adamopoulos et al., 2009; Mahmud and Feely, 2003; Vlachopoulos et al., 2004). In a recent in vivo study, we showed that cigarette smoke exposure significantly increased ($P < .05$) pulse propagation velocity (PPV) in the abdominal aorta and PWV in the carotid artery in Apoe$^{-/-}$ mice exposed to cigarette smoke (Szostak et al., 2020b). We also showed that the PPV and PWV changes were significantly smaller in mice exposed to EVP aerosols than in those exposed to cigarette smoke

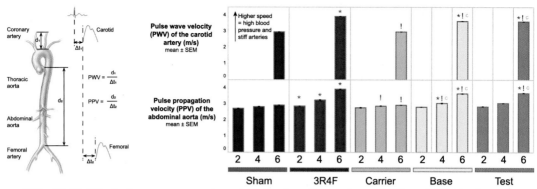

FIG. 18.21 Effect of e-vapor aerosols and 3R4F cigarette smoke on PWV and PPV in Apoe$^{-/-}$ mice. Left panel. Schematic representation of PWV and PPV acquisition area. Right panel. Carotid artery PWV at 6 months (n = 10−12) and abdominal aorta PPV at 2, 4, and 6 months (n = 8−12) of exposure. The study design and exposure conditions are described in Fig. 18.20. *, $P < .05$ versus sham; !, $P < .05$ versus test; c, $P < .05$ versus carrier; b, $P < .05$ versus base. *3R4F*, 3R4F cigarette; *PPV*, pulse propagation velocity; *PWV*, pulse wave velocity; *SEM*, standard error of the mean. (Adapted from Szostak, J., Wong, E.T., Titz, B., Lee, T., Wong, S.K., Low, T., Lee, K.M., Zhang, J., Kumar, A., Schlage, W.K., Guedj, E., Phillips, B., Leroy, P., Buettner, A., Xiang, Y., Martin, F., Sewer, A., Kuczaj, A., Ivanov, N.V., Luettich, K., Vanscheeuwijck, P., Peitsch, M.C., Hoeng, J., 2020b. A 6-month systems toxicology inhalation study in ApoE$^{-/-}$ mice demonstrates reduced cardiovascular effects of E-vapor aerosols compared to cigarette smoke. Am. J. Physiol. Heart Circ. Physiol. https://doi.org/10.1152/ajpheart.00613.2019.)

(Fig. 18.21). These in vivo observations might be more reflective of the known acute effects of cigarette smoking and nicotine on PWV than the long-term effects of cigarette smoking and ENDP use.

18.6.3 Does Switching From Cigarette Smoking to ENDP Use Improve Proatherogenic Lipid Profile?

The results of human clinical studies showed an increase in high-density lipoprotein cholesterol levels following switching from cigarette smoking to THS use for 3−6 months (Haziza et al., 2019b; Lüdicke et al., 2018b, 2019) (Chapter 17). This improvement in plasma lipoprotein profile among the study participants who switched to THS use was furthermore supported by an increase in Apolipoprotein A1 concentration and a slight decrease in both Apolipoprotein B and low-density lipoprotein cholesterol levels in these subjects. Preclinical studies demonstrated that cigarette smoke exposure for 3−6 months caused a significant increase in total cholesterol (28% and 8%), chylomicron cholesterol (87% and 29%), and very low-density lipoprotein cholesterol (41% and 11%), respectively (Szostak et al., 2020b) (Chapter 15). In contrast, EVP aerosol−exposed animals showed lipid levels similar or slightly lower than those in sham-exposed animals (Szostak et al., 2020a, b).

18.6.4 Does Switching From Cigarette Smoking to ENDP Use Reduce the Progression of Atherosclerotic Plaque?

As outlined earlier, Apoe$^{-/-}$ mice are commonly used as a model for atherogenesis (Veniant et al., 2001) and have been valuable tools for investigating smoking-related atherosclerosis (Boue et al., 2012; Lietz et al., 2013; Lo Sasso et al., 2016a). In this mouse model, cigarette smoke exposure consistently accelerated the development of atherosclerotic plaque in previous studies. In contrast, ENDP aerosols did not cause an increase in plaque growth above that observed with air exposure (Figs. 18.22 and 18.23) (Phillips et al., 2016, 2019a, b; Szostak et al., 2020b) (Chapter 15). Furthermore, mice first exposed to cigarette smoke and then switched to either air or the aerosol of THS displayed a similar reduction in plaque growth rate (Phillips et al., 2016) (Fig. 18.22). These results are causally consistent with the observation that the mechanism involved in monocyte−endothelial cell interaction, a key early event in the development of atherosclerosis (Kalra et al., 1994), was significantly less affected by THS aerosol than cigarette smoke (Phillips et al., 2016) (Fig. 18.24). These observations made in an animal model are also consistent with the results of the previously described in vitro study which showed

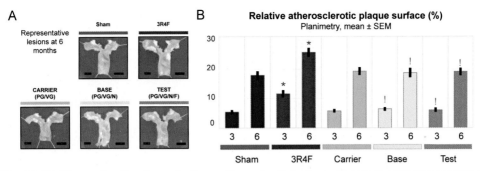

FIG. 18.22 Atherosclerotic plaque in the aortic arch—Data from microcomputed tomography at month 7. **(A)** Representative images of atherosclerotic lesions in the aortic arch, with measurements acquired by planimetry at 6 months postexposure. **(B)** Relative atherosclerotic plaque surface area in the aortic arch, evaluated by planimetry (n = 19–20). The study design and exposure conditions are described in Fig. 18.20. *, $P < .05$ versus sham; !, $P < .05$ significant versus the test group. F, flavor mix; N, nicotine; PG, propylene glycol; 3R4F, 3R4F cigarette smoke; SEM, standard error of the mean; VG, vegetable glycerin. (Adapted from Szostak, J., Wong, E.T., Titz, B., Lee, T., Wong, S.K., Low, T., Lee, K.M., Zhang, J., Kumar, A., Schlage, W.K., Guedj, E., Phillips, B., Leroy, P., Buettner, A., Xiang, Y., Martin, F., Sewer, A., Kuczaj, A., Ivanov, N.V., Luettich, K., Vanscheeuwijck, P., Peitsch, M.C., Hoeng, J., 2020b. A 6-month systems toxicology inhalation study in ApoE$^{-/-}$ mice demonstrates reduced cardiovascular effects of E-vapor aerosols compared to cigarette smoke. Am. J. Physiol. Heart Circ. Physiol. https://doi.org/10.1152/ajpheart.00613.2019.)

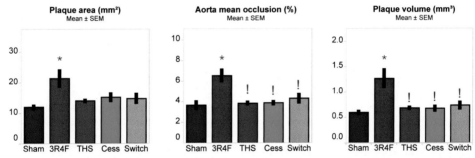

FIG. 18.23 Atherosclerotic plaque in the aortic arch—Data from microcomputed tomography at month 7. *, $P < .05$ versus sham; !, $P < .05$ versus 3R4F. Study design and exposure conditions are described in Fig. 18.8. Cess, cessation; 3R4F, 3R4F cigarette; THS, tobacco heating system. (Adapted from Phillips, B., Veljkovic, E., Boué, S., Schlage, W.K., Vuillaume, G., Martin, F., Titz, B., Leroy, P., Buettner, A., Elamin, A., Oviedo, A., Cabanski, M., De León, H., Guedj, E., Schneider, T., Talikka, M., Ivanov, N.V., Vanscheeuwijck, P., Peitsch, M.C., Hoeng, J., 2016. An 8-month systems toxicology inhalation/cessation study in Apoe$^{-/-}$ mice to investigate cardiovascular and respiratory exposure effects of a candidate modified risk tobacco product, THS 2.2, compared with conventional cigarettes. Toxicol. Sci. 149, 411–432. https://doi.org/10.1093/toxsci/kfv243.)

that, relative to cigarette smoke, THS aerosol had a significantly reduced effect on human monocyte adhesion to endothelial cells (Poussin et al., 2016) (Chapter 13).

18.6.5 Summary and Conclusions for CVD

In summary, the results of available comparative in vitro, in vivo, and clinical studies showed with remarkable consistency that, relative to cigarette smoke, ENDP aerosols had a significantly reduced effect on

endpoints relevant to CVD. Furthermore, an in vivo study showed that switching from cigarette smoke to ENDP aerosol exposure led to a reduction in CVD-related endpoints similar to the reduction induced by switching to air exposure. Finally, clinical studies showed that switching completely from cigarette smoking to ENDP use led to positive changes in the BoPHs associated with CVD. This is because ENDPs emit on average over 90% lower levels of toxicants than cigarettes, which leads to a coherent reduction in toxicant

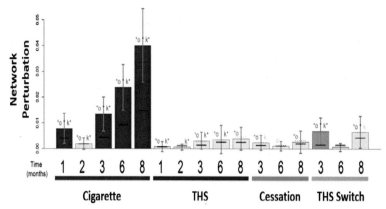

FIG. 18.24 Perturbation of the monocyte–endothelial cell interaction network, determined on the basis of expression of genes involved in promoting the adhesion of monocytes to endothelial cells. Study design and exposure conditions are described in Fig. 18.8. *Gray bars* indicate nonsignificant network perturbations, as described in Martin et al. (2014). *SEM*, standard error of the mean; *THS*, tobacco heating system.

exposure. Therefore, switching completely from cigarette smoking to ENDP use is likely to reduce the risk of CVD.

18.7 OVERALL CONCLUSIONS

The integrated review of the available study results presented above provides a solid scientific basis to conclude that ENDPs, which avoid the combustion of tobacco, are valuable tools in the efforts to reduce the harm caused by cigarette smoking and have the potential to reduce the risk of smoking-related diseases if used instead of cigarettes. These studies, which rely on the fundamental principles of toxicology and epidemiology outlined in Chapter 3, do not, however, provide hard clinical outcomes from long-term ENDP users at the population level. As stated at the beginning of this chapter, today's evaluation of ENDPs can only rely on the mechanistic basis of smoking-related diseases as enunciated by the CELSD (Chapter 3). Although these approaches are highly predictive for the overall harm reduction potential of ENDPs, definitive quantification of residual risk will have to come from long-term and large randomized clinical studies aimed at measuring hard clinical endpoints. Furthermore, long-term epidemiological data will be needed to understand the effect of ENDPs on smoking-related morbidity and mortality at the population level.

REFERENCES

Abbas, T., Keaton, M.A., Dutta, A., 2013. Genomic instability in cancer. Cold Spring Harb. Perspect. Biol. 5, a012914. https://doi.org/10.1101/cshperspect.a012914.

Adamopoulos, D., Argacha, J.-F., Gujic, M., Preumont, N., Degaute, J.-P., van de Borne, P., 2009. Acute effects of nicotine on arterial stiffness and wave reflection in healthy young non-smokers. Clin. Exp. Pharmacol. Physiol. 36, 784–789. https://doi.org/10.1111/j.1440-1681.2009.05141.x.

Adams, K.F., Koch, G., Chatterjee, B., Goldstein, G.M., O'Neil, J.J., Bromberg, P.A., Sheps, D.S., 1988. Acute elevation of blood carboxyhemoglobin to 6% impairs exercise performance and aggravates symptoms in patients with ischemic heart disease. J. Am. Coll. Cardiol. 12, 900–909. https://doi.org/10.1016/0735-1097(88)90452-4.

Adriaens, K., Gucht, D.V., Baeyens, F., 2018. IQOSTM vs. e-cigarette vs. Tobacco cigarette: a direct comparison of short-term effects after overnight-abstinence. Int. J. Environ. Res. Publ. Health 15. https://doi.org/10.3390/ijerph15122902.

Allred, E.N., Bleecker, E.R., Chaitman, B.R., Dahms, T.E., Gottlieb, S.O., Hackney, J.D., Pagano, M., Selvester, R.H., Walden, S.M., Warren, J., 1989. Short-term effects of carbon monoxide exposure on the exercise performance of subjects with coronary artery disease. N. Engl. J. Med. 321, 1426–1432. https://doi.org/10.1056/NEJM198911233212102.

Ambrose, J.A., Barua, R.S., 2004. The pathophysiology of cigarette smoking and cardiovascular disease: an update. J. Am. Coll. Cardiol. 43, 1731–1737. https://doi.org/10.1016/j.jacc.2003.12.047.

Anderson, C., Majeste, A., Hanus, J., Wang, S., 2016. E-cigarette aerosol exposure induces reactive oxygen species, DNA damage, and cell death in vascular endothelial cells. Toxicol. Sci. 154, 332–340. https://doi.org/10.1093/toxsci/kfw166.

Apte, R.N., Krelin, Y., Song, X., Dotan, S., Recih, E., Elkabets, M., Carmi, Y., Dvorkin, T., White, R.M., Gayvoronsky, L., Segal, S., Voronov, E., 2006. Effects of micro-environment- and malignant cell-derived interleukin-1 in carcinogenesis, tumour invasiveness and tumour-host interactions. Eur. J. Cancer 42, 751–759. https://doi.org/10.1016/j.ejca.2006.01.010.

Arunachalam, G., Sundar, I.K., Hwang, J.-W., Yao, H., Rahman, I., 2010. Emphysema is associated with increased inflammation in lungs of atherosclerosis-prone mice by cigarette smoke: implications in comorbidities of COPD. J. Inflamm. 7, 34. https://doi.org/10.1186/1476-9255-7-34.

Ashley, D.L., Burns, D., Djordjevic, M., Dybing, E., Gray, N., Hammond, S.K., Henningfield, J., Jarvis, M., Reddy, K.S., Robertson, C., Zaatari, G., Regulation, W.H.O.S.G. on T.P., 2008. The scientific basis of tobacco product regulation. World Health Organ. Tech. Rep. Ser. 1–277, 1 p following 277.

Ather, J.L., Martin, R.A., Ckless, K., Poynter, M.E., 2014. Inflammasome activity in non-microbial lung inflammation. J. Environ. Immunol. Toxicol. 1, 108–117.

Awji, E.G., Seagrave, J.C., Tesfaigzi, Y., 2015. Correlation of cigarette smoke-induced pulmonary inflammation and emphysema in C3H and C57Bl/6 mice. Toxicol. Sci. 147, 75–83. https://doi.org/10.1093/toxsci/kfv108.

Baby, M.K., Muthu, P.K., Johnson, P., Kannan, S., 2014. Effect of cigarette smoking on nasal mucociliary clearance: A comparative analysis using saccharin test. Lung India 31 (1), 39–42. https://doi.org/10.4103/0970-2113.125894.

Balkwill, F., Mantovani, A., 2001. Inflammation and cancer: back to Virchow? Lancet 357, 539–545. https://doi.org/10.1016/S0140-6736(00)04046-0.

Barbato, A., D'Elia, L., Perna, L., Molisso, A., Iacone, R., Strazzullo, P., Galletti, F., 2019. Increased microalbuminuria risk in male cigarette smokers: results from the "Olivetti Heart Study" after 8 years follow-up. Kidney Blood Press. Res. 44, 33–42. https://doi.org/10.1159/000498830.

Barnes, P.J., 2004. Mediators of chronic obstructive pulmonary disease. Pharmacol. Rev. 56, 515–548. https://doi.org/10.1124/pr.56.4.2.

Beane, J., Sebastiani, P., Liu, G., Brody, J.S., Lenburg, M.E., Spira, A., 2007. Reversible and permanent effects of tobacco smoke exposure on airway epithelial gene expression. Genome Biol. 8, R201. https://doi.org/10.1186/gb-2007-8-9-r201.

Beatrice, F., Massaro, G., 2019. Exhaled carbon monoxide levels in forty resistant to cessation male smokers after six months of full switch to electronic cigarettes (e-Cigs) or to A tobacco heating systems (THS). Int. J. Environ. Res. Publ. Health 16. https://doi.org/10.3390/ijerph16203916.

Beineke, P., Fitch, K., Tao, H., Elashoff, M.R., Rosenberg, S., Kraus, W.E., Wingrove, J.A., 2012. A whole blood gene expression-based signature for smoking status. BMC Med. Genom. 5, 58.

Bekki, K., Inaba, Y., Uchiyama, S., Kunugita, N., 2017. Comparison of chemicals in mainstream smoke in heat-not-burn tobacco and combustion cigarettes. J. UOEH 39, 201–207.

Belcastro, V., Poussin, C., Xiang, Y., Giordano, M., Tripathi, K.P., Boda, A., Boué, S., Guarracino, M., Martin, F., Peitsch, M.C., Hoeng, J., Romero, R., Tarca, A.L., Duan, Z., Yang, H., Gong, X., Wang, P., Zhang, C., Yang, W., Sarac, O.S., Bilgen, I., Balci, A.T., Kumar, R., Dhanda, S.K., 2018. The sbv IMPROVER systems toxicology computational challenge: identification of

human and species-independent blood response markers as predictors of smoking exposure and cessation status. Comput. Toxicol. 5, 38–51. https://doi.org/10.1016/j.comtox.2017.07.004.

Bell, M.L., Peng, R.D., Dominici, F., Samet, J.M., 2009. Emergency hospital admissions for cardiovascular diseases and ambient levels of carbon monoxide: results for 126 United States urban counties, 1999–2005. Circulation 120, 949–955. https://doi.org/10.1161/CIRCULATIONAHA.109.851113.

Belushkin, M., Tafin Djoko, D., Esposito, M., Korneliou, A., Jeannet, C., Lazzerini, M., Jaccard, G., 2020. Selected harmful and potentially harmful constituents levels in commercial e-cigarettes. Chem. Res. Toxicol. 33, 657–668. https://doi.org/10.1021/acs.chemrestox.9b00470.

Benowitz, N.L., 2010. Nicotine addiction. N. Engl. J. Med. 362, 2295–2303.

Biondi-Zoccai, G., Sciarretta, S., Bullen, C., Nocella, C., Violi, F., Loffredo, L., Pignatelli, P., Perri, L., Peruzzi, M., Marullo, A.G.M., De Falco, E., Chimenti, I., Cammisotto, V., Valenti, V., Coluzzi, F., Cavarretta, E., Carrizzo, A., Prati, F., Carnevale, R., Frati, G., 2019. Acute effects of heat-not-burn, electronic vaping, and traditional tobacco combustion cigarettes: the Sapienza University of Rome-vascular assessment of proatherosclerotic effects of smoking (SUR-VAPES) 2 randomized trial. J. Am. Heart Assoc. 8, e010455. https://doi.org/10.1161/JAHA.118.010455.

Bitzer, Z.T., Goel, R., Trushin, N., Muscat, J., Richie, J.P., 2020. Free radical production and characterization of heat-not-burn cigarettes in comparison to conventional and electronic cigarettes. Chem. Res. Toxicol. https://doi.org/10.1021/acs.chemrestox.0c00088.

Boue, S., Tarasov, K., Janis, M., Lebrun, S., Hurme, R., Schlage, W., Lietz, M., Vuillaume, G., Ekroos, K., Steffen, Y., Peitsch, M.C., Laaksonen, R., Hoeng, J., 2012. Modulation of atherogenic lipidome by cigarette smoke in apolipoprotein E-deficient mice. Atherosclerosis 225, 328–334. https://doi.org/10.1016/j.atherosclerosis.2012.09.032.

Boue, S., De Leon, H., Schlage, W.K., Peck, M.J., Weiler, H., Berges, A., Vuillaume, G., Martin, F., Friedrichs, B., Lebrun, S., Meurrens, K., Schracke, N., Moehring, M., Steffen, Y., Schueller, J., Vanscheeuwijck, P., Peitsch, M.C., Hoeng, J., 2013. Cigarette smoke induces molecular responses in respiratory tissues of ApoE(-/-) mice that are progressively deactivated upon cessation. Toxicology 314, 112–124. https://doi.org/10.1016/j.tox.2013.09.013.

Braakhuis, H.M., Park, M.V.D.Z., Gosens, I., De Jong, W.H., Cassee, F.R., 2014. Physicochemical characteristics of nanomaterials that affect pulmonary inflammation. Part. Fibre Toxicol. 11, 18. https://doi.org/10.1186/1743-8977-11-18.

Breheny, D., Oke, O., Pant, K., Gaça, M., 2017. Comparative tumor promotion assessment of e-cigarette and cigarettes using the in vitro Bhas 42 cell transformation assay. Environ. Mol. Mutagen. 58, 190–198. https://doi.org/10.1002/em.22091.

Breheny, D., Adamson, J., Azzopardi, D., Baxter, A., Bishop, E., Carr, T., Crooks, I., Hewitt, K., Jaunky, T., Larard, S., Lowe, F., Oke, O., Taylor, S., Santopietro, S., Thorne, D., Zainuddin, M., Gaça, M.D., Liu, C., Murphy, J., Proctor, C.J., 2019. In Vitro Toxicological and Biological

Responses of Aerosols from a Novel Hybrid Tobacco Product as Compared with Two Tobacco Heating Products and a Reference Cigarette [WWW Document]. https://doi.org/10.26126/intervals.6t2ejz.1.

Brusselle, G.G., Bracke, K.R., Maes, T., D'hulst, A.I., Moerloose, K.B., Joos, G.F., Pauwels, R.A., 2006. Murine models of COPD. Pulm. Pharmacol. Therapeut. 19, 155–165. https://doi.org/10.1016/j.pupt.2005.06.001.

Caponnetto, P., Maglia, M., Prosperini, G., Busà, B., Polosa, R., 2018. Carbon monoxide levels after inhalation from new generation heated tobacco products. Respir. Res. 19, 164. https://doi.org/10.1186/s12931-018-0867-z.

Carter, B.D., Abnet, C.C., Feskanich, D., Freedman, N.D., Hartge, P., Lewis, C.E., Ockene, J.K., Prentice, R.L., Speizer, F.E., Thun, M.J., Jacobs, E.J., 2015. Smoking and mortality–beyond established causes. N. Engl. J. Med. 372, 631–640. https://doi.org/10.1056/NEJMsa1407211.

Celermajer, D.S., Sorensen, K.E., Georgakopoulos, D., Bull, C., Thomas, O., Robinson, J., Deanfield, J.E., 1993. Cigarette smoking is associated with dose-related and potentially reversible impairment of endothelium-dependent dilation in healthy young adults. Circulation 88, 2149–2155. https://doi.org/10.1161/01.cir.88.5.2149.

Center for Tobacco Products, 2019. Harmful and Potentially Harmful Constituents in Tobacco Products and Tobacco Smoke: Established List. [WWW Document]. FDA. Accessed 2.14.20. http://www.fda.gov/tobacco-products/rules-regulations-and-gu idance/harmful-and-potentially-harmful-constituents-tobacco-products-and-tobacco-smoke-established-list.

Choi, S., Chang, J., Kim, K., Park, S.M., Lee, K., 2018. Effect of smoking cessation and reduction on the risk of cancer in Korean men: a population based study. Cancer Res. Treat. 50, 1114–1120. https://doi.org/10.4143/crt.2017.326.

Church, T.R., Anderson, K.E., Caporaso, N.E., Geisser, M.S., Le, C.T., Zhang, Y., Benoit, A.R., Carmella, S.G., Hecht, S.S., 2009. A prospectively measured serum biomarker for a tobacco-specific carcinogen and lung cancer in smokers. Cancer Epidemiol. Biomarkers Prev. 18, 260–266. https://doi.org/10.1158/1055-9965.EPI-08-0718.

Churg, A., Tai, H., Coulthard, T., Wang, R., Wright, J.L., 2006. Cigarette smoke drives small airway remodeling by induction of growth factors in the airway wall. Am. J. Respir. Crit. Care Med. 174, 1327–1334. https://doi.org/10.1164/rccm.200605-585OC.

Churg, A., Cosio, M., Wright, J.L., 2008. Mechanisms of cigarette smoke-induced COPD: insights from animal models. Am. J. Physiol. Lung Cell Mol. Physiol. 294, L612–L631. https://doi.org/10.1152/ajplung.00390.2007.

Churg, A., Zhou, S., Wang, X., Wang, R., Wright, J.L., 2009. The role of interleukin-1beta in murine cigarette smoke-induced emphysema and small airway remodeling. Am. J. Respir. Cell Mol. Biol. 40, 482–490. https://doi.org/10.1165/rcmb.2008-0038OC.

Churg, A., Sin, D.D., Wright, J.L., 2011. Everything prevents emphysema: are animal models of cigarette smoke-induced chronic obstructive pulmonary disease any use?

Am. J. Respir. Cell Mol. Biol. 45, 1111–1115. https://doi.org/10.1165/rcmb.2011-0087PS.

Cibella, F., Campagna, D., Caponnetto, P., Amaradio, M.D., Caruso, M., Russo, C., Cockcroft, D.W., Polosa, R., 2016. Lung function and respiratory symptoms in a randomized smoking cessation trial of electronic cigarettes. Clin. Sci. 130, 1929–1937. https://doi.org/10.1042/CS20160268.

Coussens, L.M., Werb, Z., 2002. Inflammation and cancer. Nature 420, 860–867. https://doi.org/10.1038/nature01322.

Cozzani, V., Barontini, F., McGrath, T., Mahler, B., Nordlund, M., Smith, M., Schaller, J.P., Zuber, G., 2020. An experimental investigation into the operation of an electrically heated tobacco system. Thermochim. Acta 684, 178475. https://doi.org/10.1016/j.tca.2019.178475.

Csordas, A., Bernhard, D., 2013. The biology behind the atherothrombotic effects of cigarette smoke. Nat. Rev. Cardiol. 10, 219–230. https://doi.org/10.1038/nrcardio.2013.8.

Dalrymple, A., Badrock, T.C., Terry, A., Barber, M., Hall, P.J., Thorne, D., Gaca, M.D., Coburn, S., Proctor, C., 2018. Assessment of enamel discoloration in vitro following exposure to cigarette smoke and emissions from novel vapor and tobacco heating products. Am. J. Dent. 31, 227–233.

de-Torres, J.P., Wilson, D.O., Sanchez-Salcedo, P., Weissfeld, J.L., Berto, J., Campo, A., Alcaide, A.B., García-Granero, M., Celli, B.R., Zulueta, J.J., 2015. Lung cancer in patients with chronic obstructive pulmonary disease. Development and validation of the COPD Lung Cancer Screening Score. Am. J. Respir. Crit. Care Med. 191, 285–291. https://doi.org/10.1164/rccm.201407-1210OC.

Doll, R., Peto, R., 1978. Cigarette smoking and bronchial carcinoma: dose and time relationships among regular smokers and lifelong non-smokers. J. Epidemiol. Community Health 32, 303–313. https://doi.org/10.1136/jech.32.4.303.

Dostert, C., Pétrilli, V., Van Bruggen, R., Steele, C., Mossman, B.T., Tschopp, J., 2008. Innate immune activation through Nalp3 inflammasome sensing of asbestos and silica. Science 320, 674–677. https://doi.org/10.1126/science.1156995.

Durham, A.L., Adcock, I.M., 2015. The relationship between COPD and lung cancer. Lung Cancer 90, 121–127. https://doi.org/10.1016/j.lungcan.2015.08.017.

Eltom, S., Belvisi, M.G., Stevenson, C.S., Maher, S.A., Dubuis, E., Fitzgerald, K.A., Birrell, M.A., 2014. Role of the inflammasome-caspase1/11-IL-1/18 axis in cigarette smoke driven airway inflammation: an insight into the pathogenesis of COPD. PLoS One 9, e112829. https://doi.org/10.1371/journal.pone.0112829.

Fariss, M.W., Gilmour, M.I., Reilly, C.A., Liedtke, W., Ghio, A.J., 2013. Emerging mechanistic targets in lung injury induced by combustion-generated particles. Toxicol. Sci. 132, 253–267. https://doi.org/10.1093/toxsci/kft001.

Farsalinos, K.E., Le Houezec, J., 2015. Regulation in the face of uncertainty: the evidence on electronic nicotine delivery systems (e-cigarettes). Risk Manag. Healthc. Policy 8, 157.

Farsalinos, K.E., Yannovits, N., Sarri, T., Voudris, V., Poulas, K., Leischow, S.J., 2018. Carbonyl emissions from a novel heated tobacco product (IQOS): comparison with an e-cigarette and a tobacco cigarette. Addiction 113, 2099−2106. https://doi.org/10.1111/add.14365.

Faux, S.P., Tai, T., Thorne, D., Xu, Y., Breheny, D., Gaca, M., 2009. The role of oxidative stress in the biological responses of lung epithelial cells to cigarette smoke. Biomarkers 14 (Suppl. 1), 90−96. https://doi.org/10.1080/13547500902965047.

Flanders, W.D., Lally, C.A., Zhu, B.-P., Henley, S.J., Thun, M.J., 2003. Lung cancer mortality in relation to age, duration of smoking, and daily cigarette consumption: results from Cancer Prevention Study II. Cancer Res. 63, 6556−6562.

Forster, M., Fiebelkorn, S., Yurteri, C., Mariner, D., Liu, C., Wright, C., McAdam, K., Murphy, J., Proctor, C., 2018. Assessment of novel tobacco heating product THP1.0. Part 3: comprehensive chemical characterisation of harmful and potentially harmful aerosol emissions. Regul. Toxicol. Pharmacol. 93, 14−33. https://doi.org/10.1016/j.yrtph.2017.10.006.

Fry, J.S., Lee, P.N., Forey, B.A., Coombs, K.J., 2013. How rapidly does the excess risk of lung cancer decline following quitting smoking? A quantitative review using the negative exponential model. Regul. Toxicol. Pharmacol. 67, 13−26. https://doi.org/10.1016/j.yrtph.2013.06.001.

Gale, N., McEwan, M., Eldridge, A.C., Fearon, I.M., Sherwood, N., Bowen, E., McDermott, S., Holmes, E., Hedge, A., Hossack, S., Wakenshaw, L., Glew, J., Camacho, O.M., Errington, G., McAughey, J., Murphy, J., Liu, C., Proctor, C.J., 2019. Changes in biomarkers of exposure on switching from a conventional cigarette to tobacco heating products: a randomized, controlled study in healthy Japanese subjects. Nicotine Tob. Res. 21, 1220−1227. https://doi.org/10.1093/ntr/nty104.

Gasse, P., Mary, C., Guenon, I., Noulin, N., Charron, S., Schnyder-Candrian, S., Schnyder, B., Akira, S., Quesniaux, V.F.J., Lagente, V., Ryffel, B., Couillin, I., 2007. IL-1R1/MyD88 signaling and the inflammasome are essential in pulmonary inflammation and fibrosis in mice. J. Clin. Invest. 117, 3786−3799. https://doi.org/10.1172/JCI32285.

Geiss, O., Bianchi, I., Barrero-Moreno, J., 2016. Correlation of volatile carbonyl yields emitted by e-cigarettes with the temperature of the heating coil and the perceived sensorial quality of the generated vapours. Int. J. Hyg Environ. Health 219, 268−277. https://doi.org/10.1016/j.ijheh.2016.01.004.

Surgeon General, 2010. In: How Tobacco Smoke Causes Disease: The Biology and Behavioral Basis for Smoking-Attributable Disease: A Report of the Surgeon General. Publications and Reports of the Surgeon General, Atlanta (GA).

George, J., Hussain, M., Vadiveloo, T., Ireland, S., Hopkinson, P., Struthers, A.D., Donnan, P.T., Khan, F., Lang, C.C., 2019. Cardiovascular effects of switching from tobacco cigarettes to electronic cigarettes. J. Am. Coll. Cardiol. 74, 3112−3120. https://doi.org/10.1016/j.jacc.2019.09.067.

Gillman, I.G., Kistler, K.A., Stewart, E.W., Paolantonio, A.R., 2016. Effect of variable power levels on the yield of total aerosol mass and formation of aldehydes in e-cigarette

aerosols. Regul. Toxicol. Pharmacol. 75, 58−65. https://doi.org/10.1016/j.yrtph.2015.12.019.

Goniewicz, M.L., Knysak, J., Gawron, M., Kosmider, L., Sobczak, A., Kurek, J., Prokopowicz, A., Jablonska-Czapla, M., Rosik-Dulewska, C., Havel, C., Jacob 3rd, P., Benowitz, N., 2014. Levels of selected carcinogens and toxicants in vapour from electronic cigarettes. Tob. Control 23, 133−139. https://doi.org/10.1136/tobaccocontrol-2012-050859.

Goniewicz, M.L., Gawron, M., Smith, D.M., Peng, M., Jacob, P., Benowitz, N.L., 2017. Exposure to nicotine and selected toxicants in cigarette smokers who switched to electronic cigarettes: a longitudinal within-subjects observational study. Nicotine Tob. Res. 19, 160−167. https://doi.org/10.1093/ntr/ntw160.

Gonzalez-Suarez, I., Sewer, A., Walker, P., Mathis, C., Ellis, S., Woodhouse, H., Guedj, E., Dulize, R., Marescotti, D., Acali, S., Martin, F., Ivanov, N.V., Hoeng, J., Peitsch, M.C., 2014. Systems biology approach for evaluating the biological impact of environmental toxicants in vitro. Chem. Res. Toxicol. 27, 367−376. https://doi.org/10.1021/tx400405s.

Gonzalez-Suarez, I., Martin, F., Marescotti, D., Guedj, E., Acali, S., Johne, S., Dulize, R., Baumer, K., Peric, D., Goedertier, D., Frentzel, S., Ivanov, N.V., Mathis, C., Hoeng, J., Peitsch, M.C., 2016. In vitro systems toxicology assessment of a candidate modified risk tobacco product shows reduced toxicity compared to that of a conventional cigarette. Chem. Res. Toxicol. 29, 3−18. https://doi.org/10.1021/acs.chemrestox.5b00321.

Grivennikov, S.I., Greten, F.R., Karin, M., 2010. Immunity, inflammation, and cancer. Cell 140, 883−899. https://doi.org/10.1016/j.cell.2010.01.025.

Hanahan, D., Weinberg, R.A., 2011. Hallmarks of cancer: the next generation. Cell 144, 646−674. https://doi.org/10.1016/j.cell.2011.02.013.

Haswell, L.E., Baxter, A., Banerjee, A., Verrastro, I., Mushonganono, J., Adamson, J., Thorne, D., Gaça, M., Minet, E., 2017. Reduced biological effect of e-cigarette aerosol compared to cigarette smoke evaluated in vitro using normalized nicotine dose and RNA-seq-based toxicogenomics. Sci. Rep. 7, 888. https://doi.org/10.1038/s41598-017-00852-y.

Haswell, L.E., Corke, S., Verrastro, I., Baxter, A., Banerjee, A., Adamson, J., Jaunky, T., Proctor, C., Gaça, M., Minet, E., 2018. In vitro RNA-seq-based toxicogenomics assessment shows reduced biological effect of tobacco heating products when compared to cigarette smoke. Sci. Rep. 8, 1145. https://doi.org/10.1038/s41598-018-19627-0.

Haziza, C., de La Bourdonnaye, G., Skiada, D., Ancerewicz, J., Baker, G., Picavet, P., Lüdicke, F., 2016. Evaluation of the Tobacco Heating System 2.2. Part 8: 5-Day randomized reduced exposure clinical study in Poland. Regul. Toxicol. Pharmacol. 81 (Suppl. 2), S139−S150. https://doi.org/10.1016/j.yrtph.2016.11.003.

Haziza, C., de La Bourdonnaye, G., Donelli, A., Poux, V., Skiada, D., Weitkunat, R., Baker, G., Picavet, P., Lüdicke, F., 2019a. Reduction in exposure to selected harmful and potentially harmful constituents approaching those observed upon smoking abstinence in smokers switching to the menthol tobacco heating system 2.2 for three months (Part 1). Nicotine Tob. Res. https://doi.org/10.1093/ntr/ntz013.

Haziza, C., de La Bourdonnaye, G., Donelli, A., Skiada, D., Poux, V., Weitkunat, R., Baker, G., Picavet, P., Lüdicke, F., 2019b. Favorable changes in biomarkers of potential harm to reduce the adverse health effects of smoking in smokers switching to the menthol tobacco heating system 2.2 for three months (Part 2). Nicotine Tob. Res. https://doi.org/10.1093/ntr/ntz084.

Hecht, S.S., 2012. Lung carcinogenesis by tobacco smoke. Int. J. Cancer 131, 2724–2732. https://doi.org/10.1002/ijc.27816.

Hecht, S.S., Murphy, S.E., Stepanov, I., Nelson, H.H., Yuan, J.-M., 2013. Tobacco smoke biomarkers and cancer risk among male smokers in the Shanghai cohort study. Cancer Lett. 334, 34–38. https://doi.org/10.1016/j.canlet.2012.07.016.

Hedblad, B., Ogren, M., Engström, G., Wollmer, P., Janzon, L., 2005. Heterogeneity of cardiovascular risk among smokers is related to degree of carbon monoxide exposure. Atherosclerosis 179, 177–183. https://doi.org/10.1016/j.atherosclerosis.2004.10.005.

Hedblad, B., Engström, G., Janzon, E., Berglund, G., Janzon, L., 2006. COHb% as a marker of cardiovascular risk in never smokers: results from a population-based cohort study. Scand. J. Publ. Health 34, 609–615. https://doi.org/10.1080/14034940600590523.

Helfinger, V., Schröder, K., 2018. Redox control in cancer development and progression. Mol. Aspects Med. 63, 88–98. https://doi.org/10.1016/j.mam.2018.02.003.

Hoeng, J., Maeder, S., Vanscheeuwijck, P., Peitsch, M.C., 2019. Assessing the lung cancer risk reduction potential of candidate modified risk tobacco products. Intern. Emerg. Med. 14, 821–834. https://doi.org/10.1007/s11739-019-02045-z.

Hogg, J.C., Chu, F., Utokaparch, S., Woods, R., Elliott, W.M., Buzatu, L., Cherniack, R.M., Rogers, R.M., Sciurba, F.C., Coxson, H.O., Paré, P.D., 2004. The nature of small-airway obstruction in chronic obstructive pulmonary disease. N. Engl. J. Med. 350, 2645–2653. https://doi.org/10.1056/NEJMoa032158.

Inaba, Y., Chen, J.A., Bergmann, S.R., 2010. Prediction of future cardiovascular outcomes by flow-mediated vasodilatation of brachial artery: a meta-analysis. Int. J. Cardiovasc. Imag. 26, 631–640. https://doi.org/10.1007/s10554-010-9616-1.

Inoue-Choi, M., Hartge, P., Park, Y., Abnet, C.C., Freedman, N.D., 2019. Association between reductions of number of cigarettes smoked per day and mortality among older adults in the United States. Am. J. Epidemiol. 188, 363–371. https://doi.org/10.1093/aje/kwy227.

Iskandar, A.R., Titz, B., Sewer, A., Leroy, P., Schneider, T., Zanetti, F., Mathis, C., Elamin, A., Frentzel, S., Schlage, W.K., Martin, F., Ivanov, N.V., Peitsch, M.C., Hoeng, J., 2017a. Systems toxicology meta-analysis of in vitro assessment studies: biological impact of a candidate modified-risk tobacco product aerosol compared with cigarette smoke on human organotypic cultures of the aerodigestive tract. Toxicol. Res. (Camb.) 6, 631–653. https://doi.org/10.1039/c7tx00047b.

Iskandar, A.R., Martinez, Y., Martin, F., Schlage, W.K., et al., 2017b. Comparative effects of a candidate modified-risk tobacco product Aerosol and cigarette smoke on human organotypic small airway cultures: a systems toxicology approach. Toxicol. Res. (Camb.) 6, 930–946. https://doi.org/10.1039/c7tx00152e.

Iskandar, A.R., Zanetti, F., Kondylis, A., Martin, F., Leroy, P., Majeed, S., Steiner, S., Xiang, Y., Ortega Torres, L., Trivedi, K., Guedj, E., Merg, C., Frentzel, S., Ivanov, N.V., Doshi, U., Lee, K.M., McKinney, W.J., Peitsch, M.C., Hoeng, J., 2019a. A lower impact of an acute exposure to electronic cigarette aerosols than to cigarette smoke in human organotypic buccal and small airway cultures was demonstrated using systems toxicology assessment. Intern. Emerg. Med. 14, 863–883. https://doi.org/10.1007/s11739-019-02055-x.

Iskandar, A.R., Zanetti, F., Marescotti, D., Titz, B., Sewer, A., Kondylis, A., Leroy, P., Belcastro, V., Torres, L.O., Acali, S., Majeed, S., Steiner, S., Trivedi, K., Guedj, E., Merg, C., Schneider, T., Frentzel, S., Martin, F., Ivanov, N.V., Peitsch, M.C., Hoeng, J., 2019b. Application of a multilayer systems toxicology framework for in vitro assessment of the biological effects of classic tobacco e-liquid and its corresponding aerosol using an e-cigarette device with MESH™ technology. Arch. Toxicol. 93, 3229–3247. https://doi.org/10.1007/s00204-019-02565-9.

Ito, S., Matsumura, K., Ishimori, K., Ishikawa, S., 2020. In vitro long-term repeated exposure and exposure switching of a novel tobacco vapor product in a human organotypic culture of bronchial epithelial cells. J. Appl. Toxicol. https://doi.org/10.1002/jat.3982.

Jaccard, G., Djoko, D., Moennikes, O., Jeannet, C., Kondylis, A., Belushkin, M., 2019. Comparative Assessment of HPHC Yields in THS 2.2 and Commercial Cigarettes [WWW Document]. https://doi.org/10.26126/intervals.pz63pp.1.

Jorgensen, E.D., Zhao, H., Traganos, F., Albino, A.P., Darzynkiewicz, Z., 2010. DNA damage response induced by exposure of human lung adenocarcinoma cells to smoke from tobacco- and nicotine-free cigarettes. Cell Cycle 9, 2170–2176. https://doi.org/10.4161/cc.9.11.11842.

Kalra, V.K., Ying, Y., Deemer, K., Natarajan, R., Nadler, J.L., Coates, T.D., 1994. Mechanism of cigarette smoke condensate induced adhesion of human monocytes to cultured endothelial cells. J. Cell. Physiol. 160, 154–162. https://doi.org/10.1002/jcp.1041600118.

Kawanishi, S., Ohnishi, S., Ma, N., Hiraku, Y., Murata, M., 2017. Crosstalk between DNA damage and inflammation in the multiple steps of carcinogenesis. Int. J. Mol. Sci. 18 https://doi.org/10.3390/ijms18081808.

Knoke, J.D., Shanks, T.G., Vaughn, J.W., Thun, M.J., Burns, D.M., 2004. Lung cancer mortality is related to age in addition to duration and intensity of cigarette smoking: an analysis of CPS-I data. Cancer Epidemiol. Biomarkers Prev. 13, 949–957.

Koblizek, V., Tomsova, M., Cermakova, E., Papousek, P., et al., 2011. Impairment of nasal mucociliary clearance in former smokers with stable chronic obstructive pulmonary disease relates to the presence of a chronic bronchitis phenotype. Rhinology 49 (4), 397–406. https://doi.org/10.4193/Rhino11.051.

Kuschner, W.G., D'Alessandro, A., Wong, H., Blanc, P.D., 1996. Dose-dependent cigarette smoking-related inflammatory responses in healthy adults. Eur. Respir. J. 9, 1989–1994. https://doi.org/10.1183/09031936.96.09101989.

Laugesen, M., 2015. Nicotine and toxicant yield ratings of electronic cigarette brands in New Zealand. N. Z. Med. J. 128, 77–82.

Lee, J., Taneja, V., Vassallo, R., 2012. Cigarette smoking and inflammation: cellular and molecular mechanisms. J. Dent. Res. 91, 142–149. https://doi.org/10.1177/0022034511421200.

Lee, C.-H., Hyun, M.K., Jang, E.J., Lee, N.R., Kim, K., Yim, J.-J., 2013. Inhaled corticosteroid use and risks of lung cancer and laryngeal cancer. Respir. Med. 107, 1222–1233. https://doi.org/10.1016/j.rmed.2012.12.002.

Lee, K.M., Hoeng, J., Harbo, S., Kogel, U., Gardner, W., Oldham, M., Benson, E., Talikka, M., Kondylis, A., Martin, F., Titz, B., Ansari, S., Trivedi, K., Guedj, E., Elamin, A., Ivanov, N.V., Vanscheeuwijck, P., Peitsch, M.C., McKinney, W.J., 2018. Biological changes in C57BL/6 mice following 3 weeks of inhalation exposure to cigarette smoke or e-vapor aerosols. Inhal. Toxicol. 30, 553–567. https://doi.org/10.1080/08958378.2019.1576807.

Li, X., Luo, Y., Jiang, X., Zhang, H., Zhu, F., Hu, S., Hou, H., Hu, Q., Pang, Y., 2018. Chemical analysis and simulated pyrolysis of tobacco heating system 2.2 compared to conventional cigarettes. Nicotine Tob. Res. https://doi.org/10.1093/ntr/nty005.

Liang, X., Wang, J., Guan, R., Zhao, L., Li, D., Long, Z., Yang, Q., Xu, J., Wang, Z., Xie, J., Lu, W., 2018. Limax extract ameliorates cigarette smoke-induced chronic obstructive pulmonary disease in mice. Int. Immunopharmacol. 54, 210–220. https://doi.org/10.1016/j.intimp.2017.11.004.

Lietz, M., Berges, A., Lebrun, S., Meurrens, K., Steffen, Y., Stolle, K., Schueller, J., Boue, S., Vuillaume, G., Vanscheeuwijck, P., Moehring, M., Schlage, W., De Leon, H., Hoeng, J., Peitsch, M., 2013. Cigarette-smoke-induced atherogenic lipid profiles in plasma and vascular tissue of apolipoprotein E-deficient mice are attenuated by smoking cessation. Atherosclerosis 229, 86–93. https://doi.org/10.1016/j.atherosclerosis.2013.03.036.

Lighty, J.S., Veranth, J.M., Sarofim, A.F., 2000. Combustion aerosols: factors governing their size and composition and implications to human health. J. Air Waste Manag. Assoc. 50, 1565–1618. https://doi.org/10.1080/10473289.2000.10464197. Discussion 1619-1622.

Lindner, K., Ströbele, M., Schlick, S., Webering, S., Jenckel, A., Kopf, J., Danov, O., Sewald, K., Buj, C., Creutzenberg, O., Tillmann, T., Pohlmann, G., Ernst, H., Ziemann, C., Hüttmann, G., Heine, H., Bockhorn, H., Hansen, T., König, P., Fehrenbach, H., 2017. Biological effects of carbon black nanoparticles are changed by surface coating with polycyclic aromatic hydrocarbons. Part. Fibre Toxicol. 14, 8. https://doi.org/10.1186/s12989-017-0189-1.

Lo Sasso, G., Schlage, W.K., Boué, S., Veljkovic, E., Peitsch, M.C., Hoeng, J., 2016a. The Apoe(-/-) mouse model: a suitable model to study cardiovascular and respiratory diseases in the context of cigarette smoke exposure and harm reduction. J. Transl. Med. 14, 146. https://doi.org/10.1186/s12967-016-0901-1.

Lo Sasso, G., Titz, B., Nury, C., Boué, S., Phillips, B., Belcastro, V., Schneider, T., Dijon, S., Baumer, K., Peric, D., Dulize, R., Elamin, A., Guedj, E., Buettner, A., Leroy, P., Kleinhans, S., Vuillaume, G., Veljkovic, E., Ivanov, N.V., Martin, F., Vanscheeuwijck, P., Peitsch, M.C., Hoeng, J., 2016b. Effects of cigarette smoke, cessation and switching to a candidate modified risk tobacco product on the liver in Apoe-/- mice–a systems toxicology analysis. Inhal. Toxicol. 28, 226–240. https://doi.org/10.3109/08958378.2016.1150368.

Lüdicke, F., Picavet, P., Baker, G., Haziza, C., Poux, V., Lama, N., Weitkunat, R., 2018a. Effects of switching to the tobacco heating system 2.2 menthol, smoking abstinence, or continued cigarette smoking on biomarkers of exposure: a randomized, controlled, open-label, multicenter study in sequential confinement and ambulatory settings (Part 1). Nicotine Tob. Res. 20, 161–172. https://doi.org/10.1093/ntr/ntw287.

Lüdicke, F., Picavet, P., Baker, G., Haziza, C., Poux, V., Lama, N., Weitkunat, R., 2018b. Effects of switching to the menthol tobacco heating system 2.2, smoking abstinence, or continued cigarette smoking on clinically relevant risk markers: a randomized, controlled, open-label, multicenter study in sequential confinement and ambulatory settings (Part 2). Nicotine Tob. Res. 20, 173–182. https://doi.org/10.1093/ntr/ntx028.

Lüdicke, F., Ansari, S.M., Lama, N., Blanc, N., Bosilkovska, M., Donelli, A., Picavet, P., Baker, G., Haziza, C., Peitsch, M., Weitkunat, R., 2019. Effects of switching to a heat-not-burn tobacco product on biologically relevant biomarkers to assess a candidate modified risk tobacco product: a randomized trial. Cancer Epidemiol. Biomarkers Prev. 28, 1934–1943. https://doi.org/10.1158/1055-9965.EPI-18-0915.

Madison, M.C., Landers, C.T., Gu, B.-H., Chang, C.-Y., Tung, H.-Y., You, R., Hong, M.J., Baghaei, N., Song, L.-Z., Porter, P., Putluri, N., Salas, R., Gilbert, B.E., Levental, I., Campen, M.J., Corry, D.B., Kheradmand, F., 2019. Electronic cigarettes disrupt lung lipid homeostasis and innate immunity independent of nicotine. J. Clin. Invest. 129, 4290–4304. https://doi.org/10.1172/JCI128531.

Mahmud, A., Feely, J., 2003. Effect of smoking on arterial stiffness and pulse pressure amplification. Hypertension 41, 183–187. https://doi.org/10.1161/01.hyp.0000047464.66901.60.

Mallock, N., Böss, L., Burk, R., Danziger, M., Welsch, T., Hahn, H., Trieu, H.-L., Hahn, J., Pieper, E., Henkler-Stephani, F., Hutzler, C., Luch, A., 2018. Levels of selected analytes in the emissions of "heat not burn" tobacco products that are relevant to assess human health risks. Arch. Toxicol. 92, 2145–2149. https://doi.org/10.1007/s00204-018-2215-y.

Mantovani, A., 2010. Molecular pathways linking inflammation and cancer. Curr. Mol. Med. 10, 369–373. https://doi.org/10.2174/156652410791316968.

Martin, F., Sewer, A., Talikka, M., Xiang, Y., Hoeng, J., Peitsch, M.C., 2014. Quantification of biological network perturbations for mechanistic insight and diagnostics using two-layer causal models. BMC Bioinformatics 15, 238. https://doi.org/10.1186/1471-2105-15-238.

Martin, F., Talikka, M., Hoeng, J., Peitsch, M.C., 2015. Identification of gene expression signature for cigarette smoke exposure response–from man to mouse. Hum. Exp. Toxicol. 34, 1200–1211. https://doi.org/10.1177/0960327115600364.

Martin, F., Talikka, M., Ivanov, N.V., Haziza, C., Hoeng, J., Peitsch, M.C., 2016. Evaluation of the tobacco heating system 2.2. Part 9: application of systems pharmacology to identify exposure response markers in peripheral blood of smokers switching to THS2.2. Regul. Toxicol. Pharmacol. 81 (Suppl. 2), S151–S157. https://doi.org/10.1016/j.yrtph.2016.11.011.

Martin, F., Talikka, M., Ivanov, N.V., Haziza, C., Hoeng, J., Peitsch, M.C., 2019. A meta-analysis of the performance of a blood-based exposure response gene signature across clinical studies on the tobacco heating system 2.2 (THS 2.2). Front. Pharmacol. 10, 198. https://doi.org/10.3389/fphar.2019.00198.

Martin, F., Talikka, M., Poussin, C., Belcastro, V., Boue, S., Haziza, C., Ivanov, N.V., Peitsch, M.C., Hoeng, J., 2020. Development, Application, and Crowd-Sourced Verification of a Gene-Based Signature for Evaluation of RRPs: Application to THS 2.2. https://doi.org/10.26126/intervals.mnrkj5.1 [WWW Document].

Mathis, C., Poussin, C., Weisensee, D., Gebel, S., Hengstermann, A., Sewer, A., Belcastro, V., Xiang, Y., Ansari, S., Wagner, S., Hoeng, J., Peitsch, M.C., 2013. Human bronchial epithelial cells exposed in vitro to cigarette smoke at the air-liquid interface resemble bronchial epithelium from human smokers. Am. J. Physiol. Lung Cell Mol. Physiol. 304, L489–L503. https://doi.org/10.1152/ajplung.00181.2012.

McNeil, A., 2012. Reducing Harm from Nicotine Use. Fifty Years Since Smoking and Health. Progress, Lessons and Priorities for a Smoke-free UK. London.

Messner, B., Bernhard, D., 2014. Smoking and cardiovascular disease: mechanisms of endothelial dysfunction and early atherogenesis. Arterioscler. Thromb. Vasc. Biol. 34, 509–515. https://doi.org/10.1161/ATVBAHA.113.300156.

Miyata, S., Noda, A., Ito, Y., Iizuka, R., Shimokata, K., 2015. Smoking acutely impaired endothelial function in healthy college students. Acta Cardiol. 70, 282–285. https://doi.org/10.1080/ac.70.3.3080632.

Moretto, N., Facchinetti, F., Southworth, T., Civelli, M., Singh, D., Patacchini, R., 2009. alpha,beta-Unsaturated aldehydes contained in cigarette smoke elicit IL-8 release in pulmonary cells through mitogen-activated protein kinases. Am. J. Physiol. Lung Cell Mol. Physiol. 296, L839–L848. https://doi.org/10.1152/ajplung.90570.2008.

Nakamura, A.J., Rao, V.A., Pommier, Y., Bonner, W.M., 2010. The complexity of phosphorylated H2AX foci formation and DNA repair assembly at DNA double-strand breaks. Cell Cycle 9, 389–397. https://doi.org/10.4161/cc.9.2.10475.

National Center for Chronic Disease Prevention and Health Promotion (US) Office on Smoking and Health, 2014. The Health Consequences of Smoking-50 Years of Progress: A Report of the Surgeon General.

Ogunwale, M.A., Li, M., Ramakrishnam Raju, M.V., Chen, Y., Nantz, M.H., Conklin, D.J., Fu, X.-A., 2017. Aldehyde detection in electronic cigarette aerosols. ACS Omega 2, 1207–1214. https://doi.org/10.1021/acsomega.6b00489.

Orth, S.R., 2004. Effects of smoking on systemic and intrarenal hemodynamics: influence on renal function. J. Am. Soc. Nephrol. 15 (Suppl. 1), S58–S63. https://doi.org/10.1097/01.asn.0000093461.36097.d5.

Oviedo, A., Lebrun, S., Kogel, U., Ho, J., Tan, W.T., Titz, B., Leroy, P., Vuillaume, G., Bera, M., Martin, F., Rodrigo, G., Esposito, M., Dempsey, R., Ivanov, N.V., Hoeng, J., Peitsch, M.C., Vanscheeuwijck, P., 2016. Evaluation of the Tobacco Heating System 2.2. Part 6: 90-day OECD 413 rat inhalation study with systems toxicology endpoints demonstrates reduced exposure effects of a mentholated version compared with mentholated and non-mentholated cigarette smoke. Regul. Toxicol. Pharmacol. 81 (Suppl. 2), S93–S122. https://doi.org/10.1016/j.yrtph.2016.11.004.

O'Callaghan, D.S., O'Donnell, D., O'Connell, F., O'Byrne, K.J., 2010. The role of inflammation in the pathogenesis of non-small cell lung cancer. J. Thorac. Oncol. 5, 2024–2036. https://doi.org/10.1097/jto.0b013e3181f387e4.

O'Connell, G., Graff, D.W., D'Ruiz, C.D., 2016. Reductions in biomarkers of exposure (BoE) to harmful or potentially harmful constituents (HPHCs) following partial or complete substitution of cigarettes with electronic cigarettes in adult smokers. Toxicol. Mech. Methods 26, 443–454. https://doi.org/10.1080/15376516.2016.1196282.

Parris, B.A., O'Farrell, H.E., Fong, K.M., Yang, I.A., 2019. Chronic obstructive pulmonary disease (COPD) and lung cancer: common pathways for pathogenesis. J. Thorac. Dis. 11, S2155–S2172. https://doi.org/10.21037/jtd.2019.10.54.

Penning, T.M., 2014. Human aldo-keto reductases and the metabolic activation of polycyclic aromatic hydrocarbons. Chem. Res. Toxicol. 27, 1901–1917. https://doi.org/10.1021/tx500298n.

Perotin, J.M., Coraux, C., Lagonotte, E., Birembaut, P., et al., 2018. Alteration of primary cilia in COPD. Eur. Respir. J. 52 (1), 1800122. https://doi.org/10.1183/13993003.00122-2018.

Phillips, B., Veljkovic, E., Peck, M.J., Buettner, A., Elamin, A., Guedj, E., Vuillaume, G., Ivanov, N.V., Martin, F., Boué, S., Schlage, W.K., Schneider, T., Titz, B., Talikka, M., Vanscheeuwijck, P., Hoeng, J., Peitsch, M.C., 2015. A 7-month cigarette smoke inhalation study in C57BL/6 mice demonstrates reduced lung inflammation and emphysema following smoking cessation or aerosol exposure from a prototypic modified risk tobacco product. Food Chem. Toxicol. 80, 328–345. https://doi.org/10.1016/j.fct.2015.03.009.

Phillips, B., Veljkovic, E., Boué, S., Schlage, W.K., Vuillaume, G., Martin, F., Titz, B., Leroy, P., Buettner, A., Elamin, A., Oviedo, A., Cabanski, M., De León, H., Guedj, E., Schneider, T., Talikka, M., Ivanov, N.V., Vanscheeuwijck, P., Peitsch, M.C., Hoeng, J., 2016. An 8-month systems toxicology inhalation/cessation study in Apoe$^{-/-}$ mice to investigate cardiovascular and respiratory exposure effects of a candidate modified risk tobacco product, THS 2.2, compared with conventional cigarettes. Toxicol. Sci. 149, 411–432. https://doi.org/10.1093/toxsci/kfv243.

Phillips, B., Szostak, J., Titz, B., Schlage, W., Guedj, E., Leroy, P., Vuillaume, G., Martin, F., Buettner, A., Elamin, A., Sewer, A., Sierro, N., Choukrallah, M.-A., Schneider, T., Ivanov, N.V., Vanscheeuwijck, P., Peitsch, M.C., Hoeng, J., 2019a. 6-month Systems Toxicology Inhalation/Cessation Study With CHTP 1.2 and THS 2.2 in Apoe⁻/⁻ Mice [WWW Document]. https://doi.org/10.26126/intervals.w6y4a5.1.

Phillips, B., Szostak, J., Titz, B., Schlage, W.K., Guedj, E., Leroy, P., Vuillaume, G., Martin, F., Buettner, A., Elamin, A., Sewer, A., Sierro, N., Choukrallah, M.A., Schneider, T., Ivanov, N.V., Teng, C., Tung, C.K., Lim, W.T., Yeo, Y.S., Vanscheeuwijck, P., Peitsch, M.C., Hoeng, J., 2019b. A six-month systems toxicology inhalation/cessation study in ApoE⁻/⁻ mice to investigate cardiovascular and respiratory exposure effects of modified risk tobacco products, CHTP 1.2 and THS 2.2, compared with conventional cigarettes. Food Chem. Toxicol. 126, 113–141. https://doi.org/10.1016/j.fct.2019.02.008.

Polosa, R., Morjaria, J.B., Prosperini, U., Busà, B., Pennisi, A., Malerba, M., Maglia, M., Caponnetto, P., 2020a. COPD smokers who switched to e-cigarettes: health outcomes at 5-year follow up. Ther. Adv. Chronic Dis. 11. https://doi.org/10.1177/2040622320961617.

Polosa, R., Emma, R., Cibella, F., Caruso, M., Conte, G., Benfatto, F., Ferlito, S., et al., 2020b. Saccharin transit time in exclusive e-cigarette and heated tobacco product users: a cross-sectional study. medRxiv. https://doi.org/10.1101/2020.10.21.20216630.

Porta, C., Larghi, P., Rimoldi, M., Totaro, M.G., Allavena, P., Mantovani, A., Sica, A., 2009. Cellular and molecular pathways linking inflammation and cancer. Immunobiology 214, 761–777. https://doi.org/10.1016/j.imbio.2009.06.014.

Poussin, C., Gallitz, I., Schlage, W.K., Steffen, Y., Stolle, K., Lebrun, S., Hoeng, J., Peitsch, M.C., Lietz, M., 2014. Mechanism of an indirect effect of aqueous cigarette smoke extract on the adhesion of monocytic cells to endothelial cells in an in vitro assay revealed by transcriptomics analysis. Toxicol. In Vitro 28, 896–908. https://doi.org/10.1016/j.tiv.2014.03.005.

Poussin, C., Laurent, A., Peitsch, M.C., Hoeng, J., De Leon, H., 2015. Systems biology reveals cigarette smoke-induced concentration-dependent direct and indirect mechanisms that promote monocyte-endothelial cell adhesion. Toxicol. Sci. 147, 370–385. https://doi.org/10.1093/toxsci/kfv137.

Poussin, C., Laurent, A., Peitsch, M.C., Hoeng, J., De Leon, H., 2016. Systems toxicology-based assessment of the candidate modified risk tobacco product THS2.2 for the adhesion of monocytic cells to human coronary arterial endothelial cells. Toxicology 339, 73–86. https://doi.org/10.1016/j.tox.2015.11.007.

Poussin, C., Belcastro, V., Martin, F., Boué, S., Peitsch, M.C., Hoeng, J., 2017. Crowd-sourced verification of computational methods and data in systems toxicology: a case study with a heat-not-burn candidate modified risk tobacco product. Chem. Res. Toxicol. 30, 934–945. https://doi.org/10.1021/acs.chemrestox.6b00345.

Poussin, C., Kramer, B., Lanz, H.L., Van den Heuvel, A., Laurent, A., Olivier, T., Vermeer, M., Peric, D., Baumer, K., Dulize, R., Guedj, E., Ivanov, N.V., Peitsch, M.C., Hoeng, J., Joore, J., 2020. 3D human microvessel-on-a-chip model for studying monocyte-to-endothelium adhesion under flow - application in systems toxicology. ALTEX 37, 47–63. https://doi.org/10.14573/altex.1811301.

Pratte, P., Cosandey, S., Goujon Ginglinger, C., 2017. Investigation of solid particles in the mainstream aerosol of the tobacco heating system THS2.2 and mainstream smoke of a 3R4F reference cigarette. Hum. Exp. Toxicol. 36, 1115–1120. https://doi.org/10.1177/0960327116681653.

Pratte, P., Cosandey, S., Ginglinger, C., 2019. Investigation of Solid Particles in the Mainstream Aerosol of THS 2.2 and 3R4F. https://doi.org/10.26126/intervals.5nmtfe.1 [WWW Document].

Pryor, W.A., Church, D.F., Evans, M.D., Rice, W.Y., Hayes, J.R., 1990. A comparison of the free radical chemistry of tobacco-burning cigarettes and cigarettes that only heat tobacco. Free Radic. Biol. Med. 8, 275–279. https://doi.org/10.1016/0891-5849(90)90075-t.

Rahman, M.M., Laher, I., 2007. Structural and functional alteration of blood vessels caused by cigarette smoking: an overview of molecular mechanisms. Curr. Vasc. Pharmacol. 5, 276–292. https://doi.org/10.2174/157016107782023406.

Ras, R.T., Streppel, M.T., Draijer, R., Zock, P.L., 2013. Flow-mediated dilation and cardiovascular risk prediction: a systematic review with meta-analysis. Int. J. Cardiol. 168, 344–351. https://doi.org/10.1016/j.ijcard.2012.09.047.

Ridker, P.M., MacFadyen, J.G., Thuren, T., Everett, B.M., Libby, P., Glynn, R.J., CANTOS Trial Group, 2017. Effect of interleukin-1β inhibition with canakinumab on incident lung cancer in patients with atherosclerosis: exploratory results from a randomised, double-blind, placebo-controlled trial. Lancet 390, 1833–1842. https://doi.org/10.1016/S0140-6736(17)32247-X.

Rodriguez-Portelles, A., Rodriguez-Leyva, D., 2019. Endothelial and left ventricular diastolic function in young adults exposed to tobacco. Can. J. Physiol. Pharmacol. 97, 1006–1011. https://doi.org/10.1139/cjpp-2019-0187.

Rogers, D.F., 2007. Physiology of airway mucus secretion and pathophysiology of hypersecretion. Respir. Care 52, 1134–1146. Discussion 1146-1149.

Sahu, D., Kannan, G.M., Vijayaraghavan, R., 2014. Carbon black particle exhibits size dependent toxicity in human monocytes. Int. J. Inflamm. 2014, 827019. https://doi.org/10.1155/2014/827019.

Schaller, J.-P., Keller, D., Poget, L., Pratte, P., Kaelin, E., McHugh, D., Cudazzo, G., Smart, D., Tricker, A.R., Gautier, L., 2016. Evaluation of the tobacco heating system 2.2. Part 2: chemical composition, genotoxicity, cytotoxicity, and physical properties of the aerosol. Regul. Toxicol. Pharmacol. 81, S27–S47.

Schaller, J.P., Keller, D., Poget, L., Pratte, P., Kaelin, E., McHugh, D., Cudazzo, G., Smart, D., Tricker, A., Gautier, L., Yerly, M., Reis Pires, R., Le Bouhellec, S., Ghosh, D., Hofer, I., Garcia, E., Vanscheeuwijck, P., Maeder, S., 2019a. THS 2.2 Regular: Chemical Composition and Physical Properties of the Aerosol in Comparison with the Mainstream Smoke of 3R4F. https://doi.org/10.26126/intervals.82hxcs.1 [WWW Document].

Schaller, J.P., Keller, D., Poget, L., Pratte, P., Kaelin, E., McHugh, D., Cudazzo, G., Smart, D., Tricker, A., Gautier, L., Yerly, M., Reis Pires, R., Le Bouhellec, S., Ghosh, D., Hofer, I., Garcia, E., Vanscheeuwijck, P., Maeder, S., 2019b. THS 2.2 Menthol: Chemical Composition of Aerosol in Comparison with the Mainstream Smoke Constituents of 3R4F. https://doi.org/10.26126/intervals.25g5qb.1 [WWW Document].

Schmidt, K.M.T., Hansen, K.M., Johnson, A.L., Gepner, A.D., Korcarz, C.E., Fiore, M.C., Baker, T.B., Piper, M.E., Stein, J.H., 2019. Longitudinal effects of cigarette smoking and smoking cessation on aortic wave reflections, pulse wave velocity, and carotid artery distensibility. J. Am. Heart Assoc. 8, e013939. https://doi.org/10.1161/JAHA.119.013939.

Sethi, G., Shanmugam, M.K., Ramachandran, L., Kumar, A.P., Tergaonkar, V., 2012. Multifaceted link between cancer and inflammation. Biosci. Rep. 32, 1–15. https://doi.org/10.1042/BSR20100136.

Sharman, A., Nurmagambetov, T., 2020. Changes in respiratory function and physical capacity among smokers after switching to IQOS: One year follow-up. Glob. J. Respir. Care 6, 22–29. https://doi.org/10.12974/2312-5470.2020.06.03.

Shein, M., Jeschke, G., 2019. Comparison of free radical levels in the aerosol from conventional cigarettes, electronic cigarettes, and heat-not-burn tobacco products. Chem. Res. Toxicol. 32, 1289–1298. https://doi.org/10.1021/acs.chemrestox.9b00085.

Silkoff, P.E., Erzurum, S.C., Lundberg, J.O., George, S.C., Marczin, N., Hunt, J.F., Effros, R., Horvath, I., American Thoracic Society, HOC Subcommittee of the Assembly on Allergy, Immunology, and Inflammation, 2006. ATS workshop proceedings: exhaled nitric oxide and nitric oxide oxidative metabolism in exhaled breath condensate. Proc. Am. Thorac. Soc. 3, 131–145. https://doi.org/10.1513/pats.200406-710ST.

Sleiman, M., Logue, J.M., Montesinos, V.N., Russell, M.L., Litter, M.I., Gundel, L.A., Destaillats, H., 2016. Emissions from electronic cigarettes: key parameters affecting the release of harmful chemicals. Environ. Sci. Technol. 50, 9644–9651. https://doi.org/10.1021/acs.est.6b01741.

Smith, M.R., Clark, B., Lüdicke, F., Schaller, J.-P., Vanscheeuwijck, P., Hoeng, J., Peitsch, M.C., 2016. Evaluation of the tobacco heating system 2.2. Part 1: description of the system and the scientific assessment program. Regul. Toxicol. Pharmacol. 81 (Suppl. 2), S17–S26. https://doi.org/10.1016/j.yrtph.2016.07.006.

Song, M.-A., Freudenheim, J.L., Brasky, T.M., Mathe, E.A., McElroy, J.P., Nickerson, Q.A., Reisinger, S.A., Smiraglia, D.J., Weng, D.Y., Ying, K.L., Wewers, M.D., Shields, P.G., 2020. Biomarkers of exposure and effect in the lungs of smokers, nonsmokers, and electronic cigarette users. Cancer Epidemiol. Biomarkers Prev. 29, 443–451. https://doi.org/10.1158/1055-9965.EPI-19-1245.

Spira, A., Beane, J., Shah, V., Liu, G., Schembri, F., Yang, X., Palma, J., Brody, J.S., 2004. Effects of cigarette smoke on the human airway epithelial cell transcriptome. Proc. Natl. Acad. Sci. U.S.A. 101, 10143–10148. https://doi.org/10.1073/pnas.0401422101.

Stanley, P.J., Wilson, R., Greenstone, M.A., MacWilliam, L., Cole, P.J., 1986. Effect of cigarette smoking on nasal mucociliary clearance and ciliary beat frequency. Thorax 41 (7), 519–523. https://doi.org/10.1136/thx.41.7.519.

Stepanov, I., Sebero, E., Wang, R., Gao, Y.-T., Hecht, S.S., Yuan, J.-M., 2014. Tobacco-specific N-nitrosamine exposures and cancer risk in the Shanghai Cohort Study: remarkable coherence with rat tumor sites. Int. J. Cancer 134, 2278–2283. https://doi.org/10.1002/ijc.28575.

Stephens, W.E., 2017. Comparing the cancer potencies of emissions from vapourised nicotine products including e-cigarettes with those of tobacco smoke. Tob. Control. https://doi.org/10.1136/tobaccocontrol-2017-053808.

Stinn, W., Berges, A., Meurrens, K., Buettner, A., Gebel, S., Lichtner, R.B., Janssens, K., Veljkovic, E., Xiang, Y., Roemer, E., Haussmann, H.-J., 2013a. Towards the validation of a lung tumorigenesis model with mainstream cigarette smoke inhalation using the A/J mouse. Toxicology 305, 49–64. https://doi.org/10.1016/j.tox.2013.01.005.

Stinn, W., Buettner, A., Weiler, H., Friedrichs, B., Luetjen, S., van Overveld, F., Meurrens, K., Janssens, K., Gebel, S., Stabbert, R., Haussmann, H.-J., 2013b. Lung inflammatory effects, tumorigenesis, and emphysema development in a long-term inhalation study with cigarette mainstream smoke in mice. Toxicol. Sci. 131, 596–611. https://doi.org/10.1093/toxsci/kfs312.

Stoeger, T., Reinhard, C., Takenaka, S., Schroeppel, A., Karg, E., Ritter, B., Heyder, J., Schulz, H., 2006. Instillation of six different ultrafine carbon particles indicates a surface area threshold dose for acute lung inflammation in mice. Environ. Health Perspect. 114, 328–333. https://doi.org/10.1289/ehp.8266.

Sturla, S.J., Boobis, A.R., FitzGerald, R.E., Hoeng, J., Kavlock, R.J., Schirmer, K., Whelan, M., Wilks, M.F., Peitsch, M.C., 2014. Systems toxicology: from basic research to risk assessment. Chem. Res. Toxicol. 27, 314–329. https://doi.org/10.1021/tx400410s.

Sultana, R., Nessa, A., Yeasmin, F., Nasreen, S., Khanam, A., 2019. Study on blood pressure in male cigarette smokers. Mymensingh Med. J. 28, 582–585.

Szostak, J., Wong, E., Titz, B., Lee, T., Zhang, J., Kumar, A., Schlage, W.K., Guedj, E., Phillips, B., Leroy, P., Buettner, A., Martin, F., Sewer, A., Kuczaj, A.K., Ivanov, N.V., Luettich, K., Vanscheeuwijck, P., Peitsch, M.C., Hoeng, J., Yang, X., 2020a. Impact of E-Vapor Aerosols on the Cardiovascular and Respiratory Systems in ApoE⁻/⁻ Mice. https://doi.org/10.26126/intervals.8lafdu.1 [WWW Document].

Szostak, J., Wong, E.T., Titz, B., Lee, T., Wong, S.K., Low, T., Lee, K.M., Zhang, J., Kumar, A., Schlage, W.K., Guedj, E., Phillips, B., Leroy, P., Buettner, A., Xiang, Y., Martin, F., Sewer, A., Kuczaj, A., Ivanov, N.V., Luettich, K., Vanscheeuwijck, P., Peitsch, M.C., Hoeng, J., 2020b. A 6-

month systems toxicology inhalation study in ApoE[-/-] mice demonstrates reduced cardiovascular effects of E-vapor aerosols compared to cigarette smoke. Am. J. Physiol. Heart Circ. Physiol. https://doi.org/10.1152/ajpheart.00613.2019.

Takahashi, Y., Kanemaru, Y., Fukushima, T., Eguchi, K., Yoshida, S., Miller-Holt, J., Jones, I., 2019. Novel Tobacco Vapor Product Aerosol: Chemistry Analysis and in Vitro Toxicological Evaluation in Comparison with 3R4F Cigarette Smoke [WWW Document]. https://doi.org/10.26126/intervals.v2ubz6.1.

Taylor, M., Jaunky, T., Hewitt, K., Breheny, D., Lowe, F., Fearon, I.M., Gaca, M., 2017. A comparative assessment of e-cigarette aerosols and cigarette smoke on in vitro endothelial cell migration. Toxicol. Lett. 277, 123–128. https://doi.org/10.1016/j.toxlet.2017.06.001.

Taylor, M., Thorne, D., Carr, T., Breheny, D., Walker, P., Proctor, C., Gaça, M., 2018. Assessment of novel tobacco heating product THP1.0. Part 6: a comparative in vitro study using contemporary screening approaches. Regul. Toxicol. Pharmacol. 93, 62–70. https://doi.org/10.1016/j.yrtph.2017.08.016.

Tayyarah, R., Long, G.A., 2014. Comparison of select analytes in aerosol from e-cigarettes with smoke from conventional cigarettes and with ambient air. Regul. Toxicol. Pharmacol. 70, 704–710. https://doi.org/10.1016/j.yrtph.2014.10.010.

Titz, B., Sewer, A., Luettich, K., Wong, E., Guedj, E., Nury, C., Schneider, T., Xiang, Y., Trivedi, K., Vuillaume, G., Leroy, P., Büttner, A., Martin, F., Ivanov, N., Vanscheeuwijck, P., Hoeng, J., Peitsch, M.C., 2020. Respiratory effects of exposure to aerosol from the candidate modified-risk tobacco product THS 2.2 in an 18-month systems toxicology study with A/J mice. Toxicol. Sci. Submitted.

Tobacco Advisory Group of the Royal College of Physicians, 2016. Nicotine without Smoke—Tobacco Harm Reduction. London.

Uchiyama, S., Senoo, Y., Hayashida, H., Inaba, Y., Nakagome, H., Kunugita, N., 2016. Determination of chemical compounds generated from second-generation E-cigarettes using a sorbent cartridge followed by a two-step Elution method. Anal. Sci. 32, 549–555. https://doi.org/10.2116/analsci.32.549.

Valavanidis, A., Vlachogianni, T., Fiotakis, K., Loridas, S., 2013. Pulmonary oxidative stress, inflammation and cancer: respirable particulate matter, fibrous dusts and ozone as major causes of lung carcinogenesis through reactive oxygen species mechanisms. Int. J. Environ. Res. Publ. Health 10, 3886–3907. https://doi.org/10.3390/ijerph10093886.

van der Toorn, M., Slebos, D.-J., de Bruin, H.G., Gras, R., Rezayat, D., Jorge, L., Sandra, K., van Oosterhout, A.J.M., 2013. Critical role of aldehydes in cigarette smoke-induced acute airway inflammation. Respir. Res. 14, 45. https://doi.org/10.1186/1465-9921-14-45.

van der Plas, A., Pouly, S., Blanc, N., Haziza, C., de la Bourdonnaye, G., Titz, B., Hoeng, J., Ivanov, N., Taranu, B., Heremanns, A., 2020. Impact of switching to a heat-not-burn tobacco product on CYP1A2 activity. Toxicol. Rep. https://doi.org/10.1016/j.toxrep.2020.10.017. In press.

van der Toorn, M., Frentzel, S., De Leon, H., Goedertier, D., Peitsch, M.C., Hoeng, J., 2015. Aerosol from a candidate modified risk tobacco product has reduced effects on chemotaxis and transendothelial migration compared to combustion of conventional cigarettes. Food Chem. Toxicol. 86, 81–87. https://doi.org/10.1016/j.fct.2015.09.016.

van der Toorn, M., Sewer, A., Marescotti, D., Johne, S., Baumer, K., Bornand, D., Dulize, R., Merg, C., Corciulo, M., Scotti, E., Pak, C., Leroy, P., Guedj, E., Ivanov, N., Martin, F., Peitsch, M., Hoeng, J., Luettich, K., 2018. The biological effects of long-term exposure of human bronchial epithelial cells to total particulate matter from a candidate modified-risk tobacco product. Toxicol. In Vitro 50, 95–108. https://doi.org/10.1016/j.tiv.2018.02.019.

Veniant, M.M., Withycombe, S., Young, S.G., 2001. Lipoprotein size and atherosclerosis susceptibility in Apoe(-/-) and Ldlr(-/-) mice. Arterioscler. Thromb. Vasc. Biol. 21, 1567–1570.

Vink, J.M., Jansen, R., Brooks, A., Willemsen, G., van Grootheest, G., de Geus, E., Smit, J.H., Penninx, B.W., Boomsma, D.I., 2017. Differential gene expression patterns between smokers and non-smokers: cause or consequence? Addict. Biol. 22, 550–560. https://doi.org/10.1111/adb.12322.

Vlachopoulos, C., Kosmopoulou, F., Panagiotakos, D., Ioakeimidis, N., Alexopoulos, N., Pitsavos, C., Stefanadis, C., 2004. Smoking and caffeine have a synergistic detrimental effect on aortic stiffness and wave reflections. J. Am. Coll. Cardiol. 44, 1911–1917. https://doi.org/10.1016/j.jacc.2004.07.049.

Voronov, E., Shouval, D.S., Krelin, Y., Cagnano, E., Benharroch, D., Iwakura, Y., Dinarello, C.A., Apte, R.N., 2003. IL-1 is required for tumor invasiveness and angiogenesis. Proc. Natl. Acad. Sci. U.S.A. 100, 2645–2650. https://doi.org/10.1073/pnas.0437939100.

Walser, T., Cui, X., Yanagawa, J., Lee, J.M., Heinrich, E., Lee, G., Sharma, S., Dubinett, S.M., 2008. Smoking and lung cancer: the role of inflammation. Proc. Am. Thorac. Soc. 5, 811–815. https://doi.org/10.1513/pats.200809-100TH.

Ween, M.P., Whittall, J.J., Hamon, R., Reynolds, P.N., Hodge, S.J., 2017. Phagocytosis and inflammation: exploring the effects of the components of E-cigarette vapor on macrophages. Physiol. Rep. 5 https://doi.org/10.14814/phy2.13370.

Willum-Hansen, T., Staessen, J.A., Torp-Pedersen, C., Rasmussen, S., Thijs, L., Ibsen, H., Jeppesen, J., 2006. Prognostic value of aortic pulse wave velocity as index of arterial stiffness in the general population. Circulation 113, 664–670. https://doi.org/10.1161/CIRCULATIONAHA.105.579342.

Winkelmann, B.R., von Holt, K., Unverdorben, M., 2009. Smoking and atherosclerotic cardiovascular disease: Part I: atherosclerotic disease process. Biomarkers Med. 3, 411–428. https://doi.org/10.2217/bmm.09.32.

Witschi, H., 2005. A/J mouse as a model for lung tumorigenesis caused by tobacco smoke: strengths and weaknesses. Exp. Lung Res. 31, 3–18. https://doi.org/10.1080/01902140490494959.

Wong, E.T., Kogel, U., Veljkovic, E., Martin, F., Xiang, Y., Boue, S., Vuillaume, G., Leroy, P., Guedj, E., Rodrigo, G., Ivanov, N.V., Hoeng, J., Peitsch, M.C., Vanscheeuwijck, P., 2016. Evaluation of the tobacco heating system 2.2. Part 4: 90-day OECD 413 rat inhalation study with systems toxicology endpoints demonstrates reduced exposure effects compared with cigarette smoke. Regul. Toxicol. Pharmacol. 81 (Suppl. 2), S59–S81. https://doi.org/10.1016/j.yrtph.2016.10.015.

Wong, E., Luettich, K., Krishnan, S., Wong, S.K., Lim, S.K., Yeo, D., Büttner, A., Leroy, P., Vuillaume, G., Boué, S., Hoeng, J., Vanscheeuwijck, P., Peitsch, M.C., 2020. Reduced chronic toxicity and carcinogenicity in A/J mice in response to life-time exposure to aerosol from a heated tobacco product compared with cigarette smoke. Toxicol. Sci. kfaa131. https://doi.org/10.1093/toxsci/kfaa131.

Yaghi, A., Zaman, A., Cox, G., Dolovich, M.B., 2012. Ciliary beating is depressed in nasal cilia from chronic obstructive pulmonary disease subjects. Respir. Med. 106 (8), 1139–1147. https://doi.org/10.1016/j.rmed.2012.04.001.

Yang, I.A., Relan, V., Wright, C.M., Davidson, M.R., Sriram, K.B., Savarimuthu Francis, S.M., Clarke, B.E., Duhig, E.E., Bowman, R.V., Fong, K.M., 2011. Common pathogenic mechanisms and pathways in the development of COPD and lung cancer. Expert Opin. Ther. Targets 15, 439–456. https://doi.org/10.1517/14728222.2011.555400.

Yoshida, T., Tuder, R.M., 2007. Pathobiology of cigarette smoke-induced chronic obstructive pulmonary disease. Physiol. Rev. 87, 1047–1082. https://doi.org/10.1152/physrev.00048.2006.

You, R., Lu, W., Shan, M., Berlin, J.M., Samuel, E.L., Marcano, D.C., Sun, Z., Sikkema, W.K., Yuan, X., Song, L., Hendrix, A.Y., Tour, J.M., Corry, D.B., Kheradmand, F., 2015. Nanoparticulate carbon black in cigarette smoke induces DNA cleavage and Th17-mediated emphysema. Elife 4, e09623. https://doi.org/10.7554/eLife.09623.

Yuan, J.-M., Nelson, H.H., Carmella, S.G., Wang, R., Kuriger-Laber, J., Jin, A., Adams-Haduch, J., Hecht, S.S., Koh, W.-P., Murphy, S.E., 2017. CYP2A6 genetic polymorphisms and biomarkers of tobacco smoke constituents in relation to risk of lung cancer in the Singapore Chinese Health Study. Carcinogenesis 38, 411–418. https://doi.org/10.1093/carcin/bgx012.

Yuki, D., Takeshige, Y., Nakaya, K., Futamura, Y., 2018. Assessment of the exposure to harmful and potentially harmful constituents in healthy Japanese smokers using a novel tobacco vapor product compared with conventional cigarettes and smoking abstinence. Regul. Toxicol. Pharmacol. 96, 127–134. https://doi.org/10.1016/j.yrtph.2018.05.001.

Zanetti, F., Zhao, X., Pan, J., Peitsch, M.C., Hoeng, J., Ren, Y., 2019. Effects of cigarette smoke and tobacco heating aerosol on color stability of dental enamel, dentin, and composite resin restorations. Quintessence Int. 50, 156–166. https://doi.org/10.3290/j.qi.a41601.

Zha, L., Sobue, T., Kitamura, T., Kitamura, Y., Sawada, N., Iwasaki, M., Sasazuki, S., Yamaji, T., Shimazu, T., Tsugane, S., 2019. Changes in smoking status and mortality from all causes and lung cancer: a longitudinal analysis of a population-based study in Japan. J. Epidemiol. 29, 11–17. https://doi.org/10.2188/jea.JE20170112.

Zhang, R., Dai, Y., Zhang, X., Niu, Y., Meng, T., Li, Y., Duan, H., Bin, P., Ye, M., Jia, X., Shen, M., Yu, S., Yang, X., Gao, W., Zheng, Y., 2014. Reduced pulmonary function and increased pro-inflammatory cytokines in nanoscale carbon black-exposed workers. Part. Fibre Toxicol. 11, 73. https://doi.org/10.1186/s12989-014-0073-1.

Zhao, H., Albino, A.P., Jorgensen, E., Traganos, F., Darzynkiewicz, Z., 2009. DNA damage response induced by tobacco smoke in normal human bronchial epithelial and A549 pulmonary adenocarcinoma cells assessed by laser scanning cytometry. Cytometry A 75, 840–847. https://doi.org/10.1002/cyto.a.20778.

Zhao, X., Zanetti, F., Majeed, S., Pan, J., Malmstrom, H., Peitsch, M.C., Hoeng, J., Ren, Y., 2017. Effects of cigarette smoking on color stability of dental resin composites. Am. J. Dent. 30, 316–322.

Zhao, X., Zanetti, F., Majeed, S., Pan, J., Malmstrom, H., Peitsch, M.C., Hoeng, J., 2019a. Effects of 3R4F Smoke and THS 2.2 Aerosol on the Properties of Dental Resin Composites [WWW Document]. https://doi.org/10.26126/intervals.rg5ari.1.

Zhao, X., Zanetti, F., Wang, L., Pan, J., Majeed, S., Malmstrom, H., Peitsch, M.C., Hoeng, J., Ren, Y., 2019b. Effects of different discoloration challenges and whitening treatments on dental hard tissues and composite resin restorations. J. Dent. 89, 103182. https://doi.org/10.1016/j.jdent.2019.103182.

Zhao, X., Zanetti, F., Majeed, S., Pan, J., Malmstrom, H., Peitsch, M.C., Hoeng, J., Ren, Y., 2020a. Effect of 3R4F Smoke and THS 2.2 Aerosol on the Color Stability of Teeth. [WWW Document]. https://doi.org/10.26126/intervals.lypmh2.1.

Zhao, X., Zanetti, F., Wang, L., Pan, J., Majeed, S., Malmstrom, H., Peitsch, M.C., Hoeng, J., Ren, Y., 2020b. Effects of Cigarette Smoke and Electronic Cigarette Aerosol on the Coloration of Dental Hard Tissues and Composite Resin Restorations [WWW Document]. https://doi.org/10.26126/intervals.hdw42q.1.

Zhu, S.-H., Lee, M., Zhuang, Y.-L., Gamst, A., Wolfson, T., 2012. Interventions to increase smoking cessation at the population level: how much progress has been made in the last two decades? Tob. Control 21, 110–118. https://doi.org/10.1136/tobaccocontrol-2011-050371.

CHAPTER 19

Passive Exposure to ENDP Aerosols

PATRICK PICAVET • CHRISTELLE HAZIZA • CATHERINE GOUJON-GINGLINGER •
MANUEL C. PEITSCH

19.1 INTRODUCTION

In the context of tobacco harm reduction, it is paramount to understand not only the risk reduction potential of electronic nicotine delivery products (ENDPs) (Chapter 2) for smokers but also the impact of ENDP use on passively exposed bystanders, who neither smoke nor use any other tobacco- or nicotine-containing product.

It is well established that ambient air pollution contributes substantially to the global burden of disease (Cohen et al., 2017). Hence, better air quality will, in line with the principle of toxicology (Chapter 3), lead to net population health benefits (Cohen et al., 2017). Clearly, the primary goal of air quality guidelines and legislation is to guarantee the best possible air quality in all types of environments (Chapter 8).

The central tenet of tobacco harm reduction is that ENDPs emit substantially reduced levels of toxicants, which leads to a reduction in toxicant exposure when smokers completely switch to ENDP use instead of continuing to smoke cigarettes (Chapter 17). Furthermore, the degree of exposure reduction should be coherent with the degree of reduction in toxicant emissions (Chapter 4) by ENDPs, as demonstrated for an electrically heated tobacco product (Chapter 17). This is the first causal link in the causal chain of events linking smoking to disease (CELSD) (Chapter 3). This first causal link in the CELSD also applies to passive exposure, in that a reduction in ambient toxicant concentration should lead to a coherent reduction in toxicant exposure of passively exposed individuals.

It is well understood that indoor cigarette smoking leads to a significant increase in several environmental toxicants (Chapter 8) and, therefore, smoking negatively affects indoor air quality (IAQ). In contrast, indoor use of ENDPs was shown to have, in principle, a significantly lower effect than cigarette smoking on IAQ in both controlled and more real-life settings (Chapter 8). Importantly, the effects of ENDP use on IAQ were coherent with the reduced toxicant emissions of the tested products (Chapter 8). The purpose of this chapter is to answer the question whether the reduced impact of ENDPs on IAQ also leads to reduced exposure of nonsmokers and non-ENDP users (bystanders) to cigarette smoke (CS) toxicants and, thereby, verify the first causal link in the CELSD in the context of environmental exposure.

Passive exposure to CS has been shown to lead to an increase in exposure to the harmful and potentially harmful constituents (HPHCs) of CS (Ballbè et al., 2014; Goniewicz et al., 2011; Kaplan et al., 2019; Martínez-Sánchez et al., 2014; Radwan et al., 2013). Most studies have used metabolites of nicotine (e.g., cotinine) and/or tobacco-specific nitrosamines (TSNAs), such as total 4-(methylnitrosamino)-1-(3-pyridyl)-1-butanol (tNNAL), as specific biomarkers of passive CS exposure (Goniewicz et al., 2011).

In an observational study conducted with volunteers (bystanders who neither smoke nor use e-vapor products [EVPs]) who live with cigarette smokers or EVP users, passive exposure to EVP aerosols was shown to lead to reduced salivary and urinary cotinine levels relative to passive exposure to CS. This study also showed that passive exposure to EVP aerosols led to higher levels of both salivary and urinary cotinine than living in a home where no tobacco- or nicotine-containing products are used (Ballbè et al., 2014). More recently, a pilot study assessing the effects of passive EVP aerosol exposure showed that four out of six non-EVP users living with EVP users had quantifiable levels of urinary tNNAL (Martínez-Sánchez et al., 2019). Furthermore, the levels of tNNAL in all six non-EVP users were coherent with the urinary levels of tNNAL in the EVP user they lived with (Martínez-Sánchez et al., 2019).

To assess the effects of passive exposure to a specific ENDP aerosol on the body's exposure to HPHCs, it is necessary to conduct a passive exposure study in a controlled setting, where several IAQ parameters and biomarkers of exposure (BoExps) to HPHCs are

Toxicological Evaluation of Electronic Nicotine Delivery Products. https://doi.org/10.1016/B978-0-12-820490-0.00005-5

measured during the same event. Furthermore, to understand the actual effects of passive exposure, it is important to compare them with the background effects when no such exposure occurs. Philip Morris International (PMI) conducted such a study to assess the impact of using the Tobacco Heating System 2.2 (THS) on IAQ and, in turn, assess the effects of this impact on BoExps in volunteers who neither smoke nor use any other nicotine-containing product. This passive exposure study was conducted in Japan (ClinicalTrials.gov Identifier: NCT03550989).

Prior to this, PMI had conducted studies under different simulated environments to measure the impact of indoor use of THS on IAQ (Chapter 8). These studies have shown that, out of many markers typical of environmental tobacco smoke (ETS), only nicotine and acetaldehyde were quantifiable in the air following indoor use of THS (Chapter 8) (Mitova et al., 2016, 2019a,b, 2020). These studies also showed that the concentrations of these substances were far lower than the thresholds defined by existing air quality guidelines (Chapter 8). The concentrations of all other measured ETS markers were at background levels, indicating that THS is not a source of ETS and, on the basis of existing IAQ guidelines, has no negative impact on overall air quality when used in an indoor environment (Chapter 8).

19.2 PASSIVE EXPOSURE STUDY WITH THS

This was a noninterventional observational study designed to determine the impact of THS use on IAQ and, in turn, the effects of passive exposure to environmental THS aerosol on BoExps among nonsmokers. The study was conducted in a real-life restaurant setting in Japan, where THS use, but not smoking, was allowed.

19.2.1 Study Objectives

The primary objective of this study was to estimate the mean changes in the spot urine levels of BoExps to nicotine and TSNAs in the study participants caused by passive exposure to THS aerosol.

The study also evaluated the impact of THS use on IAQ by measuring the environmental concentrations of selected CS constituents that are representative of ETS (Chapter 8).

19.2.2 Study Design, Population, and Methods

The study consisted of a series of 4-h dinner events (Fig. 19.1) where food and beverages were served. Several days could pass between events, when the restaurant was used for normal business. First, two nonexposure events (N-EEs) were conducted to measure the background effects of the study population on IAQ and BoExps. Cigarette smoking and use of any other nicotine product was prohibited during all N-EEs. Second, four exposure events (EEs) were conducted to measure the effects of THS use on IAQ and BoExps. During EEs, a predefined number of participants (23% of all participants) who normally use THS is real life were permitted to use THS.

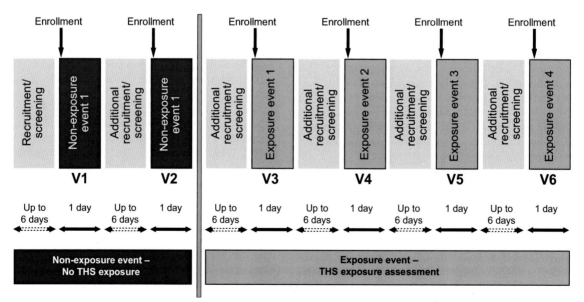

FIG. 19.1 Study flow chart of the THS passive exposure study conducted in Japan.

Three groups of participants with the following characteristics were enrolled in this study:

(1) **Nonsmokers** (defined as having abstained from using any nicotine- and/or tobacco-containing product for at least 12 months on the basis of self-reporting)

(2) **Cigarette smokers** (defined as having used at least 100 cigarettes in their lifetime, using >1 cigarette daily, with >95% of all tobacco/nicotine product use involving cigarettes)

(3) **THS users** (defined as having used at least 100 THS tobacco sticks in their lifetime, using >1 THS tobacco stick daily, with >95% of all tobacco/nicotine product use involving THS tobacco sticks)

The study participants were healthy, as self-reported. Self-reported pregnant or breast-feeding female participants were excluded from the study. Nonsmokers who either lived in a household with users of tobacco- or nicotine-containing products or were exposed to tobacco- or nicotine-containing product use at the workplace were also excluded from participation in the study.

After screening, enrolled study participants were selected to participate in a maximum of one 4-h N-EE, where no tobacco or nicotine product use was allowed, and in no more than one 4-h EE, where THS use was allowed. In the N-EEs (n = 141), on the basis of their self-reported smoking status, participants were assigned to the THS passive users group (22%), cigarette smokers group (22%), or nonsmokers group (56%). The same applied to the EEs (n = 260), with the exception that THS users were assigned to either the THS active users group or THS passive users group. Assignment to either of these two groups was performed automatically, with the THS active users group being filled first to ensure the required sample size for the events. This resulted in 54% of the EE participants being nonsmokers; 17% were cigarette smokers, while 17% were THS passive users, and 23% were assigned to the THS active users group. The baseline demographic characteristics of the study participants are presented in Fig. 19.2.

During the dinner events, a fixed menu of food, with nonalcoholic and alcoholic beverages typically served in Japanese restaurants, ensured homogeneity in the types of potential confounders of both IAQ endpoints and BoExps in the participant groups. Appetizers served at all events included carpaccio, cheese, fruits, and prosciutto. Side dishes included vegetable, potato, and rice salads. Entrees included chirashi-sushi, sashimi, penne, and spaghetti. The study personnel recorded the overall amounts of consumed food (per food type) and beverages (alcoholic and nonalcoholic).

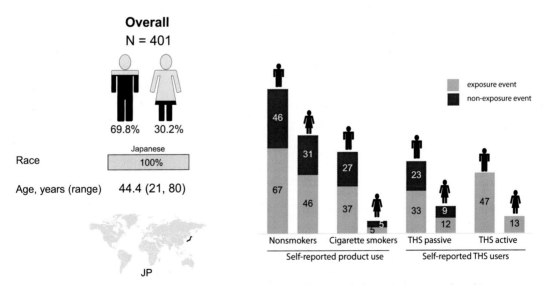

FIG. 19.2 Summary of study demographics. Participants who attended an event were assigned to a user group as described in the text. Participants may be counted twice (for each event type) if they attended more than one event. No use of tobacco- or nicotine-containing products was allowed during the nonexposure event; in the exposure event, nonsmokers, THS passive users, and cigarette smokers did not use any tobacco- or nicotine-containing products for the duration of the event; THS active users, THS users using THS for the duration of the exposure event; THS passive users, THS users not using THS for the duration of the exposure event.

Information on tobacco- and nicotine-containing product use and health status was assessed through questionnaires at enrollment and prior to each event. THS use at each EE was recorded by study personnel who collected used THS tobacco sticks at approximately 1-h intervals and evaluated the total number of tobacco sticks used per participant.

19.2.3 Product Adherence

Interpretation of results in exposure studies, as presented here, relies strongly on the accuracy of self-reported product use history and compliance. For this reason, urine specimens collected as described above were also used to confirm the self-reported nonsmoking status of the invited participants. tNNAL values over 75.9 pg/mL were used to exclude participants in the self-reported nonsmoking group from the compliant use population (Berg et al., 2012).

Furthermore, study personnel were always present during the dinner events to ensure that product use among the study participants was in compliance with the requirements of the study protocol.

19.2.4 BoExp Measurements

During these events, IAQ measurements were performed for up to 3 h prior to the start of the event (baseline assessment) and for 3 h after the last participant had entered the event for an hour. Urine samples were collected to determine BoExp levels in each participant, with the first sample collected prior to a participant entering the event hall and the second urine sample collected prior to the participant leaving the event, with a minimum exposure time of 2 h per study participant.

The level of nicotine exposure was assessed by the urinary levels of nicotine equivalents (NEQs) (Chapter 17). Exposure to TSNAs was assessed by measuring the urinary levels of tNNAL, the BoExp to 4-methylnitrosamino-1-(3-pyridyl)-1-butanone (NNK) and total N-nitrosonornicotine (tNNN), the BoExp to N-nitrosonornicotine (NNN).

19.2.5 Statistical Approach and Sample Size

Three analysis sets were defined for analysis of study results:
(1) **Enrolled participant set** (all enrolled participants who signed the informed consent form [ICF]).
(2) **Compliant exposure set** (all enrolled participants who signed the ICF, participated in an N-EE or EE, provided two urine samples [one prior to the start of event and one after a minimum 2 h of participation in the event], and were compliant with the event exposure groups [nonexposure or passive exposure]).

(3) **Active exposure set** (all enrolled participants who signed the ICF, participated as THS active users in an EE event, provided two urine samples [one prior to the start of the event and one after a minimum of 2 h after the start of active exposure], and were compliant with the active exposure group).

The tested urinary BoExps were adjusted for creatinine. In the primary analysis, the levels of the urinary BoExps (NEQ, tNNAL, and tNNN) and their changes from baseline to the end of the study were modeled by using a linear model in the compliant exposure set.

Furthermore, a mixed model analysis was performed that used the change from baseline as a dependent variable and included the following covariates in the model: baseline levels, sex, event type (N-EE or EE), duration of exposure, product use status, and product use status by event type for all BoExps. In addition, an air quality covariate related to each BoExp was included in the model, depending on the endpoint.

Appropriate contrasts were constructed to determine the effect of passive exposure to THS aerosol during the EEs on the mean change in the levels of urinary BoExp (together with the 95% confidence intervals [CIs]) in nonsmokers. Other contrasts could be constructed to determine the changes in urinary BoExps in participants with other product use statuses (cigarette smokers and THS passive users) after passive exposure to the THS. In addition, an estimate statement was added to calculate the ratio of geometric means between the exposure and nonexposure group for each product use group. The least squares (LS) means and corresponding CIs were exponentiated, back-transformed to the original scale, and reported as geometric means with CIs.

The sample size for the EEs and N-EEs was based on the expected change in exposure of a nonsmoker when exposed passively to CS, as documented in the literature. Furthermore, variability in exposure levels and method was considered for estimating the sample size needed.

19.3 PASSIVE EXPOSURE STUDY RESULTS

To our knowledge, this was the first study of its kind. The purpose of the study was to determine whether nonsmokers passively exposed to environmental THS aerosol would show higher levels of BoExps to CS constituents' representative of ETS than nonsmokers not passively exposed to THS aerosol. In addition, the study also investigated the impact of passive exposure to THS on cigarette smokers and THS users who did not use any tobacco- or nicotine-containing product during the events. This study provides insights into the background nicotine and TSNA exposure of nonsmokers, smokers, and THS users and whether passive exposure to THS aerosol has a measurable additive effect among these groups. Furthermore, IAQ was assessed during the events (Chapter 8) to understand and characterize the potential source of exposure (i.e., THS use versus background exposure in the building, study participants, food, or beverages) and, with the data on BoExp levels in the participants, to describe how environmental concentrations of nicotine and TSNAs translate into measurable human exposure.

This study provides important insights into whether THS has a negative impact on bystanders when they are passively exposed to THS in day-to-day life and, therefore, is an essential part of risk reduction assessment of a new, potentially less harmful product.

19.3.1 Nicotine Exposure

Although not the primary cause of smoking-related diseases, nicotine is addictive and not risk free (McNeill et al., 2018). The main source of exposure to nicotine is the use of tobacco- and nicotine-containing products, even though nicotine is also known to be present at low levels in certain foods (Domino et al., 1993). Nicotine is, therefore, an important compound and marker of ETS.

As outlined in Chapter 8, IAQ measurements performed during the study showed that the nicotine levels during the N-EEs were between 0.10 and 0.18 $\mu g/m^3$, whereas the highest average nicotine concentration recorded in the air during any of the EEs was about 1.5 $\mu g/m^3$, with a maximum of 2.26 $\mu g/m^3$. During the EEs, THS active users consumed a total of 187 THS tobacco sticks, on average.

19.3.2 Nicotine Exposure During Nonexposure Events

The results of the study showed that, during the N-EEs, exposure to nicotine was detected at baseline and at the end of the events in all groups, including the nonsmokers group.

At baseline, the average nicotine exposure levels were about 100 times lower in the nonsmokers group (NEQ, 0.03845 mg/g creatinine) than in the cigarette smokers group (NEQ, 4.159 mg/g creatinine) or THS passive users group (NEQ, 5.695 mg/g creatinine).

At the end of the N-EEs, the nicotine exposure levels in the nonsmokers group showed an increase (NEQ, 0.06876 mg/g creatinine; relative change, 78.85%), which was still about 100 times lower in nonsmokers than in the other groups.

In the control groups (THS passive users and cigarette smokers groups), nicotine exposure had increased by 31.96% and 29.52%, respectively (Fig. 19.3 and Table 19.1).

19.3.3 Nicotine Exposure During Exposure Events

During the EEs, nicotine was detected in the urine of nonsmokers at baseline at levels (NEQ, 0.04078 mg/g creatinine) that were, on average, about 100 times lower than the baseline levels in the cigarette smokers (NEQ, 3.051 mg/g creatinine), THS passive users (NEQ, 5.277 mg/g creatinine), and THS active users (NEQ, 4.683 mg/g creatinine) groups.

In spite of the passive exposure to THS aerosol, the nicotine exposure pattern at the end of the EEs in the nonsmokers group (NEQ, 0.6205 mg/g creatinine; relative change, 53.63%) remained similar to that observed in the same group at the end of the N-EEs. The NEQ levels were still 100 times lower in the nonsmokers group than in the other groups.

Nicotine exposure remained comparable to baseline in the cigarette smokers and THS passive users groups. The increase in nicotine levels of 79.53% in the THS active users group was expectedly more marked, as these participants had used THS during the EEs (Fig. 19.3 and Table 19.1).

The results of the statistical modeling, after adjustings for IAQ conditions to determine the effect of passive exposure to THS aerosol on the mean change in nicotine levels in the nonsmokers group, showed that nicotine exposure in this group increased with a comparable magnitude during both N-EEs and EEs (geometric LS mean of NEQ change, 1.35 and 1.20, respectively). There was no meaningful difference in the change in nicotine exposure from baseline between the two types of events in the nonsmokers group (geometric LS mean ratio, 0.89). The ressults for the cigarette smokers and THS passive users groups were comparable.

19.3.4 Exposure to TSNAs

TSNAs are notable and specific markers of ETS exposure. For this reason, NNK and NNN were monitored in the air during all dinner events. However, the levels of these TSNAs in the air were below the limit of quantification (BLQ) during the N-EEs and, more importantly, during the EEs. Consequently, the urinary levels of tNNAL and tNNN in the nonsmokers group were not quantifiable in any of the events. The levels of tNNAL and tNNN at baseline in both the N-EEs and EEs were higher in the cigarette smokers group than in the THS passive users and THS active users groups.

19.3.5 Exposure to TSNAs During Nonexposure Events

The levels of urinary BoExps to NNK and NNN (tNNAL and tNNN, respectively) in the study participants were assessed in urine samples collected at baseline and at

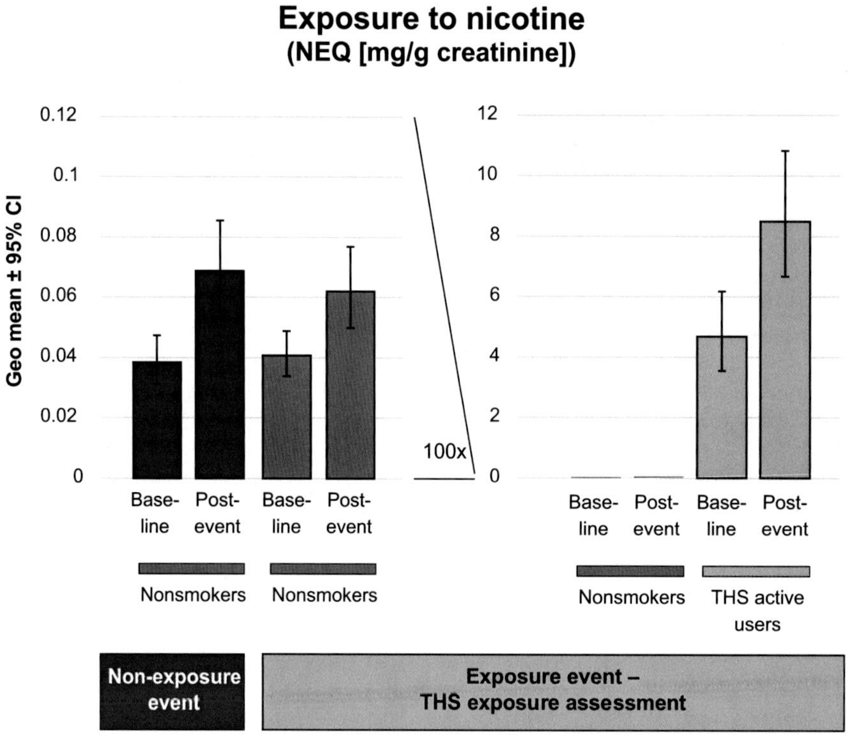

Exposure to nicotine
(NEQ [mg/g creatinine])

FIG. 19.3 Urinary biomarkers of exposure to nicotine (NEQ). *CI*, confidence interval; *Geo*, geometric; *NEQ*, nicotine equivalents.

the end of the dinner events. In the nonsmokers group, tNNAL and tNNN were not quantifiable in urinary samples at baseline or at the end of the N-EEs (96%−100% of samples BLQ).

At baseline, the levels of urinary tNNAL in the THS passive users group (20.55 ng/g creatinine) were lower than those in the cigarette smokers group (69.65 ng/g creatinine). In the cigarette smokers and THS passive users group, the levels of tNNAL at the end of the N-EEs remained comparable to the baseline levels.

In the cigarette smokers and THS passive users groups, the levels of tNNN at the end of the N-EEs were slightly increased from baseline but remained comparable to the baseline levels overall. Both at baseline and the end of the N-EEs, the tNNN levels were higher in the cigarette smokers group (3.945 and 4.008 ng/g creatinine, respectively) than in the THS passive users group (1.493 and 3.093 ng/g creatinine, respectively).

19.3.6 Exposure to TSNAs During Exposure Events

The urinary levels of tNNAL and tNNN were not quantifiable in the nonsmokers group at baseline or at the end of the EEs, even though THS use was allowed (96% of samples BLQ).

The levels of tNNAL in the THS passive users group did not increase from baseline to the end of the EEs, while those in the cigarette smokers group did. At the end of the events, the levels in the THS active users group were increased from baseline relative to those in the THS passive users group (Table 19.2).

The levels of tNNAL both at baseline and at the end of the event were higher in the cigarette smokers group (48.57 and 58.74 ng/g creatinine, respectively) than in the THS active users (21.50 and 30.45 ng/g creatinine, respectively) and THS passive users (19.68 and 20.31 ng/g creatinine, respectively) groups.

The results of tNNAL exposure in the cigarette smokers group showed comparable ratios of exposure between the baseline and end-of-event measurements across the different event types (ratio EE vs. N-EE, 0.94). However, tNNAL exposure in the THS passive exposure group was lower during the EEs than during the N-EEs (ratio EE vs. N-EE, 0.83).

At baseline, the levels of tNNN were the highest in the cigarette smokers group (2.694 ng/g creatinine), followed by the THS passive users group (1.753 ng/g creatinine) and the THS active users group (0.9088 ng/g creatinine). Similarly, at the end of the EEs, the levels of tNNN were also the highest in the cigarette smokers

TABLE 19.1
Summary of Urinary Biomarkers of Exposure—Nicotine Equivalents—Compliant Exposure Set.

			SELF-REPORTED PRODUCT USE		SELF-REPORTED THS USERS	
BoExp	**Event type**	**Time**	**Nonsmoker**	**Cigarette smoker**	**THS passive user**	**THS active user**
Creatinine-adjusted	Nonexposure	Baseline	0.03845 (107.6) [n = 70]	4.159 (316.9) [n = 27]	5.695 (82.2) [n = 27]	NA
		Final	0.06876 (118.3) [n = 73]	5.175 (316.5) [n = 30]	6.821 (91.3) [n = 31]	NA
		Relative change	78.85 (107.9) [n = 69]	29.52 (46.5) [n = 26]	31.96 (44.9) [n = 27]	NA
	Exposure	Baseline	0.04078 (126.2) [n = 112]	3.051 (447.0) [n = 38]	5.277 (111.0) [n = 44]	4.683 (144.0) [n = 59]
		Final	0.06205 (166.7) [n = 112]	2.889 (663.8) [n = 42]	5.974 (94.8) [n = 45]	8.499 (119.0) [n = 60]
		Relative change	53.63 (109.7) [n = 111]	5.668 (38.4) [n = 38]	10.22 (31.5) [n = 44]	79.53 (56.2) [n = 59]
Unadjusted	Nonexposure	Baseline	0.03433 (50.0) [n = 72]	4.158 (305.7) [n = 30]	6.199 (103.5) [n = 31]	NA
		Final	0.03388 (42.7) [n = 74]	2.203 (280.0) [n = 31]	3.349 (117.7) [n = 31]	NA
		Relative change	−1.126 (11.8) [n = 72]	−43.97 (128.0) [n = 30]	−45.97 (97.9) [n = 31]	NA
	Exposure	Baseline	0.03817 (102.7) [n = 113]	3.324 (735.8) [n = 42]	5.833 (146.3) [n = 45]	5.852 (160.8) [n = 60]
		Final	0.03709 (84.7) [n = 112]	2.120 (586.8) [n = 42]	4.089 (163.6) [n = 45]	4.916 (148.6) [n = 60]
		Relative change	−2.987 (17.5) [n = 112]	−36.21 (77.1) [n = 42]	−29.89 (119.2) [n = 45]	−15.99 (87.8) [n = 60]

All BoExp values are log-transformed (base e) prior to analysis. Presented values are in original scale after exponentiation. Values below the lower limit of quantification (LLOQ) were set to LLOQ/2. Values above the upper limit of quantification (ULOQ) were set to ULOQ. Statistics are presented as geometric mean (and geometric CV%); for relative change, geometric RC% (and geometric CV%) are presented. Baseline observation recorded prior to entering the event room. Creatinine-adjusted, NEQ/creatinine in mg/g creatinine. Final observation recorded when exiting the event room. *NA*, not applicable; *NEQ*, nicotine equivalents; *relative change*, change from baseline as the ratio ln(final)−ln(baseline); *unadjusted*, NEQ in μg/mL.

group (3.992 ng/g creatinine), but this time followed by the THS active users group (2.347 ng/g creatinine) and the THS passive users group (2.034 ng/g creatinine). The levels of tNNN increased in the cigarette smokers and THS active users groups from baseline to the end of the EEs. In comparison, only a moderate increase was observed in the THS passive users group (Table 19.3).

19.4 CONCLUSION

This chapter provides important insights into the potential impact of THS use on bystanders when they are passively exposed to THS aerosol in daily life. It is important to note that the purpose of this chapter was to evaluate the causal link between the reduced impact of THS use on IAQ (relative to cigarette smoking) (Chapter 8) and the level of exposure to aerosol constituents in bystanders who neither smoke nor use any other form of tobacco- or nicotine-containing products. The purpose was not to establish evidence to support changes in existing public smoking bans in any country.

The IAQ measurements were performed during all events of the study to understand and characterize the potential source of exposure (i.e., THS use versus

TABLE 19.2
Summary of Urinary Biomarkers of Exposure—tNNAL—Compliant Exposure Set.

			SELF-REPORTED PRODUCT USE		SELF-REPORTED THS USERS	
BoExp	Event type	Time	Nonsmoker	Cigarette smoker	THS passive	THS active
Creatinine-adjusted	Nonexposure	Baseline	NR (NR) [n = 74]	69.65 (129.8) [n = 27]	20.55 (116.2) [n = 28]	NA
		Final	NR (NR) [n = 75]	81.64 (81.6) [n = 26]	27.41 (101.4) [n = 31]	NA
		Relative change	NR (NR) [n = 0]	8.124 (18.0) [n = 20]	15.86 (34.3) [n = 18]	NA
	Exposure	Baseline	NR (NR) [n = 113]	48.57 (126.0) [n = 38]	19.68 (78.3) [n = 44]	21.50 (124.3) [n = 59]
		Final	NR (NR) [n = 113]	58.74 (81.7) [n = 42]	20.31 (81.6) [n = 45]	30.45 (90.9) [n = 58]
		Relative change	NR (NR) [n = 4]	2.785 (16.8) [n = 31]	−5.229 (22.1) [n = 32]	22.23 (30.3) [n = 42]
Unadjusted	Nonexposure	Baseline	NR (NR) [n = 74]	63.67 (177.2) [n = 30]	17.79 (172.2) [n = 31]	NA
		Final	NR (NR) [n = 75]	28.35 (198.2) [n = 31]	9.951 (181.9) [n = 31]	NA
		Relative change	NR (NR) [n = 74]	−51.72 (145.2) [n = 30]	−44.06 (111.0) [n = 31]	NA
	Exposure	Baseline	NR (NR) [n = 113]	43.53 (223.1) [n = 42]	17.83 (132.1) [n = 45]	18.84 (192.6) [n = 60]
		Final	NR (NR) [n = 113]	25.55 (271.0) [n = 42]	11.53 (146.7) [n = 45]	12.51 (208.4) [n = 60]
		Relative change	NR (NR) [n = 113]	−41.31 (71.5) [n = 42]	−35.30 (107.2) [n = 45]	−33.59 (83.4) [n = 60]

All BoExp values are log-transformed (base e) prior to analysis. Presented values are in original scale after exponentiation. Values below the lower limit of quantification (LLOQ) were set to LLOQ/2. Values above the upper limit of quantification (ULOQ) were set to ULOQ. Statistics are presented as geometric mean (and geometric CV%); for relative change, geometric RC% (and geometric CV%) are presented. Baseline observation recorded prior to entering the event room. Creatinine-adjusted, tNNAL/creatinine in ng/g creatinine. Final observation recorded when exiting the event room. *NA*, not applicable; *NR*, not reported; *relative change*, change from baseline as the ratio ln(final)−ln(baseline); *tNNAL*, total 4-(methylnitrosamino)-1-(3-pyridyl)-1-butanol; *Unadjusted*, tNNAL in pg/mL.

background exposure to the building, study participants, food, or beverages) and, with the data on BoExp levels in the participants, to describe how changes in IAQ translate into measurable exposure in humans.

First, the IAQ measurements showed that, during N-EEs, when the use of tobacco- or nicotine-containing products was not allowed—which was strictly enforced—nicotine levels were very low and increased only marginally (by 0.07 μg/m^3, on average) between background and the end of the events. During these events, human nicotine exposure (NEQ) was detected at baseline and at the end of the events across all study groups. In nonsmokers, the levels of nicotine exposure increased slightly from baseline to the end of the N-EEs, but were 100 times lower, on average, than those in the other study groups. That nicotine exposure in nonsmokers was measurable at baseline and increased during the N-EEs is best explained by the presence of study participants who used tobacco- or nicotine-containing products in their daily life. These participants may have exhaled nicotine absorbed from smoking or using THS before entering the event hall. Moreover, as shown by various studies, nicotine may be found on surfaces or clothes worn by smokers

TABLE 19.3
Summary of Primary Urinary Biomarkers of Exposure—tNNN—Compliant Exposure Set.

| BoExp | Event type | Time | SELF-REPORTED PRODUCT USE | | SELF-REPORTED THS USERS | |
			Nonsmoker	Cigarette smoker	THS passive	THS active
Creatinine-adjusted	Nonexposure	Baseline	NR (NR) [n = 74]	3.945 (85.4) [n = 27]	1.493 (134.8) [n = 27]	NA
		Final	NR (NR) [n = 75]	4.008 (176.9) [n = 25]	3.093 (202.7) [n = 29]	NA
		Relative change	NR (NR) [n = 0]	16.77 (83.8) [n = 19]	69.47 (253.5) [n = 21]	NA
	Exposure	Baseline	NR (NR) [n = 112]	2.694 (146.7) [n = 38]	1.753 (83.9) [n = 44]	0.9088 (169.7) [n = 58]
		Final	NR (NR) [n = 113]	3.992 (178.2) [n = 42]	2.034 (223.7) [n = 45]	2.347 (142.3) [n = 56]
		Relative change	NR (NR) [n = 2]	42.95 (133.1) [n = 31]	17.69 (139.8) [n = 40]	143.5 (127.7) [n = 51]
Unadjusted	Nonexposure	Baseline	NR (NR) [n = 74]	2.945 (271.5) [n = 30]	1.494 (155.0) [n = 31]	NA
		Final	NR (NR) [n = 75]	1.818 (173.2) [n = 31]	1.259 (251.6) [n = 31]	NA
		Relative change	NR (NR) [n = 74]	−39.36 (94.3) [n = 30]	−15.77 (102.3) [n = 31]	NA
	Exposure	Baseline	NR (NR) [n = 112]	2.247 (287.7) [n = 41]	1.566 (126.6) [n = 45]	0.9520 (170.5) [n = 59]
		Final	NR (NR) [n = 113]	1.591 (335.9) [n = 42]	1.187 (194.5) [n = 45]	1.380 (138.3) [n = 59]
		Relative change	NR (NR) [n = 112]	−27.38 (83.9) [n = 41]	−24.19 (102.8) [n = 45]	45.00 (94.5) [n = 59]

All BoExp values are log-transformed (base e) prior to analysis. Presented values are in original scale after exponentiation. Values below the lower limit of quantification (LLOQ) were set to LLOQ/2. Values above the upper limit of quantification (ULOQ) were set to ULOQ. Statistics are presented as geometric mean (and geometric CV%); for relative change, geometric RC% (and geometric CV%) are presented. Baseline observation recorded prior to entering the event room. Creatinine-adjusted, tNNN/creatinine in ng/g creatinine. Final observation recorded when exiting the event room. *NA*, not applicable; *NR*, not reported; *relative change*, change from baseline as the ratio ln(final)−ln(baseline); *tNNN*, total N-nitrosonornicotine; *Unadjusted*, tNNN in pg/mL.

(Bahl et al., 2014; Benton et al., 2010), which might have contributed, in part, to the presence of nicotine during N-EEs. Finally, exposure to nicotine through food consumption may have also contributed to these observations (Domino et al., 1993). These results show that exposure to low levels of nicotine exists in the current environment.

Second, the IAQ measurements showed that, during the EEs, when 23% of the participants were allowed to use THS, the highest average nicotine concentrations reached 1.5 μg/m³ (maximum of 2.26 μg/m³ in any event). These levels are in line with those of the IAQ assessment conducted under simulated conditions (Chapter 8) (Mitova et al., 2016, 2019a) and were far below the 500 μg/m³ limit of existing air quality guidelines (EU-OSHA, n.d.; "OSHA Annotated PELs | Occupational Safety and Health Administration," n.d.). Furthermore, 3-ethenylpyridine, a marker of thermal degradation of nicotine, was not measurable during any of the events. Nicotine exposure (NEQ) of nonsmokers during these EEs was similar, and not higher, to that during the N-EEs. This result is not surprising, considering the low nicotine concentrations in the air and human respiratory frequency and volume. Indeed, assuming that nonsmokers take 16 breaths per min and have a tidal volume of 0.84 L, the total inhaled volume during a 4-h event is 3226 L. With environmental nicotine concentrations of 1.5 and 2.26 $\mu g/m^3$, a nonsmoker would inhale 4.84 and 7.29 μg nicotine, respectively. This represents, respectively, 0.37% and 0.56% of the nicotine delivered by a single THS tobacco stick (Chapter 4).

In summary, after adjustment for multiple variables, including cumulative product use, the changes in nicotine exposure during the EEs showed that nonsmokers passively exposed to THS aerosol do not have an increase in nicotine exposure relative to nonsmokers not passively exposed to THS aerosol. Furthermore, the use of THS did not negatively impact IAQ, as measured by nicotine in air, considering existing IAQ guidelines.

Third, the absence of quantifiable levels of TSNAs (NNN and NNK), two potent tobacco-specific carcinogenic HPHCs, in the air during the N-EEs and, more importantly, during the EEs further strengthens the conclusion that THS use does not negatively impact IAQ. Consistent with these results, the urinary levels of their BoExp, tNNAL, and tNNN were not quantifiable in nonsmokers at baseline or at the end of any event. These results can be attributed to the previously reported significant reduction of TSNAs in THS aerosol (Chapter 4) (Schaller et al., 2016) and to the reduction in exposure observed in PMI's reduced exposure clinical studies (Haziza et al., 2016; Lüdicke et al., 2018) (Chapter 17). Moreover, the urinary levels of tNNN and tNNAL were significantly lower in THS passive and active users than in cigarette smokers, irrespective of the event type. These results add to the already published results on the exposure reduction that is achievable by switching from cigarette smoking to THS use (Haziza et al., 2016; Lüdicke et al., 2018) (Chapter 17).

REFERENCES

Bahl, V., Jacob, P., Havel, C., Schick, S.F., Talbot, P., 2014. Thirdhand cigarette smoke: factors affecting exposure and remediation. PLoS One 9, e108258. https://doi.org/10.1371/journal.pone.0108258.

Ballbè, M., Martínez-Sánchez, J.M., Sureda, X., Fu, M., Pérez-Ortuño, R., Pascual, J.A., Saltó, E., Fernández, E., 2014. Cigarettes vs. e-cigarettes: passive exposure at home measured by means of airborne marker and biomarkers. Environ. Res. 135, 76–80. https://doi.org/10.1016/j.envres.2014.09.005.

Benton, M., Chua, M.J., Gu, F., Rowell, F., Ma, J., 2010. Environmental nicotine contamination in latent fingermarks from smoker contacts and passive smoking. Forensic Sci. Int. 200, 28–34. https://doi.org/10.1016/j.forsciint.2010.03.022.

Berg, C.J., Schauer, G.L., Ahluwalia, J.S., Benowitz, N.L., 2012. Correlates of NNAL levels among nondaily and daily smokers in the college student population. Curr. Biomark. Find. 2012 https://doi.org/10.2147/CBF.S34642.

Cohen, A.J., Brauer, M., Burnett, R., Anderson, H.R., Frostad, J., Estep, K., Balakrishnan, K., Brunekreef, B., Dandona, L., Dandona, R., Feigin, V., Freedman, G., Hubbell, B., Jobling, A., Kan, H., Knibbs, L., Liu, Y., Martin, R., Morawska, L., Pope, C.A., Shin, H., Straif, K., Shaddick, G., Thomas, M., van Dingenen, R., van Donkelaar, A., Vos, T., Murray, C.J.L., Forouzanfar, M.H., 2017. Estimates and 25-year trends of the global burden of disease attributable to ambient air pollution: an analysis of data from the Global Burden of Diseases Study 2015. Lancet Lond. Engl. 389, 1907–1918. https://doi.org/10.1016/S0140-6736(17)30505-6.

Domino, E.F., Hornbach, E., Demana, T., 1993. The nicotine content of common vegetables. NEJM 329, 437. https://doi.org/10.1056/NEJM199308053290619.

EU-OSHA, n.d. Exposure to Chemical Agents and Chemical Safety - Safety and Health at Work. https://osha.europa.eu/en/legislation/guidelines/exposure_chemical_agents. (Accessed 30 June 20).

Goniewicz, M.L., Eisner, M.D., Lazcano-Ponce, E., Zielinska-Danch, W., Koszowski, B., Sobczak, A., Havel, C., Jacob, P., Benowitz, N.L., 2011. Comparison of urine cotinine and the tobacco-specific nitrosamine metabolite 4-(methylnitrosamino)-1-(3-pyridyl)-1-butanol (NNAL) and their ratio to discriminate active from passive smoking. Nicotine Tob. Res. Off. J. Soc. Res. Nicotine Tob. 13, 202–208. https://doi.org/10.1093/ntr/ntq237.

Haziza, C., de La Bourdonnaye, G., Merlet, S., Benzimra, M., Ancerewicz, J., Donelli, A., Baker, G., Picavet, P., Lüdicke, F., 2016. Assessment of the reduction in levels of exposure to harmful and potentially harmful constituents in Japanese subjects using a novel tobacco heating system compared with conventional cigarettes and smoking abstinence: a randomized controlled study in confinement. Regul. Toxicol. Pharmacol. RTP 81, 489–499. https://doi.org/10.1016/j.yrtph.2016.09.014.

Kaplan, B., Sussan, T., Rule, A., Moon, K., Grau-Perez, M., Olmedo, P., Chen, R., Carkoglu, A., Levshin, V., Wang, L., Watson, C., Blount, B., Calafat, A.M., Jarrett, J., Caldwell, K., Wang, Y., Breysse, P., Strickland, P., Cohen, J., Biswal, S., Navas-Acien, A., 2019. Waterpipe tobacco smoke: characterization of toxicants and exposure biomarkers in a cross-sectional study of waterpipe employees. Environ. Int. 127, 495–502. https://doi.org/10.1016/j.envint.2019.03.074.

Lüdicke, F., Picavet, P., Baker, G., Haziza, C., Poux, V., Lama, N., Weitkunat, R., 2018. Effects of switching to the tobacco heating system 2.2 menthol, smoking abstinence, or continued cigarette smoking on biomarkers of exposure: a randomized, controlled, open-label, multicenter study in sequential confinement and ambulatory settings (part 1). Nicotine Tob. Res. Off. J. Soc. Res. Nicotine Tob. 20, 161–172. https://doi.org/10.1093/ntr/ntw287.

Martínez-Sánchez, J.M., Ballbè, M., Pérez-Ortuño, R., Fu, M., Sureda, X., Pascual, J.A., Peruga, A., Fernández, E., 2019.

Secondhand exposure to aerosol from electronic cigarettes: pilot study of assessment of tobacco-specific nitrosamine (NNAL) in urine. Gac. Sanit. 33, 575–578. https://doi.org/10.1016/j.gaceta.2018.07.016.

Martínez-Sánchez, J.M., Sureda, X., Fu, M., Pérez-Ortuño, R., Ballbè, M., López, M.J., Saltó, E., Pascual, J.A., Fernández, E., 2014. Secondhand smoke exposure at home: assessment by biomarkers and airborne markers. Environ. Res. 133, 111–116. https://doi.org/10.1016/j.envres.2014.05.013.

McNeill, A., Brose, L., Calder, R., Bauld, L., Robson, D., 2018. Evidence Review of E-Cigarettes and Heated Tobacco Products 2018. A Report Commissioned by Public Health England. Lond. Public Health Engl.

Mitova, M.I., Campelos, P.B., Goujon-Ginglinger, C.G., Maeder, S., Mottier, N., Rouget, E.G.R., Tharin, M., Tricker, A.R., 2016. Comparison of the impact of the Tobacco Heating System 2.2 and a cigarette on indoor air quality. Regul. Toxicol. Pharmacol. 80, 91–101. https://doi.org/10.1016/j.yrtph.2016.06.005.

Mitova, M.I., Bielik, N., Campelos, P.B., Cluse, C., Goujon-Ginglinger, C.G., Jaquier, A., Gomez Lueso, M., Maeder, S., Pitton, C., Poget, L., Polier-Calame, J., Rotach, M., Rouget, E.G.R., Schaller, M., Tharin, M., Zaugg, V., 2019a. Air quality assessment of the Tobacco Heating System 2.2 under simulated residential consditions. Air Qual. Atmos. Health 12, 807–823. https://doi.org/10.1007/s11869-019-00697-6.

Mitova, M.I., Campelos, P., Goujon Ginglinger, C., Maeder, S., Mottier, N., Rouget, E.G.R., Tharin, M., Tricker, A.R., 2019b.

Impact of THS 2.2-generated Environmental Aerosol on Indoor Air Quality in Comparison with Smoke from a Commercial Cigarette. https://doi.org/10.26126/intervals.3tirx2.1.

Mitova, M., Bielik, N., Campelos, P., Cluse, C., Goujon-Gingliger, C., Jaquier, A., Gomez Lueso, M., Maeder, S., Pitton, C., Poget, L., Polier-Calame, J., Rotach, M., Rouget, E., Schaller, M., Tharin, M., Zaugg, V., 2020. Air Quality Assessment of Tobacco Heating System 2.2 under Simulated Residential Conditions. https://doi.org/10.26126/INTERVALS.4ZJDZR.1.

OSHA Annotated PELs | Occupational Safety and Health Administration, n.d. https://www.osha.gov/dsg/annotated-pels/index.html. (Accessed 30 June 20).

Radwan, G., Hecht, S.S., Carmella, S.G., Loffredo, C.A., 2013. Tobacco-specific nitrosamine exposures in smokers and nonsmokers exposed to cigarette or waterpipe tobacco smoke. Nicotine Tob. Res. 15, 130–138. https://doi.org/10.1093/ntr/nts099.

Schaller, J.-P., Keller, D., Poget, L., Pratte, P., Kaelin, E., McHugh, D., Cudazzo, G., Smart, D., Tricker, A.R., Gautier, L., Yerly, M., Reis Pires, R., Le Bouhellec, S., Ghosh, D., Hofer, I., Garcia, E., Vanscheeuwijck, P., Maeder, S., 2016. Evaluation of the Tobacco Heating System 2.2. Part 2: chemical composition, genotoxicity, cytotoxicity, and physical properties of the aerosol. Regul. Toxicol. Pharmacol. RTP 81 (Suppl. 2), S27–S47. https://doi.org/10.1016/j.yrtph.2016.10.001.

CHAPTER 20

Residual Risk of Nicotine

CAROLE MATHIS • DANIEL J. SMART • WENHAO XIA • BLAINE W. PHILLIPS •
MANUEL C. PEITSCH • JUSTYNA SZOSTAK • CARINE POUSSIN •
KARSTA LUETTICH

20.1 INTRODUCTION

As outlined in Chapter 1, the potential public health benefit of electronic nicotine delivery products (ENDPs) depends on their potential to reduce smoking-related disease risk and their acceptability as alternatives to cigarettes by adult smokers. ENDPs are only intended for current adult smokers or users who would otherwise continue to use tobacco- or nicotine-containing products.

Previous chapters have summarized nonclinical (Chapters 13–15) and clinical (Chapter 17) evidence demonstrating that switching completely from cigarette smoking to using ENDPs that emit significantly lower levels of toxicants (Chapters 4, 6–7) has the potential to reduce the risk of smoking-related disease relative to continued cigarette smoking. Because ENDPs deliver nicotine, it is also important to consider the residual health risks presented by continued nicotine exposure.

Dissociating the health effects strictly attributable to nicotine from those presented by the other chemicals typically delivered by nicotine-delivery products is challenging. Indeed, most products that deliver nicotine, with the exception of nicotine replacement therapies (NRTs) such as nicotine patches and gums, also deliver varying levels of known toxicants, including tobacco-specific nitrosamines (TSNAs), polycyclic aromatic hydrocarbons, and carbonyls. Nevertheless, clinical and epidemiological studies on NRTs and smokeless tobacco (SLT) products, such as Swedish *snus*, provide important insights into the long-term health effects of nicotine dissociated from those of cigarette smoke.

The biological effects of nicotine have been studied in many nonclinical studies, both in vivo and in vitro. Unfortunately, only few of these in vivo studies have followed well-established international guidelines[1] and

---

adequately measured nicotine uptake in blood. While inhalation studies are best suited for gaining insights into the effects of nicotine in the context of ENDP assessment, only few such studies have been reported, and nicotine was mostly administered orally (p.o.), subcutaneously (s.c.), or intraperitoneally (i.p.) in these studies.

Furthermore, few in vitro studies have used nicotine concentrations or doses that are relevant to human exposure. Indeed, many in vitro studies have employed nicotine concentrations well above the blood nicotine concentration reached by human smokers, which is approximately 22 ng/mL nicotine (136 nM), with a maximum of 35 ng/mL nicotine (216 nM) over a 24-h period (Benowitz et al., 1983; Hukkanen et al., 2005). Moreover, nicotine patch users have an average plasma nicotine concentration of 10–16 ng/mL (62–100 nM), with a maximum of 16–18 ng/mL (100–111 nM) over a 24-h period, depending on the patch used (DeVeaugh-Geiss et al., 2010). While studies with higher nicotine concentrations may inform on the potential mechanistic effects of nicotine, they are of limited relevance when assessing the health risks presented by nicotine.

These shortcomings make the interpretation of most nonclinical studies with nicotine difficult and limit the translation of their findings to humans.

Here, we summarize the available epidemiological and clinical studies on STLs and NRTs as well as in vivo and in vitro studies that have examined the mechanisms and biological processes modulated by nicotine in the context of smoking-related diseases.

20.2 NICOTINE AND CARDIOVASCULAR DISEASE

20.2.1 Introduction

Nicotine has been reported as having various effects on the cardiovascular system. After binding to nicotinic cholinergic receptors present in the autonomic ganglia

---

[1]https://www.oecd.org/env/ehs/testing/
oecdguidelinesforthetestingofchemicals.htm.

Toxicological Evaluation of Electronic Nicotine Delivery Products. https://doi.org/10.1016/B978-0-12-820490-0.00022-5

513

and adrenal glands, nicotine triggers the release of cate-cholamines such as norepinephrine and epinephrine, which stimulate the sympathetic nervous system and, subsequently, hemodynamics, depending on the plasma nicotine levels (St Helen et al., 2016; Yan and D'Ruiz, 2015). Sympathetic activation raises the heart rate and blood pressure, potentially promoting ischemia, arrhythmias (Benowitz, 2003), and atherosclerosis (Libby et al., 2016). In humans, isolating the effects of nicotine from those of other components contained in tobacco products remains challenging and necessitates investigation of the conditions in which individuals are exposed to nicotine-containing products, but without combustion. In this context, we reviewed the current clinical and epidemiological evidence on the impact of SLT products, e-vapor products (EVPs), and NRTs on cardiovascular disease (CVD) effects and risks. We also summarized the mechanistic evidence from in vivo and in vitro studies that have investigated the effects of nicotine on the cardiovascular system and development of CVDs, such as atherosclerosis and abdominal aneurysms, in animal models. We carefully captured the nicotine concentrations or doses at which effects were reported, in order to evaluate their relevance and allow better interpretability with respect to human exposure.

20.2.2 Does Nicotine Cause CVD?

20.2.2.1 Epidemiological and clinical evidence

20.2.2.1.1 Smokeless tobacco products. Approximately 25% of the total tobacco consumption worldwide is in the form of SLT (FCTC WHO, 2019; Mehrotra et al., 2019), and 82% percent of global SLT users live in Southeast Asia (Mehrotra et al., 2019; Sinha et al., 2018). In India, the number of SLT users surpasses that of smokers, and SLT consumption is common in some countries in Central Asia and Africa, in Sweden in Europe, and in the United States (US).

Unlike cigarettes, which are consumed through inhalation of smoke generated by burning tobacco, SLT products are consumed p.o. through application to the gums (e.g., snus and tobacco tooth powders) or nasal inhalation (e.g., snuff) without combustion, although they still deliver nicotine and other compounds. Chemical analyses of SLT products have demonstrated the presence of different classes of compounds, including potent carcinogens such as polycyclic aromatic hydrocarbons, inorganic metals, and TSNAs. The levels of these toxicants in SLT products vary greatly worldwide, depending on the type of tobacco plant, agricultural methods, pesticides, harvesting techniques, processing methods, and storage conditions (Mehrotra et al., 2019).

The possible association between SLT product use and CVD is based on the presence of nicotine (Asplund et al., 2003). Nicotine concentrations can vary depending on the SLT product, with concentrations ranging from an average of 9.9 mg/g chewing tobacco to 16.8 mg/g dry snuff (Djordjevic and Doran, 2009). Nicotine released from SLT products is absorbed through the mucous membranes of the mouth or nose and passes into the bloodstream. The level of nicotine in the blood of SLT users has been reported to be similar to that of smokers, although it remains high in the blood for a longer period (Benowitz et al., 1988; Digard et al., 2013).

Several reviews, including metaanalyses of epidemiological, case-control, and cross-sectional studies, have evaluated the risk of ischemic heart disease (IHD)/coronary heart disease (CHD) and stroke incidence and/or mortality associated with the use of SLT. Overall, the reviews/metaanalyses referenced in this chapter cover more than 50 studies from 1980 to 2017 (Table 20.1). They report the relative risk (RR) or odds ratios (ORs) estimated from a different number of studies or study estimates, depending on data availability and inclusion/exclusion criteria considered for the metaanalysis (Table 20.2).

20.2.2.1.1.1 IHD and stroke. Multiple metaanalyses have reported no significant overall higher risk of IHD in SLT users, with pooled-analysis OR or RR values ranging from 0.99 (95% confidence interval [CI], 0.89−1.10) to 1.19 (95% CI, 0.88−1.49) (Table 20.2). However, a positive association has been demonstrated between SLT use and IHD mortality, with RR or OR values ranging from 1.10 (95% CI, 1.00−1.20) to 1.15 (95% CI, 1.01−1.30). Boffetta and Straif also reported a nonsignificant overall higher risk of stroke associated with SLT use, but a significantly higher overall risk of mortality from stroke, with an RR of 1.40 (95% CI, 1.28−1.54) (Boffetta and Straif, 2009).

Subgroup analysis of the different evaluated risks demonstrated major regional differences (Table 20.2). SLT use was found to be significantly associated with a higher risk of IHD in the American regions/USA and Asian regions and in a multicountry study, while the RR/OR risk values obtained for the South East Asian region and European region/Sweden were not significant. In contrast, the risk of fatal CHD was significant and the highest in European SLT users (in comparison with American and Southeast Asian SLT users), which suggests that SLT products used in Europe may have a more deleterious effect on CHD outcome than those used in the Americas or Southeast Asia. Regional disparities were also observed in the risk of stroke or stroke mortality, which was reported to be significantly increased in

TABLE 20.1

Overview of the Epidemiological, Case-Control, and Cross-Sectional Studies Covered in the Reviews and Metaanalyses Cited in This Chapter, That Have Evaluated the Risk of IHD/CHD and Stroke Incidence and/or Mortality Associated With the Use of SLT Products; the Results of These Studies Are Recapitulated in Table 20.2.

Study	Year	Region	Product Type	Clarke et al. (2019) RE	Gupta et al. (2018) MA	Gupta et al. (2019) RE	Rostron et al. (2018) MA	Sinha et al. (2018) MA	Vidyasagaran et al. (2016) MA	Boffetta and Straif (2009) MA
		Publication type								
Accortt NA	2002	American region	SLT		Yes	Yes	Yes	Yes	Yes	Yes
Agasche A	2010	South East Asian region	Chewing			Yes				
Alexander M	2013	Eastern Mediterranean region	Naswar Tobacco chewing		Yes				Yes	
Arefalk G	2012	European region	Snus	Yes		Yes	Yes			
Arefalk G	2014	European region	Snus				Yes			
Asplund K	2003	European region	Snuff	Yes		Yes	Yes		Yes	Yes
Ayo-Yusuf OA	2008	African region	Snuff			H				
Bhadoria AS	2014	South East Asian region	Chewing			H				
Bolinder G	1992	European region	SLT			H				
Bolinder G	1994	European region	SLT/Snus	Yes	Yes	Yes	Yes		Yes	
Choudhury SA	2017	South East Asian region	SLT			H				
Etemadi A	2017	Eastern Mediterranean region	Nass chewing		Yes	Yes				
Gajalakshmi V	2015	South East Asian region	Tobacco chewing		Yes	Yes		Yes		

Continued

TABLE 20.1

Overview of the Epidemiological, Case-Control, and Cross-Sectional Studies Covered in the Reviews and Metaanalyses Cited in This Chapter, That Have Evaluated the Risk of IHD/CHD and Stroke Incidence and/or Mortality Associated With the Use of SLT Products; the Results of These Studies Are Recapitulated in Table 20.2.—cont'd

Study	Year	Region	Product Type	Clarke et al. (2019)	Gupta et al. (2018)	Gupta et al. (2019)	Rostron et al. (2018)	Sinha et al. (2018)	Vidyasagaran et al. (2016)	Boffetta and Straif (2009)
			Publication type	RE	MA	RE	MA	MA	MA	MA
Gupta PC	1984	South East Asian region - India	SLT							
Gupta PC	2007	South East Asian region	Chewing			H				
Gupta PC	2005	South East Asian region	Mishri and others/Chewing		Yes	Yes		Yes	Yes	
Haglund B	2007	European region	Snuff	Yes	Yes	Yes		Yes	Yes	Yes
Hansson J	2009	European region	Snus	Yes		Yes	Yes			
Hansson J	2012	European region	Snus	Yes			Yes			
Hansson J	2014	European region	Snus	Yes		Yes	Yes			
Hazarika NC	2004	South East Asian region	Chewing			H				
Henley SJ	2005	American region	Tobacco chewing/Snuff		Yes	Yes	Yes	Yes	Yes	Yes
Henley SJ	2007	American region	Spit tobacco				Yes			
Hergens MP	2007	European region	Snuff	Yes	Yes	Yes	Yes	Yes	Yes	Yes
Hergens MP	2005	European region	Snuff	Yes	Yes	Yes	Yes	Yes	Yes	Yes
Hergens MP	2008	European region	Snuff	Yes		Yes|H	Yes	Yes	Yes	Yes
Huhtasaari F	1992	European region	Snuff	Yes	Yes	Yes	Yes		Yes	Yes

Author	Year	Region	Product						
Huhtasaari F	1999	European region	Snuff	Yes	Yes	Yes	Yes	Yes	Yes
Islam SM	2015	South East Asian region	SLT					H	
Ismail IM	2016	South East Asian region	SLT					H	
Janzon E	2009	European region	Snuff				Yes	Yes	Yes
Johansson SE	2005	European region	Snus		Yes		Yes		Yes
Johansson SE	2007	European region	Snuff					Yes	
Kannan A	2009	South East Asian region	Chewing					H	
Khanam MA	2015	South East Asian region	Chewing					H	Yes
Mateen F	2012	South East Asian region	Tobacco powder		Yes				
Mushtaq N	2010	American region	SLT				Yes		
Pandey A	2009	South East Asian region	SLT					H	
Rahman MA	2008	South East Asian region	Dried tobacco leaves		Yes				Yes
Rahman MA	2012	South East Asian region	Jarda, sada pata, gul		Yes				Yes
Ram RV	2012	South East Asian region	SLT				Yes		
Roosaar A	2008	European region	Snus			Yes			
Sen A	2015	South East Asian region	SLT					H	
Shah SM	2001	Eastern Mediterranean region	Snuff					H	
Teo KK	2006	Multicountry (INTERHEART study)	Chewing		Yes				Yes

Continued

TABLE 20.1

Overview of the Epidemiological, Case-Control, and Cross-Sectional Studies Covered in the Reviews and Metaanalyses Cited in This Chapter, That Have Evaluated the Risk of IHD/CHD and Stroke Incidence and/or Mortality Associated With the Use of SLT Products; the Results of These Studies Are Recapitulated in Table 20.2.—cont'd

Study	Year	Region	Product Type	Clarke et al. (2019)	Gupta et al. (2018)	Gupta et al. (2019)	Rostron et al. (2018)	Sinha et al. (2018)	Vidyasagaran et al. (2016)	Boffetta and Straif (2009)
			Publication type	RE	MA	RE	MA	MA	MA	MA
Timberlake DS	2017	American region	Smokeless tobacco, snuff and tobacco chewing			Yes	Yes			
Vendhan G	2015	South East Asian region	Tobacco chewing						Yes	
Wennberg P	2007	European region	Snuff	Yes	Yes	Yes	Yes	Yes	Yes	Yes
Wu F	2015	South East Asian region	SLT					Yes		
Yatsuya H	2010	American region	SLT				Yes			

H, hypertension; *SLT*, smokeless tobacco; *Yes*, associated with ischemic heart disease and/or stroke; *RE*, Review; *MA*, Metaanalysis.

From Boffetta, P., Straif, K., 2009. Use of smokeless tobacco and risk of myocardial infarction and stroke: systematic review with meta-analysis. BMJ. 339, b3060. Clarke, E., Thompson, K., Weaver, S., Thompson, J., O'connell, G., 2019. Snus: a compelling harm reduction alternative to cigarettes. Harm Reduct. J. 16(1), 62. Gupta, R., Gupta, S., Sharma, S., Sinha, D.N. and Mehrotra, R., 2018. A systematic review on association between smokeless tobacco & cardiovascular diseases. Indian J Med Res. 148(1), 77—89. Gupta, R., Gupta, S., Sharma, S., Sinha, D.N., Mehrotra, R., 2019. Risk of coronary heart disease among smokeless tobacco users: results of systematic review and meta-analysis of global data. Nicotine and Tob. Res. 21(1), 25—31. Rostron, B.L., Chang, J.T., Anic, G.M., Tanwar, M., Chang, C.M., Corey, C.G., 2018. Smokeless tobaccc use and circulatory disease risk: a systematic review and meta-analysis. Open Heart. 5(2), e000846. Sinha, D.N., Gupta, P.C., Kumar, A., Bhartiya, D., Agarwal, N., Sharma, S., et al., 2018. The poorest of poor suffer the greatest burden from smokeless tobacco use: a study from 140 countries. Nicotine Tob. Res. 20(12), 1529—1532. Vidyasagaran, A.L., Siddiqi, K., Kanaan, M., 2016. Use of smokeless tobacco and risk of cardiovascular disease: A systematic review and meta-analysis. Eur. J. Prev. Cardiol. 23(18), 1970—1981.

TABLE 20.2
Smokeless Tobacco Use and Cardiovascular Outcomes.

CVD Outcome	Analysis	Region/Product	MetaAnalysis	Estimate Type	Estimates	95% CI	n*	Comment
IHD/CHD	Overall		Gupta et al. (2019)	OR	1.05	0.96–1.15	20	Any**
			Gupta et al. (2019)	OR	1.19	0.88–1.49	8	Nonfatal CHD
			Vidyasagaran et al. (2016)	OR	1.14	0.92–1.42	15	
			Boffetta and Straif (2009)	RR	0.99	0.89–1.10	9	Any
	Region-wise	AMR (USA)	Rostron et al. (2018)	**RR**	**1.17**	**1.08–1.27**	**3**	
		AMR (USA)	Boffetta and Straif (2009)	**RR**	**1.11**	**1.04–1.19**	**3**	
		SEAR	Gupta et al. (2019)	OR	1.30	0.39–2.21	3	Nonfatal CHD
		ASIA	Vidyasagaran et al. (2016)	**OR**	**1.40**	**1.01–1.95**	**4**	
		EMAR	Gupta et al. (2019)	**OR**	**1.59**	**1.34–1.83**	**1**	Nonfatal CHD
		EUR	Gupta et al. (2019)	OR	0.92	0.81–1.03	3	Nonfatal CHD
		EUR (Sweden)	Rostron et al. (2018)	RR	1.04	0.93–1.16	3	
		EUR	Vidyasagaran et al. (2016)	OR	0.91	0.83–1.01	10	
		EUR (Sweden)	Boffetta and Straif (2009)	RR	0.87	0.75–1.02	6	
	Multicountry		Gupta et al. (2019)	**OR**	**2.23**	**1.17–3.29**	**1**	Nonfatal CHD
		52 countries	Vidyasagaran et al. (2016)	**OR**	**2.23**	**1.41–3.53**	**1**	
	Product-wise	Snuff	Gupta et al. (2019)	OR	0.96	0.86–1.06	7	
		Chewing tobacco	Gupta et al. (2019)	OR	1.13	0.92–1.33	7	
	Switching from TS to SLT	AMR (USA)	Rostron et al. (2018)	**RR**	**1.13**	**1.00–1.29**	**1**	

Continued

TABLE 20.2
Smokeless Tobacco Use and Cardiovascular Outcomes.—cont'd

CVD Outcome	Analysis	Region/Product	MetaAnalysis	Estimate Type	Estimates	95% CI	n*	Comment
IHD/CHD mortality	Overall		Gupta et al. (2019)	OR	1.10	1.00–1.20	11	
			Sinha et al. (2018)	OR	1.10	1.04–1.17	17	
			Vidyasagaran et al. (2016)	OR	1.15	1.01–1.30	12	
			Boffetta and Straif_2009	RR	1.13	1.06–1.21	8	
	Region-wise	AMR	Gupta et al. (2019)	OR	1.04	0.83–1.24	2	
		AMR	Sinha et al. (2018)	OR	1.16	1.00–1.34	4	
		AMR	Vidyasagaran et al. (2016)	OR	1.03	0.83–1.27	5	
		AMR (USA)	Boffetta and Straif (2009)	RR	1.11	1.04–1.19	3	
		SEAR	Gupta et al. (2019)	OR	1.03	0.86–1.19	2	
		SEAR	Sinha et al. (2018)	OR	1.06	0.97–1.16	7	
		ASIA	Vidyasagaran et al. (2016)	OR	1.05	0.76–1.47	2	
		EMAR	Gupta et al. (2019)	OR	1.13	0.84–1.41	1	
		EUR	Gupta et al. (2019)	OR	1.30	1.14–1.47	6	
		EUR	Sinha et al. (2018)	OR	1.16	1.05–1.28	6	
		EUR (Sweden)	Vidyasagaran et al. (2016)	OR	1.38	1.13–1.67	5	
		EUR (Sweden)	Boffetta and Straif (2009)	RR	1.27	1.07–1.52	5	
	Product-wise	Snuff	Gupta et al. (2019)	OR	1.37	1.14–1.61	4	
		Chewing tobacco	Gupta et al. (2019)	OR	1.07	0.91–1.23	Not reported	
Stroke	Overall		Boffetta and Straif (2009)	RR	1.19	0.97–1.47	6	Any
	Region-wise	AMR (USA)	Rostron et al. (2018)	RR	1.28	1.01–1.62	3	

Endpoint	Subgroup	Region	Study	Type	Estimate	95% CI	No.	SLT use
		AMR (USA)	Boffetta and Straif (2009)	**RR**	**1.39**	**1.22–1.60**	**3**	Any
		EUR (Sweden)	Vidyasagaran et al. (2016)	OR	1.01	0.90–1.13	4	
		EUR (Sweden)	Rostron et al. (2018)	RR	1.04	0.92–1.17	1	
		EUR (Sweden)	Boffetta and Straif (2009)	RR	1.02	0.93–1.13	3	Any
Switching from TS to SLT		AMR (USA)	Rostron et al. (2018)	**OR**	**1.24**	**1.01–1.53**	**1**	
Stroke mortality	Overall		Sinha et al. (2018)	**OR**	**1.37**	**1.24–1.51**	**12**	
			Vidyasagaran et al. (2016)	**OR**	**1.39**	**1.29–1.49**	**12**	
			Boffetta and Straif (2009)	**RR**	**1.40**	**1.28–1.54**	**5**	
	Region-wise	AMR	Sinha et al. (2018)	**OR**	**1.44**	**1.30–1.59**	**4**	
		AMR	Vidyasagaran et al.	**OR**	**1.42**	**1.29–1.57**	**5**	
		AMR (USA)	Boffetta and Straif (2009)	**RR**	**1.39**	**1.22–1.60**	**3**	
		ASIA	Vidyasagaran et al. (2016)	**OR**	**1.34**	**1.18–1.52**	**4**	
		SEAR	Sinha et al. (2018)	**OR**	**1.37**	**1.14–1.64**	**6**	
		EUR	Sinha et al. (2018)	OR	1.25	0.91–1.70	2	
		EUR	Vidyasagaran et al.	OR	1.28	0.98–1.68	3	
		EUR (Sweden)	Boffetta and Straif (2009)	RR	1.25	0.91–1.70	2	
All circulatory disease	Region-wise	AMR (USA)	Rostron et al. (2018)	RR	1.14	0.55–2.39	1	
		EUR (Sweden)	Rostron et al. (2018)	RR	1.15	0.97–1.37	1	

*, Number of study estimates or studies; **, Same result after adjustment for smoking; Bold numbers indicate significant OR or RR. AMR, American region; EMAR, Eastern Mediterranean region; EUR, European region; IHD/CHD, ischemic heart disease/coronary heart disease; OR, odds ratio; RR, risk ratio or relative risk; SLT, smokeless tobacco; SEAR, South East Asian region; TS, tobacco smoking.

American and Asian SLT users but not significantly increased in European SLT users. These regional differences have been attributed to the variations in the chemical composition of the products used in these regions. SLT products from different geographical regions are manufactured under different conditions and frequently contain substances other than tobacco (IARC Working Group on the Evaluation of Carcinogenic Risks to Humans, 2007).

Product-wise analysis showed no significant positive association between chewing tobacco and fatal CHD (RR, 1.07; 95% CI, 0.91–1.23), while it revealed a significant positive association of fatal CHD with snuff/snus use (RR, 1.37; 95% CI, 1.14–1.61) (Gupta et al., 2019). This latter observation is supported by a study that showed a reduction in postmyocardial infarction mortality risk in snus quitters (Hergens et al., 2007). Further studies are required to confirm this association between fatal CHD and snuff/snus use. The lower mortality from smoking-related diseases among Swedish men who consume snus (Peto et al., 1992; SCENIHR (Scientific Committee on Emerging and Newly-Identified Health Risks), 2008), which is also supported by epidemiological evidence, suggests that snus may be a less harmful alternative to cigarettes. Snus is the most commonly used SLT product in Sweden, accounting for 20% of oral tobacco use in the European Union (EU), which has resulted in the lowest prevalence of daily cigarette use in the EU at 5% (Clarke et al., 2019). The health benefits of completely switching from cigarette smoking to snus use are similar to those reported for smoking cessation (Ramström et al., 2016). The Scientific Committee on Emerging and Newly Identified Health Risks concluded that snus use provides an overall risk reduction close to 50% for CVD relative to cigarette smoking (SCENIHR (Scientific Committee on Emerging and Newly-Identified Health Risks), 2008). The concentrations of numerous harmful chemicals, such as TSNAs, in Swedish snus have diminished over the past two decades because of improvements and standardization in production and processing techniques (Rutqvist et al., 2011). For example, the TSNA levels in Swedish Match's snus products have dropped from 15 to 20 µg/g dry weight in 1984 to 1–2 µg/g in 2010. These TSNA levels follow the US Food and Drug Administration's (FDA) proposed product standard, which recommends limiting the level of N-nitrosonornicotine in SLT to no more than 1 µg/g tobacco dry weight for reducing tobacco-related harm (Berman and Hatsukami, 2018).

20.2.2.1.1.2 Other CVD risk factors. Several studies have investigated the impact of SLT on heart function and blood pressure. Studies on the effects of SLT products such as snuff (Hergens et al., 2008; Hirsch et al.,

1992; Rohani and Agewall, 2004), gutka (Raghavendra et al., 2013), and maras powder (Akcay et al., 2015) have reported significant increases in resting blood pressure and heart rate, with lower delta heart rate (Raghavendra et al., 2013), changes in other heart function parameters, and altered pulse and blood pressure after use (Bolinder and de Faire, 1998; Bolinder et al., 1992; Gupta et al., 2018; Hergens et al., 2008; Hirsch et al., 1992; Rohani and Agewall, 2004; Sundstrom et al., 2012).

The impact of snus use on cardiovascular function was demonstrated by a study which showed a decrease in resting heart rate in habitual snus users who had quit the product for 6 weeks relative to subjects who continued to use it, although the results showed no significant differences in blood pressure (Bjorkman et al., 2017). Some studies have reported an acute increase in heart rate and blood pressure concomitant with an elevation in plasma epinephrine levels after administration of snuff (Wolk et al., 2005). Other studies reporting an association of SLT use with hypertension indicate that recurrent use of SLT products results in a sustained moderate nicotine level in the blood, causing sympathetic nervous system activation and increased blood pressure (Hergens et al., 2008). A positive association between serum cotinine and blood pressure reported in SLT users indicates an effect of nicotine (Bolinder and de Faire, 1998).

There are several limitations worth noting when interpreting these results:

- There was no systematic adjustment for smoking across the studies and a lack of adequate adjustment for potential confounding risk factors (e.g., body mass index, blood pressure, cholesterol levels, and other disease-specific risks) in many studies, which may have affected the results.
- Many studies lacked information on some important confounders like alcohol intake, medical history, and changes in tobacco product use.
- The studies were generally based on self-reporting, with no biochemical confirmation for quantifying SLT exposure.
- The heterogeneity in SLT types depending on the regions (e.g., snus in Sweden and chewing tobacco in Asia) was not accounted for.
- The heterogeneous numbers of studies per region make it challenging to compare the estimates (e.g., the low number of studies from the African and Western Pacific regions despite a high prevalence of SLT use in some areas of these regions).

Therefore, additional well-designed and multicountry studies with uniform methodologies and relevant confounder adjustments are necessary to evaluate the effects of SLT use on CVD risk. These studies should address the study limitations listed above and (i) adjust for smoking, (ii) properly account for confounders, (iii) correlate health effects with product-specific nicotine and toxicant contents, and (iv) verify self-reported product use patterns with biomarkers of exposure that discriminate cigarette smoking from SLT, NRT, and EVP use.

Despite these limitations, the metaanalyses and study reviews listed in Table 20.1 indicate that SLT products may increase the risk of death after myocardial infarction or stroke, but their use is not associated with an increased risk of myocardial infarction or stroke. Metaanalyses conducted by regional groups have highlighted variations in the results from European, American, and Southeastern Asian SLT users that may be explained by various factors, such as region-wise differences in the SLT products used and their chemical composition, the heterogeneity in the methodologies used for conducting the studies, other cardiovascular risk factors, and a lack of systematic information on and adjustment for confounding risk factors. None of these studies can isolate the effects of nicotine from those of the other compounds contained in SLT products. However, according to reports on snus (Asplund et al., 2003; Haglund et al., 2007; Hansson et al., 2014), nicotine is unlikely to contribute significantly to the pathophysiology of stroke. Nevertheless, nicotine may account for the sympathetic nervous system activation and blood pressure and heart rate increases recorded after SLT use, which may or may not translate to a higher risk of CVDs or adverse events in the long term.

20.2.2.1.2 E-vapor products. EVPs have evolved rapidly since their introduction in 2006 (Chapter 2). Yet all EVPs vaporize an e-liquid by activation of a heating system, typically a coil, triggered by airflow. E-liquids are mixtures of propylene glycol (PG) and vegetable glycerol (VG) in various proportions, water, nicotine, and flavors (Bhatnagar et al., 2014). Most EVPs have been reported to deliver not only nicotine but also other compounds such as carbonyls (Belushkin et al., 2020), metals, flavors, and other chemicals possibly generated by the thermal decomposition of e-liquid ingredients (Khlystov and Samburova, 2016; Ogunwale et al., 2017; Wang et al., 2017b) (Chapter 4). Emission of these compounds by EVPs depends on various parameters, such as the power applied to the heating device, PG/VG ratio, flavors present in the liquid, and efficiency/efficacy of the vaporization system (Bekki et al., 2014; Kosmider et al., 2014).

Carbonyls such as acrolein, formaldehyde, and acetaldehyde have been shown to induce oxidative stress and inflammation processes that accelerate atherosclerosis (McEvoy et al., 2015; Shields et al., 2017; Zirak et al., 2019). In rodents, elevated carbonyls levels cause an increase in number and activation of platelets, decrease in the number and function of myocardial mitochondria, and decrease in left ventricular end-systolic pressure and heart rate (Hom et al., 2016; Jin et al., 2014; Qasim et al., 2018; Takeshita et al., 2009). Metals have been reported in EVP vapors; however, their concentrations tend to fall below the regulatory limits for daily occupational exposure (Farsalinos et al., 2015). Flavors are a key ingredient of e-liquids and, hence, EVP vapors. Although many of these chemicals are safe when ingested, uncertainties about their effects following chronic inhalation persist because of limited data (Sears et al., 2017) (Chapter 16). Certain flavors have been described to trigger cytotoxicity and inflammatory responses in cells such as monocytes and endothelial cells, leading to dysfunction when tested in the form of e-liquids and in the lungs following inhalation (Fetterman et al., 2018; Muthumalage et al., 2019).

Given the potential negative impact the EVP-derived compounds mentioned above have on the cardiovascular system, either individually or in combination through additive and/or synergistic effects, it is challenging to isolate the effects of nicotine alone. Clinical studies have been conducted to evaluate the impact of acute and chronic EVP use on CVD risk factors. A subset of studies included groups of subjects who used EVPs with or without nicotine or used EVP devices with varying percentages of nicotine in the same solvent vehicles, providing an opportunity to estimate potential nicotine effects.

20.2.2.1.2.1 Effects of EVP use on heart rate and blood pressure

20.2.2.1.2.1.1 Acute effects. Several studies investigated the acute effects of electronic cigarette (e-cigarette) use on heart rate and blood pressure. A metaanalysis of 11 studies reported significant acute effects of EVP use on heart rate and systolic and diastolic blood pressure, with mean differences of 2.27 bpm ($P < .0001$), 2.02 mmHg ($P < .042$), and 2.01 mmHg ($P < .004$), respectively (Skotsimara et al., 2019). In their metaanalysis, Garcia et al. specifically focused on comparing the acute effects of EVP use and cigarette smoking on autonomic cardiovascular activity (Garcia et al., 2020). The overall mean differences between cigarette smoking and EVP use reported for heart rate and systolic and diastolic pressure were 3.06 bpm ($P < .00001$), 1.58 mmHg ($P = .025$), and 1.57 mmHg ($P = .01$), respectively. Therefore, most (Biondi-Zoccai et al., 2019; Farsalinos et al., 2014; Kerr et al., 2019; Vansickel et al., 2010; Yan and D'Ruiz, 2015), though not all (Franzen et al., 2018; Ikonomidis et al., 2018; Vlachopoulos et al., 2016), studies indicate that the effects of EVP use on acute cardiovascular autonomic functions are smaller than those of cigarette smoking. It is important to note that most studies did not confirm whether the levels of nicotine exposure were comparable between tobacco smokers and EVP users. Only Yan and colleagues monitored the delivery of nicotine in plasma by five different EVPs (two commercial and three noncommercial products) and a commercial cigarette brand. They reported significantly lower levels of nicotine in EVP users than in cigarette smokers after 1.5 h of product use and, to some extent, a positive correlation with heart rate change from baseline, but no correlation with a significant increase in systolic blood pressure (Yan and D'Ruiz, 2015).

Some clinical studies specifically addressed the question of the effect of nicotine on the autonomic cardiovascular nervous system and hemodynamics in the context of EVP use by comparing the acute effects of EVPs that contain and do not contain nicotine (summarized in Garcia et al., 2020, Supplementary File 1, Table 2). These studies adopted a randomized crossover design separated by washout periods varying from 48 h to 4 weeks. The participants were healthy and young (24–26 years old) and either occasional/active cigarette smokers or nonsmokers (including former and never-smokers). The concentrations of nicotine used were variable. Four studies included sham-vaping controls, which involved vaping without an e-liquid or with the device switched off. Only Franzen and colleagues included a session on exposure to cigarettes (Franzen et al., 2018). Some studies used flavors, such as menthol and tobacco, while others did not. The e-liquids contained 49.4%–55% PG and 35%–50% VG. The vaping protocols differed from one study to another, with the total numbers of puffs ranging from 10 to 30. Systolic blood pressure, diastolic blood pressure, and heart rate measurements were common to all studies. Some studies additionally measured heart rate variability, flow-mediated dilatation (FMD; endothelium-dependent vasodilation), skin microcirculatory blood flow, levels/activity of oxidative stress markers (e.g., myeloperoxidase, protein-bound 3-chlorotyrosine, homocitrulline, and paraoxonase-1), and nicotine or cotinine levels in blood. In general, the measurements were performed at baseline and after

exposure, starting from 5 min after exposure to up to 4 h postexposure, including measurements at regular intervals. The overall pooled mean differences in heart rate and systolic and diastolic blood pressure between EVP users exposed and not exposed to nicotine were 6.44 bpm (95% CI, 3.52–9.36; $P < .00001$), 3.73 mmHg (95% CI, 0.59–6.87; $P = .02$), and 3.25 mmHg (95% CI, 1.21–5.30; $P = .0018$), respectively (Fig. 20.1). The authors concluded that the inhaled nicotine, but not the non-nicotine constituents in the EVP aerosol, caused the acute sympathomimetic effects of EVP use. The increase in nicotine plasma levels immediately after EVP use was directly related to the increase in cardiac sympathetic activity in one study (Moheimani et al., 2017b) but not correlated with changes in heart rate and blood pressure in another (Chaumont et al., 2018). Franzen and coworkers did not measure plasma nicotine levels (Franzen et al., 2018), and Cossio and colleagues did not observe an increase in plasma nicotine levels (Cossio et al., 2020).

20.2.2.1.2.1.2 Chronic effects. A cross-sectional case-control study by Moheimani and coworkers revealed that chronic EVP users exhibited increased heart rate variability (measured to determine cardiac sympathetic to parasympathetic balance) and enhanced systemic oxidative stress relative to similarly aged controls (nonusers). There were no significant differences in resting heart rate or blood pressure between the two groups (Moheimani et al., 2017b). Similarly, in their 3.5-year prospective observational study, Polosa and colleagues found no differences in heart rate or blood pressure in EVP users compared with baseline (no vaping 60 min before measurements) or age- and sex-matched never-smokers over time. Of note, three of the nine EVP users in this study consumed products without nicotine (Polosa et al., 2017).

In healthy subjects used to cigarette smoking or EVP use, Boas and coworkers showed that the ^{18}F-fluorodeoxyglucose uptake levels in the spleen and aortic tissue in EVP users was intermediate to those in nonuser controls and cigarette smokers, indicating that the splenocardiac axis (the inflammatory signaling network underlying acute cardiac ischemia and characterized by sympathetic nerve stimulation of hematopoietic tissues) seems to be activated by EVP use, albeit to a lower extent than by smoking (Boas et al., 2017).

20.2.2.1.2.1.3 Effect of switching from cigarette smoking to EVP use. Most, but not all, studies investigating the potential health effects of switching from chronic cigarette smoking to EVP use showed decreases in systolic (pooled mean difference, -7.00; $P < .0001$) and diastolic (pooled mean difference, -3.65;

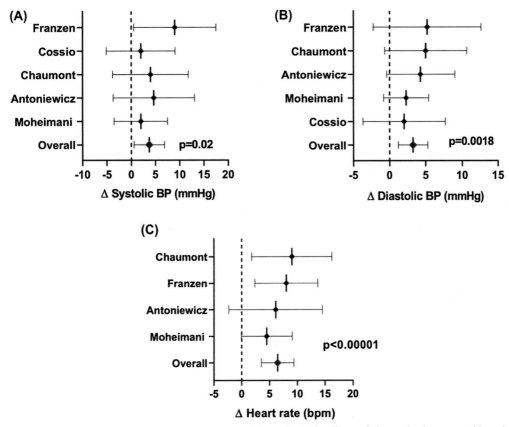

FIG. 20.1 Summary of the comparison of the acute hemodynamic effects of electronic cigarettes with and without nicotine.   Data from five acute studies revealed that the effects of EVPN on SBP **(A)**, DBP **(B)**, and HR **(C)** were significantly lower than those of EVP0. The forest plot entry for each study is the mean differences between EVPN and EVP0, with the corresponding lower and upper 95% confidence bounds. The plots to the right of the vertical line of no effect indicate that the effects of EVPN are worse than those of EVP0. *DBP*, diastolic blood pressure; *EVP*, e-vapor product; *EVPN*, EVP with nicotine; *EVP0*, EVP without nicotine; *HR*, heart rate; *SBP*, systolic blood pressure; *TC*, tobacco cigarette. (From Garcia, P.D., Gornbein, J.A. and Middlekauff, H.R., 2020. Cardiovascular autonomic effects of electronic cigarette use: a systematic review. Clin. Auton. Res. 1–13. DOI: 10.1007/s10286-020-00683-4.)

$P = .001$) blood pressure, later confirmed to be statistically significant in a metaanalysis (Skotsimara et al., 2019), but not in heart rate (pooled mean difference, -0.03; $P = .983$) (Farsalinos et al., 2016; George et al., 2019; Ikonomidis et al., 2018; Polosa et al., 2016; Veldheer et al., 2019). It is important to note that a non-negligible proportion of cigarette smokers were reported to not have fully switched to EVP use in two of the five studies (George et al., 2019; Veldheer et al., 2019).

In summary, the acute sympathoexcitatory effects of EVPs, as measured by increases in heart rate variability, heart rate, and blood pressure, can be attributed to nicotine and not to the non-nicotine constituents present in EVP aerosol. The acute

sympathetic activity observed with EVP use is reduced relative to tobacco smoking. In long-term studies, EVP users may have chronically elevated cardiac sympathetic activity relative to non-EVP users. However, this activity does not translate into clinically detectable higher heart rate or blood pressure. When switching to EVPs, cigarette smokers show a small decrease in blood pressure, but not in heart rate. However, these findings have to be interpreted with caution, by taking into account several limitations:

- Increases in plasma nicotine levels after EVP use were not systematically measured or confirmed in negative studies.
- Nicotine concentration in plasma was not systematically determined in cigarette smokers and switchers

to EVPs, which make comparison of exposure to nicotine challenging.

- There is a high degree of uncertainty around EVP aerosol exposure. In some studies, participants may have been too inexperienced with EVPs to obtain effective nicotine delivery, particularly with early-generation devices. Additionally, there is limited comparability between nicotine exposure in cigarette smokers and EVP users.
- Study protocols, populations, and EVP devices and e-liquids were largely heterogeneous. The lack of a standardized protocol may have compromised the reproducibility and comparability between studies.
- Heart rate and blood pressure were measured as surrogates. No study measured the direct autonomic cardiovascular effects of EVP use.
- Many studies focused on acute EVP use, which may only have limited value when drawing conclusions about longer-term autonomic effects.
- In general, the studies had low statistical power.
- None of the studies considered subjects with CVD. Therefore, there was no possibility to examine the potential of EVP use to modulate the risk of adverse cardiovascular events.

20.2.2.1.2.2 Effects of EVP use on myocardial function. In a study on the acute effects of EVP use on left ventricular function compared with those of smoking, Farsalinos and coworkers performed echocardiography measurements in 36 healthy heavy smokers before and after they smoked one cigarette and 40 EVP users before and after they used a device (e-liquid nicotine concentration, 11 mg/mL) for 7 min (Farsalinos et al., 2014). The results showed that, although acute smoking causes a delay in myocardial relaxation, EVP use has no immediate effects on myocardial function.

20.2.2.1.2.3 Effects of EVP use on arterial stiffness, endothelial function, and oxidative stress. Enhanced arterial stiffness is associated with an increased risk of cardiovascular events such as myocardial infarction and stroke (Mitchell et al., 2010). Various studies investigated the impact of EVP use on arterial stiffness and showed that arterial stiffness, as reflected by pulse wave velocity (PWV) measurements, increases and peaks within 15–20 min of consuming a nicotine-containing EVP but not in the case of a control EVP without nicotine (Antoniewicz et al., 2019; Franzen et al., 2018). Other studies also reported an increase in PWV just after EVP use (Fetterman et al., 2020); however, this was not as prompt as and to a lesser extent than that after cigarette smoking (Carnevale et al., 2016; Vlachopoulos et al., 2016). Carnevale and coworkers

also showed that smoking one cigarette or inhaling 9 puffs from an EVP (16 mg nicotine/250 puffs) caused a significant increase in the levels of soluble NADPH oxidase 2 (NOX2)-derived peptide and 8-iso-prostaglandin F2α and a significant decrease in nitric oxide (NO) bioavailability and vitamin E levels, all of which are indicative of oxidative stress; the effects of the EVP were less pronounced than those of cigarettes. Endothelial cells from cigarette smokers and EVP users were shown to be less responsive to the calcium ionophore A23187, producing lower levels of NO than cells from nonsmokers (Fetterman et al., 2020). An increase in circulating endothelial progenitor cells, which are thought to contribute to vascular maintenance (Balbarini and Di Stefano, 2008), was also reported in healthy volunteers after e-cigarette use (Antoniewicz et al., 2016). Additionally, after 1 month of switching to EVP use, endothelial function (i.e., FMD) and arterial stiffness (i.e., PWV) improved in chronic smokers, with a more pronounced effect in women and the most compliant participants who switched to EVPs (George et al., 2019). Together, these results indicate that switching from tobacco smoking to EVP use may reduce the harm for the vascular endothelium.

20.2.2.1.3 Nicotine replacement therapy. Cigarettes deliver nicotine, which is addictive. Therefore, pharmacological intervention in the form of NRT is regarded as the first-line therapy to help smokers overcome withdrawal symptoms during cessation. The routes of administration of nicotine in NRT include transdermal, inhalation, and buccal modes through nicotine patches, nicotine inhalers/nasal sprays, and nicotine gum/lozenges, respectively.

Randomized case-control and long-term longitudinal clinical studies and metaanalyses have been conducted to evaluate the impact of NRT in cessation trials for CVD patients (Joseph et al., 1996; Mills et al., 2014; Murray et al., 1996; US Department of Health and Human Services, 1989). The results of a randomized clinical trial by Joseph and coworkers showed no significant increase in cardiovascular events with transdermal nicotine relative to a placebo in 584 smokers with preexisting high-risk CVD (Joseph et al., 1996). In another study, myocardial perfusion in smokers noticeably improved with nicotine patch treatment, although the plasma nicotine and cotinine levels were higher in the treated group than in the untreated group (Mahmarian et al., 1997). In the 5-year Lung Health Study, 5887 adult smokers with early chronic obstructive pulmonary disease (COPD) were randomly assigned to three groups: special intervention with double-blind assignment to either bronchodilator (ipratropium bromide) or placebo inhaler (a combined total of 3923 participants) therapy or usual care (1964 participants). The participants in the special intervention groups were encouraged to quit smoking and received nicotine gum (Nicorette; 2 mg/piece, ad libitum) together with standard cognitive-behavioral strategies. The participants were monitored at regular intervals, and smoking status was confirmed by measuring exhaled CO. After study completion, approximately 5% of the participants in the special intervention group who did not succeed in quitting still used nicotine gum (between six and eight pieces per day). Importantly, the study found no association between the rate of hospitalization for adverse cardiovascular events or CVD-related death and long-term nicotine gum use (Murray et al., 1996).

A metaanalysis including 21 randomized clinical trials with NRTs reported an elevated risk of CVD events with NRT (RR, 2.29; 95% CI, 1.39–3.82), which was mainly driven by less serious events, such as tachycardia (Mills et al., 2014). In contrast, there was no clear evidence of increased relative risk of serious adverse cardiovascular events, including cardiovascular death, nonfatal myocardial infarction, and nonfatal stroke, in NRT users (RR: 1.95, 95% CI 0.26–4.30). Smoking is known to activate the sympathetic nervous system, resulting in an increased myocardial workload followed by enhanced heart rate and blood pressure (Smith and Fischer, 2001). Several studies have reported the lower sympathoexcitatory effects of NRT gums and patches compared with cigarettes in long-term smokers, despite the former having greater autonomic effects than a placebo patch (Blann et al., 1997; Lucini et al., 1998; Zevin et al., 1998).

A 12-month longitudinal study reported the beneficial effects of smoking cessation aided by NRT on vascular endothelial function, arterial stiffness, and plasma levels of soluble intercellular adhesion molecule 1 (sICAM-1) and interleukin (IL)-1β inflammatory markers after 3 months, with the effects reaching statistical significance after 12 months; in contrast, these parameters continued deteriorating in subjects who continued smoking (Xue et al., 2019). Additional evidence supports the fact that NRT use in the form of a patch or gum by smokers does not result in platelet aggregation or the thrombotic effects associated with smoking (Benowitz and Jacob, 1993; Mundal et al., 1995).

Altogether, these results indicate that smoking cessation therapies such as NRT do not raise the risk of serious cardiovascular events in healthy smokers or smokers with known CVD (Benowitz et al., 2018; Ford and Zlabek,

2005), and they even show a beneficial impact on vascular endothelial function and systemic inflammation when compared with continued smoking (Xue et al., 2019). These observations also support the idea that chemicals resulting from combustion—such as carbon monoxide, which reduces the availability of myocardial oxygen (Mall et al., 1985; Smith and Fischer, 2001)—rather than nicotine may be the principal contributors to serious smoking-related cardiovascular events.

20.2.2.2 Mechanistic evidence

Many in vivo and in vitro studies have attempted to understand the effects of nicotine on CVD. However, it should be noted that many of these in vivo studies were conducted in animals on a high-fat diet (HFD), which causes vascular inflammation by the release of proinflammatory mediators, such as tumor necrosis factor (TNF)-α and IL-1β, and accelerates the formation of atherosclerotic plaque (Ren et al., 2018; Wang et al., 2017a; Wang et al., 2019; Wu et al., 2018). Furthermore, nicotine uptake was generally not verified by blood nicotine and/or cotinine levels. Finally, it is important to note that many in vitro studies exposed cells and tissues to nicotine concentrations above the blood nicotine concentrations reached by human smokers (see Section 20.1 Introduction) and are, therefore, of limited relevance when assessing the risk of nicotine on CVD development.

20.2.2.2.1 Does nicotine impact the levels of lipids in blood?. Low-density lipoprotein (LDL) cholesterol and triglycerides are well-established mediators of atherosclerosis and a key target for primary and secondary prevention (Sandesara et al., 2019). LDL and triglycerides directly contribute to intimal cholesterol deposition and are involved in activation and enhancement of several proinflammatory, proapoptotic, and procoagulant pathways (Nordestgaard, 2016; Toth, 2016). Clinical and preclinical research suggests a strong association between high levels of total cholesterol, LDL, very low-density lipoprotein (VLDL), and triglycerides and atherosclerosis development.

With the recent global growth in EVP use, current research is increasingly focused on the effects of nicotine on the primary causes of CVD. In a previous study, nicotine administered in the form of a gum, at 16 mg per day for 2 weeks, did not significantly affect the lipid profiles—that is, the levels of triglycerides, total high-density lipoprotein (HDL) or LDL cholesterol, or apolipoproteins A1 or—in healthy nonsmoking men (Quensel et al., 1989). In smokers who abstained from smoking for 6 weeks, nicotine administration via patch (22 mg/day) did not lead to HDL cholesterol normalization in one study (Moffatt et al., 2000), while it did in another study (Allen et al., 1994). Importantly, switching from cigarette smoking to using an electrically heated tobacco product (EHTP), the Tobacco Heating System 2.2 (THS), led to a significant positive change in HDL cholesterol level at equivalent nicotine exposure (Ludicke et al., 2019) (Chapter 17).

In nonclinical studies, nicotine supplementation (6 mg/kg/day) through a liquid diet increased LDL cholesterol and decreased HDL cholesterol levels in squirrel monkeys (Cluette-Brown et al., 1986). In rats, daily s.c. administration of 0.6—2 mg/kg nicotine for 21 days or 2 months increased the total, LDL, and VLDL cholesterol and triglyceride levels and decreased HDL cholesterol levels (Chakkarwar, 2011; Joukar et al., 2012; Latha et al., 1993; Michael and Olatunji, 2018; Nacerai et al., 2017). Albino Swiss mice exposed to nicotine via a patch (21 mg/24 h) for 30 days had increased total cholesterol levels (Nieradko-Iwanicka et al., 2019). In C57BL/6 mice, however, no major change in serum lipids was observed after a 2-week exposure to 0.5 mg/L nicotine in drinking water (Hashimoto et al., 2018). In our inhalation study, no major impact on lipid metabolism was observed in apolipoprotein E-deficient ($Apoe^{-/-}$) mice exposed to EVP aerosols (Szostak et al., 2020).

Cholinergic regulation may stimulate adipose tissue lipolysis (Andersson and Arner, 1995, 2001; Arner and Bulow, 1993) and cause augmentation of plasma-free fatty acid concentrations, which is strongly associated with an increase in triglyceride and a decrease in HDL cholesterol levels (Andersson and Arner, 2001; Ryden and Arner, 2017). However, to date, no consistent effect of nicotine on lipid dysregulation has been identified (Table 20.3).

20.2.2.2.2 Does nicotine modify the activity of platelets and promote coagulation?.

In CVD development, platelets are known to play a vital role in favor of coagulation. By aggregating themselves and releasing various bioactive substances, such as growth factors, lysophospholipids, and chemokines, platelets contribute to the thromboembolic complications of atherosclerosis: heart attack, stroke, and peripheral vascular disease (Packham, 1994). Exposure to mainstream and sidestream cigarette smoke increases platelet aggregation and activity in humans (Beswick et al., 1991; Csordas and Bernhard, 2013; Renaud et al., 1984; Rubenstein et al., 2004). In studies involving exposure of platelet-rich plasma, nicotine had no major impact on platelet aggregation or function (Brinson, 1974;

Hom et al., 2016; Ljungberg et al., 2013; Nowak et al., 1996; Schedel et al., 2016). In contrast, Whiss and coworkers showed that nicotine infusion in healthy subjects (who were habituated to nicotine use but had not used it in the last 36 h) caused an increase in collagen-induced platelet aggregation and surface expression of P-selectin as soon as the plasma cotinine concentrations were maximal (Whiss et al., 2000). In other studies, a very high concentration of nicotine (10 µM) was required to induce 5-hydroxytryptamine release and platelet aggregation in platelet-rich plasma (Ljungberg et al., 2013; Pfueller et al., 1988). Importantly, this nicotine concentration is three orders of magnitude higher than that achieved by smokers, which strongly limits the relevance of these studies to human physiology.

Hom and coworkers found that, in contrast to exposure to cigarette smoke and e-vapor extracts with and without nicotine, pure nicotine exposure (50 nM) did not have a major effect on platelet activation (Hom et al., 2016). Wei and colleagues analyzed the impact of nicotine on the expression of thrombomodulin (TM). TM plays an anticoagulant role not only by inhibiting thrombin but also by accelerating the production of activated protein C, which has anticoagulant properties. The authors showed that nicotine does not influence TM mRNA and protein expression, suggesting that nicotine does not affect coagulation (Wei et al., 2018). However, Ramachandran and coworkers showed a 75% reduction in the shear-dependent rate of platelet activation in response to treatment with nicotine added to nicotine-free cigarette smoke extracts (Ramachandran et al., 2004).

In summary, the role of nicotine in coagulation is still poorly understood and deserves further investigations (Table 20.4) (Gahring and Rogers, 2005; Schedel et al., 2011).

20.2.2.2.3 Does nicotine alter endothelial function?.

Endothelial dysfunction is characterized by the reduced bioavailability of NO, which affects vascular integrity. Endothelial cells maintain the integrity of the vessel wall, and endothelial cell injury or dysfunction is an initiator of atherosclerosis (Davies, 2009). Cigarette smoking dysregulates NO pathways, causes vascular inflammation and oxidative stress, and thus leads to atherosclerosis and CVD (Davies, 2009; Golbidi et al., 2020). In normal vasculature, NO production helps preserve vascular integrity and leads to vascular relaxation. GTP cyclohydrolase I (GTPCH1) and tetrahydrobiopterin (BH4) are critical determinants of the activation of the

TABLE 20.3
Effects of Nicotine or ENDPs on the Lipid Profile.

Reference	Study Type	Species	Experimental Model	Treatment (Route)	Dose	Duration	Effects on Biological Processes and Molecular Mechanisms
Nacerai et al. (2017)	In vivo	Rat	Male albino	Nicotine tartrate (s.c.)	1 mg/kg/day	8 w	↑ LDL, ↑ TG, ↑TC, ↑ LDH, ↑ plasma MDA
Cluette-Brown et al. (1986)	In vivo	Monkey	Male squirrel monkey	Nicotine (p.o.)	6 mg/kg/day	24 m	↑ LDL, ↑ total lipids, ↑ LPL
Michael et al. (2020)	In vivo	Rat	Female Wistar	Nicotine (p.o.)	1 mg/kg/day	6 w	↑ Aldosterone and corticosterone, ↑ TG/HDL and TC/HDL ratios, ↑ MDA, ↑ PAI-1, ↓ NO
Joukar et al. (2012)	In vivo	Rat	Male Wistar	Nicotine (s.c.)	2 mg/kg/day	4 w	↑ Lipid profile, ↑ TC, HDL, VLDL and TG, ↑ TG/HDL, ↑ TAC (heart)
Chakkarwar (2011)	In vivo	Rat	Male Wistar	Nicotine (i.p.)	2 mg/kg/day	4 w	↑ Cholesterol, ↑ TG, ↓ HDL
Hashimoto et al. (2018)	In vivo	Mouse	Male C57BL/6	Nicotine (p.o.)	0.5 mg/L/day	2 w	No change in lipid metabolism; no change in glucose, TC and TG
Nieradko-Iwanicka et al. (2019)	In vivo	Mouse	Swiss Albino	Nicotine (t.d.)	21 mg/day	30 d	↑ TC

↑ and ↓ indicate a significant decrease or increase. *d*, day; *h*, hour; *HDL*, high-density lipoprotein; *LDH*, lactate dehydrogenase; *LDL*, low-density lipoprotein; *LPL*, lipoprotein lipase; *m*, month; *MDA*, malondialdehyde; *NO*, nitric oxide; *p.o.*, oral; *PAI-1*, plasminogen activator inhibitor-1; *s.c.*, subcutaneous; *t.d.*, transdermal; *TAC*, total antioxidant capacity; *TC*, total cholesterol; *TG*, triglycerides, *VLDL*, very low-density lipoprotein; *w*, week.
From Chakkarwar, V.A., 2011. Fenofibrate attenuates nicotine-induced vascular endothelial dysfunction in the rat. Vascul. Pharmacol. 55(5–6), 163–168. Cluette-Brown, J., Mulligan, J., Doyle, K., Hagan, S., Osmolski, T., Hojnacki, J., 1986. Oral nicotine induces an atherogenic lipoprotein profile. Proc. Soc. Exp. Biol. Med. 182(3), 409–413. Hashimoto, K., Zaima, N., Sekiguchi, H., Kugo, H., Miyamoto, C., Hoshino, K., et al., 2018. Dietary DNA attenuates the degradation of elastin fibers in the aortic wall in nicotine-administrated mice. J. Nutr. Sci. Vitaminol. (Tokyo). 64(4), 271–276. Joukar, S., Shahouzehi, B., Najafipour, H., Gholamhoseinian, A., Joukar, F., 2012. Ameliorative effect of black tea on nicotine induced cardiovascular pathogenesis in rat. Excli J. 11, 309–317. Michael, O.S., Dibia, C.L., Adeyanju, O.A., Olaniyi, K.S., Areola, E.D., Olatunji, L.A., 2020. Estrogen-progestin oral contraceptive and nicotine exposure synergistically confers cardio-renoprotection in female Wistar rats. Biomed. Pharmacother. 129, 110387. Nacerai, H., Gregory, T., Sihem, B., Salah, A., Souhila, A.B., 2017. Green tea beverage and epigallocatecihin gallate attenuate nicotine cardiocytotoxicity in rat. Acta Pol. Pharm. 74(1), 277–287. Nieradko-Iwanicka, B., Pietraszek, D., Pośnik, K. and Borzęcki, A., 2019. Prolonged exposure to transdermal nicotine improves memory in male mice, but impairs biochemical parameters in male and female mice. Ann. Agric. Environ. Med. 26(1), 62–66.

NO pathway (Alkaitis and Crabtree, 2012). BH4 or GTPCH1 deficiency causes a decrease in the dimerization of endothelial NO synthase (eNOS) and, consequently, eNOS activation. Uncoupled eNOS produces a superoxide instead of NO, leading to alteration of endothelial function (Alkaitis and Crabtree, 2012; Forstermann and Munzel, 2006; Wang et al., 2008).

In vitro and in vivo studies have shown that nicotine exposure may affect endothelial function. In human umbilical vein endothelial cells treated with nicotine for 48 h, the GTPCH1 protein level is decreased in a significant and dose-dependent manner, with the effects starting to be seen at nicotine concentrations of just 10 nM (Li et al., 2018). In $Apoe^{-/-}$ mice on an HFD, 100 mg/L nicotine in drinking water causes a reduction

TABLE 20.4
Effects of Nicotine on Platelets and Coagulation.

Reference	Study Type	Species	Experimental Model	Treatment (Route)	Dose	Duration	Diseases, Biological Processes, and Molecular Mechanisms
Whiss et al. (2000)	In vivo	Human	Healthy nonsmoker	Nicotine (i.v.)	0.028 mg/kg	2 h	↑ Platelet aggregation; ↓ nitrites
Wei et al. (2018)	In vitro	Human	Human umbilical vein endothelial cells (HUVECs)	Nicotine	1 p.m., 0.1, 10 nM, 1 μM	0, 6, 10, 12, 24 h	No effect on TM and EPCR expression
Hom et al. (2016)	In vitro	Human	Platelet-rich plasma	ENDP aerosol extract	1.2% and 1.8%, 12 and 18 mg	0, 30, 60, 120 min	No effect on platelet aggregation, ↑ platelet activity; ↑ CD62
Hom et al. (2016)	In vitro	Human	Platelet-rich plasma	Nicotine	50 nM	0, 30, 60, 120 min	No effect on the deposition of C1q, C3b, C4d and C5b-9
Ramachandran et al. (2004)	In vitro	Human	Platelets	Nicotine	50 nM	21 min	↓ Platelet activation
Pfueller et al. (1988)	In vitro	Human	Platelet-rich plasma	Nicotine	10 mM	1–60 min	↑ Platelet aggregation
Ljungberg et al. (2013)	In vitro	Human	Platelet-rich plasma	Nicotine	0.1, 1, 10 μM	60 min	No effect of low doses on platelet aggregation; ↑ Platelet aggregation at high dose (10 μM)
Nowak et al. (1996)	In vivo	Human	Healthy nonsmoker	Nicotine (i.v.)	0.25 μg/kg/min, 0.5 μg/kg/min	30 min	No effect of low dose; ↓ platelet aggregation during infusion with high dose
Brinson (1974)	In vitro	Human	Platelet-rich plasma	Nicotine	5 × 10-3M	5 min	↓ Platelet adhesion

↑ and ↓ indicate a significant decrease or increase. * Human-relevant nicotine concentration: The average plasma nicotine concentration in smokers is approximately 22 ng/mL (136 nM) over a 24-h period. *5-HT*, 5-hydroxytryptamine (serotonin); *ADP*, adenosine diphosphate; *C1q*, complement component C1q; *C3b*, complement component 3b; *C4d*, complement component C4d; *C5b-9*; complement membrane attack complex; *CD62*, cluster of differentiation 62 (selectin); *ENDP*, electronic nicotine delivery product; *EPCR*, endothelial protein C receptor; *h*, hour; *HUVEC*, human umbilical vein endothelial cell; *i.v.*, intravenous; *m*, month; *TM*, thrombomodulin; *w*, week.

From Brinson, K., 1974. Effect of nicotine on human blood platelet aggregation. Atherosclerosis. 20(1), 137–140. Hom, S., Chen, L., Wang, T., Ghebrehiwet, B., Yin, W., Rubenstein, D.A., 2016. Platelet activation, adhesion, inflammation, and aggregation potential are altered in the presence of electronic cigarette extracts of variable nicotine concentrations. Platelets. 27(7), 694–702. Ljungberg, L.U., Persson, K., Eriksson, A.C., Green, H., Whiss, P.A., 2013. Effects of nicotine, its metabolites and tobacco extracts on human platelet function in vitro. Toxicol. In Vitro. 27(2), 932–938. Nowak, J., Andersson, K., Benthin, G., Chen, J., Karlberg, K.E., Sylven, C., 1996. Effect of nicotine infusion in humans on platelet aggregation and urinary excretion of a major thromboxane metabolite. Acta Physiol. Scand. 157(1), 101–107. Pfueller, S.L., Burns, P., Mak, K., Firkin, B.G., 1988. Effects of nicotine on platelet function. Haemostasis. 18(3), 163–169. Ramachandran, J., Rubenstein, D., Bluestein, D., Jesty, J., 2004. Activation of platelets exposed to shear stress in the presence of smoke extracts of low-nicotine and zero-nicotine cigarettes: the protective effect of nicotine. Nicotine Tob. Res. 6(5), 835–841. Wei, Y., Lai, B., Liu, H., Li, Y., Zhen, W., Fu, L., 2018. Effect of cigarette smoke extract and nicotine on the expression of thrombomodulin and endothelial protein C receptor in cultured human umbilical vein endothelial cells. Mol Med Rep. 17(1), 1724–1700. Whiss, P.A., Lundahl, T.H., Bengtsson, T., Lindahl, T.L., Lunell, E. and Larsson, R., 2000. Acute effects of nicotine infusion on platelets in nicotine users with normal and impaired renal function. Toxicol. Appl. Pharmacol. 163(2), 95–104.

in serum NO levels, GTPCH1 expression in the aorta, and endothelial relaxation (Li et al., 2018). In rat mesenteric arteries, treatment for 24 h with nicotine concentrations exceeding the maximum human exposure by several orders of magnitude (i.e., 0.01, 0.1, or 1 mM) significantly inhibited acetylcholine-induced endothelium-dependent relaxation in a concentration-dependent manner (Luo et al., 2006). This finding was replicated in rats receiving 2 mg/kg/day nicotine i.p. for 4 weeks and was accompanied by reductions in serum and aortic nitrite/nitrate levels and NOS and superoxide dismutase (SOD) activities (Balakumar et al., 2008; Kaur et al., 2010; Luo et al., 2006). However, a 30-min incubation of the rat aortic ring with nicotine at excessive concentrations (i.e., 0.01, 0.1, or 1 mM) caused impairment of endothelium-dependent vasorelaxation only at the highest dose and to a lesser extent than incubation with cigarette sidestream smoke (Argacha et al., 2008).

Inflammation, as well as ROS production, alters BH4 production, leading to eNOS uncoupling. Endothelial NOS uncoupling increases superoxide production, resulting in an additional decrease in BH4 and NO availability. ROS generation could also lead to BH4 oxidation, causing 7,8-dihydrobiopterin (BH2) production, thereby reducing the availability of BH4 as an eNOS cofactor (Alkaitis and Crabtree, 2012; Laursen et al., 2001). Multiple studies showed that nicotine exposure increases inflammation and endothelial permeability, induces apoptosis, and decreases tight junctions and tubulins, causing endothelium reorganization and endothelial dysfunction (Barber et al., 2017; Jiang et al., 2006; Lee et al., 2015; Liu et al., 2017b; Rothig et al., 2012; Wu et al., 2018; Zhang et al., 2019b). In rats, nicotine treatment (0.01–2 mg/kg/day for 4 weeks) increased endothelial dysfunction and decreased eNOS expression, NO availability, and vascular relaxation (Balakumar et al., 2008; Chakkarwar, 2011; Jiang et al., 2006; Kaur et al., 2010; Kim et al., 2017; Liu et al., 2017a; Luo et al., 2006; Si et al., 2017; Zeinivand et al., 2013). Nicotine treatment (100 mg/L for 12 weeks) also reduced serum NO levels and vascular relaxation and accelerated atherosclerosis progression in $Apoe^{-/-}$ mice on an HFD (Li et al., 2018). In our study, exposure of $Apoe^{-/-}$ mice (fed a normal diet) to nicotine-containing EVP aerosols for 3 or 6 months led to an increase in pulse wave and pulse propagation velocities, while exposure to an EVP aerosol without nicotine did not (Szostak et al., 2020). This indicates that long-term exposure to nicotine can lead to endothelial dysfunction and arterial rigidity, but to a lesser extent than long-term cigarette smoke exposure (Chapter 15).

Altogether, these studies have shown that nicotine exerts a physiological impact on endothelium-dependent relaxation by modulating BH4, GTPCH1, eNOS, inflammation, oxidative stress, and endothelial integrity. While some of the specific mechanisms impacted by nicotine require further investigation, these studies have shown that nicotine may affect endothelial function (Table 20.5).

20.2.2.2.4 Does nicotine promote atherosclerosis and aortic aneurysm?. Atherosclerosis is a chronic inflammatory disease. Lipid infiltration, ROS formation, and inflammation are critical pathological mechanisms involved in atherosclerosis development. Additionally, a proatherogenic lipid profile mediated by high levels of LDL and VLDL contributes strongly to atherosclerosis progression. However, no consistent nicotine effects on lipid profile have been identified (see Section 20.2.2.2.1).

Several in vivo studies have attempted to elucidate whether nicotine plays a role in atherosclerosis and aortic aneurysm (Table 20.6). Many of these studies employed $Apoe^{-/-}$ mice, which develop atherosclerosis in response to cigarette smoke and HFD (Lo Sasso et al., 2016) and experience a substantial decrease in atherosclerosis development upon calorie restriction (Yang et al., 2020). Importantly, HFD leads to inflammation, which is a fundamental mechanism involved in many diseases, including CVD (Duan et al., 2018), and several in vivo studies have demonstrated that an HFD increases oxidative stress, proinflammatory mediator release, and atherosclerotic plaque size (Liu et al., 2017a; Wu et al., 2018). In these studies, nicotine treatment of animals on an HFD potentiated the release of proinflammatory mediators and accelerated atherosclerotic plaque growth, but nicotine had only limited effects on animals fed a normal diet. Furthermore, daily treatment of HFD-fed $Apoe^{-/-}$ mice with 2 mg/kg nicotine for 12 weeks doubled atherosclerotic plaque size relative to vehicle treatment (Ren et al., 2018); this was similar to the effect seen after daily administration of nicotine in drinking water for 20 weeks (Heeschen et al., 2001). Interestingly, in other $Apoe^{-/-}$ mouse studies, concomitant HFD was also required in addition to nicotine, to elicit atherosclerosis progression (Wang et al., 2017a; Wang et al., 2019; Wu et al., 2018). Exposure of $Apoe^{-/-}$ mice fed an HFD to EVP aerosol (e-liquid nicotine concentration, 2.4%) for 12 weeks also increased atherosclerotic plaque size in one study (Espinoza-Derout et al., 2019). In contrast, in $Apoe^{-/-}$ mice fed a normal diet, exposure to human-relevant doses of nicotine-containing EVP aerosols did not accelerate atherosclerosis development (Szostak et al., 2020)

TABLE 20.5
Effects of Nicotine on Endothelial Function.

Reference	Study Type	Species	Experimental Model	Treatment Route	Dose	Duration	Biological Processes and Molecular Mechanisms
Szostak et al. (2020)	In vivo	Mice	ApoE−/−	ENDS aerosol (inhalation)	35 μg/L for 3 h/d, 5d/w	3 and 6 m	↑ Pulse wave velocity, ↑ pulse propagation velocity, ↑MPI
Luo et al. (2006)	In vivo	Rats	Sprague–Dawley	Nicotine (i.p.)	2 mg/kg/d	4 w	↓ Endothelium-dependent relaxation, ↓ nitrite/nitrate, nitric oxide (NO) synthase (NOS), and superoxide dismutase (SOD) activities in aorta and serum
Balakumar et al. (2008)	In vivo	Rats	Wistar	Nicotine (i.p.)	2 mg/kg/d	4 w	↓ Endothelium-dependent relaxation, ↑ TBARS, ↑ Oxidative stress
Jiang et al. (2006)	In vivo	Rats	Sprague–Dawley	Nicotine (p.o.)	5 mg/kg/d	4 w	↓ Endothelium-dependent relaxation, ↓DDAH, ↑ADMA, ↑ alpha7 nAChR
Kaur et al. (2010)	In vivo	Rats	Wistar	Nicotine (i.p.)	2 mg/kg/d	4 w	↓ Endothelium-dependent relaxation, ↑ TBARS, ↑ superoxide anion
Si et al. (2017)	In vivo	Rats	Sprague–Dawley	Nicotine (p.o.)	0.6 mg/kg/d	28 d	↓ Endothelium-dependent relaxation, ↑ SBP, ↑ Heart Rate, ↑ Elastic lamelles, ↑ IMT, ↓ SOD, ↓GSH, ↑TBARS
Zhang Y. et al. (2019)	In vivo	Mice	Male Nlrp3+/+ and Nlrp3−/− (C57BL/6 J)	Nicotine (i.p.)	2 mg/kg/d	2 w	↓ Endothelial permeability, ↓ ZO-1 and ZO-2, ↑ Nlrp3 inflammasome activity, IL–1β
Li et al. (2018)	In vivo	Mice	ApoE−/−	Nicotine (p.o.) + HFD	100 mg/L	12 w	↓ Endothelium-dependent relaxation, ↓ serum NO, ↑ serum MDA, ↑ 4-HNE in aortic plaques

Study	Type	Species	Model/Cell type	Treatment	Concentration	Duration	Findings
Liu et al. (2017)	In vivo	Rats	Sprague–Dawley	Nicotine (p.o) + HFD	100 mg/mL	20 w	↓ Endothelium-dependent relaxation, ↑SBP, ↑eNOS uncoupling, and ↑ atherosclerosis; ↑ O2, ↑ ROS, ↑ CRP, ↑ CD36, TNFα and IL1β in HFD, ↑ CXCL9, interferon γ, IL4, and IL6, ↑ SBP, ↓ eNOS, ↓ Ach-relaxation, ↑ SBP, ↓ eNOS, ↓ Ach-relaxation
Kim et al. (2017)	In vivo	Rats	Sprague–Dawley	Nicotine (p.o.)	0.8 mg/kg	Single dose	↓ Endothelium-dependent relaxation, ↑ LDH, ↑ SBP
Chakkarwar (2011)	In vivo	Rats	Wistar	Nicotine (i.p.)	2 mg/kg/d	4 w	↓ Endothelium dependant relaxation; ↓ eNOS gene expression, ↑p22phox(435), ↓ nitrites in serum and aorta, ↑ TBARS and superoxide anion in serum
Jiang et al. (2006)	In vitro	Human	Human umbilical vein endothelial cells (HUVECs)	Nicotine	10 µM	48 h	↑ ADMA, ↑ LDH, ↑ alpha7 nAChR
(Zhang S. et al., 2001)	In vitro	Human	Primary human coronary artery endothelial cells (HCAEC)	Nicotine	0.1, 10 nM	24 h	↑Ang-I, ↑VCAM-1, ↑t-PA, ↑PAI-1, ↑vWF, ↑eNOS, and ↑ ACE
Zhang Y. et al. (2019)	In vitro	Mice	MVECs (mouse microvascular endothelial cells)	Nicotine	50, 100 nM	24 h	↓ ZO-1 and ZO-2, ↑ Nlrp3 inflammasome activity, IL-1β
Wu et al. (2018)	In vitro	Human	Human aortic endothelial cells	Nicotine	1 µM	24 h	↑ Caspase-1, IL-1β, and IL-18, ↑ NLRP3, ↑ ROS, ↑ LDH
Li et al. (2018)	In vitro	Human	HUVECs	Nicotine	0.01, 0.1, 1 µM	48 h	↓BH4, ↓GTPCH1, ↓ NO, ↑ ROS (all: strongest effect with highest dose)
Lee et al. (2015)	In vitro	Human	HUVECs	Nicotine + shear stress	0.1 µM	12 h	↑ Reorganization of endothelial cytoskeleton, ↓ actin and α-tubulin

Continued

TABLE 20.5
Effects of Nicotine on Endothelial Function.—cont'd

Reference	Study Type	Species	Experimental Model	Treatment Route	Dose	Duration	Biological Processes and Molecular Mechanisms
Rothig et al. (2012)	In vitro	Rats	Coronary endothelial cells	Nicotine	0.1 nM–1 µM	24, 48 h	↑ PTHrP (0.1, 1, 30 nM for 24 h), ↑p-p38 (30 nM for 15–60 min), ↓ Bcl2 (1 µM, 48 h)
Wang et al. (2006)	In vitro	Human	HUVECs	Nicotine	5, 10 µM	15 min	↑ VCAM1 and E-selectin,↑ Ca^{2+},↑ p-p38 and p-ERK1/2

↑ and ↓ indicate a significant decrease or increase. *ACE*, angiotensin-converting enzyme; *Ach*, acetylcholine; *ADMA*, asymmetric dimethylarginine; *Ang*, angiotensin; *BH4*, tetrahydrobiopterin; *BP*, blood pressure; Ca^{2+}, calcium; *CCR*, C-C chemokine receptor; *CD14L*, cluster of differentiation 14 ligand; *CD35*, complement C3b/C4b receptor 1; *CD36*, cluster of differentiation 36; *CRP*, C-reactive protein; *Cx*, connexin; *CXCL*, chemokine (C-X-C motif) ligand; *DDAH*, dimethylarginine dimethylaminohydrolase; *eNOS*, endothelial nitric oxide synthase; *EPCR*, endothelial protein C receptor; *EVP*, e-vapor product; *GSH*, glutathione; *h*, hour; *HFD*, high-fat diet; *HGMB*, high mobility group box; *HR*, heart rate; *IFN*, interferon; *IL*, interleukin; *IMT*, intimal media thickness; *i.p.*, intraperitoneal; *LDH*, lactate dehydrogenase; *m*, month; *MAPK*, mitogen-activated protein kinase; *MCP*, monocyte chemoattractant protein; *MIF*, macrophage migration inhibitory factor; *MPI*, myocardial performance index; *nAChR*, nicotinic acetylcholine receptor; *NLRP3*, NOD-, LRR- and pyrin domain-containing protein 3; *NO*, nitric oxide; *PAI-1*, plasminogen activator inhibitor-1; *p.o.*, oral; *PTHrP*, parathyroid hormone-related protein; *ROS*, reactive oxygen species; *SBP*, systolic blood pressure; *s.c*, subcutaneous; *SIRT*, sirtuin; *SOD*, superoxide dismutase; *TBARS*, thiobarbituric acid reactive substances; *TM*, thrombomodulin; *TNF*, tumor necrosis factor; *t-PA*, tissue plasminogen activator; *VCAM*, vascular cell adhesion molecule; *VEGF*, vascular endothelial growth factor; *vWF*, von Willebrand factor; *w*, week; *ZO*, zona occludens (tight junction protein).

From Balakumar, P., Sharma, R., Singh, M., 2008. Benfotiamine attenuates nicotine and uric acid-incuced vascular endothelial dysfunction in the rat. Pharmacol. Res. 58(5–6), 356–363. Chakkarwar, V.A., 2011. Fenofibrate attenuates nicotine-induced vascular endothelial dysfunction in the rat. Vascul. Pharmacol. 55(5–6), 163–168. Jiang, D.J., Jia, S.J., Yan, J., Zhou, Z., Yuan, Q. and Li, Y.J., 2006. Involvement of DDAH/ADMA/NOS pathway in nicotine-induced endothelial dysfunction. Biochem. Biophys. Res. Commun. 349(2), 683–693. Kaur, J., Reddy, K. and Balakumar, P., 2010. The novel role of fenofibrate in preventing nicotine-and sodium arsenite-induced vascular endothelial dysfunction in the rat. Cardiovasc. Toxicol. 10(3), 227–238. Kim, J.R., Kang, P., Lee, H.S., Kim, K.Y. and Seol, G.H., 2017. Cardiovascular effects of linalyl acetate in acute nicotine exposure. Environ. Health Prev. Med. 22(1), 42. Lee, Y.H., Chen, R.S., Chang, N.C., Lee, K.R., Huang, C.T., Huang, Y.C., et al., 2015. Synergistic impact of nicotine and shear stress induces cytoskeleton collapse and apoptosis in endothelial cells. Ann. Biomed. Eng. 43(9), 2220–2230. Li, J., Liu, S., Cao, G., Sun, Y., Chen, W., Dong, F., et al., 2018. Nicotine induces endothelial dysfunction and promotes atherosclerosis via GTPCH1. J. Cell Mol. Med. 22(11), 5406–5417. Liu, C., Zhou, M.S., Li, Y., Wang, A., Chadipiralla, K., Tian, R., et al., 2017. Oral nicotine aggravates endothelial dysfunction and vascular inflammation in diet-induced obese rats: role of macrophage TNFalpha. PLoS One. 12(12), e0188439. Luo, H.L., Zang, W.J., Lu, J., Yu, X.J., Lin, Y.X., Cao, Y.X., 2006. The protective effect of captopril on nicotine-induced endothelial dysfunction in rat. Basic Clin. Pharmacol. Toxicol. 99(3), 237–245. Rothig, A., Schreckenberg, R., Weber, K., Conzelmann, C., Da Costa Rebelo, R.M. and Schluter, K.D., 2012. Effects of nicotine on PTHrP and PTHrP receptor expression in rat coronary endothelial cells. Cell Physiol. Biochem. 29(3–4), 485–492. Si, L.Y., Kamisah, Y., Ramalingam, A., Lim, Y.C., Budin, S.B. and Zainalabidin, S., 2017. Roselle supplementation prevents nicotine-induced vascular endothelial dysfunction and remodeling in rats. Appl. Physiol. Nutr. Metab. 42(7), 735–772. Szostak, J., Wong, E.T., Titz, B., Lee, T., Wong, S.K., Low, T., et al., 2020. A 6-month systems toxicology inhalation study in ApoE(−/−) mice demonstrates reduced cardiovascular effects of E-vapor aerosols compared with cigarette smoke. Am. J. Physiol. Heart Circ. Physiol. 318(3), H604-H631. Wang, Y., Wang, Z., Zhou, Y., Liu, L., Zhao, Y., Yao, C., et al., 2006. Nicotine stimulates adhesion molecular expression via calcium influx and mitogen-activated protein kinases in human endothelial cells. Int. J. Biochem. Cell Biol. 38(2), 170–182. Wu, X., Zhang, H., Qi, W., Zhang, Y., Li, J., Li, Z., et al., 2018. Nicotine promotes atherosclerosis via ROS-NLRP3-mediated endothelial cell pyroptosis. Cell Death Dis. 9(2), 171. Zhang, S., Day, I. and Ye, S., 2001. Nicotine induced changes in gene expression by human coronary artery endothelial cells. Atherosclerosis. 154(2), 277–283. Zhang, Y., Chen, Y., Zhang, Y., Li, P.L. and Li, X., 2019. Contribution of cathepsin B-dependent Nlrp3 inflammasome activation to nicotine-induced endothelial barrier dysfunction. Eur. J. Pharmacol. 865, 172795.

TABLE 20.6
Effects of Nicotine on Atherosclerosis, Aortic Aneurysm.

Reference	Study Type	Species	Experimental Model	Treatment (Route)	Dose	Duration	Biological Processes and Molecular Mechanisms
Guo et al. (2016)	In vivo	Mouse	C57Bl/6J	Nicotine (s.c.) + AngII	1.5 and 5 mg/kg/d	28 d	↑ Incidence of AAA, ↑ abdominal aortic diameter (AAD), ↑ MMP2, MMP9, MCP-1 and RANTES in AAA tissues
Guo et al. (2016)	In vitro	Mouse	Mouse aortic vascular smooth muscle (MOVAS) cells	Nicotine	0.5, 5, 50, 500 ng/mL	3 h	↑ MCP-1 and RANTES (strongest effect with 0.5 and 5 ng/mL; higher doses were inhibitory)
Wang S. et al. (2012)	In vivo	Mouse	ApoE−/− or ApoE−/−+AMPKa1−/− model of AAA	Nicotine + AngII	1 and 5 mg/kg/d	6 w	↑ Incidence of AAA, ↑ AAD, ↑ elastin degradation, ↑ MMP-2 protein and activity, 3-NT and MDA in aortic tissues, ↑ TNA-α, IFN-γ, and IL-6 in serum
Maegdefessel et al. (2012)	In vivo	Mouse	C57BL/6 porcine pancreatic elastase (PPE) model of AAA	Nicotine (s.c.) + PPE	2.2 mg/kg/d	28 and 60 d	↑ Incidence of AAA, ↑ miR-21, ↓ Pten, ↑ Mac-1-positive cells (activated monocytes/macrophages) and Mcp-1, Il-6, Cxcl1 and Cxcl12 in aortic tissues
Maegdefessel et al. (2012)	In vivo	Mouse	ApoE−/− model of AAA	Nicotine (s.c.) + AngII	2.2 mg/kg/d	14 and 28 d	↑ Incidence of AAA, ↑ AAD, ↑ miR-21, ↓ Pten
Maegdefessel et al. (2012)	In vitro	Human	Primary human aortic endothelial cells (hAECs), aortic smooth muscle cells (hASMCs), and aortic fibroblasts (hAFBs)	Nicotine hydrogen tartrate	10 nM	48 h	↑ miR-21 (all cell types), ↓Pten (hASMCs)
Wagenhäuser et al. (2018)	In vivo	Mouse	C57BL/6	Nicotine (s.c.)	25 mg/kg/d	10 and 40 d	↑ Increased aortic stiffness (pulse wave velocity), ↑ MMP-2 and MMP-9 protein and activity in aortic tissues, ↑ elastin thinning and fragmentation

Continued

TABLE 20.6
Effects of Nicotine on Atherosclerosis, Aortic Aneurysm.—cont'd

Reference	Study Type	Species	Experimental Model	Treatment (Route)	Dose	Duration	Biological Processes and Molecular Mechanisms
Wang Z. et al. (2019)	In vivo	Mouse	ApoE−/−	Nicotine (s.c.) − HFD	2 mg/kg/d	12 w	↑ Atherosclerotic plaque size, ↑ number of vascular smooth muscle cells and autophagy in atherosclerotic lesions
Szostak et al. (2020)	In vivo	Mouse	ApoE−/−	ENDS aerosol (inhalation)	35 µg/L for 3 h/d, 5d/w	3 and 6 m	No change on atherosclerotic plaque size
Wang C. et al. (2017)	In vivo	Mouse	ApoE−/−	Nicotine (p.o.) + HFD	100 µg/mL	12 w	↑ Atherosclerotic plaque size, ↓ collagen and smooth muscle cell content of atherosclerotic lesions, ↑ macrophage number and lipid content of atherosclerotic lesions, ↑ mast cell activation
Espinoza-Derout et al. (2019)	In vivo	Mouse	ApoE−/−	ENDS aerosol (inhalation) + HFD	2.4% nicotine in e-liquid; 24 vaping episodes 30 min each/d	12 w	↑ Atherosclerotic lesion size, ↑ serum free fatty acids, changes in genes associated with metabolism, circadian rhythm, and inflammation
Ren et al. (2018)	In vivo	Mouse	ApoE−/−	Nicotine (i.p.) + HFD	2 mg/kg/d	12 w	↑ Atherosclerotic lesion size, ↑ macrophage number, collagen and lipid content of atherosclerotic lesions, ↑α1nACHR in atherosclerotic lesions, ↑ calpain-1, MMP-2 and MMP-9, IL-6, TNF-α and IL-10 in aortic tissues ↑TC, ↑TG, ↑ LDL
Ren et al. (2018)	In vitro	Mouse	MOVAS (Mouse Aortic VSMCs) and RAW264.7	Nicotine	0.5 ng/mL	24 h	↑ Cell migration and proliferation, ↑ calpain-1, MMP-2 and MMP-9

Study		Species	Model	Dose	Duration	Results
Wu et al. (2018)	In vivo	Mouse	ApoE−/− mice	Nicotine (p.o.) + HFD	100 µg/mL	12 w	↑ Atherosclerotic lesion size, ↑ lipid content of atherosclerotic lesions, ↑ NLRP3, ASC, caspase-1, IL-1β, and IL-18 in aortic tissues
Hashimoto et al. (2018)	In vivo	Mouse	C57BL/6 mice	Nicotine (p.o.)	0.5 mg/L	2 w	↑ Vascular elastin degradation, ↓ vascular collagen content, ↑ CD68, MCP-1 and MMP-2 in intima-media and adventitia
Colombo et al. (2013)	In vivo	Mouse	C57Bl/6 mice	Nicotine (s.c.) +ANG II	5 mg/kg/d	4 w	↑ BP, ↑LVSP, ↑ aortic thickness, ↑ MMP2 activity in cardiac tissue

↑ and ↓ indicate a significant decrease or increase. *3-NT*, 3-nitrotyrosine; *AAA*, abdominal aortic aneurysm; *AMPK*, 5′-AMP-activated protein kinase; *Ang*, angiotensin; *ASC*, apoptosis-associated speck-like protein containing a CARD; *BP*, blood pressure; *CD68*, cluster of differentiation 68; *CXCL*, chemokine (C-X-C motif) ligand; *EC*, endothelial cell; *EHTP*, electrically heated tobacco product; *EPC*, endothelial progenitor cell; *ERK*, extracellular signal-regulated kinase; *EVP*, e-vapor product; *h*, hour; *HFD*, high-fat diet; *HUVEC*, human umbilical vein endothelial cell; *ICAM*, intercellular adhesion molecule; *IFN*, interferon; *IKK*, IκB kinase; *IL*, interleukin; *iRANTES*, Regulated upon Activation, Normal T Cell Expressed and Presumably Secreted; *IκB*, nuclear factor of kappa light polypeptide gene enhancer in B-cells inhibitor; *JNK*, c-Jun N-terminal kinase; *m*, month; *MCP*, monocyte chemoattractant protein; *MDA*, malondialdehyde; *miR*, microRNA; *MMP*, matrix metalloproteinase; *mTOR*, mammalian target of rapamycin; *NFκB*, nuclear factor kappa-light-chain-enhancer of activated B cells; *NLRP3*, NOD-, LRR- and pyrin domain-containing protein 3; *OPN*, osteopontin; *PKC*, protein kinase C; *p.o.*, oral; *PPE*, porcine pancreatic elastase; *PTEN*, phosphatase and tensin homolog; *ROS*, reactive oxygen species; *s.c.*, subcutaneous; *SM*, smooth muscle protein; *SMA*, smooth muscle actin; *SMC*, smooth muscle cells; *STAT*, signal transducer and activator of transcription; *TNF*, tumor necrosis factor; *VCAM*, vascular cell adhesion molecule; *VLA*, very late antigen; *VSMC*, vascular smooth muscle cell; *w*, week.

From Colombo, E.S., Davis, J., Makvandi, M., Aragon, M., Lucas, S.N., Paffett, M.L., et al., 2013. Effects of nicotine on cardiovascular remodeling in a mouse model of systemic hypertension. Cardiovasc. Toxicol. 13(4), 364–369. Espinoza-Derout, J., Hasan, K.M., Shao, X.M., Jordan, M.C., Sims, C., Lee, D.L., et al., 2019. Chronic intermittent electronic cigarette exposure induces cardiac dysfunction and atherosclerosis in apolipoprotein-E knockout mice. Am. J. Physiol. Heart Circ. Physiol. 317(2), H445-H459. Guo, Z.Z., Cao, Q.A., Li, Z.Z., Liu, L.P., Zhang, Z., Zhu, Y.J., et al., 2018. SP600125 attenuates nicotine-related aortic aneurysm formation by inhibiting matrix metalloproteinase production and cc chemokine-mediated macrophage migration. Mediators Inflamm. 2016, 9142425. Hashimoto, K., Zaima, N., Sekiguchi, H., Kugo, H., Miyamoto, C., Hoshino, K., et al., 2018. Dietary DNA attenuates the degradation of elastin fibers in the aortic wall in nicotine-administrated mice. J. Nutr. Sci. Vitaminol. (Tokyo). 64(4), 271–276. Maegdefessel, L., Azuma, J., Toh, R., Deng, A., Merk, D.R., Raiesdana, A., et al., 2012. MicroRNA-21 blocks abdominal aortic aneurysm development and nicotine-augmented expansion. Sci. Transl. Med. 4(122), 122ra122. Ren, A., Wu, H., Liu, L., Guo, Z., Cao, Q., Dai, Q., 2018. Nicotine promotes atherosclerosis development in apolipoprotein E-deficient mice through α1-nAChR. J. Cell Physiol. Epub ahead of print 2018/12/27. DOI: 10.1002/jcp.27728. Szostak, J., Wong, E.T., Titz, B., Lee, T., Wong, S.K., Low, T., et al., 2020. A 6-month systems toxicology inhalation study in ApoE(−/−) mice demonstrates reduced cardiovascular effects of E-vapor aerosols compared with cigarette smoke. Am. J. Physiol. Heart Circ. Physiol. 318(3), H604–H631. Wagenhäuser, M.U., Schellinger, I.N., Yoshino, T., Toyama, K., Kayama, Y., Deng, A., et al., 2018. Chronic nicotine exposure induces murine aortic remodeling and stiffness segmentation-implications for abdominal aortic aneurysm susceptibility. Front. Physiol. 9, 1459. Wang, C., Chen, H., Zhu, W., Xu, Y., Liu, M., Zhu, L., et al., 2017. Nicotine accelerates atherosclerosis in apolipoprotein E-deficient mice by activating α7 nicotinic acetylcholine receptor on mast cells. Arterioscler Thromb. Vasc. Biol. 37(1), 53–65. Wang, S., Zhang, C., Zhang, M., Liang, B., Zhu, H., Lee, J., et al., 2012. Activation of AMP-activated protein kinase alpha2 by nicotine instigates formation of abdominal aortic aneurysms in mice in vivo. Nat. Med. 18(6), 902–910. Wang, Z., Liu, B., Zhu, J., Wang, D., Wang, Y., 2019. Nicotine-mediated autophagy of vascular smooth muscle cell accelerates atherosclerosis via nAChRs/ROS/NF-κB signaling pathway. Atherosclerosis. 284, 1–10. Wu, X., Zhang, H., Qi, W., Zhang, Y., Li, J., Li, Z., et al., 2018. Nicotine promotes atherosclerosis via ROS-NLRP3-mediated endothelial cell pyroptosis. Cell Death Dis. 9(2), 171.

(Chapter 15). Furthermore, in *Apoe*$^{-/-}$ mice fed a normal diet, cigarette smoke exposure accelerated atherosclerotic plaque formation, while exposure to human-relevant doses of an EHTP aerosol failed to have the same effect (Phillips et al., 2016, 2019) (Chapter 15).

In summary, nicotine, on its own, does not seem to accelerate the growth of atherosclerotic plaque in vivo, but it may potentiate the effects of a concomitant proinflammatory condition, such as those arising from an HFD. This may explain, at least in part, why SLT use is associated not with an overall higher risk of IHD and stroke but with a higher risk of mortality from both diseases (Section 20.2.2.1.1).

Several studies found that smoking increases the risk of abdominal aortic aneurysm (AAA) (Sakalihasan et al., 2018). Aortic aneurysms are localized dilatations of the aorta that exceed the normal diameter by 50% or >3 cm. Rupture of an aortic aneurysm can cause massive internal bleeding and is usually fatal; 80% of those reaching a hospital and 50% of those undergoing surgery for ruptured aortic aneurysms die as a consequence (Nordon et al., 2011; Verhoeven et al., 2008).

Proinflammatory mediators and proteases secreted by inflammatory cells play a critical role in AAA (Biros et al., 2012; Lu et al., 2012; Pagano et al., 2009; Xiong et al., 2009). A mouse model of AAA was developed by infusing *Apoe*$^{-/-}$ mice with angiotensin II, which leads to medial accumulation of macrophages in regions of elastin degradation, followed by expansion of the abdominal aortic diameter (AAD) and, eventually, aneurysmal rupture in some of the animals (Rateri et al., 2011; Saraff et al., 2003). In this mouse model, cigarette smoke increased the incidence of AAA as well as matrix metalloproteinase (MMP) gene expression and activity in the abdominal aorta (Stolle et al., 2010). This result is further supported by the absence of AAA in all our *Apoe*$^{-/-}$ mouse inhalation studies (all animals were on a normal diet) involving cigarette smoke and ENDP aerosol exposure (a total of over 4000 animals exposed over a 5-year period), where nicotine was delivered at doses ranging from 6 to 8 mg/kg/day. In these studies, the plasma nicotine concentrations in ENDP aerosol—exposed *Apoe*$^{-/-}$ mice ranged from 100 ng/mL to 130 ng/mL—that is, 3- to 4-fold the plasma nicotine concentrations in human smokers.

Another in vivo model for AAA uses C57BL/6 mice infused with porcine pancreatic elastase. In this model, cigarette smoke exposure also promoted aneurysm growth (Bergoeing et al., 2007; Jin et al., 2012). In both animal models, nicotine exposure led to an increase in AAD expansion (Colombo et al., 2013; Guo et al., 2016; Hashimoto et al., 2018; Maegdefessel et al., 2012; Wagenhäuser et al., 2018; Wang et al., 2012).

In summary, cigarette smoke and nicotine may potentiate the effects of hypertension in AAA (Table 20.6).

20.2.2.2.5 Does nicotine alter heart function?. In clinical studies, EVP users present mild cardiac dysfunction with increases in heart rate and systolic and diastolic blood pressure (Chaumont et al., 2018; Farsalinos et al., 2014; Franzen et al., 2018; Moheimani et al., 2017a). Studies in *Apoe*$^{-/-}$ mice have highlighted that exposure to nicotine-containing EVP aerosols decreases left ventricular fractional shortening, the ejection fraction, left ventricular systolic pressure, and left ventricular diastolic pressure and increases contraction velocity, indicating functional impairment of systodiastolic function (Espinoza-Derout et al., 2019; Szostak et al., 2020). Similarly, reduced ventricular function has also been observed in mice receiving 6 mg/kg/day nicotine s.c. for 4 months or 2 mg/kg/day i.p. for 10 days and in rats receiving 0.6 mg/kg/day nicotine i.p. for 28 days (Gaffin et al., 2011; Hu et al., 2011; Ramalingam et al., 2019).

Some studies have suggested a dysregulation of oxidative stress mechanisms in response to nicotine or ENDP aerosol exposure (Espinoza-Derout et al., 2019; Guo et al., 2019; Li et al., 2019; Nacerai et al., 2017; Zhou et al., 2010), while others have not (Phillips et al., 2016, 2019; Szostak et al., 2020). Importantly, induction of cardiac cell apoptosis and oxidative stress by nicotine requires that C56BL/6 mice be on an HFD (Sinha-Hikim et al., 2017) (Table 20.7).

20.2.3 Conclusions for CVD

This review indicates that, while nicotine exerts effects on the cardiovascular system, these effects may primarily impact/worsen preexisting conditions. Indeed, nicotine, on its own, does not seem to accelerate the growth of atherosclerotic plaque in vivo, but it may potentiate the effects of a concomitant proinflammatory condition, such as that arising from an HFD. This is consistent with the observation that an HFD is needed to elicit oxidative stress and cardiac cell apoptosis (Sinha-Hikim et al., 2017). Furthermore, studies have consistently shown that nicotine affects endothelial function and may lead to arterial stiffness over time. Moreover, clinical and in vivo studies consistently have shown that nicotine exposure affects blood pressure and systodiastolic function.

Taken together, these observations may explain, at least in part, why SLT use is associated not with an overall higher risk of IHD and stroke (Section 20.2.2) but with a higher risk of mortality from both diseases (Section 20.2.2).

The overviews of the published studies reported in Tables 20.4—20.7 highlight the heterogeneity in

TABLE 20.7
Effects of Nicotine on Heart Function.

Reference	Study Type	Species	Experimental Model	Treatment (Route)	Dose	Duration	Effect on Biological Processes and Molecular Mechanisms
(Nacerai et al., 2017)	In vivo	Rat	Male albino	Nicotine (s.c.)	1 mg/kg	8 w	↑ Cardiac and blood MDA, ↑ HSP70, Gpr78, CHOP and AIF in cardiac tissue
(Espinoza-Derout et al., 2019)	In vivo	Mouse	ApoE-/-	EVP aerosol (inhalation)	2.4% nicotine in e-liquid; 24 vaping episodes for 30 min each/d	12 w	↓ LVEF, ↓ LVFS
(Sinha-Hikim et al., 2017)	In vivo	Mouse	C57BL6	Nicotine (i.p.) + HFD	1.5 mg/kg/d	16 w	↑ Cardiomyocyte apoptosis, ↓ p-AMPK and ↑ 4-HNE, caspase-3 and caspase-9 in ventricular tissue
(Ramalingam et al., 2019)	In vivo	Rat	Sprague-Dawley	Nicotine (i.p.)	0.6 mg/kg/d	28 d	↑ Heart weight, ↑ SBP, ↓ LVSP, ↓LVDP, ↓ dL/dt, ↑ AngII in plasma and LV tissues, ↑ cardiomyocyte size, ↑collagen content, 3-NT, IL6, IL10, TNFα and ANXA1 in LV tissues, ↓ GSH : GSSG in LV tissues
(Hu et al., 2011)	In vivo	Mouse	Wild-type friend virus B (FVB)	Nicotine (i.p.)	2 mg/kg/d	10 d	↓LVFS, ↓ dL/dt, ↓ peak shortening, ↑ RT90, ↑myocardial fibrosis, ↑ cardiomyocyte ROS and caspase-3
(Gaffin et al., 2011)	In vivo	Mouse	FVB/N expressing α-tropomyosin D175N mutation	Nicotine tartrate (s.c.)	6 mg/kg/d	4 m	↑ +dp/dt, no effect on cardiac morphology
(Szostak et al., 2020)	In vivo	Mouse	ApoE-/-	EVP aerosol (inhalation)	35 µg/L for 3h/d, 5d/w	6 m	↑ Isovolumic relaxation time, ↑ MPI

nonclinical research methodology used to investigate the effects of nicotine and ENDPs on the cardiovascular system. The main limitation of most reported in vivo studies is the absence of appropriate controls and verification of nicotine uptake though measurement of blood nicotine and cotinine concentrations. The main limitation of a large number of the reported in vitro studies is that the nicotine concentrations used in these studies exceeded the plasma nicotine concentrations observed in smokers or EVP users (Fig. 20.2).

20.3 NICOTINE AND LUNG CANCER
20.3.1 Introduction
Lung cancer is the most common cancer in the world today, and more people die from lung cancer than any other type of cancer.[2] Almost all lung cancers are carcinomas and are distinguished by their histological appearance as non–small-cell lung cancer (NSCLC) or small-cell lung cancer (SCLC). SCLCs, which account for up to 15% of all lung cancers, are fast-growing and aggressive tumors thought to arise from neuroendocrine cells predominantly in the large airways (Riaz et al., 2012; Rosti et al., 2006). NSCLC, with 85% prevalence, is the most common type of lung cancer (Molina et al., 2008) and can be further categorized into adenocarcinoma, squamous cell carcinoma (SCC), and large-cell carcinoma. While SCCs typically arise in the lung epithelium lining the large airways, large-cell carcinomas and adenocarcinomas originate in the peripheral lung epithelium.

There is overwhelming evidence that tobacco smoking is the major cause of lung cancer in most human populations, and a number of epidemiological studies have demonstrated an increased risk of lung cancer in smokers (Doll and Hill, 2004; Doll and Peto, 1981; Harris et al., 2004; Wakai et al., 2006; Zhang Hong and Cai, 2003). This increased lung cancer risk is seen for all major histological types but appears to be the greatest for SCC, followed by SCLC and adenocarcinoma (Parkin et al., 2004).

Direct damage to DNA by ROS and reactive nitrogen species (RNS) is an accepted explanation for the initiation of events that ultimately lead to lung cancer (Halliwell, 2007). Oxidative damage to other macromolecules can also promote mutagenesis, particularly when proteins involved in DNA replication or repair or lipids are affected. Ensuing wide-spread mutations and deregulation of DNA repair and signal transduction pathways through modification of histones and

gene methylation patterns are common features of lung cancers (Alexandrov et al., 2016; Hecht, 2012). Many of these mechanisms, eventually culminating in carcinogenesis, have been linked to a multitude of constituents in cigarette smoke, including nicotine. Dissociating the biological effects of nicotine from those of cigarettes smoke is challenging, and, hence, the contribution of nicotine to lung carcinogenesis remains a matter of debate.

20.3.2 Does Nicotine Cause Lung Cancer?
While the International Agency for Research on Cancer (IARC) has not evaluated nicotine for carcinogenic potential, there is conflicting evidence from the scientific literature that both supports and refutes the notion that it is a lung carcinogen. Here, we review this evidence—derived from clinical, in vivo, and in vitro studies—to provide a comprehensive view on the available data, which may shed further light on the potential role of nicotine in the development of lung cancer. In particular, the nonclinical data can potentially reveal whether nicotine initiates, promotes, and/or facilitates the progression of the disease. Convincing and physiologically relevant evidence supporting these three main stages of carcinogenicity would result in a significant "complete carcinogen" classification (i.e., sufficient to induce lung cancer of its own accord), whereas a more limited dataset may preclude unequivocal conclusions and act as a trigger for further research.

20.3.2.1 Epidemiological evidence
There is little clinical evidence that would allow for a reasonable, balanced debate on the question of whether nicotine is causally linked to lung cancer. Very often, study data are confounded by cigarette smoking or consumption of other tobacco products, such as snuffs, snus, and other SLT products, which expose the user to more chemicals than just nicotine. Although consumption of SLT products is associated with a lower risk of lung cancer development than cigarette smoking, the risk reduction appears to depend on the type of product used and the geographical specifics of consumption. In Indian SLT product users, for example, the adjusted hazard ratio (HR) for lung cancer was 1.59 (95% CI, 0.87–2.90) users relative to never-users (Pednekar et al., 2011). In the Agricultural Health Study, exclusive ever-use of SLT, such as chewing tobacco or snuff, was significantly associated with lung cancer (HR, 2.21; 95% CI, 1.11–4.42), though the adjusted HR in smokers was much higher relative to never-smokers (15.48; 95% CI, 11.95–20.06) (Andreotti et al., 2017). Epidemiological data on snus use in Scandinavian countries, on the other hand, has

---

[2]http://www.cdc.gov/cancer/lung/basic_info/index.htm.

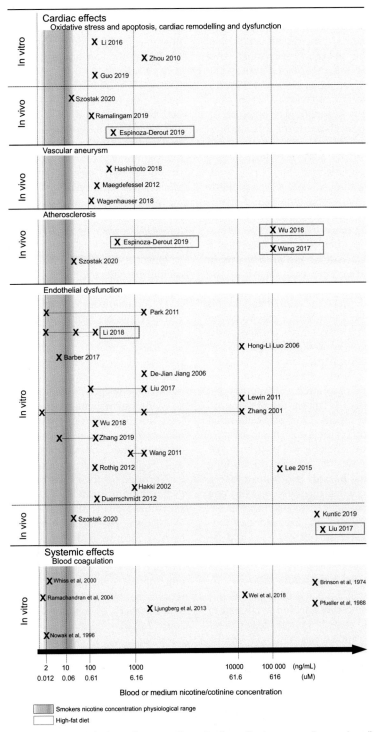

FIG. 20.2 Overview of nonclinical studies reporting nicotine effects on cardiovascular disease–related endpoints in vivo and in vitro.   The location of each reference on the x-axis reflects the range of nicotine concentrations tested where the effects were observed. Type of studies (in vivo/in vitro) are indicated on the left side. The grey area indicates the physiological range of nicotine concentration measured in the biological samples of smokers.

indicated a negligible effect on lung cancer risk in ever-users relative to never-users (Boffetta et al., 2005; Luo et al., 2007). Furthermore, it should be noted that, unlike cigarette smoking, using Swedish snus is not associated with a significant risk of oral cancer—RR values of 1.0 (95% CI, 0.7–1.3) to 1.01 (95% CI, 0.71–1.45)—or esophageal or stomach cancer (Boffetta et al., 2008; Lee, 2011; Lee and Hamling, 2009). Together, these data suggest that it is the inhalation of cigarette smoke and/or exposure to tobacco-related carcinogens, such as TSNAs, that ultimately lead to lung cancer and not exposure to nicotine.

The largest and only study to date to examine the link between nicotine alone and lung cancer risk is the Lung Health Study (Murray et al., 2009). Of the originally enrolled 5807 participants, 3923 were randomized to a smoking intervention (Lung Health Study 1). Approximately half of the participants in this subgroup (n = 1936) were encouraged to use nicotine gum (Nicorette 2 mg) liberally for up to 6 months, and, after 2.5 years, the participants in this group were asked to stop using NRT. Detailed cancer data were collected after 5 years and for an additional 5 years (Lung Cancer Substudy). Subsequently, in 3320 smoking intervention participants without cancer diagnosis, all-cause hospitalizations and emergency room visits were monitored for another 3.5 years (Lung Health Study 3). During the observation period, 75 cases of lung cancer, 33 of gastrointestinal tract cancer, and 203 of cancer from all causes were recorded. While cigarette smoking was clearly linked to lung cancer, NRT use was not associated with lung cancer (Cox proportional hazards regression models, adjusted for age, sex, baseline cigarettes per day, and lifetime pack-years of smoking). No relationship between cigarette smoking or NRT use and gastrointestinal cancer or cancer from all causes could be established (Murray et al., 2009).

20.3.2.2 Nonclinical carcinogenicity studies

It is accepted that almost all human carcinogens identified to date also cause cancer in at least one laboratory animal species (Boorman et al., 1994), and current integrative risk assessment approaches still rely on the 2-year rodent bioassay to identify cancer hazards. However, the rodent carcinogenicity bioassay is also fraught with limitations, particularly when working with weak genotoxins or attempting to translate the dose–response relationships to humans, with cancer-associated endpoints often only observed at maximally tolerated doses (Omenn, 2001). In addition, very few carcinogenicity studies have replicated human nicotine

use. Instead, they have administered nicotine to animals via routes that have resulted in markedly different pharmacokinetics and ensuing local tissue and plasma levels that often are not physiologically relevant (Matta et al., 2007).

In a 2-year inhalation study involving exposure of female Sprague Dawley rats to 0.5 mg/m^3 nicotine for 20 h/day and for 5 d/week, tumors were seen in 36% and 24% of animals in the nicotine and control groups, respectively. Among these tumors, fibroadenomas of the mammary gland were the most common but were considered to be age-related rather than linked to nicotine exposure. Other tumors, such as those of the anterior pituitary gland, ovaries, and skin, occurred only in nicotine-exposed animals and at a low frequency. Lung tumors were not detected in this inhalation study (Waldum et al., 1996).

Other studies with cancer-relevant endpoints administered nicotine at different doses via different routes and for varying durations. Differences in study design make comparisons across studies challenging. In addition, the majority of these studies are not aligned with OECD (Organisation for Economic Co-operation and Development) test guideline recommendations (OECD, 2018c,d) for group size, dose selection, and endpoints with respect to carcinogenicity studies, making the results, overall, less informative for evaluating the carcinogenic potential of nicotine. Nevertheless, prominent among these studies are a handful of mouse studies in which nicotine was administered in drinking water. For example, in one study, female and male Swiss mice were exposed to 0.5 and 0.7 mg/mL/day nicotine for their lifetime. There were no increases in lung tumor incidence or tumor incidence at organ sites other than the lungs (Toth, 1982). In another study in A/J mice, chronic nicotine administration (0.2 mg/mL/day nicotine hydrogen tartrate for 46 weeks) did not increase lung tumor multiplicity or size and also did not affect 4-(methylnitrosamino)-1-(3-pyridyl)-1-butanone (NNK)-induced tumorigenesis (Murphy et al., 2011). The latter finding is also in line with earlier observations that consumption of approximately 20 mg/kg/day nicotine in drinking water for 2–12 weeks did not promote lung tumor growth or progression in AB6F1 and Kras$^{LA2/+}$ mice, in AB6F1 mice bearing various allograft tumors (Maier et al., 2011), or in nude ovariectomized mice with A549 xenograft tumors (Jarzynka et al., 2006). However, in other studies, prolonged oral or transdermal administration of high doses of nicotine (20–25 mg/kg/day) seemed to promote the growth of tumor allografts, which is most likely due to the proangiogenic properties of nicotine, which stimulates neovascularization and thereby promotes tumor growth (Heeschen et al., 2001; Natori et al., 2003). Nicotine also seems to promote the growth of tumors induced in mice injected with a very high dose (100 mg/kg) of NNK (Davis et al., 2009; Iskandar et al., 2013). This single dose of NNK used in mice represents a dose of 8.1 mg/kg for a 60-kg human and, considering that commercial cigarettes emit NNK at an average of 128 ng/stick (Chapter 4), would represent the NNK emitted by 3.8 million cigarettes, which is equivalent to >500 years of smoking 20 cigarettes per day.

Thompson et al. reported three pheochromocytomas, four epidermoid carcinomas of the skin, one leukemia, and one fibrosarcoma but no lung tumors in rats that received 1 mg/kg/day nicotine s.c. for 22 months. The authors surmised that the tumors were age-related rather than treatment-related (Thompson et al., 1973). Galitovskiy and colleagues also did not observe lung tumors but found rhabdomyosarcomas and uterine myoleiosarcomas in A/J mice chronically treated with 3 mg/kg/day nicotine s.c. for 24 months (Galitovskiy et al., 2012). These types of tumors are common and develop spontaneously in this mouse strain (Sher et al., 2011; Sundberg et al., 1991), although the authors did not acknowledge this fact. Furthermore, the authors did also not report the high frequency of spontaneous lung tumors in untreated, aged A/J mice observed in many other studies (Landau et al., 1998; Stinn et al., 2013; Stoner and Shimkin, 1982; Wong et al., 2020). In female *Rag2*-knockout mice bearing B16 melanoma xenografts and treated with 13 mg/kg/day nicotine s.c. for 3 weeks, tumor burden and tumor size were significantly reduced relative to untreated controls (Hao et al., 2013).

More recently, our group published the results of an inhalation study in which A/J mice were exposed to the aerosol of THS, which is an EHTP (Chapter 15). In this study, exposure to THS aerosol did not increase the incidence or multiplicity of lung adenomas or adenocarcinomas relative to sham-exposed animals, even at nicotine doses of 10 mg/kg/day (Wong et al., 2020). Furthermore, the tumors in the THS aerosol—exposed female mice were the same size as those that spontaneously developed in sham-exposed animals, while, in male mice, the tumors in the THS exposure group were smaller than those in the sham-exposed animals. However, cigarette smoke exposure at a nicotine dose corresponding to 5 mg/kg/day led to an increase in the incidence and multiplicity of lung tumors (Wong et al., 2020).

In summary, the effects of nicotine on carcinogenicity were assessed in many diverse animal studies. Most of the studies reported unequivocal noncarcinogenic findings, while a few revealed that the angiogenic properties of nicotine may cause an increase in the size of tumor allografts. The preponderance of "negative"—that is, noncarcinogenic—results presumably brought a halt to further, unwarranted investigations, while, for the "positive" (carcinogenic) results, the evidence remains circumstantial, as it was obtained with unrealistically high doses of nicotine in mice bearing a tumor allograft. Taken together, the evidence indicates that nicotine does not cause lung cancer on its own in animal models.

20.3.2.3 Mechanistic evidence

Nicotine exerts its pharmacological effects through nicotinic acetylcholine receptors (nAChRs), prototypic ligand-gated ion channels which are activated by the endogenous agonists acetylcholine and choline and exogenous ligands (among others). Nicotinic acetylcholine receptors are pentamers formed by α ($\alpha1-\alpha10$), β ($\beta1-\beta4$), and other (δ, γ, and ε) subunits. The composition of nAChRs in a given biological system is heterogeneous, which confers the receptors diverse functions upon activation. More specifically, neuronal nAChR subtypes are constructed from combinations of nine α ($\alpha2-\alpha10$) and three β ($\beta2-\beta4$) subunits. In non-neural tissues, lymphocytes express the $\alpha3\beta4$, $\alpha4\beta2$, and $\alpha7$ receptor subtypes, and macrophages express the $\alpha4\beta2$ and $\alpha7$ receptor subtypes; $\alpha3$, $\alpha7$, $\alpha9$, $\beta2$, and $\beta4$ subunits are detected in the skin; $\alpha3$, $\alpha5$, $\alpha7$, $\beta2$, and $\beta4$ in the lungs; $\alpha3$, $\alpha5$, $\alpha7$, $\alpha10$, $\beta2$, and $\beta4$ in vascular endothelial cells; and $\alpha2$, $\alpha3$, $\alpha4$, $\alpha5$, $\alpha7$, and $\alpha10$ in vascular smooth muscles (reviewed in Gotti and Clementi, 2004).

Agonist/neurotransmitter binding increases the opening probability of the nAChR channel pore, allowing cations (Na^+, K^+, or Ca^{2+}, depending on the receptor type) to cross and, ultimately, result in membrane depolarization (Albuquerque et al., 2009). It is typically the Ca^{2+} influx that directly or indirectly triggers downstream signaling, including activation of the protein kinase C (PKC), the phosphatidylinositol 3-kinase/protein kinase B (PI3K/Akt), extracellular signal-regulated kinase (ERK), mitogen-activated protein kinase kinase (MEK), and janus kinase (JAK) signaling pathways (Dani, 2015; Veljkovic et al., 2018). Because these pathways are implicated in lung carcinogenesis (Ciuffreda et al., 2014; Fan et al., 2013; Fumarola et al., 2014), it is critical to understand how nicotine may affect them in lung cells. In addition, nAChRs are expressed on many different cell types, some of which compose or populate the lungs, including immune cells; therefore, the varying actions of nicotine on other mechanisms, such as inflammation, immune surveillance, and angiogenesis, also need to be considered.

Using a published framework for evaluating the mechanistic data related to nicotine's effects on various aspects of lung carcinogenesis, we reviewed the available evidence with respect to the 10 key characteristics of carcinogens outlined by Smith and colleagues (Smith et al., 2016). In particular, this review focuses on evidence that helps determine if nicotine

- is electrophilic or can be metabolically activated
- is genotoxic
- alters DNA repair or causes genomic instability
- induces epigenetic alterations
- induces oxidative stress
- induces chronic inflammation
- is immunosuppressive
- modulates receptor-mediated effects
- causes immortalization
- alters cell proliferation, cell death, or nutrient supply

20.3.2.3.1 Is nicotine electrophilic, or can it be metabolically activated?. The metabolism of nicotine is well understood and extensively detailed in the literature. More than 80% of absorbed nicotine undergoes metabolism in the liver, primarily by cytochrome P450 (CYP) 2A6, UDP-glucuronosyltransferase, and FMO3, a flavin-containing monooxygenase. As much as 85%–90% of nicotine is metabolized in the liver by CYP2A6, before elimination via renal excretion (Benowitz et al., 2009). Of note in the context of carcinogenesis, it is hypothesized that nicotine metabolism can give rise to reactive intermediates that can form DNA adducts. This has been described in one study, in which γ-OH-1,N^2-cyclic 1,N^2-propanodeoxuguanosine and O^6-methyl-deoxyguanosine adducts were found in the lungs, bladder, and heart DNA of male FVBN mice and in human BEAS-2B bronchial epithelial cells and UROtsa urothelial cells exposed to e-cigarette–derived aerosol (Lee et al., 2018). The authors hypothesized that nitrosation of nicotine leads to formation of nitrosamine ketone, which is further metabolized to the ultimate genotoxin and methylating agent methyldiazohydroxide. However, this study has been criticized both for its inadequate experimental design and failure to demonstrate that the DNA adducts do indeed derive from nicotine and not from lipid peroxidation by-products (Li et al., 2018; Queimado et al., 2018). Considering that inclusion of S9 metabolic fractions in in vitro genotoxicity tests such as the Ames assay does not lead to positive results, it seems unlikely that nicotine or its reactive metabolites exhibit notable electrophilicity. Moreover, even though another study reported the presence of DNA adducts in the liver of nicotine-exposed mice, neither the nature of these adducts was clarified nor did the study include

appropriate controls (i.e., DNA adduct content in nonexposed mice) (Cheng et al., 2003). Therefore, the question of whether nicotine exposure and subsequent metabolism directly give rise to a biologically relevant quantity of DNA adducts has yet to be satisfactorily answered.

20.3.2.3.2 Is nicotine genotoxic?. Genotoxicity refers to the damage caused by chemicals or electromagnetic radiation to DNA. Such damage can manifest itself as gene mutations or structural and numerical changes at the chromosomal level or other forms of damage, including covalent binding of the genotoxin to DNA (DNA adduct formation) and DNA breakage. There is a well-defined battery of in vitro genotoxicity assays that forms a core part of human hazard assessment and which have been used to assess whether or not nicotine has the potential to cause mutations or other forms of DNA damage.

A few studies have reported nonmutagenic findings in the bacterial reverse mutation (Ames) test for treatment with 0.49–1 mg nicotine per plate (Doolittle et al., 1995; Florin et al., 1980; Riebe et al., 1982). Interestingly, these studies used the liver S9 metabolic fraction; therefore, the results imply that S9-mediated metabolism of nicotine does not produce metabolites that are mutagenic in bacteria. Similar results were reported in nicotine studies involving other bacterial assays. Yim and Hee found no genotoxic effects associated with a 40-h nicotine treatment at concentrations ranging from 0.015 to 123 mM in a *Vibrio fischeri*–based assay, both in the absence and presence of an S9 fraction (Yim and Hee, 1995). However, Riebe et al. noted positive findings of reparable DNA damage in an assay conducted in *Escherichia coli* by using 10 µg nicotine per plate (Riebe et al., 1982).

Additional data on several other genotoxicity endpoints are derived from mammalian cell–based assays and are, at times, contradictory. For example, Riebe and Westphal found a weak increase in sister chromatid exchange (SCE) in Chinese hamster ovary (CHO) cells after a 1-h exposure to nicotine at concentrations >7.7 mM; but, this increase was only statistically significant at the highest concentration tested (35 mM) (Riebe and Westphal, 1983). At lower nicotine concentrations and similar exposure duration, neither Doolittle et al. nor Altmann et al. found an increase in CHO cell SCE (Altmann et al., 1984; Doolittle et al., 1995). In contrast, statistically significantly increased SCE frequencies were reported in CHO cells exposed to nicotine concentrations of 0.9–3.9 mM for 48 h (Trivedi et al., 1990, 1993) and in human lymphocytes following exposure to 0.001–1 mM nicotine for 24 h (Ginzkey et al., 2013).

Exposure of human gingival fibroblasts to 1 µM nicotine for 72 h significantly increased micronucleus (MN) formation (Argentin and Cicchetti, 2004), as did treatment of human lymphocytes with 0.1 and 1 mM nicotine (Ginzkey et al., 2013) and treatment of human primary parotid gland cells with 0.01 mM nicotine (Ginzkey et al., 2014a) for 24 h. The lowest nicotine concentration that produced a statistically significant increase in MN in rat peripheral blood cells was 3 mM (Muthukumaran et al., 2008; Sudheer et al., 2007a), which was at least one order magnitude higher than the concentrations that caused a significant increase in MN frequency in human cells. These results suggest that cells might have different sensitivities to nicotine in terms of MN induction, depending on their species of origin.

Chromosomal aberrations (CAs) were increased in a significant and concentration-dependent manner in CHO cells after 24-h nicotine treatment at concentrations above 2.3 mM, whereas no effects were observed after a shorter exposure (2 or 4 h) followed by a 24-h recovery period (Trivedi et al., 1990, 1993). Significant dose-dependent increases in CAs were also observed after a 1-h treatment of human lymphocytes and human primary parotid gland cells with nicotine (0.001–1 mM) (Ginzkey et al., 2013, 2014a). In addition, there were significant increases in both structural and numerical aberrations after treatment of human fetal cells with a single concentration of nicotine (15 µM) (Demirhan et al., 2011). However, Mailhes et al. exposed mouse oocytes to 1–10 mM nicotine for 16 h and found no significant changes in chromosome aneuploidy (Mailhes et al., 2000).

The comet assay has also been extensively used to study the effects of nicotine on DNA strand breaks in cell cultures, and the results vary widely. A single treatment of rat peripheral blood lymphocytes with 3 mM nicotine for 1 h significantly increased the DNA damage parameters measured by this assay, including %tail length, tail moment, %tail DNA, and olive tail moment (OTM) (Muthukumaran et al., 2008; Sudheer et al., 2007a). No changes in OTM were noted after nicotine treatment (1–100 µM, 24 h) of human OEC-M1 oral epidermal carcinoma cells at pH 6.5, whereas treatment with 1 and 10 µM nicotine at pH 8.0 induced a significant increase in DNA damage, although not in a concentration-dependent manner (Wu et al., 2005). This pH effect was not reproduced by Kleinsasser et al. in human tonsillar tissue cells and lymphocytes; however, exposure to 0.125–4 mM nicotine for 1 h did

significantly increase OTM in both cell types in a concentration-dependent manner (Kleinsasser et al., 2005). This is in contrast to the findings of Ginzkey et al. showing that nicotine treatment (0.001–1 mM) did not induce any DNA damage in human lymphocytes, even after a 24-h exposure (Ginzkey et al., 2013). Sassen et al. exposed human nasal epithelial mini-organ cultures (MOCs) to nicotine for 1 h every other day for 3 days and found that a single 1-h treatment with 2 and 4 mM nicotine on day 1 resulted in a concentration-dependent increase in OTM values. However, subsequent exposure of the same MOC on the following interval days did not further increase DNA damage at either concentration (Sassen et al., 2005). Ginzkey and coworkers also treated human nasal MOCs with nicotine (0.001 and 1 mM), but continuously for 3 weeks rather than intermittently, and found significant increases in OTM after 1 week of exposure at both concentrations, although there was no concentration dependency. This effect decreased after 2 and 3 weeks, without significant DNA migration (Ginzkey et al., 2014b). Another study from the same group also investigated the time-dependent genotoxic effects of nicotine in human parotid gland tissue MOCs. Treatment with 2 mM nicotine for 1, 2, or 3 consecutive 1-h periods resulted in significant DNA damage (increased %tail DNA), independent of exposure time (Ginzkey et al., 2010). Two studies on nicotine treatment of human primary salivary gland cells at various concentrations (0.001–4 mM, 1 h) reported significant DNA damage, as evidenced by increased % tail DNA and OTM measurements (Ginzkey et al., 2009, 2014a). Furthermore, treatment with the lowest nicotine concentration assessed (0.1 µM) in human leukocytes actually reduced DNA damage below background levels, but exposure to 10- and 100-fold higher concentrations (1 and 10 µM) induced significant increases in both %tail DNA and OTM (Sobkowiak et al., 2014).

Aside from DNA adducts, other forms of DNA damage were also assessed in several animal studies following nicotine treatment. None of these studies delivered nicotine via the inhalation route; the most common administration routes were s.c. injection and oral gavage. The endpoints assessed included MN formation, DNA breaks as revealed by the comet assay, and CA.

Adler and Attia treated male Swiss albino mice with single doses of nicotine (1 or 2 mg/kg) by oral administration and sampled bone marrow at 24 h (low dose) or at 6, 12, and 18 h (high dose) after treatment (Adler and Attia, 2003). In this study, nicotine treatment did not increase the frequency of micronucleated polychromatic erythrocytes (MNPCEs). A follow-up study with male and female mice, an extended dose range (4, 8, and 16 mg/kg), and posttreatment sampling time intervals (18, 24, 30, 36, and 48 h) (Attia, 2007) showed that nicotine did not affect the number of MNPCEs at the selected doses at two of the earlier sampling time points (18 or 24 h), despite exerting evident acute toxicity. In the 36- and 48-h samples, 8 and 16 mg/kg nicotine caused significantly increased MNPCE frequencies in both sexes, which was accompanied by significantly greater bone marrow toxicity in both male and female mice. In rats, long-term nicotine treatment via s.c. injection at a maximal tolerated dose of 2.5 mg/kg/day for 5 d/week and for 22 weeks also significantly increased MN frequency in peripheral blood cells (Muthukumaran et al., 2008; Sudheer et al., 2007a). Similarly, the mean MN frequency in peripheral blood cells was significantly increased in male and female mice at 24 h following administration of 15 mg/kg nicotine by oral gavage. The authors reported no sex difference in this toxicological endpoint, but noted that the number of mice in each group was rather small (three animals per sex per group) (Kahl et al., 2012). A recent study at PMI confirmed that high nicotine concentrations (>3.94 mM) induce DNA damage (as micronuclei) in CHO cells. However, complementary mechanistic data suggest that this was driven by a lysosomotropic mode of action, which is not likely to be physiologically relevant for ENDP users (Smart et al., 2019).

Nicotine administered by i.p. injection at doses of 5, 7.5, or 10 mg/kg did not affect the frequency of aneuploidy in ICR mouse oocytes in vivo (Mailhes et al., 2000). However, when administered orally (p.o.) at 0.77 or 1.1 mg/kg, nicotine caused CA in bone marrow cells in mice, although it is difficult to draw further conclusions from this study because of the small number of doses examined and lack of a time–response effect (Sen et al., 1991).

Nicotine exposure significantly increased the frequencies of several comet assay parameters, including tail length, tail moment, %DNA in tail, and olive tail moment, in peripheral blood in rats (Muthukumaran et al., 2008; Sudheer et al., 2007b). It also significantly increased the damage index (number of cells multiplied with the number of damage class categorized by the length of DNA tails from the comet assay) and damage frequency (number of cells with tail vs. those without in each sample) in the blood of exposed mice (Kahl et al., 2012). This study reported no sex difference; however, again, the group sizes were small (three animals per sex per group).

Together, the results from these studies indicate that nicotine is nonmutagenic but may exert apparent clastogenic effects at high concentrations. Importantly, the concentrations needed to observe clastogenicity by far exceed the physiological nicotine exposure in humans, and it is, therefore, unlikely that nicotine consumption via ENDPs leads to DNA damage.

20.3.2.3.3 Does nicotine alter DNA repair or cause genomic instability?

DNA damage can arise spontaneously, through endogenous ROS produced by the mitochondrial electron transport chain during normal cellular respiration, by replication errors, or through the action of environmental stressors such as genotoxic agents. Most damage to DNA can be repaired, and, unless there are serious perturbations in the DNA damage response pathways, a certain degree of DNA damage can be tolerated. Although in vivo studies on the effects of nicotine on DNA repair are scarce, one report provided indirect evidence on the base excision repair pathway in nicotine-exposed mice. The plasma and bronchoalveolar lavage fluid (BALF) levels of 8-hydroxy-2'-deoxyguanosine (8-OHdG)—a marker of oxidative DNA damage which may contribute to carcinogenesis by giving rise to mutations and/or modulating gene expression (Valavanidis et al., 2013)—were significantly higher in C57BL/6 mice that received a single dose of 2 μg nicotine via nebulization than in controls, indicating that induced 8-OHdG lesions were excised from DNA by repair systems active in the animals (Schweitzer et al., 2015). 8-OHdG levels were also increased in the culture medium of OCE-M1 cells treated with 1–100 μM nicotine for 24 h at pH 8.0, but without dose-dependency (Wu et al., 2005).

Because of the paucity of studies on systematic evaluation of the effects nicotine might have on DNA repair, there is currently insufficient evidence to conclusively (dis)prove that nicotine impairs DNA repair.

20.3.2.3.4 Does nicotine induce epigenetic alterations?

The term "epigenetic alterations" refers to changes in the heritable phenotype that do not involve alterations of the genetic information (i.e., the DNA sequence) but rather include DNA modifications by, for example, methylation, chromatin modification, and regulation of gene activity by microRNA (miRNA) or noncoding RNA (ncRNA). Koturbash et al. noted that *"epigenetic alterations may be early indicators of genotoxic and non-genotoxic carcinogenic exposure"* and proposed their inclusion in evaluation *"of the carcinogenic potential of environmental chemical and physical agents"* (Koturbash et al., 2011).

To date, only a few studies have investigated the effects of nicotine on miRNA in human cell cultures.

MicroRNA (MIR)1305 expression was increased in periodontal ligament–derived stem cells upon nicotine exposure (0.5–2 μM) for 3 days, while, in contrast, miR-439 expression was decreased in nicotine-treated head and neck cancer cells (Kumar et al., 2017). In normal human bronchial epithelial cells exposed to nicotine-containing e-vapor, MIR29a-5p, MIR140-5p, MIR374a-5p, MIR26a2-5p, and MIR147-5p levels were all increased; however, the expression of both MIR941 and MIR589-5p was decreased (Solleti et al., 2017). The implications of these changes to the miRNA transcriptome are currently unknown. Individual reports ascribe various tumor-suppressing and tumor-promoting properties to some of these miRNA, most likely because miRNAs have multiple targets, and, therefore, changes in their expression affect a multitude of different signaling pathways.

It should be noted that in vitro and in vivo inhalation studies comparing the effects of cigarette smoke with those of THS aerosol have shown that THS aerosol has a much reduced, if not negligible, effect on miRNA expression at equivalent nicotine exposure (Phillips et al., 2019; Sewer et al., 2016; Titz et al., 2020). Furthermore, unlike cigarette smoke, THS aerosol has a significantly reduced effect on DNA methylation (Choukrallah et al., 2019; Phillips et al., 2019). While these studies indicate that nicotine does not substantially affect miRNA expression or DNA methylation, additional studies for exploring the effects of pure nicotine on global DNA modifications and miRNA expression are needed to definitively conclude whether nicotine is an epigenetic modifier.

20.3.2.3.5 Does nicotine cause oxidative stress?.

Oxidative stress results from an imbalance between the levels of ROS and antioxidants. ROS and other reactive species act directly on cellular macromolecules, damaging lipids, proteins, and DNA. Direct damage to DNA by ROS and RNS is accepted as an explanation for the initiation of events that can ultimately lead to lung cancer (Halliwell, 2007). It is well known that interaction of DNA with hydroxyl radicals leads to the formation of mutagenic purines and pyrimidines such as 8-OHdG, one of the most abundant and readily formed oxidized DNA bases (Valavanidis et al., 2009), which can induce G:T transversions—the most frequent mutations in human cancers (Pilger and Rüdiger, 2006). Similarly, an attack on DNA by RNS can result in deamination of nucleobases and the formation of oxidative lesions with promutagenic characteristics (Ohshima and Bartsch, 1994). Oxidative damage to proteins can also promote

mutagenesis, particularly when proteins involved in DNA replication or repair, such as proliferating cell nuclear antigen (PCNA) and growth arrest and DNA-damage-inducible protein 45 (Gadd45), are affected (Fayolle et al., 2008; Kinoshita et al., 2007). Furthermore, oxidative modification of signal transducers such as protein kinases can lead to their constitutive activation, accelerating transition through the cell cycle and promoting proliferation (Matés et al., 2008). Finally, ROS also act on lipids, causing their peroxidation and, in the process, generating a number of highly reactive intermediary carbonyl compounds that can form DNA adducts and, thus, give rise to mutagenic lesions (Fearon et al., 2011).

Most in vivo studies support the notion that nicotine causes oxidative stress, mostly indirectly by negatively modulating cellular antioxidant defenses or by inducing oxidative modifications in proteins and lipids. For example, significant decreases in SOD, catalase (CAT), glutathione peroxidase (GPx), and glutathione reductase levels and/or activities were reported in the lungs or blood of rats that received various doses of nicotine s.c., i.p., or p.o. for 2–18 weeks (Chattopadhyay et al., 2010; Dhouib et al., 2015; Erat et al., 2007; Oyeyipo et al., 2014; Piubelli et al., 2005). Malondialdehyde or thiobarbituric acid reactive substance (TBARS) levels were also increased in rats and mice in response to subchronic and chronic nicotine exposure (Ateyya et al., 2016; Da Silva et al., 2010; El-Sokkary et al., 2007; Ijomone et al., 2014; Jain and Flora, 2012; Muthukumaran et al., 2008; Oyeyipo et al., 2014; Piubelli et al., 2005; Yildiz et al., 1999). Additionally, nicotine treatment resulted in oxidative stress, as evidenced by an increase in the levels of 3-nitrotyrosine, a marker of protein nitroxidation, in POII hamster cheek pouch cells and mouse and rat lungs (Barley et al., 2004; Bodas et al., 2016; El-Sokkary et al., 2007). Despite the consistency in these results, nicotine doses and administration routes were often not comparable among the studies, and at least one study found the responses to be dependent on the age of the animals (Jain and Flora, 2012).

However, a large number of in vitro studies support the view that nicotine exposure causes oxidative stress, with concordant findings on increased levels of 3-nitrotyrosine in HCPC-1 Syrian hamster oral epidermoid carcinoma cells (Banerjee et al., 2007) and lipid peroxidation markers (e.g., TBARS and malondialdehyde) in cultured rat peripheral blood lymphocytes and CHO cells (Sudheer et al., 2007a, 2007b; Yildiz et al., 1999). In addition, a number of studies revealed antioxidant system impairments, including decreased glutathione levels and SOD and CAT activities, in murine cell cultures (Erat et al., 2007; Mahapatra et al., 2009; Sudheer et al., 2007a, 2007b; Yildiz et al., 1999) and increased ROS loads in several mammalian cell lines, including mouse MLE-12 and rat lung epithelial cells, hamster oral epithelial cells, human bronchial epithelial BEAS-2B cells, primary alveolar type II cells, periodontal ligament and endothelial cells, and gingival fibroblasts (Argentin and Cicchetti, 2004; Banerjee et al., 2007; Guo et al., 2005; Lee et al., 2009; Schweitzer et al., 2015; Zanetti et al., 2014). Nicotine treatment also induced the Nrf2 antioxidant system in human periodontal ligament cells and increased heme oxygenase-1 and NAD(P)H quinone dehydrogenase 1 activities in a concentration- and time-dependent manner (Lee et al., 2009). Of note, nicotine-induced oxidative stress in vitro was decreased when cell cultures were pre- or co-treated with antioxidant chemicals such as *N*-acetylcysteine and vitamin C or antioxidant enzymes (Argentin and Cicchetti, 2004; Kahl et al., 2012; Lee et al., 2009; Wu et al., 2005; Yildiz, 2004), which lends additional mechanistic support for nicotine-induced oxidative stress.

20.3.2.3.6 Does nicotine induce chronic inflammation?.

It is now accepted that inflammation plays an integral role in all stages of tumorigenesis (Grivennikov et al., 2010). Inflammation can be triggered by various insults, such as tissue injury, infection, and cellular stress. This first-line defense mechanism rapidly triggers the release of proinflammatory substances (including cytokines, free radicals, hormones, and other small molecules) to combat the stressor by initiating inflammation-resolving processes, such as the adaptive immune response, thus facilitating immune cell trafficking (Berridge, 2012). Various transcription factors, including nuclear factor kappa B (NF-κB), activator protein 1 (AP-1), and early growth response 1 (Egr-1), induce the expression of gene products integral to the inflammatory response and thus control the production of inflammatory mediators while also indirectly contributing to the activation of the cells involved (Deng et al., 2009). While this acute inflammatory response can lead to pathological consequences, it is, in itself, not a disease but a means to maintaining homeostasis, and how the response is eventually executed typically depends on the original trigger. If the acute inflammation is not resolved and both innate and adaptive immune responses persist, chronic inflammation may ensue (Coussens and Werb, 2002; Ward, 2010). This persistent inflammatory response is known to not only alter the pro- and

antiinflammatory activities of cells within the inflamed pulmonary environment but also contribute to, for example, DNA damage through interaction with ROS that are chronically produced by immune cells (Curtis et al., 2007; Hodge et al., 2007). This inextricably links oxidative stress to inflammation and carcinogenesis. It is, therefore, not surprising to find that nicotine has also been studied with respect to its effect on inflammation pathways and immune cell function (Ashraf-Uz-Zaman et al., 2020; Reuter et al., 2010; Yang et al., 2011).

There are multiple reports of nicotine-induced lung inflammation in rats and mice, as evidenced by increased BALF cell counts and histological findings of immune cell infiltrates, independent of how much and by what route nicotine was administered (Demiralay et al., 2007; Garcia-Arcos et al., 2016; Valença et al., 2004; Yokohira et al., 2012). However, others have found no change in BALF cell counts in rats or mice receiving nicotine via inhalation, i.p. injection, intranasal instillation, s.c. injection, or osmotic minipump for varying durations (Blanchet et al., 2004; Mabley et al., 2011; Phillips et al., 2015; Xu and Cardell, 2017). This discordance between results is also reflected in the BALF cytokine levels in nicotine-exposed rats and mice: IL-1β, IL-6, macrophage inhibitory protein (Mip)-1α, chemokine (C-X-C motif) ligand (Cxcl)-10, and Cxcl2 levels were increased in rats whole-body exposed to nicotine-containing e-vapor (Garcia-Arcos et al., 2016), but no changes were seen in rats nose-only exposed to nebulized nicotine (Phillips et al., 2015). Furthermore, in contrast to cigarette smoke, THS aerosol did not trigger significant lung inflammation, as assessed by BALF cell counts and cytokine levels, across a broad range of rat and mouse inhalation studies (Oviedo et al., 2016; Phillips et al., 2019, 2016; Wong et al., 2016a, 2020). Of note, nicotine was also reported to prevent the influx of immune cells into the lungs as well as cytokine/chemokine production, essentially suppressing proinflammatory responses to treatment with lipopolysaccharide (LPS), bacteria, allergens, or hydrochloric acid (Blanchet et al., 2004; Mabley et al., 2011; Mishra et al., 2008; Ni et al., 2011; Su et al., 2007; Xu and Cardell, 2017).

Such immune responses are rarely reproducible in vitro, predominantly because multicell culture systems, such as those combining primary lung with immune cells, are difficult to generate and maintain. Nevertheless, in vitro studies in human primary and immortalized bronchial epithelial cells and organotypic lung epithelial cultures have indicated that nicotine exposure can elicit an epithelial proinflammatory response, as evidenced by increased production of cytokines and chemokines, such as IL-1α, IL-1β, IL-6, IL-8, and granulocyte/macrophage colony-stimulating factor (GM-CSF) (Balharry et al., 2008; Garcia-Arcos et al., 2016; Klapproth et al., 1998; Li et al., 2010, 2011; Tsai et al., 2006). Interestingly, these effects were not always significant or dose-dependent, and at least one study has suggested that there is a threshold concentration above which they became apparent (Klapproth et al., 1998). It is also worth noting that proinflammatory responses could be abrogated by coincubation with (+)-tubocurarine, a potent nAChR antagonist (Klapproth et al., 1998), or specific inhibitors of ERK1/2 (PD98059) and the c-Jun N-terminal kinase (JNK) (SP600125) (Tsai et al., 2006), suggesting that activation of nAChR-mediated signaling cascades is involved in nicotine exposure-related lung inflammation. Importantly, the antiinflammatory effects seen in vivo could also be confirmed in vitro in LPS-treated human primary and immortalized bronchial epithelial cells and at concentrations similar to those that resulted in increased cytokine production in other studies (Li et al., 2010, 2011), indicating that nicotine is capable of eliciting both pro- and antiinflammatory effects.

Because nAChRs are also expressed on immune cells such as neutrophils, macrophages, and lymphocytes (Gotti and Clementi, 2004; Kawashima et al., 2015; Safronova et al., 2016), it is reasonable to assume that nicotine can directly modulate their proliferation, differentiation, survival, and function. Indeed, nicotine exposure prolonged neutrophil survival and induced chemotaxis but did not affect neutrophil oxidative burst or degranulation (Aoshiba et al., 1996; Garcia-Arcos et al., 2016; Totti et al., 1984; Vukelic et al., 2013; Wongtrakool et al., 2007). In human peripheral blood mononuclear cells (PBMCs), nicotine exposure led to a slight increase in the production of proinflammatory cytokines such as IL-6, IL-10, IL-12, and TNF-α (Matsunaga et al., 2001). Rat NR8383 macrophages responded to nicotine treatment with elevated MIP-1α production (Chong et al., 2002).

Furthermore, treatment with nicotine modulated macrophage maturation and activation (Blanchet et al., 2004; St-Pierre et al., 2016; Takahashi et al., 2006) as well as the expression of peroxisome proliferator–activated receptor (PPAR)-γ, a key regulator of monocyte-to-macrophage differentiation and macrophage activation (Heming et al., 2018), in human monocyte–derived macrophages (Amoruso et al., 2007). In addition, treatment with nicotine had a range of different effects on human dendritic cells, including reduced CD1a expression and LPS-induced TNF-α and IL-10 production (Yanagita et al., 2012), hinting at a negative impact of nicotine on dendritic cell function.

However, in line with the reports on its antiinflammatory effects in rodent lungs and human lung epithelial cells, nicotine treatment also decreased LPS-stimulated cytokine/chemokine production in mouse AMJ2-C11 macrophages (Blanchet et al., 2004), human U937 monocyte-like cells (Sugano et al., 1998), and human dendritic cells (Vassallo et al., 2008).

Finally, other markers of inflammation were also modulated by nicotine treatment. For example, NF-κB was activated in gingival fibroblasts, murine lung fibroblasts, and human bronchial epithelial cells, as evidenced by increased NF-κB inhibitor (I-κBα) degradation (Nakao et al., 2009) or increased nuclear translocation of p65 and/or NF-κB transcriptional activity (Martínez-García et al., 2008; Wongtrakool et al., 2014). In addition, nicotine exposure increased prostaglandin E2 (PGE2) release and/or cyclooxygenase 2 (Cox-2) mRNA expression in gingival fibroblasts (Nakao et al., 2009). It also caused an increase in LPS-stimulated dendritic cells (Vassallo et al., 2008) and mouse tracheal rings (10 μM; 4 days) (Xu et al., 2014). A study of the global proteomic changes in rats following nicotine exposure revealed increased serum levels of contrapsin-like protease inhibitor 1, decreased serum levels of inter-alpha trypsin inhibitor 4 and alpha-1 macroglobulin, and decreased PBMC levels of vimentin and fibrinogen, all of which, the authors suggested, are indicative of a suppressed inflammatory response (Piubelli et al., 2005).

The evidence from in vivo and in vitro studies seems to indicate that nicotine can, in principle, trigger an inflammatory response at high doses. However, when nicotine is delivered to the lungs at concentrations equivalent to those delivered by ENDPs, it does not elicit a significant inflammatory response (Lee et al., 2018c; Phillips et al., 2015, 2019, 2016; Wong et al., 2016a, 2020).

20.3.2.3.7 Is nicotine immunosuppressive?.
Partial or complete suppression of immune activity is referred to as immunosuppression. In the context of carcinogenesis, immunosuppression is closely linked to chronic inflammation, and it impairs normal immune cell function, facilitates the accumulation and activation of immune suppressor cells (myeloid-derived suppressor cells, regulatory T cells, etc.), and prevents immune surveillance (Grivennikov et al., 2010; Wang and DuBois, 2015).

Although nicotine consistently attenuates the antibody-forming cell response in rats (Geng et al., 1996, 1995; Kalra et al., 2004), data from animal studies of other immune functions are more contradictory. For example, there is evidence both for and against the notion that nicotine can inhibit T-cell proliferation, activation, and differentiation (De Rosa et al., 2009; Geng et al., 1996, 1995; Kalra et al., 2002; Kalra et al., 2004). Specifically, there was no change in T-cell numbers in rats that received nicotine at 1 mg/kg/day by i.p. or s.c. injection for 3−4 weeks; however, T-cell proliferation in response to concanavalin A (Con A), a potent mitogen, was markedly reduced (Geng et al., 1995). Similar observations were also made in rats that received two to four times more nicotine transdermally via a patch (Kalra et al., 2004) as well as in rats that self-administered much lower concentrations of nicotine intravenously between 40 and 50 times per day for 5 weeks (Kalra et al., 2002). Con A-stimulated peripheral lymphocytes from rats acutely exposed to 1 mg/kg nicotine by i.p. injection exhibited decreased T-cell proliferation at 2 h postexposure but not at 24 h postexposure, and nicotine treatment had no effect on splenic T-cell proliferation. Chronic nicotine treatment for up to 21 days, on the other hand, inhibited both peripheral and splenic T-cell proliferation (Singh et al., 2000). In PBMCs from healthy subjects, nicotine treatment reduced phytohemagglutinin-stimulated T cell proliferation, albeit not significantly, in one study (De Rosa et al., 2009), but showed no effect (Oloris et al., 2010) or even caused apoptosis at concentrations exceeding 200 μM (Liu et al., 2014) in other studies. In addition to the above-described modulation of neutrophil, macrophage, and dendritic cell functions, these nicotine effects on T cells point to a broad nicotine-mediated impairment of immune cell function, although no study has replicated these findings with inhaled nicotine. In summary, the role of nicotine in immunosuppression is still unclear and needs further research, especially in the context of ENDP aerosol inhalation.

20.3.2.3.8 Does nicotine modulate receptor-mediated effects?.
Nicotine modulates the expression patterns of various nAChR subunits (muscle-type and neuronal) that are expressed in a wide range of mouse, rat, monkey, and human lung epithelial, endothelial, and immune cells (Carlisle et al., 2004; De Rosa et al., 2009; Gundavarapu et al., 2012; Lam et al., 2015; Li et al., 2017; Liu et al., 2014; Martínez-García et al., 2008; Matsunaga et al., 2001; Nishioka et al., 2010; Oloris et al., 2010; Plummer et al., 2005; Proskocil et al., 2004; Rehan et al., 2005; Roman et al., 2004; St-Pierre et al., 2016; Wang et al., 2013; West et al., 2003). In addition, upon binding to nAChRs, nicotine activates receptor-mediated signaling. Receptor activation has been evidenced in, for example, BEAS-2B cells by significant dose-dependent increases in Ca^{2+} influx, which could be inhibited by the nAChR

antagonist α-bungarotoxin but not by hexamethonium (Carlisle et al., 2004). Downstream receptor−mediated signaling, such as modulation of ERK1/2 and/or Akt, has been described in rat lung epithelial and airway smooth muscle cells, primary rat tracheal fibroblasts, rat PC12 pheochromocytoma cells, mouse Raw264.7 macrophages and El4 T cells, NIH/3T3 fibroblasts, primary mouse lung fibroblasts, mouse LA4 and Cl25 lung adenoma cells, human normal oral keratinocytes, immortalized skin keratinocytes (HaCaT), bronchial epithelial and small airway epithelial cells, endothelial progenitor cells, and various human cancer cell lines (lungs: PC9 and HCC827; breast: MCF-7 and MDA-MB-231; oral: OEC-M1, SCC40, and PCI15a) (Carlisle et al., 2004; Chu et al., 2005; Clark et al., 2010; Guo et al., 2017; He et al., 2014; Hong et al., 2017; JunHui et al., 2009; Maier et al., 2011; Mishra et al., 2008; Nakada et al., 2012; Nishioka et al., 2010; Roman et al., 2004; Tsai et al., 2006; Wang et al., 2012; West et al., 2003; Wu et al., 2009; Xu et al., 2010). Activation of the protein kinase C (PKC) pathway in response to nicotine treatment in mouse NIH/3T3 fibroblasts, primary lung fibroblasts and LA4 lung adenoma cells, primary rat tracheal fibroblasts, rat lung epithelial cells, human WI38 embryonic lung fibroblasts, and BEAS-2B cells has also been reported (Carlisle et al., 2004; Chu et al., 2005; Guo et al., 2005; Roman et al., 2004; Sakurai et al., 2011). In addition, multiple studies have found increased epidermal growth factor receptor (EGFR) phosphorylation and heparin-binding EGF-like growth factor (HB-EGF) secretion in normal human bronchial epithelial cells and human cancer cells following nicotine treatment (Khalil et al., 2013; Li et al., 2015; Martínez-García et al., 2008; Wang et al., 2013; Ye et al., 2004). Other regulators such as PPAR-γ, telomerase reverse transcriptase (TERT), sirtuin 1 (SIRT1), and PTHrP were modulated by nicotine in mouse endothelial progenitor cells (Li et al., 2017) and human WI38 embryonic lung fibroblasts (Rehan et al., 2005). Although these latter findings are derived from single reports that lack independent verification, these in vitro results indicate that nicotine may affect several classical signaling pathways that have been associated with benzo[a]pyrene (Jin et al., 2018). However, these pathways do not seem to be affected significantly in the upper airways of A/J mice exposed to THS aerosol (Titz et al., 2020).

20.3.2.3.9 Does nicotine cause immortalization?.
As a result of telomere length restriction, primary cells normally reach senescence after a limited number of population doublings (also known as the Hayflick limit)

before they ultimately die. However, cancer cells overcome these natural barriers to carcinogenesis—escaping both senescence and crisis—by possessing alterations in cell cycle regulators that govern the exit to G1 (such as p16, p53, and pRb) and/or by reexpressing telomerase (Campisi, 2013; Hanahan and Weinberg, 2011; Newbold, 2002; Yeager et al., 1998). Cells transformed in this way are capable of proliferating indefinitely and are insensitive to exogenous stimuli that may limit their growth and survival.

Only a small number of studies have examined whether nicotine may have an effect on telomere length or cause senescence directly. A concentration-dependent increase in telomerase activity and inhibition of senescence was seen in human endothelial progenitor cells treated with 0.1−100 nM nicotine for 1 week, and both effects could be abolished by pretreatment with the nAChR antagonist mecamylamine (JunHui et al., 2009). Inhibition of senescence was also seen in endothelial progenitor cells in mice that received nicotine via drinking water for 1 month, but not after longer exposure durations (Li et al., 2017). However, a 6-h treatment of BEAS-2B cells with a single, very high dose of nicotine (5 mM) increased the number of senescent cells and enhanced both apoptosis and autophagy (Bodas et al., 2016).

With respect to endpoints related to cell transformation—that is, the transition from normal to tumorigenic cell—nicotine has been shown to affect both cell differentiation and contact inhibition. For example, West and coworkers reported loss of contact inhibition and decreased anoikis in human bronchial and small airways epithelial cells following nicotine treatment (West et al., 2003). Daily nicotine treatment for a week induced the differentiation of human bronchial epithelial cells to neuronal-like cells, which was accompanied by increased EGFR activation, adhesion to extracellular matrix proteins, MMP-2 and MMP-9 activities, and NF-κB nuclear translocation (Martínez-García et al., 2008). Concentration-dependent decreases in epithelial thickness and increased expression of differentiation-specific proteins, such as cytokeratins, involucrin, and profilaggrin/filaggrin, have been seen in oral mucosal and epidermal keratinocytes and in reconstructed epidermis treated with nicotine for 2 weeks (Kwon et al., 1999). Nicotine also induced epithelial−mesenchymal transition in human bronchial epithelial cells through activation of Wnt3a/beta-catenin signaling (Zou et al., 2013) as well as anchorage-independent growth in soft agar in normal and immortalized human oral keratinocytes and BEAS-2B cells (Gemenetzidis et al., 2009; Lee et al., 2018). Together,

these studies provide some insights into nicotine's role in senescence and epithelial remodeling. Although the dose ranges for nicotine were not dissimilar among these studies, the treatment durations varied greatly—from 1 h to several weeks—and independent verification of these results is currently lacking. Therefore, it is not possible to conclude whether or not nicotine causes immortalization and malignant cell transformation.

20.3.2.3.10 Does nicotine alter cell proliferation, cell death, or nutrient supply?. Sustained growth and the ability to escape cell death mechanisms, invariably linked to epigenetic and genetic changes and immortalization, are hallmarks of cancer cells and may pose higher demands on nutrient supply (Hanahan and Weinberg, 2011). A large number of studies reported that nicotine increases proliferation of mouse, rat, and human epithelial, endothelial, and smooth muscle cells as well as breast cancer and lung cancer cells (Arredondo et al., 2001; Dasgupta et al., 2009; Davis et al., 2009; Greene et al., 2010; He et al., 2014; Heeschen et al., 2001; Hong et al., 2017; JunHui et al., 2009; Lee et al., 2005; Li et al., 2010, 2017; Maier et al., 2011; Nishioka et al., 2011; Novak et al., 2000; Wang et al., 2014; Yu et al., 2006). This effect was dose-dependent in some studies, and a treatment duration-dependent effect was observed in mouse endothelial progenitor and human bronchial epithelial 16HBE cells (Hong et al., 2017; Li et al., 2010, 2017). The maximal effective concentrations were between 10 and 100 nM in mouse and human endothelial cells (Heeschen et al., 2001; Yu et al., 2006) and between 10 and 20 μM in human smooth muscle and epithelial cells (Hong et al., 2017; Li et al., 2010). There is, however, evidence to suggest that nicotine has no effect on the proliferation of some specific cell types—such as T cells (Oloris et al., 2010), periodontal ligament−derived stem cells (Zhuo and Hui-Li, 2017), BEAS-2B cells (Novak et al., 2000), and A549 cells (Jarzynka et al., 2006)—and that it even inhibits the proliferation of A549 cells (Gao et al., 2016), oral keratinocytes, and oral cancer cells (Lee et al., 2005). The latter finding appears to be in conflict with the nicotine-mediated increases in the expression of proliferation markers Ki-67, PCNA, p21, and cyclin D1 in human primary oral keratinocytes at similar concentrations, even though these effects were proven to be nAChR-dependent, because they were abrogated by cotreatment of the cells with mecamylamine (Arredondo et al., 2001).

Deregulation of cell growth mechanisms and evasion of cell cycle regulators by tumor cells go hand-in-hand with resistance to cell death signals

(Hanahan and Weinberg, 2011). Inhibition/suppression of apoptosis by nicotine was observed in mouse thymocytes (Wright et al., 1993), transformed hamster oral epithelial cells and rat fibroblasts (Banerjee et al., 2007), human neutrophils (Aoshiba et al., 1996), normal human bronchial and small airway epithelial cells (West et al., 2003), and mouse and human cancer cells (Wright et al., 1993). Chernyavsky and coworkers observed that nicotine inhibited staurosporine-induced cytochrome C release from mitochondria isolated from human bronchial epithelial BEAS-2B cells (Chernyavsky et al., 2015). Jalili et al. reported a significant decrease in proapoptotic marker gene expression in the lungs of mice treated with 2.5 mg/kg nicotine i.p. daily for 4 weeks (Jalili et al., 2017).

In contrast, increased apoptosis following nicotine treatment was seen in mouse MLE-12 (Zanetti et al., 2014) and human BEAS-2B cells (Bodas et al., 2016), mouse peritoneal macrophages (Mahapatra et al., 2009), unstimulated human T cells (Oloris et al., 2010), and primary mouse alveolar type II cells (Zanetti et al., 2014). Nicotine treatment also increased Fas ligand mRNA expression and apoptosis in anti-CD3-stimulated T cells (Oloris et al., 2010). However, nicotine had no effect on apoptosis in human parotid gland MOCs (Ginzkey et al., 2014a), salivary gland epithelial cells (Ginzkey et al., 2009), lymphocytes (Ginzkey et al., 2013), and BEAS-2B cells (Ginzkey et al., 2012; Zanetti et al., 2014). In addition, necrosis was not seen in nicotine-treated human lymphocytes (Ginzkey et al., 2013) but was increased in periodontal ligament cells following nicotine treatment (Lee et al., 2009).

Together, these results provide some evidence that nicotine inhibits or prevents cell death, particularly in immortalized or cancer cell lines, but not consistently across normal airway cell types. Therefore, it is still unclear whether nicotine enables lung cells to bypass cell death.

20.3.3 Conclusions for Lung Cancer

Epidemiological evidence on the potential involvement of nicotine in lung cancer development is scarce, and the only available large-scale study on NRT use indicates that nicotine does not likely contribute to lung cancer risk. The low cancer risk associated with nicotine is also supported by epidemiological data showing that using Swedish snus is associated neither with a significant risk of oral cancer nor with a significant risk of esophageal or stomach cancer.

In vivo studies show that nicotine alone does not increase the incidence and multiplicity of lung tumors, but it may increase the neovascularization of tumor allografts at high doses. Genotoxicity tests confirm that

nicotine is not mutagenic, although it appears to elicit a clastogenic effect at very high doses. Less clarity exists on nicotine's effects on DNA repair systems and epigenetic changes, even though exposure to ENDP aerosols has minimal effects on miRNA expression and DNA methylation. Similarly, even though nicotine interferes with immune cell function, it is not clear whether this is directly linked to immunosuppression in the lungs and the consequent escape of tumor cells from immune surveillance. However, the evidence suggests that nicotine may cause oxidative stress and enhance inflammation, even though these mechanisms are not substantially activated by ENDP aerosols in vivo or at human-relevant doses in vitro.

It is important to note that many in vitro studies and all in vivo studies did not provide information on concentration—/dose—response relationships, and few studies reported on temporal relationships with the outcome of interest. The nicotine concentrations in many studies were high, far exceeding those in smokers, thus limiting their relevance to human exposure (Fig. 20.3). In addition, with a few exceptions, in vitro studies were acute exposures, whereas human nicotine users may be exposed repeatedly over a prolonged period. Nicotine appears to change the pattern of nAChR expression dynamically in some cell types, particularly with prolonged exposure. The interplay among the various nAChRs seems to be rather complex, and nicotine effects may vary depending on the cellular context. Again, this causes uncertainty in extrapolating the available information to human exposure scenarios.

Equally important is that not all the studies included appropriate statistical analyses. Some laboratory animal studies were conducted with as little as two animals per group, rendering them devoid of any statistical power. Rodent carcinogenicity studies designed and conducted on the basis of OECD test guidelines (OECD, 2018c,d), with the inhalation route for nicotine administration, would be a means to producing high-quality data that may ultimately help elucidate the role of nicotine in lung carcinogenesis. However, such studies are demanding in terms of resources and fraught with their own limitations, including the translatability of the findings in rodents to humans. This, together with the desire to minimize animal use in research in the spirit of the 3R principles, has driven the quest for alternative approaches. Yet, many cellular and molecular biological studies have their own caveats. Because of the complexity of the disease, in vitro models are not well suited for drawing conclusions about the role of nicotine in lung cancer in humans; but, they may provide useful mechanistic insights into how nicotine

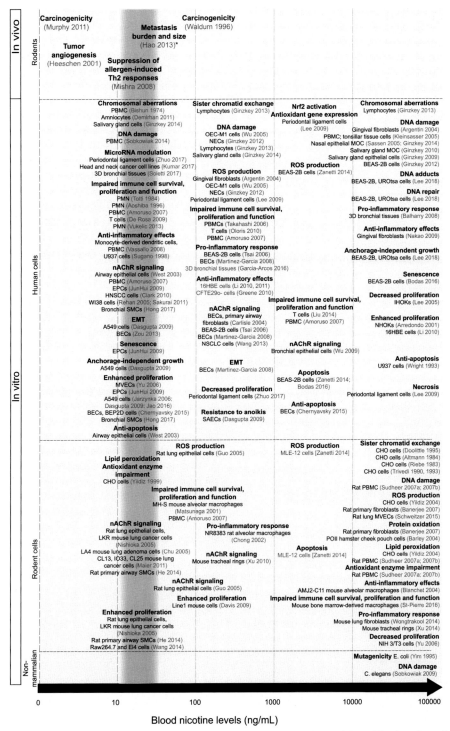

FIG. 20.3 Summary of nicotine effects on endpoints linked to carcinogenicity. The location of each reference on the x-axis reflects the range of nicotine concentrations tested for which the effects were observed. Species and type of studies (in vivo/in vitro) are indicated on the left side. The dark gray area

modulates key biological processes underlying the pathogenesis of lung cancer. Although the available data indicate that nicotine may cause oxidative stress and inflammation, the available evidence neither sufficiently nor conclusively supports a role for nicotine in lung carcinogenesis. According to this assessment, nicotine is unlikely to be a complete lung carcinogen, and additional research is required to further elucidate how these phenomena can impact disease development.

20.4 NICOTINE, REPRODUCTION, AND DEVELOPMENT

20.4.1 Introduction

Cigarette smoking is well known to be associated with an increased risk of adverse pregnancy outcomes. It is, therefore, always recommended for pregnant women to stop smoking. Because some smokers find long-term smoking abstinence difficult, pregnant smokers are increasingly turning to ENDPs that emit significantly lower levels of toxicants, including carbon monoxide—a volatile gas potentially associated with embryonic/fetal hypoxia (Ion and Bernal, 2015)—with the hope of reducing the toxicant exposure associated with cigarette smoking during their pregnancy. Still, the presence of nicotine in all ENDPs raises concerns about the safety of their use during pregnancy for both mother and child. The following section reviews the current knowledge on the potential effects of nicotine exposure on development, highlighting the gaps that still exist.

20.4.2 Nicotine Exposure and Its Impact during Pregnancy

20.4.2.1 Epidemiological evidence

A recent review estimated that 52.9% (95% CI, 45.6—60.3) of women who smoked daily continued to smoke daily during pregnancy, with the proportion ranging from 30.6% (95% CI, 25.6—36.4) in Europe to 79.6% (95% CI, 44.2—100.0) in the Western Pacific Region (Lange et al., 2018). Quitting smoking and minimizing secondhand smoke exposure are highly

recommended for pregnant women to prevent a number of complications, such as ectopic pregnancy, placental abruption, and placenta previa, as well as a range of poor fetal outcomes, such as stillbirth, growth restriction, and fetal morbidity. Smoking tobacco during pregnancy has been associated with a higher risk of preterm birth, low birth weight, and sudden infant death syndrome in addition to oral cleft malformations (U.S. Department of Health and Human Services, 2014). Life-long implications for the fetus postdelivery have been also reported, with an increased incidence of respiratory illnesses such as wheezing and asthma (Gilliland et al., 2001; Lannero et al., 2006; Skorge et al., 2005) and reduced lung function (Gilliland et al., 2000).

A range of noncombustible tobacco products (e.g., snus, snuff, chewing tobacco, and heated tobacco products) and nicotine delivery products, including NRTs (e.g., patches, gums, and lozenges) and EVPs, have been available on the market as potentially less risky alternatives for adult smokers, and their use has been rising among pregnant women (Cardenas et al., 2019b; Kurti et al., 2017; Obisesan et al., 2020). According to analytical chemistry evidence, most of the potentially harmful exposures observed with cigarette smoking (e.g., carbon monoxide exposure) are absent or strongly reduced with these alternative products. However, it is not yet clear what the pregnancy risks from using such products are compared with those associated with cigarette smoking. In a 2016 report, the World Health Organization mentioned the health risks linked to electronic nicotine delivery systems, particularly those due to the related nicotine exposure. They wrote that: "*In addition to dependence, nicotine can have adverse effects on the development of the fetus during pregnancy and may contribute to cardiovascular disease. Although nicotine itself is not a carcinogen, it may function as a 'tumor promoter' and seems to be involved in the biology of malignant diseases, as well as of neurodegeneration. Fetal and adolescent nicotine exposure may have long-term consequences for brain development, potentially leading to learning and anxiety disorders. The evidence is sufficient to warn children and adolescents, pregnant women, and women of reproductive age against*

---

indicates the range of nicotine concentrations measured in blood samples from smokers. *3D*, 3-dimensional; *BEC*, bronchial epithelial cell; *CHO*, Chinese hamster ovary; *EPC*, endothelial progenitor cell; *HNSCC*, head and neck squamous cell carcinoma; *IHOK*, immortalized human oral keratinocytes; *MOC*, mini-organ culture; *MVEC*, microvascular endothelial cells; *NEC*, nasal epithelial cell; *NHOK*, normal human oral keratinocytes; *PBMC*, peripheral blood mononuclear cell; *PMN*, polymorphonuclear cell; *SAEC*, small airway epithelial cell; *SMC*, smooth muscle cell.

ENDS use and nicotine" (WHO, 2016). Nicotine is classified by the FDA as a Pregnancy Category D drug, which
implies that nicotine exposes the user to some risk during pregnancy. This rating requires that the risks associated with nicotine exposure be outweighed by the risks
of the medical problem if left untreated. Because of the
category D status of NRTs, grant agencies have been hes-
itant to fund efficacy studies on NRTs for smoking cessation during pregnancy (Dempsey and Benowitz, 2001).

The epidemiological evidence on nicotine harm during pregnancy is debatable, as epidemiological studies
never solely measure the effects of nicotine. In fact,
most of the scientific evidence supporting the detrimental effects of nicotine exposure during embryo—fetal
development is derived from a large number of preclinical studies providing both in vitro and in vivo toxicological evidence. A recent review by Glover and Phillips
summarizes the epidemiological evidence about the
pregnancy outcome effects (such as gestation term, birth
weight, stillbirth, malformations, preeclampsia, cardiovascular and respiratory outcomes, newborn colic, and
neurobehavioral effects) of all smoke-free nicotine and
tobacco products (Glover and Phillips, 2020). By reviewing 21 studies on the use of NRT (12 studies), Swedish
snus (7 studies), Alaskan iq'milk (1 study), and e-
cigarettes (1 study) during pregnancy, the authors
concluded that the risks from smoke-free nicotine and
tobacco products, while lower than those from smoking,
are nonzero. The authors highlighted the difficulty in
assessing the impact of smoke-free product exposure
on pregnancy relative to cigarette smoke exposure, which
represents a more homogenous exposure (except for intensity). Another review summarized nine epidemiological studies (three of which were also included in the
Glover and Phillips review) that assessed the impact of
SLT use during pregnancy on birth weight, preterm birth,
stillbirth, and smallness for gestational age (SGA) (Inamdar et al., 2015). Although most of these studies showed
a significant association between SLT use and adverse
health effects in newborns, the authors acknowledged
the limitations of this metaanalysis. Indeed, some of
these studies did not measure or report any confounders,
such as smoking, alcohol use, substance and drug abuse,
and underlying maternal health conditions. In addition,
there were no biochemical measures to confirm exposure
to SLT, and the type and use of these products varied
among the participants, including variations in tobacco
content, nicotine doses, and frequency of use. Another
potential confounding effect, which was not considered
in these studies, was the impact of the other ingredients
in some of these SLT products (betel leaf, areca nut,
slaked lime, catechu, etc.). A third integrative review of

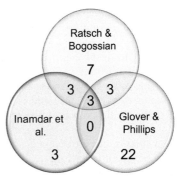

FIG. 20.4 Overlapping epidemiological studies on
pregnancy outcomes in smoke-free nicotine and tobacco
product users (Glover and Phillips, 2020; Inamdar et al., 2015;
Ratsch and Bogossian, 2014).

the literature on SLT use in pregnancy by Ratsch and
Bogossian discussed seven additional studies not
included in the other reviews (Ratsch and Bogossian,
2014) (Fig. 20.4). Again, this metaanalysis highlighted
various flaws, such as the small numbers of participants
(which did not allow for sufficient statistical power for
estimating risks) and lack of confounding variable control and precise measures of exposure. Nevertheless, the
authors still recognized that maternal SLT use may not
be safe because it can increase the rates of stillbirth, result
in low birth weight, and impact the male-to-female live
birth ratio.

When looking specifically at the impact of EVP use
on pregnancy and reproductive outcomes, Cardenas
et al. pointed out the lack of studies on this topic (Cardenas et al., 2019b). Shortly thereafter, the same authors reported the first cohort study on assessing the
impact of EVP use on birth weight and SGA in 248 pregnant women with a prevalence of current EVP use of
6.8% (95% CI, 4.4%–10.2%) (Cardenas et al.,
2019a). Participants were included if they had no underlying medical conditions, comorbidities, or ante-
natal complications. The EVP user or smoking status
was derived from a self-administered questionnaire
and by measuring biomarkers of exposure (such as salivary cotinine, exhaled carbon monoxide, and hair nicotine). They found that women who used only EVPs had
a five times higher risk of SGA than nonexposed women
(Cardenas et al., 2019a).

20.4.3 Nicotine Exposure during Pregnancy and Postnatal Development

Most of the effects of in utero nicotine exposure on
offspring phenotype are derived from animal studies
and in vitro experiments and suggest a potential risk

for the developing fetus, including defects in the immune system, neural development, and respiratory and cardiac functions.

Before discussing in detail the in vitro and in vivo evidence supporting nicotine as a developmental toxicant, we need to ask what we know about its exposure during pregnancy (Table 20.8) and the potential biological mechanisms that can be impacted by such exposure.

Nicotine is a small molecule and considered a systemic drug that can readily cross the placental barrier and concentrate in the fetal serum and amniotic fluid (Jordanov, 1990; Lambers and Clark, 1996; Luck et al., 1985). During the second trimester of gestation, nicotine concentrations in amniotic fluid collected from pregnant smokers ranged from 1.5 to 23.0 ng/mL (i.e., 9.2–141.8 nM). At birth, placental nicotine concentrations were between 3.3 and 28 ng/g (Luck et al., 1985). In a more recent study, the concentrations of nicotine in amniotic fluid from pregnant smokers

(whose smoking status was confirmed by maternal urine measurements) at the time of delivery ranged from 0 to 370 nM (Kohler et al., 2010). The plasma nicotine and cotinine concentrations associated with NRT use (such as transdermal patches and nicotine gums) during pregnancy have been determined in very few studies. Oncken et al. measured the plasma nicotine concentrations in pregnant smokers (during the second trimester of gestation) who were randomized to a transdermal 21-mg nicotine patch or to smoking ad libitum for 8 h (Oncken et al., 1997). All participants smoked approximately 20 cigarettes per day. The plasma nicotine concentrations in pregnant patch users were in the same range (12.5–19.5 ng/mL or 77–120.2 nM) as those in smoking expectant mothers. In another study on pregnant women, the use of nicotine gum resulted in a plasma nicotine concentration of 7.6–16.2 ng/mL (i.e., 46.8–100 nM) at 30 min after the start of chewing (Manning and Feyerabend, 1976). Nicotine was also detected in the milk of

TABLE 20.8
Nicotine Concentrations in Various Biological Samples and at Different Time Points During Pregnancy in Smokers and NRT Users (Not Comprehensive).

Exposure	Sample Type	Time at Sample Collection	Nicotine Concentration		Reference
			nM	ng/g	
Cigarette smoke	Amniotic fluid	Second trimester of gestation	9.2–141.8	N/A	Luck et al. (1985)
	Maternal serum		6.2–111		
Cigarette smoke	Amniotic fluid	At birth	0–370	N/A	Kohler et al. (2010)
Cigarette smoke	Amniotic fluid	Second trimester of gestation	0–191	N/A	Van Vunakis et al. (1974)
Cigarette smoke	Placenta	At birth	N/A	3.3–28	Luck et al. (1985)
	Umbilical vein serum		3.1–154	N/A	
	Maternal serum		10.5–57.9		
Cigarette smoke	Breast milk	After birth, between 0.25 and 4 h after smoking	12.3–382.2	N/A	Luck and Nau (1984)
	Maternal serum		6.2–172.6		
Transdermal, 21-mg nicotine patch	Maternal plasma	Third trimester of gestation	77–120.2	N/A	Oncken et al. (1997)
4-mg nicotine gum	Maternal plasma	Third trimester of gestation, 30 min after onset of chewing or after smoking	46.8	N/A	Manning and Feyerabend (1976)
8-mg nicotine gum			100		
Cigarette smoke			61		

N/A, not applicable.

breastfeeding smoking mothers, and breast milk is thus an additional source of exposure for the infant (Luck and Nau, 1984; Napierala et al., 2016).

Interestingly, nicotine and cotinine clearance in pregnant smokers was 60% and 140% higher, respectively, than in nonpregnant smokers (Dempsey et al., 2002). Estrogen levels are thought to influence CYP2A6 and UGT2B10 enzymatic activity. Estrogen levels rise during pregnancy and are 5- to 20-fold higher at the early and late stages of pregnancy, respectively, compared with prepregnancy estrogen levels. This change leads to accelerated nicotine clearance through an increase in the rate of nicotine C-oxidation and N-glucuronidation (Taghavi et al., 2018). In addition, the mean salivary cotinine concentration per cigarette smoked was higher in smokers postpartum than during pregnancy (3.5 vs. 9.9 ng/mL), which is in line with the higher cotinine clearance observed during pregnancy (Rebagliato et al., 1998). On the other hand, the half-life of nicotine in newborns was three to four times longer than that in adults, whereas no such difference was observed for cotinine (Dempsey et al., 2000). This could be due to differences in nicotine and cotinine clearance arising from differences in hepatic blood flow. In humans, hepatic blood flow reaches adult levels a week after birth, because of the increased blood flow in the portal vein and gradual closure of the ductus venosus. This developmental process is completed by the 18th day in human neonates, which implies that nicotine clearance would be increased within the first weeks of life. Another explanation may come from the metabolizing enzymes responsible for nicotine and cotinine clearance. In neonates, CYP2B6 expression is lower than that in adults and older children (Benowitz et al., 2009; Tateishi et al., 1997).

20.4.4 Nicotine Receptors and Nicotine Effects on Development

Nicotine is a known ligand of nAChRs (Henderson and Lester, 2015), which are normally activated by endogenous agonists such as acetylcholine. Nicotine can compete for the binding sites of nAChRs and induce responses that could have pathological effects. nAChRs are expressed during fetal development in various organs/tissues such as the nervous system, lungs, and placenta. At the early stages of brain development, nAChRs are already functional and could be activated/desensitized by nicotine, leading to potential adverse effects (England et al., 2017). Indeed, nAChRs are known to regulate critical steps of brain maturation during prenatal (e.g., development of catecholamine and brainstem autonomic nuclei), early postnatal

(e.g., neocortex, hippocampus, and cerebellum development), and adolescent (e.g., limbic system development and late monoamine maturation) periods (Dwyer et al., 2009). In non-neuronal cells, the signaling cascades induced by activation of nAChRs are still not well understood. However, nAChRs in non-neuronal cells have been shown to be associated with proliferation, migration, and adhesion, all of which are key processes in placental development (Suter and Aagaard, 2020). In humans, analysis of nAChR subunit mRNA expression by RT-PCR has indicated the presence of α2–7 and α9–10 subunits in term placenta samples (Lips et al., 2005). Immunofluorescence studies have detected these subunits in syncytiotrophoblasts and cytotrophoblasts, terminal villi, mesenchymal cells, and Hofbauer cells (Lips et al., 2005). In addition, the expression of nAChR subunits was altered in the term placenta of smoking mothers relative to nonsmoking mothers (Machaalani et al., 2014).

20.4.5 Developmental Effects of Nicotine Exposure in Animal Models

20.4.5.1 Caenorhabditis elegans

Caenorhabditis elegans (*C. elegans*) are roundworms (nematodes) native to soil environments. They have been used as a model system for developmental biology for many reasons, including the ease of expansion of *C. elegans* populations and the possibility of genetic analysis and lineage tracing during development (Brenner, 1974). In particular, *C. elegans* was one of the first organisms with a complete developmental fate map (the entire lineage of all 959 somatic cells was determined) (Sulston and Horvitz, 1977). *C. elegans* is grown on supplemented agar plates (i.e., nematode growth media plates with sodium chloride, agar, peptone, cholesterol, and potassium phosphate). Alternatively, a liquid medium may be preferred, typically a supplemented LB broth (Stiernagle, 1999). In either case, the growth medium may be supplemented with proteins (growth factors) or small molecules, such as nicotine. Note that, because of the thick cuticular exoskeleton of *C. elegans*, it is thought that the drug concentrations in the nematode are lower than those in the growth medium (Matta et al., 2007). Another important point to consider for translatability to humans is the absence of lungs and a circulatory system in *C. elegans*.

Important for translatability with human nicotine receptor signaling and effects is the fact that *C. elegans* expresses nicotinic receptors throughout its life cycle, including during the formative larval stages. The receptors are localized at multiple sites, including the body wall muscles and sensory arbor, which implicates receptor function in locomotion and nociception, respectively (Rose et al., 2013). Typically, nicotine may be administered to *C. elegans* at concentrations up to 10 mM (acute), which results in spastic paralysis (Lewis et al., 1980; Taki et al., 2014a), though there are examples where the nematodes have been cultured in nicotine concentrations as high as 30 mM (Waggoner et al., 2000). Behavioral changes in *C. elegans* have been noted when grown in medium supplemented with nicotine levels as low as 2 μM.

One of the worm behaviors that involves nAChR activity is egg laying, which requires a set of eight specialized vulval muscles. These muscles are highly innervated by cholinergic motor neurons (Kim et al., 2001). Nicotine was reported to impact egg laying behavior after chronic exposure (30 mM), shortening egg laying clusters and increasing intercluster timing (Waggoner et al., 2000). In synchronized stage L3 worms grown in liquid medium (K-medium) with different nicotine concentrations (6.2–194.5 μM) for 24 h, chronic exposure to 61.7 μM nicotine resulted in earlier and increased egg production (~10%) relative to controls; however, lower concentrations of nicotine had no effect (Smith et al., 2013).

miRNA analysis of nematodes (L1–L4 stage, post-embryonic stage, and after synchronization and hatching) transferred to treatment plates containing 20 μM or 20 mM nicotine for a 30-h incubation period identified 40 differentially expressed miRNAs. Enrichment analyses indicated involvement of these miRNAs in multiple regulatory pathways, including biological regulation, response to stimulus, immune processes, and cellular and metabolic processes. The results suggest that nicotine-induced miRNA expression patterns mediate "regulatory hormesis," which may manifest itself as behavioral and physiological phenotypes (Taki et al., 2014b). In addition, nicotine treatment also had an effect on the offspring of the treated worms: There was a dose-dependent effect on dysregulation of miRNA expression in the F1 generation, which faded with each successive generation. Functional analysis indicated perturbation of the same type of biological processes as those seen in the nicotine-treated parental population (F0); but, these similarities were much more prominent between the F0 and F2 than between the F0 and F1 generations. The authors hypothesized that the nicotine-induced changes in miRNA expression patterns in the offspring may be representative of generation-specific phenotypes brought on by adaptation and withdrawal (Taki et al., 2014a).

20.4.5.2 Xenopus

Xenopus laevis, the African clawed frog, is an amphibian model system for the study of developmental biology as well as developmental toxicity. *Xenopus* embryos undergo cleavage, gastrulation, and organogenesis in a manner similar to that in mammalian development. Therefore, the organism provides a developmentally relevant model. In addition, the frog-embryo teratogenesis assay xenopus (FETAX) offers several unique advantages over other reproductive toxicology assays, including lower cost and duration of the tests, higher number of compounds that can be tested simultaneously, and moderated animal welfare concerns relative to the tests that use rodents. For these reasons, FETAX has been used as a surrogate for mammalian tests for assessing the teratogenic potential of test compounds. In a study that compared the performance of FETAX and mammalian embryofetal developmental toxicity tests, FETAX predicted the dysmorphogenic potential of 47 of 58 compounds, showing a predictivity of 81% (Leconte and Mouche, 2013). While the *Xenopus* oocyte has been frequently used as an experimental tool for expression of exogenous recombinant nAChRs, endogenous expression of nAChRs, particularly of the γ- and ε-subunits, has also been reported in *Xenopus* embryos and implicated in *Xenopus* muscle development (Baldwin et al., 1988; Owens and Kullberg, 1989; Sullivan et al., 1999).

The developmental and reproductive toxicological (DART) aspects of nicotine and EVP aerosol exposure have been assessed in *Xenopus*. Administration of nicotine or nicotine-containing aerosols was normally realized by diluting pure nicotine or aerosols in the FETAX solution in which the *Xenopus* embryos were incubated (Dawson et al., 1988; Kennedy et al., 2017; Mouche et al., 2017). Mouche et al. established the nicotine LC_{50} (50% lethal dose) for *Xenopus* embryos at 1 mM, and the nicotine EC_{50} (half maximal effective concentration) for embryo malformation at 287 μM (Mouche et al., 2017). The teratogenic index (i.e., the ratio of LC_{50} to EC_{50}) was 3.51, which indicated that nicotine presented teratogenic potential. When exposed to low concentrations of nicotine (1.2–4.7 μM), *Xenopus* embryos readily developed malformations, including incomplete mouth development, gill hyperplasia, and skeletal kinking. At higher nicotine concentrations (>430 μM), the head and brain size were reduced, the gut poorly coiled, and the heart swollen. Further increases in nicotine concentrations to >528 μM resulted in smaller sized or incompletely developed eyes (Dawson et al., 1988). Importantly, these effects were induced by nicotine doses that are much higher than those observed in humans (Table 20.8). Exposure to diluted aerosols generated from an e-liquid containing only nicotine (at sublethal concentrations), PG, and VG had only minor effects on craniofacial development at nicotine concentrations up to 0.18 mg/mL. Of note, diluted aerosols from various commercially available flavored (and nicotine-containing) e-liquids amplified the craniofacial defects subtly but differentially, depending on the flavor additives. Importantly, facial abnormalities were also seen following exposure to nicotine-free aerosol, suggesting that exposure to the various e-liquid components, rather than nicotine alone, was responsible for the observed effects (Kennedy et al., 2017).

Importantly, developmental effects in *Xenopus* embryos were induced by high micromolar concentrations of nicotine, while the reported serum nicotine levels in human newborns of smoking mothers were orders of magnitude smaller than these, ranging from 3 to 150 nM (Luck et al., 1985). Hence, translation of these effects to humans is not appropriate.

20.4.5.3 Zebrafish

Danio rerio, more commonly known as zebrafish, is a freshwater fish which is frequently used as a model system in biomedical research, including developmental biology and toxicology. Because of the highly conserved developmental process across vertebrates, zebrafish development is comparable to that of mammalians. In fact, the OECD has developed test guideline 236 (TG236) for testing the acute developmental toxicity of chemicals in zebrafish (OECD, 2013).

Developmental toxicity of nicotine has been previously evaluated in zebrafish, partly because of this organism expresses various nAChR subtypes. Consistent with mammalian data, nicotine strongly bound to zebrafish α4β2 nAChR, while it had only a relatively weak binding affinity to zebrafish α7 nAChR and was largely inactive to other zebrafish nAChRs (Papke et al., 2012). These comparable binding affinities of nicotine make its toxicological evaluation in zebrafish mechanistically relevant to that in other mammalian systems. Similar to that in *Xenopus*, exposure of zebrafish embryos to nicotine or nicotine-containing aerosols was achieved by diluting nicotine or nicotine-containing aerosols in water or other appropriate zebrafish media, in which the embryos were placed. The nicotine concentrations were between 6.8 and 40 μM (Folkesson et al., 2016; Palpant et al., 2015; Parker and Connaughton, 2007). Chronic exposure to nicotine did not inhibit the hatching rate of fertilized zebrafish eggs, per se; but, it delayed the onset of hatching in a dose-dependent manner. At concentrations ≥20 μM, nicotine not only significantly restricted the growth of zebrafish larvae—manifested by reduced notochord length, eye diameter, and dry weight—but also adversely affected body morphology and swimming behaviors. Additionally, treatment with up to 40 μM nicotine dramatically decreased the survival of larval zebrafish by approximately 70% (Parker and Connaughton, 2007). Similarly, inhibition of larval zebrafish survival by diluted cigarette smoke, e-cigarette aerosols, and snuff extract containing a high concentration of nicotine was also revealed (Folkesson et al., 2016; Palpant et al., 2015). In addition, exposure to these aerosols or tobacco product extracts comprising a mixture of many components in addition to nicotine also affected heart morphogenesis and function. However, these cardiac effects were seemingly unrelated to nicotine, as exposure to nicotine alone did not result in heart defects (Palpant et al., 2015). Apart from its effects on survival, general growth, and cardiac development, chronic nicotine exposure, also dose-dependent (up to 33 μM), delayed the differentiation of spinal motor neuron development (Svoboda et al., 2002), which was likely the mechanism underlying the abnormal swimming behaviors induced by nicotine (Parker and Connaughton, 2007; Svoboda et al., 2002). The observation that nAChR antagonists methyllycaconitine and dihydro-β-erythroidine almost completely blocked the nicotine effects on zebrafish spinal motoneuron differentiation highlighted the involvement of nicotine binding to nAChRs (Svoboda et al., 2002). Taken together, the results of evaluation of nicotine exposure in zebrafish not only supported its detrimental effects on embryonic/fetal development but also identified organs or organ systems that are particularly vulnerable to nicotine exposure. It is, however, also important to understand that direct translation of these developmental effects in zebrafish to humans is not straightforward, particularly when dosing is considered. While these effects were generally induced by micromolar concentrations of nicotine in zebrafish, the reported serum nicotine levels in the newborns of smoking mothers were orders of magnitude smaller than these, ranging from 3 to 150 nM (Luck et al., 1985). Hence, translation of these effects to humans is not appropriate.

20.4.5.4 Rodents

Rodent species, such as mice and rats, are the current standard test systems for reproductive and developmental toxicity testing recommended by various regulatory bodies (ICH, 2017; OECD, 2018a,b, 2019; U.S.

Environmental Protection Agency, 1996). Considering the history of nicotine use and its societal prevalence, it is surprising that a comprehensive study on the reproductive and developmental toxicity of nicotine has so far not been conducted in accordance with the pertinent ICH (International Council for Harmonisation) or OECD test guidelines. Nevertheless, an extensive number of studies have focused on the effects of nicotine, administered via various routes, on very specific reproductive and developmental aspects in rodents, ranging from male/female fertility and embryonic/fetal development to postnatal development of various organs and systems. Together, these studies have provided insights into the reproductive and developmental toxicity of nicotine and will be discussed in the following sections on the basis of the individual aspect(s) they have addressed.

20.4.5.4.1 Impact of nicotine on male fertility and reproduction. Male infertility is a complex and multifactorial disease, the reason for which can be categorized into deficits in sperm production, blockage of sperm transport, and ejaculation disorders (Mayo Clinic). The average nicotine concentration in the seminal plasma of smokers was $67.7 + 37$ nM ($N = 44$ smokers), which suggests direct exposure of testicular cells and a potential effect on spermatogenesis (Pacifici et al., 1993). Thus, queries on the effects of nicotine have been primarily focused on spermatogenesis.

Chronic exposure to nicotine (2 mg/kg/day; s.c.; for 30 days) reduced the sperm count in male rats, implying disruption of spermatogenesis (Dhawan and Sharma, 2002). Others have made similar observations despite differences in routes of administration (i.p. and p.o.) and/or doses of nicotine (ranging from 0.4 to 2 mg/kg/day for 1–3 months) (Aydos et al., 2001; Kavitharaj and Vijayammal, 1999; Oyeyipo et al., 2011). This nicotine effect on spermatogenesis seemed to be mainly caused by reduced steroidogenesis and, more specifically, reduced production of androgens in the testes, downstream of the interaction between nicotine and the hypothalamic–pituitary gland–gonadal axis (Biswas et al., 1979; Jana et al., 2010; Patra et al., 1979). This notion was further supported by a study which showed that chronic administration of nicotine (0.5 and 1 mg/kg/day; i.p.; for 2 weeks) in young adult rats decreased the levels of serum gonadotropic hormones (i.e., luteinizing hormone and follicle-stimulating hormone) and reduced the number of androgen-secreting Leydig cells (Guo et al., 2017). Together, the reductions in gonadotropic hormone

levels and androgen-secreting cells contributed to a decrease in serum testosterone levels. Apart from its effects on spermatogenesis, nicotine also decreased libido in male rats (Dhawan and Sharma, 2002; Oyeyipo et al., 2013), presumably as a result of the decreased androgen levels, because the key function of androgens is the regulation of sexual behaviors (Robbins, 1996). Disruption of the differentiation, maturation, and survival of Leydig cells by chronic administration of nicotine (2 mg/kg; i.p.; for 5 weeks) was also reported in mice (Wu et al., 2019; Zhao et al., 2018), consistent with previous findings that nicotine treatment inhibited steroidogenesis in murine Leydig cells in vitro (Patterson et al., 1990). In line with the nicotine effects on Leydig cells, Reddy et al. reported that chronic administration of nicotine (2–6 mg/kg; i.p.; for 15 days) in adult mice reduced testes weight and spermatocyte and spermatid numbers, suggesting interrupted spermatogenesis in the nicotine-treated mice (Reddy et al., 1998).

20.4.5.4.2 Impact of nicotine on female fertility and early pregnancy. Female reproduction involves the sequential processes of ovulation, fertilization of the ovum by sperm in the fallopian tubes, and implantation and growth of the zygote in the uterus. To occur correctly, this complex process requires endocrine homeostasis and development and maturation of functional reproductive organs. Conversely, disruption of hormone balance and malformation and malfunction of reproductive organs will lead to defects in the overall reproduction process, resulting in infertility (Mayo Clinic).

The female reproductive system may be less sensitive to nicotine than the male reproductive system, probably because of the faster metabolism of nicotine and cotinine in women than in men. This is thought to be linked to estrogenic action (Benowitz et al., 2006). Still, the impact of nicotine on female fertility is not clear, although it may be plausible, because cotinine was measured in the follicular fluid of female smokers (710.4 ± 128.2 ng/mL or 379 ± 0.79 μM; mean ± standard error of the mean) (Zenzes et al., 1996).

The impact of nicotine administration on the continuum of events from ovulation to implantation started to be described decades ago and was mainly attributed to its neuroendocrine-disrupting effects, which resulted from the effects of nicotine on the hypothalamic–pituitary–ovarian axis (Weathersbee, 1980). Supporting this notion, Blackburn et al. revealed that subacute administration of nicotine (6.25 μg/kg; i.p.; twice daily, three times a day, or four times a day for 2 days) in immature female rats dose-dependently depleted the number of oocytes in the fallopian tube and reduced serum estradiol levels (Blackburn et al., 1994). Conversely, in proestrus rats, stimulation of nAChRs by direct microinjection of nicotine (200 μM) into the suprachiasmatic nucleus in the hypothalamus stimulated estradiol secretion and increased the numbers of growing ovarian follicles and shed ova (Vieyra et al., 2019). Therefore, the estrogen- and oocyte-depleting effects of chronic (or repeated) nicotine administration should not be confused with the transient luteinizing hormone—stimulating effect of acute nicotine treatment, which is largely due to the instant release of reservoir luteinizing hormone from the pituitary gland upon acute nicotine stimulation. Additionally, high-dose nicotine exposure (5 mg/kg or 2 mg per rat; s.c.; twice daily, for up to 5 days) of mated female rats during the preimplantation period (i.e., days 1—5 following detection of a vaginal plug) also affected the cleavage of fertilized ova and subsequent implantation of the blastocysts in the uterine horns (Card and Mitchell, 1979; Yoshinaga et al., 1979). Such a detrimental effect of nicotine on implantation during early pregnancy was also observed in mice exposed to e-cigarette aerosols generated from a liquid formulation with nicotine (2.4% w/v) dissolved in a PG/VG (55:45 ratio) mixture (Wetendorf et al., 2019).

20.4.5.4.3 Impact of nicotine on embryonic—fetal and postnatal development.

The effects of prenatal (i.e., in utero) and/or lactation nicotine exposure on pre- and postnatal development of the offspring have been documented in an extensive number of reports. One of the most readily observable effects of in utero nicotine exposure on fetal development is restriction of fetal growth, manifested by lower fetal body weight and reduced crown—rump length (Orzabal et al., 2019). A similar observation was also made in rat fetuses exposed to cigarette smoke during pregnancy (Carmines et al., 2003), although it is noteworthy that the serum nicotine level in affected dams was approximately 13 times higher than that measured in the Orzabal et al. study (2.1 vs. 0.16 μM nicotine). The underlying mechanism was postulated to be nicotine-induced uteroplacental insufficiency, that is, insufficient blood/nutritional supply to the fetus via the uterus and placenta due to nicotine's vasoconstricting effects (Dempsey and Benowitz, 2001). Apart from the growth retardation, other development defects in various offspring organs/

systems, such as the skeletal, circulatory, respiratory, and central nervous systems, were also associated with maternal exposure to nicotine during pregnancy and/ or lactation period. These results will, therefore, be discussed according to the specific organ system.

20.4.5.4.3.1 Placenta. Nicotine is a binding ligand of nAChRs (e.g., α4 and α7 subunits), which are known to be expressed in human and rat placenta (Lips et al., 2005). Acetylcholine, the endogenous ligand of nAChRs, is an important placental signaling molecule which regulates—through activation of nAChRs—various key functions such as nutrient uptake, blood flow, and fluid volume in placental vessels and placental vascularization (Lips et al., 2005). It is, therefore, a concern that chronic nicotine exposure during pregnancy may have a direct impact on placental development and normal physiological function via overstimulation of nAChRs.

The effects of nicotine on placental development were investigated in rats treated with 1 mg/kg nicotine from 2 weeks prior to mating until gestation day (GD) 15. Nicotine negatively impacted trophoblast interstitial invasion, increased placental hypoxia, reduced labyrinth vascularization, and decreased the expression levels of key transcription factors (including heart and neural crest derivatives expressed 1 [Hand1] and glial cells missing transcription factor 1 [Gcm1]) and local and circulating endocrine gland—derived vascular endothelial growth factor (EG-VEGF), a placental angiogenic factor (Holloway et al., 2014). In another study, rats that received 1 mg/kg nicotine s.c. BID from GD9 to GD20 had increased levels of corticosterone in the placenta. The corticosterone levels in fetal serum were also increased in the prenatal exposure group relative to controls. In addition, the morphology of the placenta in nicotine-treated animals was disrupted, with irregular syncytial nodes in the labyrinth zone, reduced thickness of the labyrinth zone, and increased thickness of the junctional zone; additionally, nicotine treatment was associated with reduced fetal body weight (Zhou et al., 2018). The expression levels of α4 and β2 nAChR subunits in the placenta were increased in the nicotine-exposed group, as were the levels of ERK1/2 and ETS Like-1 (Elk-1) phosphorylation. The authors suggested that prenatal nicotine exposure inhibits placental corticosteroid 11-β-dehydrogenase isozyme 2 (11β-HSD2) expression (which was decreased in the nicotine-exposed group) via activation of nAChRs and the ERK1/2/Elk-1 pathway. The reduced expression of 11β-HSD2 may then attenuate the inactivation of maternal glucocorticoids, which, in turn, would affect both fetal and placental development (Zhou et al., 2018). The same group also reported increased serum levels of total, HDL, and LDL cholesterol in pregnant rats injected daily with 2 mg/kg nicotine from GD9 to GD20, whereas the total and HDL cholesterol levels were decreased in female fetal rats. Finally, they showed that the expression of placental cholesterol transporters was perturbed upon prenatal nicotine exposure (Zhang et al., 2018).

20.4.5.4.3.2 Central nervous system. The development of the central nervous system (CNS) involves complex molecular and cellular mechanisms, continuing through pre- and postnatal stages. Neurotransmitters and their respective receptors are present early during neurodevelopment and play crucial roles in neurogenesis and synaptogenesis (Ruediger and Bolz, 2007). Therefore, perturbations of neurotransmission at critical developmental stages by exogenous neurotoxicants, including nicotine, impose detrimental effects on neural cell proliferation and differentiation as well as neural circuit formation (Slikker et al., 2005). Oral administration of nicotine (approximately 30–40 mg/kg/day via sucrose-sweetened drinking water) in pregnant mice from GD14 until parturition significantly depleted glutamatergic neurons in the median prefrontal cortex, which was mainly subsequent to the impaired proliferation of neuronal progenitors in the ventricular and subventricular zones. The fact that the α7 nAChR antagonist methyllycaconitine, but not the α4β2 antagonist dihydro-β-erythroidine, could rescue the prenatal nicotine exposure–induced impairment of neurogenesis suggested the involvement of α7 nAChRs (Aoyama et al., 2016). Using a similar exposure regimen, Heath and colleagues demonstrated that maternal exposure to nicotine during pregnancy and the nursing period significantly affected corticothalamic neuronal circuit development, and this effect involved α4β2 nAChRs (Heath et al., 2010). Alternatively, s.c. nicotine infusion by using osmotic minipumps (about 4 mg/kg/day) in pregnant rats from GD7 until parturition significantly reduced the neuronal density in the dentate gyrus in the hippocampus in the offspring (Wang and Gondre-Lewis, 2013). Taken together, it is conceivable that nAChR activation by exogenous nicotine at an inappropriate time during pre- and postnatal development may exert toxic effects on CNS development. Importantly, these adverse events in CNS development were subsequently associated with behavioral abnormalities, including cognitive impairment and increased anxiety and depression-like behaviors during adolescence and in adulthood (Aoyama

et al., 2016; Heath et al., 2010; Lee et al., 2016; Santiago and Huffman, 2014; Zhang et al., 2019a). Notably, these alterations in CNS development and behaviors in the offspring are very often sex-specific, highlighting an interaction between prenatal nicotine exposure and sex hormone stimulation in neurodevelopment (Cross et al., 2017).

20.4.5.4.3.3 Respiratory system. Perinatal insults, including intrauterine growth restriction, preterm birth, maternal exposure to toxins, and dietary deficiencies, are commonly associated with developmental defects and malfunctions of the fetal respiratory system, particularly the lungs (Stocks et al., 2013). The effects of in utero nicotine exposure of pregnant mice and rats on fetal lung development have also been documented. In rats, maternal exposure to nicotine (2 mg/kg/day; s.c.; QD) from GD3 to GD21 transiently decreased vascular endothelial growth factor receptor (VEGFR)-2 mRNA expression and increased the volume fraction of alveolar walls in the neonatal lungs on postnatal day 1. These effects gradually diminished with postnatal development (Jiang et al., 2012). In contrast, Maritz and Windvogel reported that nicotine administration (1 mg/kg/day; s.c.; QD) during the gestation and lactation periods permanently decreased the number and internal surface area of alveoli in the neonatal lungs (Maritz and Windvogel, 2003). In a more recent study in mice, preconception exposure (at 12 days before mating) plus exposure during gestation to cinnamon-flavored e-liquid aerosols significantly increased the tissue fraction, as revealed by morphometric measurements of the neonatal lungs on postnatal day 28; this was coupled with the downregulation of genes linked to lung organogenesis (Noël et al., 2020). Of note, prolonged nicotine exposure mimicked absence of α7 nAChRs in knockout mice, despite an increase in nAChR expression in the fetal lung epithelium. Both studies that reported this phenomenon also reported lung basal epithelial cell hyperplasia (Maouche et al., 2009, 2013). This suggested that chronic exposure to nicotine desensitized the lung nAChRs. Taken together, these studies indicate the adverse effects of prenatal nicotine exposure on fetal lung development, involving the downregulation of α7 nAChR functions which, in turn, regulate the differentiation and function of the lung epithelium.

20.4.5.4.3.4 Other systems. Besides its effects on fetal CNS and respiratory system development, prenatal nicotine exposure was also implied in the defective development of other organs and systems. Xiao et al. showed that chronic administration of nicotine (2 mg/kg/day; s.c.) in pregnant rats from GD9 to GD20 induced bone dysplasia and suppressed osteogenic differentiation in male offspring through promotion of angiotensin-converting enzyme expression and activation of the renin—angiotensin system via modulation of α4β2 nAChRs (Xiao et al., 2019). Similar to the observations in zebrafish, fetal cardiac development in rodents was also subject to the regulation of prenatal nicotine exposure. Pregnant rats that continuously received nicotine by s.c. infusion via an osmotic minipump (6 mg/kg/day) during GD7 to GD21 gave birth to offspring with significantly greater cardiomyocyte cell width, lower cardiomyocyte nucleus numbers, higher β-myosin heavy chain and transforming growth factor (TGF-β1) expression, and higher collagen deposition in the heart, indicating nicotine-induced cardiac remodeling in fetal rats (Chou and Chen, 2014). Additionally, repeated maternal nicotine exposure during pregnancy (2 mg/kg/day; s.c.; from GD9 to GD20) decreased estradiol synthesis and reduced testicular steroidogenesis in female and male offspring, respectively, indicating the effects of nicotine on the development of the offspring reproductive systems (Fan et al., 2019; Zhang et al., 2020).

20.4.5.5 Nonhuman primates
At birth, rodent lungs are relatively immature compared to human and nonhuman primate (NHP) lungs. Therefore, NHPs are valuable models for studying fetal lung development in response to chronic in utero nicotine exposure. Maternal exposure to 1 mg/kg/day nicotine s.c. (via osmotic minipump) during pregnancy altered fetal lung development in rhesus monkeys. Immunohistochemistry analyses showed that prenatal nicotine exposure significantly increased α7 nAChR expression in the fetal lung, which was correlated with elevated collagen expression around large airways and vessels and implied an increased risk for development of pulmonary hypertension in the fetuses (Sekhon et al., 1999, 2004).

20.4.6 Developmental and Reproductive Toxicology of Nicotine in Vitro
The effects of nicotine on DART endpoints have been evaluated by using a multitude of in vitro approaches for over 30 years. During this period, five broad DART categories have been studied in vitro: (1) embryonic development; (2) effects on fetal cells; (3) effects on the placenta; (4) effects on cells of the reproductive system and in vitro reproduction processes; and (5) effects on neurological development. These will be reviewed and discussed further here.

20.4.6.1 Embryonic development
The impact of nicotine on embryonic development in mammals has, in general, been studied in embryos of different developmental stages cultured in vitro as well as, in more recent times, in embryonic stem cells (ESCs). The development of early-stage embryos (e.g., 2—16 cells) to more advanced stages was suppressed following exposure to nicotine at concentrations ≥1 mM (Balling and Beier, 1985; Liu et al., 2008a, 2008b). In contrast, a number of studies have reported that nicotine concentrations below 1 mM had no adverse effects on the developmental progression of mouse, bovine, and rabbit embryos in vitro (Baldwin and Racowsky, 1987; Balling and Beier, 1985; Gu et al., 2013; Li et al., 2009).

The effects of nicotine on later-stage mammalian embryos have also been investigated, but at nicotine concentrations that are far from physiologically relevant. E8.5 (embryonic day 8.5) mouse embryos cultured in 1 mM nicotine for 48 h developed severe morphological anomalies and manifested oxidative cellular damage (Lin et al., 2013, 2014). Murine embryos at the same developmental stage were malformed and displayed evidence of open neural tube and/or caudal regression upon exposure to ≥3 μM nicotine for 48 h (Zhao and Reece, 2005). Moreover, fusion of palatal shelves in E13.5 mouse embryos was inhibited following a 72-h culture with 600 μM of nicotine, possibly via downregulation of the PI3K pathway (Kang and Svoboda, 2003). Rat embryos cultured in nicotine (0.61—2.46 mM) were also smaller in size than their nonexposed counterparts and displayed signs of microcephaly and cleft palate—malformations which were postulated to be brought on by cellular membrane damage (Joschko et al., 1991). Early chick embryos exposed in ovo to nicotine (<2 μM) ostensibly developed normally in terms of viability, weight, and length relative to controls. However, these embryos exhibited apparent altered axial rotation, probably as a result of incomplete closing of the neural tube in the cervical region (Bohn et al., 2017). In addition to gross developmental changes, localized effects on embryonic lung development have also been studied. Explanted embryonic murine lungs cultured in the presence of 1 μM nicotine branched markedly more than controls and expressed increased levels of surfactant proteins (SP) A and C, factors that may lead to respiratory distress syndrome and airway disease (Wongtrakool et al., 2007; Wuenschell et al., 1998). Interestingly, these enhanced levels of branching and SP expression were blocked by the nicotinic antagonists

D-tubocurarine and α-bungarotoxin, indicating that α7 nAChR signaling likely drove these effects (Wuenschell et al., 1998). Moreover, exposure of mouse lung buds to nicotine decreased BAX (BCL2 associated X), calcyclin, and osteopontin expression—changes that are thought to play a role in stimulation of branching morphogenesis (Wuenschell et al., 2004).

Experiments in human ESCs (hESCs) are fewer in number but have largely employed more physiologically relevant concentrations of nicotine for studying its DART-related effects. While cardiac-directed differentiation of hESCs was unaffected following their culture in <10 μM nicotine (Zdravkovic et al., 2008), similar nicotine concentrations in e-cigarette and cigarette smoke extracts reportedly had a significant negative impact on pluripotency and survival markers (Palpant et al., 2015). Nicotine treatment (<5 μM) delayed the differentiation of hESCs to mesodermal and endodermal lineages and also caused perturbations in three major signaling pathways (the Notch, canonical Wnt, and TGF-β pathways) that regulate stem cell pluripotency and differentiation (Liszewski et al., 2012). Furthermore, treatment with 10 μM nicotine degraded mitofusin in the human multipotent embryonal carcinoma cell line NT2/D1 and, consequently, induced mitochondrial dysfunction and cell growth inhibition (Hirata et al., 2016). In addition, while NHP ESCs appeared normal histologically and could apparently differentiate into fibroblasts in the presence of 100 nM nicotine, the treated cells showed altered gene expression, including that of N-myc, which is hypothesized to ultimately lead to disruption of organogenesis (Ben-Yehudah et al., 2013).

20.4.6.2 Fetal cells

The effects of nicotine on developmental processes that are active in postembryonic but prenatal mammals have been studied in isolated fetal cells grown in the presence of nicotine in vitro. Human amniocytes cultured in nicotine-containing medium (0.16 μM) developed significant chromosomal abnormalities relative to control cells; these data imply that nicotine may have aneugenic properties (Demirhan et al., 2011). Baseline production of 6-keto-prostaglandin F1α and thromboxane B2 was unaffected in fetal specimens that were collected from the umbilical arteries of infants born to healthy, nonsmoking women and cultured in the presence of nicotine at concentrations >60 mM (Ylikorkala et al., 1985). However, in the same study, thromboxane A2 synthesis in fetal platelets was found

to be inhibited by nicotine concentrations between 0.06 and 3 mM; but, the authors concluded that nicotine was unlikely to be the root cause of the maternal-smoking induced changes in fetal prostacyclin formation (Ylikorkala et al., 1985).

In rats, nicotine (≤100 μM) treatment affected the normal functioning of fetal growth plate chondrocytes (e.g., cartilaginous matrix synthesis; effects mediated via downregulation of insulin-like growth factor [IGF]-1 signaling) as well as lung alveolar type II cells (e.g., surfactant synthesis)—factors which are hypothesized to contribute to the intrauterine origins of osteoporosis/osteoarthritis and lung disease, respectively (Deng et al., 2013; Rehan et al., 2007). Interestingly, when another model of fetal development, namely human hepatoblasts (both male and female) produced from pluripotent stem cells, was grown in the presence of the major nicotine metabolite cotinine (1—300 nM for 8 days), no effects on ATP synthesis were observed, although caspase 3/7 and CYP1A2 and CYP3A activities were perturbed (Lucendo-Villarin et al., 2017).

20.4.6.3 Placenta

Placenta functionality in the presence of nicotine has been studied primarily by using human ex vivo cultures. While nicotine (≤1.6 μM) had no effects on placental microvascular function in an in vitro perfusion system (Bainbridge and Smith, 2006), placental transport of arginine (but not alanine and glutamine) was significantly reduced in its presence (0.8 μM), and this was postulated to play a role in interference in fetal growth (Pastrakuljic et al., 2000). Nicotine at concentrations of 2.5—20 μM was also shown to block the active uptake of α-aminoisobutyric acid in human placental villous slices and may, therefore, contribute to intrauterine fetal growth retardation (Fisher et al., 1984). Following exposure to 0.23—6 μM nicotine, cytotrophoblasts isolated from anchoring chorionic villi exhibited reduced passage through the cell cycle as well as suppressed invasion capabilities due to the lack of synthesis/activation of the invasion mediator 92-kDa type IV collagenase. These results suggest that nicotine can potentially perturb placental development (Genbacev et al., 1995, 2000).

Nicotine's effects on induction of preterm labor and spontaneous abortions through modulation of phospholipid metabolism and prostaglandin production were investigated in perfused cotyledons of human placenta. While nicotine (12 μM) prevented PGE2-induced umbilical perfusion pressure and activated phospholipase A2, its major metabolite, cotinine (11 µM), enhanced PGE2 levels and potentiated the effects of PGE2 on placental vascular resistance to decrease fetal blood flow through the placenta, which may subsequently impact successful perinatal outcome (Sastry et al., 1999). In contrast, nicotine (1 nM–100 µM) demonstrated no modulatory activities on placental choline acetyltransferase activity and was, therefore, considered not likely to affect nitric oxide signaling or its consequent processes (Wessler et al., 2003).

Two studies employed alternative biological models, namely immortalized cell lines, to study the effects of nicotine on placental cell growth and functionality. Rat choriocarcinoma (RCHO-1) cells exposed to 1 µM–1 mM nicotine showed reduced propensities for migration, invasion, and differentiation, and these effects were purportedly driven via dysregulated nAChR and MMP-9 expression (Holloway et al., 2014). In a follow-up study in RCHO-1 cells, nicotine (10–100 µM) caused a dose-dependent increase in the phosphorylation of PERK (protein kinase R-like ER kinase) and eIF2a (eukaryotic translation initiation factor 2A), both markers of endoplasmic reticulum (ER) stress, via activation of nAChRs (Wong et al., 2016b).

20.4.6.4 Cells of the reproductive system and in vitro reproduction processes

Nicotine-induced effects on male and female gametes as well as other cells of the reproductive system have been extensively studied in vitro. Direct exposure of murine spermatozoa to 0.5 and 5 mM nicotine for 30 min during the capacitation maturation step did not affect their motility or DNA integrity significantly (Gu et al., 2013). Other studies in mouse oocytes cultured in >1 mM nicotine reported conflicting findings on meiotic maturation and ploidy status (Mailhes et al., 2000; Zenzes and Bielecki, 2004). In addition, maturation of oocytes isolated from another rodent, the hamster, was impaired following culture in ≥5 mM nicotine (Racowsky et al., 1989). In oocyte–cumulus complexes isolated from large antral porcine follicles, hyaluronic acid and progesterone synthesis were suppressed by nicotine exposure (2, 20, and 200 µM). These effects may affect intrafollicular processes that are responsible for normal ovulation (Vrsanska et al., 2003). Similar to the findings in hamsters, the maturation rate of bovine oocytes cultured in ≥2 mM nicotine was markedly reduced relative to controls (Liu et al., 2008a).

Potential endocrine-disrupting properties were observed in male rats, as testosterone biosynthesis in isolated Leydig cells exposed to nicotine (and cotinine) was significantly impaired (Yeh et al., 1989). Exposure to nicotine concentrations at 6, 60, and 600 µM were inducing additional endocrine-disrupting effects in bovine theca interna and granulosa cells by reducing their ability to produce androstenedione and estradiol (Sanders et al., 2002). Moreover, the functionality of human granulosa cells in the presence of 6 µM nicotine was adversely affected, as aromatase was inhibited in a concentration-dependent manner (Barbieri et al., 1986), while progesterone and estradiol production was modulated (Bodis et al., 1997).

Nicotine (1–100 µM) also provoked norepinephrine release in the uterine horn in mice and inhibited electricity-induced contractions (Medina et al., 1992). In contrast, nicotine potentiated the contractility of rabbit myometrium strips (≥100 µM) and isolated sheep uterine arteries (≥0.01 µM) and was, therefore, postulated to contribute to the failure of quiescence and impairment of vascular function in the uterus (Nas et al., 2007; Xiao et al., 2007).

The impact of nicotine on the efficiency of parthenogenetic activation (PA) and in vitro fertilization (IVF) has been evaluated in two mammalian species. PA of bovine oocytes matured in 10 and 50 µM nicotine resulted in blastocyst development rates comparable with those in controls (Li et al., 2009). Similar findings were also reported in a related bovine study with nicotine concentrations of 0.01–0.5 mM; however, higher concentrations (2.5 and 5 mM) significantly decreased the cleavage rates (Liu et al., 2008b). In mice, the rates of successful oocyte IVF were reduced relative to controls when spermatozoa were exposed to 0.5 and 5 mM nicotine for 30 min prior to attempted fertilization (Gu et al., 2013). Collectively, the findings from these studies suggest that nicotine, particularly at high concentrations, can potentially interfere with reproduction-related processes in mammalian cells in vitro.

20.4.6.5 Neurological development

The effects of nicotine on neurological development in vitro have mainly been studied in rat models. E9.5 rat embryos exposed in vitro to 10 and 100 µM nicotine for 48 h exhibited evidence of forebrain, midbrain, and hindbrain cytotoxicity, and these pathologies reportedly occurred prior to dysmorphogenesis (Roy et al., 1998). The same researchers published their findings on rat neural stem cells derived from E14 neuroepithelium, which indicated that nicotine (30 and 100 µM) can suppress the expression of the glial phenotype without affecting the neuronal phenotype (Slotkin et al., 2016). Other rat studies that employed CNS preparations from neonatal animals exposed to nicotine in utero revealed that this type of developmental exposure altered the cholinergic control of respiratory frequency and GABAergic neurotransmission and also disrupted dendritic arborization patterns in hypoglossal motor neurons (Powell et al., 2016; Wollman et al., 2016). In addition, brainstem slices derived from rats exposed to nicotine prenatally exhibited exaggerated bradycardia-related effects during hypoxia, an effect which is hypothesized to play a causal role in sudden infant death syndrome in humans (Neff et al., 2004). In brain slices from the other rodent species studied in this context, the mouse, prenatal nicotine exposure suppressed AMPA (α-amino-3-hydroxy-5-methyl-4-isoxazolepropionic acid) and NMDA (N-methyl-D-aspartate) receptor-mediated effects within the laterodorsal tegmental nucleus, the reward-related brain region, and was, therefore, suggested to contribute to an increased likelihood of nicotine consumption by the offspring in later life (McNair and Kohlmeier, 2015).

20.4.7 Conclusions for Reproduction and Development

There are no epidemiological data on the potential impact of nicotine exposure solely on pregnancy outcomes. Three metaanalyses of epidemiological studies on the adverse effects reported after nicotine-containing product use during pregnancy were published. They concluded that there is no zero risk for the use of smoke-free nicotine and tobacco products during pregnancy. Even though the data obtained in these studies are debatable because of confounding effects, small numbers of participants, missing biomarkers of exposure measurements, and a high variability among the products and their usage, it must always be recommended to avoid nicotine exposure during pregnancy. This conclusion is also largely supported by a vast number of in vivo and in vitro studies that highlight various adverse effects, sometimes supported by mechanistic evidence, in different tissues/organs during development (the placenta, lungs, CNS, etc.). While these studies help increase public awareness of the potential health risks of nicotine to human reproduction and development, it is also important to acknowledge their limitations. First, the majority of the mammalian studies used bolus or continuous parenteral administration (e.g., via osmotic pumps) of nicotine, which resulted in distinct nicotine kinetics relative to that in humans who receive nicotine from ENDPs by inhalation. Second, the nicotine concentrations used in *C. elegans*, *Xenopus*, and zebrafish research are often very high (Fig. 20.5)

and exceed by far the plasma nicotine concentrations that can be achieved in human users. The same limitation applies to many in vitro studies. Because of these caveats, direct translation of DART findings for nicotine from animal models to humans is inappropriate. Future studies that consider the human route of administration and realistically achievable human equivalent doses will be helpful for further assessing the risk of ENDP use in reproduction and development.

20.5 CONCLUSIONS

In the context of tobacco harm reduction (Chapter 1), McNeil noted that *"Since nicotine itself is not a highly hazardous drug, encouraging smokers to obtain nicotine from sources that do not involve tobacco combustion is a potential means to reduce the morbidity and mortality they sustain, without the need to overcome their addiction to nicotine"* (McNeil, 2012). In addition, the Tobacco Advisory Group of the United Kingdom Royal College of Physicians stated that *"as most of the harm caused by smoking arises not from nicotine but from other components of tobacco smoke, the health and life expectancy of today's smokers could be radically improved by encouraging as many as possible to switch to a smoke-free source of nicotine"* (Royal College of Physicians of London. Tobacco Advisory Group, 2007). While recognizing the primacy of complete cessation of all tobacco and nicotine use as the ultimate goal to prevent harm from smoking, the report argued that promoting widespread substitution of cigarettes and other tobacco combustion products would, for smokers who made the change, achieve much the same thing. Therefore, harm reduction, as a complement to conventional tobacco control policies, could offer a means to prevent millions of deaths among tobacco smokers.

This review highlights that there are still many gaps in our understanding of the biological effects of nicotine at doses relevant to human nicotine exposure. Nevertheless, the currently available evidence on the effects of nicotine and cigarette smoke shows that *"most of the harm caused by smoking arises not from nicotine but from other components of tobacco smoke"* (Royal College of Physicians of London. Tobacco Advisory Group, 2007) and that *"nicotine is not a highly hazardous substance"* (McNeil, 2012). However, for smokers, quitting tobacco and nicotine use altogether is the best option. Furthermore, this review further emphasizes that nicotine-containing products should not be used during pregnancy, breastfeeding and development, or by people who have or are at risk of heart disease.

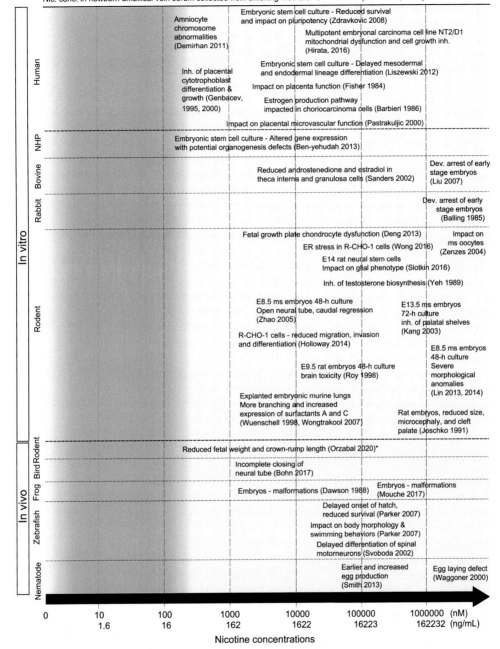

FIG. 20.5 Summary of developmental effects observed following nicotine exposure in both in vivo and in vitro DART models. The location of each reference on the x-axis reflects the range of nicotine concentrations tested where the effects were observed. Species and type of studies (in vivo/in vitro) are indicated on the left side of the figure. The dark gray area indicates the range of nicotine concentrations measured in various sample types during pregnancy in smoking mothers, as indicated at the top of the figure. * This reference (in bold) is the only in vivo study for which nicotine levels in dam sera (measured at GD11) were available, and it is also a study that assessed the impact of e-cigarette aerosol exposure. All other in vivo rodent studies mentioned in the text did not measure nicotine concentrations in exposed dams/fetuses and, thus, are not shown here. *Dev.*, development; *ER*, endoplasmic reticulum; *Inh*, inhibition; *ms*, mouse; *NHP*, nonhuman primates.

REFERENCES

Adler, I.-D., Attia, S., 2003. Nicotine is not clastogenic at doses of 1 or 2 mg/kg body weight given orally to male mice. Mutat. Res. Genet. Toxicol. Environ. Mutagen 542 (1), 139–142.

Akcay, A., Aydin, M.N., Acar, G., Mese, B., Cetin, M., Akgungor, M., et al., 2015. Evaluation of left atrial mechanical function and atrial conduction abnormalities in Maras powder (smokeless tobacco) users and smokers. Cardiovasc. J. Afr. 26 (3), 114–119.

Albuquerque, E.X., Pereira, E.F., Alkondon, M., Rogers, S.W., 2009. Mammalian nicotinic acetylcholine receptors: from structure to function. Physiol. Rev. 89 (1), 73–120.

Alexandrov, L.B., Ju, Y.S., Haase, K., Van Loo, P., Martincorena, I., Nik-Zainal, S., et al., 2016. Mutational signatures associated with tobacco smoking in human cancer. Science 354 (6312), 618–622.

Alkaitis, M.S., Crabtree, M.J., 2012. Recoupling the cardiac nitric oxide synthases: tetrahydrobiopterin synthesis and recycling. Curr. Heart Fail. Rep. 9 (3), 200–210.

Allen, S.S., Hatsukami, D., Gorsline, J., 1994. Cholesterol changes in smoking cessation using the transdermal nicotine system. Transdermal Nicotine Study Group. Prev. Med. 23 (2), 190–196.

Altmann, H., Weniger, P., Dolejs, I., 1984. Influence of nicotine on DNA metabolism. Klin. Wochenschr. 62, 101–104.

Amoruso, A., Bardelli, C., Gunella, G., Fresu, L.G., Ferrero, V., Brunelleschi, S., 2007. Quantification of PPAR-γ protein in monocyte/macrophages from healthy smokers and non-smokers: a possible direct effect of nicotine. Life Sci. 81 (11), 906–915.

Andersson, K., Arner, P., 1995. Cholinoceptor-mediated effects on glycerol output from human adipose tissue using in situ microdialysis. Br. J. Pharmacol. 115 (7), 1155–1162.

Andersson, K., Arner, P., 2001. Systemic nicotine stimulates human adipose tissue lipolysis through local cholinergic and catecholaminergic receptors. Int. J. Obes. Relat. Metab. Disord. 25 (8), 1225–1232.

Andreotti, G., Freedman, N.D., Silverman, D.T., Lerro, C.C., Koutros, S., Hartge, P., et al., 2017. Tobacco use and cancer risk in the agricultural health study. Cancer Epidemiol. Biomarkers Prev. 26 (5), 769–778.

Antoniewicz, L., Bosson, J.A., Kuhl, J., Abdel-Halim, S.M., Kiessling, A., Mobarrez, F., et al., 2016. Electronic cigarettes increase endothelial progenitor cells in the blood of healthy volunteers. Atherosclerosis 255, 179–185.

Antoniewicz, L., Brynedal, A., Hedman, L., Lundback, M., Bosson, J.A., 2019. Acute effects of electronic cigarette inhalation on the vasculature and the conducting airways. Cardiovasc. Toxicol. 19 (5), 441–450.

Aoshiba, K., Nagai, A., Yasui, S., Konno, K., 1996. Nicotine prolongs neutrophil survival by suppressing apoptosis. J. Lab. Clin. Med. 127 (2), 186–194.

Aoyama, Y., Toriumi, K., Mouri, A., Hattori, T., Ueda, E., Shimato, A., et al., 2016. Prenatal nicotine exposure impairs the proliferation of neuronal progenitors, leading to fewer glutamatergic neurons in the medial prefrontal cortex. Neuropsychopharmacology 41 (2), 578–589.

Argacha, J.F., Fontaine, D., Adamopoulos, D., Ajose, A., Borne, P.V.D., Fontaine, J., et al., 2008. Acute effect of sidestream cigarette smoke extract on vascular endothelial function. J. Cardiovasc. Pharmacol. 52 (3).

Argentin, G., Cicchetti, R., 2004. Genotoxic and antiapoptotic effect of nicotine on human gingival fibroblasts. Toxicol. Sci. 79 (1), 75–81.

Arner, P., Bulow, J., 1993. Assessment of adipose tissue metabolism in man: comparison of Fick and microdialysis techniques. Clin. Sci. 85 (3), 247–256.

Arredondo, J., Nguyen, V.T., Chernyavsky, A.I., Jolkovsky, D.L., Pinkerton, K.E., Grando, S.A., 2001. A receptor-mediated mechanism of nicotine toxicity in oral keratinocytes. Lab. Invest. 81 (12), 1653.

Ashraf-Uz-Zaman, M., Bhalerao, A., Mikelis, C.M., Cucullo, L., German, N.A., 2020. Assessing the current state of lung cancer chemoprevention: a comprehensive overview. Cancers 12 (5), 1265.

Asplund, K., 2003. Smokeless tobacco and cardiovascular disease. Prog. Cardiovasc. Dis. 45 (5), 383–394.

Asplund, K., Nasic, S., Janlert, U., Stegmayr, B., 2003. Smokeless tobacco as a possible risk factor for stroke in men: a nested case-control study. Stroke 34 (7), 1754–1759.

Ateyya, H., Nader, M.A., Attia, G.M., El-Sherbeeny, N.A., 2016. Influence of alpha-lipoic acid on nicotine-induced lung and liver damage in experimental rats. Can. J. Physiol. Pharmacol. 95 (5), 492–500.

Attia, S.M., 2007. The genotoxic and cytotoxic effects of nicotine in the mouse bone marrow. Mutat. Res. Genet. Toxicol. Environ. Mutagen 632 (1), 29–36.

Aydos, K., Guven, M.C., Can, B., Ergun, A., 2001. Nicotine toxicity to the ultrastructure of the testis in rats. BJU Int. 88 (6), 622–626.

Bainbridge, S.A., Smith, G.N., 2006. The effect of nicotine on in vitro placental perfusion pressure. Can. J. Physiol. Pharmacol. 84 (8–9), 953–957.

Balakumar, P., Sharma, R., Singh, M., 2008. Benfotiamine attenuates nicotine and uric acid-induced vascular endothelial dysfunction in the rat. Pharmacol. Res. 58 (5–6), 356–363.

Balbarini, A., Di Stefano, R., 2008. Circulating endothelial progenitor cells—characterisation, function and relationship with cardiovascular risk factors. Eur. Cardiol. 4, 16–19.

Baldwin, K.V., Racowsky, C., 1987. Nicotine and cotinine effects on development of two-cell mouse embryos in vitro. Reprod. Toxicol. 1 (3), 173–178.

Baldwin, T.J., Yoshihara, C.M., Blackmer, K., Kintner, C.R., Burden, S.J., 1988. Regulation of acetylcholine receptor transcript expression during development in *Xenopus laevis*. J. Cell Biol. 106 (2), 469–478.

Balharry, D., Sexton, K., Bérubé, K.A., 2008. An in vitro approach to assess the toxicity of inhaled tobacco smoke components: nicotine, cadmium, formaldehyde and urethane. Toxicology 244 (1), 66–76.

Balling, R., Beier, H.M., 1985. Direct effects of nicotine on rabbit preimplantation embryos. Toxicology 34 (4), 309–313.

Banerjee, A.G., Gopalakrishnan, V.K., Vishwanatha, J.K., 2007. Inhibition of nitric oxide-induced apoptosis by nicotine in oral epithelial cells. Mol. Cell. Biochem. 305 (1–2), 113–121.

Barber, K.E., Ghebrehiwet, B., Yin, W., Rubenstein, D.A., 2017. Endothelial cell inflammatory reactions are altered in the presence of E-cigarette extracts of variable nicotine. Cell. Mol. Bioeng. 10 (1), 124–133.

Barbieri, R.L., Mcshane, P.M., Ryan, K.J., 1986. Constituents of cigarette smoke inhibit human granulosa cell aromatase. Fertil. Steril. 46 (2), 232–236.

Barley, R.D., Pollock, S., Shallow, M.C., Peters, E., Lam, E.W., 2004. Tobacco-related-compound-induced nitrosative stress injury in the hamster cheek pouch. J. Dent. Res. 83 (12), 903–908.

Bekki, K., Uchiyama, S., Ohta, K., Inaba, Y., Nakagome, H., Kunugita, N., 2014. Carbonyl compounds generated from electronic cigarettes. Int. J. Environ. Res. Publ. Health 11 (11), 11192–11200.

Belushkin, M., Tafin Djoko, D., Esposito, M., Korneliou, A., Jeannet, C., Lazzerini, M., et al., 2020. Selected harmful and potentially harmful constituents levels in commercial e-cigarettes. Chem. Res. Toxicol. 33 (2), 657–668.

Ben-Yehudah, A., Campanaro, B.M., Wakefield, L.M., Kinney, T.N., Brekosky, J., Eisinger, V.M., et al., 2013. Nicotine exposure during differentiation causes inhibition of N-myc expression. Respir. Res. 14, 119.

Benowitz, N.L., 2003. Cigarette smoking and cardiovascular disease: pathophysiology and implications for treatment. Prog. Cardiovasc. Dis. 46 (1), 91–111.

Benowitz, N.L., Hukkanen, J., Jacob 3rd, P., 2009. Nicotine chemistry, metabolism, kinetics and biomarkers. Handb. Exp. Pharmacol. (192), 29–60. https://doi.org/10.1007/978-3-540-69248-5_2. Epub ahead of print 2009/02/03.

Benowitz, N.L., Jacob, P., 1993. Nicotine and cotinine elimination pharmacokinetics in smokers and nonsmokers. Clin. Pharmacol. Therapeut. 53 (3), 316–323.

Benowitz, N.L., Kuyt, F., Jacob, P., Jones, R.T., Osman, A.L., 1983. Cotinine disposition and effects. Clin. Pharmacol. Therapeut. 34 (5), 604–611.

Benowitz, N.L., Lessov-Schlaggar, C.N., Swan, G.E., Jacob 3rd, P., 2006. Female sex and oral contraceptive use accelerate nicotine metabolism. Clin. Pharmacol. Ther. 79 (5), 480–488.

Benowitz, N.L., Pipe, A., West, R., Hays, J.T., Tonstad, S., Mcrae, T., et al., 2018. Cardiovascular safety of varenicline, bupropion, and nicotine patch in smokers: a randomized clinical trial. JAMA Intern. Med. 178 (5), 622–631.

Benowitz, N.L., Porchet, H., Sheiner, L., Jacob 3rd, P., 1988. Nicotine absorption and cardiovascular effects with smokeless tobacco use: comparison with cigarettes and nicotine gum. Clin. Pharmacol. Ther. 44 (1), 23–28.

Bergoeing, M.P., Arif, B., Hackmann, A.E., Ennis, T.L., Thompson, R.W., Curci, J.A., 2007. Cigarette smoking increases aortic dilatation without affecting matrix metalloproteinase-9 and -12 expression in a modified mouse model of aneurysm formation. J. Vasc. Surg. 45 (6), 1217–1227.

Berman, M.L., Hatsukami, D.K., 2018. Reducing tobacco-related harm: FDA's proposed product standard for smokeless tobacco. Tobac. Contr. 27 (3), 352–354.

Berridge, M., 2012. Cell Stress, Inflammatory Responses and Cell Death. Cell Signalling Biology. Portland Press.

Beswick, A., Renaud, S., Yarnell, J.W., Elwood, P.C., 1991. Platelet activity in habitual smokers. Thromb. Haemostasis 66 (6), 739–740.

Bhatnagar, A., Whitsel, L.P., Ribisl, K.M., Bullen, C., Chaloupka, F., Piano, M.R., et al., 2014. Electronic cigarettes: a policy statement from the American Heart Association. Circulation 130 (16), 1418–1436.

Biondi-Zoccai, G., Sciarretta, S., Bullen, C., Nocella, C., Violi, F., Loffredo, L., et al., 2019. Acute effects of heat-not-burn, electronic vaping, and traditional tobacco combustion cigarettes: the sapienza university of rome-vascular assessment of proatherosclerotic effects of smoking (SUR - VAPES) 2 randomized trial. J. Am. Heart Assoc. 8 (6), e010455.

Biros, E., Walker, P.J., Nataatmadja, M., West, M., Golledge, J., 2012. Downregulation of transforming growth factor, beta receptor 2 and Notch signaling pathway in human abdominal aortic aneurysm. Atherosclerosis 221 (2), 383–386.

Biswas, N.M., Patra, P.B., Sanyal, S., Deb, C., 1979. Andrenogonadal interactions in nicotine-induced alteration of steroidogenesis in male rat. Andrologia 11 (3), 227–233.

Bjorkman, F., Edin, F., Mattsson, C.M., Larsen, F., Ekblom, B., 2017. Regular moist snuff dipping does not affect endurance exercise performance. PLoS One 12 (7), e0181228.

Blackburn, C.W., Peterson, C.A., Hales, H.A., Carrell, D.T., Jones, K.P., Urry, R.L., et al., 1994. Nicotine, but not cotinine, has a direct toxic effect on ovarian function in the immature gonadotropin-stimulated rat. Reprod. Toxicol. 8 (4), 325–331.

Blanchet, M.-R., Israël-Assayag, E., Cormier, Y., 2004. Inhibitory effect of nicotine on experimental hypersensitivity pneumonitis in vivo and in vitro. Am. J. Respir. Crit. Care Med. 169 (8), 903–909.

Blann, A.D., Steele, C., Mccollum, C.N., 1997. The influence of smoking and of oral and transdermal nicotine on blood pressure, and haematology and coagulation indices. Thromb. Haemostasis 78 (3), 1093–1096.

Boas, Z., Gupta, P., Moheimani, R.S., Bhetraratana, M., Yin, F., Peters, K.M., et al., 2017. Activation of the "splenocardiac axis" by electronic and tobacco cigarettes in otherwise healthy young adults. Phys. Rep. 5 (17).

Bodas, M., Van Westphal, C., Carpenter-Thompson, R., Mohanty, D.K., Vij, N., 2016. Nicotine exposure induces bronchial epithelial cell apoptosis and senescence via ROS mediated autophagy-impairment. Free Radic. Biol. Med. 97, 441–453.

Bodis, J., Hanf, V., Torok, A., Tinneberg, H.R., Borsay, P., Szabo, I., 1997. Influence of nicotine on progesterone and estradiol production of cultured human granulosa cells. Early Pregnancy 3 (1), 34–37.

Boffetta, P., Aagnes, B., Weiderpass, E., Andersen, A., 2005. Smokeless tobacco use and risk of cancer of the pancreas and other organs. Int. J. Cancer 114 (6), 992–995.

Boffetta, P., Hecht, S., Gray, N., Gupta, P., Straif, K., 2008. Smokeless tobacco and cancer. Lancet Oncol. 9 (7), 667–675.

Boffetta, P., Straif, K., 2009. Use of smokeless tobacco and risk of myocardial infarction and stroke: systematic review with meta-analysis. Br. Med. J. 339, b3060.

Bohn, N., Humphrey, V., Omelchenko-Comer, N., 2017. Effects of nicotine on chicken embryonic development. West Virginia Acad. Sci. 89 (2), 12–17.

Bolinder, G., De Faire, U., 1998. Ambulatory 24-h blood pressure monitoring in healthy, middle-aged smokeless tobacco users, smokers, and nontobacco users. Am. J. Hypertens. 11 (10), 1153–1163.

Bolinder, G.M., Ahlborg, B.O., Lindell, J.H., 1992. Use of smokeless tobacco: blood pressure elevation and other health hazards found in a large-scale population survey. J. Intern. Med. 232 (4), 327–334.

Boorman, G.A., Maronpot, R.R., Eustis, S.L., 1994. Rodent carcinogenicity bioassay: past, present, and future. Toxicol. Pathol. 22 (2), 105–111.

Brenner, S., 1974. The genetics of *Caenorhabditis elegans*. Genetics 77 (1), 71–94.

Brinson, K., 1974. Effect of nicotine on human blood platelet aggregation. Atherosclerosis 20 (1), 137–140.

Campisi, J., 2013. Aging, cellular senescence, and cancer. Annu. Rev. Physiol. 75, 685–705.

Card, J.P., Mitchell, J.A., 1979. The effects of nicotine on implantation in the rat. Biol. Reprod. 20 (3), 532–539.

Cardenas, V.M., Cen, R., Clemens, M.M., Moody, H.L., Ekanem, U.S., Policherla, A., et al., 2019a. Use of electronic nicotine delivery systems (ENDS) by pregnant women I: risk of small-for-gestational-age birth. Tob. Induc. Dis. 17, 44.

Cardenas, V.M., Fischbach, L.A., Chowdhury, P., 2019b. The use of electronic nicotine delivery systems during pregnancy and the reproductive outcomes: a systematic review of the literature. Tob. Induc. Dis. 17, 52.

Carlisle, D.L., Hopkins, T.M., Gaither-Davis, A., Silhanek, M.J., Luketich, J.D., Christie, N.A., et al., 2004. Nicotine signals through muscle-type and neuronal nicotinic acetylcholine receptors in both human bronchial epithelial cells and airway fibroblasts. Respir. Res. 5 (1), 27.

Carmines, E.L., Gaworski, C.L., Faqi, A.S., Rajendran, N., 2003. In utero exposure to 1R4F reference cigarette smoke: evaluation of developmental toxicity. Toxicol. Sci. 75 (1), 134–147.

Carnevale, R., Sciarretta, S., Violi, F., Nocella, C., Loffredo, L., Perri, L., et al., 2016. Acute impact of tobacco vs electronic cigarette smoking on oxidative stress and vascular function. Chest 150 (3), 606–612.

Chakkarwar, V.A., 2011. Fenofibrate attenuates nicotine-induced vascular endothelial dysfunction in the rat. Vasc. Pharmacol. 55 (5–6), 163–168.

Chattopadhyay, K., Mondal, S., Chattopadhyay, B., Ghosh, S., 2010. Ameliorative effect of sesame lignans on nicotine toxicity in rats. Food Chem. Toxicol. 48 (11), 3215–3220.

Chaumont, M., De Becker, B., Zaher, W., Culie, A., Deprez, G., Melot, C., et al., 2018. Differential effects of E-cigarette on microvascular endothelial function, arterial stiffness and oxidative stress: a randomized crossover trial. Sci. Rep. 8 (1), 10378.

Cheng, Y., Li, H., Wang, H., Sun, H., Liu, Y., Peng, S., et al., 2003. Inhibition of nicotine-DNA adduct formation in mice by six dietary constituents. Food Chem. Toxicol. 41 (7), 1045–1050.

Chernyavsky, A.I., Shchepotin, I.B., Galitovkiy, V., Grando, S.A., 2015. Mechanisms of tumor-promoting activities of nicotine in lung cancer: synergistic effects of cell membrane and mitochondrial nicotinic acetylcholine receptors. BMC Cancer 15 (1), 152.

Chong, I.-W., Lin, S.-R., Hwang, J.-J., Huang, M.-S., Wang, T.-H., Hung, J.-Y., et al., 2002. Expression and regulation of the macrophage inflammatory protein-1alpha gene by nicotine in rat alveolar macrophages. Eur. Cytokine Netw. 13 (2), 242–249.

Chou, H.C., Chen, C.M., 2014. Maternal nicotine exposure during gestation and lactation induces cardiac remodeling in rat offspring. Reprod. Toxicol. 50, 4–10.

Choukrallah, M.A., Sierro, N., Martin, F., Baumer, K., Thomas, J., Ouadi, S., et al., 2019. Tobacco heating system 2.2 has a limited impact on DNA methylation of candidate enhancers in mouse lung compared with cigarette smoke. Food Chem. Toxicol. 123, 501–510.

Chu, M., Guo, J., Chen, C.-Y., 2005. Long-term exposure to nicotine, via ras pathway, induces cyclin D1 to stimulate G1 cell cycle transition. J. Biol. Chem. 280 (8), 6369–6379.

Ciuffreda, L., Cesta Incani, U., S Steelman, L., L Abrams, S., Falcone, I., Del Curatolo, A., et al., 2014. Signaling intermediates (MAPK and PI3K) as therapeutic targets in NSCLC. Curr. Pharmaceut. Des. 20 (24), 3944–3957.

Clark, C.A., Mceachern, M.D., Shah, S.H., Rong, Y., Rong, X., Smelley, C.L., et al., 2010. Curcumin inhibits carcinogen and nicotine-induced Mammalian target of rapamycin pathway activation in head and neck squamous cell carcinoma. Cancer Prev. Res. (Phila) 12, 1586–1595. https://doi.org/10.1158/1940-6207.CAPR-09-0244.

Clarke, E., Thompson, K., Weaver, S., Thompson, J., O'connell, G., 2019. Snus: a compelling harm reduction alternative to cigarettes. Harm Reduct. J. 16 (1), 62.

Cluette-Brown, J., Mulligan, J., Doyle, K., Hagan, S., Osmolski, T., Hojnacki, J., 1986. Oral nicotine induces an atherogenic lipoprotein profile. Proc. Soc. Exp. Biol. Med. 182 (3), 409–413.

Colombo, E.S., Davis, J., Makvandi, M., Aragon, M., Lucas, S.N., Paffett, M.L., et al., 2013. Effects of nicotine on cardiovascular remodeling in a mouse model of systemic hypertension. Cardiovasc. Toxicol. 13 (4), 364–369.

Cossio, R., Cerra, Z.A., Tanaka, H., 2020. Vascular effects of a single bout of electronic cigarette use. Clin. Exp. Pharmacol. Physiol. 47 (1), 3–6.

Coussens, L.M., Werb, Z., 2002. Inflammation and cancer. Nature 420 (6917), 860.

Cross, S.J., Linker, K.E., Leslie, F.M., 2017. Sex-dependent effects of nicotine on the developing brain. J. Neurosci. Res. 95 (1–2), 422–436.

Csordas, A., Bernhard, D., 2013. The biology behind the atherothrombotic effects of cigarette smoke. Nat. Rev. Cardiol. 10 (4), 219–230.

Curtis, J.L., Freeman, C.M., Hogg, J.C., 2007. The immunopathogenesis of chronic obstructive pulmonary disease: insights from recent research. Proc. Am. Thorac. Soc. 4 (7), 512−521.

Da Silva, F.R., Erdtmann, B., Dalpiaz, T., Nunes, E., Rosa, D.P.D., Porawski, M., et al., 2010. Effects of dermal exposure to *Nicotiana tabacum* (Jean Nicot, 1560) leaves in mouse evaluated by multiple methods and tissues. J. Agric. Food Chem. 58 (17), 9868−9874.

Dani, J.A., 2015. Neuronal nicotinic acetylcholine receptor structure and function and response to nicotine. Int. Rev. Neurobiol. 3−19.

Dasgupta, P., Rizwani, W., Pillai, S., Kinkade, R., Kovacs, M., Rastogi, S., et al., 2009. Nicotine induces cell proliferation, invasion and epithelial-mesenchymal transition in a variety of human cancer cell lines. Int. J. Canc. 124 (1), 36−45.

Davies, P.F., 2009. Hemodynamic shear stress and the endothelium in cardiovascular pathophysiology. Nat. Clin. Pract. Cardiovasc. Med. 6 (1), 16−26.

Davis, R., Rizwani, W., Banerjee, S., Kovacs, M., Haura, E., Coppola, D., et al., 2009. Nicotine promotes tumor growth and metastasis in mouse models of lung cancer. PLoS One 4 (10), e7524.

Dawson, D.A., Fort, D.J., Smith, G.J., Newell, D.L., Bantle, J.A., 1988. Evaluation of the developmental toxicity of nicotine and cotinine with frog embryo teratogenesis assay: Xenopus. Teratog. Carcinog. Mutagen. 8 (6), 329−338.

De Rosa, M.J., Dionisio, L., Agriello, E., Bouzat, C., Del Carmen Esandi, M., 2009. Alpha 7 nicotinic acetylcholine receptor modulates lymphocyte activation. Life Sci. 85 (11−12), 444−449.

Demiralay, R., Gursan, N., Erdem, H., 2007. The effects of erdosteine, N-acetylcysteine and vitamin E on nicotine-induced apoptosis of cardiac cells. J. Appl. Toxicol. 27 (3), 247−254.

Demirhan, O., Demir, C., Tunc, E., Nandiklioglu, N., Sutcu, E., Sadikoglu, N., et al., 2011. The genotoxic effect of nicotine on chromosomes of human fetal cells: the first report described as an important study. Inhal. Toxicol. 23 (13), 829−834.

Dempsey, D., Jacob 3rd, P., Benowitz, N.L., 2000. Nicotine metabolism and elimination kinetics in newborns. Clin. Pharmacol. Ther. 67 (5), 458−465.

Dempsey, D., Jacob 3rd, P., Benowitz, N.L., 2002. Accelerated metabolism of nicotine and cotinine in pregnant smokers. J. Pharmacol. Exp. Therapeut. 301 (2), 594−598.

Dempsey, D.A., Benowitz, N.L., 2001. Risks and benefits of nicotine to aid smoking cessation in pregnancy. Drug Saf. 24 (4), 277−322.

Deng, X., Luyendyk, J.P., Ganey, P.E., Roth, R.A., 2009. Inflammatory stress and idiosyncratic hepatotoxicity: hints from animal models. Pharmacol. Rev. 61 (3), 262−282.

Deng, Y., Cao, H., Cu, F., Xu, D., Lei, Y., Tan, Y., et al., 2013. Nicotine-induced retardation of chondrogenesis through down-regulation of IGF-1 signaling pathway to inhibit matrix synthesis of growth plate chondrocytes in fetal rats. Toxicol. Appl. Pharmacol. 269 (1), 25−33.

Deveaugh-Geiss, A.M., Chen, L.H., Kotler, M.L., Ramsay, L.R., Durcan, M.J., 2010. Pharmacokinetic comparison of two nicotine transdermal systems, a 21-mg/24-hour patch and a 25-mg/16-hour patch: a randomized, open-label, single-dose, two-way crossover study in adult smokers. Clin. Therapeut. 32 (6), 1140−1148.

Dhawan, K., Sharma, A., 2002. Prevention of chronic alcohol and nicotine-induced azospermia, sterility and decreased libido, by a novel tri-substituted benzoflavone moiety from *Passiflora incarnata* Linneaus in healthy male rats. Life Sci. 71 (26), 3059−3069.

Dhouib, H., Jallouli, M., Draief, M., Bouraoui, S., El-Fazâa, S., 2015. Oxidative damage and histopathological changes in lung of rat chronically exposed to nicotine alone or associated to ethanol. Pathol. Biol. 63 (6), 258−267.

Digard, H., Proctor, C., Kulasekaran, A., Malmqvist, U., Richter, A., 2013. Determination of nicotine absorption from multiple tobacco products and nicotine gum. Nicotine Tob. Res. 15 (1), 255−261.

Djordjevic, M.V., Doran, K.A., 2009. Nicotine content and delivery across tobacco products. Handb. Exp. Pharmacol. (192), 61−82. https://doi.org/10.1007/978-3-540-69248-5_3. Epub ahead of print 2009/02/03.

Doll, R., Hill, A.B., 2004. The mortality of doctors in relation to their smoking habits: a preliminary report. 1954. Br. Med. J. 328 (7455), 1529−1533 discussion 1533.

Doll, R., Peto, R., 1981. The causes of cancer: quantitative estimates of avoidable risks of cancer in the United States today. J. Natl. Cancer Inst. 66 (6), 1191−1308.

Doolittle, D.J., Winegar, R., Lee, C.K., Caldwell, W.S., Hayes, A.W., Donald Debethizy, J., 1995. The genotoxic potential of nicotine and its major metabolites. Mutat. Res. Genet. Toxicol. 344 (3−4), 95−102.

Duan, Y., Zeng, L., Zheng, C., Song, B., Li, F., Kong, X., et al., 2018. Inflammatory links between high fat diets and diseases. Front. Immunol. 9, 2649.

Dwyer, J.B., Mcquown, S.C., Leslie, F.M., 2009. The dynamic effects of nicotine on the developing brain. Pharmacol. Ther. 122 (2), 125−139.

El-Sokkary, G.H., Cuzzocrea, S., Reiter, R.J., 2007. Effect of chronic nicotine administration on the rat lung and liver: beneficial role of melatonin. Toxicology 239 (1−2), 60−67.

England, L.J., Aagaard, K., Bloch, M., Conway, K., Cosgrove, K., Grana, R., et al., 2017. Developmental toxicity of nicotine: a transdisciplinary synthesis and implications for emerging tobacco products. Neurosci. Biobehav. Rev. 72, 176−189.

Erat, M., Ciftci, M., Gumustekin, K., Gul, M., 2007. Effects of nicotine and vitamin E on glutathione reductase activity in some rat tissues in vivo and in vitro. Eur. J. Pharmacol. 554 (2−3), 92−97.

Espinoza-Derout, J., Hasan, K.M., Shao, X.M., Jordan, M.C., Sims, C., Lee, D.L., et al., 2019. Chronic intermittent electronic cigarette exposure induces cardiac dysfunction and atherosclerosis in apolipoprotein-E knockout mice. Am. J. Physiol. Heart Circ. Physiol. 317 (2), H445−H459.

Fan, C., Li, Y., Jia, J., 2013. Protein kinase Cs in lung cancer: a promising target for therapies. J. Cancer Res. Therapeut. 9 (5), 74.

Fan, G., Zhang, Q., Wan, Y., Lv, F., Chen, Y., Ni, Y., et al., 2019. Decreased levels of H3K9ac and H3K27ac in the promotor region of ovarian P450 aromatase mediated low estradiol synthesis in female offspring rats induced by prenatal nicotine exposure as well as in human granulosa cells after nicotine treatment. Food Chem. Toxicol. 128, 256−266.

Farsalinos, K., Cibella, F., Caponnetto, P., Campagna, D., Morjaria, J.B., Battaglia, E., et al., 2016. Effect of continuous smoking reduction and abstinence on blood pressure and heart rate in smokers switching to electronic cigarettes. Intern. Emerg. Med. 11 (1), 85−94.

Farsalinos, K.E., Tsipras, D., Kyrzopoulos, S., Savvopoulou, M., Voudris, V., 2014. Acute effects of using an electronic nicotine-delivery device (electronic cigarette) on myocardial function: comparison with the effects of regular cigarettes. BMC Cardiovasc. Disord. 14, 78.

Farsalinos, K.E., Voudris, V., Poulas, K., 2015. Are metals emitted from electronic cigarettes a reason for health concern? A risk-assessment analysis of currently available literature. Int. J. Environ. Res. Publ. Health 12 (5), 5215−5232.

Fayolle, C., Pourchet, J., De Fromentel, C.C., Puisieux, A., Doré, J.-F., Voeltzel, T., 2008. Gadd45a activation protects melanoma cells from ultraviolet B-induced apoptosis. J. Invest. Dermatol. 128 (1), 196−202.

FCTC WHO, 2019. Global Progress Report on Implementation of the WHO Framework Convention on Tobacco Control. World Health Organization, 2018, Geneva, Switzerland.

Fearon, I.M., Phillips, G., Carr, T., Taylor, M., Breheny, D., Faux, P.S., 2011. The role of oxidative stress in smoking-related diseases. Mini-Rev. Org. Chem. 8 (4), 360−371.

Fetterman, J.L., Keith, R.J., Palmisano, J.N., Mcglasson, K.L., Weisbrod, R.M., Majid, S., et al., 2020. Alterations in vascular function associated with the use of combustible and electronic cigarettes. J. Am. Heart Assoc. 9 (9), e014570.

Fetterman, J.L., Weisbrod, R.M., Feng, B., Bastin, R., Tuttle, S.T., Holbrook, M., et al., 2018. Flavorings in tobacco products induce endothelial cell dysfunction. Arterioscler. Thromb. Vasc. Biol. 38 (7), 1607−1615.

Fisher, S.E., Atkinson, M., Van Thiel, D.H., 1984. Selective fetal malnutrition: the effect of nicotine, ethanol, and acetaldehyde upon in vitro uptake of alpha-aminoisobutyric acid by human term placental villous slices. Dev. Pharmacol. Ther. 7 (4), 229−238.

Florin, I., Rutberg, L., Curvall, M., Enzell, C.R., 1980. Screening of tobacco smoke constituents for mutagenicity using the Ames' test. Toxicology 15 (3), 219−232.

Folkesson, M., Sadowska, N., Vikingsson, S., Karlsson, M., Carlhäll, C.J., Länne, T., et al., 2016. Differences in cardiovascular toxicities associated with cigarette smoking and snuff use revealed using novel zebrafish models. Biol. Open 5 (7), 970−978.

Ford, C.L., Zlabek, J.A., 2005. Nicotine replacement therapy and cardiovascular disease. Mayo Clin. Proc. 80 (5), 652−656.

Forstermann, U., Munzel, T., 2006. Endothelial nitric oxide synthase in vascular disease: from marvel to menace. Circulation 113 (13), 1708−1714.

Franzen, K.F., Willig, J., Cayo Talavera, S., Meusel, M., Sayk, F., Reppel, M., et al., 2018. E-cigarettes and cigarettes worsen peripheral and central hemodynamics as well as arterial

stiffness: a randomized, double-blinded pilot study. Vasc. Med. 23 (5), 419−425.

Fumarola, C., Bonelli, M.A., Petronini, P.G., Alfieri, R.R., 2014. Targeting PI3K/AKT/mTOR pathway in non small cell lung cancer. Biochem. Pharmacol. 90 (3), 197−207.

Gaffin, R.D., Chowdhury, S.A., Alves, M.S., Dias, F.A., Ribeiro, C.T., Fogaca, R.T., et al., 2011. Effects of nicotine administration in a mouse model of familial hypertrophic cardiomyopathy, alpha-tropomyosin D175N. Am. J. Physiol. Heart Circ. Physiol. 301 (4), H1646−H1655.

Gahring, L.C., Rogers, S.W., 2005. Neuronal nicotinic acetylcholine receptor expression and function on nonneuronal cells. AAPS J. 7 (4), E885−E894.

Galitovskiy, V., Chernyavsky, A.I., Edwards, R.A., Grando, S.A., 2012. Muscle sarcomas and alopecia in A/J mice chronically treated with nicotine. Life Sci. 91 (21−22), 1109−1112.

Gao, T., Zhou, X.-L., Liu, S., Rao, C.-X., Shi, W., Liu, J.-C., 2016. In vitro effects of nicotine on the non-small-cell lung cancer line A549. J. Pakistan Med. Assoc. 66 (4), 368−372.

Garcia-Arcos, I., Geraghty, P., Baumlin, N., Campos, M., Dabo, A.J., Jundi, B., et al., 2016. Chronic electronic cigarette exposure in mice induces features of COPD in a nicotine-dependent manner. Thorax 71 (12), 1119−1129.

Garcia, P.D., Gornbein, J.A., Middlekauff, H.R., 2020. Cardiovascular autonomic effects of electronic cigarette use: a systematic review. Clin. Auton. Res. 1−13. https://doi.org/10.1007/s10286-020-00683-4.

Gemenetzidis, E., Bose, A., Riaz, A.M., Chaplin, T., Young, B.D., Ali, M., et al., 2009. FOXM1 upregulation is an early event in human squamous cell carcinoma and it is enhanced by nicotine during malignant transformation. PLoS One 4 (3), e4849.

Genbacev, O., Bass, K.E., Joslin, R.J., Fisher, S.J., 1995. Maternal smoking inhibits early human cytotrophoblast differentiation. Reprod. Toxicol. 9 (3), 245−255.

Genbacev, O., Mcmaster, M.T., Lazic, J., Nedeljkovic, S., Cvetkovic, M., Joslin, R., et al., 2000. Concordant in situ and in vitro data show that maternal cigarette smoking negatively regulates placental cytotrophoblast passage through the cell cycle. Reprod. Toxicol. 14 (6), 495−506.

Geng, Y., Savage, S.M., Razani-Boroujerdi, S., Sopori, M.L., 1996. Effects of nicotine on the immune response. II. Chronic nicotine treatment induces T cell anergy. J. Immunol. 156 (7), 2384−2390.

Geng, Y.M., Savage, S.M., Johnson, L.J., Seagrave, J., Sopori, M.L., 1995. Effects of nicotine on the immune response. I. Chronic exposure to nicotine impairs antigen receptor-mediated signal transduction in lymphocytes. Toxicol. Appl. Pharmacol. 135 (2), 268−278.

George, J., Hussain, M., Vadiveloo, T., Ireland, S., Hopkinson, P., Struthers, A.D., et al., 2019. Cardiovascular effects of switching from tobacco cigarettes to electronic cigarettes. J. Am. Coll. Cardiol. 74 (25), 3112−3120.

Gilliland, F.D., Berhane, K., Mcconnell, R., Gauderman, W.J., Vora, H., Rappaport, E.B., et al., 2000. Maternal smoking during pregnancy, environmental tobacco smoke exposure and childhood lung function. Thorax 55 (4), 271−276.

Gilliland, F.D., Li, Y.F., Peters, J.M., 2001. Effects of maternal smoking during pregnancy and environmental tobacco smoke on asthma and wheezing in children. Am. J. Respir. Crit. Care Med. 163 (2), 429−436.

Ginzkey, C., Friehs, G., Koehler, C., Hackenberg, S., Hagen, R., Kleinsasser, N.H., 2013. Assessment of nicotine-induced DNA damage in a genotoxicological test battery. Mutat. Res. 751 (1), 34−39.

Ginzkey, C., Friehs, G., Koehler, C., Hackenberg, S., Voelker, H.U., Richter, E., et al., 2010. Nicotine and methyl methane sulfonate in mini organ cultures of human parotid gland tissue. Toxicol. Lett. 197 (2), 69−74.

Ginzkey, C., Kampfinger, K., Friehs, G., Kohler, C., Hagen, R., Richter, E., et al., 2009. Nicotine induces DNA damage in human salivary glands. Toxicol. Lett. 184 (1), 1−4.

Ginzkey, C., Steussloff, G., Koehler, C., Burghartz, M., Scherzed, A., Hackenberg, S., et al., 2014a. Nicotine derived genotoxic effects in human primary parotid gland cells as assessed in vitro by comet assay, cytokinesis-block micronucleus test and chromosome aberrations test. Toxicol. In Vitro 28 (5), 838−846.

Ginzkey, C., Steussloff, G., Koehler, C., Hackenberg, S., Richter, E., Hagen, R., et al., 2014b. Nicotine causes genotoxic damage but is not metabolized during long-term exposure of human nasal miniorgan cultures. Toxicol. Lett. 229 (1), 303−310.

Ginzkey, C., Stueber, T., Friehs, G., Koehler, C., Hackenberg, S., Richter, E., et al., 2012. Analysis of nicotine-induced DNA damage in cells of the human respiratory tract. Toxicol. Lett. 208 (1), 23−29.

Glover, M., Phillips, C.V., 2020. Potential effects of using noncombustible tobacco and nicotine products during pregnancy: a systematic review. Harm Reduct. J. 17 (1), 16.

Golbidi, S., Edvinsson, L., Laher, I., 2020. Smoking and endothelial dysfunction. Curr. Vasc. Pharmacol. 18 (1), 1−11.

Gotti, C., Clementi, F., 2004. Neuronal nicotinic receptors: from structure to pathology. Prog. Neurobiol. 74 (6), 363−396.

Greene, C.M., Ramsay, H., Wells, R.J., O'neill, S.J., Mcelvaney, N.G., 2010. Inhibition of toll-like receptor 2-mediated interleukin-8 production in cystic fibrosis airway epithelial cells via the α7-nicotinic acetylcholine receptor. Mediat. Inflamm. 2010, 423241.

Grivennikov, S.I., Greten, F.R., Karin, M., 2010. Immunity, inflammation, and cancer. Cell 140 (6), 883−899.

Gu, Y.H., Li, Y., Huang, X.F., Zheng, J.F., Yang, J., Diao, H., et al., 2013. Reproductive effects of two neonicotinoid insecticides on mouse sperm function and early embryonic development in vitro. PLoS One 8 (7), e70112.

Gundavarapu, S., Wilder, J.A., Mishra, N.C., Rir-Sima-Ah, J., Langley, R.J., Singh, S.P., et al., 2012. Role of nicotinic receptors and acetylcholine in mucous cell metaplasia, hyperplasia and airway mucus formation in vitro and in vivo. J. Allergy Clin. Immunol. 130 (3), 770−780.e711.

Guo, H., Tian, L., Zhang, J.Z., Kitani, T., Paik, D.T., Lee, W.H., et al., 2019. Single-cell RNA sequencing of human embryonic stem cell differentiation delineates adverse effects of nicotine on embryonic development. Stem Cell Rep. 12 (4), 772−786.

Guo, J., Chu, M., Abbeyquaye, T., Chen, C.-Y., 2005. Persistent nicotine treatment potentiates amplification of the dihydrofolate reductase gene in rat lung epithelial cells as a consequence of ras activation. J. Biol. Chem. 280 (34), 30422−30431.

Guo, X., Wang, H., Wu, X., Chen, X., Chen, Y., Guo, J., et al., 2017. Nicotine affects rat leydig cell function in vivo and vitro via down-regulating some key steroidogenic enzyme expressions. Food Chem. Toxicol. 110, 13−24.

Guo, Z.Z., Cao, Q.A., Li, Z.Z., Liu, L.P., Zhang, Z., Zhu, Y.J., et al., 2016. SP600125 attenuates nicotine-related aortic aneurysm formation by inhibiting matrix metalloproteinase production and CC chemokine-mediated macrophage migration. Mediat. Inflamm. 2016, 9142425.

Gupta, R., Gupta, S., Sharma, S., Sinha, D.N., Mehrotra, R., 2018. A systematic review on association between smokeless tobacco & cardiovascular diseases. Indian J. Med. Res. 148 (1), 77−89.

Gupta, R., Gupta, S., Sharma, S., Sinha, D.N., Mehrotra, R., 2019. Risk of coronary heart disease among smokeless tobacco users: results of systematic review and meta-analysis of global data. Nicotine Tob. Res. 21 (1), 25−31.

Haglund, B., Eliasson, M., Stenbeck, M., Rosen, M., 2007. Is moist snuff use associated with excess risk of IHD or stroke? A longitudinal follow-up of snuff users in Sweden. Scand. J. Publ. Health 35 (6), 618−622.

Halliwell, B., 2007. Oxidative stress and cancer: have we moved forward? Biochem. J. 401 (1), 1−11.

Hanahan, D., Weinberg, R.A., 2011. Hallmarks of cancer: the next generation. Cell 144 (5), 646−674.

Hansson, J., Galanti, M.R., Hergens, M.P., Fredlund, P., Ahlbom, A., Alfredsson, L., et al., 2014. Snus (Swedish smokeless tobacco) use and risk of stroke: pooled analyses of incidence and survival. J. Intern. Med. 276 (1), 87−95.

Hao, J., Shi, F.-D., Abdelwahab, M., Shi, S.X., Simard, A., Whiteaker, P., et al., 2013. Nicotinic receptor β2 determines NK cell-dependent metastasis in a murine model of metastatic lung cancer. PLoS One 8 (2), e57495.

Harris, J.E., Thun, M.J., Mondul, A.M., Calle, E.E., 2004. Cigarette tar yields in relation to mortality from lung cancer in the cancer prevention study II prospective cohort, 1982−8. Br. Med. J. 328 (7431), 72.

Hashimoto, K., Zaima, N., Sekiguchi, H., Kugo, H., Miyamoto, C., Hoshino, K., et al., 2018. Dietary DNA attenuates the degradation of elastin Fibers in the aortic wall in nicotine-administrated mice. J. Nutr. Sci. Vitaminol. 64 (4), 271−276.

He, F., Li, B., Zhao, Z., Zhou, Y., Hu, G., Zou, W., et al., 2014. The pro-proliferative effects of nicotine and its underlying mechanism on rat airway smooth muscle cells. PLoS One 9 (4), e93508.

Heath, C.J., King, S.L., Gotti, C., Marks, M.J., Picciotto, M.R., 2010. Cortico-thalamic connectivity is vulnerable to nicotine exposure during early postnatal development through α4/β2/α5 nicotinic acetylcholine receptors. Neuropsychopharmacology 35 (12), 2324−2338.

Hecht, S.S., 2012. Lung carcinogenesis by tobacco smoke. Int. J. Cancer 131 (12), 2724−2732.

Heeschen, C., Jang, J.J., Weis, M., Pathak, A., Kaji, S., Hu, R.S., et al., 2001. Nicotine stimulates angiogenesis and promotes tumor growth and atherosclerosis. Nat. Med. 7 (7), 833.

Heming, M., Gran, S., Jauch, S.-L., Fischer-Riepe, L., Russo, A., Klotz, L., et al., 2018. Peroxisome proliferator-activated receptor-γ modulates the response of macrophages to lipopolysaccharide and glucocorticoids. Front. Immunol. 9, 893.

Henderson, B.J., Lester, H.A., 2015. Inside-out neuropharmacology of nicotinic drugs. Neuropharmacology 96 (Pt B), 178–193.

Hergens, M.P., Alfredsson, L., Bolinder, G., Lambe, M., Pershagen, G., Ye, W., 2007. Long-term use of Swedish moist snuff and the risk of myocardial infarction amongst men. J. Intern. Med. 262 (3), 351–359.

Hergens, M.P., Lambe, M., Pershagen, G., Ye, W., 2008. Risk of hypertension amongst Swedish male snuff users: a prospective study. J. Intern. Med. 264 (2), 187–194.

Hirata, N., Yamada, S., Asanagi, M., Sekino, Y., Kanda, Y., 2016. Nicotine induces mitochondrial fission through mitofusin degradation in human multipotent embryonic carcinoma cells. Biochem. Biophys. Res. Commun. 470 (2), 300–305.

Hirsch, J.M., Hedner, J., Wernstedt, L., Lundberg, J., Hedner, T., 1992. Hemodynamic effects of the use of oral snuff. Clin. Pharmacol. Ther. 52 (4), 394–401.

Hodge, S., Hodge, G., Ahern, J., Jersmann, H., Holmes, M., Reynolds, P.N., 2007. Smoking alters alveolar macrophage recognition and phagocytic ability: implications in chronic obstructive pulmonary disease. Am. J. Respir. Cell Mol. Biol. 37 (6), 748–755.

Holloway, A.C., Salomon, A., Soares, M.J., Garnier, V., Raha, S., Sergent, F., et al., 2014. Characterization of the adverse effects of nicotine on placental development: in vivo and in vitro studies. Am. J. Physiol. Endocrinol. Metab. 306 (4), E443–E456.

Hom, S., Chen, L., Wang, T., Ghebrehiwet, B., Yin, W., Rubenstein, D.A., 2016. Platelet activation, adhesion, inflammation, and aggregation potential are altered in the presence of electronic cigarette extracts of variable nicotine concentrations. Platelets 27 (7), 694–702.

Hong, W., Peng, G., Hao, B., Liao, B., Zhao, Z., Zhou, Y., et al., 2017. Nicotine-induced airway smooth muscle cell proliferation involves TRPC6-dependent calcium influx via α7 nAChR. Cell. Physiol. Biochem. 43 (3), 986–1002.

Hu, N., Guo, R., Han, X., Zhu, B., Ren, J., 2011. Cardiac-specific overexpression of metallothionein rescues nicotine-induced cardiac contractile dysfunction and interstitial fibrosis. Toxicol. Lett. 202 (1), 8–14.

Hukkanen, J., Jacob, P., Benowitz, N.L., 2005. Metabolism and disposition kinetics of nicotine. Pharmacol. Rev. 57 (1), 79–115.

IARC Working Group on the Evaluation of Carcinogenic Risks to Humans, 2007. Smokeless tobacco and some tobacco-specific N-nitrosamines. IARC Monogr. Eval. Carcinog. Risks Hum. 89, 1–592.

ICH, 2017. Guideline S5(R3): Detection of Toxicity to Reproduction for Human Pharmaceuticals.

Ijomone, O.M., Olaibi, O.K., Nwoha, P.U., 2014. Effects of chronic nicotine administration on body weight, food intake and nitric oxide concentration in female and male rats. Pathophysiology 21 (3), 185–190.

Ikonomidis, I., Vlastos, D., Kourea, K., Kostelli, G., Varoudi, M., Pavlidis, G., et al., 2018. Electronic cigarette smoking increases arterial stiffness and oxidative stress to a lesser extent than a single conventional cigarette: an acute and chronic study. Circulation 137 (3), 303–306.

Inamdar, A.S., Croucher, R.E., Chokhandre, M.K., Mashyakhy, M.H., Marinho, V.C., 2015. Maternal smokeless tobacco use in pregnancy and adverse health outcomes in newborns: a systematic review. Nicotine Tob. Res. 17 (9), 1058–1066.

Ion, R., Bernal, A.L., 2015. Smoking and preterm birth. Reprod. Sci. 22 (8), 918–926.

Iskandar, A.R., Liu, C., Smith, D.E., Hu, K.-Q., Choi, S.-W., Ausman, L.M., et al., 2013. β-Cryptoxanthin restores nicotine-reduced lung SIRT1 to normal levels and inhibits nicotine-promoted lung tumorigenesis and emphysema in A/J mice. Cancer Prev. Res. (Phila). 6 (4), 309–320. https://doi.org/10.1158/1940-6207.CAPR-12-0368.

Jain, A., Flora, S., 2012. Dose related effects of nicotine on oxidative injury in young, adult and old rats. J. Environ. Biol. 33 (2), 233.

Jalili, C., Salahshoor, M.R., Moradi, M.T., Ahookhash, M., Taghadosi, M., Sohrabi, M., 2017. Expression changes of apoptotic genes in tissues from mice exposed to nicotine. Asian Pac. J. Cancer Prev. 18 (1), 239.

Jana, K., Samanta, P.K., De, D.K., 2010. Nicotine diminishes testicular gametogenesis, steroidogenesis, and steroidogenic acute regulatory protein expression in adult albino rats: possible influence on pituitary gonadotropins and alteration of testicular antioxidant status. Toxicol. Sci. 116 (2), 647–659.

Jarzynka, M.J., Guo, P., Bar-Joseph, I., Hu, B., Cheng, S.-Y., 2006. Estradiol and nicotine exposure enhances A549 bronchioloalveolar carcinoma xenograft growth in mice through the stimulation of angiogenesis. Int. J. Oncol. 28 (2), 337–344.

Jiang, D.J., Jia, S.J., Yan, J., Zhou, Z., Yuan, Q., Li, Y.J., 2006. Involvement of DDAH/ADMA/NOS pathway in nicotine-induced endothelial dysfunction. Biochem. Biophys. Res. Commun. 349 (2), 683–693.

Jiang, J.S., Chou, H.C., Yeh, T.F., Chen, C.M., 2012. Maternal nicotine effects on vascular endothelial growth factor expression and morphometry in rat lungs. Early Hum. Dev. 88 (7), 525–529.

Jin, J., Arif, B., Garcia-Fernandez, F., Ennis, T.L., Davis, E.C., Thompson, R.W., et al., 2012. Novel mechanism of aortic aneurysm development in mice associated with smoking and leukocytes. Arterioscler. Thromb. Vasc. Biol. 32 (12), 2901–2909.

Jin, X., Liu, X., Zhang, Z., Guan, Y., Xv, R., Li, J., 2018. Identification of key pathways and genes in lung carcinogenesis. Oncol. Lett. 16 (4), 4185–4192.

Jin, Y.Z., Wang, G.F., Wang, Q., Zhang, X.Y., Yan, B., Hu, W.N., 2014. Effects of acetaldehyde and L-carnitine on morphology and enzyme activity of myocardial mitochondria in rats. Mol. Biol. Rep. 41 (12), 7923–7928.

Jordanov, J.S., 1990. Cotinine concentrations in amniotic fluid and urine of smoking, passive smoking and non-smoking pregnant women at term and in the urine of their neonates on 1st day of life. Eur. J. Pediatr. 149 (10), 734—737.

Joschko, M.A., Dreosti, I.E., Tulsi, R.S., 1991. The teratogenic effects of nicotine in vitro in rats: a light and electron microscope study. Neurotoxicol. Teratol. 13 (3), 307—316.

Joseph, A.M., Norman, S.M., Ferry, L.H., Prochazka, A.V., Westman, E.C., Steele, B.G., et al., 1996. The safety of transdermal nicotine as an aid to smoking cessation in patients with cardiac disease. N. Engl. J. Med. 335 (24), 1792—1798.

Joukar, S., Shahouzehi, B., Najafipour, H., Gholamhoseinian, A., Joukar, F., 2012. Ameliorative effect of black tea on nicotine induced cardiovascular pathogenesis in rat. EXCLI J. 11, 309—317.

Junhui, Z., Xiaojing, H., Binquan, Z., Xudong, X., Junzhu, C., Guosheng, F., 2009. Nicotine-reduced endothelial progenitor cell senescence through augmentation of telomerase activity via the PI3K/Akt pathway. Cytotherapy 11 (4), 485—491.

Kahl, V.F., Reyes, J.M., Sarmento, M.S., Da Silva, J., 2012. Mitigation by vitamin C of the genotoxic effects of nicotine in mice, assessed by the comet assay and micronucleus induction. Mutat. Res. Genet. Toxicol. Environ. Mutagen 744 (2), 140—144.

Kalra, R., Singh, S.P., Kracko, D., Matta, S.G., Sharp, B.M., Sopori, M.L., 2002. Chronic self-administration of nicotine in rats impairs T cell responsiveness. J. Pharmacol. Exp. Therapeut. 302 (3), 935—939.

Kalra, R., Singh, S.P., Pena-Philippides, J.C., Langley, R.J., Razani-Boroujerdi, S., Sopori, M.L., 2004. Immunosuppressive and anti-inflammatory effects of nicotine administered by patch in an animal model. Clin. Diagn. Lab. Immunol. 11 (3), 563—568.

Kang, P., Svoboda, K.K., 2003. Nicotine inhibits palatal fusion and modulates nicotinic receptors and the PI-3 kinase pathway in medial edge epithelia. Orthod. Craniofac. Res. 6 (3), 129—142.

Kaur, J., Reddy, K., Balakumar, P., 2010. The novel role of fenofibrate in preventing nicotine-and sodium arsenite-induced vascular endothelial dysfunction in the rat. Cardiovasc. Toxicol. 10 (3), 227—238.

Kavitharaj, N.K., Vijayammal, P.L., 1999. Nicotine administration induced changes in the gonadal functions in male rats. Pharmacology 58 (1), 2—7.

Kawashima, K., Fujii, T., Moriwaki, Y., Misawa, H., Horiguchi, K., 2015. Non-neuronal cholinergic system in regulation of immune function with a focus on α7 nAChRs. Int. Immunopharm. 29 (1), 127—134.

Kennedy, A.E., Kandalam, S., Olivares-Navarrete, R., Dickinson, A.J.G., 2017. E-cigarette aerosol exposure can cause craniofacial defects in Xenopus laevis embryos and mammalian neural crest cells. PLoS One 12 (9), e0185729.

Kerr, D.M.I., Brooksbank, K.J.M., Taylor, R.G., Pinel, K., Rios, F.J., Touyz, R.M., et al., 2019. Acute effects of electronic and tobacco cigarettes on vascular and respiratory function in healthy volunteers: a cross-over study. J. Hypertens. 37 (1), 154—166.

Khalil, A.A., Jameson, M.J., Broaddus, W.C., Lin, P.S., Chung, T.D., 2013. Nicotine enhances proliferation, migration, and radioresistance of human malignant glioma cells through EGFR activation. Brain Tumor Pathol. 30 (2), 73—83.

Khlystov, A., Samburova, V., 2016. Flavoring compounds dominate toxic aldehyde production during E-cigarette vaping. Environ. Sci. Technol. 50 (23), 13080—13085.

Kim, J., Poole, D.S., Waggoner, L.E., Kempf, A., Ramirez, D.S., Treschow, P.A., et al., 2001. Genes affecting the activity of nicotinic receptors involved in Caenorhabditis elegans egg-laying behavior. Genetics 157 (4), 1599—1610.

Kim, J.R., Kang, P., Lee, H.S., Kim, K.Y., Seol, G.H., 2017. Cardiovascular effects of linalyl acetate in acute nicotine exposure. Environ. Health Prev. Med. 22 (1), 42.

Kinoshita, A., Wanibuchi, H., Wei, M., Yunoki, T., Fukushima, S., 2007. Elevation of 8-hydroxydeoxyguanosine and cell proliferation via generation of oxidative stress by organic arsenicals contributes to their carcinogenicity in the rat liver and bladder. Toxicol. Appl. Pharmacol. 221 (3), 295—305.

Klapproth, H., Racké, K., Wessler, I., 1998. Acetylcholine and nicotine stimulate the release of granulocyte-macrophage colony stimulating factor from cultured human bronchial epithelial cells. N. Schmied. Arch. Pharmacol. 357 (4), 472—475.

Kleinsasser, N.H., Sassen, A.W., Semmler, M.P., Harreus, U.A., Licht, A.K., Richter, E., 2005. The tobacco alkaloid nicotine demonstrates genotoxicity in human tonsillar tissue and lymphocytes. Toxicol. Sci. 86 (2), 309—317.

Kohler, E., Avenarius, S., Rabsilber, A., Gerloff, C., Jorch, G., 2010. Nicotine and its metabolites in amniotic fluid at birth—assessment of prenatal tobacco smoke exposure. Hum. Exp. Toxicol. 29 (5), 385—391.

Kosmider, L., Sobczak, A., Fik, M., Knysak, J., Zaciera, M., Kurek, J., et al., 2014. Carbonyl compounds in electronic cigarette vapors: effects of nicotine solvent and battery output voltage. Nicotine Tob. Res. 16 (10), 1319—1326.

Koturbash, I., Beland, F.A., Pogribny, I.P., 2011. Role of epigenetic events in chemical carcinogenesis—a justification for incorporating epigenetic evaluations in cancer risk assessment. Toxicol. Mech. Methods 21 (4), 289—297.

Kumar, A.S., Jagadeeshan, S., Pitani, R.S., Ramshankar, V., Venkitasamy, K., Venkatraman, G., et al., 2017. Snail-modulated microRNA 493 forms a negative feedback loop with the insulin-like growth factor 1 receptor pathway and blocks tumorigenesis. Mol. Cell Biol. 37 (6), e00510—00516.

Kurti, A.N., Redner, R., Lopez, A.A., Keith, D.R., Villanti, A.C., Stanton, C.A., et al., 2017. Tobacco and nicotine delivery product use in a national sample of pregnant women. Prev. Med. 104, 50—56.

Kwon, O.S., Chung, J.H., Cho, K.H., Suh, D.H., Park, K.C., Kim, K.H., et al., 1999. Nicotine-enhanced epithelial differentiation in reconstructed human oral mucosa in vitro. Skin Pharmacol. Physiol. 12 (4), 227—234.

Lam, D.C.-L., Luo, S.Y., Fu, K.-H., Lui, M.M.-S., Chan, K.-H., Wistuba, I.I., et al., 2015. Nicotinic acetylcholine receptor expression in human airway correlates with lung function. Am. J. Physiol. Lung Cell Mol. Physiol. 310 (3), L232—L239.

Lambers, D.S., Clark, K.E., 1996. The maternal and fetal physiologic effects of nicotine. Semin. Perinatol. 20 (2), 115—126.

Landau, J.M., Wang, Z.-Y., Yang, G.-Y., Ding, W., Yang, C.S., 1998. Inhibition of spontaneous formation of lung tumors and rhabdomyosarcomas in A/J mice by black and green tea. Carcinogenesis 19 (3), 501—507.

Lange, S., Probst, C., Rehm, J., Popova, S., 2018. National, regional, and global prevalence of smoking during pregnancy in the general population: a systematic review and meta-analysis. Lancet Glob. Health 6 (7), e769—e776.

Lannero, E., Wickman, M., Pershagen, G., Nordvall, L., 2006. Maternal smoking during pregnancy increases the risk of recurrent wheezing during the first years of life (BAMSE). Respir. Res. 7, 3.

Latha, M.S., Vijayammal, P.L., Kurup, P.A., 1993. Effect of nicotine administration on lipid metabolism in rats. Indian J. Med. Res. 98, 44—49.

Laursen, J.B., Somers, M., Kurz, S., Mccann, L., Warnholtz, A., Freeman, B.A., et al., 2001. Endothelial regulation of vasomotion in apoE-deficient mice: implications for interactions between peroxynitrite and tetrahydrobiopterin. Circulation 103 (9), 1282—1288.

Leconte, I., Mouche, I., 2013. Frog embryo teratogenesis assay on *Xenopus* and predictivity compared with in vivo mammalian studies. Methods Mol. Biol. 947, 403—421.

Lee, H.-J., Guo, H.-Y., Lee, S.-K., Jeon, B.-H., Jun, C.-D., Lee, S.-K., et al., 2005. Effects of nicotine on proliferation, cell cycle, and differentiation in immortalized and malignant oral keratinocytes. J. Oral Pathol. Med. 34 (7), 436—443.

Lee, H.-J., Pi, S.-H., Kim, Y., Kim, H.-S., Kim, S.-J., Kim, Y.-S., et al., 2009. Effects of nicotine on antioxidant defense enzymes and RANKL expression in human periodontal ligament cells. J. Periodontol. 80 (8), 1281—1288.

Lee, H.-W., Park, S.-H., Weng, M.-W., Wang, H.-T., Huang, W.C., Lepor, H., et al., 2018. E-cigarette smoke damages DNA and reduces repair activity in mouse lung, heart, and bladder as well as in human lung and bladder cells. Proc. Natl. Acad. Sci. U. S. A. 115 (7), E1560—E1569.

Lee, H., Chung, S., Noh, J., 2016. Maternal nicotine exposure during late gestation and lactation increases anxiety-like and impulsive decision-making behavior in adolescent offspring of rat. Toxicol. Res. 32 (4), 275—280.

Lee, K.M., Hoeng, J., Harbo, S., Kogel, U., Gardner, W., Oldham, M., et al., 2018c. Biological changes in C57BL/6 mice following 3 weeks of inhalation exposure to cigarette smoke or e-vapor aerosols. Inhal. Toxicol. 30 (13—14), 553—567.

Lee, P.N., 2011. Summary of the epidemiological evidence relating snus to health. Regul. Toxicol. Pharmacol. 59 (2), 197—214.

Lee, P.N., Hamling, J., 2009. Systematic review of the relation between smokeless tobacco and cancer in Europe and North America. BMC Med. 7, 36.

Lee, Y.H., Chen, R.S., Chang, N.C., Lee, K.R., Huang, C.T., Huang, Y.C., et al., 2015. Synergistic impact of nicotine and shear stress induces cytoskeleton collapse and

apoptosis in endothelial cells. Ann. Biomed. Eng. 43 (9), 2220—2230.

Lewis, J., Wu, C.-H., Levine, J., Berg, H., 1980. Levamisole-resitant mutants of the nematode *Caenorhabditis elegans* appear to lack pharmacological acetylcholine receptors. Neuroscience 5 (6), 967—989.

Li, G.P., Yang, S., Liu, Y., Sessions, B.R., White, K.L., Bunch, T.D., 2009. Nicotine combined with okadaic acid or taxol adversely affects bovine oocyte maturation and subsequent embryo development. Fertil. Steril. 92 (2), 798—805.

Li, H., Wang, S., Takayama, K., Harada, T., Okamoto, I., Iwama, E., et al., 2015. Nicotine induces resistance to erlotinib via cross-talk between α 1 nAChR and EGFR in the non-small cell lung cancer xenograft model. Lung Cancer 88 (1), 1—8.

Li, J., Liu, S., Cao, G., Sun, Y., Chen, W., Dong, F., et al., 2018. Nicotine induces endothelial dysfunction and promotes atherosclerosis via GTPCH1. J. Cell Mol. Med. 22 (11), 5406—5417.

Li, Q., Zhou, X., Kolosov, V.P., Perelman, J.M., 2010. Nicotine suppresses inflammatory factors in HBE16 airway epithelial cells after exposure to cigarette smoke extract and lipopolysaccharide. Transl. Res. 156 (6), 326—334.

Li, Q., Zhou, X.D., Kolosov, V.P., Perelman, J.M., 2011. Nicotine reduces TNF-α expression through a α7 nAChR/MyD88/NF-κB pathway in HBE16 airway epithelial cells. Cell. Physiol. Biochem. 27 (5), 605—612.

Li Volti, G., Polosa, R., Caruso, M., 2018. Assessment of E-cigarette impact on smokers: the importance of experimental conditions relevant to human consumption. Proc. Natl. Acad. Sci. U. S. A. 115 (14), E3073—E3074.

Li, W., Du, D.-Y., Liu, Y., Jiang, F., Zhang, P., Li, Y.-T., 2017. Long-term nicotine exposure induces dysfunction of mouse endothelial progenitor cells. Exp. Therapeut. Med. 13 (1), 85—90.

Li, Z., Xu, W., Su, Y., Gao, K., Chen, Y., Ma, L., et al., 2019. Nicotine induces insulin resistance via downregulation of Nrf2 in cardiomyocyte. Mol. Cell. Endocrinol. 495, 110507.

Libby, P., Nahrendorf, M., Swirski, F.K., 2016. Leukocytes link local and systemic inflammation in ischemic cardiovascular disease: an expanded "cardiovascular continuum". J. Am. Coll. Cardiol. 67 (9), 1091—1103.

Lin, C., Yon, J.M., Hong, J.T., Lee, J.K., Jeong, J., Baek, I.J., et al., 2014. 4-O-methylhonokiol inhibits serious embryo anomalies caused by nicotine via modulations of oxidative stress, apoptosis, and inflammation. Birth Defects Res. B Dev. Reprod. Toxicol. 101 (2), 125—134.

Lin, C., Yon, J.M., Jung, A.Y., Lee, J.G., Jung, K.Y., Lee, B.J., et al., 2013. Antiteratogenic effects of beta-carotene in cultured mouse embryos exposed to nicotine. Evid. Based Complement Alternat. Med. 2013, 575287.

Lips, K.S., Bruggmann, D., Pfeil, U., Vollerthun, R., Grando, S.A., Kummer, W., 2005. Nicotinic acetylcholine receptors in rat and human placenta. Placenta 26 (10), 735—746.

Liszewski, W., Ritner, C., Aurigui, J., Wong, S.S., Hussain, N., Krueger, W., et al., 2012. Developmental effects of tobacco smoke exposure during human embryonic stem cell differentiation are mediated through the transforming growth factor-beta superfamily member, Nodal. Differentiation 83 (4), 169−178.

Liu, C., Zhou, M.S., Li, Y., Wang, A., Chadipiralla, K., Tian, R., et al., 2017a. Oral nicotine aggravates endothelial dysfunction and vascular inflammation in diet-induced obese rats: role of macrophage TNFalpha. PLoS One 12 (12), e0188439.

Liu, X., Wang, C.N., Qiu, C.Y., Song, W., Wang, L.F., Liu, B., 2017b. Adipocytes promote nicotine-induced injury of endothelial cells via the NF-kappaB pathway. Exp. Cell Res. 359 (1), 251−256.

Liu, Y., Li, G.P., Rickords, L.F., White, K.L., Sessions, B.R., Aston, K.I., et al., 2008a. Effect of nicotine on in vitro maturation of bovine oocytes. Anim. Reprod. Sci. 103 (1−2), 13−24.

Liu, Y., Li, G.P., Sessions, B.R., Rickords, L.F., White, K.L., Bunch, T.D., 2008b. Nicotine induces multinuclear formation and causes aberrant embryonic development in bovine. Mol. Reprod. Dev. 75 (5), 801−809.

Liu, Z., Han, B., Li, P., Wang, Z., Fan, Q., 2014. Activation of α7nAChR by nicotine reduced the Th17 response in CD4+ T lymphocytes. Immunol. Invest. 43 (7), 667−674.

Ljungberg, L.U., Persson, K., Eriksson, A.C., Green, H., Whiss, P.A., 2013. Effects of nicotine, its metabolites and tobacco extracts on human platelet function in vitro. Toxicol. In Vitro 27 (2), 932−938.

Lo Sasso, G., Schlage, W.K., Boué, S., Veljkovic, E., Peitsch, M.C., Hoeng, J., 2016. The Apoe(-/-) mouse model: a suitable model to study cardiovascular and respiratory diseases in the context of cigarette smoke exposure and harm reduction. J. Transl. Med. 14 (1), 146.

Lu, H., Rateri, D.L., Bruemmer, D., Cassis, L.A., Daugherty, A., 2012. Novel mechanisms of abdominal aortic aneurysms. Curr. Atherosclerosis Rep. 14 (5), 402−412.

Lucendo-Villarin, B., Filis, P., Swortwood, M.J., Huestis, M.A., Meseguer-Ripolles, J., Cameron, K., et al., 2017. Modelling foetal exposure to maternal smoking using hepatoblasts from pluripotent stem cells. Arch. Toxicol. 91 (11), 3633−3643.

Lucini, D., Bertocchi, F., Malliani, A., Pagani, M., 1998. Autonomic effects of nicotine patch administration in habitual cigarette smokers: a double-blind, placebo-controlled study using spectral analysis of RR interval and systolic arterial pressure variabilities. J. Cardiovasc. Pharmacol. 31 (5), 714−720.

Luck, W., Nau, H., 1984. Nicotine and cotinine concentrations in serum and milk of nursing smokers. Br. J. Clin. Pharmacol. 18 (1), 9−15.

Luck, W., Nau, H., Hansen, R., Steldinger, R., 1985. Extent of nicotine and cotinine transfer to the human fetus, placenta and amniotic fluid of smoking mothers. Dev. Pharmacol. Ther. 8 (6), 384−395.

Ludicke, F., Ansari, S.M., Lama, N., Blanc, N., Bosilkovska, M., Donelli, A., et al., 2019. Effects of switching to a heat-not-burn tobacco product on biologically relevant biomarkers to assess a candidate modified risk tobacco product: a randomized trial. Cancer Epidemiol. Biomarkers Prev. 28 (11), 1934−1943.

Luo, H.L., Zang, W.J., Lu, J., Yu, X.J., Lin, Y.X., Cao, Y.X., 2006. The protective effect of captopril on nicotine-induced endothelial dysfunction in rat. Basic Clin. Pharmacol. Toxicol. 99 (3), 237−245.

Luo, J., Ye, W., Zendehdel, K., Adami, J., Adami, H.O., Boffetta, P., et al., 2007. Oral use of Swedish moist snuff (snus) and risk for cancer of the mouth, lung, and pancreas in male construction workers: a retrospective cohort study. Lancet 369 (9578), 2015−2020.

Mabley, J., Gordon, S., Pacher, P., 2011. Nicotine exerts an anti-inflammatory effect in a murine model of acute lung injury. Inflammation 34 (4), 231−237.

Machaalani, R., Ghazavi, E., Hinton, T., Waters, K.A., Hennessy, A., 2014. Cigarette smoking during pregnancy regulates the expression of specific nicotinic acetylcholine receptor (nAChR) subunits in the human placenta. Toxicol. Appl. Pharmacol. 276 (3), 204−212.

Maegdefessel, L., Azuma, J., Toh, R., Deng, A., Merk, D.R., Raiesdana, A., et al., 2012. MicroRNA-21 blocks abdominal aortic aneurysm development and nicotine-augmented expansion. Sci. Transl. Med. 4 (122), 122ra122.

Mahapatra, S.K., Chakraborty, S.P., Majumdar, S., Bag, B.G., Roy, S., 2009. Eugenol protects nicotine-induced superoxide mediated oxidative damage in murine peritoneal macrophages in vitro. Eur. J. Pharmacol. 623 (1−3), 132−140.

Mahmarian, J.J., Moye, L.A., Nasser, G.A., Nagueh, S.F., Bloom, M.F., Benowitz, N.L., et al., 1997. Nicotine patch therapy in smoking cessation reduces the extent of exercise-induced myocardial ischemia. J. Am. Coll. Cardiol. 30 (1), 125−130.

Maier, C.R., Hollander, M.C., Hobbs, E.A., Dogan, I., Linnoila, R.I., Dennis, P.A., 2011. Nicotine does not enhance tumorigenesis in mutant K-Ras−Driven mouse models of lung cancer. Cancer Prev. Res. 4 (11), 1743−1751.

Mailhes, J.B., Young, D., Caldito, G., London, S.N., 2000. Sensitivity of mouse oocytes to nicotine-induced perturbations during oocyte meiotic maturation and aneuploidy in vivo and in vitro. Mol. Hum. Reprod. 6 (3), 232−237.

Mall, T., Grossenbacher, M., Perruchoud, A.P., Ritz, R., 1985. Influence of moderately elevated levels of carboxyhemoglobin on the course of acute ischemic heart disease. Respiration 48 (3), 237−244.

Manning, F.A., Feyerabend, C., 1976. Cigarette smoking and fetal breathing movements. Br. J. Obstet. Gynaecol. 83 (4), 262−270.

Maouche, K., Medjber, K., Zahm, J.-M., Delavoie, F., Terryn, C., Coraux, C., et al., 2013. Contribution of α7 nicotinic receptor to airway epithelium dysfunction under nicotine exposure. Proc. Natl. Acad. Sci. U. S. A. 110 (10), 4099−4104.

Maouche, K., Polette, M., Jolly, T., Medjber, K., Cloëz-Tayarani, I., Changeux, J.-P., et al., 2009. {alpha}7 nicotinic acetylcholine receptor regulates airway epithelium differentiation by controlling basal cell proliferation. Am. J. Pathol. 175 (5), 1868−1882.

Maritz, G.S., Windvogel, S., 2003. Chronic maternal nicotine exposure during gestation and lactation and the development of the lung parenchyma in the offspring. Response to nicotine withdrawal. Pathophysiology 10 (1), 69–75.

Martínez-García, E., Irigoyen, M., Ansó, E., Martínez-Irujo, J.J., Rouzaut, A., 2008. Recurrent exposure to nicotine differentiates human bronchial epithelial cells via epidermal growth factor receptor activation. Toxicol. Appl. Pharmacol. 228 (3), 334–342.

Matés, J.M., Segura, J.A., Alonso, F.J., Márquez, J., 2008. Intracellular redox status and oxidative stress: implications for cell proliferation, apoptosis, and carcinogenesis. Arch. Toxicol. 82 (5), 273–299.

Matsunaga, K., Klein, T.W., Friedman, H., Yamamoto, Y., 2001. Involvement of nicotinic acetylcholine receptors in suppression of antimicrobial activity and cytokine responses of alveolar macrophages to *Legionella pneumophila* infection by nicotine. J. Immunol. 167 (11), 6518–6524.

Matta, S.G., Balfour, D.J., Benowitz, N.L., Boyd, R.T., Buccafusco, J.J., Caggiula, A.R., et al., 2007. Guidelines on nicotine dose selection for in vivo research. Psychopharmacology 190 (3), 269–319.

Mayo Clinic, Female Infertility: Symptoms & Causes. Available at: https://www.mayoclinic.org/diseases-conditions/female-infertility/symptoms-causes/syc-20354308.

Male Infertility: Symptoms and Causes. Available at: https://www.mayoclinic.org/diseases-conditions/male-infertility/symptoms-causes/syc-20374773.

Mcevoy, J.W., Nasir, K., Defilippis, A.P., Lima, J.A., Bluemke, D.A., Hundley, W.G., et al., 2015. Relationship of cigarette smoking with inflammation and subclinical vascular disease: the Multi-Ethnic Study of Atherosclerosis. Arterioscler. Thromb. Vasc. Biol. 35 (4), 1002–1010.

Mcnair, L.F., Kohlmeier, K.A., 2015. Prenatal nicotine is associated with reduced AMPA and NMDA receptor-mediated rises in calcium within the laterodorsal tegmentum: a pontine nucleus involved in addiction processes. J. Dev. Orig. Health Dis. 6 (3), 225–241.

Mcneil, A., 2012. Reducing harm from nicotine use. In: Fifty Years since Smoking and Health. Progress, Lessons and Priorities for a Smoke-Free UK. Royal College of Physicians, London.

Medina, J.L., Navarrete, C., Lama, C., Roa, A., Cruz, M.A., Rudolph, M.I., 1992. Nicotine stimulates adrenergic terminals and inhibits contractions of mouse uterine horns. Gen. Pharmacol. 23 (3), 493–496.

Mehrotra, R., Yadav, A., Sinha, D.N., Parascandola, M., John, R.M., Ayo-Yusuf, O., et al., 2019. Smokeless tobacco control in 180 countries across the globe: call to action for full implementation of WHO FCTC measures. Lancet Oncol. 20 (4), e208–e217.

Michael, O.S., Olatunji, L.A., 2018. Nicotine exposure suppresses hyperinsulinemia and improves endothelial dysfunction mediators independent of corticosteroids in insulin-resistant oral contraceptive-treated female rats. Drug Chem. Toxicol. 41 (3), 314–323.

Mills, E.J., Thorlund, K., Eapen, S., Wu, P., Prochaska, J.J., 2014. Cardiovascular events associated with smoking cessation pharmacotherapies: a network meta-analysis. Circulation 129 (1), 28–41.

Mishra, N.C., Langley, R.J., Singh, S.P., Peña-Philippides, J.C., Koga, T., Razani-Boroujerdi, S., et al., 2008. Nicotine primarily suppresses lung Th2 but not goblet cell and muscle cell responses to allergens. J. Immunol. 180 (11), 7655–7663.

Mitchell, G.F., Hwang, S.J., Vasan, R.S., Larson, M.G., Pencina, M.J., Hamburg, N.M., et al., 2010. Arterial stiffness and cardiovascular events: the Framingham heart study. Circulation 121 (4), 505–511.

Moffatt, R.J., Biggerstaff, K.D., Stamford, B.A., 2000. Effects of the transdermal nicotine patch on normalization of HDL-C and its subfractions. Prev. Med. 31 (2 Pt 1), 148–152.

Moheimani, R.S., Bhetraratana, M., Peters, K.M., Yang, B.K., Yin, F., Gornbein, J., et al., 2017a. Sympathomimetic effects of acute E-cigarette use: role of nicotine and non-nicotine constituents. J. Am. Heart Assoc. 6 (9).

Moheimani, R.S., Bhetraratana, M., Yin, F., Peters, K.M., Gornbein, J., Araujo, J.A., et al., 2017b. Increased cardiac sympathetic activity and oxidative stress in habitual electronic cigarette users: implications for cardiovascular risk. JAMA Cardiol. 2 (3), 278–284.

Molina, J.R., Yang, P., Cassivi, S.D., Schild, S.E., Adjei, A.A., 2008. Non-small cell lung cancer: epidemiology, risk factors, treatment, and survivorship. Mayo Clin. Proc. 83 (5), 584–594.

Mouche, I., Malésic, L., Gillardeaux, O., 2017. FETAX assay for evaluation of developmental toxicity. Methods Mol. Biol. 1641, 311–324.

Mundal, H.H., Hjemdahl, P., Gjesdal, K., 1995. Acute effects of low dose nicotine gum on platelet function in non-smoking hypertensive and normotensive men. Eur. J. Clin. Pharmacol. 47 (5), 411–416.

Murphy, S.E., Von Weymarn, L.B., Schutten, M.M., Kassie, F., Modiano, J.F., 2011. Chronic nicotine consumption does not influence 4-(methylnitrosamino)-1-(3-pyridyl)-1-butanone–induced lung tumorigenesis. Cancer Prev. Res. 4 (11), 1752–1760.

Murray, R.P., Bailey, W.C., Daniels, K., Bjornson, W.M., Kurnow, K., Connett, J.E., et al., 1996. Safety of nicotine polacrilex gum used by 3,094 participants in the lung health study. Lung Health Study Research Group. Chest 109 (2), 438–445.

Murray, R.P., Connett, J.E., Zapawa, L.M., 2009. Does nicotine replacement therapy cause cancer? Evidence from the lung health study. Nicotine Tob. Res. 11 (9), 1076–1082.

Muthukumaran, S., Sudheer, A.R., Menon, V.P., Nalini, N., 2008. Protective effect of quercetin on nicotine-induced prooxidant and antioxidant imbalance and DNA damage in Wistar rats. Toxicology 243 (1–2), 207–215.

Muthumalage, T., Lamb, T., Friedman, M.R., Rahman, I., 2019. E-cigarette flavored pods induce inflammation, epithelial barrier dysfunction, and DNA damage in lung epithelial cells and monocytes. Sci. Rep. 9 (1), 19035.

Nacerai, H., Gregory, T., Sihem, B., Salah, A., Souhila, A.B., 2017. Green tea beverage and epigallocatecihin gallate attenuate nicotine cardiocytotoxicity in rat. Acta Pol. Pharm. 74 (1), 277–287.

Nakada, T., Kiyotani, K., Iwano, S., Uno, T., Yokohira, M., Yamakawa, K., et al., 2012. Lung tumorigenesis promoted by anti-apoptotic effects of cotinine, a nicotine metabolite through activation of PI3K/Akt pathway. J. Toxicol. Sci. 37 (3), 555−563.

Nakao, S., Ogata, Y., Sugiya, H., 2009. Nicotine stimulates the expression of cyclooxygenase-2 mRNA via NFκB activation in human gingival fibroblasts. Arch. Oral Biol. 54 (3), 251−257.

Napierala, M., Mazela, J., Merritt, T.A., Florek, E., 2016. Tobacco smoking and breastfeeding: effect on the lactation process, breast milk composition and infant development. A critical review. Environ. Res. 151, 321−338.

Nas, T., Barun, S., Ozturk, G.S., Vural, I.M., Ercan, Z.S., Sarioglu, Y., 2007. Nicotine potentiates the electrical field stimulation-evoked contraction of non-pregnant rabbit myometrium. Tohoku J. Exp. Med. 211 (2), 187−193.

Natori, T., Sata, M., Washida, M., Hirata, Y., Nagai, R., Makuuchi, M., 2003. Nicotine enhances neovascularization and promotes tumor growth. Mol. Cell. 16 (2).

Neff, R.A., Simmens, S.J., Evans, C., Mendelowitz, D., 2004. Prenatal nicotine exposure alters central cardiorespiratory responses to hypoxia in rats: implications for sudden infant death syndrome. J. Neurosci. 24 (42), 9261−9268.

Newbold, R.F., 2002. The significance of telomerase activation and cellular immortalization in human cancer. Mutagenesis 17 (6), 539−550.

Ni, Y.F., Tian, F., Lu, Z.F., Yang, G.D., Fu, H.Y., Wang, J., et al., 2011. Protective effect of nicotine on lipopolysaccharide-induced acute lung injury in mice. Respiration 81 (1), 39−46.

Nieradko-Iwanicka, B., Pietraszek, D., Pośnik, K., Borzęcki, A., 2019. Prolonged exposure to transdermal nicotine improves memory in male mice, but impairs biochemical parameters in male and female mice. Ann. Agric. Environ. Med. 26 (1), 62−66.

Nishioka, T., Guo, J., Yamamoto, D., Chen, L., Huppi, P., Chen, C.Y., 2010. Nicotine, through upregulating pro-survival signaling, cooperates with NNK to promote transformation. J. Cell. Biochem. 109 (1), 152−161.

Nishioka, T., Yamamoto, D., Zhu, T., Guo, J., Kim, S.-H., Chen, C.Y., 2011. Nicotine overrides DNA damage-induced G1/S restriction in lung cells. PLoS One 6 (4), e18619.

Noël, A., Hansen, S., Zaman, A., Perveen, Z., Pinkston, R., Hossain, E., et al., 2020. In utero exposures to electronic-cigarette aerosols impair the Wnt signaling during mouse lung development. Am. J. Physiol. Lung Cell Mol. Physiol. 318 (4), L705−L722.

Nordestgaard, B.G., 2016. Triglyceride-rich lipoproteins and atherosclerotic cardiovascular disease: new insights from epidemiology, genetics, and biology. Circ. Res. 118 (4), 547−563.

Nordon, I.M., Hinchliffe, R.J., Loftus, I.M., Thompson, M.M., 2011. Pathophysiology and epidemiology of abdominal aortic aneurysms. Nat. Rev. Cardiol. 8 (2), 92−102.

Novak, J., Escobedo-Morse, A., Kelley, K., Boose, D., Kautzman-Eades, D., Meyer, M., et al., 2000. Nicotine effects on proliferation and the bombesin-like peptide autocrine system in human small cell lung carcinoma SHP77 cells in culture. Lung Cancer 29 (1), 1−10.

Nowak, J., Andersson, K., Benthin, G., Chen, J., Karlberg, K.E., Sylven, C., 1996. Effect of nicotine infusion in humans on platelet aggregation and urinary excretion of a major thromboxane metabolite. Acta Physiol. Scand. 157 (1), 101−107.

Obisesan, O.H., Osei, A.D., Uddin, S.M.I., Dzaye, O., Cainzos-Achirica, M., Mirbolouk, M., et al., 2020. E-cigarette use patterns and high-risk behaviors in pregnancy: behavioral risk factor surveillance system, 2016−2018. Am. J. Prev. Med. https://doi.org/10.1016/j.amepre.2020.02.015.

OECD, 2013. Test No. 236: Fish Embryo Acute Toxicity (FET) Test.

OECD, 2018a. Test No. 414: Prenatal Developmental Toxicity Study. https://doi.org/10.1787/9789264070820-en.

OECD, 2018b. Test No. 443: Extended One-Generation Reproductive Toxicity Study.

OECD, 2018c. Test No. 451: Carcinogenicity Studies.

OECD, 2018d. Test No. 453: Combined Chronic Toxicity/Carcinogenicity Studies.

OECD, 2019. Test No. 415: One-Generation Reproduction Toxicity Study.

Ogunwale, M.A., Li, M., Ramakrishnam Raju, M.V., Chen, Y., Nantz, M.H., Conklin, D.J., et al., 2017. Aldehyde detection in electronic cigarette aerosols. ACS Omega 2 (3), 1207−1214.

Ohshima, H., Bartsch, H., 1994. Chronic infections and inflammatory processes as cancer risk factors: possible role of nitric oxide in carcinogenesis. Mutat. Res. Fund Mol. Mech. Mutagen 305 (2), 253−264.

Oloris, S.C., Frazer-Abel, A.A., Jubala, C.M., Fosmire, S.P., Helm, K.M., Robinson, S.R., et al., 2010. Nicotine-mediated signals modulate cell death and survival of T lymphocytes. Toxicol. Appl. Pharmacol. 242 (3), 299−309.

Omenn, G.S., 2001. Assessment of human cancer risk: challenges for alternative approaches. Toxicol. Pathol. 29 (1_suppl), 5−12.

Oncken, C.A., Hardardottir, H., Hatsukami, D.K., Lupo, V.R., Rodis, J.F., Smeltzer, J.S., 1997. Effects of transdermal nicotine or smoking on nicotine concentrations and maternal-fetal hemodynamics. Obstet. Gynecol. 90 (4 Pt 1), 569−574.

Orzabal, M.R., Lunde-Young, E.R., Ramirez, J.I., Howe, S.Y.F., Naik, V.D., Lee, J., et al., 2019. Chronic exposure to e-cig aerosols during early development causes vascular dysfunction and offspring growth deficits. Transl. Res. 207, 70−82.

Oviedo, A., Lebrun, S., Kogel, U., Ho, J., Tan, W.T., Titz, B., et al., 2016. Evaluation of the tobacco heating system 2.2. Part 6: 90-day OECD 413 rat inhalation study with systems toxicology endpoints demonstrates reduced exposure effects of a mentholated version compared with mentholated and non-mentholated cigarette smoke. Regul. Toxicol. Pharmacol. 81 (Suppl. 2), S93−s122.

Owens, J., Kullberg, R., 1989. In vivo development of nicotinic acetylcholine receptor channels in Xenopus myotomal muscle. J. Neurosci. 9 (3), 1018−1028.

Oyeyipo, I.P., Raji, Y., Bolarinwa, A.F., 2013. Nicotine alters male reproductive hormones in male albino rats: the role of cessation. J. Hum. Reprod. Sci. 6 (1), 40−44.

Oyeyipo, I.P., Raji, Y., Bolarinwa, A.F., 2014. Nicotine alters serum antioxidant profile in male albino rats. N. Am. J. Med. Sci. 6 (4), 168.

Oyeyipo, I.P., Raji, Y., Emikpe, B.O., Bolarinwa, A.F., 2011. Effects of nicotine on sperm characteristics and fertility profile in adult male rats: a possible role of cessation. J. Reproduction Infertil. 12 (3), 201–207.

Pacifici, R., Altieri, I., Gandini, L., Lenzi, A., Pichini, S., Rosa, M., et al., 1993. Nicotine, cotinine, and trans-3-hydroxycotinine levels in seminal plasma of smokers: effects on sperm parameters. Ther. Drug Monit. 15 (5), 358–363.

Packham, M.A., 1994. Role of platelets in thrombosis and hemostasis. Can. J. Physiol. Pharmacol. 72 (3), 278–284.

Pagano, M.B., Zhou, H.F., Ennis, T.L., Wu, X., Lambris, J.D., Atkinson, J.P., et al., 2009. Complement-dependent neutrophil recruitment is critical for the development of elastase-induced abdominal aortic aneurysm. Circulation 119 (13), 1805–1813.

Palpant, N.J., Hofsteen, P., Pabon, L., Reinecke, H., Murry, C.E., 2015. Cardiac development in zebrafish and human embryonic stem cells is inhibited by exposure to tobacco cigarettes and e-cigarettes. PLoS One 10 (5), e0126259.

Papke, R.L., Ono, F., Stokes, C., Urban, J.M., Boyd, R.T., 2012. The nicotinic acetylcholine receptors of zebrafish and an evaluation of pharmacological tools used for their study. Biochem. Pharmacol. 84 (3), 352–365.

Parker, B., Connaughton, V.P., 2007. Effects of nicotine on growth and development in larval zebrafish. Zebrafish 4 (1), 59–68.

Parkin, M., Tyczynski, J.E., Boffetta, P., Samet, J., Shields, P., Caporaso, N., 2004. Lung cancer epidemiology and etiology. In: Travis, W.D., Brambilla, E., Müller-Hermelink, H.K., et al. (Eds.), Pathology and Genetics of Tumours of the Lung, Pleura,Thymus and Heart. IARC Press, Lyon, pp. 12–15.

Pastrakuljic, A., Derewlany, L.O., Knie, B., Koren, G., 2000. The effects of cocaine and nicotine on amino acid transport across the human placental cotyledon perfused in vitro. J. Pharmacol. Exp. Therapeut. 294 (1), 141–146.

Patra, P.B., Sanyal, S., Biswas, N.M., 1979. Possible alpha-adrenergic involvement in nicotine induced alteration of spermatogenesis in rat. Andrologia 11 (4), 273–278.

Patterson, T.R., Stringham, J.D., Meikle, A.W., 1990. Nicotine and cotinine inhibit steroidogenesis in mouse leydig cells. Life Sci. 46 (4), 265–272.

Pednekar, M.S., Gupta, P.C., Yeole, B.B., Hébert, J.R., 2011. Association of tobacco habits, including bidi smoking, with overall and site-specific cancer incidence: results from the Mumbai cohort study. Cancer Causes Contr. 22 (6), 859–868.

Peto, R., Lopez, A.D., Boreham, J., Thun, M., Heath Jr., C., 1992. Mortality from tobacco in developed countries: indirect estimation from national vital statistics. Lancet 339 (8804), 1268–1278.

Pfueller, S.L., Burns, P., Mak, K., Firkin, B.G., 1988. Effects of nicotine on platelet function. Haemostasis 18 (3), 163–169.

Phillips, B., Esposito, M., Verbeeck, J., Boué, S., Iskandar, A., Vuillaume, G., et al., 2015. Toxicity of aerosols of nicotine and pyruvic acid (separate and combined) in Sprague–Dawley rats in a 28-day OECD 412 inhalation study and assessment of systems toxicology. Inhal. Toxicol. 27 (9), 405–431.

Phillips, B., Szostak, J., Titz, B., Schlage, W.K., Guedj, E., Leroy, P., et al., 2019. A six-month systems toxicology inhalation/cessation study in ApoE(-/-) mice to investigate cardiovascular and respiratory exposure effects of modified risk tobacco products, CHTP 1.2 and THS 2.2, compared with conventional cigarettes. Food Chem. Toxicol. 126, 113–141.

Phillips, B., Veljkovic, E., Boué, S., Schlage, W.K., Vuillaume, G., Martin, F., et al., 2016. An 8-month systems toxicology inhalation/cessation study in Apoe-/- mice to investigate cardiovascular and respiratory exposure effects of a candidate modified risk tobacco product, THS 2.2, compared with conventional cigarettes. Toxicol. Sci. 149 (2), 411–432.

Pilger, A., Rüdiger, H., 2006. 8-Hydroxy-2′-deoxyguanosine as a marker of oxidative DNA damage related to occupational and environmental exposures. Int. Arch. Occup. Environ. Health 80 (1), 1–15.

Piubelli, C., Cecconi, D., Astner, H., Caldara, F., Tessari, M., Carboni, L., et al., 2005. Proteomic changes in rat serum, polymorphonuclear and mononuclear leukocytes after chronic nicotine administration. Proteomics 5 (5), 1382–1394.

Plummer, H.K., Dhar, M., Schuller, H.M., 2005. Expression of the α7 nicotinic acetylcholine receptor in human lung cells. Respir. Res. 6 (1), 29.

Polosa, R., Cibella, F., Caponnetto, P., Maglia, M., Prosperini, U., Russo, C., et al., 2017. Health impact of E-cigarettes: a prospective 3.5-year study of regular daily users who have never smoked. Sci. Rep. 7 (1), 13825.

Polosa, R., Morjaria, J.B., Caponnetto, P., Battaglia, E., Russo, C., Ciampi, C., et al., 2016. Blood pressure control in smokers with arterial hypertension who switched to electronic cigarettes. Int. J. Environ. Res. Publ. Health 13 (11).

Powell, G.L., Gaddy, J., Xu, F., Fregosi, R.F., Levine, R.B., 2016. Developmental nicotine exposure disrupts dendritic arborization patterns of hypoglossal motoneurons in the neonatal rat. Dev. Neurobiol. 76 (10), 1125–1137.

Proskocil, B.J., Sekhon, H.S., Jia, Y., Savchenko, V., Blakely, R.D., Lindstrom, J., et al., 2004. Acetylcholine is an autocrine or paracrine hormone synthesized and secreted by airway bronchial epithelial cells. Endocrinology 145 (5), 2498–2506.

Qasim, H., Karim, Z.A., Silva-Espinoza, J.C., Khasawneh, F.T., Rivera, J.O., Ellis, C.C., et al., 2018. Short-term E-cigarette exposure increases the risk of thrombogenesis and enhances platelet function in mice. J. Am. Heart Assoc. 7 (15).

Queimado, L., Wagener, T., Ganapathy, V., 2018. Electronic cigarette aerosols induce DNA damage and reduce DNA repair: consistency across species. Proc. Natl. Acad. Sci. U. S. A. 115 (24), E5437–E5438.

Quensel, M., Agardh, C.D., Nilsson-Ehle, P., 1989. Nicotine does not affect plasma lipoprotein concentrations in healthy men. Scand. J. Clin. Lab. Invest. 49 (2), 149−153.

Racowsky, C., Hendricks, R.C., Baldwin, K.V., 1989. Direct effects of nicotine on the meiotic maturation of hamster oocytes. Reprod. Toxicol. 3 (1), 13−21.

Raghavendra, T., Pakkala, A., Ganashree, C.P., 2013. Acute effect of Gutkha chewing on cardiopulmonary efficiency in short term users. J. Alcohol. Drug Depend. 1, 3. https://doi.org/10.4172/2329-6488.1000115.

Ramachandran, J., Rubenstein, D., Bluestein, D., Jesty, J., 2004. Activation of platelets exposed to shear stress in the presence of smoke extracts of low-nicotine and zero-nicotine cigarettes: the protective effect of nicotine. Nicotine Tob. Res. 6 (5), 835−841.

Ramalingam, A., Budin, S.B., Mohd Fauzi, N., Ritchie, R.H., Zainalabidin, S., 2019. Angiotensin II type I receptor antagonism attenuates nicotine-induced cardiac remodeling, dysfunction, and aggravation of myocardial ischemia-reperfusion injury in rats. Front. Pharmacol. 10, 1493.

Ramström, L., Borland, R., Wikmans, T., 2016. Patterns of smoking and snus use in Sweden: implications for public health. Int. J. Environ. Res. Publ. Health 13 (11).

Rateri, D.L., Howatt, D.A., Moorleghen, J.J., Charnigo, R., Cassis, L.A., Daugherty, A., 2011. Prolonged infusion of angiotensin II in apoE(-/-) mice promotes macrophage recruitment with continued expansion of abdominal aortic aneurysm. Am. J. Pathol. 179 (3), 1542−1548.

Ratsch, A., Bogossian, F., 2014. Smokeless tobacco use in pregnancy: an integrative review of the literature. Int. J. Publ. Health 59 (4), 599−608.

Rebagliato, M., Bolumar, F., Florey Cdu, V., Jarvis, M.J., Perez-Hoyos, S., Hernandez-Aguado, I., et al., 1998. Variations in cotinine levels in smokers during and after pregnancy. Am. J. Obstet. Gynecol. 178 (3), 568−571.

Reddy, S., Londonkar, R., Ravindra, Reddy, S., Patil, S.B., 1998. Testicular changes due to graded doses of nicotine in albino mice. Indian J. Physiol. Pharmacol. 42 (2), 276−280.

Rehan, V.K., Wang, Y., Sugano, S., Romero, S., Chen, X., Santos, J., et al., 2005. Mechanism of nicotine-induced pulmonary fibroblast transdifferentiation. Am. J. Physiol. Lung Cell Mol. Physiol. 289 (4), L667−L676.

Rehan, V.K., Wang, Y., Sugano, S., Santos, J., Patel, S., Sakurai, R., et al., 2007. In utero nicotine exposure alters fetal rat lung alveolar type II cell proliferation, differentiation, and metabolism. Am. J. Physiol. Lung Cell Mol. Physiol. 292 (1), L323−L333.

Ren, A., Wu, H., Liu, L., Guo, Z., Cao, Q., Dai, Q., 2018. Nicotine promotes atherosclerosis development in apolipoprotein E-deficient mice through α1-nAChR. J. Cell. Physiol. https://doi.org/10.1002/jcp.27728. Epub ahead of print 2018/12/27.

Renaud, S., Blache, D., Dumont, E., Thevenon, C., Wissendanger, T., 1984. Platelet function after cigarette smoking in relation to nicotine and carbon monoxide. Clin. Pharmacol. Ther. 36 (3), 389−395.

Reuter, S., Gupta, S.C., Chaturvedi, M.M., Aggarwal, B.B., 2010. Oxidative stress, inflammation, and cancer: how are they linked? Free Radic. Biol. Med. 49 (11), 1603−1616.

Riaz, S.P., Lüchtenborg, M., Coupland, V.H., Spicer, J., Peake, M.D., Møller, H., 2012. Trends in incidence of small cell lung cancer and all lung cancer. Lung Cancer 75 (3), 280−284.

Riebe, M., Westphal, K., 1983. Studies on the induction of sister-chromatid exchanges in Chinese hamster ovary cells by various tobacco alkaloids. Mutat. Res. Genet. Toxicol. 124 (3−4), 281−286.

Riebe, M., Westphal, K., Fortnagel, P., 1982. Mutagenicity testing, in bacterial test systems, of some constituents of tobacco. Mutat. Res. Genet. Toxicol. 101 (1), 39−43.

Robbins, A., 1996. Androgens and male sexual behavior from mice to men. Trends Endocrinol. Metabol. 7 (9), 345−350.

Rohani, M., Agewall, S., 2004. Oral snuff impairs endothelial function in healthy snuff users. J. Intern. Med. 255 (3), 379−383.

Roman, J., Ritzenthaler, J.D., Gil-Acosta, A., Rivera, H.N., Roser-Page, S., 2004. Nicotine and fibronectin expression in lung fibroblasts: implications for tobacco-related lung tissue remodeling. FASEB.J. 18 (12), 1436−1438.

Rose, J.K., Miller, M.K., Crane, S.A., Hope, K.A., Pittman, P.G., 2013. Parental and larval exposure to nicotine modulate spontaneous activity as well as cholinergic and GABA receptor expression in adult C. elegans. Neurotoxicol. Teratol. 39, 122−127.

Rosti, G., Bevilacqua, G., Bidoli, P., Portalone, L., Santo, A., Genestreti, G., 2006. Small cell lung cancer. Ann. Oncol. 17 (Suppl. 2), ii5−ii10.

Rothig, A., Schreckenberg, R., Weber, K., Conzelmann, C., Da Costa Rebelo, R.M., Schluter, K.D., 2012. Effects of nicotine on PTHrP and PTHrP receptor expression in rat coronary endothelial cells. Cell. Physiol. Biochem. 29 (3−4), 485−492.

Roy, T.S., Andrews, J.E., Seidler, F.J., Slotkin, T.A., 1998. Nicotine evokes cell death in embryonic rat brain during neurulation. J. Pharmacol. Exp. Therapeut. 287 (3), 1136−1144.

Royal College of Physicians of London. Tobacco Advisory Group, 2007. Harm Reduction in Nicotine Addiction: Helping People Who Can't Quit. Royal College of Physicians of London.

Rubenstein, D., Jesty, J., Bluestein, D., 2004. Differences between mainstream and sidestream cigarette smoke extracts and nicotine in the activation of platelets under static and flow conditions. Circulation 109 (1), 78−83.

Ruediger, T., Bolz, J., 2007. Neurotransmitters and the development of neuronal circuits. Adv. Exp. Med. Biol. 621, 104−115.

Rutqvist, L.E., Curvall, M., Hassler, T., Ringberger, T., Wahlberg, I., 2011. Swedish snus and the GothiaTek® standard. Harm Reduct. J. 8, 11.

Ryden, M., Arner, P., 2017. Subcutaneous adipocyte lipolysis contributes to circulating lipid levels. Arterioscler. Thromb. Vasc. Biol. 37 (9), 1782−1787.

Safronova, V.G., Vulfius, C.A., Shelukhina, I.V., Mal'tseva, V.N., Berezhnov, A.V., Fedotova, E.I., et al., 2016. Nicotinic receptor involvement in regulation of functions of mouse neutrophils from inflammatory site. Immunobiology 221 (7), 761−772.

Sakalihasan, N., Michel, J.B., Katsargyris, A., Kuivaniemi, H., Defraigne, J.O., Nchimi, A., et al., 2018. Abdominal aortic aneurysms. Nat. Rev. Dis. Primers 4 (1), 34.

Sakurai, R., Cerny, L.M., Torday, J.S., Rehan, V.K., 2011. Mechanism for nicotine-induced up-regulation of Wnt signaling in human alveolar interstitial fibroblasts. Exp. Lung Res. 37 (3), 144−154.

Sanders, S.R., Cuneo, S.P., Turzillo, A.M., 2002. Effects of nicotine and cotinine on bovine theca interna and granulosa cells. Reprod. Toxicol. 16 (6), 795−800.

Sandesara, P.B., Virani, S.S., Fazio, S., Shapiro, M.D., 2019. The forgotten lipids: triglycerides, remnant cholesterol, and atherosclerotic cardiovascular disease risk. Endocr. Rev. 40 (2), 537−557.

Santiago, S.E., Huffman, K.J., 2014. Prenatal nicotine exposure increases anxiety and modifies sensorimotor integration behaviors in adult female mice. Neurosci. Res. 79, 41−51.

Saraff, K., Babamusta, F., Cassis, L.A., Daugherty, A., 2003. Aortic dissection precedes formation of aneurysms and atherosclerosis in angiotensin II-infused, apolipoprotein E-deficient mice. Arterioscler. Thromb. Vasc. Biol. 23 (9), 1621−1626.

Sassen, A.W., Richter, E., Semmler, M.P., Harreus, U.A., Gamarra, F., Kleinsasser, N.H., 2005. Genotoxicity of nicotine in mini-organ cultures of human upper aerodigestive tract epithelia. Toxicol. Sci. 88 (1), 134−141.

Sastry, B.V.R., Hemontolor, M.E., Olenick, M., 1999. Prostaglandin E2 in human placenta: its vascular effects and activation of prostaglandin E2 formation by nicotine and cotinine. Pharmacology 58 (2), 70−86.

Scenihr (Scientific Committee on Emerging and Newly-Identified Health Risks), 2008. Scientific Opinion on the Health Effects of Smokeless Tobacco Products.

Schedel, A., Kaiser, K., Uhlig, S., Lorenz, F., Sarin, A., Starigk, J., et al., 2016. Megakaryocytes and platelets express nicotinic acetylcholine receptors but nicotine does not affect megakaryopoiesis or platelet function. Platelets 27 (1), 43−50.

Schedel, A., Thornton, S., Schloss, P., Klüter, H., Bugert, P., 2011. Human platelets express functional α7-nicotinic acetylcholine receptors. Arterioscler. Thromb. Vasc. Biol. 31 (4), 928−934.

Schweitzer, K.S., Chen, S.X., Law, S., Van Demark, M., Poirier, C., Justice, M.J., et al., 2015. Endothelial disruptive proinflammatory effects of nicotine and e-cigarette vapor exposures. Am. J. Physiol. Lung Cell Mol. Physiol. 309 (2), L175−L187.

Sears, C.G., Hart, J.L., Walker, K.L., Robertson, R.M., 2017. Generally recognized as safe: uncertainty surrounding E-cigarette flavoring safety. Int. J. Environ. Res. Publ. Health 14 (10).

Sekhon, H.S., Jia, Y., Raab, R., Kuryatov, A., Pankow, J.F., Whitsett, J.A., et al., 1999. Prenatal nicotine increases pulmonary alpha7 nicotinic receptor expression and alters fetal lung development in monkeys. J. Clin. Invest. 103 (5), 637−647.

Sekhon, H.S., Proskocil, B.J., Clark, J.A., Spindel, E.R., 2004. Prenatal nicotine exposure increases connective tissue expression in foetal monkey pulmonary vessels. Eur. Respir. J. 23 (6), 906−915.

Sen, S., Sharma, A., Talukder, G., 1991. Inhibition of clastogenic effects of nicotine by chlorophyllin in mice bone marrow cells in vivo. Phytother Res. 5 (3), 130−133.

Sewer, A., Kogel, U., Talikka, M., Wong, E.T., Martin, F., Xiang, Y., et al., 2016. Evaluation of the tobacco heating system 2.2 (THS2.2). Part 5: microRNA expression from a 90-day rat inhalation study indicates that exposure to THS2.2 aerosol causes reduced effects on lung tissue compared with cigarette smoke. Regul. Toxicol. Pharmacol. 81 (Suppl. 2), S82−s92.

Sher, R.B., Cox, G.A., Mills, K.D., Sundberg, J.P., 2011. Rhabdomyosarcomas in aging A/J mice. PLoS One 6 (8), e23498.

Shields, P.G., Berman, M., Brasky, T.M., Freudenheim, J.L., Mathe, E., Mcelroy, J.P., et al., 2017. A review of pulmonary toxicity of electronic cigarettes in the context of smoking: a focus on inflammation. Cancer Epidemiol. Biomarkers Prev. 26 (8), 1175−1191.

Si, L.Y., Kamisah, Y., Ramalingam, A., Lim, Y.C., Budin, S.B., Zainalabidin, S., 2017. Roselle supplementation prevents nicotine-induced vascular endothelial dysfunction and remodelling in rats. Appl. Physiol. Nutr. Metabol. 42 (7), 765−772.

Singh, S.P., Kalra, R., Puttfarcken, P., Kozak, A., Tesfaigzi, J., Sopori, M.L., 2000. Acute and chronic nicotine exposures modulate the immune system through different pathways. Toxicol. Appl. Pharmacol. 164 (1), 65−72.

Sinha-Hikim, I., Friedman, T.C., Falz, M., Chalfant, V., Hasan, M.K., Espinoza-Derout, J., et al., 2017. Nicotine plus a high-fat diet triggers cardiomyocyte apoptosis. Cell Tissue Res. 368 (1), 159−170.

Sinha, D.N., Gupta, P.C., Kumar, A., Bhartiya, D., Agarwal, N., Sharma, et al., 2018. The poorest of poor suffer the greatest burden from smokeless tobacco use: a study from 140 countries. Nicotine Tob. Res. 20 (12), 1529−1532.

Skorge, T.D., Eagan, T.M., Eide, G.E., Gulsvik, A., Bakke, P.S., 2005. The adult incidence of asthma and respiratory symptoms by passive smoking in uterus or in childhood. Am. J. Respir. Crit. Care Med. 172 (1), 61−66.

Skotsimara, G., Antonopoulos, A.S., Oikonomou, E., Siasos, G., Ioakeimidis, N., Tsalamandris, S., et al., 2019. Cardiovascular effects of electronic cigarettes: a systematic review and meta-analysis. Eur. J. Prev. Cardiol. 26 (11), 1219−1228.

Slikker Jr., W., Xu, Z.A., Levin, E.D., Slotkin, T.A., 2005. Mode of action: disruption of brain cell replication, second messenger, and neurotransmitter systems during development leading to cognitive dysfunction–developmental neurotoxicity of nicotine. Crit. Rev. Toxicol. 35 (8−9), 703−711.

Slotkin, T.A., Skavicus, S., Card, J., Levin, E.D., Seidler, F.J., 2016. Diverse neurotoxicants target the differentiation of embryonic neural stem cells into neuronal and glial phenotypes. Toxicology 372, 42–51.

Smart, D.J., Helbling, F.R., Verardo, M., Mchugh, D., Vanscheeuwijck, P., 2019. Mode-of-action analysis of the effects induced by nicotine in the in vitro micronucleus assay. Environ. Mol. Mutagen. 60 (9), 778–791.

Smith, C.J., Fischer, T.H., 2001. Particulate and vapor phase constituents of cigarette mainstream smoke and risk of myocardial infarction. Atherosclerosis 158 (2), 257–267.

Smith Jr., M.A., Zhang, Y., Polli, J.R., Wu, H., Zhang, B., Xiao, P., et al., 2013. Impacts of chronic low-level nicotine exposure on Caenorhabditis elegans reproduction: identification of novel gene targets. Reprod. Toxicol. 40, 69–75.

Smith, M.T., Guyton, K.Z., Gibbons, C.F., Fritz, J.M., Portier, C.J., Rusyn, I., et al., 2016. Key characteristics of carcinogens as a basis for organizing data on mechanisms of carcinogenesis. Environ. Health Perspect. 124 (6), 713.

Sobkowiak, R., Musidlak, J., Lesicki, A., 2014. In vitro genoprotective and genotoxic effect of nicotine on human leukocytes evaluated by the comet assay. Drug Chem. Toxicol. 37 (3), 322–328.

Solleti, S.K., Bhattacharya, S., Ahmad, A., Wang, Q., Mereness, J., Rangasamy, T., et al., 2017. MicroRNA expression profiling defines the impact of electronic cigarettes on human airway epithelial cells. Sci. Rep. 7, 1081.

St-Pierre, S., Jiang, W., Roy, P., Champigny, C., Leblanc, É., Morley, B.J., et al., 2016. Nicotinic acetylcholine receptors modulate bone marrow-derived pro-inflammatory monocyte production and survival. PLoS One 11 (2), e0150230.

St Helen, G., Havel, C., Dempsey, D.A., Jacob 3rd, P., Benowitz, N.L., 2016. Nicotine delivery, retention and pharmacokinetics from various electronic cigarettes. Addiction 111 (3), 535–544.

Stiernagle, T., 1999. Maintenance of C. elegans, 2, pp. 51–67.

Stinn, W., Berges, A., Meurrens, K., Buettner, A., Gebel, S., Lichtner, R.B., et al., 2013. Towards the validation of a lung tumorigenesis model with mainstream cigarette smoke inhalation using the A/J mouse. Toxicology 305, 49–64.

Stocks, J., Hislop, A., Sonnappa, S., 2013. Early lung development: lifelong effect on respiratory health and disease. Lancet Respir. Med. 1 (9), 728–742.

Stolle, K., Berges, A., Lietz, M., Lebrun, S., Wallerath, T., 2010. Cigarette smoke enhances abdominal aortic aneurysm formation in angiotensin II-treated apolipoprotein E-deficient mice. Toxicol. Lett. 199 (3), 403–409.

Stoner, G.D., Shimkin, M.B., 1982. Strain A mouse lung tumor bioassay. J. Am. Coll. Toxicol. 1 (1), 145–169.

Su, X., Lee, J.W., Matthay, Z.A., Mednick, G., Uchida, T., Fang, X., et al., 2007. Activation of the α7 nAChR reduces acid-induced acute lung injury in mice and rats. Am. J. Respir. Cell Mol. Biol. 37 (2), 186–192.

Sudheer, A.R., Muthukumaran, S., Devipriya, N., Menon, V.P., 2007a. Ellagic acid, a natural polyphenol protects rat peripheral blood lymphocytes against nicotine-induced cellular and DNA damage in vitro: with the comparison of N-acetylcysteine. Toxicology 230 (1), 11–21.

Sudheer, A.R., Muthukumaran, S., Kalpana, C., Srinivasan, M., Menon, V.P., 2007b. Protective effect of ferulic acid on nicotine-induced DNA damage and cellular changes in cultured rat peripheral blood lymphocytes: a comparison with N-acetylcysteine. Toxicol In Vitro 21 (4), 576–585.

Sugano, N., Shimada, K., Ito, K., Murai, S., 1998. Nicotine inhibits the production of inflammatory mediators in U937 cells through modulation of nuclear factor-kB activation. Biochem. Biophys. Res. Commun. 252 (1), 25–28.

Sullivan, M.P., Owens, J.L., Kullberg, R.W., 1999. Role of M2 domain residues in conductance and gating of acetylcholine receptors in developing Xenopus muscle. J. Physiol. 515 (Pt 1), 31.

Sulston, J.E., Horvitz, H.R., 1977. Post-embryonic cell lineages of the nematode, Caenorhabditis elegans. Dev. Biol. 56 (1), 110–156.

Sundberg, J.P., Adkison, D.L., Bedigian, H.G., 1991. Skeletal muscle rhabdomyosarcomas in inbred laboratory mice. Vet. Pathol. 28 (3), 200–206.

Sundstrom, D., Waldenborg, M., Emilsson, K., 2012. Acute effects on the ventricular function in Swedish snuffers: an echocardiographic study. Clin. Physiol. Funct. Imag. 32 (2), 106–113.

Suter, M.A., Aagaard, K.M., 2020. The impact of tobacco chemicals and nicotine on placental development. Prenat. Diagn. https://doi.org/10.1002/pd.5660.

Svoboda, K.R., Vijayaraghavan, S., Tanguay, R.L., 2002. Nicotinic receptors mediate changes in spinal motoneuron development and axonal pathfinding in embryonic zebrafish exposed to nicotine. J. Neurosci. 22 (24), 10731–10741.

Szostak, J., Wong, E.T., Titz, B., Lee, T., Wong, S.K., Low, T., et al., 2020. A 6-month systems toxicology inhalation study in ApoE(-/-) mice demonstrates reduced cardiovascular effects of E-vapor aerosols compared with cigarette smoke. Am. J. Physiol. Heart Circ. Physiol. 318 (3), H604–H631.

Taghavi, T., Arger, C.A., Heil, S.H., Higgins, S.T., Tyndale, R.F., 2018. Longitudinal influence of pregnancy on nicotine metabolic pathways. J. Pharmacol. Exp. Therapeut. 364 (2), 238–245.

Takahashi, H.K., Iwagaki, H., Hamano, R., Yoshino, T., Tanaka, N., Nishibori, M., 2006. Effect of nicotine on IL-18-initiated immune response in human monocytes. J. Leukoc. Biol. 80 (6), 1388–1394.

Takeshita, D., Nakajima-Takenaka, C., Shimizu, J., Hattori, H., Nakashima, T., Kikuta, A., et al., 2009. Effects of formaldehyde on cardiovascular system in in situ rat hearts. Basic Clin. Pharmacol. Toxicol. 105 (4), 271–280.

Taki, F.A., Pan, X., Lee, M.-H., Zhang, B., 2014a. Nicotine exposure and transgenerational impact: a prospective study on small regulatory microRNAs. Sci. Rep. 4 (1), 1–15.

Taki, F.A., Pan, X., Zhang, B., 2014b. Chronic nicotine exposure systemically alters microRNA expression profiles during post-embryonic stages in Caenorhabditis elegans. J. Cell. Physiol. 229 (1), 79–89.

Tateishi, T., Nakura, H., Asoh, M., Watanabe, M., Tanaka, M., Kumai, T., et al., 1997. A comparison of hepatic cytochrome P450 protein expression between infancy and postinfancy. Life Sci. 61 (26), 2567–2574.

Thompson, J.H., Irwin, F.D., Kanematsu, S., Seraydarian, K., Suh, M., 1973. Effects of chronic nicotine administration and age in male fischer-344 rats. Toxicol. Appl. Pharmacol. 26 (4), 606–620.

Titz, B., Sewer, A., Luettich, K., Wong, E.T., Guedj, E., Nury, C., et al., 2020. Respiratory effects of exposure to aerosol from the candidate modified-risk tobacco product THS 2.2 in an 18-month systems toxicology study with A/J mice. Toxicol. Sci. https://doi.org/10.1093/toxsci/kfaa132. Epub ahead of print 2020/08/12.

Toth, B., 1982. Effects of long term administration of nicotine hydrochloride and nicotinic acid in mice. Anticancer Res. 2 (1–2), 71.

Toth, P.P., 2016. Triglyceride-rich lipoproteins as a causal factor for cardiovascular disease. Vasc. Health Risk Manag. 12, 171–183.

Totti, N., Mccusker, K.T., Campbell, E.J., Griffin, G.L., Senior, R.M., 1984. Nicotine is chemotactic for neutrophils and enhances neutrophil responsiveness to chemotactic peptides. Science 223 (4632), 169–171.

Trivedi, A., Dave, B., Adhvaryu, S., 1990. Assessment of genotoxicity of nicotine employing in vitro mammalian test system. Cancer Lett. 54 (1–2), 89–94.

Trivedi, A., Dave, B., Adhvaryu, S., 1993. Genotoxic effects of nicotine in combination with arecoline on CHO cells. Cancer Lett. 74 (1), 105–110.

Tsai, J.-R., Chong, I.-W., Chen, C.-C., Lin, S.-R., Sheu, C.-C., Hwang, J.-J., 2006. Mitogen-activated protein kinase pathway was significantly activated in human bronchial epithelial cells by nicotine. DNA Cell Biol. 25 (5), 312–322.

U.S. Department of Health and Human Services, 2014. The Health Consequences of Smoking-50 Years of Progress: A Report of the Surgeon General. Centers for Disease Control, Atlanta (GA).

U.S. Environmental Protection Agency, 1996. EPA/630/R-96/009: Guidelines for Reproductive Toxicity Risk Assessment.

Us Department of Health and Human Services, 1989. The Surgeon General's 1989 Report on Reducing the Health Consequences of Smoking: 25 Years of Progress. A report of the Surgeon General.

Valavanidis, A., Vlachogianni, T., Fiotakis, C., 2009. 8-hydroxy-2'-deoxyguanosine (8-OHdG): a critical biomarker of oxidative stress and carcinogenesis. J. Environ. Sci. Health C 27 (2), 120–139.

Valavanidis, A., Vlachogianni, T., Fiotakis, K., Loridas, S., 2013. Pulmonary oxidative stress, inflammation and cancer: respirable particulate matter, fibrous dusts and ozone as major causes of lung carcinogenesis through reactive oxygen species mechanisms. Int. J. Environ. Res. Publ. Health 10 (9), 3886–3907.

Valença, S.S., Da Fonseca, A.D.S., Da Hora, K., Santos, R., Porto, L.C., 2004. Lung morphometry and MMP-12 expression in rats treated with intraperitoneal nicotine. Exp. Toxicol. Pathol. 55 (5), 393–400.

Van Vunakis, H., Langone, J.J., Milunsky, A., 1974. Nicotine and cotinine in the amniotic fluid of smokers in the second trimester of pregnancy. Am. J. Obstet. Gynecol. 120 (1), 64–66.

Vansickel, A.R., Cobb, C.O., Weaver, M.F., Eissenberg, T.E., 2010. A clinical laboratory model for evaluating the acute effects of electronic "cigarettes": nicotine delivery profile and cardiovascular and subjective effects. Cancer Epidemiol. Biomarkers Prev. 19 (8), 1945–1953.

Vassallo, R., Kroening, P.R., Parambil, J., Kita, H., 2008. Nicotine and oxidative cigarette smoke constituents induce immune-modulatory and pro-inflammatory dendritic cell responses. Mol. Immunol. 45 (12), 3321–3329.

Veldheer, S., Yingst, J., Midya, V., Hummer, B., Lester, C., Krebs, N., et al., 2019. Pulmonary and other health effects of electronic cigarette use among adult smokers participating in a randomized controlled smoking reduction trial. Addict. Behav. 91, 95–101.

Veljkovic, E., Xia, W., Phillips, B., Wong, E.T., Ho, J., Casado, A.O., et al., 2018. Nicotine and Other Tobacco Compounds in Neurodegenerative and Psychiatric Diseases: Overview of Epidemiological Data on Smoking and Preclinical and Clinical Data on Nicotine. Academic Press.

Verhoeven, E.L., Kapma, M.R., Groen, H., Tielliu, I.F., Zeebregts, C.J., Bekkema, F., et al., 2008. Mortality of ruptured abdominal aortic aneurysm treated with open or endovascular repair. J. Vasc. Surg. 48 (6), 1396–1400.

Vieyra, E., Ramirez, D.A., Linares, R., Rosas, G., Dominguez, R., Morales-Ledesma, L., 2019. Stimulation of nicotinic receptors in the suprachiasmatic nucleus results in a higher number of growing follicles and ova shed. Exp. Physiol. 104 (8), 1179–1189.

Vlachopoulos, C., Ioakeimidis, N., Abdelrasoul, M., Terentes-Printzios, D., Georgakopoulos, C., Pietri, P., et al., 2016. Electronic cigarette smoking increases aortic stiffness and blood pressure in young smokers. J. Am. Coll. Cardiol. 67 (23), 2802–2803.

Vrsanska, S., Nagyova, E., Mlynarcikova, A., Fickova, M., Kolena, J., 2003. Components of cigarette smoke inhibit expansion of oocyte-cumulus complexes from porcine follicles. Physiol. Res. 52 (3), 383–387.

Vukelic, M., Qing, X., Redecha, P., Koo, G., Salmon, J.E., 2013. Cholinergic receptors modulate immune complex–induced inflammation in vitro and in vivo. J. Immunol. 1203467.

Wagenhäuser, M.U., Schellinger, I.N., Yoshino, T., Toyama, K., Kayama, Y., Deng, A., et al., 2018. Chronic nicotine exposure induces murine aortic remodeling and stiffness segmentation-implications for abdominal aortic aneurysm susceptibility. Front. Physiol. 9, 1459.

Waggoner, L.E., Dickinson, K.A., Poole, D.S., Tabuse, Y., Miwa, J., Schafer, W.R., 2000. Long-term nicotine adaptation in *Caenorhabditis elegans* involves PKC-dependent changes in nicotinic receptor abundance. J. Neurosci. 20 (23), 8802–8811.

Wakai, K., Inoue, M., Mizoue, T., Tanaka, K., Tsuji, I., Nagata, C., et al., 2006. Tobacco smoking and lung cancer risk: an evaluation based on a systematic review of epidemiological evidence among the Japanese population. Jpn J. Clin. Oncol. 36 (5), 309–324.

Waldum, H.L., Nilsen, O.G., Nilsen, T., Rørvik, H., Syversen, U., Sandvik, A.K., et al., 1996. Long-term effects of inhaled nicotine. Life Sci. 58 (16), 1339–1346.

Wang, C., Chen, H., Zhu, W., Xu, Y., Liu, M., Zhu, L., et al., 2017a. Nicotine accelerates atherosclerosis in apolipoprotein E-deficient mice by activating α7 nicotinic acetylcholine receptor on mast cells. Arterioscler. Thromb. Vasc. Biol. 37 (1), 53–65.

Wang, D., Dubois, R.N., 2015. Immunosuppression associated with chronic inflammation in the tumor microenvironment. Carcinogenesis 36 (10), 1085–1093.

Wang, H., Gondre-Lewis, M.C., 2013. Prenatal nicotine and maternal deprivation stress de-regulate the development of CA1, CA3, and dentate gyrus neurons in hippocampus of infant rats. PLoS One 8 (6), e65517.

Wang, P., Chen, W., Liao, J., Matsuo, T., Ito, K., Fowles, J., et al., 2017b. A device-independent evaluation of carbonyl emissions from heated electronic cigarette solvents. PLoS One 12 (1), e0169811.

Wang, S., Takayama, K., Tanaka, K., Takeshita, M., Nakagaki, N., Ijichi, K., et al., 2013. Nicotine induces resistance to epidermal growth factor receptor tyrosine kinase inhibitor by α1 nicotinic acetylcholine receptor–mediated activation in PC9 cells. J. Thorac. Oncol. 8 (6), 719–725.

Wang, S., Xu, J., Song, P., Wu, Y., Zhang, J., Chul Choi, H., et al., 2008. Acute inhibition of guanosine triphosphate cyclohydrolase 1 uncouples endothelial nitric oxide synthase and elevates blood pressure. Hypertension 52 (3), 484–490.

Wang, S., Zhang, C., Zhang, M., Liang, B., Zhu, H., Lee, J., et al., 2012. Activation of AMP-activated protein kinase alpha2 by nicotine instigates formation of abdominal aortic aneurysms in mice in vivo. Nat. Med. 18 (6), 902–910.

Wang, Y.Y., Liu, Y., Ni, X.Y., Bai, Z.H., Chen, Q.Y., Zhang, Y., et al., 2014. Nicotine promotes cell proliferation and induces resistance to cisplatin by α7 nicotinic acetylcholine receptor-mediated activation in Raw264. 7 and El4 cells. Oncol. Rep. 31 (3), 1480–1488.

Wang, Z., Liu, B., Zhu, J., Wang, D., Wang, Y., 2019. Nicotine-mediated autophagy of vascular smooth muscle cell accelerates atherosclerosis via nAChRs/ROS/NF-κB signaling pathway. Atherosclerosis 284, 1–10.

Ward, P.A., 2010. Acute and Chronic Inflammation. Fundamentals of Inflammation, pp. 1–16.

Weathersbee, P.S., 1980. Nicotine and its influence on the female reproductive system. J. Reprod. Med. 25 (5), 243–250.

Wei, Y., Lai, B., Liu, H., Li, Y., Zhen, W., Fu, L., 2018. Effect of cigarette smoke extract and nicotine on the expression of thrombomodulin and endothelial protein C receptor in cultured human umbilical vein endothelial cells. Mol. Med. Rep. 17 (1), 1724–1730.

Wessler, I., Schwarze, S., Brockerhoff, P., Bittinger, F., Kirkpatrick, C.J., Kilbinger, H., 2003. Effects of sex hormones, forskolin, and nicotine on choline acetyltransferase activity in human isolated placenta. Neurochem. Res. 28 (3–4), 489–492.

West, K.A., Brognard, J., Clark, A.S., Linnoila, I.R., Yang, X., Swain, S.M., et al., 2003. Rapid Akt activation by nicotine and a tobacco carcinogen modulates the phenotype of normal human airway epithelial cells. J. Clin. Invest. 111 (1), 81–90.

Wetendorf, M., Randall, L.T., Lemma, M.T., Hurr, S.H., Pawlak, J.B., Tarran, R., et al., 2019. E-cigarette exposure delays implantation and causes reduced weight gain in female offspring exposed in utero. J. Endocr. Soc. 3 (10), 1907–1916.

Whiss, P.A., Lundahl, T.H., Bengtsson, T., Lindahl, T.L., Lunell, E., Larsson, R., 2000. Acute effects of nicotine infusion on platelets in nicotine users with normal and impaired renal function. Toxicol. Appl. Pharmacol. 163 (2), 95–104.

WHO, 2016. Electronic Nicotine Delivery Systems and Electronic Non-Nicotine Delivery Systems (ENDS/ENNDS) Report.

Wolk, R., Shamsuzzaman, A.S., Svatikova, A., Huyber, C.M., Huck, C., Narkiewicz, K., et al., 2005. Hemodynamic and autonomic effects of smokeless tobacco in healthy young men. J. Am. Coll. Cardiol. 45 (6), 910–914.

Wollman, L.B., Haggerty, J., Pilarski, J.Q., Levine, R.B., Fregosi, R.F., 2016. Developmental nicotine exposure alters cholinergic control of respiratory frequency in neonatal rats. Dev. Neurobiol. 76 (10), 1138–1149.

Wong, E.T., Kogel, U., Veljkovic, E., Martin, F., Xiang, Y., Boue, S., et al., 2016a. Evaluation of the tobacco heating system 2.2. Part 4: 90-day OECD 413 rat inhalation study with systems toxicology endpoints demonstrates reduced exposure effects compared with cigarette smoke. Regul. Toxicol. Pharmacol. 81 (Suppl. 2), S59–s81.

Wong, E.T., Luettich, K., Krishnan, S., Wong, S.K., Lim, W.T., Yeo, D., et al., 2020. Reduced chronic toxicity and carcinogenicity in A/J mice in response to life-time exposure to aerosol from a heated tobacco product compared with cigarette smoke. Toxicol. Sci. https://doi.org/10.1093/toxsci/kfaa131. Epub ahead of print 2020/08/12.

Wong, M.K., Holloway, A.C., Hardy, D.B., 2016b. Nicotine directly induces endoplasmic reticulum stress response in rat placental trophoblast giant cells. Toxicol. Sci. 151 (1), 23–34.

Wongtrakool, C., Grooms, K., Bijli, K.M., Crothers, K., Fitzpatrick, A.M., Hart, C.M., 2014. Nicotine stimulates nerve growth factor in lung fibroblasts through an NFκB-dependent mechanism. PLoS One 9 (10), e109602.

Wongtrakool, C., Roser-Page, S., Rivera, H.N., Roman, J., 2007. Nicotine alters lung branching morphogenesis through the alpha7 nicotinic acetylcholine receptor. Am. J. Physiol. Lung Cell Mol. Physiol. 293 (3), L611–L618.

Wright, S., Zhong, J., Zheng, H., Larrick, J., 1993. Nicotine inhibition of apoptosis suggests a role in tumor promotion. FASEB.J. 7 (11), 1045–1051.

Wu, H.-J., Chi, C.-W., Liu, T.-Y., 2005. Effects of pH on nicotine-induced DNA damage and oxidative stress. J. Toxicol. Environ. Health A. 68 (17–18), 1511–1523.

Wu, H.-T., Ko, S.-Y., Fong, J.H.-J., Chang, K.-W., Liu, T.-Y., Kao, S.-Y., 2009. Expression of phosphorylated Akt in oral carcinogenesis and its induction by nicotine and alkaline stimulation. J. Oral Pathol. Med. 38 (2), 206–213.

Wu, J., Xu, W., Zhang, D., Dai, J., Cao, Y., Xie, Y., et al., 2019. Nicotine inhibits murine Leydig cell differentiation and maturation via regulating Hedgehog signal pathway. Biochem. Biophys. Res. Commun. 510 (1), 1–7.

Wu, X., Zhang, H., Qi, W., Zhang, Y., Li, J., Li, Z., et al., 2018. Nicotine promotes atherosclerosis via ROS-NLRP3-mediated endothelial cell pyroptosis. Cell Death Dis. 9 (2), 171.

Wuenschell, C., Kunimi, M., Castillo, C., Marjoram, P., 2004. Nicotine-responsive genes in cultured embryonic mouse lung buds: interaction of nicotine and superoxide dismutase. Pharmacol. Res. 50 (3), 341–350.

Wuenschell, C.W., Zhao, J., Tefft, J.D., Warburton, D., 1998. Nicotine stimulates branching and expression of SP-A and SP-C mRNAs in embryonic mouse lung culture. Am. J. Physiol. 274 (1), L165–L170.

Xiao, D., Huang, X., Yang, S., Zhang, L., 2007. Direct effects of nicotine on contractility of the uterine artery in pregnancy. J. Pharmacol. Exp. Therapeut. 322 (1), 180–185.

Xiao, H., Wen, Y., Pan, Z., Shangguan, Y., Magdalou, J., Wang, H., et al., 2019. Nicotine exposure during pregnancy programs osteopenia in male offspring rats via alpha4-beta2-nAChR-p300-ACE pathway. FASEB J. 33 (11), 12972–12982.

Xiong, W., Mactaggart, J., Knispel, R., Worth, J., Persidsky, Y., Baxter, B.T., 2009. Blocking TNF-alpha attenuates aneurysm formation in a murine model. J. Immunol. 183 (4), 2741–2746.

Xu, Y., Cardell, L.-O., 2017. Long-term nicotine exposure dampens LPS-induced nerve-mediated airway hyperreactivity in murine airways. Am. J. Physiol. Lung Cell Mol. Physiol. 313 (3), L516–L523.

Xu, Y., Zhang, Y., Cardell, L.-O., 2010. Nicotine enhances murine airway contractile responses to kinin receptor agonists via activation of JNK- and PDE4-related intracellular pathways. Respir. Res. 11 (1), 13.

Xu, Y., Zhang, Y., Cardell, L.-O., 2014. Nicotine exaggerates LPS-induced airway hyperreactivity via JNK-mediated up-regulation of toll-like receptor 4. Am. J. Respir. Cell Mol. Biol. 51 (3), 370–379.

Xue, C., Chen, Q.Z., Bian, L., Yin, Z.F., Xu, Z.J., Zhang, A.L., et al., 2019. Effects of smoking cessation with nicotine replacement therapy on vascular endothelial function, arterial stiffness, and inflammation response in healthy smokers. Biosci. Rep. 70 (8), 719–725.

Yan, X.S., D'ruiz, C., 2015. Effects of using electronic cigarettes on nicotine delivery and cardiovascular function in comparison with regular cigarettes. Regul. Toxicol. Pharmacol. 71 (1), 24–34.

Yanagita, M., Kobayashi, R., Kojima, Y., Mori, K., Murakami, S., 2012. Nicotine modulates the immunological function of dendritic cells through peroxisome proliferator-activated receptor-γ upregulation. Cell. Immunol. 274 (1–2), 26–33.

Yang, I.A., Relan, V., Wright, C.M., Davidson, M.R., Sriram, K.B., Savarimuthu Francis, S.M., et al., 2011. Common pathogenic mechanisms and pathways in the development of COPD and lung cancer. Expert Opin. Ther. Targets 15 (4), 439–456.

Yang, J., Zeng, P., Liu, L., Yu, M., Su, J., Yan, Y., et al., 2020. Food with calorie restriction reduces the development of atherosclerosis in apoE-deficient mice. Biochem. Biophys. Res. Commun. 524 (2), 439–445.

Ye, Y.N., Liu, E.S.L., Shin, V.Y., Wu, W.K.K., Luo, J.C., Cho, C.H., 2004. Nicotine promoted colon cancer growth via epidermal growth factor receptor, c-Src, and 5-lipoxygenase-mediated signal pathway. J. Pharmacol. Exp. Therapeut. 308 (1), 66–72.

Yeager, T.R., Devries, S., Jarrard, D.F., Kao, C., Nakada, S.Y., Moon, T.D., et al., 1998. Overcoming cellular senescence in human cancer pathogenesis. Genes Dev. 12 (2), 163–174.

Yeh, J., Barbieri, R.L., Friedman, A.J., 1989. Nicotine and cotinine inhibit rat testis androgen biosynthesis in vitro. J. Steroid Biochem. 33 (4A), 627–630.

Yildiz, D., 2004. Comparison of pure nicotine and smokeless tobacco extract induced formation of 8-OH-dG. Toxicol. Mech. Methods 14 (4), 253–256.

Yildiz, D., Liu, Y.-S., Ercal, N., Armstrong, D.W., 1999. Comparison of pure nicotine-and smokeless tobacco extract-induced toxicities and oxidative stress. Arch. Environ. Contam. Toxicol. 37 (4), 434–439.

Yim, S.H., Hee, S.S.Q., 1995. Genotoxicity of nicotine and cotinine in the bacterial luminescence test. Mutat. Res. Environ. Mutagen Relat. Subj. 335 (3), 275–283.

Ylikorkala, O., Viinikka, L., Lehtovirta, P., 1985. Effect of nicotine on fetal prostacyclin and thromboxane in humans. Obstet. Gynecol. 66 (1), 102–105.

Yokohira, M., Nakano, Y., Hashimoto, N., Yamakawa, K., Ninomiya, F., Kishi, S., et al., 2012. Toxicity of nicotine by repeated intratracheal instillation to f344 rats. J. Toxicol. Pathol. 25 (4), 257–263.

Yoshinaga, K., Rice, C., Krenn, J., Pilot, R.L., 1979. Effects of nicotine on early pregnancy in the rat. Biol. Reprod. 20 (2), 294–303.

Yu, R., Wu, M., Lin, S., Talbot, P., 2006. Cigarette smoke toxicants alter growth and survival of cultured mammalian cells. Toxicol. Sci. 93 (1), 82–95.

Zanetti, F., Giacomello, M., Donati, Y., Carnesecchi, S., Frieden, M., Barazzone-Argiroffo, C., 2014. Nicotine mediates oxidative stress and apoptosis through cross talk between NOX1 and Bcl-2 in lung epithelial cells. Free Radic. Biol. Med. 76, 173–184.

Zdravkovic, T., Genbacev, O., Larocque, N., Mcmaster, M., Fisher, S., 2008. Human embryonic stem cells as a model system for studying the effects of smoke exposure on the embryo. Reprod. Toxicol. 26 (2), 86–93.

Zeinivand, M., Rahmani, M.R., Allatavakoli, M., Shamsizadeh, A., Hassanshahi, G., Rezazadeh, H., et al., 2013. Effect of co-administration of morphine and nicotine on cardiovascular function in two-kidney one clip hypertensive (2K1C) rats. Bosn. J. Basic Med. Sci. 13 (3), 140–145.

Zenzes, M.T., Bielecki, R., 2004. Nicotine-induced disturbances of meiotic maturation in cultured mouse oocytes: alterations of spindle integrity and chromosome alignment. Tob. Induc. Dis. 2 (3), 151–161.

Zenzes, M.T., Reed, T.E., Wang, P., Klein, J., 1996. Cotinine, a major metabolite of nicotine, is detectable in follicular fluids of passive smokers in in vitro fertilization therapy. Fertil. Steril. 66 (4), 614−619.

Zevin, S., Jacob 3rd, P., Benowitz, N.L., 1998. Dose-related cardiovascular and endocrine effects of transdermal nicotine. Clin. Pharmacol. Ther. 64 (1), 87−95.

Zhang, H., Cai, B., 2003. The impact of tobacco on lung health in China. Respirology 8 (1), 17−21.

Zhang, C., Fan, S.J., Sun, A.B., Liu, Z.Z., Liu, L., 2019a. Prenatal nicotine exposure induces depression-like behavior in adolescent female rats via modulating neurosteroid in the hippocampus. Mol. Med. Rep. 19 (5), 4185−4194.

Zhang, G., Zhou, J., Huang, W., Yu, L., Zhang, Y., Wang, H., 2018. Placental mechanism of prenatal nicotine exposure-reduced blood cholesterol levels in female fetal rats. Toxicol. Lett. 296, 31−38.

Zhang, Q., Pei, L.G., Liu, M., Lv, F., Chen, G., Wang, H., 2020. Reduced testicular steroidogenesis in rat offspring by prenatal nicotine exposure: epigenetic programming and heritability via nAChR/HDAC4. Food Chem. Toxicol. 135, 111057.

Zhang, Y., Chen, Y., Zhang, Y., Li, P.L., Li, X., 2019b. Contribution of cathepsin B-dependent Nlrp3 inflammasome activation to nicotine-induced endothelial barrier dysfunction. Eur. J. Pharmacol. 865, 172795.

Zhao, X., Xu, W., Wu, J., Zhang, D., Abou-Shakra, A., Di, L., et al., 2018. Nicotine induced autophagy of Leydig cells rather than apoptosis is the major reason of the decrease of serum testosterone. Int. J. Biochem. Cell Biol. 100, 30−41.

Zhao, Z., Reece, E.A., 2005. Nicotine-induced embryonic malformations mediated by apoptosis from increasing intracellular calcium and oxidative stress. Birth Defects Res. B Dev. Reprod. Toxicol. 74 (5), 383−391.

Zhou, J., Liu, F., Yu, L., Xu, D., Li, B., Zhang, G., et al., 2018. nAChRs-ERK1/2-Egr-1 signaling participates in the developmental toxicity of nicotine by epigenetically down-regulating placental 11beta-HSD2. Toxicol. Appl. Pharmacol. 344, 1−12.

Zhou, X., Sheng, Y., Yang, R., Kong, X., 2010. Nicotine promotes cardiomyocyte apoptosis via oxidative stress and altered apoptosis-related gene expression. Cardiology 115 (4), 243−250.

Zhuo, C., Hui-Li, L., 2017. Restoration of miR-1305 relieves the inhibitory effect of nicotine on periodontal ligament-derived stem cell proliferation, migration, and osteogenic differentiation. J. Oral Pathol. Med. 46 (4), 313−320.

Zirak, M.R., Mehri, S., Karimani, A., Zeinali, M., Hayes, A.W., Karimi, G., 2019. Mechanisms behind the atherothrombotic effects of acrolein, a review. Food Chem. Toxicol. 129, 38−53.

Zou, W., Zou, Y., Zhao, Z., Li, B., Ran, P., 2013. Nicotine-induced epithelial-mesenchymal transition via Wnt/β-catenin signaling in human airway epithelial cells. Am. J. Physiol. Lung Cell Mol. Physiol. 304 (4), L199−L209.

CHAPTER 21

Conclusions and Outlook

JULIA HOENG • MANUEL C. PEITSCH

21.1 INTRODUCTION

The purpose of tobacco harm reduction (THR) is to accelerate the reduction in smoking-related population harm, recognizing that millions of smokers would otherwise continue to smoke. It does so by complementing measures for reducing smoking prevalence—especially those that deter initiation and encourage cessation—with measures that reduce exposure to toxicants in smokers who would otherwise not quit smoking. The goal is to provide these smokers with alternative products that emit significantly lower levels of toxicants than cigarettes and are, therefore, less harmful than cigarettes. Electronic nicotine delivery products (ENDPs) are intended to be such alternatives. However, it is well understood that these products are not risk-free and deliver nicotine, which is addictive. For this reason, ENDPs are only intended for current adult smokers or users who would otherwise continue to use tobacco- or nicotine-containing products.

For an ENDP to qualify as a less harmful alternative to cigarettes, it is of utmost importance that it has been scientifically proven to emit and expose users to significantly lower level of toxicants and to cause significantly less adverse effects than cigarettes. In the context of the ENDP assessment framework (Chapter 3), it means that the effects of switching from cigarette smoking to ENDP use must approach those of cessation. Because smoking cessation is the most effective way to reduce the risk of smoking-related harm and disease, it is the "gold standard" for scientific assessment of ENDPs (Institute of Medicine, 2012). Furthermore, the scientific assessment of an ENDP should not uncover new adverse health effects.

After a brief introduction to THR and the key parameters of the equation that influence harm reduction policies (Chapter 1), this book summarizes current scientific evidence showing that ENDPs, briefly defined in Chapter 2, have the potential to be less harmful than cigarettes. While much of the evidence is based on the assessment of an electrically heated tobacco product (EHTP)—Tobacco Heating System 2.2, developed and assessed

by Philip Morris International—the evidence presented in this book reflects the collective outcome of scientifically sound and rigorous studies conducted within an ENDP assessment framework built on the basis of two key principles (Chapter 3): (i) the well-known and well-documented epidemiology of smoking and cessation and (ii) the fundamental principle (or the Natural Law) of toxicology. Importantly, the principle and mechanisms of toxicology explain the known epidemiology of smoking and smoking cessation and can be expressed as a causal chain of events that link smoking to disease (CELSD) (Chapter 3) (Fig. 20.1). The CELSD serves as a guide upon which a comprehensive assessment program for ENDPs can be developed (Chapter 3) (Fig. 20.1). Such an assessment program is enabled by modern systems toxicology approaches (Hoeng et al., 2012; Sturla et al., 2014) (Chapter 9)—derived from the fundamental principles of systems biology (Ideker et al., 2001)—that can be applied to varying degrees to in vitro, in vivo, and clinical studies. Importantly, such a systems-based approach provides a sound scientific basis for addressing some of the key challenges faced in the assessment of ENDPs (Chapter 3):

A. The most prevalent smoking-related diseases generally occur after decades of smoking, and the reduction in excess risk following smoking cessation and, a fortiori, switching to ENDPs is slow and depends upon an individual's smoking history.

B. Smoking affects several organ systems and multiple biological mechanisms so that no single endpoint can inform, on its own, about the relative risk of ENDPs in comparison with that of cigarettes.

21.2 CONCLUSIONS OF THE TOXICOLOGICAL ASSESSMENT OF ENDPS

The totality of the scientific evidence available for the assessed ENDPs shows that they emit reduced levels of toxicants, which leads to reduced toxicant exposure,

Toxicological Evaluation of Electronic Nicotine Delivery Products. https://doi.org/10.1016/B978-0-12-820490-0.00013-4

which, in turn, leads to reduced toxicity and, consequently, reduced adverse health effects (Fig. 21.1). The evidence is remarkably consistent across all sound scientific studies and coherent along the CELSD (Fig. 21.1). This is not surprising given the natural law of toxicology and the epidemiology of smoking and cessation (Chapter 3).

21.2.1 Emission of Toxicants

The central tenet of THR is that ENDPs must be designed to and actually emit significantly lower levels

of toxicants than cigarettes. This is the first event in the CELSD (Chapter 3). Therefore, as outlined in Chapter 2, the fundamental design objective of ENDPs is to reduce and, to the extent possible, eliminate the emission of toxicants while maintaining a satisfactory level of nicotine delivery and product features that enable smokers who would not quit to completely switch to ENDPs. In fact, ENDPs that avoid combustion of tobacco have been shown to emit significantly lower levels of toxicants than cigarettes. This covers not only

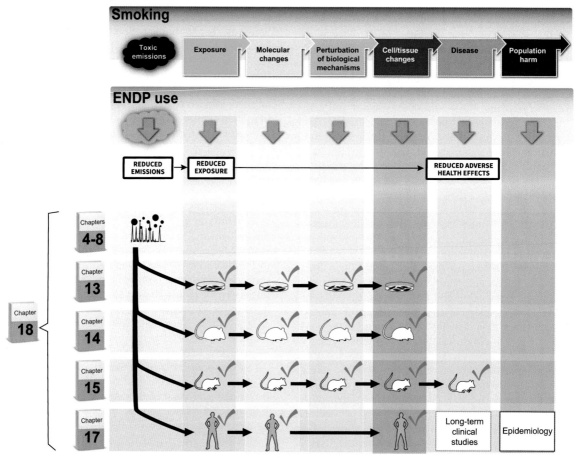

FIG. 21.1 The totality of the scientific evidence mapped to the CELSD. The available, sound scientific evidence regarding aerosol chemistry and physics (Chapters 4–8), in vitro toxicology (Chapter 13), in vivo toxicology (Chapter 14), animal models of disease (Chapter 15), and clinical studies (Chapter 17) is reviewed in the context of the main smoking-related diseases (Chapter 18). The reduction in toxicant emissions by ENDPs leads to a coherent reduction in toxicant exposure. This reduction in toxicant exposure leads to a coherent reduction in all events along the CELSD that is consistent across all studies and mechanisms activated by cigarette smoke exposure. Long-term clinical studies (orange box) are necessary to further substantiate and quantify the disease risk reduction potential in humans, and epidemiological studies are needed to quantify the net population benefits of ENDPs. *Black arrows*, causally coherent link; *green tick marks*, reduced effect of ENDP aerosol relative to cigarette smoke; *CELSD*, causal chain of events linking smoking to disease; *ENDP*, electronic nicotine delivery product.

the harmful and potentially harmful constituents of cigarette smoke listed by authorities (Chapter 4) but also a much broader range of substances (Chapter 6), including carbon-based solid nanoparticles and free radicals (Chapter 7). Moreover, the reduction in toxicant emissions by ENDPs also leads, in principle, to a reduced impact on indoor air quality relative to cigarettes, when used by consumers in both experimental and real-world environments (Chapter 8). ENDPs also generate aerosols that are respirable but may dissipate more quickly than cigarette smoke (Chapter 5).

21.2.2 Exposure to Toxicants

A significant reduction in toxicant emission by ENDPs should lead to an equally significant reduction in toxicant exposure. This is the second event in the CELSD (Chapter 3). Studies in animal models of disease (Chapter 15) and, most importantly, human subjects (Chapter 17) have consistently shown that switching from cigarette smoking to the investigated ENDPs led to reduced toxicant exposure relative to cigarette smoking. These exposure reductions were consistent across all studies and, importantly, coherent with the degree of reduction in toxicant emissions by the tested ENDP. In studies that included a smoking abstinence arm, switching achieved an exposure reduction that approached that of cessation, which is the maximum exposure reduction a smoker can achieve (Chapter 17). Furthermore, the significantly lower impact of ENDP use on indoor air quality (relative to cigarette smoking) (Chapter 8) also leads to a significantly lower exposure to cigarette smoke—specific constituents in bystanders (Chapter 19).

21.2.3 Aerosol Toxicity

A significant reduction in toxicant exposure leads to an equally significant reduction in molecular changes and, hence, reduces the amplitude of perturbation of the biological mechanisms that cause changes at the cellular and tissue level. The reduction of such changes, in turn, causes a reduction in physiological changes. These causally linked events of the CELSD have been assessed in vitro, in vivo, and in clinical studies (Chapter 3). Nonclinical studies aimed at comparing the effects of ENDP aerosols with those of cigarette smoke and fresh air are collectively known as toxicology studies and must be conducted by following international guidelines and sound scientific principles. They should also employ validated measurement methods. Importantly, nonclinical studies should be designed to compare the effects of an ENDP aerosol with those of cigarette smoke and fresh air and, when feasible, also compare the effects of switching from cigarette smoke to ENDP aerosol

exposure with those of continued cigarette smoke exposure and cessation in vivo (Phillips et al., 2016) and in vitro (Ito et al., 2020). Such "switching studies" are the closest analog to the human situation, as ENDPs are intended for smokers who do not quit. Furthermore, it is crucial that nonclinical model systems be exposed to cigarette smoke and ENDP aerosol concentrations that are reflective of realistic human exposure (Chapters 10 and 11). In fact, particular care has to be given to aerosol generation and exposure in nonclinical studies to ensure that study results can be linked to a well-understood exposure concentration (Chapter 12) and are relevant for human translation (Chapter 10). Clinical studies should also follow accepted international guidelines and be designed to compare the effects of switching to an ENDP with those of continued smoking and cessation. Importantly, clinical studies should monitor product use and exposure by using biomarkers of exposure to allow objective assessment of product use by study participants and, thereby, account for the effects of dual use.

Studies conducted by following these principles have shown that the aerosols generated by the investigated ENDPs are less toxic than cigarette smoke in vitro (Chapter 13) and in vivo (Chapters 14 and 15) across a wide range of biological mechanisms and endpoints at the cellular, tissue, and physiological levels. These studies have also shown that the effects of switching approach those of cessation in vitro (Ito et al., 2020) and in vivo (Phillips et al., 2016) (Chapter 15). Moreover, a 6-month clinical study conducted with an ENDP has shown that switching from cigarette smoking to ENDP use led to positive changes in a number of biomarkers of potential harm (BoPHs) (Chapter 17) that are aligned with the effects of smoking cessation.

Importantly, the totality of the evidence shows that the reduced effects of the assessed ENDP aerosols, relative to those of cigarette smoke, are consistent across a broad range of biological mechanisms known to be affected by cigarette smoke. Furthermore, the observed reductions in toxicity were coherent with the reduced levels of toxicants emitted by the tested ENDPs (relative to cigarettes) and the ensuing reductions in toxicant exposure. These results are in full agreement with the fundamental principle of toxicology and the epidemiology of smoking and cessation (Chapter 3).

Finally, the totality of the evidence available to date does not indicate that switching from cigarette smoking to ENDP use leads to new identifiable health risks when ENDPs are designed to heat tobacco or an e-liquid and only contain ingredients—such as nicotine, glycerin, propylene glycol, and small amounts of flavoring substances—that have been shown to cause little toxicity on their own (Chapter 16).

21.2.4 ENDP Aerosols and Disease Manifestations In Vivo

Epidemiological evidence shows that smoking-related diseases generally occur after decades of smoking and that the reduction in excess risk following smoking cessation is slow (Chapter 3). This means that clinical health outcome studies that aim to assess the reduction in disease risk associated with switching from cigarette smoking to ENDP use are difficult to execute in a premarket setting. The use of animal models of disease is a way to address this challenge, as they permit the long-term and life-long studies necessary for observing the disease manifestations caused by cigarette smoke exposure. By applying a systems-based approach to toxicology, studies in animal models of disease can also be ideal for collecting a broad and diverse dataset relevant to all events of the CELSD (Chapters 3 and 9). Therefore, combining systems toxicology with animal models of disease enables comprehensive evaluation of the effects of an ENDP aerosol relative to those of cigarette smoke across all causally linked events of the CELSD, from exposure to disease manifestation, at the molecular, mechanistic, cell, tissue, and physiological levels (Chapter 15). However, it is crucial to understand the similarities and differences between these animal models and human biology to ensure proper species translation (Chapter 10).

Studies conducted with animal models of disease consistently show that the aerosols generated by the investigated ENDPs cause fewer disease manifestations than cigarette smoke (Chapters 15 and 18). These studies also reveal the remarkable consistency of the reduced effects of ENDP aerosols relative to cigarette smoke across all steps of the CELSD, in complete alignment with the fundamental principle of toxicology and the epidemiology of smoking and cessation.

21.3 OUTLOOK

Although toxicological evaluation of ENDPs has made great progress in recent years, many questions remain to be answered and require more research, possibly by using new approaches. This section mentions just a few of them.

21.3.1 Long-term Human Studies and Epidemiology

The final demonstration of the risk reduction potential of ENDPs will undoubtedly come from long-term studies in human populations (Fig. 21.1). Furthermore, such studies are necessary to confirm that ENDPs do not cause novel health risks that are not associated with cigarette smoking and, ultimately, to quantify the true health risks associated with long-term use of nicotine dissociated from smoke and other potential toxicants (Chapter 20). Epidemiological studies might also provide insights into the effects of product use patterns on net population benefits.

First, disease risk reduction studies could be conducted on the major smoking-related diseases—cardiovascular disease (CVD), chronic obstructive pulmonary disease (COPD), and lung cancer—to assess the effects of switching to an ENDP relative to those of continued smoking and cessation. Such studies are complex and will need to account for factors such as adherence to the use of a specific ENDP as well as changes in lifestyle and product use patterns during the course of the studies. While these studies will take time, there are already some encouraging signs emerging from an exploratory analysis of a 12-month extension of a 6-month switching study conducted with a specific ENDP (Chapter 17) (Ansari et al., 2019). This analysis showed that study subjects with mild to moderate COPD who predominantly used the investigated ENDP displayed more pronounced positive changes (shifting in the direction of smoking cessation) in BoPHs than the predominantly healthy general study population. The BoPHs included in this analysis, relevant to respiratory and CVD mechanisms, were forced expiratory volume in 1 s (FEV$_1$), white blood cell counts, and soluble intercellular adhesion molecule 1 and 8-epi-prostaglandin F2α levels.

In addition to long-term clinical studies in the major smoking-related diseases, there are also emerging opportunities to conduct more short-term human harm reduction studies. For instance, Crohn's disease (CD) is worsened by smoking (Berkowitz et al., 2018; Chong et al., 2019), and smoking cessation has been shown to reduce disease severity within a reasonable time frame (Cosnes et al., 2001; Lewis et al., 2007). There is also emerging data showing that use of e-vapor products (EVPs) might lead to a less severe form of the disease in CD patients (Chong et al., 2019). Furthermore, it has been shown that cigarette smokers have a higher risk of bone fracture (Kanis et al., 2005; Shen et al., 2015; Ward and Klesges, 2001; Wu et al., 2016), and smoking cessation improves bone density over time (Ward and Klesges, 2001). Additionally, in vivo studies conducted in mice have shown that cigarette smoke significantly deteriorates bone integrity and biomechanical properties (Akhter et al., 2005; Reumann et al., 2020) and reduces callus formation during bone healing (El-Zawawy et al., 2006). Conversely, exposure to the aerosol of certain EVPs was shown to have a significantly reduced effect on bone integrity and biomechanical properties relative to cigarette smoke (Reumann et al., 2020). Taken together, CD and bone fracture and healing may represent opportunities for further assessing the harm reduction potential of ENDPs.

Second, epidemiological studies can be conducted once ENDPs have been adopted by a sizable portion of smokers and have been available in the market long enough to have a measureable effect on smoking-related disease incidence and related mortality. For such studies to be feasible, however, recording of specific product use, at least at a category level, is a prerequisite. Under current practices, tobacco users are generally recorded as "smoker," "former smoker," "nonsmoker," and, in some cases, "smokeless tobacco user." These categories are not sufficient to enable epidemiological studies on ENDPs, and it is necessary to include additional use categories reflective of available ENDPs to assess their population-level effect and, thereby, verify the predictions of various population health impact models (Lee et al., 2020).

Ecological studies have been used to assess the impact of air pollution on population health. In cases where a measurable change in air pollution was induced by a specific event, such studies could effectively assess the impact of changes in air pollution on several population health parameters. For example, several studies reported on the health impact of the air pollution changes induced by pollution control policies during the 2008 Olympic Games in Beijing (Schleicher et al., 2011). These studies showed, for instance, that the reduction in air pollution due to the air quality control measures implemented for the duration of the games led to a temporarily decreased risk of CVD mortality (Su et al., 2015), and asthma (Li et al., 2010) as well as an increase in birth weight (Huang et al., 2015; Rich et al., 2015). Such ecological studies could also be performed in an attempt to correlate the effect of ENDP market introductions with potential health effects at the population level. Possibly the most striking example of a shift in product use prevalence (from cigarettes to ENDPs) caused by the market introduction of ENDPs has recently been observed in Japan, where an accelerated decline in cigarette sales was associated with the market introduction and increasing sales of EHTPs and hybrid products (Cummings et al., 2020). This shift in product use prevalence offers a unique "natural experiment" for assessing the effect of ENDPs on public health parameters. For example, these products emit very low levels of carbon monoxide (CO) relative to cigarettes (Chapters 4 and 17), and, as CO is a key cardiovascular toxicant that

has been associated with CVD (Liu et al., 2018; Yang et al., 1998), one would expect to observe a measurable reduction in hospitalization for cardiovascular events in Japan. Therefore, conducting such studies will help generate early insights into the actual population harm reduction potential of ENDPs.

21.3.2 Product Innovation

As outlined at the beginning of this book (Chapter 1, Section 1.5.2.1), product innovation is faced with a multiobjective optimization challenge, which involves minimizing product harm while maximizing product acceptance by smokers who would not otherwise quit. At the same time, the product should be as minimally attractive as possible to former and never smokers, including youth. These challenges define the role of product innovation by setting the objectives for product developers. First and foremost, future ENDPs should be further optimized from a toxicological perspective. This means that developers should aim to further reduce toxicant emissions and, importantly, ensure that flavors and other ingredients are selected from a list of substances that have been adequately assessed to understand their maximum allowable use levels through inhalation (Chapter 16). Second, products should be further developed to improve smoker acceptance and, thereby, increase their likelihood of switching if they do not quit. Third, systems for preventing youth access should be developed and embedded with the ENDPs to minimize unintended consequences. However, developing an ENDP with zero risk that is acceptable to all smokers remains a utopia. Therefore, ENDPs will never be risk-free. They deliver nicotine, which is addictive.

21.3.3 Further Nonclinical Assessment Studies

To date, the evidence from scientifically sound nonclinical studies does not indicate that ENDPs will cause new toxic effects that are not already known to be associated with cigarette smoking and/or nicotine. This evidence is based on the observation that switching from cigarette smoking to ENDP use leads to a consistent reduction in the perturbation of all biological mechanisms affected by cigarette smoke exposure. This is coherent with the reduction in toxicant exposure induced by switching. However, it is necessary to further study the effects of ENDPs, and especially their ingredients, to evaluate their residual long-term risk. This need is accentuated given the diversity of ENDPs that are emerging on the market. For instance, long-term use of ENDPs should be assessed for reproductive toxicological effects in comparison with cigarette smoking, and flavoring substances and other ingredients should be assessed for allergic sensitization before being used in ENDPs. Furthermore, novel in vitro approaches should be developed with the aim of extending the battery of available in vitro model systems (Chapter 13) and covering a broader spectrum of pathophysiological mechanisms that are relevant to ENDP assessment, thereby reducing the need for animal testing (see below).

21.3.4 Development of Novel Approaches for ENDP Assessment

Toxicological assessment of ENDPs relies heavily on rodent studies, including rats and mice. While the former are mainly used for studies aligned with regulatory guidelines for safety toxicology (Chapter 14), the latter are mostly used as animal models of disease (Chapter 15). While species translation has its challenges (Chapters 10 and 15), comparison of the effects of cigarette smoke with those of ENDP aerosols in animal models remains invaluable because of the fact that cigarette smoke affects a very broad range of biological mechanisms, many of which involve multiple cell types and organs. However, this is not a sustainable approach, and the aim is to gradually replace animal testing with alternative methods that are relevant to human health and biology.

Therefore, the need for ENDP assessment drives novel developments in a number of areas, such as new analytical chemistry methodologies for determining the composition of ENDP aerosols (Knorr et al., 2019) as well as new physicochemical approaches (Sosnowski et al., 2019) and adverse outcome pathways of defined disease mechanisms (Lowe et al., 2017; Luettich et al., 2017) for evaluating the effects of these aerosols on biological systems. The assessment needs also drive developments at the interface between engineering and in vitro research (Hoeng et al., 2020; Marx et al., 2020; Schimek et al., 2020). These developments are enabled by advances in three-dimensional printing and microfluidics as well as by the development of complex in vitro cultures involving multiple cell types (Marescotti et al., 2019) and organotypic tissue cultures that mimic human airway epithelia and the response of human airways to cigarette smoke (Mathis et al., 2013). This has led to the recent development of microphysiological systems that can be used to assess the effects of ENDP aerosols on mechanisms relevant to CVDs (Poussin et al., 2020) and liver toxicity (Bovard et al., 2017, 2018; Schimek et al., 2020) as well as a novel in vitro aerosol exposure system that can, like the human respiratory tract, actively breathe, operate medical inhalers,

and take puffs from tobacco products (Steiner et al., 2020). Furthermore, high-content screening has recently been adapted to organotypic airway epithelial cultures grown at the air–liquid interface (Marescotti et al., 2020), an example of how measurement methods can be adapted to modern in vitro model systems relevant to ENDP assessment. These developments represent only the beginning of a research and development journey that will eventually make animal models obsolete in ENDP assessment.

21.4 OVERALL CONCLUSIONS

The studies reported in this book demonstrate that ENDPs designed to minimize the emission of toxicants, when they do, are less harmful than cigarettes and, therefore, have the potential to reduce the risk of smoking-related disease in smokers who switch to them completely. Needless to say, any claim that switching to a specific ENDP presents less risk of harm than continued smoking should be adequately substantiated. Finally, it is important to remember that studies also show that ENDP aerosols are not devoid of toxicants and that ENDPs are, therefore, not risk-free.

The conclusions of the overall toxicological assessment of ENDPs reported here should inform science-based THR policies, risk-proportionate regulation, and marketing and sales practices (Chapter 1). Indeed, ENDPs are not for people who have never smoked or who have quit smoking. Moreover, it is clear that ENDPs are not an alternative to quitting, and the best choice is undoubtedly to quit tobacco and/or nicotine use altogether. However, for those smokers who would otherwise continue to smoke, switching to ENDPs is a better choice than continuing to smoke cigarettes and may provide an opportunity to leave cigarettes behind for good.

REFERENCES

Akhter, M.P., Lund, A.D., Gairola, C.G., 2005. Bone biomechanical property deterioration due to tobacco smoke exposure. Calcif. Tissue Int. 77, 319–326. https://doi.org/10.1007/s00223-005-0072-1.

Ansari, S.M., Sergio, F., Medlin, L.F., Lama, N., Elamin, A., Haziza, C., 2019. Tobacco Heating System 2.2 in mild to moderate COPD subjects: an exploratory analysis. Chest 156, A465–A466. https://doi.org/10.1016/j.chest.2019.08.485.

Berkowitz, L., Schultz, B.M., Salazar, G.A., Pardo-Roa, C., Sebastián, V.P., Álvarez-Lobos, M.M., Bueno, S.M., 2018. Impact of cigarette smoking on the gastrointestinal tract inflammation: opposing effects in Crohn's disease and ulcerative colitis. Front. Immunol. 9, 74. https://doi.org/10.3389/fimmu.2018.00074.

Bovard, D., Iskandar, A., Luettich, K., Hoeng, J., Peitsch, M.C., 2017. Organs-on-a-chip: a new paradigm for toxicological assessment and preclinical drug development. Toxicol. Res. Appl. 1, 1–16. https://doi.org/10.1177/2397847317726351.

Bovard, D., Sandoz, A., Luettich, K., Frentzel, S., Iskandar, A., Marescotti, D., Trivedi, K., Guedj, E., Dutertre, Q., Peitsch, M.C., Hoeng, J., 2018. A lung/liver-on-a-chip platform for acute and chronic toxicity studies. Lab Chip 18, 3814–3829. https://doi.org/10.1039/c8lc01029c.

Chong, C., Rahman, A., Loonat, K., Sagar, R.C., Selinger, C.P., 2019. Current smoking habits in British IBD patients in the age of e-cigarettes. BMJ Open Gastroenterol. 6, e000309. https://doi.org/10.1136/bmjgast-2019-000309.

Cosnes, J., Beaugerie, L., Carbonnel, F., Gendre, J.P., 2001. Smoking cessation and the course of Crohn's disease: an intervention study. Gastroenterology 120, 1093–1099. https://doi.org/10.1053/gast.2001.23231.

Cummings, K.M., Nahhas, G.J., Sweanor, D.T., 2020. What is accounting for the rapid decline in cigarette sales in Japan? Int. J. Environ. Res. Publ. Health 17. https://doi.org/10.3390/ijerph17103570.

El-Zawawy, H.B., Gill, C.S., Wright, R.W., Sandell, L.J., 2006. Smoking delays chondrogenesis in a mouse model of closed tibial fracture healing. J. Orthop. Res. Off. Publ. Orthop. Res. Soc. 24, 2150–2158. https://doi.org/10.1002/jor.20263.

Hoeng, J., Bovard, D., Peitsch, M.C. (Eds.), 2020. Organ-on-a-Chip: Engineered Microenvironments for Safety and Efficacy Testing. Elsevier. https://doi.org/10.1016/C2018-0-01892-7.

Hoeng, J., Deehan, R., Pratt, D., Martin, F., Sewer, A., Thomson, T.M., Drubin, D.A., Waters, C.A., de Graaf, D., Peitsch, M.C., 2012. A network-based approach to quantifying the impact of biologically active substances. Drug Discov. Today 17, 413–418. https://doi.org/10.1016/j.drudis.2011.11.008.

Huang, C., Nichols, C., Liu, Y., Zhang, Y., Liu, X., Gao, S., Li, Z., Ren, A., 2015. Ambient air pollution and adverse birth outcomes: a natural experiment study. Popul. Health Metrics 13, 17. https://doi.org/10.1186/s12963-015-0050-4.

Ideker, T., Galitski, T., Hood, L., 2001. A new approach to decoding life: systems biology. Annu. Rev. Genom. Hum. Genet. 2, 343–372.

Institute of Medicine, 2012. Committee on Scientific Standards for Studies on Modified Risk Tobacco Products. Scientific Standards for Studies on Modified Risk Tobacco Products. National Academies Press.

Ito, S., Matsumura, K., Ishimori, K., Ishikawa, S., 2020. In vitro long-term repeated exposure and exposure switching of a novel tobacco vapor product in a human organotypic culture of bronchial epithelial cells. J. Appl. Toxicol. 40 (9), 1248–1258. https://doi.org/10.1002/jat.3982.

Kanis, J.A., Johnell, O., Oden, A., Johansson, H., De Laet, C., Eisman, J.A., Fujiwara, S., Kroger, H., McCloskey, E.V., Mellstrom, D., Melton, L.J., Pols, H., Reeve, J., Silman, A., Tenenhouse, A., 2005. Smoking and fracture risk: a meta-analysis. Osteoporos. Int. J. Establ. Result Coop. Eur. Found. Osteoporos. Natl. Osteoporos. Found. USA 16, 155–162. https://doi.org/10.1007/s00198-004-1640-3.

Knorr, A., Almstetter, M., Martin, E., Castellon, A., Pospisil, P., Bentley, M.C., 2019. Performance evaluation of a nontargeted platform using two-dimensional gas chromatography time-of-flight mass spectrometry integrating computer-assisted structure identification and automated semiquantification for the comprehensive chemical characterization of a complex matrix. Anal. Chem. 91, 9129–9137. https://doi.org/10.1021/acs.analchem.9b01659.

Lee, P.N., Abrams, D., Bachand, A., Baker, G., Black, R., Camacho, O., Curtin, G., Djurdjevic, S., Hill, A., Mendez, D., Muhammad-Kah, R.S., Murillo, J.L., Niaura, R., Pithawalla, Y.B., Poland, B., Sulsky, S., Wei, L., Weitkunat, R., 2020. Estimating the population health impact of recently introduced modified risk tobacco products: a comparison of different approaches. Nicotine Tob. Res., ntaa102 https://doi.org/10.1093/ntr/ntaa102.

Lewis, C.M., Whitwell, S.C.L., Forbes, A., Sanderson, J., Mathew, C.G., Marteau, T.M., 2007. Estimating risks of common complex diseases across genetic and environmental factors: the example of Crohn disease. J. Med. Genet. 44, 689–694. https://doi.org/10.1136/jmg.2007.051672.

Li, Y., Wang, W., Kan, H., Xu, X., Chen, B., 2010. Air quality and outpatient visits for asthma in adults during the 2008 Summer Olympic Games in Beijing. Sci. Total Environ. 408, 1226–1227. https://doi.org/10.1016/j.scitotenv.2009.11.035.

Liu, C., Yin, P., Chen, R., Meng, X., Wang, L., Niu, Y., Lin, Z., Liu, Y., Liu, J., Qi, J., You, J., Kan, H., Zhou, M., 2018. Ambient carbon monoxide and cardiovascular mortality: a nationwide time-series analysis in 272 cities in China. Lancet Planet. Health 2, e12–e18. https://doi.org/10.1016/S2542-5196(17)30181-X.

Lowe, F.J., Luettich, K., Talikka, M., Hoang, V., Haswell, L.E., Hoeng, J., Gaca, M.D., 2017. Development of an adverse outcome pathway for the onset of hypertension by oxidative stress-mediated perturbation of endothelial nitric oxide bioavailability. Appl. Vitro Toxicol. 3, 131–148. https://doi.org/10.1089/aivt.2016.0031.

Luettich, K., Talikka, M., Lowe, F.J., Haswell, L.E., Park, J., Gaca, M.D., Hoeng, J., 2017. The adverse outcome pathway for oxidative stress-mediated EGFR activation leading to decreased lung function. Appl. Vitro Toxicol. 3, 99–109. https://doi.org/10.1089/aivt.2016.0032.

Marescotti, D., Bovard, D., Morelli, M., Sandoz, A., Luettich, K., Frentzel, S., Peitsch, M., Hoeng, J., 2020. In vitro high-content imaging-based phenotypic analysis of bronchial 3D organotypic air-liquid interface cultures. SLAS Technol. 25, 247–252. https://doi.org/10.1177/2472630319895473.

Marescotti, D., Serchi, T., Luettich, K., Xiang, Y., Moschini, E., Talikka, M., Martin, F., Baumer, K., Dulize, R., Peric, D., Bornand, D., Guedj, E., Sewer, A., Cambier, S., Contal, S., Chary, A., Gutleb, A.C., Frentzel, S., Ivanov, N.V., Peitsch, M.C., Hoeng, J., 2019. How complex should an in vitro model be? Evaluation of complex 3D alveolar model with transcriptomic data and computational biological network models. ALTEX 36, 388–402. https://doi.org/10.14573/altex.1811221.

Marx, U., Akabane, T., Andersson, T.B., Baker, E., Beilmann, M., Beken, S., Brendler-Schwaab, S., Cirit, M., David, R.,

Dehne, E.-M., Durieux, I., Ewart, L., Fitzpatrick, S.C., Frey, O., Fuchs, F., Griffith, L.G., Hamilton, G.A., Hartung, T., Hoeng, J., Hogberg, H., Hughes, D.J., Ingber, D.E., Iskandar, A., Kanamori, T., Kojima, H., Kuehnl, J., Leist, M., Li, B., Loskill, P., Mendrick, D.L., Neumann, T., Pallocca, G., Rusyn, I., Smirnova, L., Steger-Hartmann, T., Tagle, D.A., Tonevitsky, A., Tsyb, S., Trapecar, M., Van de Water, B., Van den Eijnden-van Raaij, J., Vulto, P., Watanabe, K., Wolf, A., Zhou, X., Roth, A., 2020. Biology-inspired microphysiological systems to advance patient benefit and animal welfare in drug development. ALTEX 37, 364–394. https://doi.org/10.14573/altex.2001241.

Mathis, C., Poussin, C., Weisensee, D., Gebel, S., Hengstermann, A., Sewer, A., Belcastro, V., Xiang, Y., Ansari, S., Wagner, S., Hoeng, J., Peitsch, M.C., 2013. Human bronchial epithelial cells exposed in vitro to cigarette smoke at the air-liquid interface resemble bronchial epithelium from human smokers. Am. J. Physiol. Lung Cell Mol. Physiol. 304, L489–L503. https://doi.org/10.1152/ajplung.00181.2012.

Phillips, B., Veljkovic, E., Boué, S., Schlage, W.K., Vuillaume, G., Martin, F., Titz, B., Leroy, P., Buettner, A., Elamin, A., Oviedo, A., Cabanski, M., De León, H., Guedj, E., Schneider, T., Talikka, M., Ivanov, N.V., Vanscheeuwijck, P., Peitsch, M.C., Hoeng, J., 2016. An 8-month systems toxicology inhalation/cessation study in apoe$^{-/-}$ mice to investigate cardiovascular and respiratory exposure effects of a candidate modified risk tobacco product, THS 2.2, compared with conventional cigarettes. Toxicol. Sci. Off. J. Soc. Toxicol. 149, 411–432. https://doi.org/10.1093/toxsci/kfv243.

Poussin, C., Kramer, B., Lanz, H.L., Van den Heuvel, A., Laurent, A., Olivier, T., Vermeer, M., Peric, D., Baumer, K., Dulize, R., Guedj, E., Ivanov, N.V., Peitsch, M.C., Hoeng, J., Joore, J., 2020. 3D human microvessel-on-a-chip model for studying monocyte-to-endothelium adhesion under flow - application in systems toxicology. ALTEX 37, 47–63. https://doi.org/10.14573/altex.1811301.

Reumann, M.K., Schaefer, J., Titz, B., Aspera-Werz, R.H., Wong, E.T., Szostak, J., Häussling, V., Ehnert, S., Leroy, P., Tan, W.T., Kuczaj, A., Audretsch, C., Springer, F., Badke, A., Augat, P., Quentanilla-Fend, L., Martella, M., Lee, K.M., Peitsch, M.C., Hoeng, J., Nussler, A.K., 2020. E-vapor aerosols do not compromise bone integrity relative to cigarette smoke after 6-month inhalation in an ApoE$^{-/-}$ mouse model. Arch. Toxicol. 94, 2163–2177. https://doi.org/10.1007/s00204-020-02769-4.

Rich, D.Q., Liu, K., Zhang, J., Thurston, S.W., Stevens, T.P., Pan, Y., Kane, C., Weinberger, B., Ohman-Strickland, P., Woodruff, T.J., Duan, X., Assibey-Mensah, V., Zhang, J., 2015. Differences in birth weight associated with the 2008 Beijing olympics air pollution reduction: results from a natural experiment. Environ. Health Perspect. 123, 880–887. https://doi.org/10.1289/ehp.1408795.

Schimek, K., Frentzel, S., Luettich, K., Bovard, D., Rütschle, I., Boden, L., Rambo, F., Erfurth, H., Dehne, E.-M., Winter, A., Marx, U., Hoeng, J., 2020. Human multi-organ chip co-culture of bronchial lung culture and liver spheroids for substance exposure studies. Sci. Rep. 10, 7865. https://doi.org/10.1038/s41598-020-64219-6.

Schleicher, N., Norra, S., Dietze, V., Yu, Y., Fricker, M., Kaminski, U., Chen, Y., Cen, K., 2011. The effect of mitigation measures on size distributed mass concentrations of atmospheric particles and black carbon concentrations during the Olympic Summer Games 2008 in Beijing. Sci. Total Environ. 412–413, 185–193. https://doi.org/10.1016/j.scitotenv.2011.09.084.

Shen, G.S., Li, Y., Zhao, G., Zhou, H.B., Xie, Z.G., Xu, W., Chen, H.N., Dong, Q.R., Xu, Y.J., 2015. Cigarette smoking and risk of hip fracture in women: a meta-analysis of prospective cohort studies. Injury 46, 1333–1340. https://doi.org/10.1016/j.injury.2015.04.008.

Sosnowski, T., Jabłczyńska, K., Odziomek, M., Schlage, W.K., Kuczaj, A.K., 2019. Physico-chemical Studies of Direct Interactions between Components of Electronic Cigarette Liquid Mixtures and Lung Surfactants. https://doi.org/10.26126/intervals.h2jvit.1.

Steiner, S., Herve, P., Pak, C., Majeed, S., Sandoz, A., Kuczaj, A., Hoeng, J., 2020. Development and testing of a new-generation aerosol exposure system: the independent holistic air-liquid exposure system (InHALES). Toxicol. Vitro Int. J. Publ. Assoc. BIBRA 67, 104909. https://doi.org/10.1016/j.tiv.2020.104909.

Sturla, S.J., Boobis, A.R., FitzGerald, R.E., Hoeng, J., Kavlock, R.J., Schirmer, K., Whelan, M., Wilks, M.F., Peitsch, M.C., 2014. Systems toxicology: from basic research to risk assessment. Chem. Res. Toxicol. 27, 314–329. https://doi.org/10.1021/tx400410s.

Su, C., Hampel, R., Franck, U., Wiedensohler, A., Cyrys, J., Pan, X., Wichmann, H.-E., Peters, A., Schneider, A., Breitner, S., 2015. Assessing responses of cardiovascular mortality to particulate matter air pollution for pre-, during- and post-2008 olympics periods. Environ. Res. 142, 112–122. https://doi.org/10.1016/j.envres.2015.06.025.

Ward, K.D., Klesges, R.C., 2001. A meta-analysis of the effects of cigarette smoking on bone mineral density. Calcif. Tissue Int. 68, 259–270. https://doi.org/10.1007/BF02390832.

Wu, Z.-J., Zhao, P., Liu, B., Yuan, Z.-C., 2016. Effect of cigarette smoking on risk of hip fracture in men: a meta-analysis of 14 prospective cohort studies. PLoS One 11, e0168990. https://doi.org/10.1371/journal.pone.0168990.

Yang, W., Jennison, B.L., Omaye, S.T., 1998. Cardiovascular disease hospitalization and ambient levels of carbon monoxide. J. Toxicol. Environ. Health 55, 185–196. https://doi.org/10.1080/009841098158485.

Postface

By the time this book went into production, the US FDA has issued a modified risk tobacco product (MRTP) order for the tobacco heating system.[1] The agency found this order would be *appropriate to promote the public health and is expected to benefit the health of the population as a whole.* With this decision, the US FDA authorizes the marketing of the *IQOS* tobacco heating system with the following reduced exposure claim:

AVAILABLE EVIDENCE TO DATE:

- The IQOS system heats tobacco but does not burn it.

- This significantly reduces the production of harmful and potentially harmful chemicals.
- Scientific studies have shown that switching completely from conventional cigarettes to the IQOS system significantly reduces your body's exposure to harmful or potentially harmful chemicals.

This is a historic decision. It marks the first time that the US FDA has granted MRTP marketing orders for an innovative electronic nicotine delivery product.

---

[1]Marketed under the name *IQOS*.

Index

Note: Page numbers followed by "f" indicate figures and "t" indicate tables.

Printed in the United States
By Bookmasters